We Want To Hear From You

Please take a moment to give us feedback regarding this edition of *Cancer Management: A Multidisciplinary Approach*, 11th Edition. Please respond to the few questions below and drop this card in a mailbox. Postage is paid. Thank you for your help.

1. Would you like to continue to receive this publication in the future? YES   NO

2. Which description best reflects how you would advise a colleague regarding the Handbook?
   ___ Very valuable "must read"   ___ Helpful, read if you have time
   ___ Valuable, try to read whenever possible   ___ Not very valuable

3. How often do you use this handbook?
   ___ Several times a day   ___ Weekly   ___ Monthly
   ___ Daily   ___ Bi-weekly   ___ Other ___

4. Which of the following chapters do you find most helpful (check all that apply):

   ___ Breast Cancer   ___ Hematologic Malignancies   ___ Head & Neck Cancers
   ___ Lung Cancer   ___ Lymphomas   ___ Dermatologic Toxicities
   ___ GI Cancers   ___ Myeloma   ___ Pain Management
   ___ GU Cancers   ___ Leukemias   ___ Growth Factors
   ___ Gynecologic Cancers   ___ Brain Tumors   ___ Other (please specify) ___

5. Would you be interested in receiving this information in an electronic format? YES   NO

6. Do you have any suggestions for making this handbook more useful to you in your practice?
   _____

Print Your Name _____   Specialty _____   Years in Practice _____
                (Please Print Legibly)

Address _____   City _____   State ___ Zip ___

E-mail _____   Visit **www.cancernetwork.com** for online edition.

12/2008

About This Treatment Guide

The Oncology Group of CMPMedica, publisher of *ONCOLOGY* and *Oncology NEWS International*, and the website, **cancernetwork.com**, is pleased to present *Cancer Management: A Multidisciplinary Approach, 11th edition.*

Cancer Management: A Multidisciplinary Approach is designed to present important clinical information concisely, uniformly, and logically, emphasizing the natural history of the malignancy, screening and diagnosis, staging and prognosis, and treatment.

The fundamental principle behind this comprehensive treatment guide is the importance of a truly integrated, multidisciplinary approach to the management of the patient with cancer. Accordingly, the discussion of each disease site combines the perspectives of medical oncology, surgical oncology, and radiation oncology, as appropriate. Further, each of the book's medical editors represent a particular discipline.

The Oncology Group would like to thank the contributors and all involved in the development and production of this important handbook. In particular, we thank the book's principal editors:

> **Richard Pazdur, MD** (Medical Oncology)
> US Food and Drug Administration
>
> **Lawrence D. Wagman, MD** (Surgical Oncology)
> Center for Cancer Prevention and Treatment, St. Joseph Hospital
>
> **Kevin A. Camphausen, MD** (Radiation Oncology)
> National Cancer Institute
>
> **William J. Hoskins, MD** (Gynecologic Oncology)
> Memorial Sloan-Kettering Cancer Center

We also thank the staff of The Oncology Group and in particular wish to recognize the efforts of Angela Cibuls and Susan Reckling.

This 11th edition has been produced in an effort to keep pace with the rapidly changing field of oncology. Be sure to visit **www.cancernetwork.com**, where the full text of this edition will be made available online, with important updates as appropriate.

Please let us know how you use this book, and how we can make it even more valuable. We look forward to hearing from you.

Sincerely,

Cara H. Glynn
Sr. Editorial Director
Cara.Glynn@cmpmedica.com

Beth Scholz
Group Vice President
Beth.Scholz@cmpmedica.com

11TH EDITION

Cancer Management: A Multidisciplinary Approach

Medical, Surgical, & Radiation Oncology

Edited by

Richard Pazdur, MD
Director, Office of Oncology Drug Products
Center for Drug Evaluation and Research
US Food and Drug Administration

Lawrence D. Wagman, MD
Executive Medical Director
The Center for Cancer Prevention and Treatment
St. Joseph Hospital

Kevin A. Camphausen, MD
Chief, Radiation Oncology Branch
National Cancer Institute

William J. Hoskins, MD
Executive Director of Surgical Activities
Memorial Sloan-Kettering Cancer Center

And the publishers of the journal ONCOLOGY

CMPMedica
United Business Media

Note to the reader

The information in this volume has been carefully reviewed for accuracy of dosage and indications. Before prescribing any drug, however, the clinician should consult the manufacturer's current package labeling for accepted indications, absolute dosage recommendations, and other information pertinent to the safe and effective use of the product described. This is especially important when drugs are given in combination or as an adjunct to other forms of therapy. Furthermore, some of the medications described herein, as well as some of the indications mentioned, had not been approved by the US Food and Drug Administration at the time of publication. This possibility should be borne in mind before prescribing or recommending any drug or regimen.

> The views expressed are the result of independent work and do not necessarily represent the views or findings of the US Food and Drug Administration or the United States.

Library of Congress Catalog Card Number 2008938898
ISBN Number 9781891483622

For information on purchasing additional copies of this publication, visit www.cancernetwork.com or contact us at: Cancer Management Handbook, CMPMedica LLC, 4601 W. 6th St., Ste. B, Lawrence, KS 66049. Phone: 1-800-444-4881 or 1-785-838-7576; fax: 1-785-838-7566, or e-mail: orders@cmp.com.

CMPMedica
United Business Media

Publishers of
ONCOLOGY
ONCOLOGY Nurse Edition
Oncology NEWS International
cancernetwork.com

Contents

HEMATOLOGIC MALIGNANCIES

PALLIATIVE AND SUPPORTIVE CARE

Contributors

Thomas E. Ahlering, MD
Urology Division
University of California,
Irvine Medical Center

Steven R. Alberts, MD
Division of Medical Oncology
Mayo Clinic

Penny R. Anderson, MD
Department of Radiation Oncology
Fox Chase Cancer Center

Andrew J. Armstrong, MD
Department of Medicine
Duke University Medical Center

Al B. Benson III, MD
Division of Hematology/Oncology
Robert H. Lurie Comprehensive Cancer
Center, Feinberg School of Medicine/
Northwestern University

J. Sybil Biermann, MD
Department of Orthopaedic Surgery
University of Michigan
Comprehensive Cancer Center

Charles D. Blanke, MD
Department of Medicine
The University of British Columbia

Deborah Bradley
Division of Hematology/Oncology
University of Michigan

Ilana Braun, MD
Department of Oncologic Psychiatry
Massachusetts General Hospital

Eduardo Bruera, MD
Department of Palliative Care
and Rehabilitation Medicine
M. D. Anderson Cancer Center

Mark Buyyounouski, MD
Department of Radiation Oncology
Fox Chase Cancer Center

Emiliano Calvo, MD, PhD
Division of Medical Oncology
Centro Integral Oncológico Clara Campal

Kevin A. Camphausen, MD
Radiation Oncology Branch
National Cancer Institute

Dennis S. Chi, MD
Gynecology Service
Memorial Sloan-Kettering Cancer Center

Brian C. -H. Chiu, PhD
Department of Preventive Medicine
Northwestern University

Warren Chow, MD
Department of Medical Oncology
City of Hope National Medical Center

Deborah E. Citrin, MD
Radiation Oncology Branch
National Cancer Institute

Lawrence R. Coia, MD
Southern Ocean County
Radiation Oncology
Manahawkin, New Jersey

Jay S. Cooper, MD
Department of Radiation Oncology
Maimonides Medical Center

Jorge E. Cortes, MD
Department of Leukemia
M. D. Anderson Cancer Center

Jeffrey Crawford, MD
Department of Medical Oncology
Duke University Medical Center

Carey A. Cullinane, MD
Department of Surgical Oncology
Long Beach Memorial Medical Center

Lisa M. DeAngelis, MD
Department of Neurology
Memorial Sloan-Kettering
Cancer Center

Lawrence Driver, MD
Pain Symptom Management Section
M. D. Anderson Cancer Center

Joshua D. I. Ellenhorn, MD
Division of Surgery
City of Hope National Medical Center

Carmen P. Escalante, MD
Department of General Internal
Medicine, Ambulatory Treatment, and
Emergency Care
M. D. Anderson Cancer Center

Richard Essner, MD
Division of Surgery
John Wayne Cancer Institute

Andrew M. Evens, DO
Division of Hematology/Oncology
Robert H. Lurie Comprehensive Cancer
Center, Feinberg School of Medicine/
Northwestern University

Steven J. Feigenberg, MD
Department of Radiation Oncology
Fox Chase Cancer Center

Paul Fisher, MD
Department of Radiology
Stony Brook University Medical Center

Keith Flaherty, MD
Division of Hematology/Oncology
Abramson Cancer Center of the
University of Pennsylvania

Stephen J. Forman, MD
Division of Hematology and Bone
Marrow Transplantation
City of Hope National Medical Center

Deborah Frassica, MD
Department of Radiation Oncology
The Sidney Kimmel Comprehensive
Cancer Center at Johns Hopkins

Guillermo Garcia-Manero
Department of Leukemia
M. D. Anderson Cancer Center

Bonnie S. Glisson, MD
Department of Thoracic/
Head and Neck Medical Oncology
M. D. Anderson Cancer Center

Leo I. Gordon, MD
Division of Hematology/Oncology
Robert H. Lurie Comprehensive Cancer
Center, Feinberg School of Medicine/
Northwestern University

Richard J. Gralla, MD
Division of Hematology/Oncology
North Shore University Hospital and
LIJ Medical Center

Frederic W. Grannis, Jr., MD
Section of Thoracic Surgery
City of Hope National Medical Center

Kathryn M. Greven, MD
Department of Radiation Oncology
Wake Forest University School of
Medicine

Steven M. Grunberg, MD
Division of Medical Oncology
University of Vermont

Bruce G. Haffty, MD
Department of Radiation Oncology
UMDNJ - Robert Wood Johnson
Medical School
The Cancer Institute of New Jersey

John D. Hainsworth, MD
Department of Clinical Research
Sarah Cannon Research Institute
Nashville, Tennessee

Brent K. Hollenbeck, MD
Department of Medicine/Urology
University of Michigan Comprehensive
Cancer Center

Eric M. Horwitz, MD
Department of Radiation Oncology
Fox Chase Cancer Center

William J. Hoskins, MD
Department of Surgery
Memorial Sloan-Kettering Cancer Center

Mimi Hu, MD
Department of Endocrine Neoplasia
and Hormonal Disorders
M. D. Anderson Cancer Center

Mark Hurwitz, MD
Department of Radiation Oncology
Brigham and Women's Hospital

Maha Hussain, MD
Division of Hematology/Oncology
University of Michigan
Comprehensive Cancer Center

Jimmy J. Hwang, MD
Division of Hematology/Oncology
Lombardi Comprehensive Cancer Center
Georgetown University Medical Center

James Ito, Jr., MD
Department of Infectious Diseases
City of Hope National Medical Center

Rajesh V. Iyer, MD
Department of Radiation Oncology
Community Medical Center
Saint Barnabas Health Care System

Sundar Jagannath, MD
Myeloma and Transplant
St. Vincent's Comprehensive
Cancer Center

Ishmael Jaiyesimi, DO
Division of Hematology/Oncology
William Beaumont Hospital

Lori Jardines, MD
Department of Surgery
Albert Einstein Medical Center

Aminah Jatoi, MD
Department of Medical Oncology
Mayo Clinic

Hagop Kantarjian, MD
Department of Leukemia
M. D. Anderson Cancer Center

Aradhana Kaushal, MD
Radiation Oncology Branch
National Cancer Institute

John J. Kavanagh, MD
Department of Gynecologic Oncology
M. D. Anderson Cancer Center

Kemp H. Kernstine, MD, PhD
Department of Thoracic Surgery
City of Hope National Medical Center

Fadlo R. Khuri, MD
Department of Hematology/Oncology
Winship Cancer Institute of
Emory University

Lily Lai, MD
Division of Surgery
City of Hope National Medical Center

Mario E. Lacouture, MD
Department of Dermatology
Robert H. Lurie Comprehensive Cancer
Center, Feinberg School of Medicine/
Northwestern University

Nicole Lamanna, MD
Department of Medicine/
Leukemia Service
Memorial Sloan-Kettering Cancer Center

Jeffrey P. Lamont, MD
Department of Surgery
Baylor University Medical Center

Miriam N. Lango, MD
Department of Surgical Oncology
Fox Chase Cancer Center

Joseph Lattanzi, MD
Southern Ocean County
Radiation Oncology
Manahawkin, New Jersey

Alan List, MD
*Department of Hematologic
Malignancies
H. Lee Moffitt Cancer Center and
Research Institute*

Jay S. Loeffler, MD
*Department of Radiation Oncology
Massachusetts General Hospital*

Patrick J. Loehrer, MD
*Division of Hematology/Oncology
Indiana University Cancer Center*

Charles Loprinzi, MD
*Department of Medical Oncology
Mayo Clinic*

Robert Lustig, MD
*Department of Radiation Oncology
University of Pennsylvania*

Robert Maki, MD, PhD
*Department of Medicine
Memorial Sloan-Kettering Cancer Center*

Adam N. Mamelak, MD
*Division of Neurosurgery
Cedars-Sinai Medical Center*

Gary N. Mann, MD
*Division of Surgery
University of Washington*

Ellen Manzullo, MD
*Department of General Internal
Medicine, Ambulatory Treatment,
and Emergency Care
M. D. Anderson Cancer Center*

Maurie Markman, MD
*Department of Clinical Research
M. D. Anderson Cancer Center*

David Scott Miller, MD
*Division of Gynecologic Oncology
University of Texas Southwestern
Medical Center*

Ronald T. Mitsuyasu, MD
*Department of Medicine
UCLA CARE Center*

Judd W. Moul, MD
*Division of Urologic Surgery
Duke University Medical Center*

Benjamin Movsas, MD
*Department of Radiation Oncology
Henry Ford Health System*

Michael S. Mulligan, MD
*Department of Surgery
University of Washington*

Nikhil C. Munshi, MD
*Department of Adult Oncology
Dana-Farber Cancer Institute*

Robert J. Myerson, MD, PhD
*Department of Radiation Oncology
Washington University*

Margaret R. O'Donnell, MD
*Department of Hematology/
Hematopoietic Stem Cell Transplantation
City of Hope National Medical Center*

Bert O'Neil, MD
*Department of Medicine
University of North Carolina
at Chapel Hill*

Richard Pazdur, MD
*Office of Oncology Drug Products
Center for Drug Evaluation
and Research
US Food and Drug Administration*

Carlos A. Perez, MD
*Department of Radiation Oncology
Washington University School of
Medicine*

Louis L. Pisters, MD
*Department of Urology
M. D. Anderson Cancer Center*

Peter W. T. Pisters, MD
*Division of Surgery
M. D. Anderson Cancer Center*

Stephen P. Povoski, MD
*Division of Surgery
The Ohio State University*

Bruce G. Redman, DO
Division of Hematology/Oncology
University of Michigan Comprehensive
Cancer Center

Paul Richardson, MD
Department of Medical Oncology/
Hematologic Malignancies
Dana-Farber Cancer Institute

John Andrew Ridge, MD, PhD
Department of Surgical Oncology
Fox Chase Cancer Center

Brian I. Rini, MD
Department of Solid Tumor
Oncology and Urology
Cleveland Clinic Taussig Cancer Center

John M. Robertson, MD
Department of Radiation Oncology
William Beaumont Hospital

Steven T. Rosen, MD
Division of Hematology/Oncology
Robert H. Lurie Comprehensive Cancer
Center, Feinberg School of Medicine/
Northwestern University

Melanie Royce, MD, PhD
Division of Hematology/Oncology
University of New Mexico Cancer
Research and Treatment Center

Stephen C. Rubin, MD
Division of Gynecologic Oncology
Hospital of the University of
Pennsylvania

Paul Sabbatini, MD
Gynecologic Section
Solid Tumor Division
Memorial Sloan-Kettering
Cancer Center

Aaron Sasson, MD
Department of Surgery
University of Nebraska Medical Center

Roderich E. Schwarz, MD, PhD
Department of Surgery
University of Texas Southwestern
Medical Center

Walter Scott, MD
Department of Thoracic
Surgical Oncology
Fox Chase Cancer Center

Richard T. Silver, MD
Department of Medicine
Weill Cornell Medical College

Douglas Skarecky, BS
Department of Urology
University of California,
Irvine Medical Center

Philippe E. Spiess, MD
Department of Genitourinary Oncology
H. Lee Moffitt Cancer Center
and Research Institute

David Straus, MD
Department of Medicine
Memorial Sloan-Kettering
Cancer Center

Chris H. Takimoto, MD, PhD
Department of Pharmacology
University of Texas Health Science Center
at San Antonio

Richard Tsang, MD
Department of Radiation Oncology
Princess Margaret Hospital

Alan Valentine, MD
Department of Neuro-Oncology
M. D. Anderson Cancer Center

Rena Vassilopoulou-Sellin, MD
Department of Endocrine Neoplasia
and Hormonal Disorders
M. D. Anderson Cancer Center

Akila Viswanathan, MD
Department of Radiation Oncology
Dana-Farber Cancer Institute

Madhuri Vithala, MD
Division of Medical Oncology
University of Vermont

Lawrence D. Wagman, MD
Division of Surgery
The Center for Cancer Prevention
and Treatment, St. Joseph Hospital

Sharon M. Weinstein, MD
Department of Anesthesiology
Huntsman Cancer Institute
University of Utah

Lawrence M. Weiss, MD
Division of Pathology
City of Hope National Medical Center

Mark A. Weiss, MD
Department of Medicine/
Leukemia Service
Memorial Sloan-Kettering Cancer Center

Mitchell Weiss, MD
Department of Radiation Oncology
Monmouth Medical Center

Jeffrey Weitzel, MD
Department of Clinical Cancer Genetics
City of Hope National Medical Center

William G. Wierda, MD, PhD
Department of Leukemia
M. D. Anderson Cancer Center

Jane N. Winter, MD
Division of Hematology/Oncology
Robert H. Lurie Comprehensive Cancer
Center, Feinberg School of Medicine/
Northwestern University

Joachim Yahalom, MD
Department of Radiation Oncology
Memorial Sloan-Kettering Cancer Center

Alan W. Yasko, MD
Department of Orthopaedic Oncology
Robert H. Lurie Comprehensive Cancer
Center, Feinberg School of Medicine/
Northwestern University

Sriram Yennurajalingam, MD
Department of Palliative Care
and Rehabilitation Medicine
M. D. Anderson Cancer Center

Sally Yowell Barbour, PHARMD
Department of Medical Oncology
Duke University Medical Center

Publishing Staff

Cara H. Glynn	*Sr. Editorial Director*
Angela Cibuls	*Project Manager*
Susan Reckling	*Managing Editor*
Stacey Cuozzo	*Production Editor*
Terri Gelfand	*Sr. Editorial Coordinator*
Lisa Katz	*Creative Director*
Andrew Barkus	*Group Production Manager*
Beth Scholz	*Group Vice President*

Preface

This 11th edition of *Cancer Management: A Multidisciplinary Approach* reflects the ongoing commitment of the authors, editors, and publishers to rapidly disseminate to oncologists the most current information on the clinical management of cancer patients. The concept for this multidisciplinary text arose more than 10 years ago. We have since made every effort to update, refine, and optimize each new edition to meet the growing and changing needs of the more than 10,000 clinicians and cancer specialists who receive this publication each year, many of whom have told us they refer to this publication daily in their clinical practice.

Important updates and comprehensive revisions have been made to this latest 11th edition. Substantial changes have been made to a number of chapters, including those on breast cancer, non–small-cell lung cancer, colon, rectal, and anal cancers, and melanoma. Plus we've added a new color atlas on dermatologic toxicities associated with novel targeted therapies. And throughout the book, updates have been made to all of the chapters to reflect the latest information about cancer treatment and data on novel therapies and new and ongoing clinical trials.

This 11th volume also provides information on some of the oncology drugs that are listed below, which are newly approved or have received approval for a new indication since the last edition was published. These include: bendamustine (Treanda); bevacizumab (Avastin); bortezomib (Velcade); dalteparin (Fragmin): denileukin diftitox (Ontak); dexrazoxane (Totect); docetaxel (Taxotere); doxorubicin HCl liposome injection (Doxil); fosaprepitant dimeglumine for Injection (Emend); granisetron (Sancuso); human papillomavirus (HPV) vaccine (Gardasil); ixabepilone (Ixempra); nilotinib (Tasigna); oxymorphone HCl (Opana); pemetrexed (Alimta); romiplostim (Nplate); raloxifene hydrochloride (Evista); sorafenib (Nexavar); temsirolimus (Torisel); and topotecan (Hycamtin):

The 46 chapters and 4 Appendices in this newest edition represent the efforts of over 100 contributors from approximately 50 institutions in the United States and Canada.

Three consistent goals continue to guide our editorial policies:

- To provide practical information for physicians who manage cancer patients
- To present this information concisely, uniformly, and logically, emphasizing the natural history of the malignancy, screening and diagnosis, staging and prognosis, and treatment
- To emphasize a collaborative multidisciplinary approach to patient management that involves surgical, radiation, and medical oncologists, as well as other health care professionals, working as a cohesive team.

As with all previous editions, each chapter (as appropriate) in the current volume has been authored jointly by practicing medical, surgical, and radiation oncologists. In some cases, other specialists have been asked to contribute their expertise to a particular chapter.

All of our contributors personally manage patients using a multidisciplinary approach in their respective institutions. Thus, these chapters reflect the recommendations of practitioners cognizant that decisions and recommendations regarding therapies must be founded on evidence-based research directed at practical patient care in a cost-effective manner.

To write, edit, and publish this 1,000+-page text requires the dedication of all of the authors, as well as a professional publication staff to coordinate the technical aspects of editing and publishing. We, the authors and editors, acknowledge the following individuals at CMPMedica: Angela Cibuls, Project Manager; Susan Reckling, Managing Editor; Stacey Cuozzo, Production Editor; Andrew Barkus, Group Production Manager, Cara Glynn, Senior Editorial Director; and Beth Scholz, Group Vice President. We also thank Lisa Katz, Claudine Kiffer, Anne Landry, Andrew Nash, and Ronald Piana, for their efforts.

Richard Pazdur, MD
Director, Office of Oncology Drug Products
Center for Drug Evaluation and Research
US Food and Drug Administration

Lawrence D. Wagman, MD
Executive Medical Director
The Center for Cancer Prevention and Treatment
St. Joseph Hospital
Orange, California

Kevin A. Camphausen, MD
Chief, Radiation Oncology Branch
National Cancer Institute

William J. Hoskins, MD
Executive Director of Surgical Activities
Memorial Sloan-Kettering Cancer Center
New York, New York

CHAPTER I

Principles of surgical oncology

Lawrence D. Wagman, MD

Surgical oncology, as its name suggests, is the specific application of surgical principles to the oncologic setting. These principles have been derived by adapting standard surgical approaches to the unique situations that arise when treating cancer patients.

The surgeon is often the first specialist to see the patient with a solid malignancy, and, in the course of therapy, he or she may be called upon to provide diagnostic, therapeutic, palliative, and supportive care. In each of these areas, guiding paradigms that are unique to surgical oncology are employed.

In addition, the surgical oncologist must be knowledgeable about all of the available surgical and adjuvant therapies, both standard and experimental, for a particular cancer. This enables the surgeon not only to explain the various treatment options to the patient but also to perform the initial steps in diagnosis and treatment in such a way as to facilitate and avoid interfering with future therapeutic options.

Invasive diagnostic modalities

As the surgeon approaches the patient with a solid malignancy or abnormal nodal disease or the rare individual with a tissue-based manifestation of a leukemia, selection of a diagnostic approach that will have a high likelihood of a specific, accurate diagnosis is paramount. The advent of high-quality invasive diagnostic approaches guided by radiologic imaging modalities has limited the open surgical approach to those situations where the disease is inaccessible, a significant amount of tissue is required for diagnosis, or a percutaneous approach is too dangerous (due, for example, to a bleeding diathesis, critical intervening structures, or the potential for unacceptable complications, such as pneumothorax).

Lymph node biopsy

The usual indication for biopsy of the lymph node is to establish the diagnosis of lymphoma or metastatic carcinoma. Each situation should be approached in a different manner.

Lymphoma The goal of biopsy in the patient with an abnormal lymph node and suspected lymphoma is to make the general diagnosis and to establish the lymphoma type and subtype. Additional analyses of the cells in the node, its internal architecture, and the subpopulations of cells are critical for subsequent treatment. Although advances in immunocytochemical and histochemical analyses have been made, adequate tissue is the key element in accurate diagnosis.

Consequently, the initial diagnosis of lymphoma should be made on a completely excised node that has been minimally manipulated to ensure that there is little crush damage. When primary lymphoma is suspected, the use of needle aspiration does not consistently allow for the complete analyses described above and can lead to incomplete or inaccurate diagnosis and treatment delays.

When recurrent lymphoma is the primary diagnosis, analysis of a specific cell type is important for assessing changes in the type of lymphoma and whether a transformation has occurred. In the rare situation in which recurrent Hodgkin lymphoma is suspected, a core biopsy may be adequate if the classic Reed-Sternberg cells are identified. However, in the initial and recurrent settings, biopsy of an intact node is often required.

Carcinoma The diagnosis of metastatic carcinoma often requires less tissue than is needed for lymphoma. Fine-needle aspiration (FNA), core biopsy, or subtotal removal of a single node will be adequate in this situation. For metastatic disease, the surgeon will use a combination of factors, such as location of the node, physical examination, and symptoms, to predict the site of primary disease. When this information is communicated to the pathologist, the pathologic evaluation can be focused on the most likely sites so as to obtain the highest diagnostic yield. The use of immunocytochemical analyses can be successful in defining the primary site, even on small amounts of tissue.

Head and neck adenopathy The head and neck region is a common site of palpable adenopathy that poses a significant diagnostic dilemma. Nodal zones in this area serve as the harbinger of lymphoma (particularly Hodgkin lymphoma) and as sites of metastasis from the mucosal surfaces of the upper aerodigestive tract; nasopharynx; thyroid; lungs; and, occasionally, intra-abdominal sites, such as the stomach, liver, and pancreas.

Because treatment of these nodal metastases varies widely, and subsequent treatments may be jeopardized by inconveniently placed biopsy incisions, the surgical oncologist must consider the most likely source of the disease prior to performing the biopsy. FNA or core biopsy becomes a valuable tool in this situation, as the tissue sample is usually adequate for basic analysis (cytologic or histologic), and special studies (eg, immunocytochemical analyses) can be performed as needed.

Biopsy of a tissue-based mass

Several principles must be considered when approaching the seemingly simple task of biopsying a tissue-based mass. As each of the biopsy methods has unique risks, yields, and costs, the initial choice can be a critical factor in the timeliness and expense of the diagnostic process. It is crucial that the physician charged with making the invasive diagnosis be mindful of these factors.

Mass in the aerodigestive tract In the aerodigestive tract, biopsy of a lesion should include a representative amount of tissue taken preferably from the periphery of the lesion, where the maximum amount of viable malignant cells will be present. Because the treatment of in situ and invasive diseases varies greatly, the biopsy must be of adequate depth to determine penetration of the tumors. This is particularly true for carcinomas of the oral cavity, pharynx, and larynx.

Breast mass Although previously a common procedure, an open surgical biopsy of the breast is rarely indicated today. Palpable breast masses that are highly suspicious (as indicated by physical findings and mammography) can be diagnosed as malignant with close to 100% accuracy with FNA. However, because the distinction between invasive and noninvasive diseases is often required prior to the initiation of treatment, a core biopsy, performed either under image guidance (ultrasonography or mammography) or directly for palpable lesions, is the method of choice.

An excellent example of the interdependence of the method of tissue diagnosis and therapeutic options is the patient with a moderate-sized breast tumor considering breast conservation who chooses preoperative chemotherapy for downsizing of the breast lesion. The core biopsy method establishes the histologic diagnosis, provides adequate tissue for analyses of hormone-receptor levels and other risk factors, causes little or no cosmetic damage, does not perturb sentinel node analyses, and does not require extended healing prior to the initiation of therapy. In addition, a small radio-opaque clip can be placed in the tumor to guide the surgical extirpation. This step is important because excellent treatment responses can make it difficult for the surgeon to localize the original tumor site.

Mass in the trunk or extremities For soft-tissue or bony masses of the trunk or extremities, the biopsy technique should be selected on the basis of the planned subsequent tumor resection. The incision should be made along anatomic lines in the trunk or along the long axis of the extremity. When a sarcoma is suspected, FNA can establish the diagnosis of malignancy, but a core biopsy will likely be required to determine the histologic type and plan neoadjuvant therapy.

Preoperative evaluation

As with any surgical patient, the preoperative evaluation of the cancer patient hinges primarily on the individual's underlying medical condition(s). Because most new cancers occur in older patients, careful attention must be paid to evaluation of cardiovascular risks. Adequate information can usually be obtained from a standard history, physical examination, and electrocardiogram (ECG), but any concerns identified should be subjected to a full diagnostic work-up.

The evaluation should also include a detailed history of current and previous therapies. Many patients will be on anticoagulation, aspirin, or analgesics, all of which may impact on their perioperative management. Previous use of doxorubicin or trastuzumab (Herceptin) may be associated with cardiac dysfunction and the use of bleomycin with severe lung sensitivity to oxygen concentrations > 30%. Due to the association of bowel anastomotic perforation with the use of bevacizumab (Avastin), the timing of colonic surgery should be modified. Some of the cytotoxic agents (oxaliplatin [Eloxatin], irinotecan) used to treat colon and rectal cancers are associated with liver injury.

Prior radiation therapy is associated with fibrosis and delayed healing. An appreciation of potential postoperative problems secondary to these factors is important in planning the surgical extirpation and reconstruction. For example, in a patient who requires mastectomy after failed breast-conserving surgery, the zone of tissue damage from the original radiation therapy can be assessed by reviewing the port and boost site films or by examining the irradiated site for tattoo marks used to align the radiation field. Plans for resection of heavily irradiated tissues should be made preoperatively in concert with the reconstructive surgeon, and the relative increased risk of postoperative problems should be discussed with the patient. This evaluation should include the type of tissue to be transferred, analysis of potential donor and recipient sites and vessels, and assurance that the appropriate microvascular equipment is available, in the event that it is needed during surgery.

Pathologic confirmation of the diagnosis

The treatment of cancer is based almost exclusively on the organ of origin and, to a lesser degree, on the histologic subtype. Unless the operative procedure is being performed to make a definitive diagnosis, review of the pathologic material is needed to confirm the diagnosis preoperatively.

There are few exceptions to this doctrine, and it behooves the surgeon to have a confirmed diagnosis, including the in situ or invasive nature of the cancer, prior to performing an operation. This tenet assumes paramount importance when one is performing procedures for which there is no recourse once the specimen is removed, eg, laryngectomy, mastectomy, removal of the anal sphincter, and extremity amputation.

Ironically, in some situations, a preoperative or intraoperative diagnosis cannot be confirmed, despite the fact that the preoperative and intraoperative physical findings, laboratory data, and radiologic studies (pre- and intraoperative) overwhelmingly suggested the cancer diagnosis. The classic example of this dilemma is the jaundiced patient with a firm mass in the pancreatic head. The Whipple procedure (pancreaticoduodenectomy) causes significant morbidity but is required to make the diagnosis and treat the cancer. In any of these situations, the preoperative discussion with the patient must include the possibility that the final diagnosis may be a benign lesion.

Resection

The principles of resection for malignant disease are based on the surgical goal (complete resection vs debulking), functional significance of the involved organ or structure, and the ability to reconstruct the involved and surrounding structures. Also important are the technical abilities of the surgeon or availability of a surgical team, adequacy of neoadjuvant and adjuvant therapies, and the biologic behavior (local and systemic) of the disease. Although "operable" is used to describe the physiologic status of the patient, the definition of "resectable" varies, and this term can be defined only in the context of the aforementioned modifying parameters.

Wide excision

A wide excision includes the removal of the tumor itself and a margin of normal tissue, usually exceeding 1 cm in all directions from the tumor. The margin is variable in a large, complex (multiple tissue compartments) specimen, and the limiting point of the resection is defined by the closest approximation of cancerous tissue to the normal tissue that is excised.

Wide margins are recommended for tumors with a high likelihood of local recurrence (eg, dermatofibrosarcoma protuberans) and for tumors without any reliable adjuvant therapeutic options.

Breast The use of adjuvant radiation therapy has permitted the use of breast-conserving surgery, which limits the excision of wide margins of normal breast tissue.

Colon and rectum For carcinoma of the colon and rectum, the width of excision is defined by the longitudinal portion of the bowel and the inclusion of adjacent nodal tissue. The principles of wide resection require removal of normal bowel (including at least 5 cm of uninvolved tissue), the associated mesenteric leaf, and adjacent rectal soft tissue (mesorectum). Current guidelines require the removal of 12 to 15 nodes for evaluation.

This general principle has been modified in the distal rectum, where lateral margins are maintained using the principles of mesorectal excision, and longitudinal bowel margins of 2 cm are accepted. This modification reflects the emphasis on functional results (ie, maintenance of anal continence) and the availability of neoadjuvant (preoperative chemotherapy and irradiation) therapy to reduce the tumor size and resectability and postoperative adjuvant radiation therapy and chemotherapy to improve local control.

No touch technique

This principle is based on the concept that direct contact with and manipulation of the tumor during resection can lead to an increase in local implantation and embolization of tumor cells, respectively. Theoretically, the metastatic potential of the primary lesion would be enhanced by the mechanical extrusion of tumor cells into local lymphatic and vascular spaces. There may be some validity to this theory with respect to tumors that extend directly into the venous system (eg, renal cell tumors with extension to the vena cava) or those that extensively involve local venous drainage (eg, large hepatocellular carcinomas).

Extensive palpation and manipulation of a colorectal primary have been shown to result in direct shedding of tumor cells into the lumen of the large bowel. The traditional strategy to lessen this risk was to ligate the proximal and distal lumen of the segment containing the tumor early in the resection. These areas were then included in the resection, limiting the contact of shed tumor cells with the planned anastomotic areas.

Neither of the previous theoretical situations (ie, manipulation of the tumor and direct contact of the tumor with the anastomotic area) has been definitively tested in controlled, prospective, randomized trials. However, the risk-benefit ratio should favor adherence to the general principles of minimal tumor manipulation, protection of the anastomotic areas, and exclusion of the resection bed from potential implantation with tumor cells.

The minimally invasive surgical techniques introduced approximately 20 years ago were incorporated into the surgical procedures for a non-oncologic scenario–cholecystectomy, hiatal and inguinal hernia repair, and treatment of benign diseases of the female reproductive tract. Transfer of the technology to the oncologic setting was met with resistance, as questions of technical (number of nodes resected and less tactile input during resection) and therapeutic (local control, disease-free survival, and overall survival) equivalence were raised.

Careful clinical research has answered these initial reservations for colon cancer and to a lesser degree for rectal cancers. Results from a prospective randomized trial reported by the Laparoscopic Colectomy (LC) trial group documented that although the laparoscopic operations took longer than the open procedures (150 vs 95 minutes), there was no difference in the margins obtained, the 30-day mortality, or the complication rate. LC resulted in a shorter overall hospital stay (4 vs 5 days) and less use of parenteral narcotics (3 vs 4 days) than the open procedure. There was no difference identified for the oncologic outcomes of disease-free recurrence or overall survival.

Examples in colon cancer will serve as paradigms for the study of other tumors. The introduction of the da Vinci robotic system has opened new areas for technical investigation and evaluation of operative outcomes. Expansion of minimally invasive techniques (laparoscopic and robotic-assisted), with preservation of oncologic principles and improvement in patients' quality-of-life outcomes, will drive surgical interventions.

Lymphadenectomy

Early surgical oncologic theory proposed that breast cancer progressed from the primary site to the axillary lymph nodes to the supraclavicular nodes and nodes of the neck. This theory led to the radical surgical approach that included resection of all of the breast tissue and some or all of the above-noted draining nodal basins (ie, modified radical, radical, or extended radical mastectomy).

Absent from this approach was an appreciation of the nodes not only as a deposit of regional metastatic disease but also as a predictor of systemic disease. Modern treatment approaches view nodal dissection as having a triple purpose: the surgical removal of regional metastases, the prediction of prognosis, and the planning of adjuvant therapy.

The surgical technique and boundaries for lymphadenectomy are based on nodal basins that are defined by consistent anatomic structures. For example, dissection of the neck is defined by the mandible, anterior strap muscles of the neck, clavicle, trapezius muscle, carotid artery, vagus nerve, brachial plexus, and fascia overlying the deep muscles of the neck.

Modifications of classic techniques Each of the classic anatomic lymphadenectomies has been modified along lines that consider the predicted positivity and functional impact of the dissection. To use the example of radical neck dissection, the modifications include supraomohyoid dissection for tumors of the floor of the mouth (a high-risk zone) and sparing of the spinal accessory nerve (functional prevention of shoulder drop and loss of full abduction of the shoulder).

Sentinel node biopsy

As alluded to in the previous paragraphs, lymph node dissection has therapeutic value only in patients with positive nodes. In individuals with pathologically negative nodes, the benefit is limited to prediction of prognosis and documentation of pathologic negativity. Therefore, in the pathologically negative nodal basin, there is minimal benefit of such a dissection to outweigh the risks and untoward sequelae.

Technique The technique of sentinel node identification has been developed to address clinically negative nodal basins. With this technique, the node or nodes that preferentially drain a particular primary tumor are identified by mapping and then surgically excised. The mapping agents include radiolabeled materials and vital dyes that are specifically taken up by, and transported in, the lymphatic drainage systems. These mapping and localizing agents, used alone or in combination, are critical in defining the unique flow patterns to specific lymph node(s) and ambiguous drainage patterns (eg, a truncal melanoma that may drain to the axilla, supraclavicular, or inguinal spaces).

Unresolved issues As this field of directed diagnostic node biopsy and dissection develops, many technical issues related to the timing and location of the injection sites are being evaluated. In addition, the type of pathologic evaluation (ie, the number of sections examined per node and the use of immunohistochemical analysis) is undergoing intense scrutiny.

A study of 200 consecutive patients who had sentinel lymph node biopsies performed for breast cancer examined the concepts of injecting dye and radioactive tracer into either the breast or the overlying dermis. The authors believed that the technical aspects of intradermal injection were simpler and more easily reproduced than those of injections into the breast. Injections were performed in group 1 intraparenchymally and in group 2 intradermally. The combination of blue dye and isotope localization produced a 92% success rate in group 1 and a 100% success rate in group 2. The authors concluded that dermal and parenchymal lymphatics of the breast drain to the same lymph node and that the more simple approach of dermal injection may simplify and optimize sentinel lymph node localization.

For melanoma, for which these techniques were originally developed, researchers are studying the feasibility and clinical relevance of evaluating nodal material with polymerase chain reaction (PCR) techniques. These techniques are also being studied in breast cancer, where the clinical relevance (indication for adjuvant therapy) of micrometastases is accounted for in their size in the staging system. The significance of PCR-only metastases is highly controversial and, therefore, questions the need for this intense level of pathologic scrutiny.

Elective lymph node dissection has limited value in intermediate-thickness melanoma. In clinically node-negative patients, the use of the sentinel node technique can avoid postoperative complications, increase confidence about the better prognosis, and avoid the significant side effects of adjuvant immunologic therapy. However, the identification of histologically positive nodes via sentinel node biopsy is expected to have significant benefit in consideration of therapeutic node dissection and systemic therapies. In contrast, for patients with sentinel node-positive breast cancer, the value of completing a level I, II axillary node dissection is uncertain.

Palliation

In the continuum of care for the cancer patient, aspects of palliation, or the reduction of suffering, are delegated to the surgeon. This text includes many examples of palliative surgical procedures: venous access, surgical relief of ascites with shunt procedures, neurosurgical intervention for chronic pain, fixation of pathologic fractures, and placement of feeding tubes to deliver food and medications. The surgeon must be versed in the techniques of and indications for such interventions and discuss their risks and benefits with the patient, caregivers, and referring physician. The barriers to the initiation and practice of palliative surgery include the reluctance of patients, family, and referring physicians; health care system administrative obstacles; and cultural factors. A "therapeutic index" (time spent receiving treatment for symptoms versus time symptom free) should be constructed and discussed during the benefit/risk, informed consent process.

Resuscitation issues An ethical issue of resuscitation must be addressed when considering palliative surgical intervention. Some may take the position that if a patient is to have surgery, he or she must be willing to undergo full resuscitation if required. That tenet may be set aside in the palliative setting, in which the operative intervention is planned only to relieve suffering. In such a case, a frank discussion with the patient and appropriate family members can avoid the distressing situation of the patient being placed on unwanted, fruitless life support. Again, the surgeon is called upon not only to provide a technical service but also to achieve a comprehensive understanding of the disease process and how it affects each individual cancer patient.

SUGGESTED READING

Fortner JG: Inadvertent spread of cancer at surgery: Incidence and outcomes. J Surg Oncol 53:191–196, 1993.

Krouse RS, Nelson RA, Farrell BR, et al: Surgical palliation at a cancer center. Arch Surg 136:773–778, 2001.

McCahill LE, Krouse R, Chu D, et al: Indications and use of palliative surgery–results of Society of Surgical Oncology survey. Ann Surg Oncol 9:104–112, 2002.

McIntosh SA, Purushotham AD: Lymphatic mapping and sentinel node biopsy in breast cancer. Br J Surg 85:1347–1356, 1998.

The Clinical Outcomes of Surgical Therapy Study Group: A comparison of laparoscopically assisted and open colectomy for colon cancer. N Engl J Med 350:2050–2059, 2004.

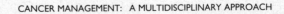

CHAPTER 2

Principles of radiation therapy

Kevin A. Camphausen, MD, and Lawrence R. Coia, MD

This chapter provides a brief overview of the principles of radiation therapy. The topics to be discussed include the physical aspects of how radiation works (ionization, radiation interactions) and how it is delivered (treatment machines, treatment planning, and brachytherapy). Recent relevant techniques of radiation oncology, such as conformal and stereotactic radiation therapy, also will be presented. These topics are not covered in great technical detail. It is hoped that a basic understanding of radiation treatment will benefit those practicing in other disciplines of cancer management. This chapter does not address the principles of radiobiology, which guide radiation oncologists in determining issues of treatment time, dose, and fractionation or in combining radiation with sensitizers, protectors, and chemotherapy or hormones.

How radiation works

IONIZING RADIATION

Ionizing radiation is energy sufficiently strong to remove an orbital electron from an atom. This radiation can have an electromagnetic form, such as a high-energy photon, or a particulate form, such as an electron, proton, neutron, or alpha particle.

High-energy photons By far, the most common form of radiation used in practice today is the high-energy photon. Photons that are released from the nucleus of a radioactive atom are known as gamma rays. When photons are created electronically, such as in a clinical linear accelerator, they are known as x-rays. Thus, the only difference between the two terms is the origin of the photon.

Inverse square law The intensity of an x-ray beam is governed by the inverse square law. This law states that the radiation intensity from a point source is inversely proportional to the square of the distance away from the radiation source. In other words, the dose at 2 cm will be one-fourth of the dose at 1 cm.

Electron volt Photon absorption in human tissue is determined by the energy of the radiation, as well as the atomic structure of the tissue in question. The basic unit of energy used in radiation oncology is the electron volt (eV); 10^3 eV = 1 keV, 10^6 eV = 1 MeV.

PHOTON-TISSUE INTERACTIONS

Three interactions describe photon absorption in tissue: the photoelectric effect, Compton effect, and pair production.

Photoelectric effect In this process, an incoming photon undergoes a collision with a tightly bound electron. The photon transfers practically all of its energy to the electron and ceases to exist. The electron departs with most of the energy from the photon and begins to ionize surrounding molecules. This interaction depends on the energy of the incoming photon, as well as the atomic number of the tissue; the lower the energy and the higher the atomic number, the more likely that a photoelectric effect will take place.

An example of this interaction in practice can be seen on a diagnostic x-ray film. Since the atomic number of bone is 60% higher than that of soft tissue, bone is seen with much more contrast and detail than is soft tissue. The energy range in which the photoelectric effect predominates in tissue is about 10–25 keV.

Compton effect The Compton effect is the most important photon-tissue interaction for the treatment of cancer. In this case, a photon collides with a "free electron," ie, one that is not tightly bound to the atom. Unlike the photoelectric effect, in the Compton interaction both the photon and electron are scattered. The photon can then continue to undergo additional interactions, albeit with a lower energy. The electron begins to ionize with the energy given to it by the photon.

The probability of a Compton interaction is inversely proportional to the energy of the incoming photon and is independent of the atomic number of the material. When one takes an image of tissue using photons in the energy range in which the Compton effect dominates (~25 keV–25 MeV), bone and soft-tissue interfaces are barely distinguishable. This is a result of the atomic number independence.

The Compton effect is the most common interaction occurring clinically, as most radiation treatments are performed at energy levels of about 6–20 MeV. Port films are films taken with such high-energy photons on the treatment machine and are used to check the precision and accuracy of the beam; because they do not distinguish tissue densities well, however, they are not equal to diagnostic films in terms of resolution.

Pair production In this process, a photon interacts with the nucleus of an atom, not an orbital electron. The photon gives up its energy to the nucleus and, in the process, creates a pair of positively and negatively charged electrons. The positive electron (positron) ionizes until it combines with a free electron. This generates two photons that scatter in opposite directions.

The probability of pair production is proportional to the logarithm of the energy of the incoming photon and is dependent on the atomic number of the material. The energy range in which pair production dominates is ≥ 25 MeV. This interaction occurs to some extent in routine radiation treatment with high-energy photon beams.

ELECTRON BEAMS

With the advent of high-energy linear accelerators, electrons have become a viable option in treating superficial tumors up to a depth of about 5 cm. Electron depth dose characteristics are unique in that they produce a high skin dose but exhibit a falloff after only a few centimeters.

Electron absorption in human tissue is greatly influenced by the presence of air cavities and bone. The dose is increased when the electron beam passes through an air space and is reduced when the beam passes through bone.

Common uses The most common clinical uses of electron beams include the treatment of skin lesions, such as basal cell carcinomas, and boosting of areas that have previously received photon irradiation, such as the postoperative lumpectomy or mastectomy scar in breast cancer patients, as well as select nodal areas in the head and neck.

MEASURING RADIATION ABSORPTION

The dose of radiation absorbed correlates directly with the energy of the beam. An accurate measurement of absorbed dose is critical in radiation treatment. The deposition of energy in tissues results in damage to DNA and diminishes or eradicates the cell's ability to replicate indefinitely.

Gray The basic unit of radiation absorbed dose is the amount of energy (joules) absorbed per unit mass (kg). This unit, known as the gray (Gy), has replaced the unit of rad used in the past (100 rads = 1 Gy; 1 rad = 1 cGy).

Exposure To measure dose in a patient, one must first measure the ionization produced in air by a beam of radiation. This quantity is known as exposure. One can then correct for the presence of soft tissue in the air and calculate the absorbed dose in Gy.

Percentage depth dose The dose absorbed by tissues due to these interactions can be measured and plotted to form a percentage depth dose curve. As energy increases, the penetrative ability of the beam increases and the skin dose decreases.

How radiation is delivered

TREATMENT MACHINES

Linear accelerators

High-energy radiation is delivered to tumors by means of a linear accelerator. A beam of electrons is generated and accelerated through a waveguide that increases their energy to the keV to MeV range. These electrons strike a tungsten target and produce x-rays.

X-rays generated in the 10–30-keV range are known as grenz rays, whereas the energy range for superficial units is about 30–125 keV. Orthovoltage units generate x-rays from 125–500 keV.

Orthovoltage units continue to be used today to treat superficial lesions; in fact, they were practically the only machines treating skin lesions before the recent emergence of electron therapy. The maximum dose from any of these low-energy units is found on the surface of patients; thus, skin becomes the dose-limiting structure when treating patients at these energies. The depth at which the dose is 50% of the maximum is about 7 cm. Table 1 lists the physical characteristics of several relevant x-ray energies.

Megavoltage units The megavoltage linear accelerator has been the standard radiotherapy equipment for the past 20 to 30 years. Its production of x-rays is identical to that of lower-energy machines. However, the energy range of megavoltage units is broad–from 4 to 20 MeV. The depth of the maximum dose in this energy range is 1.5–3.5 cm. The dose to the skin is about 30% to 40% of the maximum dose.

Most megavoltage units today also have electron-beam capabilities, usually in the energy range of about 5–20 MeV. To produce an electron beam, the tungsten target is moved away from the path of the beam. The original electron beam that was aimed at the tungsten target is now the electron beam used for treatment. Unlike that of photons, the electron skin dose is high, about 80% to 95% of the maximum dose. A rule of thumb regarding the depth of penetration of electrons is that 80% of the dose is delivered at a depth (in cm) corresponding to one-third of the electron energy (in MeV). Thus, a 12-MeV beam will deliver 80% of the dose at a depth of 4 cm.

Altering beam intensity and field size When measurements are made at the point just past the target, the beam is more intense in the center than at the edges. Optimal treatment planning is obtained with a relatively constant intensity across the width of the beam. This process is accomplished by placing a flattening filter below the target.

For the radiation beam to conform to a certain size, high atomic number collimators are installed in the machine. They can vary the field size from 4×4 cm to 40×40 cm at a distance of 100 cm from the target, which is the distance at which most treatments are performed.

TABLE 1: Depth dose characteristics for clinical radiotherapy beams

Nominal energy	Depth of maximum dose (cm)	Skin dose (%)
240 kV(p)	Surface	100
Cobalt-60	0.500	50
6 MeV	1.500	35
10 MeV	2.500	25
18 MeV	3.000	15

kV(p) = kilovolt (peak)

If it is decided that a beam should be more intense on one side than the other, high atomic number filters, known as wedges, are placed in the beam. These filters can shift the dose distribution surrounding the tumor by 15°–60°. Wedges can also be used to optimize the dose distribution if the treatment surface is curved or irregular.

Shielding normal tissue Once the collimators have been opened to the desired field size that encompasses the tumor, the physician may decide to block out some normal tissue that remains in the treatment field. This is accomplished by placing blocks (or alloy), constructed of a combination of bismuth, tin, cadmium, and lead, in the path of the beam. In this way, normal tissues are shielded, and the dose can be delivered to the tumor at a higher level than if the normal structures were in the field. These individually constructed blocks are used in both x-ray and electron treatments. A more modern technique involves multileaf collimators mounted inside the gantry. They provide computerized, customized blocking instead of having to construct a new block for each field. (See section on "Intensity-modulated radiation therapy.")

PRETREATMENT PROCEDURES

Certain imaging procedures must be performed before radiation therapy is begun.

Pretreatment CT Before any treatment planning can begin, a pretreatment CT scan is often performed. This scan allows the radiation oncologist to identify both the tumor and surrounding normal structures.

Simulation The patient is then sent for a simulation. The patient is placed on a diagnostic x-ray unit that geometrically simulates an actual treatment machine. With use of the CT information, the patient's treatment position is simulated by means of fluoroscopy. A series of orthogonal films are taken, and block templates that will shield any normal structures are drawn on the films. These films are sent to the mold room, where technicians construct the blocks to be used for treatment. CT simulation is a modern alternative to "conventional" simulation and is described later in this chapter.

Guides for treatment field placement Small skin marks, or tattoos, are placed on the patient following proper positioning in simulation. These tattoos will guide the placement of treatment fields and give the physician a permanent record of past fields should the patient need additional treatment in the future.

It is imperative that the patient be treated in a reproducible manner each day. To facilitate this, Styrofoam casts that conform to the patient's contour and place the patient in the same position for each treatment are constructed. Lasers also help line up the patient during treatment.

TREATMENT PLANNING AND DELIVERY

Determining optimal dose distribution The medical physicist or dosimetrist uses the information from CT and simulation to plan the treatment on a computer. A complete collection of machine data, including depth dose and beam profile information, is stored in the computer. The physics staff aids the radiation oncologist in deciding the number of beams (usually two to four) and angles of entry. The goal is to maximize the dose to the tumor while minimizing the dose to surrounding normal structures.

Several treatment plans are generated, and the radiation oncologist chooses the optimal dose distribution. The beam-modifying devices discussed earlier, such as blocks and wedges, may be used to optimize the dose distribution around the tumor.

Establishing the treatment plan The planning computer will calculate the amount of time each beam should be on during treatment. All pertinent data, such as beam-on time, beam angles, blocks, and wedges, are recorded in the patient's treatment chart and sent to the treatment machine. The radiation therapist will use this information, as well as any casts, tattoos, and lasers, to set up and treat the patient consistently and accurately each day.

Taking weekly port films As part of departmental quality assurance, weekly port films are taken for each beam. They ensure that the beams and blocks are consistently and correctly placed for each treatment. Port films are images generated by the linear accelerator at energies of 6–20 MeV. Because of the predominance of the Compton effect in this energy range, these images are not as detailed as those at diagnostic film energies (as mentioned earlier), but they still provide important information on treatment accuracy and ensure the quality of setup and treatment.

BRACHYTHERAPY

Brachytherapy is the term used to describe radiation treatment in which the radiation source is in contact with the tumor. This therapy contrasts with external-beam radiotherapy, in which the radiation source is 80–100 cm away from the patient.

In brachytherapy, dose distribution is almost totally dependent on the inverse square law because the source is usually within the tumor volume. Because of this inverse square dependence, the proper placement of radiation sources is crucial.

Isotopes Table 2 lists commonly used isotopes and their properties. In the past, radium was the primary isotope used in brachytherapy. Recently, because of its long half-life and high energy output, radium has been replaced with cesium (Cs), gold (Au), and iridium (Ir). These isotopes have shorter half-lives than radium and can be shielded more easily because of their lower energies.

Types of implants Brachytherapy procedures can be performed with either temporary or permanent implants. Temporary implants usually have long half-lives and higher energies than permanent implants. These sources can be manufactured in several forms, such as needles, seeds, and ribbons.

All temporary sources are inserted into catheters that are placed in the tumor during surgery. A few days after surgery, the patient is brought to the radiation clinic and undergoes pretreatment simulation. Wires with nonradioactive metal

TABLE 2: Physical characteristics of commonly used radioisotopes

Isotope	Energy (MeV)	Half-life
Radium-226	0.830	1,600 yr
Cesium-137	0.662	30 yr
Cobalt-60	1.250	5.26 yr
Iridium-192	0.380	74.2 d
Iodine-125	0.028	60.2 d
Gold-198	0.412	2.7 d
Palladium-103	0.210	17d

seeds are threaded into these catheters. Several films are taken, and the images of the seed placement can be digitized into a brachytherapy treatment planning computer.

Once the treatment plan is complete and the physician has chosen the optimal dose rate (usually 50–60 cGy/h), the sources can be implanted. The actual implantation takes place in the patient's private room. The duration of treatment is usually 1 to 3 days. The majority of temporary implants are loaded interstitially.

Common uses Interstitial low-dose–rate (LDR) brachytherapy is commonly used for cancer of the oral cavity and oropharynx and sarcoma. Prostate cancer is probably the most common site for which LDR brachytherapy "seeds" are used today. Intracavitary LDR brachytherapy is frequently used in gynecologic applications. High-dose–rate (HDR) brachytherapy is used with remote afterloading techniques, as described below.

Remote afterloading brachytherapy

Because brachytherapy requires numerous safety precautions and entails unnecessary exposure of personnel and family members to radiation, remote afterloading of temporary implants has become popular in recent years. The two types of remote afterloading that can be used for treatment are LDR and HDR sources. The most popular LDR source used today is Cs-137, which has a dose rate of about 1 cGy/min. The most widely used HDR source is Ir-192. This isotope has a dose rate of about 100 cGy/min.

General procedures The pretreatment brachytherapy procedures outlined above are also implemented in remote afterloading brachytherapy. Once the treatment plan has been approved by the physician, the patient is brought into the treatment room. The LDR cesium source or HDR iridium source is connected to the end of a cable inside its respective afterloading unit. This unit is programmed with the data from the planning computer. The cable is sent out from the unit into one of the patient's catheters. Several catheters can be connected to the unit. Each catheter is irradiated, one at a time, until the prescribed dose has been delivered.

The motor that drives the source out of the treatment unit is connected electronically to the door of the treatment room. If the treatment must be stopped for any reason, simply opening the door triggers an interlock that draws the source back into the unit. Because of this device, oncology personnel will not be exposed to any radiation should they need to see the patient during treatment. This interlock is the main safety advantage of remote afterloading over manual afterloading.

LDR treatment Uterine cancer is the most popular application for intracavitary treatment with LDR remote afterloading brachytherapy. These procedures are performed in the patient's room. The interlock is connected to the patient's door so that nurses can take vital signs and give medication and family members can visit the patient without risk of radiation exposure.

HDR treatment The most common applications of HDR brachytherapy are for tumors of the vaginal apex, esophagus, lungs, and, most recently, breasts and prostate. Most HDR treatments are performed on an outpatient basis. Allowing the patient to return home the same day after therapy is one advantage of HDR afterloading brachytherapy. Patients with prostate cancer are the exception. They may remain in the hospital for 2 to 3 days during treatment.

Recent advances in planning and treatment

CT SIMULATION

Until recently, CT and simulation were separate pretreatment procedures. Within the past decade, many cancer centers have combined CT and simulation into a single diagnostic-treatment planning unit, known as a CT simulator. The major advantage of this combination is that both procedures can be performed by one unit, and, thus, the patient does not have to make two separate visits to the clinic. Also, CT simulation is bringing the radiation clinic into the digital age, with hospitals reporting an increase in speed, efficiency, and accuracy of treatment planning and delivery.

Procedure In brief, in the first step of this new procedure, the patient is placed on the CT simulator table and undergoes a normal CT study. The physician has the capability of outlining the tumor and any normal structures on each CT slice. A computer performs a three-dimensional (3D) transformation of the CT slices and creates a digitally reconstructed radiograph (DRR).

The DRR resembles a normal diagnostic film, except that it is digital and can be manipulated to achieve better contrast and detail than regular film. The outlines of the tumor and organs are displayed on the DRR for any viewing angle. The physician can then draw blocks on the DRR with a more accurate idea of where the tumor and normal tissues actually are.

The DRR is digitized into the treatment planning computer, and any CT slices and their contours drawn by the physician are transferred as well. This DRR is either sent to the mold room for block construction or is transferred to the treatment planning software for multileaf collimator optimization. Treatment plans are generated as discussed earlier.

At the time of the patient's first treatment, DRRs and port films are digitized and saved on a local area network (LAN). Physicians can then call up these images on their desktop computers for weekly patient quality assurance.

CONFORMAL RADIATION THERAPY

Conformal radiation therapy is a geometric shaping of the radiation beam that conforms with the beam's eye view of the tumor. Conformal therapy utilizes the outlining capabilities of the CT simulator. The physician outlines the tumor volume, generates DRRs, and draws an appropriate margin from 1–2 cm around the tumor. These fields conform closely to the shape of the tumor and, thus, shield more critical structures than do normal blocks. The margin allows for setup errors of a few millimeters each day. Appropriate immobilization of the target volume must be achieved in each patient through the use of devices that constrain movement ("casts"), so that the target is accurately localized.

Films are sent to the mold room for block construction. Since the fields are "tighter" around the tumor, the prescribed dose can be increased. By increasing the dose to the tumor, local control will be improved.

INTENSITY-MODULATED RADIATION THERAPY (IMRT)

Intensity-modulated radiation therapy (IMRT), an extension of conformal therapy, allows for shaping of the intensity of the radiation beam. This is an important improvement, especially when the target is not well separated from normal tissues.

A uniform dose distribution can be created around the tumor by either modulating the intensity of the beam during its journey through the linear accelerator or using multileaf collimators. Multileaf collimators consist of 80 or more individual collimators, or "leaves," located at the head of the linear accelerator, which can be adjusted to the shape of the tumor. (For a technical description, the reader is referred to the text by Khan; see "Suggested Reading.")

Both of these methods alter the fluence (the number of x-rays per unit area) of radiation exiting the accelerator. The final result is a uniform dose distribution around the tumor and minimal dose to the surrounding normal tissues, often below tolerance levels. This improves the risk-benefit ratio.

The clinical use of IMRT has grown as computer power increases and costs decline. Preliminary clinical data have shown that prostate doses can be increased significantly without increasing the complication rate. IMRT must be administered within a closely monitored program with rigorous quality assurance, since it can potentially cause significant injury if not appropriately applied.

Several types of IMRT delivery are now becoming standard in radiation oncology clinics. Dynamic conformal therapy with multileaf collimators is being used routinely in hospitals around the country. With this approach, collimators conform to the tumor volume with the beam on while the treatment unit is rotating around the patient. This is an example of totally computer-controlled radiation delivery.

TOMOTHERAPY

Serial tomotherapy is an enhancement of the method previously described. An accelerator is equipped with mini-multileaf collimators that form a "slit" of radiation (normally 2 × 20 cm). The gantry is rotated through an entire arc around the patient while the mini-multileaf collimators are driven in and out of the field, thus modulating the intensity of the beam. The treatment couch is advanced by a few millimeters and the next arc is treated. An entire treatment is given once all the adjoining arcs have been delivered.

Instead of treating the patient on a normal linear accelerator, with helical tomotherapy the patient travels continuously through a modified CT ring. This CT ring has the capability of administering 6-mV x-rays, as in a standard linear accelerator, while at the same time performing a conventional diagnostic CT scan. Any anatomic or position changes that might require replanning can be performed before that day's treatment. Following treatment, a daily, real-time image of the dose distribution can be obtained.

PROTON THERAPY

Protons, a form of particulate radiation, have been investigated recently as a means to improve tumor control. A proton has a charge of +1, is a stable particle, and, together with the neutron, makes up the atomic nucleus.

Protons are delivered to the tumor in the same manner as are photons and electrons. The dose deposited by protons remains relatively constant as they travel through the normal tissues proximal to the target.

The kinetic energy of the protons is transferred to the tumors by electrons knocked out of atoms. These electrons ionize DNA, and their biologic effectiveness resembles that of megavoltage photons.

Bragg peak At the end of the path, biologic effectiveness increases sharply as the protons slow down and eventually stop. This increase in dose is called the Bragg peak. The size of the Bragg peak is usually smaller than the tumor, however. This problem can be resolved by scanning the Bragg peak through the tumor volume by sequentially irradiating the target with lower energies. The dose falloff of the Bragg peak is sharp enough that the normal tissues distal to the tumor receive a negligible radiation dose.

Current clinical applications Uveal melanomas and skull-base sarcomas adjacent to CNS tissues, as well as prostate cancer, are areas in which proton therapy has been under clinical study, with promising results. Clinical studies are also examining its use in non–small-cell lung, hepatocellular, and paranasal sinus carcinomas.

STEREOTACTIC RADIOSURGERY

Stereotactic radiosurgery is a 3D technique that delivers the radiation dose in one fraction. Specially designed collimators are attached to a linear accelerator, which delivers a high dose of radiation to a small volume, usually about 3 cm in diameter. Several stationary beams or multiple arc rotations concentrate the radiation dose to the lesion while sparing surrounding normal tissue.

Although it is most often used to treat lesions within the brain, it can be used for selected extracranial sites (in which case it may be referred to as "body radiosurgery").

Use in treating arteriovenous malformations Stereotactic radiosurgery is used to treat certain patients with arteriovenous malformations. These intracranial lesions arise from the abnormal development of arteries and venous sinuses. Surgical excision is the standard treatment of choice for operable lesions, but stereotactic radiosurgery has become a viable option for inoperable malformations.

Use in treating brain tumors As with conformal radiotherapy, clinical trials involving stereotactic radiosurgery for brain tumors are being conducted at major cancer centers. However, based on positive early results, many community centers have begun instituting a stereotactic radiosurgery program, either with a dedicated cobalt unit (Gamma Knife) or a linear accelerator-based system. Small (< 4 cm) tumors of the brain, whether primary, metastatic, or recurrent, may benefit from this treatment technique. The Gamma Knife is a form of stereotactic radiosurgery that uses multiple focused cobalt beams to treat lesions in the brain.

SUGGESTED READING

Chao KSC: Practical Essentials of Intensity Modulated Radiation Therapy, 2nd edition. Philadelphia, Lippincott Williams & Wilkins, 2004.

Chinnaiyan P, Allen GW, Harari PM: Radiation and new molecular agents, Part II: Targeting HDAC, HSP90, IGF-1R, P13K, and Ras. Semin Radiat Oncol 16:59–64, 2006.

Choudhury A, Cuddihy A, Bristow RG: Radiation and new molecular agents, Part I: Targeting ATM-ATR checkpoints, DNA repair, and the proteasome. Semin Radiat Oncol 16:51–58, 2006.

Coia LR, Schultheiss TE, Hanks GE: A Practical Guide to CT Simulation. Madison, Wisconsin, Advanced Medical Publishing, 1995.

Fenwick JD, Tome WA, Soisson ET, et al: Tomotherapy and other innovative IMRT delivery systems. Semin Radiat Oncol 16:199–208, 2006.

Hall EJ: Radiobiology for the Radiologist, 5th edition. Philadelphia, Lippincott Williams & Wilkins, 2000.

IMRT CWG: Intensity modulated radiotherapy: Current status and issues of interest. Int J Radiat Oncol Biol Phys 51:880–914, 2001.

Khan FM: Treatment Planning in Radiation Oncology. Baltimore, Maryland, Williams & Wilkins, 1998.

Perez CA, Brady LW: Principles and Practice of Radiation Oncology. Philadelphia, Lippincott-Raven, 1998.

Suit H: The Gray Lecture: Coming technical advances in radiation oncology. Int J Radiat Oncol Biol Phys 53:798–809, 2002.

Ten Haken RK, Lawrence TS: The clinical application of intensity-modulated radiation therapy. Semin Radiat Oncol 16:224–231, 2006.

Van Dyk J: The Modern Technology of Radiation Oncology. Madison, Wisconsin, Medical Physics Publishing, 1999.

CHAPTER 3

Principles of oncologic pharmacotherapy

Chris H. Takimoto, MD, PhD, and Emiliano Calvo, MD, PhD

The effective use of cancer chemotherapy requires a thorough understanding of the principles of neoplastic cell growth kinetics, basic pharmacologic mechanisms of drug action, pharmacokinetic and pharmacodynamic variability, and mechanisms of drug resistance. Recent scientific advances in the field of molecular oncology have led to the identification of large numbers of potential targets for novel anticancer therapies. This has resulted in a tremendous expansion of the drug development pipeline, and in the present era, the diversity of clinically useful novel anticancer therapeutic agents is growing at an unprecedented rate. However, the great enthusiasm that surrounds these new agents must be tempered by the challenges they present in optimizing their clinical use and in rationally integrating them with existing anticancer therapies. This discussion focuses on the basic principles underlying the development of modern combination chemotherapy, and it is followed by a description of the major classes of chemotherapeutic drugs and their mechanisms of action.

The cell cycle and tumor growth pattern

The growth pattern of individual neoplastic cells may greatly affect the overall biologic behavior of human tumors and their responses to specific types of cancer therapy. Tumor cells can be subdivided into three general populations: (1) cells that are not dividing and are terminally differentiated; (2) cells that continue to proliferate; and (3) nondividing cells that are currently quiescent but may be recruited into the cell cycle. The kinetic behavior of dividing cells is best described by the concept of the cell cycle.

The cell cycle is composed of four distinct phases during which the cell prepares for and undergoes mitosis. The G_1 phase consists of cells that have recently completed division and are committed to continued proliferation. After a variable period, these cells begin to synthesize DNA, marking the beginning of the S phase. After DNA synthesis is complete, the end of the S phase is followed by the premitotic rest interval called the G_2 phase. Finally, chromosome condensation occurs and the cells divide during the mitotic M phase. Resting diploid cells that are not actively dividing are described as being in the G_0 phase. The transition between cell-cycle phases is strictly regulated by specific signaling proteins; however, these cell-cycle checkpoints may become aberrant in some tumor types.

Some anticancer agents induce their cytotoxic effects during specific phases of the cell cycle. Antimetabolites, such as fluorouracil (5-FU) and methotrexate, are more active against S-phase cells, whereas the vinca alkaloids, epipodophyllotoxins, and taxanes are relatively more M-phase specific. These kinetic properties may have clinically important consequences for cancer chemotherapy. For example, cell-cycle–nonspecific agents, such as the alkylating agents and platinum derivatives, generally have linear dose-response curves (ie, increasing the dose increases cytotoxicity). In contrast, cell-cycle–specific agents will often plateau in their concentration-dependent effects because only a subset of proliferating cells remain fully sensitive to drug-induced cytotoxicity. These cell-cycle–specific agents tend to be schedule dependent, because the only way to increase the total cell kill is by extending the duration of exposure, not by increasing the dose.

In clinical practice, solid tumors typically have low growth fractions and heterogeneous doubling times; as they increase in size, tumors may outgrow their blood and nutrient supply, leading to slower growth rates. In real life, most tumors display a sigmoid-shaped Gompertzian growth pattern in which growth rates decline as tumors expand. The most rapid growth occurs at small tumor volumes, whereas larger tumors may harbor higher numbers of nonproliferating cells, potentially making them less sensitive to agents that selectively target dividing cells. This understanding of tumor growth kinetics has been used to support the development of novel clinical strategies for optimizing cancer chemotherapy. This includes the use of adjuvant chemotherapy to treat small volumes of tumor cells during times of high growth rates and the sequential administration of non–cross-resistant drug combinations.

TABLE 1: Principles for selecting agents for use in combination chemotherapy regimens

Drugs known to be active as single agents should be selected for use in combinations; preferentially drugs that induce complete remission should be included.

Drugs with different mechanisms of action and with additive or synergistic cytotoxic effects on the tumor should be combined.

Drugs with different dose-limiting toxicities should be combined, so full or nearly full therapeutic doses can be utilized.

Drugs should be used at their optimal dose and schedule.

Drugs should be given at consistent intervals, and the treatment-free period should be as short as possible to allow for recovery for the most sensitive normal tissues.

Drugs with different patterns of resistance should be used to minimize cross-resistance.

Principles of combination chemotherapy

Based upon cell kinetic and pharmacologic principles, a set of guidelines for designing modern combination chemotherapy regimens has been derived. Multiagent therapy has three important theoretical advantages over single-agent therapy. First, it can maximize cell kill while minimizing host toxicities by using agents with nonoverlapping dose-limiting toxicities. Second, it may increase the range of drug activity against tumor cells with endogenous resistance to specific types of therapy. Finally, it may also prevent or slow the development of newly resistant tumor cells. Specific principles for selecting agents for use in combination chemotherapy regimens are listed in Table 1.

DEFINITION OF RESPONSE

In clinical studies, formal response criteria have been developed and have gained wide acceptance. The National Cancer Institute (NCI) has proposed and implemented newer standard response criteria called Response Evaluation Criteria in Solid Tumors (RECIST). In contrast, the World Health Organization (WHO) has a different standard for assessing response. Major differences between these guidelines are outlined in Appendix 1.

DRUG RESISTANCE

Drug resistance to chemotherapy may arise from a variety of different mechanisms, including anatomic, pharmacologic, and genetic processes. Some of the common factors that may broadly affect tumor cell sensitivity to different classes of agents include the failure of drugs to penetrate into specific sanctuary sites, such as the brain and testes, or the development of mutations in the target proteins that render them less sensitive to specific molecular inhibitors. Another factor may be decreased drug accumulation resulting from the increased expression of drug efflux pumps in the cell membrane, such as p-glycoprotein, which is encoded for by the multidrug resistance (MDR-1) gene. This 170-kDa glycoprotein normally removes toxins or xenobiotic metabolites from cells via an energy-dependent process. High levels of MDR-1 expression in tumor cells correlate with resistance to a wide range of cytotoxic agents. Other drug efflux pumps that have been implicated in the development of broad resistance to cancer chemotherapy include the MDR-associated protein (MRP) and breast cancer resistance protein (BCRP).

Pharmacokinetic and pharmacodynamic variability

VARIABILITY IN CLEARANCE

The rational clinical use of cancer chemotherapy requires a thorough understanding of the variability in human response to drug therapy. One of the major goals of the field of clinical pharmacology is to precisely define the processes responsible for this variability in drug action. Pharmacokinetic variability can arise from interindividual differences in drug adsorption, distribution, metabolism, and excretion. All of these processes result in differences in drug delivery to its ultimate site of action. In contrast, pharmacodynamic variability arises from inherent differences in the sensitivity of target tissues to drug effects. Both kinetic and dynamic factors can complicate the treatment of individual cancer patients and must be addressed by the practicing oncologist on a daily basis. Although a formal review of drug pharmacokinetics and pharmacodynamics is not possible here, a brief discussion of the most clinically relevant points is warranted.

The most clinically useful parameter in drug therapy is clearance, because clearance reflects all the processes in the body that contribute to drug elimination. In oncology, the importance of clearance is enhanced because clearance is the only parameter that relates dose to the measured area under the concentration vs time curve (AUC), which is a useful measure of systemic drug exposure. Mathematically, clearance is defined as dose/AUC. Clearance is not a rate of drug elimination; instead it is defined as a volume of drug cleared per unit of time.

Overcoming interindividual variation in clearance is a fundamental goal of pharmacokinetic analyses. Because they tend to be highly toxic with low efficacy, anticancer drugs may have the narrowest therapeutic index of any class of agents used in clinical medicine. Thus, the ability to administer an individualized dose of drug to achieve a uniform target AUC and a uniform clinical result is often a high priority for cancer therapeutics. Because clearance defines the relationship between dose and AUC, estimating clearance prior to anticancer drug administration is extremely important. A common attempt to individualize cancer chemotherapy is to dose a drug based upon the body surface area (BSA) expressed in mg/m^2 to achieve a uniform AUC in patients with different body sizes. Inherent in this approach is the fundamental assumption that clearance is strongly correlated with BSA. However, when studied formally, the relationship between clearance and BSA is often weak and does not consistently justify the routine use of this dosing approach. Nonetheless, although the application of BSA-based dosing has been widely criticized, it still remains a common practice.

Recognizing clinical situations in which drug clearance is commonly altered, such as in patients with hepatic or renal dysfunction, is important for agents that are eliminated by these routes. For example, carboplatin is extensively cleared by glomerular filtration, and its systemic AUC in plasma ultrafiltrates is strongly correlated with pharmacodynamic effects, such as thrombocytopenia. Thus, dosing strategies that estimate the glomerular filtration rate (GFR) to achieve a targeted AUC and thereby minimize excessive toxicity in individual patients have gained wide clinical acceptance. Likewise, for hepatically metabolized drugs, doses must be adjusted in patients with liver dysfunction. However, accurately assessing hepatic drug-metabolizing capacity is more difficult than estimating the GFR. Nonetheless, guidelines for dose-adjusting agents metabolized in the liver, such as doxorubicin, have been established.

PHARMACOGENOMIC VARIABILITY

Variability in drug action may also be caused by genetic factors. The new field of pharmacogenomics attempts to define the impact of genetic differences on drug kinetics and dynamics. McLeod and Evans have defined pharmacogenomics as the field of study of "the inherited nature of interindividual differences in drug disposition and effects." Clinically relevant genetic variations have been characterized in specific drug-metabolizing enzymes, such as the cytochrome P-450 isoforms CYP2D6 and CYP2C9.

In the field of medical oncology, well-defined examples of clinically relevant pharmacogenetic differences are relatively few; however, this is an important area of ongoing research. Perhaps the best characterized example in clinical oncology is the inherited deficiency of the thiopurine methyltransferase (TPMT) enzyme that results in severe intolerance to thiopurine therapy. Another example is the inherited variation in dihydropyrimidine dehydrogenase (DPD) activity, the rate-limiting catabolic enzyme responsible for clearance of 5-FU. Genetic alterations associated with DPD deficiency have been identified in rare patients experiencing severe and fatal toxicity after treatment with standard doses of 5-FU. Finally, interindividual variation in irinotecan-induced toxicities may be partially explained by genetic polymorphisms in the gene encoding the UDP-glucuronosyltransferase (UGT) 1A1 enzyme that is involved in the clearance of the active metabolite SN-38. Also, the identification of somatic mutations in the tyrosine kinase domain of the epidermal growth factor receptor (EGFR) in non–small-cell lung cancer (NSCLC) and their correlation with response to EGFR inhibitors has become an important event in the fields of cancer genomics and therapeutics. The issue of ethnic diversity in the pathogenesis of given tumors was raised by the initial observation of a higher response to gefitinib (Iressa) and erlotinib (Tarceva) in patients of Asian origin, together with the discovery that they harbor more frequent EGFR mutations in non–small-cell lung cancer.

Pharmacodynamic polymorphisms that directly affect target tissue sensitivity to drug effects are also clinically important. For example, polymorphisms in the promoter region of the thymidylate synthase gene have been correlated with tumor response to 5-FU–based chemotherapy that targets this enzyme. In the near future, our understanding of how genetics affects a drug's pharmacokinetics may ultimately allow for the optimization of specific treatment regimens for individual patients. Likewise, our understanding of how genetics affects pharmacodynamic variation may be enhanced by powerful new technologies that can characterize the expression of literally thousands of genes within the tumor itself. The molecular profiling of tumor cells by DNA microarray techniques and other advances in biotechnology offer tremendous hope for improving our ability to treat cancer in the near future.

Molecularly targeted therapies

At the beginning of the 21st century, important and meaningful advances in anticancer therapeutics are being discovered at an unparalleled rate. Much of this progress is driven by the explosion of knowledge in the field of molecular oncology. The sequencing of the entire human genome has dramatically increased the number of promising molecular targets for new and novel anticancer treatment strategies. These advances hold great promise for developing a new generation of agents with high specificity for tumor cells (see discussion later in this chapter).

Chemotherapeutic agents classified by mechanism of action

Alkylating agents

The alkylating agents impair cell function by forming covalent bonds with the amino, carboxyl, sulfhydryl, and phosphate groups in biologically important molecules. The most important sites of alkylation are DNA, RNA, and proteins. The electron-rich nitrogen at the 7 position of guanine in DNA is particularly susceptible to alkylation.

Alkylating agents depend on cell proliferation for activity but are not cell-cycle-phase–specific. A fixed percentage of cells are killed at a given dose. Tumor resistance probably occurs through efficient glutathione conjugation or by enhanced DNA repair mechanisms. Alkylating agents are classified according to their chemical structure and mechanism of covalent bonding; this drug class includes the nitrogen mustards, nitrosoureas, and platinum complexes, among other agents (Table 2).

Nitrogen mustards The nitrogen mustards, which include such drugs as mechlorethamine (Mustargen), cyclophosphamide, ifosfamide, and chlorambucil (Leukeran), are powerful local vesicants; as such, they can cause problems ranging from local tissue necrosis to pulmonary fibrosis to hemorrhagic cystitis. The metabolites of these compounds are highly reactive in aqueous solution, in which an active alkylating moiety, the ethylene immonium ion, binds to DNA. The hematopoietic system is especially susceptible to these compounds.

Nitrosoureas The nitrosoureas are distinguished by their high lipid solubility and chemical instability. These agents rapidly and spontaneously decompose into two highly reactive intermediates: chloroethyl diazohydroxide and isocyanate. The lipophilic nature of the nitrosoureas enables free passage across membranes; therefore, they rapidly penetrate the blood-brain barrier, achieving effective CNS concentrations. Consequently, these agents are used for a variety of brain tumors.

Platinum agents Cisplatin is an inorganic heavy metal complex that has activity typical of a cell-cycle-phase–nonspecific alkylating agent. The compound produces intrastrand and interstrand DNA cross-links and forms DNA adducts, thereby inhibiting the synthesis of DNA, RNA, and proteins. Carboplatin has the same active diamine platinum moiety as cisplatin, but it is bonded to an organic carboxylate group that allows increased water solubility and slower hydrolysis to the alkylating aqueous platinum complex, thus altering toxicity

TABLE 2: Chemotherapeutic agents[a]

Alkylating agents

- **Nitrogen mustards:** chlorambucil, cyclophosphamide, estramustine, ifosfamide, mechlorethamine, melphalan
- **Aziridine:** thiotepa
- **Alkyl sulfonate:** busulfan
- **Nitrosoureas:** carmustine, lomustine, streptozocin
- **Platinum complexes:** carboplatin, cisplatin, oxaliplatin
- **Nonclassic alkylators:** altretamine, dacarbazine, procarbazine, temozolomide

Antimetabolites

- **Folate analogs:** methotrexate, pemetrexed
- **Purine analogs:** fludarabine, mercaptopurine, thioguanine
- **Adenosine analogs:** cladribine, pentostatin
- **Pyrimidine analogs:** capecitabine, cytarabine, floxuridine, fluorouracil, gemcitabine
- **Substituted urea:** hydroxyurea

Natural products

- **Antitumor antibiotics:** bleomycin, dactinomycin, daunorubicin, doxorubicin, epirubicin, idarubicin, mitoxantrone, mitomycin, valrubicin
- **Epipodophyllotoxins:** etoposide, teniposide
- **Microtubule agents:** docetaxel, paclitaxel, vinblastine, vincristine, vinorelbine
- **Camptothecin analogs:** irinotecan, topotecan
- **Enzyme:** asparaginase

Targeted agents

- **Monoclonal antibodies:** alemtuzumab, bevacizumab, cetuximab, panitumumab, rituximab, trastuzumab,
- **Molecularly targeted therapies:** bortezomib, dasatinib, erlotinib, gefitinib, imatinib, lapatinib, sorafenib, sunitinib, temsirolimus

[a]For a comprehensive table of drug information including dosages and toxicities, see Appendix 4.

profiles. Oxaliplatin (Eloxatin) is distinguished from the other platinum compounds by a di-amino-cyclohexane ring bound to the platinum molecule, which interferes with resistance mechanisms to the drug.

Antimetabolites

Antimetabolites are structural analogs of the naturally occurring metabolites involved in DNA and RNA synthesis. As the constituents of these metabolic pathways have been elucidated, a large number of structurally similar drugs that alter the critical pathways of nucleotide synthesis have been developed. Antimetabolites exert their cytotoxic activity either by competing with normal metabolites for the catalytic or regulatory site of a key enzyme or by substituting for a metabolite that is normally incorporated into DNA and RNA. Because of this mechanism of action, antimetabolites are most active when cells are in the S phase and have little effect on cells in the G_0 phase. Consequently, these drugs are most effective against tumors that have a high growth fraction.

Antimetabolites have a nonlinear dose-response curve, such that after a certain dose, no more cells are killed despite increasing doses (5-FU is an exception). The antimetabolites can be divided into folate analogs, purine analogs, adenosine analogs, pyrimidine analogs, and substituted urea.

Natural products

A wide variety of compounds possessing antitumor activity have been isolated from natural substances, such as plants, fungi, and bacteria. Likewise, selected compounds have semisynthetic and synthetic designs based on the active chemical structure of the parent compounds, and they, too, have cytotoxic effects.

Antitumor antibiotics Bleomycin preferentially intercalates DNA at guanine-cytosine and guanine-thymine sequences, resulting in spontaneous oxidation and formation of free oxygen radicals that cause strand breakage.

Anthracyclines The anthracycline antibiotics are products of the fungus *Streptomyces percetus* var *caesius.* They are chemically similar, with a basic anthracycline structure containing a glycoside bound to an amino sugar, daunosamine. The anthracyclines have several modes of action. Most notable are intercalation between DNA base pairs and inhibition of DNA–topoisomerases I and II. Oxygen free radical formation from reduced doxorubicin intermediates is thought to be a mechanism associated with cardiotoxicity.

Epipodophyllotoxins Etoposide is a semisynthetic epipodophyllotoxin extracted from the root of *Podophyllum peltatum* (mandrake). It inhibits topoisomerase II activity by stabilizing the DNA–topoisomerase II complex; this process ultimately results in the inability to synthesize DNA, and the cell cycle is stopped in the G_1 phase.

Vinca alkaloids The vinca alkaloids are derived from the periwinkle plant *Vinca rosea.* Upon entering the cell, vinca alkaloids bind rapidly to the tubulin. The binding occurs in the S phase at a site different from that associated with paclitaxel and colchicine. Thus, polymerization of microtubules is blocked, resulting in impaired mitotic spindle formation in the M phase.

Taxanes Paclitaxel and docetaxel (Taxotere) are semisynthetic derivatives of extracted precursors from the needles of yew plants. These drugs have a novel 14-member ring, the taxane. Unlike the vinca alkaloids, which cause microtubular disassembly, the taxanes promote microtubular assembly and stability, therefore blocking the cell cycle in mitosis. Docetaxel is more potent than paclitaxel in enhancing microtubular assembly and also induces apoptosis.

Camptothecin analogs include irinotecan and topotecan (Hycamtin). These semisynthetic analogs of the alkaloid camptothecin, derived from the Chinese ornamental tree *Camptotheca acuminata*, inhibit topoisomerase I and interrupt the elongation phase of DNA replication.

Targeted agents

Monoclonal antibodies Although monoclonal antibodies (MAbs) have been used in cancer therapeutics since the late 1990s, the number of new agents in this class is growing exponentially. Several unconjugated MAbs have established utility in medical oncology as highly targeted therapies. The earliest therapeutic MAb to show convincing utility in medical oncology was rituximab (Rituxan), approved in 1997 for the treatment of non-Hodgkin lymphoma. This antibody targets the CD20 antigen found on B-cell lymphocytes and can be used clinically as a single agent or in association with combination chemotherapy. Another MAb, trastuzumab (Herceptin), has shown excellent activity in combination with chemotherapy in breast cancer patients whose tumor cells overexpress the human epidermal growth factor receptor 2 (HER2) protein. Finally, alemtuzumab (Campath) is a MAb that recognizes the CD52 antigen expressed on both B-cell and T-cell lymphocytes. This agent is useful in the treatment of chemotherapy-refractory B-cell chronic lymphocytic leukemia.

In 2004, two new MAbs were approved by the US Food and Drug Administration (FDA) for the treatment of patients with advanced colorectal cancer: bevacizumab (Avastin) and cetuximab (Erbitux). Bevacizumab binds to the vascular endothelial growth factor (VEGF) and prevents ligand-induced VEGF receptor activation, which blocks the stimulation of endothelial cell growth and inhibits new blood vessel formation in tumors that secrete VEGF. Cetuximab binds the EGFR on the surface of tumor cells, ultimately leading to downregulation of this signaling pathway. This process blocks tumor growth and proliferation and can reverse tumor resistance to chemotherapeutic agents such as irinotecan. Cetuximab is now also indicated for head and neck cancer. Bevacizumab has received indications in lung and breast cancers.

Panitumumab (Vectibix), approved by the FDA in 2006, is another MAb that targets EGFR and is indicated for use in colorectal cancer that has metastasized following standard chemotherapy.

A recent randomized trial found that the addition of bevacizumab to irinotecan- and 5-FU–based chemotherapy in newly diagnosed patients with advanced colorectal cancer significantly improved the response rate (45% vs 35%; $P = .0029$), duration of response (10.4 vs 7.1 months; $P = .0014$), and median survival (20.3 vs 15.6 months; $P = .0003$) compared with placebo. Grade 3 hypertension (10.9% vs 2.3%) and GI perforations (1.5% vs 0%) were more common in the bevacizumab arm, but overall, the bevacizumab therapy was thought to be well tolerated. This was the first randomized clinical trial demonstrating a survival benefit for antiangiogenic therapy.

Small-molecule targeted therapies Molecularly targeted therapies are designed to selectively interact with specific molecular pathways within cells to achieve a rational antitumor effect. The classic rationally designed molecularly targeted agent is imatinib (Gleevec), which was identified in screening studies designed to detect inhibitors of the Bcr-Abl tyrosine kinase, present in virtually all cases of chronic myelogenous leukemia. Originally synthesized as an inhibitor of platelet-derived growth factor receptor (PDGFR), it is also a potent inhibitor of the c-*kit* tyrosine kinase. Imatinib binds to the ATP-binding site and inhibits the tyrosine kinase's ability to phosphorylate its substrates.

Gefitinib (Iressa) is another small-molecule–targeted therapy that is a signal transduction inhibitor of the EGFR tyrosine kinase. It binds noncovalently to the ATP-binding site of the intracellular domain of the EGFR protein and blocks the kinase activity. Its anticancer effects arise from the ability to interfere with EGFR-mediated signaling, which is associated with cell proliferation, angiogenesis, and cell motility.

Erlotinib (Tarceva) is an HER1/EGFR-targeted therapy that has demonstrated a significant survival benefit as second-line therapy for patients with advanced NSCLC. A randomized phase III study performed by the NCI of Canada compared erlotinib with best supportive care in patients with recurrent or refractory non–small-cell lung cancer following treatment with either one or two lines of prior chemotherapy. As reported by Shepherd et al, erlotinib was significantly better than best supportive care in terms of response rate (8.9% vs < 1%; $P < .001$), disease progression-free survival (2.23 vs 1.84 months; $P < .001$), and median survival (6.7 vs 4.7 months; $P = .001$). Rash and diarrhea were the most frequent side effects, although only 5% of patients discontinued erlotinib due to drug-related toxicities. This is the first randomized trial of an EGFR inhibitor in lung cancer demonstrating a significant survival benefit.

Another targeted therapy is the 26S proteasome inhibitor bortezomib (Velcade). The 26S proteasome is a ubiquitous multiprotein complex responsible for degrading a variety of regulatory proteins involved in cancer cell proliferation. In multiple myeloma cells, bortezomib induces apoptosis by mechanisms that are not precisely defined. One hypothesis is that the inhibition of the proteasomal degradation of I-κB, an inhibitor of the transcription factor Nuclear Factor kappa B (NF-κB), prevents the constitutive activation of NF-κB. In multiple myeloma cells, NF-κB is thought to be necessary for cell proliferation and survival.

Sunitinib (Sutent) is an oral small molecule multitargeted tyrosine kinase inhibitor with antiproliferative and antiangiogenic activity attributed to the inhibition of PDGFR, VEGFR, KIT, and FLT$_3$. In a phase II study by Motzer et al, involving 63 patients with metastatic renal cell carcinoma, sunitinib resulted in a 33% partial response rate (95% confidence interval [CI], 22% to 46%), a 37%

A randomized phase III study was launched to compare sunitinib (Sutent) vs interferon alfa in previously untreated patients with metastatic renal cell carcinoma (RCC). A total of 750 patients were randomized to sunitinib (n = 375) and interferon alfa (n = 375). Sunitinib was administered at 50 mg/d po for 4 weeks, followed by 2 weeks off treatment. The cycle was repeated. Interferon alfa was dosed at 9 MU subcutaneously 3 times a week *(Motzer RJ, Hutson TE, Tomczak P, et al: NEJM 356:115-124, 2007)*. Final analysis of overall survival, a secondary endpoint, was reported at ASCO. In patients with treatment-naive advanced RCC, treatment with sunitinib more than doubled progression-free survival compared with interferon alfa (11 months vs 5 months, $P < .000001$). The median overall survival was 26.4 months vs 21.8 months, respectively ($P = .051$). The objective response rate was 47% vs 12% ($P < .000001$). This is the first study to show a median survival of more than 2 years for patients with metastatic RCC *(Figlin RA, Hutson TE, Tomczak P, et al: J Clin Oncol 26(18S, part I):256s [abstract 5024], 2008)*.

rate of stable disease lasting at least 3 months, and a 1-year median survival of 65% (95% CI, 50% to 76%). Treatments were well tolerated, with major grade 3 or 4 toxicities consisting of lymphopenia, neutropenia, elevated amylase/lipase levels without associated pancreatitis, and fatigue or asthenia.

Sorafenib (Nexavar) is a new oral small multitargeted molecule with antiproliferative and antiangiogenic activity attributed to the inhibition of PDGFR, VEGFR, KIT, FLT[3], and, RAF-1.

Temsirolimus (Torisel) is a specific inhibitor of mTOR, a signaling protein that regulates cell growth and angiogenesis. It has been evaluated in a phase III, randomized, three-arm study versus interferon-alpha or the combination of both agents in the treatment of first-line, poor-risk patients with advanced renal cell carcinoma. Results have shown this agent to be the first to produce a significant increase in overall survival with an acceptable safety profile.

Sunitinib, sorefenib, and temsirolimus all show significant activity in advanced renal cell cancer patients, frequently producing prolonged stabilization of disease, and in the case of sunitinib, objective remissions. These targeted therapies have displaced cytokines as the gold standard for treating advanced-stage renal cell tumors.

Other newer molecularly targeted therapies include dasatinib (Sprycel), approved by the FDA for treatment of chronic myelogenous leukemia and Philadelphia-positive acute lymphoblastic leukemia, and lapatinib (Tykerb), approved by the FDA for treatment of advanced or metastatic HER2-positive breast cancer in combination with capecitabine (Xeloda).

The relevance of pharmacogenomics to molecularly targeted therapies was highlighted by the impressive finding that specific somatic mutations localizing to the ATP-binding site of the EGFR tyrosine kinase in lung tumors were associated with clinical response. In eight of nine patients with NSCLC who responded to gefitinib therapy, specific mutations were identified, whereas none was found in seven matched nonresponders. This landmark finding, coupled with what is already known about *c-kit* mutations that "drive" the proliferation of gastrointestinal stromal cell tumors in response to imatinib therapy, suggests that it may ultimately be possible to prospectively select patients with NSCLC who have a high probability of responding to EGFR tyrosine kinase inhibitors. Further studies are under way to confirm these findings and to extend the observation to other tumor types.

See Appendix 3 for a list of drugs and/or new indications recently approved for treatment of cancer and Appendix 4 for the uses, dosages, and toxicities of the chemotherapeutic agents discussed in this chapter.

SUGGESTED READING

Cunningham D, Humblet Y, Siena S, et al: Cetuximab monotherapy and cetuximab plus irinotecan in irinotecan-refractory metastatic colorectal cancer. N Engl J Med 351:337–345, 2004.

Hudes G, Carducci M, Tomczak P, et al: Temsirolimus, interferon alfa, or both for advanced renal cell cancer. N Engl J Med 356:2271–2281, 2007.

Hurwitz H, Fehrenbacher L, Novotny W, et al: Bevacizumab plus irinotecan, fluorouracil, and leucovorin for metastatic colorectal cancer. N Engl J Med 350:2335–2342, 2004.

Lynch TJ, Bell DW, Sordella R, et al: Activating mutations in the epidermal growth factor receptor underlying responsiveness of non-small-cell lung cancer to gefitinib. N Engl J Med 350:2129–2139, 2004.

McLeod HL, Evans WE: Pharmacogenomics: Unlocking the human genome for better drug therapy. Annu Rev Pharmacol Toxicol 41:101–121, 2001.

Morabito A, De Maio E, Di Maio M, et al: Tyrosine kinase inhibitors of vascular endothelial growth factor receptors in clinical trials: Current status and future directions. Oncologist 11:753–764, 2006.

Motzer RJ, Hutson TE, Tomczak P, et al: Sunitinib versus interferon alfa in metastatic renal-cell carcinoma. N Engl J Med 356:115–134, 2007.

Olopade OI, Schwartsmann G, Saijo N, et al: Disparities in cancer care: A worldwide perspective and roadmap for change. J Clin Oncol 24:2135–2136, 2006.

Paez JG, Janne PA, Lee JC, et al: EGFR mutations in lung cancer: Correlation with clinical response to gefitinib therapy. Science 304:1497–1500, 2004.

Shepherd FA, Pereira J, Ciuleanu TE, et al: Erlotinib in previously treated non–small-cell lung cancer. N Engl J Med 353:123–132, 2005.

Weinshilboum R: Inheritance and drug response. N Engl J Med 348:529–537, 2003.

CHAPTER 4

Head and neck tumors

John Andrew Ridge, MD, PhD, Bonnie S. Glisson, MD, Miriam N. Lango, MD, Steven Feigenberg, MD, and Eric M. Horwitz, MD

In 2008, it was estimated that head and neck cancers comprised 2% to 3% of all cancers in the United States and accounted for 1% to 2% of all cancer deaths. This total includes 22,900 cases of oral cavity cancer, 12,250 cases of laryngeal cancer, and 12,410 cases of pharyngeal cancer. Most patients with head and neck cancer have metastatic disease at the time of diagnosis (regional nodal involvement in 43% and distant metastasis in 10%).

Head and neck cancers encompass a diverse group of uncommon tumors that frequently are aggressive in their biologic behavior. Moreover, patients with a head and neck cancer often develop a second primary tumor. These tumors occur at an annual rate of 3% to 7%, and 50% to 75% of such new cancers occur in the upper aerodigestive tract or lungs.

The anatomy of the head and neck is complex and is divided into sites and subsites (Figure 1). Tumors of each site have a unique epidemiology, anatomy, natural history, and therapeutic approach. This chapter will review these lesions as a group and then individually by anatomic site.

Epidemiology

Gender Head and neck cancer is more common in men; 66% to 95% of cases occur in men. The incidence by gender varies with anatomic location and has been changing as the number of female smokers has increased. The male-female ratio is currently 3:1 for oral cavity and pharyngeal cancers. In patients with Plummer-Vinson syndrome, the ratio is reversed, with 80% of head and neck cancers occurring in women.

Age The incidence of head and neck cancer increases with age, especially after 50 years of age. Although most patients are between 50 and 70 years old, head and neck cancer does occur in younger patients. There are more women and fewer smokers in the younger patient group.

It is controversial whether head and neck cancer is more aggressive in younger patients or in older individuals. This "aggressiveness" probably reflects the common delay in diagnosis in the younger population, since, in most studies, younger patients do not have a worse prognosis than their older counterparts.

Race The incidence of laryngeal cancer is higher in African-Americans relative to the white, Asian, and Hispanic populations.

Additionally, in African-Americans, head and neck cancer is associated with lower survival for similar tumor stages. The overall 5-year survival rate is 56% in whites and 34% in African-Americans.

Geography There are wide variations in the incidence of head and neck cancer among different geographic regions. The risk of laryngeal cancer, for example, is two to six times higher in Bombay, India, than in Scandinavia. The higher incidence of the disease in Asia is thought to reflect the prevalence of

FIGURE 1: Anatomic sites and subsites of the head and neck. The approximate distribution of head and neck cancer is oral cavity, 44%; larynx, 31%; and pharynx, 25%.

risk factors, such as betel nut chewing and use of smokeless tobacco. In the United States, the high incidence among urban males is thought to reflect exposure to tobacco and alcohol. Among rural women, there is an increased risk of oral cancer related to the use of smokeless tobacco (snuff).

Nasopharyngeal carcinoma is another head and neck tumor with a distinct ethnic predilection. Endemic areas include southern China, northern Africa, and regions of the far Northern Hemisphere—areas in which the diet of inhabitants includes large quantities of salted meat and fish. When people from these regions migrate to areas with a lower disease incidence, their risk falls but remains elevated. Cancer of the nasopharynx in these geographic areas also has been associated with Epstein-Barr virus (EBV) infection (see section on "Etiology and risk factors").

Etiology and risk factors

Risk factors for head and neck cancer include tobacco and alcohol use, ultraviolet (UV) light exposure, viral infection, and environmental exposures.

Tobacco The incidence of head and neck tumors correlates most closely with the use of tobacco.

Cigarettes Head and neck tumors occur six times more often among cigarette smokers than nonsmokers. The age-standardized risk of mortality from laryngeal cancer appears to rise linearly with increasing cigarette smoking. For the heaviest smokers, death from laryngeal cancer is 20 times more likely than for nonsmokers. Furthermore, active smoking by head and neck cancer patients is associated with significant increases in the annual rate of second primary tumor development (compared with former smokers or those who have never smoked). Use of unfiltered cigarettes or dark, air-cured tobacco is associated with further increases in risk.

Cigars Total cigar smoking increased by nearly 50% in the United States in the 1990s. Often misperceived as posing a lower health risk than cigarette smoking, cigar smoking results in a change in the site distribution for aerodigestive tract cancer, according to epidemiologic data. Although the incidence of cancer at some sites traditionally associated with cigarette smoking (eg, larynx, lungs) is decreased in cigar smokers, the incidence of cancer is actually higher at other sites where pooling of saliva and associated carcinogens tends to occur (oropharynx, esophagus).

Smokeless tobacco Use of smokeless tobacco also is associated with an increased incidence of head and neck cancer, especially in the oral cavity. Smokeless tobacco users frequently develop premalignant lesions, such as oral leukoplakia, at the site where the tobacco quid rests against the mucosa. Over time, these lesions may progress to invasive carcinomas. The use of snuff has been associated with an increase in cancers of the gum and oral mucosa.

Alcohol Alcohol consumption, by itself, is a risk factor for the development of pharyngeal and laryngeal tumors, although it is a less potent carcinogen

FIGURE 2: Levels of the neck as determined by lymphatic drainage patterns

than tobacco. For individuals who use both tobacco and alcohol, these risk factors appear to be synergistic and result in a multiplicative increase in risk.

UV light exposure is a risk factor for the development of cancer of the lips. At least 33% of patients with lip cancer have outdoor occupations.

Occupational exposures A small group of head and neck cancers may be attributable to occupational exposures. Nasal cancer has been associated with wood dust exposure, and squamous cell cancer of the maxillary sinus, with nickel exposure. Petroleum exposure may be associated with pharyngeal cancer, but the relationship has not been proven.

Radiation exposure Exposure to radiation is clearly an important risk factor for thyroid cancer and has been associated with cancer of the salivary glands.

Viruses There is a strong link between EBV exposure and the development of nasopharyngeal cancer. The potential etiologic role of human papillomavirus (HPV) in oropharyngeal cancer is supported by a growing body of evidence. A recent case-control study of 100 patients with squamous cancer of the oropharynx documented that HPV DNA, type 16, was found in 72% of tumor specimens. Further, 64% of the patients had antibodies to HPV-16 oncoproteins. Oral infection with HPV increased the risk of oropharyngeal cancer with an odds ratio of 14.6 (95% confidence interval [CI], 6.3–36.6). This risk was independent of tobacco and alcohol use.

Diet Epidemiologic studies suggest that dietary intake of vitamin A, β-carotene, and α-tocopherol may reduce the risk of developing head and neck cancer.

Marijuana Smoking marijuana is associated with the development of head and neck cancer, but the degree of risk is unknown.

Anatomy

As mentioned previously, the anatomy of the head and neck region is complex. The anatomic sites are illustrated in Figure 1. More detailed descriptions are included below in the discussions of specific sites and subsites.

Levels of the neck

The anatomy of the neck is relevant to the treatment of all head and neck cancers. The neck may be divided into levels (Figure 2). The lymphatic drainage of the unmanipulated neck is systematic and predictable; knowledge of these drainage patterns assists the clinician in locating the primary tumor that has given rise to a neck metastasis (Table 1).

Level I includes the submental and submandibular triangles.

Level II includes the superior jugular chain nodes extending from the mandible down to the carotid bifurcation and posteriorly to the posterior border of the sternocleidomastoid muscle.

Level III consists of the jugular nodes from the carotid bulb inferiorly to the omohyoid muscle.

Level IV continues from the omohyoid muscle inferiorly to the clavicle.

Level V represents the posterior triangle bounded by the posterior border of the sternocleidomastoid anteriorly, the anterior border of the trapezius posteriorly, and the clavicle inferiorly.

Signs and symptoms

Head and neck cancer typically produces symptoms referable to the upper aerodigestive tract, including alterations in deglutition, phonation, hearing, and respiration. In particular, patients should be questioned about dysphagia, odynophagia, globus sensation, hoarseness, a change in the ability to form words, epistaxis, epiphora, otalgia, hemoptysis, stuffiness of the ears, and trismus. (Signs and symptoms of cancer at specific anatomic sites and subsites can be found in the respective discussions of these tumors.)

TABLE 1: Lymphatic drainage of the head and neck and associated sites of primary tumors

Lymphatic drainage	Likely primary sites
Level I	
Submental	Lower lip, chin, anterior oral cavity (including anterior one-third of the tongue and floor of the mouth)
Submandibular	Upper and lower lips, oral tongue, floor of the mouth, facial skin
Level II	Oral cavity and pharynx (including soft palate, base of the tongue, and piriform sinus)
Level III	Larynx, hypopharynx, and thyroid
Level IV	Larynx, hypopharynx, thyroid, cervical esophagus, and trachea
Level V	Nasopharynx, thyroid, paranasal sinuses, and posterior scalp
Supraclavicular	Infraclavicular sites (including lungs, esophagus, breasts, pancreas, GI tract, GU and gynecologic sources)

It is important to ascertain the duration and course (progression or improvement) of symptoms. Progression of disease is often noted during the evaluation and worsens the prognosis.

Screening and diagnosis

SCREENING

Molecular diagnostic techniques have shown promise as screening tools to identify neoplastic cells in saliva and sputum specimens. Nevertheless, since patients with head and neck cancer are unlikely to be engaged in the health-care system, the means by which patient screening would be achieved remains a fundamental problem.

DIAGNOSIS

The need for expeditious diagnosis of head and neck cancer and referral to a skilled head and neck specialist cannot be overemphasized, as early diagnosis can lead to a reduction in mortality. One study suggested that in the 24 months prior to the diagnosis of head and neck cancer, patients had a median of 10.5 health-care visits. These visits provide an opportunity to evaluate patients' symptoms and underscore the important role of dentists and primary care physicians in the early diagnosis of head and neck cancer.

History

Risk factors as outlined previously, including a history of tobacco and alcohol use and environmental exposures, should be reviewed. Any adult patient with symptoms referable to the upper aerodigestive tract that have lasted longer than 2 weeks or with an asymptomatic neck mass should undergo a thorough examination with a high index of suspicion for carcinoma.

Physical examination

The physical examination is the best means for detecting lesions of the upper aerodigestive tract. Frequently, the initial assessment also will indicate the severity and chronicity of the disease. Due to the frequent occurrence of multiple primary tumors in patients with a head and neck tumor, careful evaluation of the entire upper aerodigestive tract is necessary at the time of diagnosis. The examination should always follow a systematic approach.

Skin/scalp A search should be made for ulcers, nodules, and pigmented or other suspicious lesions. This part of the evaluation is frequently overlooked.

Cranial nerves A cranial nerve evaluation is essential for any patient with a head and neck tumor or neck mass (which may be a manifestation of occult cancer). This evaluation should include assessing eye motion (cranial nerves [CN] III, IV, and VI); testing sensation of the face (CN V); examining the muscles of facial expression by having the patient grin, grimace, raise eyebrows, close eyes tightly, show teeth, and puff out the cheeks (CN VII); testing of hearing (CN VIII); assessing gag reflex (CN IX); evaluating vocal cord mobility (CN X); and having the patient fully abduct the shoulder (CN XI) and protrude the tongue (CN XII). Even the slightest abnormality may be helpful in identifying a primary tumor.

Eyes/ears/nose The eyes, ears, and nose should be evaluated for any sign of mass effect, abnormal drainage/discharge, bleeding, or effusion.

Oral cavity Halitosis may be the first indication of a lesion in the upper aerodigestive tract. The teeth, gingivae, and entire mucosal surface should be inspected. (Dentures should be removed.) The lymphoid tissue of the tonsillar pillars should be inspected and any asymmetry noted. Tongue mobility also should be evaluated.

The floor of the mouth, tongue, and cheeks should be palpated using a bimanual technique (one gloved finger inside the mouth and the second hand under the mandible). Palpation should be the last step of the examination due to stimulation of the gag reflex. Worrisome lesions should be biopsied.

Neck A systematic examination of the neck consistently documents the location of any mass. Palpation is the cornerstone of the examination. It is performed by grasping the tissue and feeling the nodes between the thumb and index and long fingers. The relationship of a mass to major structures, such as the salivary gland, thyroid, and carotid sheath, should be considered.

Important qualities of a mass include location, character, tenderness, size, mobility, and associated thrill or bruit. The thyroid should be palpated.

Indirect laryngoscopy The nasopharynx, hypopharynx, and larynx should all be examined with care. The vocal cords should be visualized and their mobility evaluated. Mirror examination provides an overall impression of mobility and asymmetry, which may point to a hidden tumor.

Direct laryngoscopy Nasopharyngoscopes permit a thorough inspection of the upper aerodigestive tract in the office setting. Attention should be focused individually on the piriform sinuses, tongue base, pharyngeal walls, epiglottis, arytenoids, and true and false vocal cords. Also, any pooling of secretions should be noted.

Endoscopy Approximately 5% of patients with head and neck cancer have a synchronous primary squamous cell cancer of the head and neck, esophagus, or lungs. Examination with the patient under anesthesia with endoscopy (which may include direct laryngoscopy, esophagoscopy, and bronchoscopy) and directed biopsy should be performed in all patients with an occult primary squamous cell cancer and in many patients with a *known* head and neck primary. Examination with the patient under anesthesia also can provide information regarding the extent of the tumor.

The most common sites of silent primary tumors are the tonsils, base of the tongue, and piriform sinuses. Tumors of the nasopharynx have become easier to identify with the increased use of flexible nasopharyngoscopy. Biopsies should be performed in common areas of silent primaries in addition to the primary anatomic sites associated with lymphatic drainage of any neck mass.

Laboratory evaluation

There are no specific screening laboratory tests other than preoperative studies performed in the diagnostic evaluation of most head and neck carcinomas. EBV, anticapsid antibodies, and serum immunoglobulin G are tumor markers for nasopharyngeal carcinomas.

Diagnostic imaging

Plain x-rays Posteroanterior and lateral chest x-rays should be obtained in all adult patients to eliminate the possibility of occult lung metastasis or a second primary. A Panorex film may be helpful in delineating bony involvement in some cases of oral cavity lesions.

CT The CT scan is probably the single most informative test in the assessment of a head and neck tumor. It may delineate the extent of disease and the presence and extent of lymphatic involvement. CT scans of the chest, abdomen, and pelvis sometimes may identify the site of an occult primary tumor presenting with a node low in the neck. CT offers high spatial resolution and discriminates among fat, muscle, bone, and other soft tissues and surpasses MRI in the detection of bony erosion.

MRI may provide accurate information regarding the size, location, and soft-tissue extent of tumor. It provides limited information regarding bony involvement, unless there is gross involvement of the marrow space. Relatively greater sensitivity of MRI in relation to CT is offset by its decreased specificity. The main disadvantage of MRI is movement artifact, which is a particular problem in the larynx and hypopharynx. Gadolinium-enhanced MRI is probably superior to CT for imaging tumors of the nasopharynx and oropharynx.

PET has been evaluated in both primary and recurrent squamous cell carcinomas of the head and neck. ^{18}F-fluorodeoxyglucose (FDG) is the most commonly used PET radiotracer. It enters the cell and undergoes the first step in glycolysis to produce FDG-6-phosphate, which reflects the metabolic rate of the tissue. The metabolic rate of malignancies is higher than that of most benign tumors or normal tissues. FDG imaging therefore has the potential to distinguish between benign and malignant processes, grade tumors, identify metastases, and diagnose tumor recurrence. In head and neck cancer, FDG imaging has been useful in detecting clinically occult recurrences, although it has proved less useful in identifying an occult primary site for metastatic cervical disease.

Biopsy

Biopsies of the primary tumor often can be performed in an outpatient setting.

Punch or cup forceps biopsy is important in the diagnosis of mucosal lesions. The biopsy should be obtained at the border of the lesion away from areas of obvious necrosis.

Fine-needle aspiration (FNA) is a useful diagnostic modality. Multiple passes are made through the lesion with a fine-gauge (22-gauge) needle while suction is applied. Suction should be released before withdrawing the needle through surrounding soft tissue of the neck. FNA has an associated false-negative rate as low as 7%. The diagnostic accuracy depends on the physician's skill and the cytopathologist's experience.

Cytology is particularly useful in distinguishing a metastatic squamous cell carcinoma from other malignant histologies. However, a negative result should not be interpreted as "absence of malignancy."

Core biopsy should not be performed on a neck mass, with the rare exception of a proven lymphoma.

Open biopsy should be performed only when a diagnosis has not been made after extensive clinical evaluation and FNA is nondiagnostic. The operation should be performed only by a surgeon prepared to conduct immediate definitive surgical treatment at that time (which may entail radical neck dissection).

Pathology

Squamous cell carcinoma

More than 90% of all head and neck cancers are squamous cell carcinomas.

Histologic grade There are three histologic grades based on the amount of keratinization: A well-differentiated tumor is characterized by > 75% keratinization; a moderately differentiated tumor, by 25% to 50%; and a poorly differentiated tumor, by < 25%.

In general, the more poorly differentiated a lesion, the higher is the incidence of regional metastases and the poorer the prognosis. Histologic grade has not been a consistent predictor of clinical behavior, however. Features that predict aggressive behavior include perineural spread, lymphatic invasion, and tumor spread beyond the lymph node capsule.

Morphologic growth patterns Four morphologically distinct growth patterns have been recognized. The ulcerative type is the most common form and begins as a round or oval ulcer that is friable. Ulcerative lesions progress toward infiltration. Infiltrative lesions extend deeply into underlying tissues. The exophytic type tends to grow more superficially and metastasize later than the other types. It begins as an area of thickened epithelium.

In 2007, a case-control study providing epidemiologic evidence of a causal role for human papillomavirus (HPV) in oropharyngeal cancer was published. Oral infection with HPV-16 or any other 37 subtypes was independently associated with oropharyngeal cancer. HPV-16 was identified in 72% of oropharyngeal tumors. Patients without a history of smoking and/ or ethanol abuse were more likely to harbor oral HPV-16. Combined exposure to HPV and tobacco or alcohol was not synergistic for oropharyngeal cancer development. The development of opharyngeal cancer was associated with high-risk sexual behaviors, including a high lifetime number of sexual partners, casual sexual relations, young age at first intercourse, and infrequent condom use. An HPV vaccine may reduce the incidence of oropharyngeal cancer (*D'Souza G, Kreimer AR, Viscidi R, et al: N Engl J Med 356:1944-1956, 2007*).

Verrucous cancer is an uncommon variant that, in the United States, typically occurs in elderly patients with poor oral hygiene or ill-fitting dentures. It is characterized by a warty, bulky, elevated, fungating appearance. Verrucous cancers seldom metastasize.

The inactivation of p53, a central event in head and neck carcinogenesis, occurs by means of several prognostically significant mechanisms. Over 50% of head and neck squamous cell carcinomas have been found to harbor a mutation of the p53 gene and linked to diminished survival. HPV, which causes inactivation of p53 via elaboration of E6 and E7 oncogenes, has been identified in 35% to 75% of oropharyngeal squamous cell carcinomas and has been associated with an improved clinical outcome.

Other tumor types

Other less common head and neck cancers include mucoepidermoid carcinoma, adenoid cystic carcinoma, and adenocarcinoma, all of which may arise in the salivary glands. Head and neck cancers with neuroendocrine features include small-cell undifferentiated cancer and esthesioneuroblastoma (olfactory neuroblastoma). Both Hodgkin lymphoma and non-Hodgkin lymphoma may also be diagnosed as head and neck tumors, often involving the lymph nodes of the neck or Waldeyer's ring.

Sequence of disease progression

There is a sequence of disease progression from atypia/dysplasia through carcinoma in situ to frankly invasive cancer. Leukoplakia and erythroplakia are terms applied to clinically identifiable lesions that may harbor invasive cancer or undergo malignant transformation.

Leukoplakia results from chronic irritation of mucous membranes by carcinogens; this irritation stimulates the proliferation of white epithelial and connective tissue. Histopathologic examination reveals hyperkeratosis variably associated with underlying epithelial hyperplasia. In the absence of underlying dysplasia, leukoplakia rarely (< 5%) is associated with progression of disease to malignancy.

Erythroplakia is characterized by superficial, friable, red patches adjacent to normal mucosa. It is commonly associated with underlying epithelial dysplasia and has a much greater potential for malignancy than leukoplakia. Carcinoma is found in nearly 40% of erythroplakia.

Dysplasia is characterized by cellular atypia, loss of normal maturation, and loss of normal epithelial stratification. It is graded as mild, moderate, or severe, based on the degree of nuclear abnormality present. In the transition from mild to severe dysplasia, nuclear abnormalities become more marked, mitoses become more apparent, and these changes involve increasing depth of epithelium. The likelihood of developing a carcinoma relates to the degree of dysplasia. In the case of severe dysplasia, as many as 24% of patients may develop invasive squamous cell cancer.

Carcinoma in situ is characterized by the presence of atypical changes throughout the epithelium with complete loss of stratification. It is estimated that approximately 75% of invasive squamous cell carcinomas have an associated in situ component. Specific DNA mutations have also been identified in the sequence of disease progression from mild dysplasia to atypia to carcinoma in situ to invasive carcinoma.

Regional and distant metastases

The incidence of lymph node metastases is related to the size and thickness of the primary tumor. If the primary site is near the midline, contralateral or bilateral metastases should be anticipated. In the presence of lymph node metastases, extracapsular spread of tumor is an important prognostic factor.

Staging and prognosis

Staging system The TNM staging system of the American Joint Committee on Cancer (AJCC) maintains uniformity in the staging of head and neck tumors. The staging of primary mucosal tumors of the head and neck varies with the anatomic location and will be covered later by site. However, the staging system for metastases and stage groupings are nearly uniform for all mucosal sites.

Prognosis correlates strongly with stage at diagnosis. For many head and neck cancer sites, survival for patients with stage I disease exceeds 80%. For patients with locally advanced disease at the time of diagnosis, stages III and IV disease, survival drops below 40%. Development of nodal metastases reduces survival of a patient with a small primary tumor by ~50%. Involvement of even a single lymph node is associated with a marked decline in survival. Most patients with head and neck cancer have stage III or IV disease at diagnosis.

Pattern of relapse Despite aggressive primary treatment, the majority of relapses that occur following a head and neck cancer are within the head and neck. Locoregional relapse accounts for ~80% of primary treatment failures. Distant metastases increase as the disease progresses and most often involve the lungs, bones, and liver. By the time of death, 10% to 30% of patients will have clinically detected distant metastases.

Field cancerization is an important concept related to the natural history of head and neck cancer. This term describes the diffuse epithelial injury throughout the head and neck, lungs, and esophagus that results from chronic exposure to carcinogens.

Clinically, field cancerization is manifested by the frequent occurrence of (1) mucosal abnormalities, such as leukoplakia and dysplasia, beyond the margins of a head and neck cancer and (2) second primary tumors within this exposed field. The lifetime risk of a patient with head and neck cancer developing a new cancer is 20% to 40%. Over time, as the risk of relapse of the initial cancer declines, the development of a new cancer represents the greatest risk for these patients.

Treatment approaches

In general, head and neck tumors may be treated using a single modality for early-stage disease (stage I or II) but may require multimodality therapy for advanced disease (stage III or IV).

The best therapeutic approach for the primary tumor depends on the anatomic site. The approach to treatment of the neck also varies with the site and treatment of the primary tumor. When the primary tumor is treated with irradiation, the "at-risk" regional lymphatics are incorporated into the treatment fields. Neck dissections should remain standardized (ie, complete anatomic dissections, as opposed to "berry picking" or random biopsy) in these settings so as to avoid incomplete surgery.

Preoperative assessment Before surgical resection, preoperative assessment of the extent of disease is essential. Complete physical examination and appropriate radiologic evaluation are necessary. Direct laryngoscopy and esophagoscopy are frequently performed to determine tumor extent and to rule out the presence of a second primary tumor. A chest x-ray or CT scan may be obtained to screen for distant metastases or a primary lung cancer.

Surgical principles Classic principles of surgical oncology apply to head and neck cancer. Complete resection is necessary. Securing sufficient margins may be challenging due to the many structures in this area. Reconstruction is complex after resection of head and neck tumors, as the surgery may have an impact on appearance, speech, and swallowing. Decisions regarding the extent of resection should be made by experienced surgeons.

Surgery plus radiation therapy

The combination of radical surgery and radiation therapy has been used for several decades to treat patients with advanced head and neck cancers.

Postoperative vs preoperative radiation therapy Postoperative radiation therapy (60 to 70 Gy in 6 to 7 weeks) reduces the rate of locoregional recurrence from ~50% to 15% for tumors with pathologic features predictive of locoregional recurrence. The indications for postoperative radiation therapy are well established and include a large primary tumor (T4), close or positive margins, an involved lymph node > 3 cm or multiple involved lymph nodes, extracapsular extension, tumor fixation, and connective tissue invasion. The addition of postoperative radiation therapy reduces the risk of locoregional failure but does not decrease the risk of developing distant metastases.

Preoperative radiotherapy (45 to 50 Gy in 4 to 5 weeks) has been used for patients with advanced primary tumors, but rates of locoregional recurrence appear to be lower and complications fewer with postoperative radiation therapy. Preoperative radiotherapy is indicated for marginally resectable tumors, such as those with fixed cervical lymph nodes. In this setting, preoperative irradiation often permits resection of an otherwise unresectable tumor.

Postoperative chemotherapy/radiation therapy Two randomized clinical trials were launched to determine whether the addition of concurrent chemotherapy to radiation therapy enhanced locoregional tumor control and survival in high-risk patients with head and neck cancer following definitive surgical resection. The results of these trials were published in 2004. In the Radiation Therapy Oncology Group (RTOG) 95-01/intergroup trial, patients with high-risk features including two or more involved lymph nodes, extracapsular extension, or positive margins following definitive surgical resection were randomized to receive 6,000 to 6,600 cGy of postoperative irradiation with or without cisplatin (given on days 1, 22, and 43). With a median follow-up of 45.9 months, the estimated 2-year rate of local and regional tumor control was 82% in the combined-therapy group versus 72% in the radiotherapy group ($P= .01$). The disease-free ($P = .04$) but not overall ($P = .19$) survival was significantly longer in the combined-treatment group. The incidence of acute adverse effects (grade 3 or greater) was higher in the combined-treatment group (77% vs 34%; $P < .001$).

In the EORTC (European Organization for Research on the Treatment of Cancer) trial 22931, similar conclusions were reported. In this study, however, the overall survival rate was found to be significantly improved in the combined-therapy group compared with the radiotherapy group. After a mean of 60 months, the overall survival of 334 randomized patients was 53% in the combined-treatment group versus 40% in the radiation-alone group ($P = .02$). The discrepancy in effect on overall survival was thought to be related to different entry criteria used in the RTOG and EORTC trials.

In a comparative analysis of the two trials, extracapsular extension and/or microscopically involved surgical margins were the only risk factors for which the impact of chemoradiation therapy was significant for survival in both trials. Patients with two or more histopathologically involved lymph nodes without the presence of extracapsular extension as their only risk factor did not benefit from the addition of chemotherapy.

Curative radiation therapy

Radiation therapy with curative intent usually involves daily treatment for 6–7 weeks (total dose, 60 to 70 Gy). Although there is no tissue loss with radiation therapy, complications include dry mouth, tissue fibrosis, trismus, bone necrosis, and hypothyroidism. Some problems are common and sufficiently debilitating to warrant significant concern in treatment planning for head and neck cancer. Surgery often produces less morbidity.

Radiation fractionation

The RTOG 90-03 trial was conducted to determine the efficacy of various fractionation schemes in the treament of locally advanced head and neck cancer. Four schedules were tested: (1) standard fractionation at 2 Gy/fraction/d, 5 d/wk, to 70 Gy/35 fractions/7 wk; (2) hyperfractionation at 1.2 Gy/fraction, twice daily, 5 d/wk to 81.6 Gy/68 fractions/7 wk; (3) accelerated fractionation with split at 1.6 Gy/fraction, twice daily, 5 d/wk to 67.2 Gy/42 fractions/6 wk, including a 2-week rest after 38.4 Gy; or (4) accelerated fractionation with a concomitant boost at 1.8 Gy/fraction/d, 5 d/wk, and 1.5 Gy/fraction/d to a boost field as a second daily treatment for the last 12 treatment days to 72 Gy/42 fractions/6 wk. A total of 1,113 patients were entered in the study, with a median follow-up of 23 months.

Patients treated with both hyperfractionation and accelerated fractionation with a concomitant boost had significantly increased locoregional tumor control rates compared with patients on the other two arms. All three groups treated with the altered fractionation schemes had more acute, but not late, side effects. The study concluded that hyperfractionation and accelerated fractionation with a concomitant boost are superior to conventionally fractionated radiotherapy.

Intensity-modulated radiation therapy

Intensity-modulated radiation therapy (IMRT) is a more sophisticated approach for obtaining highly conformal radiation dose distributions needed to irradiate complex targets positioned near sensitive normal structures. Treatment planning for IMRT (also known as inverse planning) is different from that of conventional or three-dimensional cranial radiation therapy planning. The starting point with IMRT is a description of the desired dose distribution rather than the application of traditional fields and beam modifiers to generate an acceptable plan. Conventional radiation treatment utilizes relatively uniform beams of radiation (typically between 2 and 4 beams), whereas IMRT, instead of using 4 beams of 50 cGy each, could use 50 beams of 4 cGy each. Each beam direction is divided into multiple segments to modulate the radiation dose.

The role of IMRT continues to be defined, although its use should not be considered standard for all head and neck tumors. IMRT in head and neck cancer is ideal in the setting of a tumor adjacent to a critical structure (eyes, optic nerve, spinal cord, brainstem, optic chiasm), which would not otherwise be treatable adequately with conventional planning.

Various groups have examined dosimetric and quality-of-life differences between IMRT and conventional radiation techniques. The group at Memorial Sloan-Kettering Cancer Center compared its IMRT planned treatment for nasopharyngeal cancer with conventional treatment with a conformal boost. Locoregional tumor control was 97%, versus 78%, at 2 years. The University of Michigan and Washington University have reported reductions in late xerostomia with IMRT.

Chemotherapy

Induction (neoadjuvant) chemotherapy versus concomitant chemotherapy and radiation therapy A rationale for using induction chemotherapy for treating advanced-stage laryngeal cancer involves using chemotherapy as a marker of radiation sensitivity to select potentially radiocurable patients. In the VA Laryngeal Cancer Cooperative Study, the major benefit for the patients in the experimental arm was laryngeal preservation in two-thirds of patients. In this study, lack of substantial tumor response to induction chemotherapy was not associated with reduced survival. In addition, patients who failed to respond to induction chemotherapy underwent surgery, which had the advantage of not being performed in an irradiated field. In the RTOG 91-11 trial, 11 of 12 patients who refused laryngectomy for lack of a response were nevertheless salvaged with radiotherapy, suggesting response to induction chemoradiation may not predict radioresponsiveness.

The use of concurrent treatment (opposed to induction) using chemotherapy and irradiation is associated with an increased locoregional tumor control and survival. When used concurrently with radiotherapy, the function of chemotherapy is thought to "radiosensitize" the tissue in the radiation field, rather than to function as a selector of radiation response. The RTOG 91-11 trial demonstrated improved locoregional tumor control as well as an increased rate of laryngeal preservation in patients with stage III and IV resectable laryngeal cancer who underwent concurrent chemoradiation therapy (for details, see discussion later in chapter). However, the rate of mucosal toxicity in those receiving concomitant chemotherapy was double the rate in either of the other two arms. One year following treatment, 23% of patients in the concurrent treatment group tolerated only a soft or liquid diet, and 3% could not swallow at all. Patients with extensive T4 primaries, such as those with cartilage invasion or those with involvement of the tongue base, were not included in the study.

The toxicity of chemotherapeutic agents has prompted the development of molecular agents with potentially greater tumor specificity and diminished toxicity. In one study, concomitant treatment with an anti-EGFR (epidermal growth factor receptor) antibody (cetuximab [Erbitux]) improved locoregional tumor control and survival in patients with oropharyngeal, laryngeal, and hypopharyngeal cancers. With a median follow-up of 54 months, the overall survival in the combined-therapy group was 49 months, compared with 29.3 months in the radiation-alone arm ($P = .03$). Combined-modality treatment was not associated with any increased mucosal toxicity or long-term differences in measured quality of life.

Chemotherapy and survival Numerous clinical trials have shown an improvement in locoregional tumor control using concurrent chemoradiation therapy, but a survival benefit has been observed less consistently. Recently published information from an updated meta-analysis of chemotherapy in head and neck cancer reports individual patient outcomes for 50 trials of concomitant chemoradiation therapy compared with irradiation alone. It included two separate analyses of trials from 1965 to 1993 and 1994 to 2000 and combined data. The pooled hazard ratio was 0.81, with a $P < .0001$ and an absolute survival benefit of 8% at 5 years for concomitant treatment. There was no difference in survival benefit in trials from the two time periods. In contrast, neoadjuvant chemotherapy with cisplatin and fluorouracil (5-FU) prior to locoregional therapy (commonly radiation), compared with locoregional therapy, was associated with a hazard ratio of 0.9. Indirect comparison of concomitant as opposed to neoadjuvant chemotherapy yielded a hazard ratio of 0.86 ($P = .0001$), demonstrating the importance of timing with respect to the integration of chemotherapy in primary management.

In the RTOG 91-11 randomized clinical trial, chemotherapy given concurrently with irradiation, or sequentially prior to irradiation, was found to suppress the incidence of distant metastases and to improve disease-specific survival relative to irradiation alone. Overall survival, however, was not affected.

Concurrent chemoradiation therapy has been found to have greater efficacy than irradiation alone in the setting of unresectable squamous cell cancer, based on a head and neck intergroup study. In this study, 295 patients with stages III and IV head and neck cancer were randomized to participate in one of three arms: (A) radiotherapy alone to 70 Gy in 35 fractions; (B) 70 Gy in 35 fractions plus concurrent cisplatin on days 1, 22, and 43; and (C) split-course radiotherapy and 3 cycles or concurrent cisplatin/5-FU chemotherapy, with 30 Gy given with cycle 1 and 30–40 Gy given with cycle 3. Grade 3 or worse toxicity occurred in 53% of arm A patients, 86% of arm B patients, and 77% of arm C patients. The 2- and 3-year Kaplan-Meier projected survivals for arm A are 30% and 20%, compared with 43% and 37% for arm B ($P = .016$) and 40% and 27% for arm C ($P = .13$). Median survival is 12.6 months for arm A, 19.1 months for arm B, and 14.0 months for arm C. The addition of concurrent high-dose single-agent cisplatin to conventional radiotherapy significantly improved survival with acceptable toxicity. Additionally, concurrent multiagent chemotherapy did not offset the loss of efficacy resulting from split-course irradiation.

The impact of adjuvant concomitant chemotherapy and radiotherapy on survival was assessed in two similarly designed trials in high-risk postoperative head and neck cancer patients testing adjuvant chemoradiation therapy against standard postoperative radiotherapy. In the RTOG 95-01 trial, disease-free survival was significantly increased in patients treated with adjuvant chemoradiation therapy relative to those treated with radiotherapy alone, but overall survival was not affected. In the EORTC trial published at the same time as the RTOG trial, the 5-year overall survival was also significantly improved in the concomitant chemotherapy and radiotherapy group.

Induction chemotherapy in combination with concomitant chemoradiation therapy Concurrent chemoradiation therapy is the current standard of care for patients with locally advanced squamous cell carcinoma of the head and neck. Many think this paradigmatic shift has influenced patterns of failure, and distant metastasis has become more important. Several phase I/II studies have tested this approach and shown its feasibility and efficacy. In fact, now several phase III studies have demonstrated superiority (response rate and survival) of a taxane-based triplet (docetaxel [Taxotere] and cisplatin) as induction therapy as opposed to the historic standard (cisplatin and 5-FU) when combined with concurrent therapy. Although to date, there have been no data suggesting this combination is better than concurrent chemoradiation alone. Two studies are currently enrolling patients evaluating this question.

Adjuvant chemotherapy following surgery or irradiation Adjuvant chemotherapy has been given following initial surgery or radiation therapy to eliminate microscopic residual disease and distant metastases. Although this approach has resulted in a reduced rate of distant metastasis, it has not been associated with improved locoregional tumor control or survival, except in a large meta-analysis. As concomitant approaches evolve and locoregional tumor control for advanced disease becomes the rule rather than the exception, the value of additional chemotherapy (as induction or adjuvant therapy) will need to be reexplored to address the problem of distant metastasis.

Locally advanced head and neck cancer Data from prospective trials continue to support the use of altered fractionation and concurrent chemotherapy and irradiation as an alternative to surgery or conventionally fractionated irra-

In March 2006, cetuximab (Erbitux) received FDA approval for use in combination with radiotherapy (RT) for patients with squamous cell cancer of the head and neck as well as monotherapy for metastatic disease. In one study, 424 patients with locoregionally advanced head and neck cancer were randomly assigned to receive treatment with high-dose RT alone or with weekly cetuximab. The primary endpoint was the duration of control of locoregional disease; secondary endpoints included overall and progression-free survival. The median duration of locoregional tumor control was 24.4 months among patients treated with cetuximab plus RT and 14.9 months among those given RT alone (hazard ratio [HR] for locoregional progression or death, 0.68; P = .005). With a median follow-up of 54.0 months, the median duration of overall survival was 49.0 months among patients treated with combined therapy and 29.3 months among those treated with RT alone (HR for death, 0.74; P = .03). RT plus cetuximab significantly prolonged progression-free survival (HR for disease progression or death, 0.70; P = .006); (Bonner JA, Harari PM, Giralt J, et al: N Engl J Med 354:567-578, 2006).

diation alone for locally advanced cancers of the head and neck. The long-term results of RTOG 90-03, which randomized 1,113 patients with stages III and IV squamous cell carcinoma of the oral cavity, oropharynx, or supraglottic larynx and stages II to IV squamous cell carcinoma of the base of the tongue or hypopharynx to receive one of four different schedules of irradiation alone, have been reported. They included 72 Gy/42 fractions (1.8 Gy/fraction initially, followed by 1.5 Gy/fraction to a boost field for the last 12 fractions twice daily). Locoregional tumor control and disease-free survival were superior for the hyperfractionated arms and accelerated fractionation with the concomitant boost compared with the other two arms. The hyperfractionated arm demonstrated a trend toward improved overall survival.

Updated results for RTOG 99-14, a phase II prospective study designed to integrate the altered fractionated radiation regimen from RTOG 90-03 with chemotherapy, were also reported in 2005. Cisplatin was given during weeks 1, 3, and 5. Longer-term results for 76 of 84 patients were reported, and the 3-year disease-free, overall, and cause-specific survival rates were 45.8%, 57.7%, and 61.2%, respectively. The 3-year local recurrence and distant metastasis rates were 38.7% and 23.3%, respectively. Of 35 patients who were alive, 22 had a temporary feeding tube, and 17% (6 patients) still required a feeding tube at the time of their last follow-up.

RTOG 97-03, a three-arm randomized phase II trial, evaluated the feasibility of concurrent, multi-agent chemotherapy with radiation therapy. In this study, three different regi-

At ASCO 2007, investigators presented data on excision repair cross-complementation group 1 (ERCC-1) enzyme, which appears to be related to resistance to platinum-based chemotherapy as previously demonstrated in other cancer sites specifically for patients treated with head and neck cancer. In this study, patients who had low levels of ERCC-1 expression were at four times greater odds of benefiting from an objective response to chemotherapy (P = .01), which corresponds to a lower risk of cancer-related death (Mountzios G, Handra-Luca A, Hernandez J, et al: J Clin Oncol 25[18S]:6011, 2007). A second study demonstrated a 54% ERCC-1 expression rate, which similarly translates into poor outcomes in terms of progression-free survival and overall survival (Jun H, Ahn M, Kim H, et al: J Clin Oncol 25[18S]:6061, 2007).

mens of chemotherapy were used with irradiation (70 Gy/35 fractions) for oral cavity, oropharyngeal, and hypopharyngeal cancers. Arm 1 received cisplatin (10 mg/m^2) and 5-FU, (400 mg/m^2) continuous infusion daily for the final 10 days of radiotherapy. Treatment on arm 2 consisted of hydroxyurea (1 g/d), and 5-FU, (800 mg/m^2) continuous infusion delivered concurrently with radiation therapy. Arm 3 received paclitaxel (30 mg/m^2) and cisplatin (20 mg/m^2) weekly. The incidence of acute toxicity was high, with the lowest incidence of persistent feeding tube dependence in arm 3. Arm 2 was associated with a slightly higher rate of grade 4 toxicity and treatment interruption. All arms demonstrated improved survival relative to historic controls treated with radiation therapy alone.

To diminish toxicity and maximize locoregional tumor control in locally advanced oropharyngeal and laryngeal cancers, a phase II trial using taxane-based induction followed by concurrent chemoradiation therapy was conducted through the Eastern Cooperative Oncology Group (ECOG; E2399). A total of 111 patients (T2N+ or T3-4N0–3) underwent induction therapy with 2 cycles of paclitaxel (175 mg/m^2) and carboplatin followed by concurrent weekly paclitaxel (30 mg/m^2 to 70 Gy). Patients with progressive or stable disease at the primary site after induction therapy underwent surgery. Patients with primary laryngeal cancers fared significantly worse using this regimen. Patients with laryngeal cancer had a lower rate of major response to induction chemotherapy, a lower 2-year progression-free survival, and a trend toward higher distant failure than those with primary oropharyngeal cancer. The 2-year progression-free survival was 50% for patients with laryngeal cancer, compared with 75% for those with oropharyngeal cancer ($P = .05$).

Chemotherapy for recurrent or metastatic disease The combination of cisplatin/5-FU produces overall response rates of approximately 30% and survival rates of 6 months. In randomized trials comparing this combination with single-agent cisplatin, 5-FU, or methotrexate, response rates with the single agents are lower, but survival is equivalent. However, because many practitioners believe response is a surrogate for palliation, cisplatin/5-FU has been used widely in this setting.

In September 2007, docetaxel (Taxotere) in combination with cisplatin and fluorouracil (TPF) was approved by the FDA for use as induction therapy for patients with locally advanced squamous cell cancer of the head and neck. The trial that led to this indication was a multicenter open-label randomized phase III evaluation of TPF compared with PF for 3 cycles prior to chemoradiation with weekly carboplatin. A total of 501 patients with stages III–IV disease, deemed either unresectable or candidates for organ preservation, were randomized. Locoregional control was improved in the TPF arm (70% vs 62%). This translated to an improvement in overall survival with median survival rates of 71 vs 30 months and a hazard ratio for survival in the TPF arm of .70 ($P = .006$). Distant failure was similar in both arms and uncommon, observed in less than 10% of patients. Neutropenia and neutropenic fever were more common in the TPF group. With the addition of prophylactic antibiotics, the regimen was, however, safe and feasible *(Posner MR, Hershock DM, Blajman CR, et al: N Engl J Med 357:1705-1715, 2007).*

The taxanes are the most active cytotoxins yet identified in head and neck cancer, with overall response rates of approximately 35% in patients with recurrent or incurable disease. In one randomized trial, the combination of paclitaxel/cisplatin has been compared with cisplatin/5-FU in patients with recurrent disease. A total of 194 patients who were therapy-naive for recurrent disease with an ECOG performance status of 0–1 were randomized. Efficacy outcomes were similar in the two arms, with median survival rates of 8 and 9 months for arms 1 and 2, respectively. Paclitaxel/cisplatin was less toxic and more convenient, representing an effective and safe alternative to the traditional 5-FU–containing regimen.

Based on nearly universal expression of EGFR in squamous cell cancer of the head and neck, EGFR-targeted agents have been evaluated in patients with recurrent disease. Although the single agent response rates of cetuximab (monoclonal antibody), erlotinib (Tarceva), and gefitinib (Iressa; tyrosine kinase inhibitors) in this setting are only in the range of 5% to 15%, their use in combination with chemotherapy, particularly cetuximab, holds more promise. Preliminary results of the EXTREME trial, which accrued 442 patients with recurrent or metastatic squamous cell cancer of the head and neck, showed that compared with platinum-based chemotherapy alone, the combination with cetuximab improved median (7.4 months vs 10.1 months) and 1-year (31% vs 39%) survival rates, with a hazard ratio of 0.8 ($P = .036$). Similar promising, albeit preliminary, results have been reported from phase II single-arm studies of cetuximab/paclitaxel and erlotinib/docetaxel/cisplatin. Overall, these observations lend impetus to further investigation of EGFR-targeted therapy in combination with neoadjuvant chemotherapy and with chemoradiation therapy in patients with curable disease. Many such trials are ongoing.

Photodynamic therapy

Photodynamic therapy may have some promise in the treatment of mucosal dysplasia and small head and neck tumors.

Small studies of photodynamic therapy, performed at several institutions, suggest that widespread areas of carcinoma in situ or severe dysplasia, as well as cancer, are often extirpated after photodynamic therapy. Although some patients have experienced durable remissions, the long-term efficacy of this modality remains uncertain.

Pulsed dye laser therapy for early laryngeal lesions

The pulsed dye laser initially used to treat vascular lesions has recently been investigated in the treatment of respiratory papillomatosis, dysplastic cancers, and early invasive glottic carcinomas. The efficacy of the laser is mediated through its antiangiogenic properties. The treatment is nontoxic, preserves the laryngeal microarchitecture, and preserves or restores near-normal vocal quality. Additionally, this modality can be utilized in an outpatient clinic setting. Preliminary findings are favorable. At this time, however, pulsed dye laser therapy should be considered investigational.

Chemoprevention

The area of chemoprevention has received a great deal of attention in recent years, and the concept of field cancerization is important in this context. As mentioned previously, this concept refers to the diffuse epithelial injury incurred by upper aerodigestive tract mucosa due to chronic exposure to carcinogens (most commonly alcohol and tobacco). These mucosal changes increase the risk of developing premalignant lesions (leukoplakia and erythroplakia), as well as multiple primary lesions.

Retinoids (vitamin A analogues) have been investigated as chemopreventive agents in the aerodigestive tract based on their efficacy in tumor models, such as the hamster buccal pouch. Retinoids mediate changes in gene expression through interaction with nuclear retinoic acid receptors, which function as transcription factors. Nutritional epidemiology studies also have indicated that low serum levels of both carotenoids and retinoids contribute to the risk of cancer development in the epithelium of the upper aerodigestive tract.

The role of retinoids in the prevention of second primary tumors in patients treated with curative intent for an early-stage index squamous cell cancer of the head and neck has been investigated in three randomized trials. The initial study was a small, single-center phase III trial of *cis*-retinoic acid (1–2 mg/kg/d) by Hong et al. Although this study demonstrated decreased second primary tumors in the experimental arm, compliance and morbidity with this high dose were problematic. A second study using a low dose of *cis*-retinoic acid (10 mg/d) was performed by ECOG and was negative. Results from a third large, multicenter trial with an intermediate dose of 30 mg/d have been reported in abstract form and are also negative in regard to second primary prevention.

Rehabilitation

Rehabilitation also is very important in the perioperative care of patients with head and neck cancer. It includes physical and occupational therapy, speech and swallowing rehabilitation, and nutritional support. For example, resection of the spinal accessory nerve, which innervates the trapezius muscle, leads to scapular winging, inability to abduct the arm fully, and, eventually, severe pain around the shoulder. These symptoms may be ameliorated with appropriate physical therapy.

Adapting to the loss of the larynx also requires intensive rehabilitation and patient motivation. Voice rehabilitation options include esophageal speech, artificial larynges (portable, battery-operated devices), and tracheoesophageal shunts.

Nutritional support is facilitated by temporary nasoduodenal tubes or gastrostomy tubes (which impose added morbidity but are more socially acceptable and ease the patient's transition to normal activities).

TABLE 2: Types of neck dissection and structures removed in the treatment of head and neck cancer

Type of neck dissection	Structures removed
Comprehensive neck dissection	
"Classic" radical neck dissection	All lymph-bearing tissue (levels I-V), spinal accessory nerve (cranial nerve [CN] XI), sternocleidomastoid muscle, and internal jugular vein
Modified radical neck dissection	Neck dissection with sparing of one or more of the above structures
Type I	CN XI spared
Type II	CN XI and internal jugular vein spared
Type III (functional neck dissection)	All three structures spared (CN XI, internal jugular vein, and sternocleidomastoid muscle)
Selective neck dissection	Removal of lymph-bearing tissue from:
Lateral	Levels II-IV
Posterolateral	Levels II-V
Supraomohyoid	Levels I-III

From Medina JE, Rebual NM: Neck dissection, in Cummings CW, Fredrickson J, Harker LE, et al (eds): Otolaryngology: Head and Neck Surgery, pp 1649–1672. St. Louis, Mosby Yearbook, 1993.

Management of symptoms and treatment side effects

Eating problems At the time of diagnosis, many patients with head and neck cancer will have lost a significant amount of weight. Maintaining adequate nutrition is a major problem for these patients, as both the tumor and treatment side effects, such as mucositis from chemotherapy and radiation therapy, may be contributory. For patients who are unable to eat or who are being treated with aggressive concomitant chemotherapy and radiation therapy protocols, placement of a gastrostomy tube is often necessary to maintain caloric intake and adequate hydration.

Pain Clinicians must also be aware of the significant pain associated with these lesions and use narcotic analgesics appropriately to relieve discomfort.

Mucositis The use of chemotherapy concomitantly with radiation therapy increases the occurrence of mucositis.

Nephrotoxicity and ototoxicity For patients treated with cisplatin-containing regimens, renal insufficiency and ototoxicity are potential serious side effects.

Xerostomia Following radiation therapy of a head and neck cancer, xerostomia may be a significant long-term side effect. In some patients, pilocarpine (Salagen) has been useful in stimulating the production of saliva.

The use of organic thiophosphates, such as amifostine (Ethyol), in patients undergoing radiotherapy for head and neck cancer reduces the severity of late xerostomia without compromising the antitumor activity of the irradiation.

Gastroesophageal reflux Often asymptomatic or "silent" gastroesophageal reflux disease (GERD) is a common finding in patients treated for pharyngolaryngeal squamous cell carcinoma. In addition, cisplatin-containing chemotherapy may aggravate GERD.

Treatment of the neck

Either irradiation alone or radical neck dissection will control metastatic squamous cell cancer to a single small neck node more than 90% of the time if there is no extracapsular tumor spread. Hence, radiation treatment may easily provide prophylactic treatment of the neck if control of the primary tumor is undertaken with irradiation. Traditionally, if the tumor in the neck was N2 or greater, or if there was tumor beyond the confines of a node, neck dissection and irradiation were combined for optimal control of the neck tumor. The need for neck dissection in patients clinically staged N2–N3 with a complete clinical and radiographic response following radiation therapy remains under investigation.

Types of dissection

There are several approaches to the surgical treatment of the neck nodes in patients with head and neck cancer (Table 2). This discussion will be limited to two types of neck dissection: comprehensive and selective.

Comprehensive neck dissection entails complete removal of all lymphatic tissue from the neck (levels I–V). A radical neck dissection includes comprehensive node dissection with removal of the sternocleidomastoid muscle, jugular vein, and spinal accessory nerve. Modified radical neck dissection was developed to diminish the morbidity of the classic operation. The most important structure to preserve is the spinal accessory nerve.

Selective neck dissection consists of the removal of lymph node groups at highest risk of containing metastases from a primary cancer. In such procedures, the lymph nodes removed correspond to the most significant drainage basins of specific head and neck tumor sites. These are staging operations usually performed in patients with clinically N0 neck cancer. If metastases are identified, further treatment to the neck will be required. A selective neck dissection should not be employed as the sole treatment of clinically palpable disease.

Sentinel lymph node biopsy for oral cavity lesions has been evaluated. Forty patients with clinically N0 neck cancer underwent sentinel lymph node biopsy followed by complete neck dissection. A sentinel node was identified in 90% of necks, with a 97% accuracy rate in predicting the nodal status of the remainder of the neck. This finding corresponded to a sensitivity of 94% and a specificity of 100%. Although these results are encouraging, they need to be validated in a larger trial. An ongoing American College of Surgeons Oncology Group study (Z0360) is examining this technique in patients with T1 or T2, N0 oral cavity cancer. Sentinel lymph node biopsy may prove useful in small lesions without deep penetration, but it remains investigational.

Follow-up of long-term survivors

As mentioned, head and neck cancers are aggressive tumors. The majority (80%) of recurrences will develop within 2 years. Since many recurrences are treatable with curative intent, patients should be followed closely during the months following their treatment. This period coincides with the time of greatest need from the standpoint of rehabilitation.

After 2 years, second primary tumors of the head and neck and lungs become important causes of death and morbidity. Late complications of treatment such as radionecrosis, radiation-induced fibrosis, and hypothyroidism, as well as sequelae of spinal accessory nerve sacrifice or injury, may develop even after years. Complications and second primary cancers are more common in patients who continue to smoke.

Timing of follow-up evaluations Follow-up evaluations at regular intervals should be complete and should include a focused history and examination, as outlined previously. Physicians who are able to perform a head and neck examination (including laryngoscopy) should direct follow-up. After surgical treatment, this evaluation will usually require visits with the head and neck surgeon. Patients treated with irradiation should be followed by both their radiation oncologist and a head and neck surgeon or otolaryngologist.

Evaluations should be scheduled every 1 to 2 months during the first year after treatment, every 2 to 4 months during the second year, every 3 to 6 months during the third year, and every 6 months thereafter for several more years.

Imaging and laboratory studies Any mucosal abnormality should be biopsied. There are no tumor markers or other useful laboratory studies to follow. Chest x-rays should be obtained yearly. There is little justification for performing CT scans or MRI in the follow-up of asymptomatic patients. Thyroid-stimulating hormone (TSH) should be measured yearly in patients who have received irradiation to the larynx or nasopharynx.

HEAD AND NECK TUMOR REGIONS

As mentioned previously, tumors occurring at different anatomic sites and subsites of the head and neck vary considerably with regard to epidemiology, risk factors, anatomy, natural history, staging of the primary tumor, and therapy. The following sections highlight these differences.

ORAL CAVITY

Sites of the oral cavity include the lips, hard palate, floor of the mouth, buccal mucosa, and tongue. Cancers at these sites comprise < 5% of all malignancies in the United States.

Anatomy

The oral cavity extends from the cutaneous vermilion junction of the lips to the junction of the hard and soft palates above and to the line of the circumvallate papillae below. It includes the lips, buccal mucosa, upper and lower alveolar ridges, retromolar trigone, floor of the mouth, hard palate, and anterior two-thirds of the tongue (the "oral" tongue). The primary lymphatic drainage is to the submental triangle, submandibular nodes, and upper deep jugular nodes.

Natural history

The most common presenting complaint is a sore in the mouth or on the lips. One-third of patients present with a neck mass.

The differential diagnosis includes other malignancies and benign diseases or lesions. Other malignancies to be considered include salivary gland tumors, sarcoma, lymphoma, and melanoma. Benign diseases include pyogenic granu-loma, tuberculous disease, aphthous ulcers, and chancres.

Benign mucosal lesions include papillomas and keratoacanthomas, which may be exophytic or infiltrative. The exophytic lesions are less aggressive. The infiltrative papillomas and keratoacanthomas are more often associated with destruction of surrounding tissues and structures. These lesions may progress to malignancy. The TNM staging system for cancers of the lips and oral cav-ity is outlined in Table 3. T4 lesions have been divided into T4a (resectable) and T4b (unresectable) in the sixth edition of the *AJCC Cancer Staging Manual.*

Treatment

Management of cancers of the oral cavity involves surgery or radiotherapy for T1 or T2 lesions or combined-modality treatment that includes surgical resection and postoperative radiation therapy (60–70 Gy in 6–7 weeks) for advanced disease. For early-stage disease, surgery and radiotherapy are considered to have equivalent efficacy, although surgery is associated with less morbidity. Supraomohyoid neck dissection is performed in surgically treated patients with N0 necks. Bilateral neck dissection is performed if the tumor approaches the midline. Neck dissection is recommended for tumor thickness that is at least 4 mm.

TABLE 3: TNM staging system for cancers of the lips and oral cavity

Primary tumor (T)

Tx	Primary tumor cannot be assessed
T0	No evidence of primary tumor
Tis	Carcinoma in situ
T1	Tumor 2 cm or less in greatest dimension
T2	Tumor more than 2 cm but not more than 4 cm in greatest dimension
T3	Tumor more than 4 cm in greatest dimension
T4	(lip) Tumor invades through cortical bone, inferior alveolar nerve, floor of mouth, or skin of face, ie, chin or nose[a]
T4a	(oral cavity) Tumor invades adjacent structures (eg, through cortical bone, into deep [extrinsic] muscle of the tongue, maxillary sinus, or skin of face); resectable lesions
T4b	Tumor involves masticator space, pterygoid plates, or skull base and/or encases internal carotid artery; unresectable lesions

Regional lymph nodes (N)

Nx	Regional nodes cannot be assessed
N0	No regional lymph node metastasis
N1	Metastasis in a single ipsilateral lymph node, 3 cm or less in greatest dimension
N2	Metastasis in a single ipsilateral lymph node, more than 3 cm but not more than 6 cm in greatest dimension; or in multiple ipsilateral lymph nodes, none more than 6 cm in greatest dimension; or in bilateral or contralateral lymph nodes, none more than 6 cm in greatest dimension
N2a	Metastasis in a single ipsilateral lymph node, more than 3 cm but not more than 6 cm in greatest dimension
N2b	Metastasis in multiple ipsilateral lymph nodes, none more than 6 cm in greatest dimension
N2c	Metastasis in bilateral or contralateral lymph nodes, none more than 6 cm in greatest dimension
N3	Metastasis in a lymph node, more than 6 cm in greatest dimension

ORAL CAVITY SITE: LIPS

The lips are the most common site of oral cavity cancer. There are approximately 4,000 new cases per year in the United States. The lower lip is affected most often. The vast majority of patients (90%) with lip cancer are men, and 33% have outdoor occupations.

Natural history

The most frequent presentation is a slow-growing tumor of the lower lip that may bleed and hurt. Physical examination must include assessment of hypoesthesia in the distribution of the mental nerve (cutaneous sensation of the chin area). Currently, fewer than 10% of American patients with squamous cell carcinoma of the lower lip have cervical metastases.

Distant metastases (M)

Mx   Distant metastasis cannot be assessed

M0   No distant metastasis

M1   Distant metastasis

Stage grouping

Stage 0	Tis	N0	M0
Stage I	T1	N0	M0
Stage II	T2	N0	M0
Stage III	T3	N0	M0
	T1	N1	M0
	T2	N1	M0
	T3	N1	M0
Stage IVA	T4a	N0	M0
	T4a	N1	M0
	T1	N2	M0
	T2	N2	M0
	T3	N2	M0
	T4a	N2	M0
Stage IVB	Any T	N3	M0
	T4b	Any N	M0
Stage IVC	Any T	Any N	M1

From Greene FL, Page DL, Fleming ID, et al (eds): AJCC Cancer Staging Manual, 6th ed. New York, Springer-Verlag, 2002.

[a] Superficial erosion alone of bone/tooth socket by gingival primary is not sufficient to classify a tumor as T4.

Treatment

The primary tumor Patients with early-stage lip cancers are usually treated with surgery. Radiation therapy may be utilized in patients who are medically unsuited for surgery or who refuse surgical resection.

Resection involves excision with at least 0.5 cm of normal tissue circumferentially beyond the recognized border of the tumor. After the resection of larger lesions, reconstruction may pose a major challenge. Small tumors are excised with a V incision.

Patients with advanced disease (stage III or IV) are usually managed with a combination of surgery and postoperative radiation therapy (60–70 Gy in 6–7 weeks).

The neck Elective treatment of the neck is seldom recommended for patients with squamous cell carcinoma of the lower lip and a clinically negative neck because few of these patients have cervical metastases. Neck dissection is recommended only in patients with palpable cervical metastases. Neck dissection is followed by postoperative radiation therapy.

Results The cure rate for T1–T3 tumors is 90% with surgical excision alone. Smaller lesions (T1–T2) may be treated equally well with radiation therapy. Survival rates for patients with T1 and T2 lesions are 90% and 80%, respectively. Overall, younger patients have a poorer prognosis, as do those with involvement of the mandible and extension of the tumor within the oral cavity.

ORAL CAVITY SITE: TONGUE

The oral tongue (anterior two-thirds) is the site of 75% of all tongue cancers. There are approximately 7,320 new cases of oral tongue cancer each year in the United States.

Natural history

The most common presenting symptom in patients with cancer of the tongue is a persistent, nonhealing ulcer with or without associated pain. Other symptoms include difficulty with deglutition and speech. There may be a history of leukoplakia, especially in younger women.

Rate of growth Cancer of the tongue seems to grow more rapidly than other oral cavity cancers. Tongue cancers may grow in an infiltrative or exophytic fashion. The infiltrative tumors may be quite large at presentation.

Lesion thickness Thicker lesions have a worse prognosis than thin cancers, and lesion thickness is a more important prognostic factor than is simple tumor stage. The incidence of clinically occult cervical metastases to the neck is significantly higher when the tumor thickness exceeds 4 mm.

Cervical metastases occur more frequently from tongue cancer than from any other tumor of the oral cavity. At initial evaluation, 40% of patients have node metastases.

Treatment

Early-stage disease Treatment usually entails partial glossectomy. Margins should be assessed at the time of resection, as the disease spreads along muscle bundles, leading to more extensive tumor than is appreciated grossly.

Radiation therapy (60–70 Gy in 6–7 weeks) is a suitable option for small or minimally infiltrating tumors. Large, infiltrative lesions should be treated with combined-modality therapy (radiation therapy and surgical resection).

Advanced disease More advanced tumors with mandibular involvement require composite resection, including a partial glossectomy, mouth floor resection, and mandibulectomy.

The neck A selective neck dissection is often recommended for clinically N0 neck cancer. Comprehensive neck dissection is required in the presence of palpable cervical metastases.

Results Control of disease closely correlates with the extent of the primary tumor and the presence of metastases. Rates of local tumor control using radiation therapy or surgery are similar for T1 (~85%) and T2 (~80%) tumors. T3 tumors should be treated using surgery and radiation therapy. Only 10% to 15% of local recurrences are amenable to repeated resection.

Overall survival is approximately 50%. Rates of survival at 5 years by stage follow: stage I, 80%; stage II, 60%; and stages III–IV, 15% to 35%. For equivalent primary cancers, the presence of lymph node metastases decreases the survival rate by 50%.

Improved prognosis for human papillomavirus (HPV)-associated squamous cancer of the head and neck has been suggested by multiple single-institution retrospective analyses. In a phase II trial, patients with locally advanced oropharyngeal and laryngeal cancers were treated with neoadjuvant paclitaxel and carboplatin followed by radiation with weekly paclitaxel. These data, presented in abstract form, indicate 40% of evaluable cases were positive for HPV. Patients who were HPV-positive had a higher response rate to both neoadjuvant chemotherapy and chemoradiation and had improved survival. Hazard ratios for progression and death were 0.28 and 0.21, respectively, for patients with HPV-positive tumors. These preliminary prospective data are strong confirmation of previous retrospective analyses identifying HPV association as a favorable prognostic indicator, especially for oropharyngeal primary tumors (*Fakhry C, Westra W, Li S, et al: J Clin Oncol 25[18S]:6000, 2007*).

ORAL CAVITY SITE: FLOOR OF THE MOUTH

There are approximately 4,000 cases of floor of the mouth cancer in the United States annually. Mouth floor cancer accounts for 10% to 15% of all oral cavity cancers.

Pathology

Most lesions are moderately differentiated to well-differentiated squamous cell cancers and are exophytic.

Natural history

Patients usually present with a painful mass located near the oral tongue. Because these lesions do not cause pain until they are deep, they are frequently advanced at presentation.

Extension of disease into the soft tissues of the submandibular triangle is not uncommon. Fixation of the tumor to bone suggests possible mandibular involvement. A Panorex film of the mandible may reveal invasion of the mandible via direct extension (through a tooth socket) or via perineural invasion spreading along the mental nerve through the mental foramen. Changes in the mental foramen can be distinct or demonstrate slight asymmetry when compared with the contralateral anatomy. Restricted tongue mobility reflects invasion into the root of the tongue. Palpation demonstrates the depth of infiltration much better than does inspection alone.

Tumors near the midline may obstruct the duct of the submandibular gland, leading to swelling and induration in the neck, which may be difficult to distinguish from lymph node metastases. Level I nodes are the first-echelon metastatic sites.

Multifocality Multifocal cancers are more common in the floor of the mouth than in other oral cavity sites. Approximately 20% of patients with mouth floor tumors have a second primary tumor, half of which are in the head and neck.

Treatment

Early invasive lesions (T1–T2) involving the mucosa alone may be treated with either surgery or irradiation (60–70 Gy in 6–7 weeks) alone, with comparable results. Primary tumors with mandibular involvement should be surgically resected.

Cancer invades the mandible through tooth sockets. Hence, if the tumor merely abuts the mandible, a marginal mandibulectomy (which removes the bone margin but preserves continuity) may be performed. Otherwise, a segmental resection is needed. Selective neck dissection for treatment planning is advisable for thick stage I or II cancers.

Advanced disease The treatment of choice for advanced disease is combined-modality therapy with surgery and radiation therapy. Complete surgical resection may require a composite resection of the mandible, including a partial glossectomy and neck dissection for advanced primary cancers. Lesions near the midline with a clinically positive lymph node require ipsilateral comprehensive neck dissection with a contralateral selective (supraomohyoid) neck dissection. Otherwise, both sides of the neck should be treated with irradiation.

Results Overall, ~40% of patients are cured of their disease; 80% of recurrences appear within the first 2 years. Survival rates at 5 years by stage follow: stage I, 85%; stage II, 75%; stage III, 66%; and stage IV, 30%. Signs of poor prognosis include involvement of both the tongue and mandible and extension of the tumor beyond the oral cavity.

OROPHARYNX

Carcinoma of the oropharynx affects 4,000 patients in the United States annually.

Anatomy and pathology

The opening to the oropharynx is a ring bounded by the anterior tonsillar pillars (faucial arch), extending upward to blend with the uvula and inferiorly across the base of the tongue (behind the circumvallate papillae). The walls of the oropharynx are formed by the pharyngeal constrictor muscles, which overlie the cervical spine posteriorly. The superior boundary is the soft palate, which separates the oropharynx from the nasopharynx.

Subsites of the oropharynx include the base of the tongue, soft palate, tonsillar area, and posterior pharyngeal wall. The extent of a primary tumor may be difficult to assess due to its location.

The jugulodigastric nodes (levels II and III) constitute the first echelon of lymphatic drainage. Metastases may also appear in the parapharyngeal and retropharyngeal nodes and may be detected only through imaging studies.

Premalignant lesions occur in the oropharynx but are less common than in the oral cavity.

Treatment

Radiation therapy External-beam radiation therapy (65–70 Gy over 7 weeks) and interstitial irradiation have been used in the curative treatment of oropharyngeal carcinomas for over 70 years. Radiation therapy represents a reasonable alternative to surgery and may also be required following radical resection of tumors with poor pathologic features to reduce the likelihood of local recurrence.

Altered fractionation schedules (accelerated and/or hyperfractionated) have gained interest in the past several years based on both theoretical grounds and the results of mainly retrospective data. One prospective, randomized trial in patients with oropharyngeal cancer (excluding base of the tongue cancer) documented a 20% increase in locoregional tumor control and a 14% survival benefit at 5 years in patients who received 8,050 cGy in a hyperfractionated schedule, as opposed to 7,000 cGy in a conventionally fractionated schedule, specifically for intermediate-risk patients with T2 or T3 N0 or N1 squamous cell carcinomas. This improvement in outcome was not offset by any significant increase in acute or late tissue toxicity.

Local tumor control rates with radiation therapy for all primary sites (including the tonsils, soft palate, base of the tongue, and posterior oropharyngeal wall) follow: T1, 90%; T2, 80%; T3, 65%; and T4, 55%. Cancers of the tonsillar fossa are better controlled with irradiation than are cancers arising in other subsites of the oropharynx.

Chemoradiation therapy A number of studies supporting the use of multimodality therapy with radiation therapy and chemotherapy as an alternative to surgery with postoperative irradiation or irradiation alone have been published. In an intergroup trial by Adelstein et al, cisplatin (100 mg/m^2) given every 3 weeks with standard irradiation was found to be safe and effective. Induction therapy followed by concurrent chemoradiation regimens has the potential for diminishing distant failure while maintaining the local tumor control achieved via concurrent regimens. Such regimens are currently under active investigation.

Surgery Surgical extirpation of relatively inaccessible tumors in the oropharynx traditionally required radical surgery, including mandibulotomy or mandibulectomy and occasionally laryngectomy. These surgical procedures were associated with worse functional outcomes relative to nonsurgical approaches. Radical surgery, however, has been supplanted by minimally invasive approaches, facilitated by the development of endoscopes, microscopes, electrocautery devices, lasers, and laryngoscopes and retractors. Using bivalved laryngoscopes for tumor exposure, surgical resection using the carbon dioxide laser coupled to a microscope has led to complete pathologic resections and high local control rates for oropharyngeal cancer. The reported functional results have been good, with few patients requiring placement of a feeding tube or tracheotomies.

The use of the line-of-sight CO_2 laser beam has been limited by inadequate exposure of the pathologic lesion in patients with short or stiff necks, retrognathia, full dentition, trismus, or obesity. Limited access to pathology has precluded use of transoral CO_2 laser surgery in many patients. A flexible photonic bandgap fiber for the delivery of CO_2 laser energy, developed by OmniGuide Inc, allows video-assisted visualization and extirpation of previously poorly accessible pathology. Limited access has also been surmounted by the adaptation of the surgical robot for transoral applications. The daVinci Surgical System (Intuitive Surgical, Sunnyvale, CA), originally designed as a three-armed robotic device controlling "wristed" surgical microinstruments and angled telescopes, has now been FDA approved for a variety of general, cardiac, gynecologic, and urologic procedures. Improved surgical exposure to tumors in the upper aerodigestive tract have been reported relative to those obtained with more traditional transoral approaches. However, the role of minimally invasive surgery for the treatment of oropharyngeal tumors has yet to be defined.

OROPHARYNGEAL SITE: BASE OF THE TONGUE

Cancer of the base of the tongue is far less common than that of the oral tongue.

Anatomy

The base of the tongue is bordered anteriorly by the circumvallate papillae and posteriorly by the epiglottis. There is a rich lymphatic network, with metastases frequently seen in levels II–V.

Natural history

The base of the tongue is notorious for lesions that infiltrate deeply into muscle and are advanced at diagnosis. This finding is probably due to the relatively asymptomatic anatomic location. Thus, bimanual oral examination with digital palpation is a critical part of the physical examination.

Most patients present with pain and dysphagia. Other symptoms include a neck mass, weight loss, otalgia, and trismus.

All oropharyngeal cancers have a strong propensity to spread to the lymph nodes, and base of the tongue tumors are no exception. Approximately 70% of patients with T1 primary base of the tongue tumors have clinically palpable disease in the neck, and 20%–30% have palpable, bilateral lymph node metastases. The risk of nodal metastases increases with increasing T stage and approaches 85% for T4 lesions.

Treatment

Early-stage disease Stage I or II cancers may be treated equally effectively with either surgical resection or radiation therapy (65–70 Gy in 6–7 weeks) alone. If irradiation of the primary tumor is employed, both sides of the neck should be treated, even if the nodes do not seem to be involved. Surgical management of an oropharyngeal malignancy includes lymphadenectomy. For patients clinically staged N0, selective neck dissection encompassing levels II–IV is sufficient. For patients with cancers at the base of the tongue, bilateral neck dissection is required.

Advanced disease More advanced disease may require total resection of the tongue base with or without laryngectomy to ensure complete removal of disease. Total resection of the tongue base is associated with severe oropharyngeal dysphagia with aspiration, but even subtotal resection of the base of the tongue may result in significant aspiration, which is exacerbated by postoperative radiotherapy. Total laryngectomy may be the only way to isolate the airway from oral secretions and eliminate the risk of aspiration. Chemoradiation therapy via external-beam irradiation or irradiation alone combined with an implant can be curative for patients with advanced tumors of the tongue base.

Results In general, the prognosis of cancers of the tongue base is poor due to their advanced stage at presentation. The extent of nodal disease predicts survival. For T1 and T2 cancers, local tumor control rates approach 85%. The major determinant of treatment failure is the tumor's growth pattern, with a high local tumor control rate for exophytic lesions and a far worse rate for infiltrative tumors.

OROPHARYNGEAL SITE: TONSILS AND TONSILLAR PILLAR

The tonsils and tonsillar pillar are the most common locations for tumors of the oropharynx.

Natural history

Tonsillar fossa tumors tend to be more advanced and more frequently metastasize to the neck than do tonsillar pillar cancers. At presentation, 55% of patients with fossa tumors have N2 or N3 disease, and contralateral metastases are common. Symptoms include pain, dysphagia, weight loss, a mass in the neck, and trismus.

Treatment

Single-modality therapy (irradiation or surgery alone) is acceptable for T1 and T2 tumors. Irradiation alone (60–70 Gy in 6–7 weeks) may be curative for more advanced tumors, although many of these lesions will require surgery combined with irradiation. The neck should always be included in treatment planning. More advanced disease usually requires surgery combined with irradiation (60–70 Gy in 6–7 weeks). Well-lateralized cancers of the tonsillar fossa (minimal to no involvement of the soft palate or base of the tongue) may be treated with unilateral irradiation since contralateral neck failure is rare (< 10%).

HYPOPHARYNX

Hypopharyngeal cancers are approximately one-third as common as laryngeal cancers.

Anatomy

The hypopharynx (or laryngopharynx) is the entrance to the esophagus. The superior aspect (above the plane of the hyoid bone) communicates with the oropharynx, and the inferior border is situated in the plane of the lowest part of the cricoid cartilage (the esophageal inlet). The anterior surface (postcricoid area) is contiguous with the posterior surface of the larynx, adjacent to the lamina of the cricoid cartilage. The pharyngeal musculature forms the lateral and posterior walls. The piriform sinuses are within the hypopharynx on each side of the larynx.

The hypopharynx contains three subsites: the paired piriform sinuses (lateral, pear-shaped funnels); the posterior pharyngeal wall, from the level of the vallecula to the level of the cricoarytenoid joints; and the postcricoid area (pharyngoesophageal junction), which begins just below the arytenoids and extends to the inferior border of the cricoid cartilage. The piriform sinuses are composed of a medial wall, which abuts the aryepiglottic fold, and a lateral wall. Seventy percent of hypopharyngeal cancers occur in the piriform sinuses.

Natural history

Hypopharyngeal tumors produce few symptoms until they are advanced (~70% are stage III at presentation). They may cause a sore throat, otalgia, a change in voice, odynophagia, or an isolated neck mass. Subtle changes on physical examination, including pooling of secretions, should be regarded with concern.

Nodal metastases Diffuse local spread is common and is due to tumor extension within the submucosa. Abundant lymphatic drainage results in a higher incidence of lymph node metastases than with other head and neck tumors. At presentation, 70% to 80% of patients with hypopharyngeal tumors have palpable cervical lymph node metastases; in half of these patients, palpable cervical nodes are the presenting complaint. Levels II and III are most commonly involved. Bilateral metastases are seen in only 10% of patients with piriform sinus cancers but in 60% of those with postcricoid tumors.

Synchronous lesions are common. Overall, 20% to 25% of patients with hypopharyngeal cancer develop a second primary tumor within 5 years, usually in the head and neck.

Chemotherapy and external-beam radiotherapy Similar in design to the VA Cooperative Laryngeal Cancer Study, a randomized EORTC trial has shown that initial therapy with cisplatin and 5-FU, followed by definitive irradiation in patients with complete remissions (or, alternatively, surgical salvage), results in at least equivalent survival relative to immediate pharyngolaryngectomy. Of patients treated with initial chemotherapy, 28% retained a functional larynx at 3 years (approximately two-thirds of survivors).

Though directed to laryngeal cancers (rather than hypopharyngeal cancers), the RTOG 91-11 trial results have been widely interpreted as applying to hypopharyngeal cancer, increasing enthusiasm for concomitant chemoradiation therapy for patients with advanced cancers of the hypopharynx.

Transoral laser surgery for piriform sinus carcinoma Organ-sparing approaches such as transoral laser microsurgery for piriform sinus carcinomas have been used in several institutions for the past 25 years. Long-term follow-up in a retrospective review of 129 previously untreated patients has been published (Steiner et al). In this series, which included mostly advanced-stage disease, the reported 5-year local control rate was 82% for patients with stages I and II cancers and 69% for those with stages III and IV cancers. Radiation therapy was administered after surgery. Laryngeal preservation rates were comparable to the local tumor control rates. The 2-year overall survival rates were 91% for patients with stages I and II cancer and 75% for patients with stages III and IV cancer. These oncologic and functional results compare favorably with those obtained with either nonsurgical or surgical approaches requiring opening the neck and pharynx.

LARYNX

Laryngeal cancers constitute approximately 1.2% of all new cancer diagnoses in the United States. Approximately 12,250 new cases are expected in the year 2008.

TABLE 4: TNM staging system for cancers of the larynx

Primary tumor (T)

Tx	Primary tumor cannot be assessed
T0	No evidence of primary tumor
Tis	Carcinoma in situ

Glottis

T1	Tumor limited to the vocal cord(s) (may involve anterior or posterior commissure) with normal mobility
T1a	Tumor limited to one vocal cord
T1b	Tumor involves both vocal cords
T2	Tumor extends to the supraglottis and/or subglottis or with impaired vocal cord mobility
T3	Tumor limited to the larynx with vocal cord fixation
T4a	Tumor invades through the thyroid cartilage and/or invades tissues beyond the larynx (eg, trachea, soft tissues of the neck, including deep extrinsic muscle of the tongue, strap muscles, thyroid, or esophagus [resectable])
T4b	Tumor invades prevertebral space, encases carotid artery, or invades mediastinal structures (unresectable)

Supraglottis

T1	Tumor limited to one subsite of the supraglottis with normal vocal cord mobility
T2	Tumor invades mucosa of more than one adjacent subsite of the supraglottis or glottis or region outside the supraglottis (eg, mucosa of base of the tongue, vallecula, medial wall of piriform sinus) without fixation of the larynx
T3	Tumor limited to the larynx with vocal cord fixation and/or invades any of the postcricoid area or pre-epiglottic tissues
T4a	Tumor invades through the thyroid cartilage and/or invades tissues beyond the larynx (eg, trachea, soft tissues of neck [resectable], including deep extrinsic muscle of the tongue, strap muscles, thyroid, or esophagus)
T4b	Tumor invades prevertebral space, encases carotid artery, or invades mediastinal structures (unresectable)

Subglottis

T1	Tumor limited to the subglottis
T2	Tumor extends to vocal cord(s) with normal or impaired mobility
T3	Tumor limited to the larynx with vocal cord fixation
T4a	Tumor invades cricoid or thyroid cartilage and/or invades tissues beyond the larynx (eg, trachea, soft tissues of the neck, including deep extrinsic muscles of the tongue, strap muscles, thyroid, or esophagus [resectable])
T4b	Tumor invades prevertebral space, encases carotid artery, or invades mediastinal structures (unresectable)

Anatomy and pathology

Laryngeal anatomy is complex and includes cartilages, membranes, and muscles. The three subsites of the larynx are the glottis, or true vocal cords; the

Regional lymph nodes (N)

Nx   Regional lymph nodes cannot be assessed

N0   No regional lymph node metastasis

NI   Metastasis in a single ipsilateral lymph node, 3 cm or less in greatest dimension

N2   Metastasis in a single ipsilateral lymph node, more than 3 cm but not more than 6 cm in greatest dimension; or in multiple ipsilateral lymph nodes, none more than 6 cm in greatest dimension; or in bilateral or contralateral lymph nodes, none more than 6 cm in greatest dimension

    N2a   Metastasis in a single ipsilateral lymph node, more than 3 cm but not more than 6 cm in greatest dimension

    N2b   Metastasis in multiple ipsilateral lymph nodes, none more than 6 cm in greatest dimension

    N2c   Metastasis in bilateral or contralateral lymph nodes, none more than 6 cm in greatest dimension

N3   Metastasis in a lymph node(s), more than 6 cm in greatest dimension

Distant metastases (M)

Mx   Distant metastasis cannot be assessed

M0   No distant metastasis

MI   Distant metastasis

Stage grouping

Stage	T	N	M
Stage 0	Tis	N0	M0
Stage I	TI	N0	M0
Stage II	T2	N0	M0
Stage III	T3	N0	M0
	TI	NI	M0
	T2	NI	M0
	T3	NI	M0
Stage IVA	T4a	N0	M0
	T4a	NI	M0
	TI	N2	M0
	T2	N2	M0
	T3	N2	M0
	T4a	N2	M0
Stage IVB	T4b	Any N	M0
	Any T	N3	M0
Stage IVC	Any T	Any N	MI

From Greene FL, Page DL, Fleming ID, et al (eds): AJCC Cancer Staging Manual, 6th ed. New York, Springer-Verlag, 2002.

supraglottis, which includes the false cords, epiglottis, and aryepiglottic folds; and the subglottis, which is the region below the glottis and within the cricoid cartilage. The TNM staging system for cancers of the larynx is outlined in Table 4.

Treatment

Surgery Surgical treatment for laryngeal cancer includes transoral or open approaches. Treatment is dictated by the site and extent of the lesion. All or part of the larynx may need to be removed to achieve surgical control of laryngeal cancer. Decision-making for partial laryngectomy is complex and depends on the patient's overall health, the extent of local disease, the skill of the surgeon, and patient preference.

External-beam radiation therapy and chemoradiation therapy With improvements in techniques and fractionation schedules, external-beam radiation therapy, which allows for laryngeal preservation, is an option for all but the most advanced tumors.

Results As in other head and neck sites, patients with early laryngeal cancer may be treated with surgery or radiation therapy, and those with advanced-stage disease require multimodal therapy, including surgery and postoperative radiation therapy or chemotherapy and radiation therapy. For T1 and T2 tumors of the glottic or supraglottic larynx, radiation therapy is associated with local tumor control rates of 75% to 95%. Open partial laryngectomy for early laryngeal cancer is associated with local tumor control rates of 84% to 98% but requires a temporary tracheotomy and may be associated with postoperative vocal and swallowing dysfunction. Transoral laser surgery for early laryngeal cancer has yielded local tumor control rates of 82% to 100%, without significant dysphagia or a need for a temporary tracheotomy. However, transoral laser surgery requires technical expertise limited to a small number of institutions.

Select patients with T3 or T4 laryngeal cancers may be candidates for larynx preservation surgery, but most require total laryngectomy as the surgical option. The VA Cooperative Laryngeal Cancer Study was the first trial to test the efficacy of chemotherapy and radiation therapy in the management of stages III and IV laryngeal cancer, assess the possibility for laryngeal preservation using such a regimen, and compared its efficacy against the historic standard of surgery and postoperative radiation therapy. The VA Cooperative Laryngeal Cancer Study randomized patients with resectable squamous cell carcinoma of the larynx to receive either total laryngectomy followed by radiation therapy or neoadjuvant therapy with cisplatin and 5-FU followed by radiation therapy for those achieving a good response to chemotherapy.

Approximately two-thirds of patients survived 2 years following the combination of either chemotherapy plus irradiation or resection plus irradiation. Of those patients initially treated with chemotherapy and irradiation, one-third required total laryngectomy because of a lack of response to treatment; the larynx was successfully preserved in two-thirds of these patients. In this study, the increased local recurrence rate in the chemoradiation therapy group was offset by the decreased incidence of distant metastases and second primary tumors, and the 2-year survival rate was comparable between the groups. Advanced T stage was a risk factor for local failure in this study. Salvage total laryngectomy was required for 56% of T4 laryngeal cancers, suggesting that patients with bulky primary tumors may not be optimal candidates for organ-preservation therapy.

Data from the RTOG 91-11 trial demonstrated an improvement in locoregional tumor control using concurrent chemoradiation therapy relative to induction chemotherapy followed by radiotherapy or radiotherapy alone. There was no primarily surgical or altered fractionated arm in this study. This three-armed study randomized 517 patients with stages III and IV laryngeal cancer to receive one of the following regimens: induction chemotherapy (with cisplatin/5-FU) followed by radiation therapy or concurrent chemoradiotherapy (with cisplatin given on days 1, 22, and 43) or radiation therapy alone. Locoregional tumor control for the three arms was 61%, 78%, and 56%, respectively. The larynx preservation rate was 75%, 88%, and 70%, respectively. Notably, patients with T4 laryngeal cancers comprised only 10% of patients in this study, compared with 25% in the original VA Cooperative Laryngeal Cancer Study, accounting for the improved local tumor control with surgery.

The cure rate for early cancers of the larynx approaches 80% or more. Half of patients with T3 cancer are cured, whereas more than two-thirds of patients with T4 cancer will die of the disease.

LARYNGEAL SITE: SUPRAGLOTTIS

Supraglottic tumors occur less frequently than tumors of the true vocal cords. The epiglottis is the most common location for supraglottic cancers.

Natural history

Tumors close to the glottis produce symptoms earlier than tumors at other subsites. In contrast, nearly 60% of patients with supraglottic tumors have T3 or T4 primary tumors at presentation.

The supraglottis has a rich lymphatic network. There is an associated high incidence of lymph node metastases in early-stage tumors (40% for T1 tumors). The incidence of metastases in patients with clinically N0 neck cancer is about 15%. The incidence of bilateral cervical lymph node involvement is about 10%, and this rate increases to 60% for anterior tumors. The neck is a frequent site of recurrence in patients with supraglottic malignancies.

Treatment

The primary tumor Appropriate cancers may be treated with partial laryngectomy. Supraglottic laryngectomy removes the upper portion of the thyroid cartilage and its contents, including the false vocal cords, as well as the epiglottis and aryepiglottic folds. This approach preserves speech and swallowing, but more extensive resections are not well tolerated by patients with impaired lung function who are not able to tolerate the inevitable postoperative aspiration. Supracricoid partial laryngectomy is suitable for supraglottic tumors that cross the ventricle to involve the glottis. Select T3 tumors with limited pre-epiglottic space involvement may be approached with this procedure. Patients must have sufficient pulmonary reserve to be able to tolerate the chronic aspiration associated with this procedure. The local tumor control rates of transoral laser supraglottic laryngectomy are between 75% and 100% for T1 and T2 lesions in recent series and are associated with less postoperative dysphagia than open approaches. Significant technical expertise is needed, and patients must have the proper habitus to assure adequate exposure. Supraglottic laryngectomy is seldom appropriate as salvage therapy following irradiation due to complications, including swelling, difficulty swallowing, and poor wound healing. The usual salvage operation for persistent supraglottic cancer following radiation therapy is total laryngectomy. Advanced disease requires multimodal therapy, as previously discussed.

More advanced disease requires combined-modality treatment and often requires total laryngectomy. Radiation therapy may be employed with curative intent, as may induction chemotherapy followed by irradiation, as described earlier.

The neck The high incidence of cervical metastases makes treatment of the neck a necessity. About one-third of cases of clinically negative neck cancer contain involved nodes, and the incidence of recurrence in untreated patients is high. For patients undergoing surgical treatment of T1–T2 primary tumors, bilateral selective neck dissection is advisable.

Preservation of the larynx Mature data from RTOG 91-11 have been published, confirming preliminary results. A total of 547 patients were randomly assigned to undergo one of three treatments: induction therapy with cisplatin plus 5-FU followed by radiotherapy, radiotherapy with concurrent administration of cisplatin, or radiotherapy alone. The rate of locoregional tumor control was significantly better with radiotherapy and concurrent cisplatin (78% vs 61% with induction cisplatin plus 5-FU followed by radiotherapy and 56% with radiotherapy alone). Both regimens with chemotherapy had lower rates of distant metastases and resulted in better disease-free survival than radiotherapy alone. Overall survival rates were similar in all three groups.

At 2 years, the proportion of patients in whom the larynx was preserved after irradiation and concurrent cisplatin (88%) differed significantly from the proportion in the groups given induction chemotherapy followed by irradiation (75%, $P = .005$) or irradiation alone (70%, $P < .001$). The authors concluded that the combination of irradiation and concurrent cisplatin was superior to induction chemotherapy followed by irradiation or irradiation alone for laryngeal preservation and locoregional tumor control.

LARYNGEAL SITE: GLOTTIS

The glottis is the most common location of laryngeal cancer in the United States, comprising more than half of all cases.

Natural history

The cure rate for tumors of the true vocal cords is high. These cancers produce symptoms early, and, thus, most are small when detected. Approximately 60% are T1 and 20% are T2. Normal cord mobility implies invasion of disease limited to the submucosa. Deeper tumor invasion results in impaired vocal cord motion; this finding is most common in the anterior two-thirds of the vocal cord.

The true vocal cords have very little lymphatic drainage. Cervical metastases are infrequent with T1 (1%) and T2 tumors (3% to 7%).

Treatment

The primary tumor Carcinoma in situ is highly curable and may be treated equally well with microexcision, laser vaporization, or radiation therapy. Treatment decisions should be based on the extent of local disease. Serial recurrences should heighten suspicion of an invasive component, and a more aggressive approach, such as partial or total laryngectomy or irradiation, should be employed. Hypofractionated (> 2 Gy/d) radiotherapy is preferred to conventional fractionation (1.8–2 Gy). Local tumor control for T1 using surgery or irradiation is comparable, usually greater than 90%. Local tumor control for T2 glottic lesions is reported between 70% and 85% with radiotherapy and 85% and 95% with open partial laryngectomy. Partial laryngectomy can be performed in selected patients after irradiation failure of some T1–T2 glottic cancers.

Advanced T4 disease is best treated with total laryngectomy. Most T3 lesions are now being treated with concomitant chemoradiotherapy, with salvage laryngectomy required in ~20% of patients for residual/recurrent disease or laryngeal dysfunction.

The neck Due to the sparse lymphatic network and low incidence of cervical metastases, elective neck dissection is indicated only for transglottic lesions.

Results Cure rates by tumor size alone follow: T1, 90%; T2, 80%; T3, 50%; and T4, 40%. Neck involvement worsens the prognosis dramatically.

LARYNGEAL SITE: SUBGLOTTIS

Subglottic cancer is unusual, accounting for fewer than 10% of all laryngeal cancers.

Natural history

These cancers tend to be poorly differentiated, and, as the region is clinically "silent," most present as advanced lesions (~70% are T3–T4). The subglottis also has rich lymphatic drainage, and the incidence of cervical metastases is 20% to 30%.

Treatment

Partial laryngectomy is not practical for the treatment of tumors in the subglottis, and, thus, therapy usually includes total laryngectomy plus neck dissection. Combination therapy (surgery plus radiation therapy [60–65 Gy in 6–7 weeks]) is recommended for more advanced disease.

Results The cure rate for the uncommon T1 and T2 tumors is ~70%. Most failures occur in the neck. The cure rate for more advanced lesions is ~40%.

UNKNOWN HEAD AND NECK PRIMARY SITE

The cervical lymph nodes are the most common metastatic site at which squamous cell carcinoma is found.

Natural history

Most patients who present with squamous cell carcinoma involving cervical lymph nodes, especially in the upper or middle portion of the cervical chain, will have a primary site within the head and neck. When the lower cervical or supraclavicular lymph nodes are involved, a primary lung cancer should be suspected.

In the overwhelming majority of these cases, the primary lesion will be discovered based on history, physical examination, proper radiographic evaluation (CT and/or MRI), and examination with the patient under anesthesia with endoscopy (direct laryngoscopy and nasopharyngoscopy), targeted biopsies, and tonsillectomy. Esophagoscopy and bronchoscopy seldom yield a diagnosis in patients with upper cervical lymph node involvement. "Silent" primary tumors are most often discovered in the base of the tongue or within tonsillar crypts.

Treatment

A substantial percentage of patients achieve long-term disease-free survival after treatment of the involved side of the neck. Locoregional control and survival are diminished by multiple lymph nodes and the presence of extracapsular extension of disease in the involved neck.

Irradiation alone Patients with early-stage neck disease (N1 disease or small, mobile N2a disease) can often be treated with radiotherapy alone. Radiation therapy dosages and techniques should be similar to those used in patients with advanced primary head and neck cancer. The nasopharynx, and oropharynx, with or without the hypopharynx, should be included in the irradiated field.

Surgery alone When neck dissection is used at the initial treatment, a primary tumor in the head and neck subsequently becomes obvious in about 20% of patients when radiation therapy is not employed.

Irradiation alone or combined with surgery Combination therapy (surgery plus radiation therapy [60–65 Gy in 6–7 weeks]) is recommended for patients found at surgery to have multiple involved nodes or extracapsular extension or who have suspected residual microscopic disease in the neck without a clinically detectable tumor. Open nodal biopsy does not appear to compromise outcome as long as adequate radiotherapy is delivered subsequently.

In most modern series utilizing predominantly combination therapy, 5-year survival rates exceed 50%. The volume of tumor in the involved neck influences outcome, with N1 and N2 disease having a significantly higher cure rate than N3 disease or massive neck involvement. Regional relapse is usually predicted by extranodal disease.

Chemotherapy The role of chemotherapy in treating patients with an unknown primary metastatic squamous carcinoma in cervical lymph nodes remains undefined. The benefit of concurrent chemoradiation therapy of these patients is uncertain (because their primary sites are small or absent), and neck control after resection followed by irradiation, or after irradiation alone, is excellent in patients with cancers of an unknown primary site.

NASOPHARYNX

Nasopharyngeal carcinoma is uncommon in most of the world. Endemic areas include southern China, northern Africa, and regions of the far Northern Hemisphere. The incidence (per 1,000 population) ranges from 25.6 in men and 10.2 in women in Hong Kong to 0.6 in men and 0.1 in women in Connecticut.

Epidemiology and risk factors

Gender and age The incidence of nasopharyngeal cancer peaks in the fourth to fifth decades of life, and the male-female ratio is 2.2:1.0. Both patient age at disease onset and male-female ratio are lower for nasopharyngeal cancer than for other head and neck malignancies.

Risk factors Nasopharyngeal carcinoma (most notably WHO [World Health Organization] types 2 and 3 [see section on "Anatomy and pathology"]) appears to have different determinants than other head and neck cancers. They include diet, viral agents, and genetic susceptibility. Populations of endemic areas have a diet characterized by high consumption of salt-cured fish and meat. Studies reveal an association between EBV and nasopharyngeal carcinoma. Anti-EBV antibodies have been found in the sera and saliva of patients with this type of carcinoma. Major histocompatibility (MHC) profiles associated with an increased relative risk include H2, BW46, and B17 locus antigens.

TABLE 5: TNM staging system for cancers of the pharynx (including base of tongue, soft palate, and uvula)

Primary tumor (T)

Tx	Primary tumor cannot be assessed
T0	No evidence of primary tumor
Tis	Carcinoma in situ

Nasopharynx

T1	Tumor confined to the nasopharynx
T2	Tumor extends to the soft tissue of the oropharynx and/or nasal fossa
T2a	Without parapharyngeal extension[a]
T2b	With parapharyngeal extension[a]
T3	Tumor invades bony structures and/or paranasal sinuses
T4	Tumor with intracranial extension and/or involvement of cranial nerves, infratemporal fossa, hypopharynx, or orbit

Oropharynx

T1	Tumor 2 cm or less in greatest dimension
T2	Tumor more than 2 cm but not more than 4 cm in greatest dimension
T3	Tumor more than 4 cm in greatest dimension
T4a	Tumor invades the larynx, deep/extrinsic muscle of the tongue, medial pterygoid, hard palate, or mandible (resectable)
T4b	Tumor invades lateral pterygoid muscle, pterygoid plates, lateral nasopharynx, or skull base or encases carotid artery (unresectable)

Hypopharynx

T1	Tumor limited to one subsite of the hypopharynx and 2 cm or less in greatest dimension
T2	Tumor involves more than one subsite of the hypopharynx or an adjacent site or measures more than 2 cm but not more than 4 cm in greatest dimension without fixation of the hemilarynx
T3	Tumor measures more than 4 cm in greatest dimension or with fixation of the hemilarynx
T4a	Tumor invades thyroid/cricoid cartilage, hyoid bone, thyroid gland, esophagus, or central compartment soft tissue[b] (resectable)
T4b	Tumor invades prevertebral fascia, encases carotid artery, or involves mediastinal structures (unresectable)

Anatomy and pathology

The nasopharynx communicates anteriorly with the nasal cavity and inferiorly with the oropharynx. The superior border is the base of the skull. The lateral and posterior pharyngeal walls are composed of muscular constrictors. Posteriorly, the nasopharynx overlies the first and second cervical vertebrae. The eustachian tubes open into the lateral walls. The soft palate divides the nasopharynx from the oropharynx.

Cancers arising in the nasopharynx are classified using WHO criteria: type 1

Regional lymph nodes (N): Nasopharynx

Nx   Regional lymph nodes cannot be assessed
N0   No regional lymph node metastasis
N1   Unilateral metastasis in lymph node(s), 6 cm or less in greatest dimension, above the supraclavicular fossa[c]
N2   Bilateral metastasis in lymph node(s), 6 cm or less in greatest dimension, above the supraclavicular fossa[c]
N3   Metastasis in a lymph node(s) > 6 cm and/or to the supraclavicular fossa
  N3a   Greater than 6 cm in dimension
  N3b   Extension to the supraclavicular fossa[c]

Regional lymph nodes (N): Oropharynx and hypopharynx

Nx   Regional lymph nodes cannot be assessed
N0   No regional lymph node metastasis
N1   Metastasis in a single ipsilateral lymph node, 3 cm or less in greatest dimension
N2   Metastasis in a single ipsilateral lymph node, more than 3 cm but not more than 6 cm in greatest dimension; or in multiple ipsilateral lymph nodes, none more than 6 cm in greatest dimension; or in bilateral or contralateral lymph nodes, none more than 6 cm in greatest dimension
  N2a   Metastasis in a single ipsilateral lymph node, more than 3 cm but not more than 6 cm in greatest dimension
  N2b   Metastasis in multiple ipsilateral lymph nodes, none more than 6 cm in greatest dimension
  N2c   Metastasis in bilateral or contralateral lymph nodes, none more than 6 cm in greatest dimension
N3   Metastasis in a lymph node, more than 6 cm in greatest dimension

Distant metastases (M)

Mx   Distant metastasis cannot be assessed
M0   No distant metastasis
M1   Distant metastasis

[a] Parapharyngeal extension denotes posterolateral infiltration of tumor beyond the pharyngobasilar fascia.
[b] Central compartment soft tissue includes prelaryngeal strap muscles and subcutaneous fat.
[c] Midline nodes are considered ipsilateral nodes.

continued on following page

denotes differentiated squamous cell carcinoma; type 2, nonkeratinizing carcinoma; and type 3, undifferentiated carcinoma. The TNM staging system for cancers of the pharynx is outlined in Table 5.

Natural history

A mass in the neck is the presenting complaint in 90% of patients. Other presenting symptoms include a change in hearing, sensation of ear stuffiness, tinnitus, nasal obstruction, and pain.

TABLE 5: TNM staging system for cancers of the pharynx (including base of tongue, soft palate, and uvula) *(continued)*

Stage grouping: Nasopharynx

Stage 0	Tis	N0	M0
Stage I	T I	N0	M0
Stage IIA	T2a	N0	M0
Stage IIB	T I	N I	M0
	T2	N I	M0
	T2a	N I	M0
	T2b	N0	M0
	T2b	N I	M0
Stage III	T I	N2	M0
	T2a	N2	M0
	T2b	N2	M0
	T3	N0	M0
	T3	N I	M0
	T3	N2	M0
Stage IVA	T4	N0	M0
	T4	N I	M0
	T4	N2	M0
Stage IVB	Any T	N3	M0
Stage IVC	Any T	Any N	M I

Stage grouping: Oropharynx and hypopharynx

Stage 0	Tis	N0	M0
Stage I	T I	N0	M0
Stage II	T2	N0	M0
Stage III	T3	N0	M0
	T I	N I	M0
	T2	N I	M0
	T3	N I	M0
Stage IVA	T4a	N0	M0
	T4a	N I	M0
	T I	N2	M0
	T2	N2	M0
	T3	N2	M0
	T4a	N2	M0
Stage IVB	T4b	Any N	M0
	Any T	N3	M0
Stage IVC	Any T	Any N	M I

From Greene FL, Page DL, Fleming ID, et al (eds): AJCC Cancer Staging Manual, 6th ed. New York, Springer-Verlag, 2002.

Cranial nerve involvement Invasion of disease into the base of the skull is seen in ~25% of cases and may lead to cranial nerve involvement. CN VI is the first cranial nerve to be affected, followed by CN III and CN IV. Deficits are manifested by changes in ocular motion. Involvement of CN V may also occur; this is manifested by pain or paresthesia high in the neck or face.

Level V metastases Unlike malignancies of the oral cavity and oropharynx, nasopharyngeal cancers often metastasize to level V lymph nodes. Bilateral metastases are common.

CANCER MANAGEMENT: A MULTIDISCIPLINARY APPROACH

Treatment

Treatment of nasopharyngeal cancer usually involves radiation therapy (65–70 Gy) for the primary tumor and draining lymph nodes. Overall survival is 50% at 5 years. Surgical resection has high morbidity and is seldom entertained.

Nasopharyngeal cancer is distinguished from other sites of head and neck cancer by its radiosensitivity and chemosensitivity. Although advanced nodal disease can be controlled by irradiation alone in ~50% of patients, eventual distant metastasis remains a problem.

The final report of the intergroup trial 0099 confirmed that for patients with locally advanced nasopharyngeal cancer, concurrent cisplatin chemotherapy with radiation therapy (followed by systemic chemotherapy) provided a clear survival benefit compared with treatment with irradiation alone. At 5 years, patients who received combined-modality therapy had an overall survival rate of 67%, compared with 37% with radiation therapy alone ($P = .001$). Disease-free survival at 5 years was 74% for the chemoradiation therapy arm versus 46% for the radiation therapy-alone arm.

RECURRENT HEAD AND NECK CANCER

As mentioned previously, surveillance after treatment of head and neck cancer is mandatory, as early detection of second primary cancers or locoregional recurrence affords the best chance for disease control. Nearly two-thirds of patients whose head and neck cancer recurs develop a tumor at (or near) the primary site or in the neck nodes. Eighty percent of head and neck cancer recurrences eventuate within 2 years. Development of a recurrent tumor in the neck is the single most common type of treatment failure in patients with squamous cell carcinoma of the upper aerodigestive tract.

Differentiating recurrence from late complications of irradiation Differentiating between recurrent carcinoma and significant sequelae of radiotherapy is a difficult clinical problem at all sites within the head and neck. Any suspicious mucosal changes, enlarged nodes in the neck, or discrete subcutaneous nodules warrant prompt biopsy.

Candidates for surgery Different choices of first treatment (ie, surgery or radiation therapy) and the intensity of follow-up influence success in treating recurrence. Aggressive surgical intervention should be offered to two groups of patients with recurrent local or regional disease: those whose therapy is chosen with curative intent and those who have the prospect for significant palliation.

The types of recurrence that may be approached surgically with the greatest likelihood of success include (1) metastases in the neck after initial treatment limited to the primary tumor alone and (2) reappearance or persistence of cancer at a site previously treated with radiotherapy alone. Salvage resection may also be considered in other situations, however. They include the appearance of cancer in the neck after prior irradiation or neck dissection, at the margins after previous resection, and even at the base of the skull.

Although surgery is the standard of care for the treatment of recurrent disease, there is a growing body of evidence suggesting that reirradiation with concurrent chemotherapy can cure selected patients when resection is not possible. Several institutions have reported experiences retreating patients, and these results led to the development of the first multi-institution reirradiation study.

A single-arm, phase II study (RTOG 96-10) evaluated toxicity and therapeutic results for patients with recurrent squamous cell carcinoma of the head and neck. Eighty-six patients received four weekly courses of 1.5-Gy fractions twice daily with concurrent 5-FU and hydroxyurea. Each cycle was separated by 1 week of rest. The median survival was 8.1 months and the 1- and 2-year survival rates were 41.7% and 16.2%, respectively. Compared with patients who experienced early recurrences, patients whose disease recurred 3 years after the original irradiation fared better, with 1- and 2-year survival rates of 48.1% and 32.1%, respectively.

The first results for the entire cohort of patients for RTOG 99-11, the successor trial to RTOG 96-10, were presented in 2005. In this study, patients previously irradiated, with locally recurrent or second primary head and neck tumors, were treated with split-course hyperfractionated radiotherapy (60 Gy total; 1.5 Gy/fraction twice daily for 5 days every 2 weeks for 4 cycles), in combination with cisplatin (15 mg/m^2 IV daily) x 5 and paclitaxel (20 mg/m^2 IV daily x 5) every 2 weeks for 4 cycles. Granulocyte colony-stimulating factor (G-CSF) support was administered on days 6 through 13 of each 2-week cycle. Of the 105 patients enrolled, 99 were eligible for analysis, and 23% of the patients had second primary head and neck tumors. The median prior dose of radiotherapy was 65.4 Gy (range 45–75 Gy), and the median time from prior radiotherapy was 40 months.

Of eight patients with grade 5 (fatal) toxicities, five occurred during the acute period (dehydration, pneumonitis, neutropenia [2 cases], and cerebrovascular accident) and three during the late period (two of three attributable to carotid hemorrhage). Other acute toxicities included leukopenia (30% grade 3/4), anemia (21% grade 3/4), and gastrointestinal toxicity (48% grade 3/4). The median follow-up for patients was 23.6 months, and the median survival was 12.1 months.

The estimated 1- and 2-year overall survival rates were 50.2% and 25.9%, respectively. The median and 1-year progression-free survival rates were 7.8 months and 35%, respectively. Overall survival was significantly better ($P = .044$) than for the historic control in RTOG 96-10 (estimated 1- and 2-year overall survival rates 41.7% and 16.7%, respectively).

Despite significant toxicity and high mortality, hyperfractionated split-course reirradiation with concurrent cisplatin and paclitaxel chemotherapy proved feasible in this select patient population. This approach was to be tested in an RTOG 04-21, a phase III trial, which randomizes patients between this arm and chemotherapy alone, although it was closed due to a lack of accrual in early 2007.

Unless a patient cannot tolerate an operation, resection of discrete local or regional recurrent tumors should be entertained as the first course of treatment. Management of recurrences involves complex decision-making and requires familiarity with multidisciplinary care.

SUGGESTED READING

Adelstein DJ, Li Y, Adams GL, et al: An Intergroup phase III comparison of standard radiation therapy and two schedules of concurrent chemoradiotherapy in patients with unresectable squamous cell head and neck cancer. J Clin Oncol 21:92–98, 2003.

Ang KK, Harris J, Garden AS, et al: Concomitant boost radiation and concurrent cisplatin for advanced head and neck carcinomas: Radiation Therapy Oncology Group Phase II Trial 99-14. J Clin Oncol 23:3008–3015, 2005.

Bensadoun RJ, Benezery K, Dassonville O, et al: French multicenter phase III randomized study testing concurrent twice-a-day radiotherapy and cisplatin/5-fluorouracil chemotherapy (BiRCF) in unresectable pharyngeal carcinoma: Results at 2 years (FNCLCC-GORTEC). Int J Radiat Oncol Biol Phys 64:983–994, 2006.

Bernier J, Cooper JS Pajak TF, et al: Defining risk levels in locally advanced head and neck cancers: A comparative analysis of concurrent postoperative radiation plus chemotherapy trials of the EORTC (#22931) and RTOG (#9501). Head Neck 27:843–850, 2005.

Bernier J, Domenge C, Ozsahin M, et al: Postoperative irradiation with or without concomitant chemotherapy for locally advanced head and neck cancer. N Engl J Med 350:1945–1952, 2004.

Bonner JA, Harari PM, Giralt J, et al: Radiotherapy plus cetuximab for squamous-cell carcinoma of the head and neck. N Engl J Med 354:567–578, 2006.

Bourhis J, Lapeyre M, Tortochaux J, et al: Phase III randomized trial of very accelerated radiation therapy compared with conventional radiation therapy in squamous cell head and neck cancer: A GORTEC trial. J Clin Oncol 24:2873–2878, 2006.

Cooper JS, Pajak TF, Forastiere AA, et al: Postoperative concurrent radiotherapy and chemotherapy for high-risk squamous-cell carcinoma of the head and neck. N Engl J Med 350:1937–1944, 2004.

Curran D, Giralt J, Harari PM, et al: Quality of life in head and neck cancer patients after treatment with high-dose radiotherapy alone or in combination with cetuximab. J Clin Oncol 25:2191–2197, 2007.

D'Souza G, Kreimer AR, Viscidi R, et al: Case-control study of human papillomavirus and oropharyngeal cancer. N Engl J Med 356:1944–1956, 2007.

Forastiere AA, Goepfert H, Maor M, et al: Concurrent chemotherapy and radiotherapy for organ preservation in advanced laryngeal cancer. N Engl J Med 349:2091–2098, 2003.

Garden AS, Asper JA, Morrison WH, et al: Is concurrent chemoradiation the treatment of choice for all patients with stage III or IV head and neck carcinoma? Cancer 100:1171–1178, 2004.

Hitt R, Lopez-Pousa A, Martinez-Trufero J, et al: Phase III study comparing cisplatin plus fluorouracil to paclitaxel, cisplatin, and fluorouracil induction chemotherapy followed by chemoradiotherapy in locally advanced head and neck cancer. J Clin Oncol 23:8636–8645, 2005.

Hockstein NG, Nolan NP, O'Malley BW Jr, et al: Robot-assisted pharyngeal and laryngeal microsurgery: Results of robotic cadaver dissections. Laryngoscope 115:1003–1008, 2005.

Horwitz EM, Harris J, Langer CJ, et al: Combination with split course concomitant hyperfractionated re-irradiation in patients with recurrent squamous cell cancer of the head and neck: Results of RTOG 99-11. Int J Radiat Oncol Biol Phys 63(suppl 1):S72–S73, 2005.

Jun H, Ahn M, Kim H, et al: Clinical significance of ERCC1 expression in advanced squamous cell carcinoma of the head and neck treated with cisplatin-based concurrent chemoradiation. J Clin Oncol 25(18S):6061, 2007.

Lobe TE, Wright SK, Irish MS: Novel uses of surgical robotics in head and neck surgery. J Laparoendosc Adv Surg Tech A 15:647–652, 2005.

Mountzios G, Handra-Luca A, Hernandez J, et al: ERCC1 immunohistochemical expression and cancer-specific survival in patients with locally advanced squamous-cell carcinoma of the head and neck treated by cisplatin-based induction chemotherapy. J Clin Oncol 25(18S):6011, 2007.

O'Malley BW Jr, Weinstein GS, Snyder W, et al: Transoral robotic surgery (TORS) for base of tongue neoplasms. Laryngoscope 116:1465–1472, 2006.

Pignon JP, le Maitre A, Bourhis J: Meta-analyses of chemotherapy in head and neck cancer (MACH-NC): An update. Int J Radiat Oncol Biol Phys 69:S112–S114, 2007.

Posner MR, Hershock DM, Blajman CR, et al: Cisplatin and fluorouracil alone or with docetaxel in head and neck cancer. N Engl J Med 357:1705–1715, 2007.

Pradier O, Christiansen H, Schmidberger H, et al: Adjuvant radiotherapy after transoral laser microsurgery for advanced squamous carcinoma of the head and neck. Int J Radiat Oncol Biol Phys 63:1368–1377, 2005.

Terris DJ, Haus BM, Gourin CG, et al: Endo-robotic resection of the submandibular gland in a cadaver model. Head Neck 27:946–951, 2005.

Trotti A, Fu KK, Pajak TF, et al: Long-term outcomes of RTOG 90-03: A comparison of hyperfractionation and two variants of acclerated fractionation to standard fractionation radiotherapy for head and neck squamous carcinoma. Int J Radiat Oncol Biol Phys 63:S70–S71, 2005.

Urba S, Wolf G, Eisbruch A, et al: Single-cycle induction chemotherapy selects patients with advanced laryngeal cancer for combined chemoradiation: A new treatment paradigm. J Clin Oncol 24:593–598, 2006.

Vermorken J, Mesia R, Vega V, et al: Cetuximab extends survival of patients with recurrent or metastatic SCCHN when added to first line platinum based therapy: Results of a randomized phase III (EXTREME) study. J Clin Oncol 25(18S):6091, 2007.

Yom SA, Machtay M, Biel MA, et al: Survival impact of planned restaging and early surgical salvage following definitive chemoradiation for locally advanced squamous cell carcinomas of the oropharynx and hypopharynx. Am J Clin Oncol 28:385–392, 2005.

Zeitels SM, Franco RA Jr, Dailey SH, et al: Office-based treatment of glottal dysplasia and papillomatosis with the 585-nm pulsed dye laser and local anesthesia. Ann Otol Rhinol Laryngol 113:265–276, 2004.

CHAPTER 5

Thyroid and parathyroid cancers

Mimi I. Hu, MD, Rena Vassilopoulou-Sellin, MD, Robert Lustig, MD, and Jeffrey P. Lamont, MD

Endocrine malignancies, although relatively uncommon, are often difficult to diagnose and treat effectively. According to American Cancer Society (ACS) estimates, more than 35,000 new cases of endocrine neoplasms were diagnosed in the United States in 2007, and approximately 2,320 deaths resulted from these cancers. This chapter will focus on thyroid and parathyroid cancers. (A discussion of carcinoid tumors, insulinomas, gastrinomas, and other gastrointestinal neuroendocrine tumors, as well as adrenocortical cancer, can be found in chapter 14.)

THYROID CANCER

Thyroid cancer is the most common endocrine cancer. The number of deaths from thyroid cancer estimated for the year 2007 was 1,530, or 4.6% of all new thyroid cancer cases.

The prevalence rate for occult thyroid cancers found at autopsy is 5% to 10%, except in Japan and Hawaii, where the rate can be as high as 28%. Autopsy rates do not correlate with clinical incidence.

The prevalence of thyroid nodules in the general population is 4% to 7%, with nodules being more common in females than males. The prevalence of thyroid cancer in a solitary nodule or in multinodular thyroid glands is 10% to 20%; this increases with irradiation of the neck in children and older men (see section on "Etiology and risk factors").

Tumor types

Thyroid cancer is classified into four main types according to its morphology and biologic behavior: papillary, follicular, medullary, and anaplastic. Differentiated (papillary and follicular) thyroid cancers account for > 90% of thyroid malignancies and constitute approximately 0.8% of all human malignancies. Medullary thyroid cancers represent 3% to 5% of all thyroid neoplasms. About 75% of patients with medullary cancer have a sporadic form of the disease, whereas the remaining 25% have inherited disease. Anaplastic carcinoma represents < 3% of all thyroid carcinomas.

Papillary thyroid carcinoma is the most common subtype and has an excellent prognosis. Most papillary carcinomas contain varying amounts of follicular tissue. When the predominant histology is papillary, the tumor is considered to be a papillary carcinoma. Because the mixed papillary-follicular variant tends to behave like a pure papillary cancer, it is treated in the same manner and has a similar prognosis.

Papillary tumors arise from thyroid follicular cells, are unilateral in most cases, and are often multifocal within a single thyroid lobe. They vary in size from microscopic to large cancers that may invade the thyroid capsule and infiltrate into contiguous structures. Papillary tumors tend to invade the lymphatics, but vascular invasion (and hematogenous spread) is uncommon.

Up to 40% of adults with papillary thyroid cancer may present with regional lymph node metastases, usually ipsilateral. Distant metastases occur, in decreasing order of frequency, in the lungs, bones, and other soft tissues. Older patients have a higher risk for locally invasive tumors and for distant metastases. Children may present with a solitary thyroid nodule, but cervical node involvement is more common in this age group; up to 10% of children and adolescents may have lung involvement at the time of diagnosis.

Follicular thyroid carcinoma is less common than papillary thyroid cancer, occurs in older age groups, and has a slightly worse prognosis. Follicular thyroid cancer can metastasize to the lungs and bones, often retaining the ability to accumulate radioactive iodine (which can be used for therapy). Metastases may be appreciated many years after the initial diagnosis.

Follicular tumors, although frequently encapsulated, commonly exhibit microscopic vascular and capsular invasion. Microscopically, the nuclei tend to be large and have atypical mitotic figures. There is usually no lymph node involvement.

Follicular carcinoma can be difficult to distinguish from its benign counterpart, follicular adenoma. This distinction is based on the presence or absence of capsular or vascular invasion, which can be evaluated after surgical excision but not by fine-needle aspiration (FNA).

Thyroglobulin, normally synthesized in the follicular epithelium of the thyroid, is present in well-differentiated papillary and follicular carcinomas and infrequently in anaplastic carcinomas but not in medullary carcinomas. Therefore, thyroglobulin immunoreactivity is considered to be indicative of a follicular epithelial origin.

Hürthle cell carcinoma Hürthle cell, or oxyphil cell, carcinoma is a variant of follicular carcinoma. Hürthle cell carcinoma is composed of sheets of Hürthle cells and has the same criteria for malignancy as does follicular carcinoma. Hürthle cell carcinoma is thought to have a worse outcome than follicular carcinoma and is less apt to concentrate radioactive iodine.

Medullary thyroid carcinoma originates from the C cells (parafollicular cells) of the thyroid and secretes calcitonin. Secretory diarrhea and flushing, related to calcitonin secretion, can be clinical features of advanced medullary

THYROID

thyroid carcinoma. On gross examination, most tumors are firm, grayish, and gritty.

Sporadic medullary thyroid carcinoma usually presents as a solitary thyroid mass; metastases to cervical and mediastinal lymph nodes are found in half of patients and may be present at the time of initial presentation. Distant metastases to the lungs, liver, bones, and adrenal glands most commonly occur late in the course of the disease.

Hereditary medullary thyroid carcinoma presents as a bilateral, multifocal process. Histologically, hereditary medullary carcinoma of the thyroid does not differ from the sporadic form. However, the hereditary form is frequently multifocal, and it is common to find areas of C-cell hyperplasia in areas distant from the primary carcinoma. Another characteristic feature of hereditary medullary carcinoma is the presence of amyloid deposits.

Genetic factors There are three hereditary forms: familial medullary thyroid carcinoma; multiple endocrine neoplasia type 2A (MEN-2A), characterized by medullary thyroid cancer, pheochromocytomas, and hyperparathyroidism; and multiple endocrine neoplasia type 2B (MEN-2B), characterized by medullary thyroid cancer, marfanoid habitus, pheochromocytomas, and neuromas. These syndromes are associated with germ-line mutations of the *RET* proto-oncogene, which codes for a receptor tyrosine kinase (RTK). Hereditary medullary thyroid carcinoma is inherited as an autosomal-dominant trait with high penetrance and variable expression. In addition, approximately 40% of sporadic medullary thyroid carcinomas contain somatic *RET* mutations, which may represent potential therapeutic targets. (For a discussion of genetic testing to screen for *RET* mutations in MEN kindreds, see section on "Diagnostic work-up.")

Anaplastic carcinoma Anaplastic tumors are high-grade neoplasms characterized histologically by a high mitotic rate and lymphovascular invasion. Aggressive invasion of local structures is common, as are lymph node metastases. Distant metastases tend to occur in patients who do not succumb early to regional disease. Occasional cases of anaplastic carcinoma have been shown to arise from preexisting differentiated thyroid carcinoma or in a preexisting goiter.

Other tumor types Lymphomas of the thyroid account for < 5% of primary thyroid carcinomas. Other tumor types, such as teratomas, squamous cell carcinomas, and sarcomas, may also rarely cause primary thyroid cancers.

Epidemiology

Age and gender Most patients are between the ages of 25 and 65 years at the time of diagnosis of thyroid carcinoma. Women are affected more often than men (2:1 ratio for the development of both naturally occurring and radiation-induced thyroid cancer).

Etiology and risk factors

Differentiated thyroid cancer

Therapeutic irradiation External low-dose radiation therapy to the head and neck during infancy and childhood, frequently used between the 1940s and 1960s for the treatment of a variety of benign diseases, has been shown to predispose an individual to thyroid cancer. The younger a patient is at the time of radiation exposure, the higher is the subsequent risk of developing thyroid carcinoma. Also, as mentioned previously, women are at increased risk of radiation-induced thyroid cancer. There is a latency period ranging from 10 to 30 years from the time of low-dose irradiation to the development of thyroid cancer.

As little as 11 cGy and as much as 2,000 cGy of external radiation to the head and neck have been associated with a number of benign and malignant diseases. It was once thought that high-dose irradiation (> 2,000 cGy) to the head and neck did not increase the risk of neoplasia. However, it has been shown that patients treated with mantle-field irradiation for Hodgkin lymphoma are at increased risk of developing thyroid carcinoma compared with the general population, although they are more likely to develop hypothyroidism than thyroid cancer.

Radiation-associated thyroid cancer has an identical natural history and prognosis as sporadic thyroid cancer.

Other factors Besides radiation-induced thyroid cancer, there are only sparse data on the etiology of differentiated thyroid cancer. There has been intensive research on distinguishing molecular factors important for cell differentiation, growth, and motility. Considerable attention has focused on BRAF, a member of the RAF family of serine/threonine kinases that mediates cellular responses to growth-promoting signals via the RAS-RAF-MEK-MAPK signaling pathway. BRAF mutations so far have only been documented in papillary thyroid carcinoma (45%) and papillary thyroid carcinoma-derived anaplastic thyroid carcinoma (25%). Over the past few years, BRAF mutations have been implicated as potential prognostic factors and therapeutic targets.

Signs and symptoms

Most thyroid cancers present as asymptomatic thyroid nodules. Patients may feel pressure symptoms from nodules as they begin to increase in size. A change in the voice can be caused by a thyroid cancer or benign goiter. The voice change usually occurs when there is compression of the larynx or invasion of the recurrent laryngeal nerve.

On physical examination, a thyroid nodule that is hard or firm and fixed may represent a cancer. The presence of palpable enlarged nodes in the lateral neck, even in the absence of a palpable nodule in the thyroid gland, could represent metastases to the lymph nodes.

Diagnostic work-up

As mentioned previously, thyroid nodules are present in 4% to 7% of the general population and in a higher percentage of individuals who have had irradiation to the head and neck region. Most thyroid nodules are benign (colloid nodules or adenomas); therefore, it is important for the work-up to lead to surgical resection for malignant nodules and to avoid unnecessary surgery for benign lesions. Although most solid nodules are benign, thyroid carcinomas usually present as solid nodules. A cystic nodule or a "mixed" (cystic-solid) lesion is less likely to represent a carcinoma and more likely to be a degenerated colloid nodule.

> A multigene real-time polymerase chain reaction assay of six novel candidate markers (ECM1, TMPRSS4, ANGPT2, TIMP1, EFNB2, EGFR) was applied to 31 thyroid fine-needle aspiration and 95 frozen thyroid tumor samples to determine whether malignant tumors can be distinguished from benign specimens. The mRNA expression of four of the markers was found to be up-regulated in malignant tumors; each was an independent marker of malignancy. This assay may be a useful diagnostic test, especially in regard to indeterminate biopsy results (Kebebew E, Peng M, Reiff E, et al: Cancer 106:2592-2597, 2006).

History The history is very important in the evaluation of thyroid nodules. If there is a history of irradiation to the head and neck, the risk of there being cancer in the nodule is higher (as great as 50%) than in nonirradiated patients (10%–20% risk).

Age also is important in the evaluation of thyroid nodules. Nodules that occur in either the very young or the very old are more likely to be cancerous, particularly in men.

A new nodule or a nodule that suddenly begins to grow is worrisome as well.

FNA has become the initial diagnostic test for the evaluation of thyroid nodules. FNA can determine whether the lesion is cystic or solid. For solid lesions, cytology can yield one of three results: benign, malignant, or indeterminate. The accuracy of cytologic diagnosis from FNA is 70% to 80%, depending on the experience of the person performing the aspiration and the pathologist interpreting the cytologic specimen.

In a series of 98 "suspicious" FNAs, findings of cellular atypia (pleomorphism, enlarged nuclei, nuclear grooves, coarse or irregular chromatin, prominent or multiple nucleoli, or atypical or numerous mitotic figures) or follicular lesions with atypia were associated with malignancy 20% and 44% of the time, respectively. Follicular lesions without atypia have a 6.7% risk of malignancy. Core needle biopsy has been used as an alternative method for diagnosis. Some studies have shown the adequacy of sample may be greater with core biopsy than FNA. However, there are conflicting reports to whether a core biopsy offers greater accuracy in the diagnosis of a thyroid nodule. Thus, as outlined in the 2006 ATA guidelines, FNA biopsy remains the recommended procedure for evaluating thyroid nodules.

Imaging modalities Ultrasonographic and radionuclide (radioiodine and technetium) scans are also used in the evaluation of thyroid nodules.

Ultrasonography is now widely considered an essential tool in the assessment of thyroid nodules. The presence of certain features is associated with malignancy and can guide physicians in deciding which nodules should be biopsied. Although there is a decrease in cancer rate per nodule in patients with multiple nodules, the overall rate of thyroid cancer per patient is similar to that seen in patients with a solitary nodule.

Thyroid cancer is most often found in the dominant, or largest, nodule in multinodular glands; however, approximately one-third of the cases of cancer are found in nondominant nodules. Nodule size is a poor predictor for malignancy, as the likelihood of cancer has been shown to be the same regardless of nodule size.

A recent consensus statement from the Society of Radiologists in Ultrasound outlined various features of solitary nodules associated with thyroid cancer: microcalcifications, hypoechogenicity, irregular margins or no halo, solid composition, intranodule vascularity, and more tall than wide dimensions. No single feature has both high sensitivity and specificity; however, the combination of more than one factor can increase the likelihood of cancer. Other than characterization of thyroid nodules, ultrasonography can guide the FNA biopsy, which increases the diagnostic efficacy of the procedure. Additionally, ultrasonography can identify abnormal cervical lymph nodes, which should prompt a biopsy of the lymph node and possibly an ipsilateral thyroid nodule.

Thyroid isotope scans cannot differentiate absolutely a benign from a malignant nodule but can, based on the functional status of the nodule, assign a probability of malignancy. "Hot" thyroid nodules (ie, those that concentrate radioiodine) represent functioning nodules, whereas "cold" nodules are nonfunctioning lesions that do not concentrate the isotope. Most thyroid carcinomas occur in cold nodules, but only 10% of cold nodules are carcinomas. It is not necessary to operate on all cold thyroid nodules. CT or MRI scan of the neck may be appropriate in some cases.

Calcitonin level Medullary thyroid carcinomas usually secrete calcitonin, which is a specific product of the thyroid C cells (parafollicular cells). In patients who have clinically palpable medullary carcinoma, the basal calcitonin level is almost always elevated. In patients with smaller tumors or C-cell hyperplasia, the basal calcitonin level may be normal, but administration of synthetic gastrin (pentagastrin) or calcium results in marked elevation of calcitonin levels. The use of calcitonin levels as a tumor marker and stimulation screening in hereditary forms of medullary cancers has been largely replaced by genetic testing (see below).

Carcinoembryonic antigen (CEA) Serum CEA levels are elevated in patients with medullary thyroid cancer.

Ruling out pheochromocytoma Medullary thyroid carcinoma can be associated with MEN-2A, MEN-2B, or familial non-MEN. Both the MEN-2A and MEN-2B syndromes are characterized by medullary thyroid cancer and pheochromocytoma. Thus, in any patient with hereditary medullary thyroid carcinoma, it is imperative that the preoperative work-up include a determination

TABLE 1: AJCC/UICC staging of thyroid cancer

Primary tumor (T)

Tx	Primary tumor cannot be assessed
T0	No evidence of primary tumor
T1	Tumor ≤ 2 cm in greatest dimension, limited to the thyroid
T2	Tumor 2 cm to 4 cm in greatest dimension, limited to the thyroid
T3	Tumor > 4 cm in greatest dimension limited to the thyroid, or any tumor with minimal extrathyroid extension (eg, extension to sternothyroid muscle or perithyroid soft tissues)
T4a	Tumor of any size extending beyond the thyroid capsule to invade subcutaneous soft tissues, larynx, trachea, esophagus, or recurrent laryngeal nerve
T4b	Tumor invades prevertebral fascia or encases carotid artery or mediastinal vessels

Note: All categories may be subdivided: (a) solitary tumor, (b) multifocal tumor (the largest determines the classification).

Regional lymph nodes (N)

Nx	Regional lymph nodes cannot be assessed
N0	No regional lymph node metastasis
N1	Regional lymph node metastasis
N1a	Metastasis to level VI (pretracheal, paratracheal, and prelaryngeal/Delphian lymph nodes)
N1b	Metastasis to unilateral or bilateral cervical or mediastinal lymph node(s)

Distant metastasis (M)

Mx	Distant metastasis cannot be assessed
M0	No distant metastasis
M1	Distant metastasis

Stage grouping:

Papillary or follicular < 45 years old				Papillary or follicular (≥ 45 years old) or medullary (any age patient)			
Stage I	Any T	Any N	M0	Stage I	T1	N0	M0
Stage II	Any T	Any N	M1	Stage II	T2	N0	M0
Stage III				Stage III	T3	N0	M0
					T1	N1a	M0
					T2	N1a	M0
					T3	N1a	M0
Stage IVA				Stage IVA	T4a	N0	M0
					T4a	N1a	M0
					T1	N1b	M0
					T2	N1b	M0
					T3	N1b	M0
					T4a	N1b	M0
Stage IVB				Stage IVB	T4b	Any N	M0
Stage IVC				Stage IVC	Any T	Any N	M1

Stage grouping: Undifferentiated (anaplastic)[a]

Stage IV	Any T	Any N	Any M

AJCC = American Joint Committee on Cancer; UICC = International Union Against Cancer
[a] For undifferentiated cancers, all cases are classified as stage IV.
From Greene FL, Page DL, Fleming ID, et al (eds): AJCC Cancer Staging Manual, 6th ed. New York, Springer-Verlag, 2002.

of 24-hour urinary catecholamine and metanephrine levels to rule out the presence of a pheochromocytoma. Fractionated plasma metanephrine levels have been demonstrated to have a high sensitivity and may be included in the initial assessment.

Genetic testing Germ-line mutations in the *RET* proto-oncogene are responsible for familial non-MEN medullary thyroid carcinoma in addition to MEN-2A and MEN-2B. DNA analysis performed on a peripheral blood sample is a highly reliable method for identifying the presence of a *RET* mutation. Approximately 95% of patients with a *RET* mutation will eventually develop medullary carcinoma of the thyroid, thus prophylactic surgical treatment is recommended. The specific mutated codon of *RET* may correlate with the aggressiveness of medullary carcinoma of the thyroid. This should be considered when counseling affected individuals and their families regarding prophylactic thryoidectomy and the age at which to perform such surgery. Long-term data regarding the effectiveness of prophylactic thyroidectomy based on RET testing are scarce at this time. In a recent report of 50 patients (ages 19 years and younger) treated surgically after positive RET mutational analysis, 33 patients had carcinoma identified in the surgical specimen. At the time of the publication, 44 patients were found to be disease-free more than 5 years after surgery.

Recommended ages for prophylactic surgery range from within the first 6 months of life to 10 years of age depending on the mutation. The prophylactic surgical procedure of choice is total thyroidectomy with or without central lymph node dissection. Although this approach reflects general recommendations, there remain significant concerns about the ethics and safety of surgery based on genetic testing for this and many other diseases.

Periodic determinations of stimulated calcitonin levels may help make the early diagnosis of medullary thyroid carcinoma in those who do not undergo surgery but will not always prevent the development of metastatic medullary thyroid carcinoma.

Screening

At this time, no organization recommends periodic screening for thyroid cancer using neck palpation or ultrasonography in average-risk, asymptomatic adults. However, the ACS recommends examination of the thyroid during a routine checkup, since this surveillance can result in case findings.

Staging and prognosis

Unlike most other cancers, in which staging is based on the anatomic extent of disease, the American Joint Committee on Cancer (AJCC) and International Union Against Cancer (UICC) staging of thyroid cancer also takes into consideration patient age at the time of diagnosis and tumor histology (Table 1).

Differentiated thyroid cancers Recurrence and death following initial treatment of differentiated thyroid cancer can be predicted using a number of risk classification schemes. The most commonly used systems are the AMES (age, metastases, extent, and size) and AGES (age, grade, extent, and size) classifications.

Low-risk patients are generally those < 45 years of age with low-grade nonmetastatic tumors that are confined to the thyroid gland and are < 1 to 5 cm. Low-risk patients enjoy a 20-year survival rate of 97% to 100% after surgery alone.

High-risk patients are those ≥ 45 years old with a high-grade, metastatic, locally invasive tumor in the neck or with a large tumor. Large size is defined by some authors as > 1 cm and by other authors as > 2 or > 5 cm. The 20-year survival rate in the high-risk group drops to between 54% and 57%.

Intermediate-risk patients include young patients with a high-risk tumor (metastatic, large, locally invasive, or high grade) or older patients with a low-risk tumor. The 20-year survival rate in this group of patients is ~85%.

Medullary thyroid carcinoma is associated with an overall 10-year survival rate of 40% to 60%. When medullary carcinoma is discovered prior to becoming palpable, the prognosis is much better: Patients with stage I medullary tumors (ie, tumors ≤ 2 cm or nonpalpable lesions detected by screening and provocative testing) have a 10-year survival rate of 95%.

Stage II medullary cancers (tumors > 2 but < 4 cm) are associated with a survival rate of 50% to 90% at 10 years. Patients who have lymph node involvement (stages III and IVA disease) have a 10-year survival rate of 15% to 50%. Unfortunately, approximately 50% of patients have lymph node involvement at the time of diagnosis.

When there are distant metastases (stages IVB and IVC), the long-term survival rate is compromised. In patients with metastatic medullary thyroid cancer, the disease often progresses at a very slow rate, and patients may remain alive with disease for many years.

Anaplastic thyroid cancer does not have a generally accepted staging system, and all patients are classified as having stage IV disease. Anaplastic carcinoma is highly malignant and has a poor 5-year survival rate (0%–25%). Most patients die of uncontrolled local disease within several months of diagnosis.

Treatment

As most thyroid nodules are not malignant, it is important to differentiate malignant from benign lesions to determine which patients should undergo surgery. If the cytologic result from FNA indicates that the nodule is benign, which is the case most of the time, the nodule can be safely followed. The patient may be placed on thyroxine therapy to suppress thyroid-stimulating hormone (TSH) and then reevaluated in 6 months. Adequate suppression is considered to be a TSH level of 0.2 to 0.4 µU/mL for 6 months.

SURGERY

Malignant or indeterminate cytologic features are the main indications for surgery.

Malignant nodule

Differentiated thyroid cancer If the cytologic result shows a malignant lesion, thyroidectomy should be performed. There is significant debate in the literature regarding the extent of thyroid surgery for primary tumors confined to one lobe. The surgical options include total lobectomy, total lobectomy with contralateral subtotal lobectomy (subtotal thyroidectomy), or total thyroidectomy. The decision about which procedure to perform should be based on the risk of local recurrence and the anticipated use of radioactive iodine (see section on "Radioactive I-131").

Most authorities agree that a good-risk patient (age < 45 years) with a 1-cm or smaller papillary thyroid cancer should undergo ipsilateral total lobectomy alone. Most experts also agree that total thyroidectomy (or at least subtotal thyroidectomy) is appropriate for high-risk patients with high-risk tumors. Intermediate-risk patients are treated with total lobectomy alone or total (or subtotal) thyroidectomy plus postoperative radioactive iodine. Preoperative neck imaging may help plan the surgery. Patients with radiation-induced thyroid malignancies can be treated similarly, as their cancers have a similar prognosis; however, a total thyroidectomy may be preferable in these patients because of the increased risk of multicentric tumors.

The neck should be palpated intraoperatively. If positive nodes are found, a regional lymph node dissection should be performed.

Medullary carcinoma Patients with medullary thyroid cancer should be treated with total thyroidectomy and a sampling of the regional nodes. If there is involvement of the nodes, a modified neck dissection should be performed (see section on "Lymph node dissection"). If the cancer is confined to the thyroid gland, the patient is usually cured. Postoperative adjuvant external irradiation may be used in certain circumstances (see section on "External radiation therapy").

Anaplastic carcinoma A tracheostomy often is required in patients with anaplastic thyroid cancer because of compression of the trachea. If the tumor is confined to the local area, total thyroidectomy may be indicated to reduce local symptoms produced by the tumor mass. Radiation therapy is used to improve locoregional control, often together with radiosensitizing chemotherapy.

Indeterminate or suspicious nodule

The nodule that yields indeterminate or suspicious cytologic results and is cold on thyroid scanning should be removed for histologic evaluation. The initial operation performed in most patients should be total lobectomy, which entails removal of the suspicious nodule, hemithyroid, and isthmus. There is no role for nodulectomy or enucleation of thyroid nodules. The specimen can be sent for frozen-section analysis during surgery. If the diagnosis is a colloid nodule, no further resection of the thyroid is required.

Follicular lesion If frozen-section biopsy results indicate a follicular lesion in a patient who is a candidate for total thyroidectomy, and a decision cannot be made as to whether the lesion is benign or malignant, two options are available: (1) stop and wait for final confirmation of the diagnosis, which may require a future operation; or (2) proceed with subtotal or total thyroidectomy, which obviates the need for a later operation. The diagnosis of follicular carcinoma requires identification of vascular or capsular invasion, which may not be evident on frozen-section biopsy.

Hürthle cell carcinoma If the nodule is diagnosed as a Hürthle cell carcinoma, total thyroidectomy is generally recommended for all large (> 4 cm) invasive lesions. Small lesions can be managed with total lobectomy. However, controversy remains over the optimal treatment approach for this cancer.

Lymph node dissection

Therapeutic dissection Therapeutic central neck node dissection should be performed for medullary carcinomas and other thyroid neoplasms with nodal involvement. The dissection should include all the lymphatic tissue in the pretracheal area and along the recurrent laryngeal nerve and anterior mediastinum. If there are clinically palpable nodes in the lateral neck, a modified neck dissection is performed.

Prophylactic dissection There is no evidence that performing prophylactic neck dissection improves survival. Therefore, aside from patients with medullary thyroid cancer, who have a high incidence of involved nodes, only therapeutic neck dissection is indicated.

Removal of individual abnormal nodes ("berry picking") is not advised when lateral neck nodes are palpable because of the likelihood of missing involved nodes and disrupting involved lymphatic channels.

Metastatic or recurrent disease

Survival rates from the time of the discovery of metastases (lung and bone) from differentiated thyroid cancer are less favorable than those associated with local recurrence (5-year survival rates of 38% and 50%, respectively). Survival also depends on whether the metastatic lesions take up I-131.

Surgery, with or without I-131 ablation (discussed below), can be useful for controlling localized sites of recurrence. Approximately half of patients who undergo surgery for recurrent disease can be rendered free of disease with a second operation.

RADIOACTIVE I-131

Uses in papillary or follicular thyroid carcinoma

There are two basic uses for I-131 in patients diagnosed with papillary or follicular thyroid carcinoma: ablation of normal residual thyroid tissue after thyroid surgery and treatment of thyroid cancer, either residual disease in the neck or metastasis to other sites in the body. It should be emphasized that patients with medullary, anaplastic, and most Hürthle cell cancers do not benefit from I-131 therapy.

Postoperative ablation of residual thyroid tissue should be considered in high-risk patients and patients with high-risk tumors. Ablation of residual normal thyroid tissue allows for the use of I-131 scans to monitor for future recurrence, possibly destroys microscopic foci of metastatic cancer within the remnant, and improves the accuracy of thyroglobulin monitoring.

Ablation must also be accomplished in patients with regional or metastatic disease prior to the use of I-131 for treatment, as the normal thyroid tissue will preferentially take up iodine compared to the cancer. Some states permit the use of I-131 for ablation and treatment on an outpatient basis, but administration is strictly governed by national guidelines, which minimize the risk of radiation exposure to the public.

Following surgery, the patient can be treated with liothyronine for a duration of 2 weeks. The TSH level should be determined approximately 4 to 6 weeks after surgery; in patients who undergo total or subtotal thyroidectomy, TSH levels will generally be > 50 µU/mL. A postoperative iodine scan can then be performed. If this scan documents residual thyroid tissue, an ablative dose of I-131 should be given. The patient should be advised not to undergo any radiographic studies with iodine during ablation therapy and to avoid seafood and vitamins or cough syrups containing iodine. Patients are prepared with a specific diet prior to the I-131 therapy. Iodine-123 may also be used in the postoperative setting. It may produce a better image quality than I-131 scans.

For patients who have contraindications for thyroid hormone withdrawal, administration of recombinanthuman thyroid-stimulating hormone is an alternative for preparation for radioiodine ablation of a post-surgical thyroid remant.

Iodine-131 dose In general, doses of I-131 up to 75 to 100 mCi will ablate residual thyroid tissue within 6 months following ingestion. In some patients, it may take up to 1 year for complete ablation to occur. Patients should be monitored following ablation, and when they become hypothyroid, hormone replacement therapy should be given until they are clinically euthyroid and TSH is suppressed. Recently, lower doses have been found to be effective, and some authors have recommended doses between 25 and 50 mCi, assuming they achieve euthyroid levels with TSH suppression to < 0.1 µU/mL.

Follow-up I-131 scan Approximately 6 to 12 months after ablation of the thyroid remnant, a follow-up I-131 scan should be performed. Recombinant human thyrotropin alpha (Thyrogen) is now available. Patients may continue on thyroid replacement and receive two doses of thyrotropin prior to I-131 scanning; this approach can prevent the symptoms of hypothyroidism.

Treatment of residual cancer For disease in the tumor bed or lymph nodes that was not surgically resectable, an I-131 dose of 100 to 150 mCi is given. For disease in the lungs or bone, the I-131 dose is 200 mCi. Following this therapy, the patient is again put on thyroid hormone replacement, and adequate suppression is maintained by monitoring TSH levels.

Follow-up Some clinicians advocate obtaining a repeat scan in 1 year, along with a chest x-ray, and repeating this procedure yearly until a normal scan is obtained. However, the frequency of repeat scans and the dose of I-131 are rather controversial and should be guided by the individual's risk profile.

Following thyroid remnant ablation, serum thyroglobulin measurements are useful in monitoring for recurrence. Since thyroglobulin in a patient receiving thyroid hormone replacement may be suppressed, a normal test may be incorrect ~10% of the time. In general, the presence of disease is accurately predicted by a thyroglobulin value > 5 ng/mL while the patient is in the suppressed state and by a value > 10 ng/mL in the hypothyroid state. However, measurable disease may not be identified in many patients. Whether or not they should be treated on the basis of the thyroglobulin value if the I-131 scan is normal is a subject of current debate. Any rise in the thyroglobulin level from the previous value should increase the suspicion of recurrent disease.

Chest x-rays should continue to be performed at yearly intervals for at least 10 years. Neck ultrasonography is also useful to evaluate locoregional recurrence. Continued monitoring is necessary, as late recurrence can occur. It should be pointed out that certain aggressive tumors may neither be radioactive iodine–avid nor synthesize thyroglobulin. PET scanning may contribute to localization of disease in some cases and may even carry prognostic value. PET/CT may be more useful than other imaging techniques; in a recent study, additional information was obtained with PET/CT in up to 67% of cases.

Side effects and complications

Acute effects The acute side effects of I-131 therapy include painful swelling of the salivary glands and nausea. Ibuprofen or other pain relievers are usually used to decrease salivary gland discomfort. Nausea may be treated with standard antiemetics.

Rarely, in patients with significant residual thyroid tissue, radioactive iodine may cause acute thyroiditis, with a rapid release of thyroid hormone. This problem can be treated with steroids and β-blockers.

Patients must also be cautioned not to wear contact lenses for at least 3 weeks following ingestion of I-131, as the tears are radioactive and will contaminate the lenses and possibly lead to corneal ulceration.

Bone marrow suppression and leukemia are potential long-term complications of I-131 therapy but are poorly documented and appear to be extremely rare. Patients should have a CBC count performed prior to ingestion of an I-131 dose to ensure adequate bone marrow reserve. They should also have yearly blood counts. Leukemia occurs rarely with doses of I-131 < 1,000 mCi.

Pulmonary fibrosis may be seen in patients with pulmonary metastases from papillary or follicular thyroid cancer who are treated with I-131. Those with a miliary or micronodular pattern are at greater risk, as a portion of normal lung around each lesion may receive radiation, leading to diffuse fibrosis.

Effects on fertility Data have documented an increase in follicle-stimulating hormone (FSH) levels in one-third of male patients treated with I-131. Changes in FSH after one or two doses of I-131 are generally transitory, but repeated doses may lead to lasting damage to the germinal epithelium. Sperm banking should be considered in male patients likely to receive cumulative doses of I-131 higher than 500 mCi.

The effects of I-131 on female fertility have been investigated. A published article showed no significant difference in the fertility rate in women receiving radioactive iodine. However, it is generally recommended to avoid pregnancy for 1 year after therapeutic I-131 administration.

No ill effects have been noted in the offspring of treated patients.

EXTERNAL RADIATION THERAPY

Papillary or follicular thyroid cancer

There are a number of indications for external irradiation of papillary or follicular thyroid carcinoma. Surgery followed by radioactive iodine may be used for disease that extends beyond the capsule. However, if all gross disease cannot be resected, or if residual disease is not radioactive iodine–avid, external irradiation is used as part of the initial approach for locally advanced disease in older patients.

Unresectable disease External irradiation is useful for unresectable disease extending into the connective tissue, trachea, esophagus, great vessels, and anterior mediastinum. For unresected disease, doses of 6,000 to 6,500 cGy are recommended. The patient should then undergo I-131 scanning, and, if uptake is detected, a dose of I-131 should be administered.

Recurrence after resection External irradiation may also be used after resection of recurrent papillary or follicular thyroid carcinoma that no longer shows uptake of I-131. In this situation, doses of 5,000 to 6,000 cGy are delivered to the tumor bed to prevent local recurrence. Multiple-field techniques and extensive treatment planning are necessary to deliver high doses to the target volume without the risk of significant complications.

Palliation of bone metastases External radiation therapy is useful in relieving pain from bone metastasis. If the metastasis shows evidence of I-131 uptake, the patient should be given a therapeutic dose of I-131 followed by local external radiation therapy to the lesion of up to 4,000 to 5,000 cGy. The use of intravenous bisphosphonate therapy has been shown to decrease the pain of bone metastasis and improve reported quality of life.

Twice daily radiation therapy may be of benefit over once-a-day treatment for local tumor control and possibly survival *(Wang Y, Tsang R, Asa S, et al: Cancer 107:1786-1792, 2006).*

Anaplastic thyroid carcinoma

Anaplastic carcinoma of the thyroid is an exceptionally aggressive disease. It often presents as a rapidly expanding mass in the neck and may not be completely resected. External irradiation to full dose (6,000–6,500 cGy) may slow the progress of this disease but rarely controls it.

Chemoradiation therapy There are reports of the use of accelerated fractionation regimens of external irradiation (160 cGy twice daily to 5,700 cGy) with weekly doxorubicin in patients with anaplastic thyroid cancer, as well as reports of the combination of doxorubicin and cisplatin with external irradiation. These regimens have improved local tumor control but at the expense of increased toxicity. Unfortunately, the majority of patients die of progressive disease.

Medullary thyroid carcinoma

External irradiation has been used for medullary thyroid cancer in the postoperative setting. Indications include positive surgical margins, gross residual disease, or extensive lymph node metastasis. The recommended dose is 5,000 cGy in 5 weeks.

> A report from a prospective, multicenter tumor registry stratified patients with low-risk (stages I and II) and high-risk (stages III and IV) disease and evaluated overall survival, disease-specific survival, and disease-free survival. Longer overall survival in high-risk patients was associated with near-total thyroidectomy, radioactive iodine, and aggressive thyroid hormone suppression. This study demonstrated clearly that aggressive thyroid hormone suppression therapy in high-risk patients was associated with better outcomes, whereas modest suppression in stage II patients yielded similar results. Stage I patients did not appear to have any change in outcomes based on the degree of suppression (Jonklaas J, Sarlis NJ, Litofsky D, et al: Thyroid 16:1229-1242, 2006).

ROLE OF MEDICAL THERAPY

Differentiated thyroid cancer

Thyroid hormone suppression As mentioned previously, thyroid hormone is used to suppress TSH in most patients with differentiated thyroid cancer after surgery and prior to I-131 scanning and (as appropriate) treatment. Greater TSH suppression has been associated with improved progression-free survival in patients with high-risk papillary thyroid carcinoma.

Systemic chemotherapy is used for widespread disease, although reproducibly effective regimens have not been identified to date.

New therapeutic approaches Over the past few years, molecularly targeted treatments have been studied in patients with advanced thyroid carcinoma no longer responsive to radioactive iodine. They include multitargeted tyrosine kinase inhibitors, a DNA methylation inhibitor, histone deacetylase inhibitors, a proteasome inhibitor, and a heat-shock protein-90 inhibitor. These agents are still being investigated in clinical trials.

Medullary thyroid carcinoma

In patients with medullary thyroid carcinoma, the usual treatment is surgery. Various oral, small molecule tyrosine kinase inhibitors have been investigated in patients with locally advanced, metastatic, or progressive hereditary and sporadic medullary thyroid carcinomas. The responses have been variable among agents and have consisted of partial response as the best outcome. However, the development of these novel agents and others offers much promise in the targeted treatment of metastatic medullary thyroid carcinoma, which currently has no effective cure. In patients with hereditary medullary carcinoma who have a coexisting pheochromocytoma, appropriate control of catecholamine hypersecretion should precede thyroid surgery.

Anaplastic thyroid carcinoma

As mentioned previously, the usual treatment for patients with resectable or localized anaplastic thyroid cancer is surgery. Like radiotherapy, chemotherapy is an important alternative approach, but further evaluation is needed to optimize its effectiveness.

PARATHYROID CARCINOMA

Parathyroid carcinoma is a rare cause of hypercalcemia, accounting for < 2% of cases with primary hyperparathyroidism.

Epidemiology and etiology

The disease presents in midlife and occurs with similar frequency in both genders. The etiology of parathyroid carcinoma is obscure; an association with prior neck irradiation is not apparent. Parathyroid carcinoma can be associated with the hereditary hyperparathyroidism-jaw tumor syndrome, which is due to an inactivating mutation of the *HRPT2* gene that encodes the parafibromin protein. In addition, somatic mutations of the *HRPT2* gene have been demonstrated in sporadic parathyroid carcinomas (66%–100%) but have not been seen with sporadic adenomas.

Signs and symptoms

Most patients with parathyroid cancer have symptomatic moderate to severe hypercalcemia (mean serum calcium level, 15 mg/dL) and high parathyroid hormone levels. They often present with a palpable neck mass. Unlike benign hyperparathyroidism, renal and bone abnormalities are more common in patients with parathyroid cancer.

Rarely, nonfunctioning tumors may present as neck masses; their clinical course is similar to that of functioning tumors. Clinical concern about parathyroid cancer should be raised in the presence of a palpable neck mass and severe hypercalcemia, recurrent hyperparathyroidism, or associated vocal cord paralysis.

Pathology

The principal features of parathyroid cancer include a trabecular pattern, mitotic figures, thick fibrous bands, and capsular or vascular invasion of disease. Other important features include lymphatic or hematogenous metastases and histologic evidence of tumor infiltration into the surrounding tissues (including macroscopic adherence or vocal cord paralysis).

Although cytologic evidence of mitoses is necessary to establish the diagnosis of carcinoma, mitotic activity alone is an unreliable indicator of malignancy. The only reliable microscopic finding of malignancy is invasion of surrounding structures or metastasis to lymph nodes or other organs.

Vandetanib (Zactima), a RET, VEGFR and EGFR inhibitor has been studied in hereditary and sporadic medullary thyroid carcinoma at 100 mg and 300 mg daily doses (Haddad RI, Krebs AD, Vasselii J, et al: J Clin Oncol 26:6024, 2008 and Wells SA, Gosnell JE, Gagel RF, et al: J Clin Oncol 25[18S]:6018, 2007). A randomized, placebo-controlled phase III study of the 300 mg dose in hereditary/sporadic medullary thyroid cancer is ongoing. XL184, an inhibitor of RET, MET, VEGFR2, KIT, and FLT3, is currently in a phase I trial in which more than 20 patients with medullary thyroid carcinoma. Of the 10 evaluable patients on study for > 3 months, 30% achieved partial response and 70% had stable disease and all had reductions in calcitonin and CEA (Salgia R, Sherman SI, Hong DS, et al: J Clin Oncol 26:3522, 2008). Based on these encouraging results, an international, phase III trial is underway.

Treatment

Surgical treatment of primary hyperparathyroidism

The diagnosis of parathyroid carcinoma is sometimes made during surgical exploration for primary hyperparathyroidism. Most surgeons advocate identification of all four parathyroid glands. In most cases, the upper glands can be found on the posterior aspect of the upper third of the thyroid lobe, just cephalad to the inferior thyroid artery and adjacent to the recurrent laryngeal nerve as it enters the larynx.

The inferior parathyroid glands are more variable in location. Most are found on the posterior or lateral aspect of the lower pole

A series of 28 cases of parathyroid carcinoma were analyzed for the presence of MEN1 and HRPT2 mutations to identify possible molecular tools to improve the diagnosis of parathyroid carcinomas. A somatic mutation in MEN1 was found in 13% of the cancers (which is less than that seen with sporadic adenomas), and 15% demonstrated HRPT2 mutations. Further studies evaluating the diagnostic effectiveness of these molecular markers are needed (Haven CJ, van Puijenbroek M, Tan MH, et al: Clin Endocrinol [Oxf] 67:370-376, 2007).

of the thyroid gland, but the inferior parathyroid glands may be ectopically placed in the superior or true mediastinum, often within the thymus.

The inferior and, less commonly, superior glands can be located in an ectopic location in the upper or lateral neck, adjacent to the esophagus, or within the carotid sheath.

Surgical exploration for primary hyperparathyroidism Most cases of primary hyperparathyroidism are caused by a single hyperfunctioning parathyroid adenoma. If the surgeon finds one (or occasionally two) enlarged abnormal gland(s) and the remaining glands are normal, the enlarged gland should be removed.

If four enlarged glands are found, indicating the rare case of primary parathyroid hyperplasia, subtotal parathyroidectomy including 3.5 glands should be performed. Consideration should be given to transplanting the remaining gland remnant to an ectopic location that would be easily accessible to the surgeon if hyperparathyroidism recurs.

If only normal glands are found at exploration, a missed adenoma in an ectopic location should be suspected. Thorough intraoperative neck and superior mediastinal exploration should be performed, and if the missing gland cannot be found, thymectomy and hemithyroidectomy should be performed to exclude an intrathymic or intrathyroidal adenoma. Localization studies, including CT/MRI or radionuclide imaging, should precede reexploration for a missed adenoma.

Intraoperative parathyroid hormone (ioPTH) levels are increasingly used to guide surgery for primary hyperparathyroidism. A 50% or greater decrease in the ioPTH level from the preexcision value to the 10-minute postexcision value is used as a predictor of successful surgery. The advent of ioPTH monitoring, coupled with preoperative localization studies (sestamibi scanning), has facilitated less invasive surgical techniques, such as minimally invasive parathyroidectomy. This has resulted in shorter average hospitalization stays and reduced postoperative recovery times.

The use of ioPTH with parathyroid hyperplasia requires more strict evaluation of ioPTH levels. Siperstein et al performed a prospective evaluation of ioPTH and bilateral neck exploration and found that up to 15% of cases will have additional "abnormal" glands that were not predicted by ioPTH or preoperative imaging. This study demonstrates the need for long-term follow-up of patients undergoing focused parathyroid surgery.

Cinacalcet (Sensipar) has been demonstrated in an open-label, single-arm study to reduce hypercalcemia by more than 1 mg/dL in 62% of patients with parathyroid carcinoma. This study identifies this medication as a potential option in patients who fail to respond to surgical or other medical treatments (*Silverberg SJ, Rubin MR, Faiman C, et al: J Clin Endocrinol Metab* 92:3803-3808, 2007).

If parathyroid carcinoma is suspected, based on the severity of hyperparathyroidism or invasion of surrounding tissues by a firm parathyroid tumor, aggressive wide excision is indicated. This procedure should include ipsilateral thyroidectomy and en bloc excision of surrounding tissues as necessary.

Patterns of recurrence of cancer The average time from initial surgery to the first recurrence of cancer is approximately 3 years but may be as long as 10 years. The thyroid gland is the usual site of involvement, with disease "seeding" in the neck a common pattern. Other sites of involvement include the recurrent nerve, strap muscles, esophagus, and trachea.

Distant metastases can be present at the time of initial surgery, or local spread to contiguous structures in the neck may be followed subsequently by distant metastases to the lungs, bone, and liver.

In a recent analysis, 85% of patients with parathyroid carcinoma were alive 5 years after diagnosis; death usually results from complications of the hypercalcemia rather than from the tumor burden.

Treatment of isolated metastases Isolated metastases should be aggressively resected to enhance survival and control hypercalcemia.

Medical therapy

Morbidity and mortality are generally caused by the effects of unremitting hypercalcemia rather than tumor growth. Medical treatment provides temporary palliation of hypercalcemia. Drugs used include bisphosphonates, such as pamidronate (60–80 mg q4–6d) or zoledronic acid (Zometa); calcitonin, 4–8 IU/kg q6–12h; mithramycin (plicamycin [Mithracin]), 25 µg/kg q4–6d; and gallium nitrate (Ganite), 100–200 mg/m^2/d IV for 5 days. Cinacalcet (Sensipar), a calcimimetic that targets the calcium-sensing receptor on parathyroid cells and reduces parathyroid hormone secretion, is an FDA-approved oral treatment of hypercalcemia associated with parathyroid carcinoma (30 mg bid).

SUGGESTED READING

ON THYROID CARCINOMA

Bal CS, Kumar A, Pant GS: Radioiodine dose for remnant ablation in differentiated thyroid carcinoma: A randomized clinical trial in 509 patients. J Clin Endocrinol Metab 89:1666–1673, 2004.

Baudin E, Schlumberger M: New therapeutic approaches for metastatic thyroid carcinoma; Lancet Oncol 8:148–156, 2007.

Cooper DS, Doherty GM, Haugen BR, et al: Management guidelines for patients with thyroid nodules and differentiated thyroid cancer. Thyroid 16:109–142, 2006.

David A, Blotta A, Rossi R, et al: Clinical value of different responses of serum thyroglobulin to recombinant human thyrotropin in the follow-up of patients with differentiated thyroid carcinoma. Thyroid 15:267–273, 2005.

de Groot JW, Links TP, Plukker JT, et al: RET as a diagnostic and therapeutic target in sporadic and hereditary endocrine tumors. Endocr Rev 27:535–560, 2006.

Frates MC, Benson CB, Charbonneau JW, et al: Management of thyroid nodules detected at US: Society of Radiologists in Ultrasound consensus conference statement. Radiology 237:794–800, 2005.

Krassas GE, Pontikides N: Gonadal effect of radiation from 131I in male patients with thyroid carcinoma. Arch Androl 51:171–175, 2005.

Mazzaferri EL, Robbins RJ, Spencer CA, et al: A consensus report of the role of serum thyroglobulin as a monitoring method for low-risk patients with papillary thyroid carcinoma. J Clin Endocrinol Metab 88:1433–1441, 2003.

Meadows KM, Amdur RJ, Morris CG, et al: External beam radiotherapy for differentiated thyroid cancer. Am J Otolaryngol 27:24–28, 2006.

Nahas Z, Goldenberg D, Fakhry C, et al: The role of positron emission tomography/computed tomography in the management of recurrent papillary thyroid carcinoma. Laryngoscope 115:237–243, 2005.

Sampson E, Brierley JD, Le LW, et al: Clinical management and outcome of papillary and follicular (differentiated) thyroid cancer presenting with distant metastasis at diagnosis. Cancer 110:1451–1456, 2007.

Torlontano M, Attard M, Crocetti U, et al: Follow-up of low risk patients with papillary thyroid cancer: Role of neck ultrasonography in detecting lymph node metastases. J Clin Endocrinol Metab 89:3402–3407, 2004.

United States Nuclear Regulatory Commission: Medical, industrial, and acdemic uses of nuclear materials: Regulations, guidance, and communications. Available at: www.nrg.gov. Accessed September 6, 2005.

Urhan M, Dadparvar S, Mavi A, et al: Iodine-123 as a diagnostic imaging agent in differentiated thyroid carcinoma: A comparison with iodine-131 post-treatment scanning and serum thyroglobulin measurement. Eur J Nucl Med Mol Imaging 34:1012–1017, 2007.

Verburg FA, de Keizer B, Lips CJ, et al: Prognostic significance of successful ablation with radioiodine of differentiated thyroid cancer patients. Eur J Endocrinol 152:33–37, 2005.

ON PARATHYROID CARCINOMA

Busaidy N, Jimenez C, Habra MA, et al: Parathyroid carcinoma: A 22-year experience. Head Neck 26:716–726, 2004.

Grant CS, Thompson G, Farley D, et al: Primary hyperparathyroidism surgical management since the introduction of minimally invasive parathyroidectomy: Mayo Clinic experience. Arch Surg 140:472–479, 2005.

Rawat N, Khetan N, Williams DW, et al: Parathyroid carcinoma. Br J Surg 92:1345–1353, 2005.

Rolighed L, Heickendorff L, Hessov I, et al: Primary hyperparathyroidism: Intraoperative PTH measurements. Scand J Surg 93:43–47, 2004.

Siperstein A, Berber E, Mackey R, et al: Prospective evaluation of sestamibi scan, ultrasonography, and rapid PTH to predict the success of limited exploration of sporadic primary hyperparathyroidism. Surgery 136:872–880, 2004.

CHAPTER 6

Non–small-cell lung cancer

Benjamin Movsas, MD, Fadlo R. Khuri, MD, and Kemp H. Kernstine, MD, PhD

Lung cancer has been the leading cause of cancer death among men in the United States for years, and since 1988, it has become the number-one cause of cancer death among women. An estimated 220,020 new cases of lung cancer are expected in 2008, and 162,610 deaths due to this disease are expected to occur. This exceeds the combined number of deaths from the leading causes of cancer (breast, prostate, and colon cancers). It accounts for 6% of all deaths in the United States.

Lung cancer develops from pulmonary parenchymal or bronchial supportive tissues. Although multiple cell types are often found within a single lung tumor, one type usually predominates. Based on the therapeutic approach, there are two major subdivisions of lung cancer: small-cell lung cancer (SCLC), for which chemotherapy is the primary treatment, and non–small-cell lung cancer (NSCLC), which in its early stages (I and II) is treated primarily with surgery.

This chapter provides basic information on the epidemiology, etiology, screening, prevention, and signs and symptoms of lung cancer in general and then focuses specifically on the diagnosis, staging, pathology, and treatment of NSCLC and carcinoid tumors of the lungs, as well as the pulmonary evaluation of lung cancer patients and follow-up of long-term survivors.

Chapter 7 provides information on the staging, pathology and pathophysiology, and treatment of the far less common SCLC and concludes with brief discussions of mesothelioma and thymoma.

Epidemiology

Gender In the United States, the estimated number of new lung cancer cases for 2008 is 118,200 for men and 101,820 for women. Although the incidence of lung cancer had been rising in women, the rate of increase has begun to slow recently. The incidence is decreasing in men.

Age The age at which lung cancer patients are diagnosed varies widely, but the median age at diagnosis is approximately 70 years.

Race In the United States, the highest incidence of lung cancer in men and women is found in African Americans (110.6/100,000 for men and 50.3/100,000 for women) followed by Caucasians (88.8/100,000 for men and 56.2/100,000 for women).

Geography There are geographic variations in the incidence of lung cancer, with the highest rates worldwide observed in North America and Eastern Europe; in the United States, the highest rates are found in northern urban areas and along the southern coast from Texas to Florida. The state with the highest incidence of lung cancer is Kentucky, with an incidence of 137.9/100,000 in men and 73.5/100,000 in women.

Survival The overall 5-year survival rate for lung cancer is 15%, of which there has been a 1% improvement each decade for the past 30 years.

Etiology and risk factors

Cigarette smoking Approximately 87% of all cases of lung cancer are related to cigarette smoking. There is a relatively strong dose-response relationship between cigarette smoking and the development of this cancer. The greater the number of cigarettes smoked on a daily basis and the greater the number of years of smoking, the greater is the risk of lung cancer. An individual who smokes one pack of cigarettes daily has a 20-fold increased risk of lung cancer compared to a nonsmoker.

The overall incidence of cigarette smoking decreased from 1974 through 1992. Smoking cessation decreases the risk of lung cancer, but a significant decrease in risk does not occur until approximately 5 years after stopping, and the risk remains higher in former smokers than in nonsmokers for at least 25 years. The benefit of smoking cessation is greater if it occurs at a younger age.

Smoking cessation is difficult. Recent data have suggested that a variety of hereditary factors increase the risk of addiction to nicotine among some individuals. Nevertheless, millions of former smokers have quit successfully. Smoking cessation programs that address both physical withdrawal from nicotine and psychological dependence appear to be more effective than either of these approaches alone. In addition, continued efforts are needed to prevent adolescents and preadolescents from beginning to smoke or to encourage them to quit after a brief period of experimentation.

Several cancer centers have recently reported that more than half of their patients with newly diagnosed lung cancer are former smokers, having quit more than 1 year before diagnosis. Healthy ex-smokers represent a large group of individuals who may benefit from effective tools for early detection and/or chemoprevention of lung cancer.

Secondhand smoke Not only is smoking risky for those who smoke, but it also poses a hazard to nonsmokers who either live or work with smokers. It is estimated that approximately 3,000 lung cancer deaths per year in the United States are due to secondhand smoke. Individuals who live in a household with a smoker have a 30% increase in the incidence of lung cancer compared to nonsmokers who do not live in such an environment.

Asbestos exposure is another risk factor for lung cancer. Cigarette smokers who are exposed to asbestos develop lung cancer at an extremely high rate. There is a 90-fold increase compared with unexposed individuals. Exposure to asbestos is also a major risk factor for the development of mesothelioma (see discussion of this cancer in the following chapter).

Radioactive dust and radon exposure Uranium miners who have been exposed to radioactive dust and radon gas also have an increased incidence of lung cancer. Although there has been some controversy about the risk posed by exposure to residential radon gas, a study conducted in Sweden showed an increased incidence of lung cancer in individuals who were exposed to a high level of radon in their homes.

Screening and prevention

Screening

Currently, screening for lung cancer among asymptomatic individuals at elevated risk due to smoking history or occupational exposures is not recommended. An unfortunate result of this policy is that most patients present in advanced stage, and cure rates have improved little over the past 30 years. Only 7% of NSCLC patients are diagnosed in stage IA.

Three randomized screening trials conducted in the United States in the 1970s failed to show a reduction in lung cancer mortality among the smokers who were screened by sputum cytology and chest x-ray for lung cancer. Despite the fact that these American trials were not designed to evaluate chest x-ray as a screening tool, the results led most experts to conclude that screening for lung cancer was not worthwhile. In addition, most investigators recommended that research efforts and resources be allocated to the *prevention* of lung cancer. A more recent, randomized, prospective trial from Czechoslovakia showed that screening with a chest x-ray increased the diagnosis of early-stage lung cancer but failed to reduce the mortality from lung cancer.

The potential to screen for lung cancer has received renewed interest due to the superior performance of low-dose helical CT compared with chest radiography in detecting small lesions. Although there is insufficient evidence to establish policy related to routine screening for lung cancer with spiral CT, there is a growing trend toward promoting screening with this new technology to individuals at increased risk for lung cancer.

Numerous studies are currently under way to evaluate chest CT scan for lung cancer screening. Several recent reports from Japan, Germany, and the United States have documented the ability of low-dose spiral CT scans to detect lung cancer at an early stage. In some recent trials, more than 80% of lung cancers detected by screening were diagnosed in stage I.

Kaneko screened male smokers > 50 years of age. Of the 15 cancers detected by CT scan, only 4 were seen on chest x-ray; 14 of the 15 cancers were stage I, with an average diameter of 1.6 cm. Ohmatsu found 35 lung cancers (0.37% detection rate) with 9,452 CT scans. Of these cancers, 27 were stage IA. These patients had a 3-year survival rate of 83%.

The International Early Lung Cancer Action Project (I-ELCAP, http://www.ielcap.org/professionals.htm) is a single-arm prospective study that has accrued more than 35,000 study subjects in 30 sites and documented that a high percentage of lung cancers are detected in stage I, a stage in which long-term survival can reasonably be anticipated in more than 60% of patients. These studies provide early evidence to suggest that CT lung cancer population screening has the potential to reduce lung cancer mortality in the near future.

In a controversial article from I-ELCAP, Henschke et al presented the results of their low-dose CT screening trial in 31,567 high-risk participants. CT was performed every 7 to 18 months. Lung cancer was found in 484 (1.5%) of whom 412 (85%) were stage 1, with an 88% 10-year survival rate estimated in that cohort. Noncalcified pulmonary nodules were detected in 233 participants (23% [95% confidence interval (CI): 21–26]) by low-dose CT at baseline, compared with 68 (7% [95% CI: 5–9]) by chest radiography. Lung cancer was detected by CT in 27 patients (2.7% [95% CI: 1.8–3.8]) and by chest radiography in 7 patients (0.7% [95% CI: 0.3–1.3]).

Of the 27 CT-detected cancers, 26 were resectable. Stage I cancers were diagnosed in 23 of 27 patients (85%) by CT and 4 of 7 patients (57%) by chest radiography. In addition, low-dose CT detected four more nonparenchymal cases of lung cancer: two with endobronchial lesions and two in the mediastinum. These cases show an added benefit of low-dose CT over chest radiography, although the data were not included in the analysis. (The study primarily focused on malignant disease in noncalcified pulmonary nodules detected by low-dose CT or radiography.) It remains to be seen, however, whether lung cancer screening with low-dose spiral CT will reduce the lung cancer mortality of the study population or only improve the 5-year survival rate of the patients diagnosed with lung cancer.

Based on growing evidence that spiral CT may truly provide for a successful early detection strategy, the National Cancer Institute (NCI) launched the National Lung Screening Trial (NLST, http://www.nci.nih.gov/NLST) in September 2002. NLST has accrued 50,000 current and former smokers (aged 55–74) into a prospective trial, randomizing participants to receive annual spiral CT or annual chest x-rays. Survival data will not be available for a number of years.

The efficacy of lung cancer screening is also being evaluated as part of the Prostate, Lung, Colorectal, and Ovarian Cancer Screening Trial (PLCO). Men and women were randomized to receive annual chest x-ray versus usual care. Eligibility was not based on risk of lung cancer, because given the large size of the study (> 100,000 participants), it was expected that there would be appreciable numbers of current and former smokers among the participants.

In response to the I-ELCAP results, Bach et al reviewed the collective results of three prospective concurrently run randomized screening trials in 3,246 high-risk patients. They found no reduction in lung cancer deaths or advanced cancer in the screened groups.

The increased use of CT scanning in the United States, currently more than 62 million scans per year, has significantly increased the exposure to radiation in the population and may be a future health issue. The exposure to radiation from two to three CT scans in an adult is similar to that experienced by survivors of atomic bombs dropped on Japan in 1945. The risks associated with exposure to radiation are highest in children.

Biomarkers, proteomic evaluations, and circulating endothelial cells are currently under intensive investigation within and outside the Early Detection Research Network (http://edrn.nci.nih.gov/). The lack of demonstrated benefit for the earlier radiographic screening approaches should not be misinterpreted as nihilism about the early detection of lung cancer. Individuals at risk (current and former smokers) who present with symptoms consistent with lung cancer deserve appropriate evaluation. A lack of resolution of radiographic abnormalities on a chest x-ray obtained after the completion of empiric antibiotic therapy for pneumonia should prompt further evaluation for possible lung cancer.

Chemoprevention

The concept of field carcinogenesis was originally developed for the aerodigestive tract in the early 1950s. Reducing the exposure of the epithelial mucosa to carcinogens, predominately cigarette smoke, has the greatest impact on reducing the incidence of cancer in high-risk individuals.

The Finnish Alpha-Tocopherol Beta-Carotene Study evaluated 29,133 male smokers over 5 to 8 years, and there was an 18% increased incidence of lung cancer in the group taking beta-carotene. Other chemopreventative agents studied in a phase III fashion include retinol, aspirin, retinyl palmitate, etretinate, isotretinoin, α-tocopherol, 4-hydroxyphenyl retinamide, anethole dithiolethione, and N-acetylcysteine. None of them showed any preventive benefit.

Second primary lung tumors develop at a rate of 1% to 3% annually for the first 5 years following resection of stage I NSCLC.

The intergroup randomized trial that assessed the ability of 13-*cis*-retinoic acid to prevent the occurrence of a second primary cancer in patients with completely resected stage I NSCLC showed no impact of treatment on the incidence of second primary tumors. Furthermore, patients who continued to smoke and who received isotretinoin had a higher risk of recurrence of the index cancer. The early findings have demonstrated a higher-than-expected recurrence rate in patients with early-stage lung cancer who received 13-*cis*-retinoic acid and continued to smoke. Also, there was no reduction in second primary tumors in the 13-*cis*-retinoic acid-treated group. Trials using cyclooxygenase-2 (COX-2) inhibition are yet to be reported in former and current smokers. Tyrosine kinase inhibition is currently being studied to reverse bronchial premalignant lesions and Ki-67 levels in the Lung Cancer Biomarkers Chemoprevention Consortium trial.

Selenium as L-selenomethionine has been shown to inhibit cell growth, induce apoptosis in vitro, and retard carcinogenesis at higher dose levels in animal models. Epidemiologic data suggest an inverse relationship between selenium intake and lung cancer.

In a study by Clark et al designed to determine the effects of selenium on the incidence of basal or squamous cell carcinomas, nutritional supplementation with this agent showed no consequences on the incidence of skin cancer; however, secondary analyses revealed that it was associated with significantly fewer cases of lung cancer.

A phase III intergroup selenium prevention trial has been designed to follow the lung cancer isotretinoin prevention trial. To reduce the incidence of second primary tumors, this double-blind design is randomizing patients by a 2:1 ratio to receive either selenomethionine (200 µg/d) versus placebo daily for 48 months. Patients are monitored for safety, development of second primary tumors, and recurrence. There are 1,552 patients that have been entered into the run in phase, and of those 1,375 have been enrolled in the trial. Based on enrollment to date, the projected goal of 1,960 patients should be reached by February 2011.

Educational programs Although the information from the intergroup randomized chemoprevention study is being collected, it is important to continue educational efforts to prevent adolescents from smoking cigarettes and to advocate smoking cessation in active smokers. Some experts believe that educational programs must begin during childhood, probably between the ages of 6 and 10 years. Targeting children and young adults is a significant priority of any lung cancer reduction program.

Signs and symptoms

The clinical manifestations of lung cancer depend on the location and extent of the tumor. In patients who have localized disease, the most common symptoms are related to obstruction of major airways, infiltration of lung parenchyma, and invasion of surrounding structures, including the chest wall, major blood vessels, and viscera.

Cough is a major manifestation of lung cancer and is present in nearly 80% of patients with symptomatic lung cancer. It is important to remember, however, that most lung cancer patients are current or former smokers and may have a cough related to chronic irritation of the upper and/or lower airways from cigarette smoke. Therefore, smokers should be asked whether there has been a change in their cough, such as an increase in frequency or severity.

Dyspnea and hemoptysis Increasing dyspnea and hemoptysis may be signs of lung cancer, although in the case of hemoptysis, 70% of patients bleed from nonmalignant causes, mostly infection, and more frequently, bronchitis. In patients who present with hemoptysis, are older than age 40, and have a history of smoking and chronic obstructive pulmonary disease without an abnormality on chest radiograph, lung cancer should be considered in the differential diagnosis.

Pneumonia Postobstructive pneumonia secondary to partial or complete bronchial obstruction occurs relatively frequently in association with lung cancer. It is important to obtain repeat chest x-rays in adults who have been treated for pneumonia to be certain that the radiographic abnormalities have cleared completely.

Pleural effusion Lung cancer may spread to the pleural surface or may obstruct segmental or lobar lymphatics, resulting in pleural effusion and increased dyspnea.

Chest pain Approximately 5% of lung tumors invade the chest wall. The resultant pain is a better predictor of chest wall invasion than are chest CT findings. An individual who complains of persistent chest pain should have a chest x-ray to exclude the presence of peripheral lung cancer that has invaded the chest wall.

Shoulder and arm pain Apical tumors that infiltrate surrounding structures (also called Pancoast tumors) produce shoulder and/or arm pain as a result of brachial plexus compression. Tumors in the apical lung segments may be difficult to detect on a routine chest x-ray; therefore, a person who complains of persistent shoulder pain, particularly with signs of neurologic involvement, should have a CT scan of the chest to look for an apical tumor. An MRI scan of the chest apex may be beneficial. It is also important to examine the lung apex in bone films obtained to evaluate shoulder pain.

Horner's syndrome Invasion of the sympathetic ganglion by an apical lung tumor causes Horner's syndrome (ptosis, myosis, and ipsilateral anhidrosis).

Hoarseness secondary to vocal cord paresis or paralysis occurs when tumors and lymph node metastases compress, cause dysfunction in, or invade the recurrent laryngeal nerve. This situation is more common on the left side, where the recurrent laryngeal nerve passes under the aortic arch, but it may also occur with high lesions on the right side of the mediastinum.

Other symptoms of tumor compression Lung tumors may also cause dysphagia by compression or invasion of the esophagus or superior vena cava syndrome by compression or invasion of this vascular structure.

Some tumors may result in wheezing or stridor secondary to compression or invasion of the trachea and may also cause signs of cardiac tamponade secondary to involvement of the pericardial surface and subsequent accumulation of pericardial fluid.

Signs and symptoms of metastatic disease Lung cancer can metastasize to multiple sites, most commonly to bone, liver, brain, lungs (contralateral or ipsilateral), and adrenal glands.

A lung cancer patient who has brain metastases may complain of headaches or specific neurologic symptoms, or family members may notice a decrease in the patient's mental acuity. Also, metastatic lung cancer may cause spinal cord compression, resulting in a characteristic sequence of symptoms: pain, followed by motor dysfunction, and then sensory symptoms. The patient may have any or all of these symptoms.

Patients who complain of band-like pain encircling one or both sides of the trunk may have spinal cord compression. In addition, coughing and sneezing may cause significant exacerbation of pain from spinal cord compression.

Bone x-rays and/or a bone scan are warranted in lung cancer patients who complain of persistent pain in the trunk or extremities. If performed in the evaluation of lung cancer, [18]fluorodeoxyglucose (FDG)-PET supplants the need for a bone scan in most patients. PET appears to be more sensitive but less specific for bone metastases. If plain films are normal or equivocal for metastases, CT and/or MRI may be helpful to evaluate suspicious areas. MRI of the spine is the most effective way to evaluate suspected spinal cord compression.

Systemic paraneoplastic symptoms Lung cancer is commonly associated with systemic manifestations, including weight loss (with or without anorexia). In addition, patients frequently complain of fatigue and generalized weakness. SCLC is associated with hormone production, which causes endocrine syndromes in a subset of patients, such as SIADH (syndrome of inappropriate antidiuretic hormone secretion) and via secretion of ACTH (adrenocorticotropic hormone) hypercortisolism.

Specific neurologic syndromes, such as Lambert-Eaton syndrome (see chapter 44), cortical cerebellar degeneration, and peripheral neuropathy, may occur in lung cancer patients but are relatively rare.

Clubbing Although clubbing may occur in a variety of conditions, it is important for the clinician to evaluate a patient's hands. If clubbing is noted, obtaining a chest x-ray may result in the early diagnosis of lung cancer.

Hypertrophic osteoarthropathy A relatively small percentage of patients with lung cancer may present with symptomatic hypertrophic osteoarthropathy. In this syndrome, periosteal inflammation results in pain in affected areas, most commonly the ankles and knees.

Carcinoid syndrome is extremely uncommon in patients who have a bronchial carcinoid tumor. Most of these patients are asymptomatic (tumors are found by x-ray), and a few have cough from an endobronchial lesion.

TUMOR BIOLOGY

Non–small-cell tumors account for approximately 85% of all lung cancers. The three major tumor types included under this category are adenocarcinoma, squamous cell carcinoma, and large-cell carcinoma.

Staging and prognosis

Staging

2009 changes to TNM The staging of lung cancer must be conducted in a methodical and detailed manner. The TNM staging system, updated by Mountain (Table 1), applies equally well to all histologies of NSCLC, but TNM for SCLC is less helpful. Most patients have advanced disease at the time of presentation.

Stage is commonly reported as either clinical or pathologic, designated as c or p, respectively. Clinical stage is based on noninvasive (or minimally invasive) tests, whereas pathologic stage is based on tissue obtained during surgery (see section on "Diagnosis and staging evaluation").

TABLE 1: TNM staging of lung cancer[a]

Primary tumor (T)

Tx	Tumor proven by the presence of malignant cells in bronchopulmonary secretions but not visualized roentgenographically or bronchoscopically or any tumor that cannot be assessed, as in pretreatment staging
T0	No evidence of primary tumor
Tis	Carcinoma in situ
T1	Tumor ≤ 3.0 cm in greatest dimension, surrounded by lung or visceral pleura, and without evidence of invasion proximal to a lobar bronchus at bronchoscopy
T2	Tumor > 3.0 cm in greatest dimension; or tumor of any size that either invades the visceral pleura or has associated atelectasis or obstructive pneumonitis extending to the hilar region (but involving less than the entire lung). At bronchoscopy, the proximal extent of demonstrable tumor must be within a lobar bronchus or at least 2.0 cm distal to the carina
T3	Tumor of any size with direct extension into the chest wall (including superior sulcus tumors), diaphragm, or mediastinal pleura or pericardium without involving the heart, great vessels, trachea, esophagus, or vertebral body; or tumor in the main bronchus within 2 cm of, but not involving, the carina
T4	Tumor of any size with invasion of the mediastinum or involving the heart, great vessels, trachea, esophagus, vertebral body, or carina; or presence of exudative pleural effusion (whether cytology positive or negative)

Regional lymph nodes (N)

Nx	Regional lymph nodes cannot be assessed
N0	No demonstrable metastasis to regional lymph nodes
N1	Metastasis to lymph nodes in the peribronchial and/or ipsilateral hilar region, including direct extension
N2	Metastasis to ipsilateral mediastinal and subcarinal lymph nodes
N3	Metastasis to contralateral mediastinal, contralateral hilar, ipsilateral or contralateral scalene, or supraclavicular lymph nodes

Distant metastasis (M)

Mx	Distant metastasis cannot be assessed
M0	No distant metastasis
M1	Distant metastasis

Stage grouping

Occult carcinoma	Tx	N0	M0
Stage 0	Tis	N0	M0
Stage IA	T1	N0	M0
Stage IB	T2	N0	M0
Stage IIA	T1	N1	M0
Stage IIB	T2	N1	M0
	T3	N0	M0
Stage IIIA	T3	N1	M0
	T1-3	N2	M0
Stage IIIB	Any T	N3	M0
	T4	Any N	M0
Stage IV	Any T	Any N	M1

[a] See text for changes to TNM system taking effect in 2009.
From Mountain CF: Revisions in the International System for Staging Lung Cancer. Chest 111:1710–1717, 1997.

The International Association for the Study of Lung Cancer has developed changes in the TNM system (TNM 7) based on an international collection and review of 100,809 patients. These changes will take effect in early 2009. They include the following:

Change

1. T4 pleural and/or pericardial effusion and/or pleural nodules becomes M1a
2. Additional nodules in the contralateral lung are subclassified as M1a
3. Distant metastases are subclassified as M1b

Subclassify

4. T1 into T1a and T1b
   a. T1a ≤ 2 cm
   b. T1b > 2 cm and ≤ 3 cm
5. T2 into T2a and T2b
   a. T2a > 3 cm and ≤ 5 cm
   b. T2b > 5 cm and ≤ 7 cm

Reclassify

6. T2 lesions larger than 7 cm as T3
7. T4 tumors with additional nodules in the primary lobe as T3
8. M1 by additional nodules in the ipsilateral lung (different lobe) as T4

Prognostic factors

Stage The most important prognostic factor in lung cancer is the stage of disease.

Performance status and weight loss Within a given disease stage, the next most important prognostic factors are performance status and recent, unexplained weight loss. The two scales used to define performance status are the Eastern Cooperative Oncology Group (ECOG) performance status system and the Karnofsky system (see Appendix 1). Simply, patients who are ambulatory have a significantly longer survival than those who are nonambulatory. Similarly, patients who have lost > 5% of body weight during the preceding 3–6 months have a worse prognosis than patients who have not lost a significant amount of weight.

Molecular prognostic factors Several studies published over the past decade have indicated that mutations of *ras* proto-oncogenes, particularly K-*ras*, portend a poor prognosis in NSCLC, and in the case of adenocarcinomas, are more frequently found in smokers. Accordingly, selective research has focused on developing molecularly targeted therapeutic approaches to the *ras* proto-oncogenes, in particular, the farnesyl transferase inhibitors as well as epidermal growth factor receptor (EGFR) inhibitors and antiangiogenic approaches (see section on "Novel and promising agents").

Of equal relevance was the completion of large studies by Pastorino et al and Kwiatowski et al evaluating the prognostic importance of immunocytochemical and molecular pathologic markers in stage I NSCLC.

In the study by Pastorino et al, gene-expression profiles were performed in 198 tumor samples to develop a predictive model for recurrence, the lung metagene model. The model was then tested in three cohorts of stage IA patients and was found to be highly accurate in predicting the likelihood of recurrence. By identifying patients who are likely to recur, adjuvant therapy is more likely to be effective. In the study by Kwiatowski et al, gene-expression profiles were performed in 185 frozen samples and a 5-gene signature that correlated with relapse-free and overall survival was identified.

> **P**otti et al used microarray techniques to study prognosis in stage I non-small cell lung cancer. Their results indicate that the lung metagene model offers a potential mechanism to estimate a patient's risk of disease recurrence and, in principle, to affect decisions regarding the use of adjuvant chemotherapy in early-stage NSCLC *(Potti A, Mukherjee S, Petersen R, et al: N Engl J Med 355:570-580, 2006).*

The findings of these two studies suggest that pathologic invasion and extent of surgical resection may yield the most critical prognostic information, but mutation of the K-*ras* oncogene and absence of expression of the H-*ras* p21 proto-oncogene may augment the pathologic information. Further data indicate that a molecular prognostic model differentiating patients with lung cancer may be possible using proteomics or other molecular biology techniques.

Molecular profiling has been described as a means to molecularly characterize tumors and to identify the metastatic potential and regional growth character. Other molecular markers that portend a poor prognosis include reduced expression of RASSF1A and FHIT (fragile histidine triad); reduced expression of catenins and E-cadherin; reduction in tumor suppressor genes *p53*, retinoblastoma gene, *p16INK4A,* and *p15INK4B*; increased telomerase activity; overexpression of EGFR (c-ErbB-1), matrix metalloproteinase, HER2/*neu* (c-Erb-2), and vascular endothelial growth factor (VEGF); c-Met overexpression; overexpression of mutated p53; urokinase plasminogen activator overexpression; promoters of angiogenesis; reduced expression of *nm23* gene; and low KAI1/CD82.

Quality of life (QOL) The Radiation Therapy Oncology Group (RTOG) re-analyzed the results of RTOG 9801 to assess the added value of QOL as a prognostic factor for overall survival. On multivariate analysis, they found that the global QOL score superseded the classic predictors of survival (eg, Karnofsky performance status, stage, etc) in patients with locally advanced NSCLC. Patients with a global QOL score less than the median (66.7 of 100) had a 70% higher rate of death than patients with a QOL $\geq$ 66.7 ($P = .002$). Of note, patients who were married or had a partner had higher QOL scores than those who were not ($P = .004$). A clinically meaningful increase in the QOL score (of 10 points) corresponded to a decrease in the hazard of death by 10% ($P = .002$). This study highlights the "added value" of patient-reported outcomes and the need to incorporate QOL measures into clinical oncology trials.

Diagnosis and staging evaluation

History and physical examination

The diagnosis and preoperative staging of lung cancer begin with a good history and physical examination. When obtaining the history, the clinician should keep in mind the tendency for lung cancer to involve major airways and other central structures. Similarly, the patterns of metastatic dissemination and systemic manifestations must be considered when conducting the physical examination.

Patients should be questioned specifically about the presence of palpable masses, dysphagia, bone pain, headache, or changes in vision. Careful auscultation and percussion may suggest the presence of atelectasis or pleural effusion. Auscultation of the chest also may provide evidence of large airway obstruction and pulmonary consolidation. Rhonchi and wheezing may provide some helpful treatment planning information. An enlarged liver may indicate hepatic metastases.

Palpation of the neck and supraclavicular fossa Discovery of adenopathy of the neck and supraclavicular fossa may allow both diagnosis and staging, by needle or open biopsy.

Imaging studies

Chest x-rays provide initial helpful information in patients with new respiratory symptoms. Posteroanterior (PA) and lateral chest x-rays are fundamental in assessing the local extent of the primary tumor and also may provide valuable information regarding metastatic disease.

The chest x-ray should be inspected for the presence of a pleural effusion or synchronous pulmonary nodules, and the bones should be examined for evidence of osseous metastases. A widened mediastinum usually indicates metastatic disease within the mediastinal lymph nodes. Comparison with previous x-rays is helpful and well worth the effort expended in their retrieval.

Chest CT from the lower neck to the mid level of the kidneys, including the entire liver and adrenal glands with 5 to 10 mm slices, is performed routinely to further define the primary tumor and to identify lymphatic or parenchymal metastases. In a review of 20 studies that assessed the value of CT scan to determine mediastinal lymph node involvement, with an average prevalence of 28%, CT had a pooled sensitivity of 57%, a specificity of 82%, and a negative predictive value (NPV) of 83%. Benign enlargement of mediastinal nodes is more common in patients with postobstructive infection. Histologic confirmation of the presence or absence of tumor within the mediastinal lymph nodes is necessary whenever this information will change treatment recommendations. In patients who are considered surgical candidates, metastatic tumor is found in approximately 15% to 20% of mediastinal lymph nodes < 1 cm in greatest diameter.

It is important to remember that patients with persistent symptoms, such as cough and dyspnea, who have a normal chest x-ray may be harboring a central lesion that is not obvious on chest x-ray but can be easily detected by chest CT. Also, as previously mentioned, apical tumors (Pancoast tumors) may be difficult to detect on a chest radiograph but are usually readily apparent on a CT scan.

PET For lung masses, FDG accumulation on PET implies a significant likelihood of malignancy.

The maximum standardized uptake value (SUV) threshold of 2.5 within the region of interest optimizes the sensitivity and specificity of PET in assessing suspicious lung lesions larger than 1 cm. An FDG-avid lesion on PET should never be assumed to be malignant, and a PET-negative lesion is not absolutely benign. Bronchioloalveolar and carcinoid are two cell types that do not readily accumulate FDG. Furthermore, higher SUV lesions do not imply a greater likelihood of cancer; the highest SUVs have been found in inflammatory lesions, such as granulomas and infections.

A review of 18 studies of the utility of PET to assess the mediastinal lymph nodes demonstrated a pooled sensitivity of 84% and a specificity of 89%, with a positive predictive value (PPV) of 79% and an NPV of 93%. Combining the results of CT and PET, the PPV and NPV were 83% to 93% and 88% to 95%, respectively. Thus, FDG-PET is superior to CT scanning in staging the mediastinal lymph nodes. An estimated 15% to 20% of patients with a known or suspected diagnosis benefit from a preoperative FDG-PET, because previously unrecognized metastatic disease will be discovered.

Several trials have evaluated the prognostic significance of FDG uptake on PET scan in NSCLC. Utilizing multivariate Cox analysis, these studies noted that SUV, particularly when > 7 to 10, was an independent prognostic factor.

PET scanning may also prove a valuable tool for staging and evaluating patients undergoing radiation therapy and patients with NSCLC treated with chemoradiotherapy or irradiation. In a study by MacManus et al, the PET response after treatment was found to be a powerful predictor of survival.

Adrenal gland The adrenal gland may be the sole site of metastatic disease in as many as 10% of patients with NSCLC, though patients with adrenal masses should not be assumed to have metastatic disease and should not be denied a potentially curative surgery on the basis of a scan alone. Less than 1% of adrenal masses at least 1 cm in size that are negative on FDG-PET are malignant. Contrast-enhanced MRI-weighted images may assist in achieving a diagnosis. Suspicious adrenal masses should be either biopsied or resected in potentially operable patients to confirm the stage of disease.

Obtaining a tissue diagnosis

The next step is to obtain a histologic or cytologic diagnosis of the radiologically revealed lesion, although preoperative histologic diagnosis need not be obtained in a highly suspicious lung mass without evidence of distant or locoregional metastases (see below).

Central lesions Collecting sputum cytologies for 3 consecutive days provides a cytologic diagnosis for central lesions 71% of the time and for peripheral lesions 49% of the time. In clinically suspicious lung nodules/masses, a negative sputum cytology result warrants further clinical investigation. Flexible bronchoscopy is commonly required to achieve a diagnosis. For central lesions that are exophytic, at least three direct forceps biopsies should be performed to achieve a 74% sensitivity. Washings and brushings add to the sensitivity but by themselves have a sensitivity of 48% and 59%, respectively. Further improved sensitivity is obtained with bronchoscopic fluoroscopically directed transbronchial needle aspiration biopsies. For central lesions, the overall sensitivity for flexible bronchoscopy is 88% in experienced hands.

In addition, bronchoscopy may provide important staging information, such as whether the tumor involves the distal trachea or carina, and may help plan the appropriate operation (lobectomy or sleeve resection vs pneumonectomy). Determining the degree of bronchial involvement assists surgical planning. Bronchoscopy-directed biopsies should be performed to assist in determining the intended line of resection, especially when evaluating for submucosal involvement.

Peripheral lesions Bronchoscopy is less likely to yield a diagnosis in patients with peripherally located lesions. Bronchoscopic ability to make a diagnosis of malignancy in peripheral lesions is dependent upon size; for those less than 2 cm, the sensitivity is 33%, and for lesions greater than 2 cm, it is 62%. If a bronchiole is seen traversing or extending to the mass on CT, the sensitivity is reported to be twice as high, nearly 60%.

A CT-guided needle biopsy may diagnose up to 90% of peripheral lung cancers but is dependent on the quality of the CT scan and the experience of the radiologist performing the procedure. The false-negative rate is 20% to 30%. Needle biopsy is usually reserved for patients who are not candidates for an operation due to distant metastatic disease or poor health or performance status. If the patient is a candidate for surgery, resection is generally recommended for any suspicious mass whether the result of needle biopsy is positive or nondiagnostic. Therefore, for patients with a suspicious peripheral lesion that is not associated with pleural effusion, mediastinal adenopathy, or other evidence of metastatic disease, it is reasonable to proceed directly to surgery.

Mediastinoscopy Mediastinoscopy is a time-tested technique whereby the middle (cervical mediastinoscopy) and the anterior mediastinum may be assessed for direct or metastatic lymph node involvement. In the hands of a specialist, the risk of biopsy trauma to local structures (great vessels, trachea, or esophagus), bleeding, recurrent nerve paresis, infection, or death is minimal. Whole-node biopsies may be taken, achieving a great deal of information about the location, degree of nodal involvement, and lymph node capsular invasion. There is no evidence that mediastinoscopic biopsy spreads tumor within the mediastinum, worsens the prognosis, or renders eventual surgical mediastinal dissection difficult.

With the advent of the videoscopic technology, the video-assisted lymphadenectomy (VAMLA) and the transcervical extended mediastinal lymphadenectomy (TEMLA) have been described, whereby extensive mediastinal evaluation and

TABLE 2: Selective indications for mediastinoscopy

Enlarged N1, N2, or N3 lymph nodes on chest CT scan

FDG-PET–positive mediastinal disease

Centrally located tumors

T2-T4 tumors

---

lymph node resection are performed. The additional 1 to 2 hours to perform these procedures and slightly increased patient discomfort are offset by the significant improvement in the access to the nodal stations, acquisition of lymph nodes, and improved staging and therapeutic potential.

Selective indications for mediastinoscopy are listed in Table 2. To assess response to therapy, repeat mediastinoscopy has been performed with few complications. Patients with N2 disease may potentially benefit from neoadjuvant treatment. Patients with N3 disease are considered to be stage IIIB and less likely to benefit from surgical resection. There have been a few retrospective reports that have demonstrated survival from induction therapy in patients with microscopic N3 involvement.

Endobronchial ultrasonography and endoesophageal ultrasonography staging Endobronchial ultrasonography (EBUS) is a real-time means of directly evaluating mediastinal masses and lymph nodes to direct transtracheal and transbronchial fine-needle (TTNA) and core aspiration/biopsy. It provides access to all of the paratracheal, subcarinal, and proximal hilar lymph node stations. It appears to have a similar sensitivity to mediastinoscopy (85%–90%) and may reduce the need for mediastinoscopy.

Real-time transesophageal biopsies by endoesophageal ultrasonography (EUS) can be performed on mediastinal tumors and the lymph nodes with similar sensitivity and accuracy to EBUS. EUS provides access to lymph node stations in the posterior mediastinum in the mid to distal periesophageal lymph nodes, involved in 10% to 15% of patients. Both are minimal access procedures that can be performed with little risk.

Thoracentesis and thoracoscopy Individuals who have pleural effusions should undergo thoracentesis. Video-assisted thoracoscopic surgery (VATS) should be used to assess patients who have cytology-negative effusions. Sixty percent of patients with known pleural disease and effusions will have cytology-negative effusions. However, lung cancer patients with exudative cytology-negative effusions and their cytology-positive counterparts appear to have equally poor survival. VATS permits direct visualization of the pleural surface, enables direct biopsy of the pleural nodules, and also may facilitate biopsy of ipsilateral mediastinal lymph nodes. The role of VATS to assess effusions remains to be elucidated.

Measurement of serum tumor-associated antigens has no current role in the staging of NSCLC.

Diagnosis and evaluation of suspected carcinoid tumor

A carcinoid tumor of the lungs may be suspected in a patient with a slowly enlarging pulmonary mass and a prolonged history of respiratory symptoms. Patients usually have no symptoms. Most tumors are located centrally and exist endobronchially. When they occur, symptoms may include wheezing, recurrent pneumonia, dyspnea, and potentially paraneoplastic syndromes. Bronchoscopy frequently assists in diagnosing the lesion. The finding of a polypoid, pale, firm mass should not lull the bronchoscopist into taking a large-forceps biopsy. First, these masses are frequently vascular, and massive bleeding has been reported; second, the entire mass can be accidentally removed, making it difficult to identify the site of the original location of the polyp.

Given the bleeding potential, rigid bronchoscopy may be a better way to assess these lesions. Especially with cytology, carcinoid tumors may be difficult to differentiate from small-cell and atypical carcinoid tumors. Carcinoid tumor should be suspected when a small-cell tumor diagnosis by fine-needle aspiration does not respond to therapy. True carcinoids will have metastatic nodal disease in 5% to 10% of patients and have an excellent prognosis with surgical resection. Atypical carcinoid tumors are differentiated from typical tumors in that they have more than two mitotic figures per high-powered field and areas of necrosis.

Unlike its infradiaphragmatic counterpart, pulmonary carcinoid tumors rarely present with paraneoplastic syndromes, including carcinoid syndrome, acromegaly, and Cushing syndrome. Therefore, it is only necessary to measure urinary 5-hydroxyindoleacetic acid (5-HIAA) excretion prior to surgery in symptomatic patients. Less than 3% of all patients with pulmonary carcinoid tumors have detectable urinary 5-HIAA.

Intraoperative staging

Intraoperative staging is an integral part of any operation for lung cancer. In addition to the thorough visual and tactile inspection of the lungs, diaphragm, and pleura, the ipsilateral mediastinal lymph nodes must be either completely removed or at least sampled.

The American Thoracic Society has assigned numbered levels to locations in which lymph nodes are regularly found, defined by their relation to constant anatomic structures. A complete mediastinal lymph node dissection is associated with little morbidity and lengthens the operation only slightly.

Pulmonary evaluation

To determine the volume of lung that can be removed without rendering the patient a pulmonary cripple and to identify those individuals at risk for postoperative complications, each patient may undergo pulmonary function testing, spirometry, and potentially a diffusing capacity. The results of pulmonary testing should be referenced to the normal values for ethnicity, height, age, and sex rather than the absolute value.

TABLE 3: WHO and IASLC guidelines for the histologic classification of lung cancer

I	**Adenocarcinoma**
	i. Adenocarcinoma with mixed subtypes
	1. Well-differentiated fetal adenocarcinoma
	2. Mucinous adenocarcinoma
	3. Mucinous cystadenocarcinoma
	4. Clear cell adenocarcinoma
	5. Signet ring adenocarcinoma
	ii. Acinar
	iii. Papillary
	iv. Bronchioloalveolar carcinoma
	1. Mucinous
	2. Nonmucinous
	3. Mixed mucinous and nonmucinous
	v. Solid adenocarcinoma with mucin
II	**Squamous**
	i. Papillary
	ii. Small-cell
	iii. Clear cell
	iv. Basaloid
III	**Large-cell**
	i. Large-cell neuroendocrine carcinoma
	ii. Basaloid carcinoma
	iii. Lymphoepithelioma-like carcinoma
	iv. Mixed large-cell neuroendocrine carcinoma
	v. Clear cell carcinoma with rhabdoid phenotype
IV	**Adenosquamous carcinoma**
V	**Carcinomas with pleomorphic, sarcomatous characteristics**
	i. Carcinosarcoma
	ii. Pulmonary blastoma
	iii. Carcinomas with spindle and/or giant cells
	1. Giant cell carcinoma
	2. Spindle cell carcinoma
	3. Pleomorphic carcinoma
	iv. Other
VI	**Carcinoid**
	i. Typical carcinoid
	ii. Atypical carcinoid
VII	**Carcinomas of salivary gland origin**
	i. Adenoid cystic carcinoma
	ii. Mucoepidermoid carcinoma
	iii. Others
VIII	**Unclassified**

Adapted from the World Health Organization (WHO): Histologic typing of lung tumors. In: International Classification of Tumors. Geneva, Switzerland: WHO, 1991; Travis WD, Colby TV, Corrin B, et al: World Health Organization: Histological Typing of Lung and Pleural Tumours, 3rd ed. Berlin: Springer-Verlag, 1999. IASLC = International Association for the Study of Lung Cancer

Forced expiratory volume in 1 second Postoperative respiratory failure rarely occurs if the postresection forced expiratory volume in 1 second (FEV_1) is > 30% of predicted. Regardless of the extent of the scheduled resection (lobectomy or pneumonectomy), if the preoperative FEV_1 is < 60% of predicted, a split-function perfusion scan should be obtained to determine the contribution of each lung region to overall pulmonary function. This information may be critical when an unplanned pneumonectomy is required to achieve complete tumor resection.

Other pulmonary function tests A diffusing capacity of the lung for carbon monoxide (D_LCOa; a = adjusted for the patient's hemoglobin level) < 60% of the predicted value or a maximum voluntary ventilation (MVV) < 35% is associated with increased postoperative morbidity. Patients with a baseline oximetry saturation of less than 90% and those who desaturate with exercise more than 4% have a greater likelihood of postoperative complications. Arterial blood gas Pco_2 > 45 mm Hg is an independent risk factor for increased operative morbidity and mortality.

In patients with borderline lung function, further physiologic testing may be required to better estimate pulmonary reserve prior to and after surgery. Quantitative pulmonary ventilation-perfusion scanning may assist in this endeavor. The perfusion portion is used to calculate the percentage of lung to be removed and the estimated postoperative percentage of normal. An additional test is exercise pulmonary function testing. Patients are monitored for heart rate, rhythm, blood pressure, and oxygen consumption. Patients who reach their target heart rate and exercise capacity and who have a maximal oxygen consumption > 15 mL/kg/min are less likely to have a postoperative complication and mortality.

Pathology

The World Health Organization and the International Association for the Study of Lung Cancer have devised guidelines for the histologic classification of lung cancer, which are revised as necessary (Table 3). The different cell-type classifications are performed using light microscopy and do not require electron microscopy or immunohistochemistry. There are variations in the natural history of the different cell types and potential differences in response to treatment and survival. Overall, 90% to 95% of NSCLCs are adenocarcinomas, squamous, or large cell, with 3% to 4% being mixed tumors, such as adenosquamous carcinomas. Three major types of tumors are included under the NSCLC category: adenocarcinomas, squamous cell carcinomas, and large-cell carcinomas.

Adenocarcinomas are the most common type of NSCLC, accounting for approximately 30% to 40% of cases. Of all the types of lung cancer, adenocarcinomas are most likely to occur in nonsmokers or former smokers. They are also the most common tumors in women.

Typically, adenocarcinomas present as small peripheral lesions that have a high propensity to metastasize to both regional lymph nodes and distant sites. Because of the tendency of the primary tumor to occur in peripheral locations, it frequently produces no symptoms. In contrast with their metastatic lesions, the primary adenocarcinoma tumor is histologically heterogeneous in 80% of patients, consisting of numerous histologic subtypes, and is classified as "mixed-" or "indeterminate-adenocarcinoma."

Bronchioloalveolar adenocarcinoma (BAC) During the past decade, it has become apparent that the incidence of BAC is increasing. This tumor originates from type II pneumocytes, and it may present as a pneumonic infiltrate, as multiple nodules scattered throughout the lungs, and, occasionally, as a single nodule.

Squamous cell tumors comprise approximately 30% of all cases of lung cancer. These tumors tend to occur in a central location and tend to spread to regional lymph nodes; they are the most likely of all lung cancers to remain localized and to cavitate. In fact, autopsy studies have shown that about 15% to 30% of patients with squamous cell carcinoma may die of local disease without evidence of distant metastases.

Large-cell carcinomas account for approximately 10% to 15% of all lung cancers. They tend to present as relatively large peripheral lesions and, like adenocarcinomas, have a high propensity to metastasize to regional lymph nodes and distant sites.

Treatment

In operable candidates, clinically staged IA, IB, IIA, and IIB NSCLC should undergo anatomic complete surgical resection. Primarily, patients with stages IIIB and IV disease are treated nonoperatively. Although multimodality therapy is routinely recommended for stage IIIA disease, it is recommended that it be performed within a clinical trial.

SURGICAL APPROACH

The appropriate treatment of NSCLC is resection of the lobe containing the tumor. Occasionally, a bilobectomy or pneumonectomy is required. Mortality approximates 3% following lobectomy and 7% following pneumonectomy. A wedge or segmental resection has a three to five times higher incidence of local recurrence and a lower 5-year survival than a lobectomy. Therefore, if the patient can tolerate the procedure, the standard operation should be a lobectomy, rather than a wedge resection or segmentectomy. As a curative resection, segmentectomy, though, has not been sufficiently evaluated, and more recent investigation demonstrates that in selected tumors, when the bronchus and vascular supply are individually ligated with a regional node resection, survival appears to be comparable and it salvages lung parenchyma.

Evaluation of the SEER (Surveillance, Epidemiology, and End Results) database found that in stage I lung cancer, the difference in long-term survival between a wedge resection and lobectomy was neglible after 71 years of age.

A radiologic and PET evaluation has demonstrated that lesions smaller than 2 cm, peripheral ground-glass opacity with a PET maximum SUV of less than 2.5, and no evidence of metastatic disease may be considered for a more limited resection if the surgical margin is approximately the size of the lesion.

Video-assisted thoracoscopic surgery Traditionally, lung cancers have been resected through a posterolateral thoracotomy incision. Muscle-sparing incisions may reduce pain. The current trend is toward an even less invasive approach: lobectomy and lymph node dissection with VATS. This approach appears to offer the same cancer operation and survival with perhaps lower morbidity.

Two VATS methods have been described: the mass hilar ligation technique and individual ligation of the vasculature and airway. Patients with peripheral tumors up to 4 to 6 cm without clinical hilar or mediastinal adenopathy appear to be good candidates for a VATS procedure. Conversion rates to open thoracotomy are 10%, and hospital stays are usually 3 to 5 days.

The results of several VATS series show lower complication rates than reported series for thoracotomy; granted a selection bias may have occurred. One small randomized trial showed a significant benefit favoring VATS. Patients have better shoulder function, better performance on the 6-minute walk, and less impairment of vital capacity after VATS than after thoracotomy. A VATS approach may be better tolerated than other approaches for older patients.

Patients with pathologic stage IA disease have a 70% to 80% 5-year survival rate after resection, whereas 5-year survival rates are 60% in those with stage IB disease and 40% to 50% in those with stage IIA/IIB disease. Patients found to have N2 (stage IIIA) disease located at a single nodal level have a 25% to 30% 5-year survival rate. A radiological and PET evaluation has demonstrated that lesions less than 2 cm in size, peripheral ground-glass opacity with a PET max SUV of less than 2.5 and no evidence of metastatic disease may be considered for a more limited resection if the surgical margin is approximately the size of the lesion.

Mediastinal lymph node involvement The standard lung cancer operation should include sampling or dissection of mediastinal lymph nodes. The presence of metastases in any of the mediastinal lymph nodes (N2 and/or N3 disease) is indicative of advanced disease and is thought by some to represent a contraindication to surgery. Resection of mediastinal disease may have prognostic significance, implications for postoperative care, and potential therapeutic value. Some series of patients with N2 disease have shown a 5-year survival rate of 20% to 30%, but patients in these series are highly selected.

Patients with N2 disease may potentially benefit from neoadjuvant treatment. Patients with N3 disease are considered to be stage IIIB and less likely to benefit from surgical resection. There have been a few retrospective reports that have demonstrated survival from induction therapy in patients with microscopic N3 involvement. The American College of Surgeons has completed accrual to a randomized, prospective study comparing survival following mediastinal lymph node sampling versus dissection. Complications and operative mortality appear equivalent between the sampling and dissection groups. Long-term survival is under investigation. Also, clinical trials are currently testing preoperative chemotherapy and chemoradiation therapy in patients with mediastinal node involvement.

Preoperative histologic assessment of the mediastinal lymph nodes is essential if multilevel metastases are suspected, as there have been few long-term survivors among patients with metastatic disease at more than one level. Nonsurgical treatment appears preferable, or patients should be offered participation in a trial designed to assess the benefits of neoadjuvant therapy. Although patients with stage IIIB tumors are usually treated with irradiation and chemotherapy (see later discussions), the occasional patient with isolated involvement of the vena cava or atrium can undergo resection.

Carcinoid tumors Although the majority of carcinoid tumors remain localized, regional lymph node metastases are identified in 5% to 15% of patients. The surgical approach, therefore, should be similar to that used in NSCLC. If a small tumor in a proximal airway is identified and there is no histologic evidence of lymph node disease, a bronchoplastic procedure with preservation of lung tissue can sometimes be performed. Rates of survival at 10 years are > 90% for patients with stage I disease and 60% for patients with stage II disease.

ADJUVANT THERAPY

Chemotherapy

Classic postoperative adjuvant chemotherapy has been tested in three randomized trials conducted by the Lung Cancer Study Group (LCSG). For almost 20 years, the relative value of adjuvant chemotherapy for resectable NSCLC has been disputed and debated. In a randomized, prospective study involving 488 patients, Keller et al showed no benefit to adjuvant chemotherapy. The ALPI (Adjuvant Lung Project Italy) study of 1,209 patients also showed no survival benefit. In contrast, the International Adjuvant Lung Cancer Trial (IALT) randomized 1,867 patients to receive cisplatin (Platinol)-based adjuvant chemotherapy or no treatment. At 5 years, the treatment arm showed a survival advantage of 4.1% ($P = .003$), compared with the observation arm.

Two trials, the Canadian BR-10 and Cancer and Leukemia Group B (CALGB) 9633, both demonstrated clinically significant improvement in survival, with minimal chemotherapy side effects; cisplatin and vinorelbine (Navelbine) were used in the BR-10 trial and carboplatin and paclitaxel were used in CALGB 9633. These results, in combination with the recent positive findings of the adjuvant trial of UFT (a drug composed of tegafur and uracil mixed at the ratio of 1:4) in patients with stage IB NSCLC, increase the likelihood of adjuvant platinum-based therapy becoming the standard of treatment for patients with stages IB–IIIB NSCLC.

Further data from two subsequent positive adjuvant chemotherapy trials support this new standard. Based on these data, the standard of practice has shifted to chemotherapy for operable NSCLC, either adjuvant or in the induction setting. The potential benefits are higher efficacy of chemotherapy early in the natural history of disease, facilitation of subsequent local therapy, and early eradication of distant micrometastases. Despite these positive data, not all patients benefit from adjuvant chemotherapy.

Stage I disease In one trial, adjuvant therapy with 6 courses of CAP (cyclophosphamide, Adriamycin [doxorubicin], and Platinol [cisplatin]) failed to produce a significant survival advantage in patients with stage I lung cancer. The IALT demonstrated that modern adjuvant chemotherapy could be provided with a survival advantage. In patients with stage IB disease, CALGB 9335 compared postoperative carboplatin and paclitaxel with surgery alone and found a clinically significant survival advantage, with minimal morbidity. The Canadian BR-10 trial demonstrated similar results using cisplatin and vinorelbine; patients with stage II disease were included as well.

The current trend is to provide involvement in a chemopreventive clinical trial for stage IA patients. For patients with stage IB disease, platinum-based adjuvant chemotherapy (cisplatin or carboplatin combined with a taxane or vinorelbine) should be strongly considered.

Stage II/III disease In two earlier trials, postoperative adjuvant chemotherapy with 6 courses of CAP, given alone in one study and following postoperative radiation therapy in the other, resulted in a modest improvement in median survival but had no impact on long-term survival. In contrast, the IALT, ANITA (Adjuvant Navelbine International Trialist Association), CALGB 9623, and Canadian BR-10 trials demonstrated a clinically significant survival advantage, justifying consideration for adjuvant chemotherapy. There does not appear to be any survival advantage to adding adjuvant mediastinal radiotherapy to chemotherapy, unless there are particularly high risk factors for local recurrence.

Radiation therapy

A trial conducted by the LCSG showed that in patients with squamous cell carcinoma of the lungs and resected N1/N2 disease, administration of postoperative radiation reduced the risk of recurrence in the chest from 20% to 1%. Although there was no improvement in overall survival, postoperative irradiation was associated with a significant improvement in disease-free survival for patients with N2 disease. A trial by the British Medical Research Council reached similar conclusions.

A meta-analysis of nine randomized trials assessing postoperative radiation therapy in lung cancer reported a 21% increase in mortality in patients receiving this therapy. However, many of the patients in these trials had N0 disease, for whom few would advocate radiation therapy. Also, most of the patients were treated with cobalt-60 beams and technically limited treatment planning, not with modern radiation therapy techniques.

Recently, the impact of radiation therapy on survival was reanalyzed in the ANITA trial, in which postoperative radiation therapy was optional, based on each center's practice. Interestingly, in patients with N2 (mediastinal) disease, adjuvant radiation therapy improved overall survival in both arms: 21% versus 17% in the observation arms and 47% versus 34% in the adjuvant chemotherapy arms (with or without radiation therapy, respectively). Based on this descriptive analysis, radiation therapy appeared to provide a benefit in addition to adjuvant chemotherapy in patients with N2 disease (whereas the converse was true in patients with N1 disease). A randomized trial with and without postoperative radiation therapy in patients with resected N2 disease is under development in Europe.

These results created a lack of consensus about treatment recommendations, with some experts advocating the use of postoperative radiation therapy to reduce local recurrence, and others avoiding it because of the absence of an effect on survival.

At present, therefore, the appropriate role of postoperative radiation therapy remains controversial. Such therapy should be seriously considered, however, in patients at high risk for locoregional relapse (ie, those with mediastinal disease, multiple positive lymph nodes or lymph node stations, extracapsular extension, bulky nodal disease, or close or microscopically positive margins). In patients who are receiving adjuvant chemotherapy, it is reasonable to administer the chemotherapy first (as it has been associated with a survival benefit) followed by radiation therapy (for enhanced local tumor control).

Moreover, in a randomized trial by Keller et al, no benefit was shown for concurrent chemoradiation over radiation therapy when in the adjuvant setting for completely resected patients with stage II/IIIA NSCLC. An exception may be in patients with microscopic residual disease (ie, positive margins or extracapsular extension), for whom a delay in radiation therapy may be detrimental.

NEOADJUVANT CHEMOTHERAPY OR CHEMORADIATION THERAPY

During the past decade, numerous phase II trials showed that, in general, it is feasible to perform pulmonary resection following chemotherapy or chemoradiation therapy. Although surgery can be more difficult after preoperative treatment, morbidity and mortality were acceptable.

Stage IIIA/IIIB disease The greater effectiveness of current chemotherapeutic regimens to reduce disease bulk suggested that their use prior to surgery, either alone or in combination with radiation therapy, might increase both resectability and survival in patients with stage IIIA NSCLC. Multiple phase II trials have shown such an approach to be feasible; however, it is not clear that such a strategy improves median or long-term survival over best nonsurgical chemoradiotherapy among patients who initially have more than minimal N2 disease.

Current recommendations In selected patients, preoperative treatment may have a favorable effect on outcome in surgically resectable stage IIIA NSCLC. Although aggressive neoadjuvant approaches may have increased treatment-associated mortality, in experienced institutions, potential benefits seem to outweigh the risks. The results of the intergroup randomized trial comparing preoperative chemoradiation therapy with definitive chemoradiation therapy (in pathologic N2 disease) showed a significant improvement in progression-free survival (but not overall survival) in the surgical arm ($P = .02$). This approach, however, may not be optimal if a pneumonectomy is required, as this procedure was associated with a high rate of treatment-related deaths (> 20%). It is not clear whether patients with persistently positive N2 disease after neoadjuvant therapy will benefit from surgical resection.

Stages I–IIIA disease Neoadjuvant chemotherapy may even play a role in early-stage disease. A multicenter trial from France randomized 373 patients with stages I–IIIA NSCLC to undergo either surgery alone or chemotherapy (mitomycin [6 mg/m² on day 1], ifosfamide [1.5 g/m² on days 1 to 3], and cisplatin [30 mg/m² on days 1 to 3]) at 3-week intervals for 3 cycles followed by surgery. Disease-free survival was significantly longer in the patients randomized to receive neoadjuvant chemotherapy than in those treated with surgery alone ($P = .02$). The most striking benefit of chemotherapy was seen in patients who had minimal lymphadenopathy (either N0 or N1, $P = .008$). No excessive complications were seen in the chemotherapy-treated patients.

Cumulative data support a difference in treatment, but no one study is statistically significant. Pooled analyses suggest positive benefit to neoadjuvant therapy with all individual studies showing a trend towards improved overall survival, and significant differences in disease-free survival. Following on previous trials was a study presented this year by Scagliotti in which 270 patients with stage IB through IIIA NSCLC were randomized to surgery and follow-up versus induction chemotherapy with cisplatin and gemcitabine (Gemzar) followed by surgery. This trial closed early due to accrual problems, after only 270 of a projected 700 patients enrolled in this study. Overall survival at 3 years favored the chemotherapy plus surgery arm with $P = .053$. Overall survival at 3 years for the neoadjuvant arm was 67% versus 60% for surgery alone ($P = .053$). A subset analysis suggested that for stage IIB through IIIA, three year overall survival was 70% versus 40% in favor of chemotherapy ($P = .001$), whereas there was no difference for patients with stage IB through IIA who were treated. This continues to support data suggesting that for stage IIB through IIIA disease, chemotherapy, either in the adjuvant or neoadjuvant setting provides a significant survival advantage.

TREATMENT OF PATIENTS WITH MEDICALLY INOPERABLE STAGE I/II DISEASE

Some patients with resectable stage I or II NSCLC are high-risk operative candidates because of poor cardiopulmonary function or other medical problems. Other patients refuse to undergo surgery despite the recommendation of their treating physicians. In such patients, an attempt should be made to optimize pulmonary function by encouraging smoking cessation and initiating vigorous treatment with bronchodilators, corticosteroids, and antibiotics.

Radiation therapy

Several institutions have reported their experience with definitive radiation therapy for such patients. Although the results are not as good as those reported in patients selected for surgery (possibly due to differences in patient selection and between clinical versus pathologic staging), patients with medically inoperable early-stage NSCLC clearly should be offered radiation therapy, with a reasonable expectation of cure.

Radiofrequency ablation

Patients who are not operative candidates may be treated with radiofrequency ablation (RFA). There is considerable experience with RFA for cancer in other organs, and its use for lung cancer is growing. It can be performed either intra-operatively or percutaneously with CT guidance. The preliminary findings show these radiologic results: complete response (0%), partial response (50%), stable disease (30%), and disease progression (20%). In a recent study in which more than 300 intrathoracic lesions were treated in 211 sessions, pneumothoraces developed in 51% of the sessions, of which 17% required aspiration and 22% required chest tube placement.

TREATMENT OF PATIENTS WITH STAGE IIIA/IIIB DISEASE

Radiation therapy

In the past, radiation therapy was considered the standard therapy for patients with stage IIIA or IIIB disease. Long-term survival was poor, in the range of 5%, with poor local control and early development of distant metastatic disease.

Altered fractionation schedules A randomized trial compared standard daily radiation therapy (66 Gy) with a continuous hyperfractionated accelerated radiation therapy regimen [CHART] that delivered 54 Gy over 2.5 weeks. The altered fractionation schedule resulted in improved 2-year survival.

Various efforts have assessed combining altered fractionation schema with chemotherapy. Although the results of Radiation Therapy Oncology Group (RTOG) 94-10 did not favor altered fractionation (see section on "Concurrent vs sequential chemoradiation therapy"), the long-term results of another study support this strategy.

Jeremic et al compared hyperfractionated radiation therapy (bid to 69.6 Gy) and concurrent low-dose daily carboplatin/etoposide (Vepesid) with or without weekend carboplatin/etoposide in a randomized trial of approximately 200 patients. Although investigators found no benefit with the addition of weekend carboplatin/etoposide, both arms demonstrated promising median survival times of 20 and 22 months and excellent 5-year survival rates of 20% and 23%.

Conformal radiation therapy

Hayman et al reported updated results of the Michigan phase I dose-escalation trial of three-dimensional (3D) conformal radiation therapy for NSCLC. In this study, the radiation dose was escalated based on the effective volume of irradiated lung (up to 102.9 Gy). Such doses produced acceptable toxicity and no cases of isolated failures in purposely nonirradiated, clinically uninvolved nodal regions. This strategy is now being integrated with chemotherapy.

Socinski et al reported a dose-escalation radiotherapy (from 60 Gy up to 74 Gy) trial, using 3D computer-assisted planning techniques, in patients receiving induction carboplatin and paclitaxel and concurrent weekly carboplatin/paclitaxel. Ninety-seven percent (31 of 32) of the patients completed therapy to 74 Gy, as planned. The grade 3/4 esophagitis rate overall was relatively low at only 11%.

Moreover, the results found a promising median survival of 26 months and a 3-year survival of 47%.

Indeed, several analyses support the importance of radiation therapy dose escalation in stage III NSCLC. Movsas et al analyzed data from over 1,400 patients treated in nine prospective RTOG nonoperative NSCLC studies activated during the 1990s. The analysis was stratified by the presence of chemotherapy and the accrual year. On multivariate analysis, they found that a higher biologically equivalent dose (BED) significantly predicted for higher overall survival and higher locoregional tumor control. For an increase in BED of 10 Gy, there was a dramatic reduction in the hazard of death by 14%. Similarly, researchers at the University of Michigan found a significantly improved survival in patients treated with a higher BED. To test this important hypothesis prospectively, an RTOG/intergroup phase III trial has recently opened to compare concurrent chemoradiation therapy with either 60 Gy or 74 Gy.

Chemoradiation therapy

Chemoradiation therapy versus radiation therapy alone At least 11 randomized trials have compared thoracic irradiation alone with chemoradiation therapy in patients with stage III NSCLC. Several meta-analyses have demonstrated a small, but statistically significant, improvement in survival with the combined-modality regimens.

Movsas et al recently reported the long-term survival results of RTOG 9801, a phase III trial of induction paclitaxel (P) and carboplatin (C) followed by hyperfractionated radiation therapy (69.6 Gy at 1.2 Gy bid) concurrent with P/C in which patients were randomized to receive or not receive amifostine (Ethyol), a radioprotector, during chemoradiation therapy. The median survival and 5-year survival rates were 17.1 months and 17% (AM arm) versus 18.4 months and 16% (no-AM), P = .97. The rate of late radiation therapy toxicities was similar. The promising 5-year overall survival rate suggests that induction P/C followed by concurrent radiation therapy and weekly low-dose P/C is comparable to other regimens using cisplatin doublets at higher dosages every 3 to 4 weeks (Movsas B, Moughan J, Langer C, et al: J Clin Oncol 25[18S]:7529, 2007).

Concurrent versus sequential chemoradiation therapy Furuse et al evaluated mitomycin, vindesine, and Platinol (cisplatin; MVP), administered either concurrently or prior to thoracic irradiation (56 Gy), in patients with unresectable stage III NSCLC. With over 300 patients randomized, survival favored concurrent over sequential therapy (median survival, 16.5 months vs 13.3 months, and 5-year survival rates, 15.8% vs 8.9%; $P = .04$). Furuse et al also reported the patterns of failure, which demonstrated a benefit of concurrent chemoradiotherapy in improving the local relapse-free survival ($P = .04$) but not the distant relapse-free survival ($P = .6$).

Curran et al presented the long-term results of a larger randomized trial (> 600 patients) comparing sequential and concurrent chemoradiotherapy (RTOG 9410). The 4-year survival with concurrent cisplatin/vinblastine and once-daily irradiation was 21% versus 12% with sequential treatment ($P = .04$). The third treatment arm (concurrent cisplatin/oral etoposide and hyperfractionated irradiation) was intermediate, with a 4-year survival of 17%.

The role of altered radiation therapy fractionation, may deserve further study. ECOG 2597 randomized patients after induction chemotherapy (with carboplatin and paclitaxel) to receive either standard radiation therapy (64 Gy/ 2 Gy fraction) versus hyperfractionated accelerated radiation therapy (HART), 57.6 Gy delivered 1.5 Gy three times daily over 2.5 weeks. Although the study closed prematurely due to poor accrual (only 111 patients were eligible), the median survival in the investigational arm appeared promising (22 months).

Several randomized phase II trials also appear to support the use of concurrent chemoradiation therapy for locally advanced NSCLC. For example, Belani et al performed a randomized phase II study in 276 patients of three chemoradiation therapy regimens with paclitaxel, carboplatin, and thoracic irradiation in their locally advanced multimodality protocol (LAMP). They found that concurrent chemoradiation therapy followed by adjuvant chemotherapy appeared to have the best therapeutic outcome, with a median survival of 16.3 months, compared with either induction chemotherapy followed by concurrent chemoradiation therapy (median survival, 12.7 months) or sequential chemotherapy followed by irradiation (median survival, 13 months).

Similarly, in another randomized phase II study, Zatloukal et al studied 102 patients treated with concurrent chemoradiation therapy and sequential chemotherapy followed by irradiation. The chemotherapy consisted of 4 cycles of cisplatin and vinorelbine. The investigators reported a median survival in the concurrent arm of ~20 months, vs ~13 months in the other arm ($P = .02$).

Movsas et al reported the results of the first Patterns of Care Study (PCS) for lung cancer, which was conducted to determine the national patterns of radiation therapy practice in patients treated for nonmetastatic lung cancer. As supported by clinical trials, the PCS for lung cancer demonstrated that patients with clinical stage III NSCLC received chemotherapy plus radiation therapy more than radiation therapy alone ($P < .0001$). In clinical stage I NSCLC, though, radiation therapy alone was the primary treatment ($P < .0001$). Factors correlating with increased

The Hoosier Oncology Group (HOG) recently reported the results of the phase III trial of cisplatin plus etoposide plus concurrent chest radiation therapy with or without consolidation docetaxel (Taxotere; D) in patients with inoperable stage III NSCLC. In a study of 203 patients (of whom 147 were randomized to receive or not receive D) with a median follow-up of 25.6 months, they reported a median survival time in the docetaxel arm of 21.6 months versus 24.2 months in the observation arm ($P = 0.94$). They concluded that consolidation docetaxel does not further improve survival and is associated with significant toxicity (including an increased rate of hospitalization and premature deaths) and should not be used in this setting in patients with unresectable stage III NSCLC (Hanna NH, Neubauer M, Ansari R, et al: J Clin Oncol [abstract] 25[18S]:7512, 2007). Interestingly, in a randomized phase II trial of consolidation with gemcitabine (Gemzar; G) versus G + D (following chemoradiotherapy), Movsas et al reported a greater response rate and longer progression-free survival (14.6 months versus 7.1 months) with G + D versus G alone (Movsas B, Langer C, Wang LH et al: J Thorac Oncol [abstract] 2 [suppl]: 648s, 2007).

use of chemotherapy included lower age ($P < .0001$), histology (SCLC > NSCLC; $P < .0001$), increasing clinical stage ($P < .0001$), increasing Karnofsky performance status ($P < .0001$), and lack of comorbidities ($P = .0002$) but not academic versus nonacademic facilities ($P = .81$). Of all patients receiving chemotherapy, approximately three-quarters received it concurrently with radiation therapy. Only 3% of all patients were treated on Institutional Review Board–approved trials, demonstrating the need for improved accrual to clinical trials. Future PCSs will be done as part of the Quality Research in Radiation Oncology(QRRO) project.

New chemotherapeutic agents plus irradiation Several phase I/II trials evaluated carboplatin and paclitaxel given concurrently with thoracic irradiation. These studies showed acceptable toxicity and relatively high response rates, and in one of the studies, the 3-year survival rate was quite high (39%).

In addition to paclitaxel and carboplatin, many other chemotherapeutic agents with activity in NSCLC have emerged, including docetaxel (Taxotere), vinorelbine, gemcitabine, UFT, and irinotecan (Camptosar). A trial from Japan tested induction chemotherapy with irinotecan and cisplatin followed by radiation therapy with weekly irinotecan (30 mg/m² during radiation therapy). The study reported a response rate of 65% and a median survival rate of 16.5 months, with a grade 3/4 esophagitis rate of only 4%.

Typically, it can be difficult to deliver systemic doses of chemotherapy following concurrent chemoradiotherapy. However, the Southwest Oncology Group (SWOG) has reported a phase II study of concurrent chemoradiation therapy (cisplatin/etoposide) followed by consolidation docetaxel (75–100 mg/m² q21d × 3). This group of patients with pathologically documented stage IIIB NSCLC (pleural effusion excluded) had a promising median survival of 27 months. Toxicity during consolidation therapy consisted primarily of neutropenia (56% grade 4). However, as often occurs, the promising results of phase II trials are not always reproduced in larger phase III studies.

Recently, Rolland et al reported the results of a meta-analysis using individual patient data from randomized clinical trials. They showed that concomitant chemoradiation therapy, as compared with sequential chemotherapy and radiation therapy, improved survival of patients with locally advanced NSCLC, primarily due to a decrease in locoregional tumor progression. Overall, there was an absolute benefit in survival of 6% at 3 years (Rolland E, Le Pechoux C, Curran WJ, et al: Int J Radiat Onc Biol Phys [abstract] 69 [suppl]:5s, 2007).

Current treatment recommendations

At present, it is reasonable to consider concurrent chemoradiation therapy (with once-daily radiation therapy) as a new treatment paradigm in stage III (inoperable) lung cancer patients with an ECOG performance status of 0/1 who have not lost more than 5% of their usual body weight.

Novel biologic agents Recently, the results of SWOG 0023 were updated. This was a randomized phase III trial of gefitinib (Iressa) versus placebo maintenance after chemoradiation therapy followed by docetaxel in patients with stage III NSCLC. With a median follow-up of 27 months in 243 randomized patients, the median survival for the gefitinib arm (n = 118) was 23 months versus 35 months for the placebo arm (n = 125; p = .013). The authors concluded that in this unselected population, gefitinib did not improve survival. The decrease in survival was likely due to cancer, not to gefitinib toxicity.

Recently, Lu et al have reported the results of a phase III study of AE-941, a shark cartilage extract with antiangiogenic properties, with induction chemotherapy and concomitant chemoradiation therapy in patients with stage III NSCLC. This was a placebo-controlled trial, and patients received AE-941 versus placebo at the start of induction chemotherapy, which was continued after chemoradiation therapy as maintenance therapy. A total of 384 patients were enrolled over more than 5 years, and then the trial was closed due to insufficient accrual. The median survival time was 14.4 months in the AE-941 arm versus 15.6 months in the placebo arm (P = .73). They concluded that shark cartilage extract in this setting did not improve survival in patients with unresectable stage III NSCLC.

Chemoradiotherapy Blumenschein et al combined cetuximab (Erbitux) with paclitaxel and carboplatin with radiation therapy. This phase II RTOG-sponsored trial accrued a total of 87 patients with a twenty-four month overall survival of 52% and a disease control rate of 78%. The combination was well-tolerated and is being developed into a phase III trial, testing not only the addition of cetuximab, but dose escalation to 74 Gy.

TREATMENT OF PATIENTS WITH STAGE IV DISEASE

Until recently, there was considerable controversy over the value of treating stage IV NSCLC patients with chemotherapy. Treatment with older cisplatin-containing regimens, such as cisplatin/etoposide, showed only a modest effect on survival, improving median survival by approximately 6 weeks, according to a meta-analysis, and yielding a 1-year survival rate of approximately 20% (as compared with a rate of approximately 10% for supportive care).

However, several chemotherapeutic agents have produced response rates in excess of 20% in NSCLC (Table 4). The potentially useful newer agents include the taxanes (paclitaxel and docetaxel), vinorelbine, gemcitabine, and irinotecan. Several of these drugs have unique mechanisms of action. Paclitaxel and docetaxel increase polymerization of tubulin; gemcitabine is an antimetabolite; and irinotecan is a topoisomerase I inhibitor.

Furthermore, randomized trials demonstrated that a combination of a newer agent plus cisplatin significantly improves the response rate over cisplatin monotherapy (historically considered the most active agent for NSCLC). This increase in response rate translates into significant, although modest, improvement in survival.

TABLE 4: Active newer agents for NSCLC chemotherapy

Agent	Number of studies	Number of patients	Response rate (%) (range)
Irinotecan	3	150	34 (32-37)
Docetaxel	7	257	33 (21-54)
Paclitaxel	4	151	22 (10-24)
Gemcitabine	7	566	21 (20-26)
Vinorelbine	4	501	21 (12-32)

Optimal chemotherapy for advanced NSCLC

Until the early 1990s, regimens of cisplatin plus a vinca alkaloid or etoposide were most common. More recently, regimens that employ newer agents are more widely used. However, choosing one regimen from many options is a difficult task because there is no survival advantage documented for one regimen over another or standard regimen versus regimens containing newer agents.

Table 5 summarizes the results of selected randomized trials in which combination regimens containing a newer agent are compared with old "standard" regimens or regimens containing another newer agent. Subtle differences in the eligibility criteria (eg, inclusion of patients with stage III tumors or those with poor performance status) make it difficult to directly compare the trial results. Nevertheless, there is a trend indicating that regimens containing newer agents show higher response rates and also better survival outcomes in some series than do older regimens.

Vinorelbine plus cisplatin combination Vinorelbine was the first agent that demonstrated improved activity against NSCLC in combination with cisplatin. The European multicenter trial reported by LeChevalier showed the results favoring a cisplatin plus vinorelbine combination (vinorelbine, 30 mg/m² weekly; cisplatin, 120 mg/m² on days 1 and 29, then every 6 weeks) over a vindesine plus cisplatin combination (vindesine, 3 mg/m² weekly; cisplatin, 120 mg/m² on days 1 and 29, then every 6 weeks) and vinorelbine alone (30 mg/m² weekly). The median survival duration of 40 weeks in the vinorelbine/cisplatin treatment arm was significantly longer than the 32 weeks in the vindesine/cisplatin arm ($P = .04$) and 31 weeks in the vinorelbine monotherapy arm ($P < .001$). This trial, however, did not confirm the role of vinorelbine in NSCLC therapy, even though it confirmed the role of cisplatin.

To address this issue, SWOG conducted a study comparing cisplatin alone (100 mg/m² every 4 weeks) with the vinorelbine/cisplatin combination (cisplatin, 100 mg/m² every 4 weeks; vinorelbine, 25 mg/m² weekly × 3 every 4 weeks). Survival outcome was analyzed for 415 patients, 92% with stage IV tumors. The vinorelbine/cisplatin treatment significantly improved the disease progression-free (median, 2 months vs 4 months; $P = .0001$) and overall survival (median, 6 months vs 8 months; 1-year survival 20% vs 36%; $P = .0018$).

TABLE 5: Results of selected randomized trials evaluating chemotherapy regimens of newer agents in advanced NSCLC

Initial investigator	Chemotherapy regimen	No. of patients	Response rate (%)	Median survival	1-yr survival rate (%)
LeChevalier (1994)	Vinorelbine + cisplatin	206	30	40 wk	35
	Vindesine + cisplatin	200	19	32 wk	27
	Vinorelbine	206	14	31 wk	30
Bonomi (1996)	Etoposide + cisplatin	600	12	7.69 mo	31.6
	Paclitaxel + cisplatin	(total)	27	9.56 mo	36.9
	Paclitaxel + cisplatin + G-CSF		32	9.99 mo	39.1
Giaccone (1997)	Teniposide + cisplatin	157	28	9.9 mo	41
	Paclitaxel + cisplatin	152	41	9.7 mo	43
Belani (1998)	Etoposide + cisplatin	179	14	9.9 mo	37
	Paclitaxel + carboplatin	190	22	9.5 mo	32
Crino (1998)	Mitomycin + ifosfamide + cisplatin	152	28	38 wk	NA
	Gemcitabine + cisplatin	154	40	35 wk	NA
Georgoulias (1999)	Docetaxel + cisplatin	152	32	10 mo	42
	Docetaxel + gemcitabine	144	34	9 mo	34
Masuda (1999)	Irinotecan + cisplatin	378	43	50.3 wk	47.5
	Vindesine + cisplatin	(total)	31	47.4 wk	37.9
	Irinotecan		21	46.1 wk	40.7
Kelly (1999)	Paclitaxel + carboplatin	184	27	8 mo	36
	Vinorelbine + cisplatin	181	27	8 mo	33
Schiller (2000)	Paclitaxel + cisplatin	1,163	21	7.8 mo	31
	Gemcitabine + cisplatin	(total)	21	8.1 mo	36
	Docetaxel + cisplatin		17	7.4 mo	31
	Paclitaxel + carboplatin		15	8.2 mo	35
Frasci (2000)	Gemcitabine + vinorelbine	60	22	29 wk	30
	Vinorelbine	60	15	18 wk	13
Lilenbaum (2002)	Paclitaxel + carboplatin	292	29	10 mo	NA
	Paclitaxel	290	17	8.6 mo	NA

G-CSF = granulocyte colony-stimulating factor; NA = data not available

Comella et al reported interim analysis results of a phase III trial of the Southern Italy Cooperative Oncology Group. A three-drug regimen (cisplatin, gemcitabine, and vinorelbine) was associated with a substantial survival gain over the cisplatin and vinorelbine regimen (median survival time, 51 weeks and 35 weeks, respectively).

Paclitaxel plus platinum compound A number of studies demonstrate promising results with paclitaxel in combination with cisplatin or carboplatin and other agents. Two large randomized trials compared paclitaxel plus cisplatin with standard regimens. In a three-arm, randomized ECOG trial (ECOG 5592) reported by Bonomi et al, 600 eligible patients with chemotherapy-naive stage IIIB to IV NSCLC were randomly assigned to receive a combination of cisplatin (75 mg/m^2) plus etoposide (100 mg/m^2 daily on days 1 to 3) versus either low-dose (135 mg/m^2 over 24 hours) or high-dose (250 mg/m^2 over 24 hours with growth factor) paclitaxel plus cisplatin (75 mg/m^2). The response rates for the low-dose and high-dose paclitaxel arms were 26.5% and 32.1%, respectively, significantly better than the cisplatin/etoposide arm (12.0%). Superior survival was observed with the combined paclitaxel regimens (median survival time, 9.99 months; 1-year survival, 39%) compared with etoposide plus cisplatin (median survival, 8 months; 1-year survival rate, 32%; $P = .048$). Comparing survival rates for the two dose levels of paclitaxel revealed no significant differences.

In a European trial of similar design reported by Giaccone et al, cisplatin/paclitaxel improved the response rate and quality-of-life parameters. There was no improvement in overall survival, however, compared with a standard regimen of cisplatin/teniposide (Vumon).

Paclitaxel/carboplatin has been the most widely favored regimen for first-line chemotherapy in all NSCLC stages among US medical oncologists, mainly due to promising phase II trial results and the ease of administration for outpatients, with manageable toxicity profiles compared with those of cisplatin-containing regimens. One of the early phase II trials, for example, reported a response rate of 62%, a median survival duration of 53 weeks, and a 1-year survival rate of 54%. However, a randomized trial sponsored by the manufacturer of paclitaxel failed to demonstrate a survival advantage over the standard cisplatin plus etoposide regimen. Nevertheless, paclitaxel plus carboplatin may remain a community standard because a SWOG trial reported results equivalent to the time-tested vinorelbine/cisplatin regimen (see Table 5).

Combination versus single-agent chemotherapy A randomized phase III study conducted by the CALGB further supported the superiority of combination chemotherapy over single-agent therapy. Previous trials had indicated that a platinum plus a novel agent was superior to a platinum alone. Lilenbaum et al demonstrated that for patients with stage IIIB or IV NSCLC, carboplatin and paclitaxel are superior to paclitaxel alone, even for patients with an ECOG performance status of 2. This randomized trial showed a median survival advantage for the combination therapy.

Gemcitabine plus cisplatin Gemcitabine has also been approved by the US Food and Drug Administration (FDA) for use against NSCLC based on a series of successful phase II trials of cisplatin/gemcitabine and three major phase III trials. The Hoosier Oncology Group study, reported by Sandler et al, compared gemcitabine/cisplatin with cisplatin alone and showed a modest improvement in median and 1-year survival comparable to those seen in the vinorelbine trials. The Spanish and Italian trials, reported by Cardenal et al and Crino et al, compared gemcitabine plus cisplatin with standard-regimen cisplatin plus etoposide and mitomycin plus ifosfamide plus cisplatin, respectively. Although there was a significant improvement in overall response, these two studies failed to demonstrate a survival benefit.

Because gemcitabine is relatively well tolerated without dose-limiting myelosuppression, it is being evaluated for use as a single agent or in combination with other agents in older or medically compromised patients. Italian investigators report that gemcitabine combined with the vinorelbine regimen is associated with significantly better survival than single-agent vinorelbine in elderly patients with NSCLC.

Other combination regimens that contain cisplatin plus newer agents, such as docetaxel or irinotecan, also showed similar results when compared with other two-drug regimens of either two newer or two older agents.

Major randomized trials comparing cytotoxic regimens

To identify a better chemotherapy regimen for advanced-stage NSCLC, the US cooperative study groups conducted large phase III trials. The SWOG investigators compared paclitaxel/carboplatin with vinorelbine/cisplatin (the time-tested regimen in previous European and SWOG trials). A total of 404 evaluable patients were randomized to receive either paclitaxel (225 mg/m^2 over 3 hours) plus carboplatin (at an area under the curve [AUC] of 6 mg/mL/min on day 1) every 21 days or vinorelbine (25 mg/m^2 weekly) plus cisplatin (100 mg/m^2 on day 1) every 28 days. Overall response rates were 27% for both groups. The median survival times were also identical (8 months), with virtually identical 1-year survival rates (35% and 33%, respectively). Although both regimens provided effective palliation for advanced NSCLC, the investigators identified paclitaxel/carboplatin for future studies because of a favorable toxicity profile and better tolerability and compliance.

The ECOG 1594 trial compared three platinum-based regimens containing new agents in the treatment of NSCLC with a control arm of cisplatin and paclitaxel. The regimens were gemcitabine (1,000 mg/m^2 on days 1, 8, and 15) plus cisplatin (100 mg/m^2 on day 1) every 4 weeks, docetaxel (75 mg/m^2) plus cisplatin (75 mg/m^2 on day 1) every 3 weeks, and paclitaxel (225 mg/m^2 over 3 hours) plus carboplatin (at an AUC of 6 mg/mL/min on day 1) every 21 days; the reference regimen was paclitaxel (175 mg/m^2 over 24 hours) plus cisplatin (75 mg/m^2 on day 1) every 21 days.

Analysis of 1,163 eligible patients showed no statistically significant differences in overall response, median survival, and 1-year survival rates when compared with the control arm, paclitaxel and cisplatin. Gemcitabine plus cisplatin was associated with a statistically significant prolongation of time to disease progression when compared with the control arm (4.5 months vs 3.5 months; $P = .002$) but was also associated with a higher percentage of grade 4 thrombocytopenia, anemia, and renal toxicity.

Recent randomized trials have begun to suggest that differentiating treatment regimens by histology may be important. A phase III trial by Scagliotti et al randomized 1,725 patients to a combination of cisplatin and gemcitabine versus cisplatin and pemetrexed (Alimta). In patients who did not have a squamous cell histology, the combination of cisplatin and pemetrexed had a superior overall survival. On the other hand, in patients with squamous cell histol-

---

ogy, the combination of cisplatin and gemcitabine had a superior survival. These and other data suggest that pemetrexed and platinum appear to be superior in non-squamous cell populations.

Because all the regimens showed similar efficacy, quality of life becomes a critical issue in choosing a particular regimen. The decision to use one regimen over another will depend not only on ease of administration and side effects, but also on the personal preference and experience of the treating oncologist.

Second-line chemotherapy for NSCLC

Before the new generation of more effective agents became available, few, if any, significant benefits were expected from second-line chemotherapy. As a result, reports in the literature seldom address this issue specifically or systematically. The most experience with second-line chemotherapy in NSCLC is with docetaxel, which has received FDA approval for this indication based on two randomized phase III trials confirming the promising phase II results of docetaxel monotherapy in patients with advanced NSCLC previously treated with platinum-based chemotherapy.

In a multicenter US trial reported by Fossella et al, 373 patients were randomized to receive either docetaxel (100 mg/m² [D100] or 75 mg/m² [D75]) or a control regimen of vinorelbine (30 mg/m²/wk) or ifosfamide (2 g/m² × 3 days) every 3 weeks. Overall response rates were 10.8% with D100 and 6.7% with D75, each significantly higher than the 0.8% response of the control arm ($P = .001$ and $P = .036$, respectively). Although overall survival was not significantly different among the three groups, the 1-year survival was significantly higher with D75 than with the control treatment (32% vs 19%; $P = .025$).

In a phase III trial led by Hanna et al, 572 previously treated patients were randomized to receive pemetrexed with vitamin B_{12}, folic acid, and dexamethasone or docetaxel with dexamethasone. The overall response rate in the pemetrexed arm was higher, 9.1% versus 8.8%. The median disease progression–free

A recently reported phase III, open-label randomized study evaluated pemetrexed (Alimta) plus cisplatin (AC arm) vs gemcitabine (Gemzar) plus cisplatin (GC arm) in the first-line treatment of 1,725 patients with stage IIIB or IV NSCLC. Patients were randomized to receive cisplatin 75 mg/m² on d 1 and gemcitabine 1,250 mg/m² on d 1 and 8 (n = 863) or cisplatin 75 mg/m² and pemetrexed 500 mg/m² on d 1 (n = 862) every 3 wk for up to 6 cycles.

In a prespecified analysis, the impact of non–small-cell lung cancer (NSCLC) histology on overall survival was examined. Clinically relevant differences in survival according to histology were observed. In the nonsquamous cell NSCLC subgroup, the median survival was 11.0 and 10.1 months in the AC and GC groups, respectively (unadjusted hazard ratio 0.84 [95% CI = 0.74, 0.96]). However, in the squamous cell histology subgroup, the median survival was 9.4 vs 10.8 months in the AC and GC groups, respectively (unadjusted hazard ratio 1.22 [95% CI = 0.99, 1.50]).

The investigators reported that this is the first prospective phase III study in NSCLC to show survival differences based on histologic type (Scagliotti GV, Parikh P, von Pawel J, et al: J Clin Oncol 26:3543-3551, 2008).

Based on the results of this study, the FDA recently approved pemetrexed, in combination with cisplatin, in the first-line treatment of locally advanced and metastatic NSCLC, for patients with nonsquamous histology.

survival was 2.9 months for each arm, and the median survival favored pemetrexed (8.3 vs 7.9 mo). The 1-year survival for each arm was 29.7%. Adverse reactions (grade 3/4) were more severe with docetaxel.

The second trial reported by Shepherd et al compared single-agent docetaxel with best supportive care. The initial docetaxel dose was 100 mg/m^2, which was changed to 75 mg/m^2 midway through the trial because of toxicity. A total of 204 patients were enrolled; 49 received D100, 55 received D75, and 100 received best supportive care. Treatment with docetaxel was associated with significant prolongation of survival (7.0 months vs 4.6 months; log-rank test, $P = .047$) and time to disease progression (10.6 weeks vs 6.7 weeks; $P < .001$).

Hanna et al conducted a noninferiority trial to test whether pemetrexed was equivalent to docetaxel in the second-line setting. They randomized 571 patients to receive 500 mg/m^2 of pemetrexed or 75 mg/m^2 of docetaxel preceded by a vitamin B_{12} injection every 2 cycles. The median survival on the two arms was equivalent, but the pemetrexed arm had significantly less grade 3/4 neutropenia and fewer hospitalizations overall. On the basis of this study, the FDA approved pemetrexed for second-line therapy for NSCLC.

Duration of chemotherapy

The American Society of Clinical Oncology (ASCO) has recommended that no more than 8 cycles of chemotherapy be administered to patients with stage IV NSCLC. However, therapy should be individualized depending on the quality of tumor response and the patient's tolerance.

Two trials during the last 2 years have suggested that there may be some benefit to maintenance chemotherapy in patients who have response or stable disease after front-line therapy. Fidias et al suggested that adding docetaxel as maintenance therapy after platinum-based front-line chemotherapy can delay tumor progression and lead to improvements in disease-free survival. Data by Ciuleanu et al presented at the 2008 ASCO meeting utilized maintenance pemetrexed after front-line response to chemotherapy and also showed a significant improvement in progression-free survival from 2 months for placebo to 4 months for pemetrexed. In both these trials subpopulation analysis showed that certain groups of patients tend to benefit especially from maintenance chemotherapy. This phenomenon is currently being explored by investigators.

The European phase III randomized FLEX trial (First-Line Trial for Patients With EGFR-Expressing Advanced NSCLC) demonstrated a benefit for the addition of cetuximab (Erbitux) to standard platinum-based chemotherapy in patients with previously untreated advanced, EGFR-expressing NSCLC. As reported at the 2008 ASCO plenary session, all 1,125 study patients received doublet chemotherapy with cisplatin and vinorelbine, and half the patients also received cetuximab. Overall survival was significantly improved in the study arm given cetuximab (11.3 months vs 10.1 months; $P = .04$). Manageable acne-like rash was the main cetuximab-related side effect (Pirker R, Szczesna A, von Pawel J, et al: J Clin Oncol 26:[abstract 3], 2008).

Novel and promising agents

Several novel agents are being developed for the treatment of solid tumors, including lung cancer. These novel agents include signal transduction inhibitors, such as tyrosine kinase inhibitors (eg, erlotinib [Tarceva], gefitinib [Iressa]), antiangiogenic agents, including both monoclonal antibodies, such as bevacuzimab [Avastin], and small molecule tyrosine kinase inhibitors of VEGF, such as sunitinib (Sutent) and sorafenib (Nexavar), and monoclonal antibodies (C225 [antiepidermal growth factor receptor antibody] and trastuzumab [Herceptin]). Many of these novel agents are being tested in combination with chemotherapeutic agents, as their mechanisms of action suggest that they may be far more effective as chronic inhibitors of cancer progression than as classic cytotoxics.

Combinations of cetuximab with chemotherapy also appear promising. Pirker et al showed that adding cetuximab to cytotoxic chemotherapy with cisplatin and vinorelbine improved median survival from 10.1 to 11.3 months in a randomized trial of 1,125 with advanced and metastatic NSCLC. This statistically significant ($P = .044$) 1.2 month improvement in median survival was not duplicated when cetuximab was added to taxane/platinum based chemotherapy. However, in both of these studies adding cetuximab to chemotherapy improved response rate, and these data are currently being evaluated in their totality as physicians integrate this epidermal growth factor receptor into the therapeutic arm of NSCLC.

Gefitinib and erlotinib To date, most phase I studies of these various compounds have suffered from a difficulty in developing pharmacologically or molecularly driven endpoints that will serve as reasonable intermediate biomarkers of efficacy or even surrogates for toxicity. Further research has focused on the novel small molecule tyrosine kinase inhibitors erlotinib and gefitinib. Two phase II trials of gefitinib in the second- and third-line settings were conducted in Europe and Japan. Patients were randomized to receive either 250 or 500 mg/d. The drug was found to be active, with an 11% to 18% response rate, and there was no superiority for the higher dose. Similar data were seen for erlotinib.

Unfortunately, randomized combination trials of gefitinib at 250 and 500 mg/d with cytotoxic chemotherapy, either paclitaxel and carboplatin in one trial or gemcitabine and cisplatin in the other study versus placebo in frontline therapy, failed to demonstrate any survival advantage. These results have cast a pall over the development of tyrosine kinase inhibitors in combination with chemotherapy. Regardless, the question of whether or not to approve these new agents for third-line therapy of lung cancer in cisplatin/docetaxel-refractory patients remains open for debate.

The activity demonstrated by gefitinib and erlotinib as single agents in advanced NSCLC generated much optimism, including a recent trial indicating that erlotinib improved survival (by a median of 2 months) in the second- and third-line treatments of NSCLC, with a substantial increase in 1-year survival ($P < .001$). After the initial successes with chemotherapy and promising results from targeted tyrosine kinase inhibitors in stages IIIB and IV NSCLC, several large phase III trials of either gefitinib or erlotinib in combination with conventional platinum-based chemotherapy were conducted as the INTACT 1 and INTACT 2 trials or the TALENT and TRIBUTE trials.

The phase III trials of single-agent erlotinib and gefitinib, when compared with best supportive care in the second- and third-line settings, had dramatically different results. Shepherd et al conducted a randomized trial of erlotinib (150 mg/d) versus placebo in 723 patients previously treated with front- or second-line chemotherapy for NSCLC. A total of 488 patients received erlotinib and 243 received placebo.

The median overall survival significantly favored the erlotinib arm (6.7 months vs 4.7 months), with a reduction in the hazard ratio of 0.73 ($P > .001$), as did the 1-year survival rate (31% vs 21%; $P > .01$). Quality of life and median time to deterioration also significantly favored erlotinib. On the other hand, the phase III trial of gefitinib versus best supportive care in more than 1,600 patients was reported and showed no significant advantage to gefitinib at 250 mg/d in a patient population with a significant number of active smokers.

Bevacizumab When combined with chemotherapy, bevacizumab (Avastin) appears to result in a significant survival advantage for patients with advanced NSCLC. Based on promising phase II data of bevacizumab in combination with carboplatin and paclitaxel, Sandler et al randomized 878 patients to receive either bevacizumab with carboplatin and paclitaxel or carboplatin and paclitaxel alone.

The PASSPORT trial is designed to evaluate the safety of bevacizumab (Avastin) in the first- and second-line settings. The primary endpoint is safety based on the rate of grade 2 or greater central nervous system (CNS) hemorrhage. A combined report presented at ASCO 2008 included patients entered onto the PASSPORT trial (n = 65) and patients on the ATLAS trial (n = 26), which was amended to include patients with treated and controlled brain metastases. PASSPORT also allowed patients treated in either the first- or second-line setting; ATLAS included only patients treated in the first-line setting. During active treatment, no grade 2 or greater CNS hemorrhagic events were reported; one grade 2 CNS hemorrhage was reported in a patient who progressed following cessation of bevacizumab treatment. The PASSPORT trial has completed accrual with approximately 110 patients. This early analysis suggests bevacizumab is safe in the setting of brain metastases provided patients are treated effectively and definitively and that they retain good performance status *(Akerley WL, Langer CJ, Oh Y, et al: J Clin Oncol 26:[abstract 8043], 2008).*

There was a significant increase in the response rate for the combination (27.2%) with bevacizumab versus paclitaxel and carboplatin alone (10%; $P < .0001$), and both median and progression-free survival significantly favored the bevacizumab combination arm (overall survival: 12.5 months vs 10.2 months; $P = .007$; hazard ratio = 0.77; 95% confidence interval = 0.65–0.93; progression-free survival: 6.4 months vs 4.5 months; $P < .0001$; hazard ratio = 0.62; 95% confidence interval = 0.53–0.72). As in the phase II trial, this study reported a total of eight treatment-related deaths on the bevacizumab arm versus two on the paclitaxel and carboplatin arm. A second phase III randomized trial testing the value of adding bevacizumab to gemcitabine and cisplatin therapy showed an improvement in disease-free survival, but not overall survival.

Bexarotene The mechanisms of action of these new small molecules are widely divergent, and their combinations with the cytotoxics may not necessarily lead to an enhanced response rate. Khuri and colleagues demonstrated, however, that the combination of cisplatin, vinorelbine, and bexarotene (Targretin, a retinoid-X-receptor [RXR]-specific novel retinoid) resulted in substantial median and 2-year survival rates in patients with stage IIIB NSCLC with malignant pleural effusion or stage IV NSCLC. Median survival in this multicenter study was 14 months in the phase II portion; 2-year survival was 32%; and 3-year survival was 18%. The combination yielded modest response rates (25%), not markedly superior to what was expected with cisplatin and vinorelbine alone. Two phase III trials adding bexarotene to standard chemotherapy failed to show a significant overall difference in median survival. Some survival benefit was seen in those patients who developed grade 3/4 hypertriglyceridemia as a result of the bexarotene, accounting for 35% to 40% of all patients enrolled in this study.

This finding has led to an uncoupling of the requirement for higher response rates when adding cytotoxic agents to one another in the belief that doing so may lead to enhanced survival. There now appears to be a great deal of promise associated with several small molecules, either alone or combined with chemotherapy. Novel agents such as gefitinib or lonafarnib have shown promising efficacy in small trials that have included patients with NSCLC; gefitinib alone resulted in an 18% response rate in second- or third-line therapy for NSCLC in a study population recruited across several continents.

Other promising novel agents currently being investigated in lung cancer include inhibitors of the insulin-like growth factor receptor. Karp et al showed that these agents appear to be particularly promising in squamous cell lung tumors with response rates in a small study as high as 70%.

Current treatment recommendations

It is important to note that patients who have lost significant amounts of weight or who have a poor performance status are at greater risk for toxicity, including a higher likelihood of lethal toxicity, when they are treated with modest doses of chemotherapy. Based on currently available data, a reasonable approach for patients with stage IV NSCLC who have a good performance status (ECOG performance status 0/1) and have not lost a significant amount of weight (< 5% of usual weight) would be to encourage them to participate in a clinical trial. However, it would also be appropriate to treat this group of patients with etoposide plus cisplatin or with one of the newer combination regimens, such as gemcitabine/cisplatin, vinorelbine/cisplatin, paclitaxel/cisplatin, paclitaxel/carboplatin, or docetaxel/cisplatin (Tables 6 and 7).

ROLE OF PHOTODYNAMIC THERAPY

Photodynamic therapy (PDT), which combines Photofrin (a hematoporphyrin derivative in which the less active porphyrin monomers have been removed) with an argon-pumped dye laser, has been explored in a variety of different tumors, with varying results. Several investigators have reported excellent results with PDT in early-stage head and neck cancers as well as intrathoracic tumors. However, initial studies have involved a limited number of patients.

TABLE 6: Single-agent chemotherapy regimens for NSCLC

Drug	Dose and schedule
Vinorelbine	30 mg/m^2 IV weekly
LeChevalier T, Brisgand D, Douillard J-Y, et al: J Clin Oncol 12:360–367, 1994.	
Vinorelbine	For patients 70 years old or older: 30 mg/m^2 IV on days 1 and 8, every 21 days
Gridelli C, Perrone F, Cigolari S, et al: Proc Am Soc Clin Oncol [abstract] 20:308a, 2001.	
Docetaxel	75 mg/m^2 IV on day 1 every 3 weeks
Shepherd FA, Dancey J, Ramlau R, et al: J Clin Oncol 18:2095–2103, 2000.	
Pemetrexed	500 mg/m^2 IVPB every 3 weeks
Dexamethasone (4 mg by mouth twice daily) should be started a day before and a day after pemetrexed. All patients should also receive folic acid (350–1,000 mg/d) started about a week before and thereafter while taking pemetrexed. Vitamin B$_{12}$ (1,000 mg IM) should be started about 1 to 2 weeks before pemetrexed and every 9 weeks while taking pemetrexed.	
Hanna N, Shepherd F, Fossella FV, et al: J Clin Oncol [abstract] 22:1589–1597, 2004.	
Gefitinib	250 mg orally once a day
Kris MG, Natale RB, Herbst RS, et al: JAMA 290:2149–2158, 2003.	
Gemcitabine	1,000 mg/m^2 IV on days 1, 8, and 15 every 4 weeks
Vansteenkiste J, Vandebroek J, Nackaerts K, et al: Proc Am Soc Clin Oncol [abstract] 19:1910a, 2000.	

IVPB = intravenous piggy back
Table prepared by Ishmael Jaiyesimi, DO

Although this novel technique seems to be extremely promising, it appears to be applicable to a minority of patients with NSCLC. Nevertheless, PDT appears to be particularly useful for the treatment of early-stage lung cancer for a variety of reasons. First, it appears to preserve lung function and can be repeated as additional tumors appear—an important consideration as such patients appear to be at high risk for developing other new tumors. Second, this technique does not preclude ultimate surgical intervention when deemed necessary.

Results in early-stage NSCLC Perhaps most striking are the results reported by Furuse et al, who treated 54 patients with 64 early-stage lung cancers using Photofrin (2.0 mg/kg) and 630-nm illumination of 100 to 200 J/cm^2. Of 59 accessible tumors, 50 responded completely and 6 showed partial responses. Five of the complete responders developed recurrences 6 to 8 months after treatment.

The major predictor of response in this study was tumor length. The likelihood of achieving a complete response was 97.8% if the tumor was < 1 cm, as opposed to only 42.9% if the lesion was > 1 cm. The overall survival rate in these patients was 50% at 3 years.

TABLE 7: Combination chemotherapy regimens recommended for NSCLC

Regimen	Agents	Dose and schedule	Treatment interval
PT	Platinol	75 mg/m^2 IV on day 2	3 weeks
	Taxol	135 mg/m^2 IV on day 1 (24-h infusion)	
CP	Carboplatin	AUC of 6 mg/mL/min IV on day 1	
	Paclitaxel	225 mg/m^2 IV on day 1 (3-h infusion)	3 weeks
PG	Platinol	100 mg/m^2 IV on day 1	4 weeks
	Gemcitabine	1,000 mg/m^2 IV on days 1, 8, and 15	
PD	Platinol	75 mg/m^2 IV on day 1	3 weeks
	Docetaxel	75 mg/m^2 IV on day 1	
PV	Platinol	100 mg/m^2 IV on day 1	4 weeks
	Vinorelbine	25 mg/m^2 IV on days 1, 8, 15, and 22	
PCB	Paclitaxel	200 mg/m^2 IV on day 1 (3-hr infusion)	3 weeks
	Carboplatin	AUC of 6 mg/mL/min IV on day 1	
	Bevacizumab	15 mg/kg IV	

AUC = area under the curve

A similar study by Kato et al also indicated a 96.8% complete response rate for tumors < 0.5 cm but only a 37.5% rate for tumors > 2 cm. The overall 5-year survival rate for the 75 patients treated in this study was 68.4%, which is acceptable by current standards.

Results in advanced-stage NSCLC Two prospective, randomized trials (European and US/Canadian) compared PDT with the neodymium:yttrium-aluminum-garnet (Nd:YAG) laser for partially obstructive, advanced NSCLC. Investigators analyzed results from the two trials both individually and collectively. Collective analysis included data from 15 centers in Europe and 20 centers in the United States and Canada and involved a total of 211 patients. In the European trial, 40% of the patients had received prior therapy, whereas in the US/Canadian trial, all of the patients had received previous treatment.

Tumor response was similar for both therapies at 1 week. However, at 1 month, 61% and 42% of the patients treated with PDT in the European and US/Canadian trials, respectively, were still responding, compared with 36% and 19% of patients who underwent laser therapy in the two trials.

PDT also produced more dramatic improvements in dyspnea and cough than did Nd:YAG therapy in the European trial, but the two treatments had similar effects on these symptoms in the US/Canadian trial. Both sets of investigators concluded that PDT appears to be superior to laser therapy for the relief of dyspnea, cough, and hemoptysis. Also, the overall incidence of adverse reactions was similar with the two therapies (73% for PDT vs 64% for Nd:YAG therapy). Early-stage lung cancer, most specifically endobronchial squamous cell carcinoma smaller than 1 cm, is effectively treated with PDT, with a complete response rate of 75% and a recurrence rate of 30% over 5 years.

PALLIATION OF LOCAL AND DISTANT SYMPTOMS

Radiation therapy

Many patients with lung cancer experience distressing local symptoms at some time. They may arise from airway obstruction by the primary tumor, compression of mediastinal structures by nodal metastases, or metastatic involvement of distant organs. Radiation therapy is effective in palliating most local symptoms, as well as symptoms at common metastatic sites, such as bone and brain. For selected patients with a solitary brain metastasis and controlled disease in other sites, resection followed by irradiation appears to be superior to radiation therapy alone in improving both survival and quality of life. (For more information regarding management of brain metastases, see chapter 26.)

Doses In the United States, radiation oncologists often use doses of ~30 Gy in 10 fractions for palliative thoracic treatment in lung cancer. Data from the United Kingdom suggest that similar efficacy without greater toxicity may be achieved with more abbreviated schedules, such as 17 Gy in 2 fractions 1 week apart or single fractions of 10 Gy (see Table 8). Such schedules may facilitate the coordination of irradiation and chemotherapy and also reduce patient travel and hospitalization.

Recently, just over 400 patients with inoperable NSCLC (stage III/IV) were randomized to receive three different fractionation regimens (8.5 Gy × 2, 2.8 Gy × 15, or 2.0 Gy × 25). Using the EORTC (European Organization for Research on the Treatment of Cancer) Quality-of-Life Questionnaire (QLQ) C-30 with the lung cancer-specific module (LC-13), Sundstrom et al found the effect of hypofractionated irradiation (17 Gy in 2 fractions) was comparable to that with longer fractionation schemes with regard to symptom relief and survival.

TABLE 8: Percentage of patients with symptoms of NSCLC palliated by external-beam irradiation

Symptom	Standard RT (24-30 Gy in 6-10 fractions)	17 Gy in 2 fractions (first trial/second trial)	1 fraction of 10 Gy
Cough	56	65/48	56
Hemoptysis	86	81/75	72
Chest pain	80	75/59	72
Anorexia	64	68/45	55
Depression	57	72/NA	NA
Anxiety	66	71/NA	NA
Breathlessness	57	66/41	43

NA = data not available; RT = radiation therapy

Data from Bleehen NM, Girling DJ, Fayers PM, et al: Br J Cancer 63:265–270, 1991; Bleehen NM, Bolger JJ, Hasleton PS, et al: Br J Cancer 65:934–941, 1992.

Endobronchial irradiation with cobalt-60 or iridium-192 has been used to palliate symptoms arising from partial airway obstruction, including cough, dyspnea, and hemoptysis. The dosimetric advantage of being able to deliver a high radiation dose to the obstructing endobronchial tumor while sparing adjacent normal structures, such as the lungs, spinal cord, and esophagus, has clear appeal, particularly in the patient whose disease has recurred following prior external-beam irradiation. Although good rates of palliation have been reported with endobronchial irradiation, significant complications, including fatal hemoptysis, are seen in 5% to 10% of patients. It remains unclear, however, how often this complication is actually due to the irradiation or the underlying disease itself.

Endobronchial irradiation should be considered as one of several approaches (including laser excision, cryotherapy, and stent placement) used in the management of patients with symptomatic airway obstruction, and management should be individualized. All of these approaches are more suitable for partial than for complete airway obstruction.

Chemotherapy

Several trials have explored the use of chemotherapy to palliate specific symptoms in patients with lung cancer. In general, these trials have found that rates of symptomatic improvement were considerably higher than objective response rates and were not dissimilar to symptomatic response rates with local radiation therapy.

Thus, although radiation therapy remains the most appropriate modality for the treatment of such problems as superior vena cava obstruction, spinal cord compression, brain metastases, or localized bone pain, patients who have more extensive disease without these local emergencies may be considered for palliative chemotherapy, which may relieve local symptoms and prolong survival.

Bisphosphonates

Approximately 30% to 65% of patients with advanced lung cancer develop bone metastases. The median survival following development of bone metastases is 6 months. Bone disease is associated with significant morbidity, including severe pain, hypercalcemia of malignancy, pathologic fracture, and spinal cord or nerve root compression. Treatment of bone metastases may include surgical intervention, radiation therapy, and chemotherapy. Bisphosphonate treatment can decrease skeleton-related complications, delay progressive disease, and relieve bone pain.

Bisphosphonates such as clodronate, pamidronate (Aredia), and zoledronic acid (Zometa) exhibit strong affinity for the hydroxyapatite crystal of bone and preferentially accumulate at sites of active bone remodeling, where they prevent bone resorption. They provide effective treatment for hypercalcemia of malignancy and have been shown to delay the onset of progressive bone disease and relieve bone pain in studies largely performed in patients with metastases secondary to breast cancer, multiple myeloma, and prostate cancer. Nitrogen-containing bisphosphonates, such as pamidronate and zoledronic acid, appear to exert antitumor effects. Zoledronic acid has also been found to have pronounced antinociceptive effects, which have been absent with other bisphosphonates in preclinical studies. Zoledronic acid is the only bisphosphonate shown to be effective in reducing skeletal complications in patients with bone metastases from lung cancer and solid tumors other than breast and prostate cancers.

Follow-up of long-term survivors

At present, no standard follow-up protocol exists for patients with cured NSCLC or SCLC. However, long-term follow-up should at least include serial physical examinations once the patient has reached the 5-year mark. Controversy currently exists about the value of utilizing CT scanning or even chest x-rays for the long-term follow-up of these patients.

In this vein, retrospective reviews of the literature have revealed that patients with SCLC appear to have the highest rate of second primary tumor development—as high as 30%—over the course of their lifetime, with some studies reporting annual second primary tumor rates of 5% to 10%. Therefore, the concept of chemoprevention appears to have particular merit in these patients.

A randomized chemoprevention study of patients with stage I NSCLC showed a surprisingly high annual recurrence rate of 6.5% in patients with T1 tumors, as opposed to 11.2% in patients with T2 tumors. Whether retinoids are effective chemopreventive agents remains to be seen. Nevertheless, there is clearly a need for effective chemoprevention for both of these tumor subsets, as well as the establishment of consistent guidelines for routine long-term follow-up. Given the current controversy over lung cancer screening, however, it is unlikely that this issue will be resolved without the performance of another prospective screening trial.

SUGGESTED READING

American College of Chest Physicians; Health and Science Policy Committee: Diagnosis and management of lung cancer: ACCP evidence-based guidelines. Chest 123(1 suppl):D-G, 1S–337S, 2003.

Arriagade R, Bergman B, Dunant A, et al: Cisplatin-based adjuvant chemotherapy in patients with completely resected non-small-cell lung cancer. N Engl J Med 350:351–360, 2004.

Bach PB, Jett JR, Pastorino, et al: Computed tomography screening and lung cancer outcomes. JAMA 297:953–961, 2007.

Belani CP, Wang W, Johnson DH, et al: Induction chemotherapy followed by either standard thoracic radiotherapy or hyperfractionated accelerated radiotherapy for patients with unresectable stage IIIA and B NSCLC. J Clin Oncol 23:3760–3767, 2005.

Blumenschein GR Jr, Khuri FR, von Pawel J, et al: Phase III trial comparing carboplatin, paclitaxel, and bexarotene with carboplatin and paclitaxel in chemotherapy-naive patients with advanced or metastatic non–small-cell lung cancer: SPIRIT II. J Clin Oncol 26:1879–1885, 2008.

Brenner DJ, Hall EJ: Computed tomography–An increasing source of radiation exposure. N Engl J Med 357:2277–2284, 2007.

Fukuoka M, Yano S, Giaccone G, et al: Multi-institutional randomized phase II trial of gefitinib for previously treated patients with advanced non-small-cell lung cancer. J Clin Oncol 21:2237–2246, 2003.

Gandara DR, Chansky K, Albain KS, et al: Consolidation docetaxel after concurrent chemoradiotherapy in stage IIIB non–small-cell lung cancer: Phase II Southwest Oncology Group Study S9504. J Clin Oncol 21:2004–2010, 2003.

Giaccone G, Herbst RS, Manegold C, et al: Gefitinib in combinaton with gemcitabine and cisplatin in advanced non-small-cell lung cancer: A phase III–INTACT 1. J Clin Oncol 22:777–784, 2004.

Herbst RS, Giaccone G, Schiller JH, et al: Gefitinib in combination with paclitaxel and carboplatin in advanced non-small -cell lung cancer: A phase III trial–INTACT 2. J Clin Oncol 22:785–794, 2004.

I-ELCAP; Henschke CI, Yankelevitz DF, et al: Survival of patients with stage I lung cancer detected on CT screening. N Engl J Med 355:1763–1771, 2006.

Jemal A, Siegel R, Ward E, et al: Cancer statistics, 2008. CA Cancer J Clin 58:71–96, 2008.

Karp DD, Paz-Ares LG, Novello S, et al: High activity of the anti-IGF-IR antibody CP-751,871 in combination with paclitaxel and carboplatin in squamous NSCLC. J Clin Oncol 26:8015, 2008.

Kato H, Ichinose Y, Ohta M, et al: A randomized trial of adjuvant chemotherapy with uracil-tegafur for adenocarcinoma of the lung. N Engl J Med 350:1713–1721, 2004.

Kawahara M: Irinotecan in the treatment of small cell lung cancer: A review of patient safety considerations. Expert Opin Drug Saf 5:303–312, 2006.

Keller SM, Adak S, Wagner H, et al: A randomized trial of postoperative adjuvant therapy in patients with completely resected stage II or IIIA non-small-cell lung cancer. Eastern Cooperative Oncology Group. N Engl J Med 343:1217–1222, 2000.

Kris MG, Natale RB, Herbst RS, et al: Efficacy of gefitinib, an inhibitor of the epidermal growth factor receptor tyrosine kinase, in symptomatic patients with non-small cell lung cancer: A randomized trial. JAMA 290:2149–2158, 2003.

Kuzdzat J, Zielinski M, Papla B, et al: The transcervical extended mediastinal lymphadenectomy versus cervical mediastinoscopy in non-small cell lung cancer staging. Eur J Cardiothorac Surg 31:88–94, 2007.

Lilenbaum RC, Herndon J, List M, et al: Single-agent versus combination chemotherapy in advanced NSCLC: The Cancer and Leukemia Group B (study 9730). J Clin Oncol 23:190–196, 2005.

Martelli M, Clerici M, Cognetti F, et al: Adjuvant Lung Project Italy/European Organisation for Research Treatment of Cancer–Lung Cancer Cooperative Group Investigators: Randomized study of adjuvant chemotherapy for completely resected stage I, II, or IIIA non–small-cell lung cancer. J Natl Cancer Inst 95:1453–1461, 2003.

Movsas B, Moughan J, Komaki R, et al: Radiotherapy (RT) Patterns of Care Study (PCS) in lung carcinoma. J Clin Oncol 21:4553–4559, 2003.

Movsas B, Scott C, Langer C, et al: Randomization of amifostine in locally advanced NSCLC patients receiving chemotherapy and hyperfractionated radiation. Radiation Therapy Oncology Group 98-01. J Clin Oncol 23:2145–2154, 2005.

Pirker R, Szczesna A, von Pawel J, et al: FLEX: A randomized, multicenter, phase III study of cetuximab in combination with cisplatin/vinorelbine (CV) versus CV alone in the first-line treatment of patients with advanced non–small-cell lung cancer (NSCLC). J Clin Oncol 26:[abstract 3], 2008

Pisters K, Vallieres E, Bunn PA, et al: S9900: Surgery alone or surgery plus induction paclitaxel/carboplatin chemotherapy in early stage non-small cell lung cancer: Followup on a phase III trial. J Clin Oncol 25:[18S]:7520, 2007.

Ramlau R, Zatloukal P, Jassem J, et al: Randomized phase III trial comparing bexarotene (L1069-49)/cisplatin/vinorelbine with cisplatin/vinorelbine in chemotherapy-naive patients with advanced or metastatic non–small-cell lung cancer: SPIRIT I. J Clin Oncol 26:1886–1892, 2008.

Rosen LS, Bordon D, Tchekmedyian S, et al: Zoledronic acid versus placebo in the treatment of skeletal metastases in patients with lung cancer and other solid tumors: A phase III, double-blind, randomized trial–The Zoledronic Acid Lung Cancer and Other Solid Tumors Study Group. J Clin Oncol 21:3150–3157, 2003.

Sandler AB, Gray R, Brahmer J, et al: Randomized phase II/III trial of paclitaxel plus carboplatin with or without bevacizumab in patients with advanced non-squamous non-small-cell lung cancer: An Eastern Cooperative Oncology Group trial. N Engl J Med 355:2542–2550, 2006.

Scagliotti GV, Parikh P, von Pawel J, et al: Phase III study comparing cisplatin plus gemcitabine with cisplatin plus pemetrexed in chemotherapy-naive patients with advanced-stage non-small-cell lung cancer. J Clin Oncol 26:3543–3551, 2008.

Schiller JH, Harrington D, Belani CP, et al: Comparison of four chemotherapy regimens for advanced non–small-cell lung cancer. N Engl J Med 2:92–98, 2002.

Shepherd FA, Rodrigues Pereira J, Ciuleanu T, et al: Erlotinib in previously treated non-small-cell lung cancer. N Engl J Med 353:123–132, 2005.

Strauss GM: Adjuvant chemotherapy of lung cancer: Methodologic issues and therapeutic advances. Hematol Oncol Clin North Am 19:263–281, 2005.

Strauss GM, Herndon JE, Maddaus MA, et al: Adjuvant chemotherapy in stage IB non-small cell lung cancer: Update of Cancer and Leukemia Group B protocol 9633. J Clin Oncol 24[18S]:7007, 2006.

Sundstrom S, Bremnes RM, Aasebo U, et al: Hypofractionated palliative radiotherapy (17 Gy/2 fractions) in advanced NSCLC is comparable to standard fractionation for symptom control and survival: A national phase III trial. J Clin Oncol 22:801–810, 2004.

Swann RS, Machtay M, Komaki R, et al: Impact of overall treatment time during concurrent chemoradiotherapy for locally advanced NSCLC: An RTOG secondary analysis. J Clin Oncol 23[16S]:7061, 2005.

Timmerman R, McGarry R, Yiannoutsos C, et al: Excessive toxicity when treating central tumors in a phase II study of stereotactic body radiation therapy for medically inoperable early-stage lung cancer. J Clin Oncol 24:4833–4839, 2006.

Winton T, Livingston R, Johnson D, et al: Vinorelbine plus cisplatin vs. observation in resected non-small cell lung cancer. N Engl J Med 352:2589–2597, 2005.

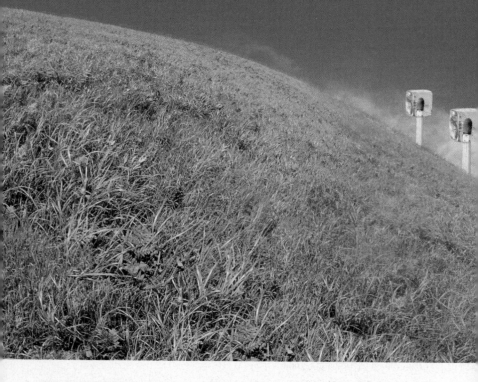

In moderate-risk* regimens

Approach chemotherapy with confidence by reducing the risk of febrile neutropenia

Neulasta® (pegfilgrastim) is indicated to decrease the incidence of infection, as manifested by febrile neutropenia, in patients with nonmyeloid malignancies receiving myelosuppressive anticancer drugs associated with a clinically significant incidence of febrile neutropenia.

Important Product Safety Information
Splenic rupture (including fatal cases), acute respiratory distress syndrome, and sickle cell crises have been reported. Allergic reactions, including anaphylaxis, have also been reported. The majority of these reactions occurred upon initial exposure. However, in rare cases, allergic reactions, including anaphylaxis, recurred within days after discontinuing anti-allergic treatment.

In a placebo-controlled trial, bone pain occurred at a higher incidence in Neulasta®-treated patients as compared to placebo-treated patients (31% vs. 26%). The most common adverse events reported in either placebo- or active-controlled trials were consistent with the underlying cancer diagnosis and its treatment with chemotherapy, with the exception of bone pain.

Please refer to brief summary of Neulasta® Prescribing Information.

*Regimens associated with ≥ 17% risk of febrile neutropenia.

Consequences of febrile neutropenia, such as hospitalization, may impact patient care

First- and subsequent-cycle Neulasta® achieved significant results in patients receiving a moderate-risk* regimen:

- 94% reduction in febrile neutropenia vs. placebo (17% vs.1%).[1,2]

- 93% reduction in febrile neutropenia–related hospitalization vs. placebo (14% vs.1%).[1,2]

Neulasta® is given once per chemotherapy cycle and should not be administered in the period between 14 days before and 24 hours after administration of cytotoxic chemotherapy.

Neulasta®
(pegfilgrastim)

Start with support

References: **1.** Vogel C, et al. *J Clin Oncol.* 2005;23:1178-1184. **2.** Neulasta® (pegfilgrastim) Prescribing Information. Thousand Oaks, Calif: Amgen.

♥ Neulasta®
(pegfilgrastim)
Start with support

BRIEF SUMMARY OF PRESCRIBING INFORMATION

INDICATIONS AND USAGE
Neulasta® is indicated to decrease the incidence of infection, as manifested by febrile neutropenia, in patients with nonmyeloid malignancies receiving myelosuppressive anticancer drugs associated with a clinically significant incidence of febrile neutropenia.

CONTRAINDICATIONS
Neulasta® is contraindicated in patients with known hypersensitivity to *E coli*-derived proteins, pegfilgrastim, Filgrastim, or any other component of the product.

WARNINGS
General
The safety and efficacy of Neulasta® for peripheral blood progenitor cell (PBPC) mobilization has not been evaluated in adequate and well-controlled studies. Neulasta® should not be used for PBPC mobilization.

Splenic Rupture
SPLENIC RUPTURE, INCLUDING FATAL CASES, HAS BEEN REPORTED FOLLOWING THE ADMINISTRATION OF NEULASTA® AND ITS PARENT COMPOUND, FILGRASTIM. PATIENTS RECEIVING NEULASTA® WHO REPORT LEFT UPPER ABDOMINAL AND/OR SHOULDER TIP PAIN SHOULD BE EVALUATED FOR AN ENLARGED SPLEEN OR SPLENIC RUPTURE.

Acute Respiratory Distress Syndrome (ARDS)
Acute respiratory distress syndrome (ARDS) has been reported in patients receiving Neulasta®, and is postulated to be secondary to an influx of neutrophils to sites of inflammation in the lungs. Patients receiving Neulasta® who develop fever, lung infiltrates, or respiratory distress should be evaluated for the possibility of ARDS. In the event that ARDS occurs, Neulasta® should be discontinued and/or withheld until resolution of ARDS and patients should receive appropriate medical management for this condition.

Allergic Reactions
Allergic reactions to Neulasta®, including anaphylaxis, skin rash, urticaria, and erythema/flushing have been reported in postmarketing experience. The majority of reported events occurred upon initial exposure. In some cases, symptoms recurred with rechallenge, suggesting a causal relationship. In rare cases, allergic reactions including anaphylaxis, recurred within days after initial anti-allergic treatment was discontinued. If a serious allergic reaction occurs, appropriate therapy should be administered, with close patient follow-up over several days. Neulasta® should be permanently discontinued in patients with serious allergic reactions.

Sickle Cell Disorders
Severe sickle cell crises have been associated with the use of Neulasta® in patients with sickle cell disorders. Severe sickle cell crises, in some cases resulting in death, have also been associated with Filgrastim, the parent compound of pegfilgrastim. Only physicians qualified by specialized training or experience in the treatment of patients with sickle cell disorders should prescribe Neulasta® for such patients, and only after careful consideration of the potential risks and benefits.

PRECAUTIONS
General
Use With Chemotherapy and/or Radiation Therapy
Neulasta® should not be administered in the period between 14 days before and 24 hours after administration of cytotoxic chemotherapy (see **DOSAGE AND ADMINISTRATION**) because of the potential for an increase in sensitivity of rapidly dividing myeloid cells to cytotoxic chemotherapy.

The use of Neulasta® has not been studied in patients receiving chemotherapy associated with delayed myelosuppression (eg, nitrosoureas, mitomycin C).

The administration of Neulasta® concomitantly with 5-fluorouracil or other antimetabolites has not been evaluated in patients. Administration of pegfilgrastim at 0, 1, and 3 days before 5-fluorouracil resulted in increased mortality in mice; administration of pegfilgrastim 24 hours after 5-fluorouracil did not adversely affect survival.

The use of Neulasta® has not been studied in patients receiving radiation therapy.

Potential Effect on Malignant Cells
Pegfilgrastim is a growth factor that primarily stimulates neutrophils and neutrophil precursors; however, the G-CSF receptor through which pegfilgrastim and Filgrastim act has been found on tumor cell lines, including some myeloid, T-lymphoid, lung, head and neck, and bladder tumor cell lines. The possibility that pegfilgrastim can act as a growth factor for any tumor type cannot be excluded. Use of Neulasta® in myeloid malignancies and myelodysplasia (MDS) has not been studied. In a randomized study comparing the effects of the parent compound of Neulasta®, Filgrastim, to placebo in patients undergoing remission induction and consolidation chemotherapy for acute myeloid leukemia, important differences in remission rate between the two arms were excluded. Disease-free survival and overall survival were comparable; however, the study was not designed to detect important differences in these endpoints.*

Information for Patients
Patients should be informed of the possible side effects of Neulasta® and be instructed to report them to the prescribing physician. Patients should be informed of the signs and symptoms of allergic drug reactions and be advised of appropriate actions. Patients should be counseled on the importance of compliance with their Neulasta® treatment, including regular monitoring of blood counts.

If it is determined that a patient or caregiver can safely and effectively administer Neulasta® (pegfilgrastim) at home, appropriate instruction on the proper use of Neulasta® (pegfilgrastim) should be provided for patients and their caregivers, including careful review of the "Information for Patients and Caregivers" insert. Patients and caregivers should be cautioned against the reuse of needles, syringes, or drug product, and be thoroughly instructed in their proper disposal. A puncture-resistant container for the disposal of used syringes and needles should be available.

Laboratory Monitoring
To assess a patient's hematologic status and ability to tolerate myelosuppressive chemotherapy, a complete blood count and platelet count should be obtained before chemotherapy is administered. Regular monitoring of hematocrit value and platelet count is recommended.

Drug Interaction
No formal drug interaction studies between Neulasta® and other drugs have been performed. Drugs such as lithium may potentiate the release of neutrophils; patients receiving lithium and Neulasta® should have more frequent monitoring of neutrophil counts.

Increased hematopoietic activity of the bone marrow in response to growth factor therapy has been associated with transient positive bone imaging changes. This should be considered when interpreting bone-imaging results.

Carcinogenesis, Mutagenesis, and Impairment of Fertility
No mutagenesis studies were conducted with pegfilgrastim. The carcinogenic potential of pegfilgrastim has not been evaluated in long-term animal studies. In a toxicity study of 6 months duration in rats given once weekly subcutaneous injections of up to 1000 mcg/kg of pegfilgrastim (approximately 23-fold higher than the recommended human dose), no precancerous or cancerous lesions were noted.

When administered once weekly via subcutaneous injections to male and female rats at doses up to 1000 mcg/kg prior to, and during mating, reproductive performance, fertility, and sperm assessment parameters were not affected.

Pregnancy Category C
Pegfilgrastim has been shown to have adverse effects in pregnant rabbits when administered subcutaneously every other day during gestation at doses as low as 50 mcg/kg/dose (approximately 4-fold higher than the recommended human dose). Decreased maternal food consumption, accompanied by a decreased maternal body weight gain and decreased fetal body weights were observed at 50 to 1000 mcg/kg/dose. Pegfilgrastim doses of 200 and 250 mcg/kg/dose resulted in an increased incidence of abortions. Increased post-implantation loss due to early resorptions was observed at doses of 200 to 1000 mcg/kg/dose, and decreased numbers of live rabbit fetuses were observed at pegfilgrastim doses of 200 to 1000 mcg/kg/dose, given every other day.

Subcutaneous injections of pegfilgrastim of up to 1000 mcg/kg/dose every other day during the period of organogenesis in rats were not associated with an embryotoxic or fetotoxic outcome. However, an increased incidence (compared to historical controls) of wavy ribs was observed in rat fetuses at 1000 mcg/kg/dose every other day. Very low levels (< 0.5%) of pegfilgrastim crossed the placenta when administered subcutaneously to pregnant rats every other day during gestation.

Once weekly subcutaneous injections of pegfilgrastim to female rats from day 6 of gestation through day 18 of lactation at doses up to 1000 mcg/kg/dose did not result in any adverse maternal effects. There were no deleterious effects on the growth and development of the offspring and no adverse effects were found upon assessment of fertility indices.

There are no adequate and well-controlled studies in pregnant women. Neulasta® should be used during pregnancy only if the potential benefit to the mother justifies the potential risk to the fetus.

Nursing Mothers
It is not known whether pegfilgrastim is excreted in human milk. Because many drugs are excreted in human milk, caution should be exercised when Neulasta® is administered to a nursing woman.

Pediatric Use
The safety and effectiveness of Neulasta® in pediatric patients have not been established. The 6 mg fixed dose single-use syringe formulation should not be used in infants, children, and smaller adolescents weighing less than 45 kg.

Geriatric Use

Of the 932 patients with cancer who received Neulasta® in clinical studies, 139 (15%) were age 65 and over, and 18 (2%) were age 75 and over. No overall differences in safety or effectiveness were observed between patients age 65 and older and younger patients.

ADVERSE REACTIONS

(See **WARNINGS**, **Splenic Rupture**, **Acute Respiratory Distress Syndrome (ARDS)**, **Allergic Reactions**, and **Sickle Cell Disorders**.)

Clinical Trial Experience

Because clinical trials are conducted under widely varying conditions, adverse reaction rates observed in the clinical trials of Neulasta® cannot be directly compared to rates in the clinical trials of other drugs and may not reflect the rates observed in practice. The adverse reaction information from clinical trials does, however, provide a basis for identifying the adverse events that appear to be related to Neulasta® use and for approximating rates.

The data described below reflect exposure to Neulasta® in 932 patients. Neulasta® was studied in placebo- and active-controlled trials (n = 467, and n = 465, respectively). The population encompassed an age range of 21 to 88 years. Ninety-two percent of patients were female. The ethnicity of the patients was as follows: 75% Caucasian, 18% Hispanic, 5% Black, and 1% Asian. Patients with solid tumors (breast [n = 823], lung and thoracic tumors [n = 53]) or lymphoma (n = 56) received Neulasta® after nonmyeloablative cytotoxic chemotherapy. Most patients received a single 100 mcg/kg (n = 259) or a single 6 mg (n = 546) dose per chemotherapy cycle over 4 cycles.

In the placebo-controlled trial, bone pain occurred at a higher incidence in Neulasta®-treated patients as compared to placebo-treated patients. The incidence of other commonly reported adverse events were similar in the Neulasta®- and placebo-treated patients, and were consistent with the underlying cancer diagnosis and its treatment with chemotherapy. The data in Table 1 reflect those adverse events occurring in at least 10% of patients treated with Neulasta® in the placebo-controlled study.

Table 1. Adverse Events Occurring in ≥10%[a] of Patients in the Placebo-Controlled Study

Event	Neulasta® (n = 467)	Placebo (n = 461)
Alopecia	48%	47%
Bone Pain[b]	31%	26%
Diarrhea	29%	28%
Pyrexia (not including febrile neutropenia)	23%	22%
Myalgia	21%	18%
Headache	16%	14%
Arthralgia	16%	13%
Vomiting	13%	11%
Asthenia	13%	11%
Peripheral Edema	12%	10%
Constipation	10%	6%

[a]Events occurring in ≥ 10% of Neulasta®-treated patients and at a higher incidence as compared to placebo-treated patients

[b]Bone pain is limited to the specified adverse event term "bone pain"

In the active controlled studies, common adverse events occurred at similar rates and severities in both treatment arms (Neulasta®, n = 465; Filgrastim, n = 331). These adverse experiences occurred at rates between 72% and 15% and included: nausea, fatigue, alopecia, diarrhea, vomiting, constipation, fever, anorexia, skeletal pain, headache, taste perversion, dyspepsia, myalgia, insomnia, abdominal pain, arthralgia, generalized weakness, peripheral edema, dizziness, granulocytopenia, stomatitis, mucositis, and neutropenic fever.

Bone Pain

The analysis of bone pain described below is based on a composite analysis using multiple, related, adverse event terms.

In the placebo-controlled study, the incidence of bone pain was 57% in Neulasta®-treated patients compared to 50% in placebo-treated patients. Bone pain was generally reported to be of mild-to-moderate severity.

Among patients experiencing bone pain, approximately 37% of Neulasta®- and 31% of placebo-treated patients utilized non-narcotic analgesics and 10% of Neulasta®- and 9% of placebo-treated patients utilized narcotic analgesics.

In the active-controlled studies, the use of non-narcotic and narcotic analgesics in association with bone pain was similar between Neulasta®- and Filgrastim-treated patients. No patient withdrew from study due to bone pain.

Laboratory Abnormalities

In clinical studies, leukocytosis (WBC counts > 100 x 10⁹/L) was observed in less than 1% of 932 patients with nonmyeloid malignancies receiving Neulasta®. Leukocytosis was not associated with any adverse effects.

Immunogenicity

As with all therapeutic proteins, there is a potential for immunogenicity. Binding antibodies to pegfilgrastim were detected using a BIAcore assay. The approximate limit of detection for this assay is 500 ng/mL. Pre-existing binding antibodies were detected in approximately 6% (51/849) of patients with metastatic breast cancer. Four of 521 pegfilgrastim-treated subjects who were negative at baseline developed binding antibodies to pegfilgrastim following treatment. None of these 4 patients had evidence of neutralizing antibodies detected using a cell-based bioassay.

The detection of antibody formation is highly dependent on the sensitivity and specificity of the assay, and the observed incidence of antibody positivity in an assay may be influenced by several factors, including sample handling, concomitant medications, and underlying disease. Therefore, comparison of the incidence of antibodies to Neulasta® with the incidence of antibodies to other products may be misleading.

Cytopenias resulting from a neutralizing antibody response to exogenous growth factors have been reported on rare occasions in patients treated with other recombinant growth factors. There is a theoretical possibility that an antibody directed against pegfilgrastim may cross-react with endogenous G-CSF, resulting in immune-mediated neutropenia. This has not been observed in clinical studies of Neulasta®.

Postmarketing Experience

The following adverse reactions have been identified during postapproval of Neulasta®. Because these reactions are reported voluntarily from a population of uncertain size, it is not always possible to reliably estimate their frequency or establish a causal relationship to drug exposure.

- splenic rupture (see **WARNINGS: Splenic Rupture**)
- acute respiratory distress syndrome (ARDS) (see **WARNINGS: Acute Respiratory Distress Syndrome**)
- allergic reactions (including anaphylaxis, skin rash, urticaria, erythema/flushing) (see **WARNINGS: Allergic Reactions**)
- sickle cell crisis (see **WARNINGS: Sickle Cell Disorders**)
- injection site pain
- Sweet's syndrome (acute febrile dermatosis)

OVERDOSAGE

The maximum amount of Neulasta® that can be safely administered in single or multiple doses has not been determined. Single subcutaneous doses of 300 mcg/kg have been administered to 8 healthy volunteers and 3 patients with non-small cell lung cancer without serious adverse effects. These patients experienced a mean maximum ANC of 55 x 10⁹/L, with a corresponding mean maximum WBC of 67 x 10⁹/L. The absolute maximum ANC observed was 96 x 10⁹/L with a corresponding absolute maximum WBC observed of 120 x 10⁹/L. The duration of leukocytosis ranged from 6 to 13 days. Leukapheresis should be considered in the management of symptomatic individuals.

DOSAGE AND ADMINISTRATION

The recommended dosage of Neulasta® is a single subcutaneous injection of 6 mg administered once per chemotherapy cycle. Neulasta® should not be administered in the period between 14 days before and 24 hours after administration of cytotoxic chemotherapy (see **PRECAUTIONS**).

The 6 mg fixed-dose formulation should not be used in infants, children, and smaller adolescents weighing less than 45 kg.

No dosing adjustment is necessary for renal dysfunction.

Neulasta® should be visually inspected for discoloration and particulate matter before administration. Neulasta® should not be administered if discoloration or particulates are observed.

Rx Only

This product, its production, and/or its use may be covered by one or more US Patents, including US Patent Nos. 5,824,784; 4,810,643; 4,999,291; 5,582,823; 5,580,755, as well as other patents or patents pending.

REFERENCE

*Heil G, Hoelzer D, Sanz MA, et al. A randomized, double-blind, placebo-controlled, phase III study of Filgrastim in remission induction and consolidation therapy for adults with de novo Acute Myeloid Leukemia. *Blood.* 1997;90:4710-4718.

v.8 Issue Date: 10/2007

Manufactured by:
Amgen Manufacturing, Limited, a subsidiary of Amgen Inc.
One Amgen Center Drive
Thousand Oaks, CA 91320-1799
©2002–2008 Amgen Inc.
All rights reserved. MC40421

CHAPTER 7

Small-cell lung cancer, mesothelioma, and thymoma

Bonnie S. Glisson, MD, Benjamin Movsas, MD, and Walter Scott, MD

As discussed in chapter 6, there are two major subdivisions of lung cancer: small-cell lung cancer (SCLC), for which chemotherapy is the primary treatment, and non–small-cell lung cancer (NSCLC). SCLC is decreasing in frequency in the United States, with recent data showing it represents only 14% of lung cancers. This chapter provides information on the staging and prognosis, pathology and pathophysiology, treatment, and follow-up of long-term survivors of SCLC and concludes with brief discussions on mesothelioma and thymoma.

Chapter 6 provides information on the epidemiology, etiology, screening and prevention, and diagnosis of lung cancer in general and covers NSCLC and carcinoid tumors of the lungs.

SMALL-CELL LUNG CANCER

Staging and prognosis

The TNM staging system, used for all NSCLC patients, does not predict well for survival in SCLC patients and is generally not utilized in SCLC, except for surgical staging (see chapter 6, Table 1). Rather, SCLC is usually described as either limited (M0) or extensive (M1), although these general terms are inadequate when evaluating the role of surgery. Patients with SCLC who have stages I–III disease, excluding those with a malignant pleural effusion, are classified as having limited disease. These patients constitute approximately one-third of all SCLC patients. The remaining SCLC patients fall into the extensive-disease category, which includes any patient with a malignant pleural effusion or any site of distant disease, such as the brain, liver, adrenal gland, bone, and bone marrow.

The staging of lung cancer must be conducted in a methodical and detailed manner to permit appropriate therapeutic recommendations and to allow comparison of treatment results from different institutions.

Stage is commonly reported as either clinical or pathologic. The former is based on noninvasive (or minimally invasive) tests, whereas the latter is based on tissue obtained during surgery (see chapter 6).

The most important prognostic factor in lung cancer is the stage of disease. Within a given disease stage, the next most important prognostic factors are performance status and recent weight loss. The two scales used to define performance status are the Eastern Cooperative Oncology Group (ECOG) performance status system and the Karnofsky performance index (see Appendix 1). In short, patients who are ambulatory have a significantly longer survival. Those who have lost ≥ 5% of body weight during the preceding 3 to 6 months have a worse prognosis.

Pathology and pathophysiology

SCLC tends to present with a large central lung mass and associated extensive hilar and mediastinal lymphadenopathy. Clinically evident distant metastases are present in approximately two-thirds of patients at diagnosis. Additionally, data from autopsy examination indicate micrometastatic disease in 63% of patients who died within 30 days of attempted curative resection of SCLC. Thus, it is a systemic disease at presentation in the majority of patients.

SCLC is a small, blue, round cell tumor that is primitive and undifferentiated at the light microscopic level. Electron microscopy demonstrates its neuroendocrine derivation by the presence of dense core granules. The immunohistochemical evidence of neuroendocrine derivation includes positive staining for chromogranin, synaptophysin, and other proteins. The APUD (amine precursor uptake and decarboxylation) machinery present in the dense core granule leads to the production of biologically active amines and promotes the synthesis of polypeptide hormones such as ADH and ACTH. Paraneoplastic syndromes due to hormone excess result. The most common of these syndromes, syndrome of inappropriate antidiuretic hormone secretion (SIADH), occurs in approximately 10% of patients with SCLC. Hypercortisolism and a Cushing's-like syndrome are more rare, seen in only 1% to 2% of patients.

Treatment

TREATMENT OF DISEASE LIMITED TO LUNG PARENCHYMA

Surgery

The majority of patients with SCLC present with advanced-stage disease. In the 5% to 10% of patients whose tumor is limited to the lung parenchyma, very often the diagnosis is established only after the lung mass has been removed. If, however, the histology has been determined by bronchoscopic biopsy or fine-needle aspiration and there is no evidence of metastatic disease following extensive scanning, examination of the bone marrow, and biopsy of the mediastinal lymph nodes, resection should be performed. Adjuvant chemotherapy is recommended because of the high likelihood of the development of distant metastases following surgery.

The surgical approach in SCLC is similar to that used in NSCLC: A lobectomy or pneumonectomy should be followed by a thorough mediastinal lymph node dissection. Tumor resection in SCLC should be limited to patients who have no evidence of mediastinal or supraclavicular lymph node metastases. Recent data suggest that patients with SCLC, presenting as a solitary pulmonary nodule and proven pathologically to be stage I, have a 5-year survival rate of ~70% when treated with resection and adjuvant chemotherapy.

TREATMENT OF DISEASE LIMITED TO THE THORAX

Approximately one-third of SCLC patients present with disease that is limited to the thorax and can be encompassed within a tolerable radiation portal. In early studies in which either radiation therapy or surgery alone was used to treat such patients, median survival was only 3 to 4 months, and the 5-year survival rate was in the range of 1% to 2%. The reason for the failure of these therapies was both rapid recurrence of intrathoracic tumor and development of distant metastasis.

Chemotherapy

During the 1970s, it became apparent that SCLC was relatively sensitive to chemotherapy. Various combination chemotherapy regimens were used to treat limited SCLC. Although none of the regimens was clearly superior, median survival was approximately 12 months, and the 2-year survival rate was approximately 10% to 15%. It appears that maintenance chemotherapy adds little to survival in patients with limited SCLC.

Chemotherapy plus thoracic irradiation

One of the major advances in treating SCLC in the past 15 years is the recognition of the value of early and concurrent thoracic chemoradiation therapy. This advance was clearly facilitated by the increase in therapeutic index when PE (cisplatin [Platinol]/etoposide) chemotherapy is given with thoracic irradiation, as opposed to older anthracycline- or alkylator-based regimens. Although the major impact from this approach is improved locoregional control, there are also hints from randomized trials that early control of disease in the chest can also reduce the risk of distant metastasis.

An intergroup trial directly compared once-daily with twice-daily fractionation (45 Gy/25 fractions/5 weeks vs 45 Gy/30 fractions/3 weeks) given at the beginning of concurrent chemoradiation therapy with PE. Initial analysis showed excellent overall results, with median survival for all patients of 20 months and a 40% survival rate to 2 years. With a minimum follow-up of 5 years, survival was significantly better in the twice-daily than in the once-daily irradiation group (26% vs 16%). The only difference in toxicity was a temporary increase in grade 3 esophagitis in patients receiving twice-daily radiation therapy.

Outcomes for patients with limited-stage SCLC have improved significantly over the past 20 years. In an analysis of phase III trials during this period, median survival was 12 months in the control arm in 26 phase III studies initiated between 1972 and 1981, compared with 17 months in studies between 1982 and 1992 ($P < .001$). Five studies demonstrated a statistically significant improvement in survival in the experimental arm compared with the control arm. Interestingly, all five studies involved some aspect of thoracic radiation therapy (three trials compared chemotherapy alone vs chemoradiation therapy; one compared early with late radiation therapy; and one compared daily vs twice-daily thoracic radiation therapy). Similarly, data from the Surveillance, Epidemiology, and End Results (SEER) database demonstrate that the 5-year survival rate has more than doubled from 1973 to 1996 (5.2% vs 12.2%; $P = .0001$).

Current recommendations Although important questions remain as to the optimal radiation doses, volumes, and timing with regard to chemotherapy, a reasonable standard is to deliver thoracic irradiation concurrently with PE chemotherapy (cisplatin [60 mg/m^2 IV on day 1] and etoposide [120 mg/m^2 IV on days 1–3]). An attempt is made to integrate thoracic irradiation as early as possible, during cycle 1 (or 2). Fried et al performed a meta-analysis evaluating early versus late timing of radiation therapy in limited-stage SCLC. Earlier radiation therapy was defined as prior to 9 weeks after initiation of chemotherapy versus late radiation therapy ($\geq$ 9 weeks). Seven trials (n = 1,542 patients) were included in the analysis. They reported a small but significant improvement in 2-year overall survival for early versus late radiation therapy (5.2%; $P = .03$). This finding is similar to the benefit of adding radiation therapy or prophylactic cranial irradiation to chemotherapy. A greater difference was evident for the subset of patients receiving early rather than late hyperfractionated radiation therapy and platinum-based chemotherapy. Hyperfractionated accelerated fractionation should be considered, given the results of the intergroup 0096 trial. An intergroup phase III study is under way to compare twice-daily radiation therapy to 45 Gy versus once-daily with radiation therapy to a higher dose (70 Gy) versus a modified regimen combining these strategies.

Irradiation can be incorporated sequentially with chemotherapy; however, this approach appears to be inferior to early concurrent therapy and should be reserved for use in those for whom concurrent approaches are predicted to be excessively toxic. Takada et al reported on a randomized trial of concurrent versus sequential thoracic radiotherapy in combination with PE in over 200 patients with limited-stage SCLC; they demonstrated a benefit to concurrent therapy, with a median survival of 27.0 months (30%, concurrent arm) versus 19.7 months (20%, sequential arm; $P = .097$). Thoracic radiation therapy consisted of 45 Gy over 3 weeks, starting either with the first cycle of PE in the concurrent arm or after the fourth cycle in the sequential arm.

Results of an intergroup trial indicate that radiation therapy strategies that increase biologic dose can improve local control and survival. Further exploration of accelerated fractionation or conventional doses > 45 Gy is warranted and is currently being investigated in prospective trials.

Komaki et al reported on a phase I dose-escalation trial of thoracic radiotherapy with concurrent chemotherapy (Radiation Therapy Oncology Group [RTOG] 9712). In this regimen, the initial (larger) radiation field was treated once a day, and the smaller boost field was treated twice daily, to a maximum tolerated dose of 61.2 Gy.

Movsas et al reported the results of the first Patterns of Care Study (PCS) for lung cancer in the United States. This study was conducted to determine the national patterns of radiotherapy practice in patients treated for nonmetastatic lung cancer in 1998–1999. As supported by clinical trials, patients with limited-stage SCLC received chemotherapy plus radiotherapy more often than radiotherapy alone (92% vs 5%; $P < .0001$). However, the median radiotherapy dose was 50 Gy, 80% at 1.8 to 2.0 Gy per fraction. Only 6% of patients received hyperfractionated (twice-daily) radiotherapy. A total of 22% received prophylactic cranial irradiation (PCI), with a median dose of 30 Gy in 15 fractions. As key studies supporting twice-daily radiotherapy in PCI and NSCLC were published in 1999, the penetration of these trials will be assessed in the next PCS lung survey.

Interestingly, Choi et al reported long-term survival data from their phase I trial assessing chemotherapy with either standard daily radiotherapy or accelerated twice-daily radiotherapy as from the Cancer and Leukemia Group B (CALGB) 8837 trial. They previously reported that the maximum tolerated dose was 45 Gy in 30 fractions for twice-daily radiotherapy and > 70 Gy in 35 fractions for once-daily radiotherapy. The 5-year survival estimated (from this phase I trial) for the twice-daily arm was 20%, versus 36% for the once-daily radiotherapy arm.

Surgery

Although surgical resection is not usually part of the standard therapy for SCLC, the Japanese Clinical Oncology Lung Cancer Study Group reported the results of a phase II trial of postoperative adjuvant PE in patients with completely resected stages I–IIIA SCLC. The 5-year survival rates (in a cohort of 62 patients) for pathologic stages I, II, and IIIA SCLC were 69%, 38%, and 40%, respectively.

The role of surgery for stage II or IIIA SCLC has evolved from a number of phase II trials and retrospective case series to include specific indications; they include resection of tumors with mixed histology (containing both SCLC and NSCLC components), salvage surgery for chemoresistant localized SCLC or local relapse after initial response to chemoradiotherapy, or second primary tumors after cure of initial SCLC. Johnson has shown that the rate of second primary NSCLC in patients treated for SCLC can be as high as 2% to greater than 10% per year.

Prospective, randomized trials are ongoing in Europe and Japan to examine the role of surgery as part of multimodality therapy for patients with stages II and IIIA SCLC.

Prophylactic cranial irradiation

Recognition that patients with SCLC were at high risk for the development of brain metastases led to the suggestion that they be given PCI to prevent the clinical manifestation of previously present but occult CNS disease. The role of PCI has been controversial. Most trials have shown a reduction in CNS relapse rates but little effect on survival with PCI. There also has been concern about the contribution of PCI to the late neurologic deterioration seen in some patients with SCLC, although recent studies show neurologic impairment in many patients with SCLC prior to any treatment.

A meta-analysis of all randomized trials of PCI in patients with SCLC who achieved a complete or near-complete response to induction chemotherapy (alone or combined with thoracic irradiation) showed a statistically significant improvement in survival in patients treated with PCI (20.7% at 3 years vs 15.3% in those not given PCI). The survival improvement with PCI was seen in all patient subgroups, regardless of age, stage of disease, type of induction treatment, or performance status. Approximately 85% of the patients included in the meta-analysis had limited disease, and recommendations for use of PCI have been applied generally to this subgroup. A recent randomized trial, however, suggests benefit for PCI in patients with responding extensive disease as well (see sidebar).

Model calculations from data on patterns of failure in patients achieving a systemic complete response suggest that the greatest gain in survival to be expected with PCI is in the range of 5%. To demonstrate this convincingly would require randomized trials of about 700 patients–substantially larger than trials conducted to date. However, the recent meta-analysis of randomized trials of PCI in SCLC patients achieving complete or near-complete response of systemic disease showed a survival improvement of this magnitude with PCI.

Current recommendations Patients should be offered PCI after completion of chemotherapy/chemoradiation therapy if they have clear regression of disease and a retained ECOG performance status of 0 to 2. It should optimally be integrated within 3 to 5 weeks of the last cycle of chemotherapy.

TABLE 1: Common chemotherapy regimens for SCLC

Drug/combination	Dose and schedule
Etoposide + cisplatin or carboplatin	
Etoposide	100-120 mg/m^2 IV on days 1-3
Cisplatin	60-75 mg/m^2 IV on day 1
	or
Etoposide	100 mg/m^2 IV on days 1-3
Carboplatin	Area under the curve of 5 mg/mL/min IV on day 1
Repeat cycle every 3 weeks.	
Irinotecan + cisplatin	
Irinotecan	60 mg/m^2 on days 1, 8, and 15
Cisplatin	60 mg/m^2 IV on day 1
Repeat cycle every 4 weeks for 4 cycles.	

Noda K, Nishiwaki Y, Kawahara M, et al: N Engl J Med 346:85–91, 2002.

Table prepared by Ishmael Jaiyesimi, DO

Radiation doses for PCI should probably be in the range of 25 to 30 Gy, with a daily fraction size of 2.0 to 2.5 Gy, although recent data suggest that such doses delay and reduce rates of CNS relapse but may not eliminate it; thus, higher doses may warrant exploration. Larger fraction sizes would be expected to produce greater toxicity. Smaller fractions given twice daily may reduce toxicity, and trials of this approach are under way.

TREATMENT OF EXTENSIVE DISEASE

As mentioned previously, two-thirds of SCLC patients have extensive disease at diagnosis. Without treatment, median survival in this group of patients is 6 to 8 weeks. Treatment with combination chemotherapy increases the median survival duration to approximately 8 to 10 months.

Induction chemotherapy

The combination of cisplatin or carboplatin/etoposide (see Table 1 for common dose ranges) is considered the standard of care in the United States at this time. This standard is primarily based on therapeutic index, as randomized trials have not demonstrated a survival benefit for this combination relative to the older regimen of cyclophosphamide, doxorubicin, and vincristine. The regimen is repeated at 3-week intervals for 4 to 6 courses. In North America, multiple randomized trials of newer cytotoxins replacing etoposide in a doublet with cisplatin, or added to the etoposide/platin base, have not provided a survival benefit. Japanese data that showed a 3.4-month survival advantage for irinotecan (Camptosar), as opposed to etoposide, with cisplatin were not confirmed in a trial in the US. A second North American study, reproducing the Japanese trial, has completed accrual and is pending analysis.

TREATMENT OF PERSISTENT DISEASE

Progressive SCLC is classified based on response and duration of response to initial induction therapy. Patients whose tumors do not regress or progress up to 60 to 90 days following the last cycle of chemotherapy are considered to have refractory disease. Conversely, patients whose tumors respond and who have an unmaintained progression-free interval longer than 60 to 90 days, are deemed to have sensitive relapse. This categorization is based on the probability of objective response to additional cytotoxic therapy, which is uncommon, typically less than 15%, in the case of platin-refractory SCLC.

Topotecan (Hycamtin) is the only drug approved by the US Food and Drug Administration (FDA) for the treatment of recurrent disease. Its initial indication in 1998 was in patients with sensitive relapse and was based on similar efficacy compared with an older three-drug regimen. A subsequent trial compared intravenous administration with oral topotecan capsules, documenting similar efficacy and tolerance. Most recently, a randomized trial of 141 patients, ECOG performance status of 0 to 2, compared oral topotecan with best supportive care. Patients with both refractory and sensitive disease were accrued. Median survival was nearly doubled on the topotecan arm, 26 versus 14 weeks ($P = .0104$), as was 6-month survival, 49% versus 26%. Benefit was seen in all subgroups analyzed, including patients with refractory cancer and an ECOG performance status of 2. Despite a low rate of response to topotecan of 7% and typical side effects, treated patients had slower deterioration of quality of life and improved symptom control. Based on these data, the FDA granted topotecan in capsule form a broad indication for treatment of recurrent SCLC in October 2007.

More limited data with irinotecan suggest its activity is probably similar to that of topotecan; however, it has never been evaluated in a randomized trial in the recurrent setting.

Other cytotoxins, known more for their efficacy in NSCLC, such as docetaxel (Taxotere) and paclitaxel, gemcitabine (Gemzar), and vinorelbine, do not have high single-agent response rates in therapy-naive SCLC and are not recognized as standard in management.

Integration of biologics in therapy

Ongoing clinical research is focused on integration of molecularly targeted therapy in an effort to make progress in treating this stubborn malignancy. At this time, data from completed trials do not indicate an active strategy with a biologic, whether in combination with induction chemotherapy, as maintenance following induction, or as single agents for recurrent disease.

High-dose chemotherapy plus bone marrow transplant (BMT) Most phase II trials using high doses of chemotherapy plus BMT appear to show no advantage to the high-dose approach over standard doses of chemotherapy.

Alternating chemotherapy regimens have been used to overcome drug resistance. In randomized trials, alternating chemotherapy regimens have shown a slight improvement in terms of median survival (4–6 weeks) when compared with a single chemotherapeutic regimen but no improvement in long-term survival.

PALLIATION OF LOCAL AND DISTANT SYMPTOMS

Radiation therapy

Many patients with lung cancer have distressing local symptoms at some point in their disease course. These symptoms may arise from airway obstruction by the primary tumor, compression of mediastinal structures by nodal metastases, or metastatic involvement of distant organs. Radiation therapy is effective in palliating most local symptoms as well as symptoms at common metastatic sites, such as bone and brain.

Doses In the United States, most radiation oncologists use doses in the range of 30 Gy in 10 fractions for palliative treatment. Data from the United Kingdom suggest that similar efficacy without greater toxicity may be achieved with more abbreviated schedules, such as 17 Gy in 2 fractions 1 week apart or single fractions of 11 Gy (see chapter 6, Table 8). Such schedules may facilitate the coordination of irradiation and chemotherapy and also may reduce patient travel and hospitalization.

Endobronchial irradiation with cobalt-60 or iridium-192 has been used to palliate symptoms arising from partial airway obstruction, including cough, dyspnea, and hemoptysis. The dosimetric advantage of being able to deliver a high radiation dose to the obstructing endobronchial tumor while sparing adjacent normal structures, such as the lungs, spinal cord, and esophagus, has clear appeal, particularly in the patient whose disease has recurred following prior external-beam irradiation. Although good rates of palliation have been reported with endobronchial irradiation, significant complications, including fatal hemoptysis, are seen in 5% to 10% of patients. Whether this represents a true treatment complication versus the underlying disease remains unclear.

Other local approaches

Endobronchial irradiation should be considered as only one of several approaches (including laser excision, cryotherapy, and stent placement) in the treatment of patients with symptomatic airway obstruction, and management should be individualized. All of these approaches are more suitable for partial than for complete airway obstruction.

Chemotherapy

Several recent trials have explored the use of chemotherapy to palliate specific symptoms in patients with lung cancer. In general, these trials have found that rates of symptomatic improvement were considerably higher than objective response rates and were not dissimilar to symptomatic response rates with local radiation therapy. Chemotherapy in the newly diagnosed patient is highly palliative for relief of symptoms related to superior vena cava syndrome, obstructive lung disease, and painful bony metastases. In the patient with recurrent disease, irradiation is more commonly associated with symptomatic relief from these localized problems. Radiation therapy remains the standard of care for even chemotherapy-naive patients with spinal cord compression or symptomatic brain metastasis.

Follow-up of long-term survivors

At present, no standard follow-up protocol exists for patients with cured SCLC or NSCLC. However, at least long-term follow-up should include serial physical examinations once the patient has reached the 5-year mark. Controversy currently exists about the value of utilizing CT scanning or even chest x-rays for the long-term follow-up of these patients.

In this vein, retrospective reviews of the literature have revealed that patients with SCLC appear to have the highest rate of second primary tumor development, as high as 30% over the course of their lifetime, with some studies reporting annual second primary tumor rates of 5% to 10%. Therefore, the concept of chemoprevention appears to have particular merit in these patients.

MESOTHELIOMA

Mesotheliomas are uncommon neoplasms derived from the cells lining the pleura and peritoneum. Currently, 2,000 to 3,000 new cases are diagnosed in the United States each year.

Epidemiology

Gender Men are affected five times more commonly than women.

Age The median age at diagnosis is 60 years.

Etiology and risk factors

Asbestos exposure The relationship between asbestos exposure and diffuse pleural mesothelioma was first reported by Wagner, who documented 33 pathologically confirmed cases from an asbestos mining region in South Africa. Selikoff and colleagues documented a 300-fold increase in mortality from mesothelioma among asbestos insulation workers in the New York metropolitan region when compared with the general population. The interval between asbestos exposure and tumor formation is commonly 3 to 4 decades.

Asbestos fibers are generally divided into two broad groups: serpentine and amphibole. The latter includes crocidolite, the most carcinogenic form of asbestos. The inability of phagocytic cells to digest the fiber appears to initiate a cascade of cellular events that results in free-radical generation and carcinogenesis.

Diagnosis

Patients with mesothelioma usually seek medical attention while the disease is limited to a single hemithorax and commonly complain of dyspnea and pain.

Dyspnea results from diffuse growth of the tumor on both the parietal and visceral pleurae, which encase the lung in a thick rind. Pain is caused by direct tumor infiltration of intercostal nerves.

Chest x-ray and CT Chest x-ray demonstrates pleural thickening, pleura-based masses, or a pleural effusion. Chest computed tomography (CT) scan more accurately portrays the extent of disease and frequently reveals chest wall invasion, as well as pericardial and diaphragmatic extension.

Thoracentesis and thoracoscopy Thoracentesis and pleural biopsy usually are sufficient to establish the diagnosis of malignancy, but a thoracoscopic or open biopsy is often required to provide enough tissue to make an accurate histologic diagnosis of mesothelioma.

Distinguishing mesothelioma from other neoplasms Light microscopy is often insufficient for differentiating among mesothelioma, metastatic adeno-carcinoma, and sarcoma. Immunohistochemistry and electron microscopy are frequently necessary to establish the diagnosis.

Although adenocarcinomas stain positive for carcinoembryonic antigen (CEA), Leu-M1, and secretory component, mesotheliomas stain negative for these markers. Mesotheliomas stain positive for cytokeratin, whereas sarcomas do not. Mesotheliomas have characteristically long microvilli that are well demonstrated by the electron microscope; adenocarcinomas have short microvilli.

Pathology

Mesotheliomas may contain both epithelial and sarcomatoid elements and are classified by the relative abundance of each component. Epithelial mesotheliomas are most common (50%), followed by mixed (34%) and sarcomatoid (16%) tumors. Survival for the epithelial type is 22 months, compared with only 6 months for patients with other types.

Staging and prognosis

The International Mesothelioma Interest Group has developed a staging system based on TNM descriptors. This was adopted by the AJCC (Table 2). Another commonly utilized staging system for mesothelioma, that of Butchart, is based on inexact descriptions of the extent of local tumor growth or distant metastases (Table 3). Other, more detailed staging systems based on TNM criteria have been proposed.

The median survival following diagnosis ranges from 9–21 months. Although autopsy series have demonstrated distant metastases in as many as 50% of patients with mesothelioma, death usually results from local tumor growth.

Position emission tomography (PET) scanning may prove to be a viable prognostic tool for malignant pleural mesothelioma.

TABLE 2: New International Staging System for Diffuse MPM

(T) Tumor

T1a   Tumor limited to the ipsilateral parietal pleura, including mediastinal and diaphragmatic pleura

        No involvement of the visceral pleura

T1b   Tumor involving the ipsilateral parietal pleura, including mediastinal and diaphragmatic pleura

        Scattered foci of tumor also involving the visceral pleura

T2   Tumor involving each of the ipsilateral pleural surfaces (parietal, mediastinal, and diaphragmatic, and visceral)

        Involvement of diaphragmatic muscle

        Confluent visceral pleural tumor (including the fissures) or extension of tumor from visceral pleura into the underlying pulmonary parenchyma

T3   Locally advanced but potentially resectable tumor; tumor involving all of the ipsilateral pleural surfaces (parietal, mediastinal, diaphragmatic, and visceral)

        Involvement of the endothoracic fascia

        Extension into mediastinal fat

        Solitary, completely resectable focus of tumor extending into the soft tissues of the chest wall

        Nontransmural involvement of the pericardium

T4   Locally advanced technically unresectable tumor; tumor involving all of the ipsilateral pleural surfaces (parietal, mediastinal, diaphragmatic, and visceral)

        Diffuse extension or multifocal masses of tumor in the chest wall, with or without associated rib destruction

        Direct transdiaphragmatic extension of tumor to the peritoneum

        Direct extension of tumor to one or more mediastinal organs

        Direct extension of tumor into the spine

        Tumor extending through to the internal surface of the pericardium with or without a pericardial effusion; or tumor involving the myocardium

(N) Lymph nodes

Nx   Regional lymph nodes cannot be assessed

N0   No regional lymph node metastases

N1   Metastases in the ipsilateral bronchopulmonary or hilar lymph nodes

N2   Metastases in subcarinal or ipsilateral mediastinal lymph nodes, including ipsilateral internal mammary nodes

N3   Metastases in contralateral mediastinal, contralateral internal mammary, and ipsilateral or contralateral supraclavicular lymph nodes

(M) Metastasis

Mx   Distant metastasis not assessable

M0   No distant metastasis

M1   Distant metastasis present

Stage

Stage I

    Ia   T1aN0M0

    Ib   T1bN0M0

Stage II   T2N0M0

Stage III   Any T3M0

        Any N1M0

        Any N2M0

Stage IV   Any T4

        Any N3

        Any M1

MPM = Malignant pleural mesothelioma

From Greene FL, Page DL, Fleming ID, et al (eds): AJCC Cancer Staging Manual, 6th ed. New York, Springer-Verlag, 2002.

TABLE 3: Staging of mesothelioma according to Butchart

Stage	Description
I	Tumor confined within the "capsule" of the parietal pleura, ie, involving only the ipsilateral pleura, lungs, pericardium, and diaphragm
II	Tumor invading the chest wall or involving mediastinal structures, eg, the esophagus, heart, opposite pleura; lymph node involvement within the chest
III	Tumor penetrating the diaphragm to involve the peritoneum; involvement of opposite pleura; lymph node involvement outside the chest
IV	Distant blood-borne metastases

Treatment

Treatment rarely results in cure and should be considered palliative.

Combined-modality treatment options include chest tube insertion and pleurodesis to control the pleural effusion. Currently, there is renewed interest in aggressive treatment that includes extrapleural pneumonectomy with concomitant resection of the diaphragm and pericardium, followed by chemotherapy and radiotherapy. Recent studies are exploring the role of postoperative intensity-modulated radiotherapy in this setting. Subtotal pleurectomy is a less extensive surgical procedure that debulks the majority of tumor, permits reexpansion of the lung, and prevents recurrence of the pleural effusion.

Chemotherapy The benefit of chemotherapy for patients who have unresectable mesothelioma was clarified in a randomized trial. This study was a single-blind, multicenter, two-arm trial with cisplatin alone in the control arm and cisplatin combined with the multitargeted antifolate pemetrexed (Alimta) in the experimental arm. The study was based on the observation that pemetrexed produced a 16% objective response rate in previous phase II evaluation. In the randomized trial, patients treated with pemetrexed and cisplatin had an estimated median survival of 12.1 months, as compared with 9.3 months in those treated with cisplatin alone. On the basis of this improvement in survival, the combination of pemetrexed and cisplatin has received an FDA indication for the treatment of unresectable mesothelioma. The same combination is undergoing further evaluation in a neoadjuvant approach in patients with resectable disease.

THYMOMA

Thymoma is a rare mediastinal tumor that occurs mainly in the anterosuperior mediastinum.

TABLE 4: World Health Organization histologic classification of thymoma

World Health Organization (WHO) classification	Histiogenetic classification (Müller-Hermelink)
A	Medullary thymoma
AB	Mixed thymoma
B1	Predominantly cortical thymoma
B2	Cortical thymoma
B3	Well-differentiated thymic carcinoma

C
   Epidermoid keratinizing
     carcinoma (squamous cell)
   Epidermoid nonkeratinizing
     carcinoma
   Lymphoepithelioma-like carcinoma
   Sarcomatoid carcinoma
   Basaloid carcinoma
   Mucoepidermoid carcinoma
   Undifferentiated carcinoma
	Thymic carcinoma

A = atrophic, similar to that of an adult thymus; B = bioactive; C = cancer (with obvious signs of cell mitoses)

Epidemiology

Gender The tumor affects both sexes equally.

Age Thymoma is most often seen in people in the fourth and fifth decades of life.

Etiology and associated syndromes

The etiology of thymoma is unknown, and the risk factors have not been identified. Thymoma is a tumor originating within the epithelial cells of the thymus. One-third to one-half of patients present with an asymptomatic anterior mediastinal mass, one-third present with local symptoms (eg, cough, chest pain, superior vena cava syndrome, and/or dysphagia), and one-third of cases are detected during the evaluation of myasthenia gravis. Distant metastases are distinctly uncommon at initial presentation of this tumor.

In addition to myasthenia gravis, which occurs in approximately 30% of patients with thymoma, a host of paraneoplastic syndromes have been seen in association with thymoma. These other syndromes, which occur in less than 5% of patients, include pure red cell aplasia, hypogammaglobulinemia, and a variety of other autoimmune disorders.

Diagnosis

The most commonly described symptoms are pleuritic chest pain or discomfort, dry cough, and dyspnea. Physical examination may reveal adenopathy, wheezing, fever, superior vena cava syndrome, vocal cord paralysis, and other paraneoplastic syndromes.

Chest x-ray and CT scan A chest x-ray provides an initial basis for diagnosis. The location, size, density, and presence of calcification within the mass can all be determined. Comparison of the film to previously obtained films is usually helpful.

Following identification of a mediastinal mass on conventional radiography, contrast-enhanced CT scanning should be performed. CT scanning can differentiate the cystic form from a solid lesion as well as the presence of fat, calcium, or fluid within the lesion. Magnetic resonance imaging (MRI) is increasingly available for use in the evaluation of mediastinal pathology, but it is less frequently utilized than CT. MRI is superior to CT scanning in defining the relationship between mediastinal masses and vascular structures and is useful in the assessment of vascular invasion by the tumor.

Invasive diagnostic tests CT-guided percutaneous needle biopsy specimens are obtained using fine-needle aspiration techniques and cytologic evaluation or with larger-core needle biopsy and histologic evaluation. Fine-needle specimens are usually adequate to distinguish carcinomatosis lesions, but core biopsies may be necessary to distinguish most mediastinal neoplasms. Immunohistochemical techniques and electron microscopy have greatly improved the ability to differentiate the cell of origin in mediastinal neoplasms. Most series reported diagnostic yields for percutaneous needle biopsy of 70% to 100%.

Mediastinoscopy is a relatively simple surgical procedure accomplished with the patient under general anesthesia. It is an adequate approach to the superior, middle, and upper posterior mediastinum, and most series report a diagnostic accuracy of 80% to 90%. Anterior mediastinotomy (Chamberlain approach) provides for direct biopsy of tissue and has a diagnostic yield of 95% to 100%. Thoracotomy is occasionally necessary to diagnose mediastinal neoplasms, but its indications have been largely supplanted by video-assisted thoracoscopic techniques, which yield 100% accuracy.

The most common tumors in the differential diagnosis of an anterior mediastinal tumor are lymphomas and germ-cell tumors. Immunohistochemical markers are helpful to differentiate thymoma from tumors originating from other cell types.

Pathology

Two of the most common classification schemes for thymoma are listed in Table 4. Verley and Hollman propose a classification system based on tumor architecture, cellular differentiation, and predominant cell type. Bernatz et al describe a simpler classification by presenting thymoma based on the percentage of epithelial cells and lymphocytes. In both of these systems, thymoma with a predominance of epithelial cells is associated with a greater increased incidence of invasion and a subsequently worse prognosis.

Staging and prognosis

The staging system proposed by Masaoka et al has been widely adopted. Stage is an independent predictor of recurrence and long-term survival. The 5-year survival rates are 96% for stage I thymoma, 86% for stage II, 69% for stage III, and 50% for stage IV.

Treatment

SURGICAL TREATMENT

All patients whose tumors are potentially resectable should undergo surgery. If the patient has evidence of myasthenia gravis, a preoperative consultation with a clinical neurologist should be considered. The incision of choice is almost always a median sternotomy, which is quick and easy to make and provides excellent exposure to the anterior mediastinum and neck. Although the surgeon is considered the best judge of a tumor's invasiveness, it is often difficult to grossly separate invasion from adherence to surrounding tissue. Experience with minimally invasive approaches (such as transcervical thymectomy) is growing; however, until longer term data become available, sternotomy should still be considered the standard surgical approach.

Complete resection of thymoma has been found to be the most significant predictor of long-term survival. Several studies have examined the extent of surgical resection on survival and disease-free survival rates. In 241 operative cases, Maggi and colleagues found an 82% overall survival rate in those whose tumors underwent complete resection and a 26% survival rate at 7 years in those undergoing biopsy alone. Other investigators reported similar results in surgical patients. Therefore, regardless of stage, tumor resectability is one of the important predictors of treatment outcome.

RADIATION TREATMENT

Thymomas are generally radiosensitive tumors, and the use of radiation therapy in their treatment is well established. It has been used to treat all stages of thymoma, either before or after surgical resection. General agreement exists regarding the postoperative treatment of invasive thymoma (stages II and III). The value of adjuvant radiation therapy for invasive thymomas is well documented and should be included in the treatment regimen regardless of the completeness of tumor resection.

CHEMOTHERAPY

Chemotherapy has been used in the treatment of invasive thymomas with increasing frequency during the past decade (Table 5). The most active agents appear to be cisplatin, doxorubicin, ifosfamide, and corticosteroids. Combina-

TABLE 5: Common chemotherapy regimens for thymoma

Regimen	Dose and schedule
CAPPr	
Cyclophosphamide	500 mg/m^2 IV on day 1
Adriamycin (doxorubicin)	20 mg/m^2/d infused continuously on days 1-3
Platinol (cisplatin)	30 mg/m^2/d IV on days 1-3
Prednisone	100 mg/d PO on days 1-5
Repeat cycle every 3-4 weeks.	

Adapted from Shin DM, Walsh GL, Komaki R, et al: Ann Intern Med 129:100–104, 1998.

Single agent	
Cisplatin	100 mg/m^2 IV on day 1
Appropriate IV prehydration, posthydration along with mannitol and electrolytes	
Repeat cycle every 3 weeks.	

Adapted from Bonomi PD, Finkelstein D, Aisner S, et al: Am J Clin Oncol 16:342–345, 1993.

Ifosfamide	1.5 g/m^2 infused continuously on days 1-5
Mesna	Continuous infusion as appropriate
Repeat cycle every 3 weeks.	

Adapted from Highley MS, Underhill CR, Parnis FX, et al: J Clin Oncol 17:2737–2744, 1999.

Table prepared by Ishmael Jaiyesimi, DO

tion chemotherapy has generally shown higher response rates and has been used in both neoadjuvant and adjuvant settings and in the treatment of metastatic or recurrent thymomas. CAP or CAPPr (cyclophosphamide, Adriamycin [doxorubicin], Platinol [cisplatin], and prednisone) regimens have been used in neoadjuvant and/or adjuvant settings. These regimens have also been used for recurrent thymoma.

Unresectable thymoma

Advanced-stage (III/IVA) thymomas are usually difficult to remove completely. Multidisciplinary approaches, including induction chemotherapy followed by surgical resection, postoperative radiation therapy, and consolidation chemotherapy, have been reported.

Induction chemotherapy consists of cyclophosphamide (500 mg/m^2 IV on day 1), doxorubicin (20 mg/m^2/d, continuous infusion, on days 1–3), cisplatin (30 mg/m^2/d IV on days 1–3), and prednisone (100 mg/d PO on days 1–5), repeated every 3–4 weeks for 3 courses. Twenty-two evaluable patients were consecutively treated from 1990 to 2000 in a prospective phase II study at M. D. Anderson Cancer Center. After induction chemotherapy, 17 of 22 patients (77%) had major responses, including 3 complete responses.

Twenty-one patients underwent surgical resection. All patients received post-operative radiation therapy and consolidation chemotherapy. With a median follow-up of 50.3 months, overall survival rates at 5 years and 7 years were 95% and 79%, respectively. The rate of disease progression-free survival was 77% at 5 and 7 years. The multidisciplinary approaches to unresectable thymoma appear to be promising.

SUGGESTED READING

ON SMALL-CELL LUNG CANCER

Blackhall FH, Shepherd FA: Small cell lung cancer and targeted therapies. Curr Opin Oncol 19:103–108, 2007.

De Ruysscher D, Pijls-Johannesma M, Bentzen SM, et al: Time between the first day of chemotherapy and the last day of chest radiation is the most important predictor of survival in limited-disease small-cell lung cancer. J Clin Oncol 24:1057–1063, 2006.

Fried DB, Morris DE, Poole C, et al: Systematic review evaluating the timing of thoracic radiation therapy in combined modality therapy for limited-stage small-cell lung cancer. J Clin Oncol 22:4837–4845, 2004.

Glisson BS: Recurrent small cell lung cancer: Update. Semin Oncol 30:72–8, 2003.

Hanna N, Bunn PA Jr, Langer C, et al: Randomized phase III trial comparing irinotecan/cisplatin with etoposide/cisplatin in patients with previously untreated extensive-stage small-cell lung cancer. J Clin Oncol 24:2038–2043, 2006.

Movsas B, Moughan J, Komaki R, et al: Radiotherapy (RT) Patterns of Care Study (PCS) in lung carcinoma. J Clin Oncol 24:4553–4559, 2003.

O'Brien ME, Ciuleanu TE, Tsekov H, et al: Phase III trial comparing supportive care alone with supportive care with oral topotecan in patients with relapsed small-cell lung cancer. J Clin Oncol 24:5441–5447, 2006.

Slotman B, Faivre-Finn C, Kramer G, et al: Prophylactic cranial irradiation in extensive small-cell lung cancer. N Engl J Med 357:664–672, 2007.

ON MESOTHELIOMA

Flores RM, Zakowski M, Venkatraman E, et al: Prognostic factors in the treatment of malignant pleural mesothelioma at a large tertiary referral center. J Thorac Oncol 2:957–965, 2007.

Hazarika M, White RM Jr, Booth BP, et al: Pemetrexed in malignant pleural mesothelioma. Clin Cancer Res 11:982–992, 2005.

ON THYMOMA

Huang J, Rizk NP, Travis WD, et al: Feasibility of multimodality therapy including extended resections in stage IVA thymoma. J Thorac Cardiovasc Surg 134:1477–1483, 2007.

Kim ES, Putnam JB, Komaki R, et al: A phase II study of a multidisciplinary approach with induction chemotherapy, followed by surgical resection, radiation therapy, and consolidation chemotherapy for unresectable malignant thymomas: Final report. Lung Cancer 44:369–379, 2004.

CHAPTER 8

Breast cancer overview
Risk factors, screening, genetic testing, and prevention

Lori Jardines, MD, Bruce G. Haffty, MD, Paul Fisher, MD,
Jeffrey Weitzel, MD, and Melanie Royce, MD, PhD

Breast cancer is the most common malignancy in women, accounting for 31% of all female cancers. Breast cancer also is responsible for 15% of cancer deaths in women, making it the number-two cause of cancer death. An estimated 182,460 new invasive breast cancer cases will be diagnosed in women in the United States in 2008, and 40,480 women will die of this cancer. There are approximately 2 million breast cancer survivors in the United States.

This chapter provides an overview of breast cancer, with discussions of epidemiology, etiology and risk factors, genetic cancer risk assessment, signs and symptoms, screening and diagnosis, prevention (including lifestyle changes and chemoprevention), staging, and prognosis. The three chapters to follow focus on the management of stages 0 and I, stage II, and stages III and IV breast cancers.

Epidemiology

Gender Breast cancer is relatively uncommon in men; the female-to-male ratio is approximately 100:1. It accounts for < 1% of all cancer cases in men, and an estimated 450 men will die of the disease in 2008. The incidence of breast cancer in men has remained relatively stable over the past decades, except in Africa, where for unclear reasons the incidence is rising. *BRCA* mutations are associated with an increased risk for breast cancer in men.

The most common presentation in men is asymmetric gynecomastia, often related to a single effect of drug therapy (such as from digoxin) or liver failure. All palpable masses in men should be carefully examined. Based upon the findings on physical examination, mammography and breast ultrasonography should be considered. Fine-needle aspiration (FNA) or core biopsy can be used to distinguish between gynecomastia and breast cancer. Core biopsy may be performed if the FNA is nondiagnostic.

Age The risk of developing breast cancer increases with age. The disease is uncommon in women younger than 40 years of age; only about 0.8% of breast cancers occur in women < 30 years old and approximately 6.5% develop in women between 30 and 40 years old.

TABLE I: Survival of women with breast cancer, according to stage, without chemotherapy

Stage	Survival rate at 8 years (%)
I	90
II	70
III	40
IV	10

Race Caucasian women have a higher overall rate of breast cancer than African-American women; however, this difference is not apparent until age 50 and is marked only after menopause. The incidence of breast cancer in American Asian and Hispanic women is approximately half that in American Caucasian women. Breast cancer risk is extremely low in Native-American women.

Geography There is at least a fivefold variation in the incidence of breast cancer among different countries, although this difference appears to be narrowing. The incidence of breast cancer is significantly lower in Japan, Thailand, Nigeria, and India than in Denmark, the Netherlands, New Zealand, Switzerland, the United Kingdom, and the United States. Women living in North America have the highest rate of breast cancer in the world. It has been suggested that these trends in breast cancer incidence may be related, in some way, to dietary influences, particularly dietary fat consumption (see section on "Etiology and risk factors").

Socioeconomic status The incidence of breast cancer is higher in women of higher socioeconomic background. This relationship is most likely related to lifestyle differences, such as age at first birth.

Disease site The left breast is involved slightly more frequently than the right, and the most common locations of the disease are the upper outer quadrant and retroareolar region. The risk of contralateral breast cancer in women with *BRCA* mutations is approximately 40% at 10 years after the initial diagnosis of breast cancer. This risk is higher in *BRCA1* than *BRCA2* mutation carriers and those first diagnosed at age < 50.

Risk for breast cancer may be reduced in women who take tamoxifen. It may also be reduced in women who undergo bilateral salpingo-oophorectomy (BSO), especially when this procedure is performed in women younger than age 50. The protective effect of BSO is pronounced among women who develop breast cancer premenopausally.

Survival Survival rates for patients with nonmetastatic breast cancer have improved in recent years (Table 1). These improvements may be secondary to advances in adjuvant chemotherapy and radiation therapy. The contribution of screening mammography to breast cancer–specific survival is variable, favoring a reduction in breast cancer mortality of up to 25% in some series. Its impact on overall survival is less certain.

Etiology and risk factors

Numerous risk factors have been associated with the development of breast cancer, including genetic, environmental, hormonal, and nutritional influences. Despite all of the available data on breast cancer risk factors, 75% of women with this cancer have no risk factors.

Genetic factors Hereditary forms of breast cancer constitute only 5% to 7% of breast cancer cases overall. However, the magnitude of the probability that a woman will develop cancer if she inherits a highly penetrant cancer gene mutation justifies the intense interest in predictive testing. Commercial testing is available for several genes (*BRCA1, BRCA2,* and *p53)* associated with a high risk for breast cancer development.

Elevated risk for breast cancer is also associated with mutations in the *PTEN* gene in Cowden's syndrome (described later), and a modest increased risk (relative risk of 3.9–6.4) may be seen in women who are heterozygous for a mutation in the *ATM* gene, which is associated with the recessive disease ataxia-telangiectasia in the homozygous state. A moderately increased risk for breast cancer (2-fold for women and 10-fold for men) has been associated with a variant (1100 delC) in the cell-cycle checkpoint kinase gene, *CHEK2,* among families without *BRCA* gene mutations.

BRCA1 gene The *BRCA1* gene is located on chromosome 17. This gene is extremely large and complex, and more than 1,000 different mutations have been discovered, distributed along the entire gene. *BRCA1* mutations are inherited in an autosomal-dominant fashion and are associated with an increased risk for breast, ovarian, and, to a lesser degree, prostate cancers. A *BRCA1* mutation carrier has a lifetime risk of developing breast cancer on the order of 56% to 85% and a 15% to 45% lifetime risk of developing ovarian cancer.

BRCA2 gene The *BRCA2* gene was localized to chromosome 13. *BRCA2* is approximately twice as large as *BRCA1* and similarly complex.

Alterations in *BRCA2* have been associated with an increased incidence of breast cancer in both women (similar to *BRCA1*) and men (6% lifetime risk). Increased risk for ovarian cancer, pancreatic cancer, prostate cancer, and melanoma has also been reported. Together, *BRCA1* and *BRCA2* account for most hereditary breast and ovarian cancer families and approximately half of hereditary breast cancer families.

The incidence of *BRCA* gene mutations in the general breast cancer population is unknown, since most of the data have come from studies of high-risk populations. In one population-based study of women with breast cancer, only 9.4% of women < 35 years of age at the time of diagnosis and 12.0% of women < 45 years old who also had a first-degree relative with breast cancer had germline *BRCA1* or *BRCA2* mutations. However, a 40-year-old woman of Ashkenazi Jewish ancestry who has breast cancer has a 20% to 30% probability of bearing one of three founder *BRCA* gene mutations, based on data from high-risk clinics, testing vendors, and Israeli series.

Masciari et al conducted a pilot trial of F¹⁸-Fluorodeoxyglucose-PET/CT screening in Li-Fraumeni syndrome (LFS). Members of LFS families with documented germline TP53 mutations or obligate carrier status, no history of cancer within 5 years of enrollment, and no symptoms of cancer or ill health were offered FDG-PET/CT scanning as a screening test. Scans were reviewed clinically, as well as centrally by an expert radiologist. Of 15 individuals, baseline FDG-PET/CT scan identified asymptomatic cancers in 3 (20%). Two individuals had papillary thyroid cancers (stages II and III) and one individual had stage II esophageal adenocarcinoma. These preliminary data provide the first evidence for a potential cancer surveillance strategy that may be worthy of further investigation for patients with LFS. Concerns about radiation exposure and other challenges inherent in screening high-risk patients will require further consideration *(Masciari S, Van den Abbeele AD, Diller LR, et al: JAMA 299:1315-1319, 2008).*

Li-Fraumeni syndrome This rare syndrome is characterized by premenopausal breast cancer in combination with childhood sarcoma, brain tumors, leukemia, and adrenocortical carcinoma. Tumors frequently occur in childhood and early adulthood and often present as multiple primaries in the same individual. Germline mutations in the *p53* gene on chromosome 17p have been documented in persons with this syndrome. Inheritance is autosomal dominant, with a penetrance of at least 50% by age 50. Given the rarity, diversity of tumor types, and age at risk spanning both child and young adulthood, coherent screening strategies beyond those for the early-onset breast cancer risk are difficult to find.

Cowden's syndrome is inherited as an autosomal-dominant trait and is notable for a distinctive skin lesion (trichilemmoma) and mucocutaneous lesions. Patients with this uncommon syndrome have a high incidence of GI polyps and thyroid disorders; lifetime estimates for breast cancer among women with this syndrome range from 25% to 50%. Germline mutations in the *PTEN* gene, located on chromosome 10q23, are responsible for this syndrome.

Family history The overall relative risk of breast cancer in a woman with a positive family history in a first-degree relative (mother, daughter, or sister) is 1.7. Premenopausal onset of the disease in a first-degree relative is associated with a threefold increase in breast cancer risk, whereas postmenopausal diagnosis increases the relative risk by only 1.5. When the first-degree relative has bilateral disease, there is a fivefold increase in risk. The relative risk for a woman whose first-degree relative developed bilateral breast cancer prior to menopause is nearly 9.

Proliferative breast disease The diagnosis of certain conditions after breast biopsy is also associated with an increased risk for the subsequent development of invasive breast cancer. They include moderate or florid ductal hyperplasia and sclerosing adenosis, which pose only a slightly increased risk of breast cancer (1.5–2.0 times); atypical ductal or lobular hyperplasia, which moderately increases risk (4–5 times); and lobular carcinoma in situ (LCIS), which markedly increases risk (8–11 times; see more detailed discussion of LCIS in chapter 9). Patients who have a family history of breast cancer along with a personal history of atypical epithelial hyperplasia have an 8-fold increase in breast cancer risk when compared with patients with a positive family history alone and an 11-fold increase in breast cancer risk when compared with patients who do not have atypical hyperplasia and have a negative family history.

Personal cancer history A personal history of breast cancer is a significant risk factor for the subsequent development of a second, new breast cancer. This risk has been estimated to be as high as 1% per year from the time of diagnosis of an initial sporadic breast cancer. Women with *BRCA*-associated cancer have a 3% to 5% per year risk of contralateral breast cancer (cumulative lifetime risk of up to 64% in high-risk cohorts). Women with a history of endometrial, ovarian, or colon cancer also have a higher likelihood of developing breast cancer than those with no history of these malignancies.

Menstrual and reproductive factors Early onset of menarche (< 12 years old) has been associated with a modest increase in breast cancer risk (twofold or less). Women who undergo menopause before age 30 have a twofold reduction in breast cancer risk when compared with women who undergo menopause after age 55. A first full-term pregnancy before age 30 appears to have a protective effect against breast cancer, whereas a late first full-term pregnancy or nulliparity may be associated with a higher risk. There is also a suggestion that lactation protects against breast cancer development.

Radiation exposure An increased rate of breast cancer has been observed in survivors of the atomic bomb explosions in Japan, with a peak latency period of 15 to 20 years. More recently, it has been noted that patients with Hodgkin's lymphoma who are treated with mantle irradiation, particularly women who are younger than age 20 at the time of radiation therapy, have an increased incidence of breast cancer.

Exogenous hormone use Epidemiologic data provide strong evidence for an association between plasma estrogens and breast cancer risk.

The 1996 large meta-analysis of the relationship between oral contraceptive use and breast cancer risk showed that a history of recent oral contraceptive use was a better predictor of breast cancer risk than duration of use. (Meta-analysis consisted of 54 earlier studies including 53,297 women with breast cancer and 100,239 women without breast cancer.) The increase in risk for cur-

Following the publication of the WHI trial results, the use of hormone replacement therapy (HRT) decreased by 38% in the United States, with approximately 20 million fewer prescriptions written in 2003 than in 2002. In the same period, an initial analysis of data from the National Cancer Institute's Surveillance, Epidemiology, and End Results (SEER) registries showed a decline (by 6.7%) in the age-adjusted incidence rate of breast cancer in the United States. Regression analysis showed that the decrease began in mid-2002 and had begun to level off by mid-2003. A comparison of incidence rates in 2001 with those in 2004 (omitting the years in which the incidence was changing) showed that the decrease in annual age-adjusted incidence was 8.6% (95% confidence interval [CI], 6.8 to 10.4). The decrease was evident only in women who were 50 years of age or older and was more evident in cancers that were estrogen receptor-positive than in those that were estrogen receptor-negative. The authors concluded that the decrease in breast cancer incidence, which is temporally related to the first report of the WHI trial results, is due in part to the ensuing drop in the use of HRT among postmenopausal women in the United States *(Ravdin PM, Cronin KA, Howlader N, et al: N Engl J Med 356:1670-1674, 2007).*

rent users was modest (24% for ever users vs never users). These data were based primarily on older high-dose and moderate-dose oral contraceptive pills and not the recently introduced low-dose pills. Therefore, it is likely that the small increase in breast cancer risk associated with the early formulations of oral contraceptives will diminish with the new low-dose pills.

In regard to hormone replacement therapy (HRT) or postmenopausal hormone use, results from the Women's Health Initiative (WHI) showed that the overall risks of estrogen plus progestin outweigh the benefits. This large randomized clinical trial sponsored by the National Institutes of Health (NIH) included more than 16,000 healthy women. Results from the WHI trial were published in 2002, after an average 5.6 years of follow-up, and included a 26% increase in risk of invasive breast cancer among women taking estrogen plus progestin, compared with women taking placebo. In addition, in women taking these hormones, there were increased risks of heart disease, stroke, and blood clots.

The NIH stopped the estrogen-alone arm of the WHI trial in March 2004. No increase in breast cancer risk was observed in the estrogen-alone arm during the study period (7 years of follow-up). The NIH concluded that estrogen alone does not appear to increase or decrease a woman's risk of heart disease, although it does appear to increase her risk of stroke and decrease her risk of hip fracture.

Alcohol Moderate alcohol intake (two or more drinks per day) appears to modestly increase breast cancer risk.

High-fat diet Diets that are high in fat have been associated with an increased risk for breast cancer. Women who have diets high in animal fat from red meat or high-fat dairy foods have an increased risk of developing breast cancer. Whether the increase in breast cancer risk is associated with the fat content or an unknown carcinogen in these foods is unclear.

Obesity Alterations in endogenous estrogen levels secondary to obesity may enhance breast cancer risk. Obesity appears to be a factor primarily in postmenopausal women.

Genetic cancer risk assessment

Genetic testing clearly has the potential to benefit carefully selected and counseled families. Education and adequately trained health care professionals are key elements in the successful integration of genetic cancer risk assessment into clinical practice.

The genetic risk assessment process begins with an evaluation of perceived risk and the impact of cancer on the patient and family. This information forms the framework for counseling.

Comprehensive personal and family histories Detailed information regarding personal, reproductive, and hormonal risk factors is noted. Family history, including age at disease onset, types of cancer, and current age or age at death, is obtained for all family members going back at least three generations.

TABLE 2: Features indicating an increased likelihood of a *BRCA* mutation

Early-onset breast cancer, especially in the setting of a limited family structure

Ovarian cancer (with or without a family history of breast or ovarian cancer)

Breast and ovarian cancers in the same woman

Bilateral breast cancer

Ashkenazi Jewish heritage

Male breast cancer

ER, PR, and HER2/*neu* negative ("triple negative") premenopausal breast cancer

---

Documentation of cancer cases is crucial to accurate risk estimation. Pathology reports, medical record notes, and death certificates may all be used in determining the exact diagnosis.

Pedigree construction and evaluation The family pedigree is then constructed and analyzed to determine whether a pattern of cancer in the family is consistent with genetic disease. Sometimes, small family structure or lack of information about the family limits assessment of a hereditary trait; other times, clues such as ancestry or early age at diagnosis influence risk assessment and the usefulness of genetic testing.

Individual risk assessment Several models are used to estimate the likelihood that a detectable *BRCA1* or *BRCA2* mutation is responsible for the disease in the family. The BRCAPRO computer program is a cancer risk assessment tool that uses a family history of breast or ovarian cancer in first- and second-degree relatives to calculate the probabilities that either a *BRCA1* or *BRCA2* mutation is responsible for the disease. It includes a Bayesian calculation (of conditional probability) to account for age-specific penetrance differences. If genetic testing is not performed or results are uninformative, the empiric breast cancer risk is estimated by the phenotype as well as the Claus model (derived from the Cancer and Hormone Study, which uses age at onset of breast cancer among first- and second-degree relatives). Personal and family characteristics that are associated with an increased likelihood of a *BRCA1* or *BRCA2* mutation are summarized in Table 2.

Education about the principles of genetics and hereditary cancer patterns is provided. Information on the application of genetic testing (appropriateness, limitations, advantages, and disadvantages) is also given.

Genetic counseling and testing Informed consent is obtained before genetic testing is performed. For individuals who decide to undergo testing, a post-test counseling session is scheduled to disclose and explain the results in person.

Customized screening and prevention recommendations Regardless of whether or not a woman undergoes genetic testing, a customized management plan is delineated, with the goal of prevention or early detection of malignancy,

Relative risks of incidence and mortality for cancer from the Million Women Study were reported in late 2007. A total of 1.2 million UK women were recruited into the Million Women Study, aged 50-64 during 1996-2001, and followed up, on average, for 5.4 years for cancer incidence and 7.0 years for cancer mortality. A total of 45,037 incident cancers and 17,203 deaths from cancer occurred over the follow-up period. Increased incidence of breast cancer was noted with increasing body mass index. For breast cancer, the effect of body mass index on risk differed significantly according to menopausal status. In postmenopausal women, the relative risk was 1.40. In addition to body mass index, calculations were adjusted for age, geographical region, socioeconomic status, age at first birth, parity, smoking status, alcohol intake, physical activity, years since menopause, and use of hormone replacement therapy *(Reeves GK, Pirie K, Beral V, et al: BMJ 335:1134, 2007).*

within the context of her personal preferences and degree of risk (Table 3).

Laboratory methods

Several techniques/strategies for detecting mutations in cancer genes have been adopted by different researchers and commercial vendors. Current technology misses 8% to 10% of pathologic alterations in *BRCA1* and *BRCA2* (generally large rearrangements).

The sole commercial vendor for *BRCA* gene testing in the United States recently added a quantitative polymerase chain reaction (PCR)-based exon dosage assay to screen for large rearrangements.

Directed assays are available for specific founder or ancestral mutations that are common in a given population. Among Ashkenazi Jews, 1 in 40 individuals bears one of three founder mutations (185delAG and 5382insC in *BRCA1* and 6174delT in *BRCA2)*; these mutations account for 25% of early-onset breast cancer in this population. Moreover, 95% of Ashkenazi Jews with a *BRCA* gene mutation will have one of the three founder mutations.

The lifetime risk of breast cancer was 82% among founder mutation carriers in a large cohort of Jewish families identified via a New York breast cancer study. The lifetime risk of ovarian cancer was 54% for *BRCA1* and 23% for *BRCA2*, similar to the risk in multiplex families from the Breast Cancer Linkage Consortium (BCLC). However, a population-based study indicated a lifetime breast cancer risk of 40% to 73%.

Limitations All of the approaches to detecting mutations have limitations. In general, discovery of an inactivating or "deleterious" mutation of either *BRCA1* or *BRCA2* indicates a high probability that a person will develop breast and/or ovarian cancer.

One of the greatest challenges is the interpretation of missense mutations. These mutations are more likely to be significant if located in an evolutionarily conserved or functionally critical region of the protein. In the absence of a clear disease association, it is often difficult to exclude the possibility that a given missense alteration simply represents a rare polymorphism. Using advanced methods, a recent study was able to characterize 133/1,433 variants as likely polymorphisms and 43 as likely deleterious; the majority would still be designated as "genetic variants of uncertain significance."

TABLE 3: Risk management options for *BRCA* mutation carriers[a]

Recommended for breast cancer detection

Monthly self-examination of the breast beginning in late teen years

Beginning at age 25 (or at least 10 years before the earliest onset cancer in the kindred):

Clinician breast examination every 6 months

Annual mammography

Consider annual breast MRI if there is significant mammographic density

Discussed as options:

Bilateral risk reduction mastectomy (total or skin-sparing)

Participation in clinical trials for chemoprevention

Recommended for ovarian cancer detection or prevention

Risk reduction salpingo-oophorectomy recommended upon completion of childbearing

Pelvic examination and Pap smear annually

Considered optional:

Serum CA-125 every 6 months

and transvaginal ultrasonography every 6 months

[a] Also offered to women at increased risk because of a positive family history of hereditary breast and ovarian cancers but for whom genotypic information is not available.

Testing strategies

In general, testing should be initiated with the youngest affected individual in a given family. Even if one is convinced that a family has hereditary breast and ovarian cancers based on clinical criteria, there is only a 50% chance that an offspring or sibling of an affected patient will have inherited the deleterious allele. Therefore, only a positive test result (detection of a known or likely deleterious mutation) is truly informative.

Until the "familial mutation" is known, a negative test result could mean either that the unaffected person being tested did not inherit the cancer susceptibility mutation or that the person inherited the disease-associated gene, but the mutation was not detectable by the methods used.

In many cases, no affected family members are available for testing. In that case, one may proceed with genetic testing of an unaffected

> Walsh et al recently demonstrated inherited genomic rearrangements of BRCA1 and BRCA2 in 35 of 300 (12%) sequence-negative high-risk families. They also highlighted other single-gene breast cancer predisposition traits in a subset of families (eg, 14 with CHEK2 mutation and 3 with TP53 mutation). In part, this prompted accelerated implementation of a commercial screen (*Walsh T, Casadei S, Coats KH, et al: JAMA 295:1379-1388, 2006*).

person, but only after she has been thoroughly counseled regarding its risks, benefits, and limitations.

Unless there is a suggestive family history, cancer susceptibility testing is not considered appropriate for screening unaffected individuals in the general population. However, it may be reasonable to test unaffected persons who are members of an ethnic group in which specific ancestral mutations are prevalent and whose family structure is limited (ie, the family is small, with few female relatives or no information due to premature death from noncancerous causes).

Impact of genetic cancer risk status on management

Data from the BCLC suggest that the cumulative risk of developing a second primary breast cancer is approximately 65% by age 70 among *BRCA* gene mutation carriers who have already had breast cancer. A large, retrospective cohort study of BRCA carriers with a history of limited-stage breast cancer indicated up to a 40% risk of contralateral breast cancer at 10 years. A subsequent study of the same cohort noted almost a 13% risk for ovarian cancer in the same interval and that that ovarian cancer was the cause of cancer death in 25% of stage I breast cancer patients with *BRCA* mutations.

Thus, knowledge of the genetic status of a woman affected with breast cancer might influence the initial surgical approach (eg, bilateral mastectomy might be recommended for a mutation carrier instead of a more conservative procedure). Moreover, since ovarian cancer risk may be markedly increased in women with *BRCA1* mutations (and to a lesser degree with *BRCA2* mutations), additional measures, such as surveillance for presymptomatic detection of early-stage tumors or consideration of oophorectomy, may be warranted.

A study of 491 BRCA carriers with stage I or II breast cancer indicated that the risk of ovarian cancer was 12.7% at 10 years for BRCA1 (6.8% for BRCA2), and ovarian cancer was the cause of death in 25% of the stage I breast cancer patients. According to data from *BRCA* carriers who underwent risk reduction salpingo-oophorectomy (RRSO), breast cancer risk may also be decreased by the reduction in ovarian hormone exposure.

Kauff et al reported their findings of a multicenter prospective analysis of RRSO to prevent BRCA-associated breast and ovarian cancers. During a median follow-up of 40 months, RRSO was associated with a 52% reduction in breast cancer risk and a 91% reduction in ovarian cancer risk, with the greatest risk reduction occurring in women with the *BRCA2* gene mutation. A total of 886 female *BRCA1* or *BRCA2* mutation carriers older than age 30 were enrolled from 1 of 11 study centers between 1994 and 2004. Women were treated with either ovarian surveillance (n = 325) or RRSO (n = 561). The investigators believe their results confirm that RRSO is highly protective against BRCA-associated breast and ovarian cancers. This protection may differ between carriers of *BRCA1* and *BRCA2* mutations.

Both retrospective and prospective data have demonstrated the efficacy (> 90% risk reduction) of bilateral mastectomy in women who are at high risk for the disease based upon *BRCA* genetic status. Women who opt for risk reduction mastectomy should be offered reconstruction. Skin-sparing mastectomy may enhance the cosmetic results of reconstruction and should be discussed with the patient's surgeon. This procedure entails removing the breast tissue (including the nipple-areolar complex).

The efficacy of bilateral risk reduction mastectomy has been confirmed in a large prospective study of 483 women with *BRCA* mutations. With a mean follow-up of 6.4 years, risk reduction mastectomy reduced the risk of breast cancer by 90% (95% in women who also underwent RRSO).

Potential benefits and risks of genetic testing

The ability to identify individuals at highest risk for cancer holds the promise of improved prevention and early detection of cancers. Patients who are *not* at high risk can be spared anxiety and the need for increased surveillance. Recent studies suggest a better emotional state among at-risk relatives who undergo testing than among those who choose not to know their status. The patient's perception of risk is often much higher than risk estimated by current models.

Potential risks Potential medical, psychological, and socioeconomic risks must be addressed in the context of obtaining informed consent for genetic testing.

Concerns about insurance Fear about adverse effects of testing on insurability remains the premier concern among patients. Close behind that is concern about the cost of analyzing large complex genes ($3,100 for full sequencing of *BRCA1* and *BRCA2* and an additional $650 if the test for genomic rearrangements is ordered a la carte).

Legal and privacy issues The legal and privacy issues surrounding genetic testing are as complex as the testing technologies. Although several state laws regarding the privacy of medical information, genetic testing, and insurance and employment discrimination have been passed, they vary widely.

The 1996 Health Insurance Portability and Accountability Act (US public law 104-191), governing group medical plans, stipulates that genetic information may not be treated as a preexisting condition in the absence of a diagnosis of the condition related to such information. It further prohibits basing rules for eligibility or costs for coverage on genetic information. However, the law does not address genetic privacy issues and does not cover individual policies. Many states have laws addressing genetic discrimination, but concerns about gaps remained. Recent Federal legislation expanded protection against genetic discrimination to include individual policies (see sidebar later in chapter).

Recommendations for genetic testing

Updated guidelines from the American Society of Clinical Oncology (ASCO) recommend that cancer predisposition testing be offered only in the following situations: (1) a person has a strong family history of cancer or early onset of disease; (2) the test can be adequately interpreted; and (3) the results will influence the medical management of the patient or family member. Recent data indicated an increased probability of detecting a *BRCA* mutation among single cases (no close relative with breast or ovarian cancer) of breast cancer in people

FIGURE 1: Malignant calcifications (comedocarcinoma) in a classic linear dot and dash configuration (BI-RAD 5 lesion). BI-RAD = Breast Imaging Reporting Data System.

FIGURE 2: Left panel: A dense mass with partially unsharp margins (BI-RAD 4 lesion), which proved to be a fibroadenoma. Right panel: A small, spiculated mass (BI-RAD 5 lesion), which has engulfed a coarse, benign calcification. This lesion proved to be an invasive ductal carcinoma, not otherwise specified (NOS). BI-RAD = Breast Imaging Reporting Data System.

FIGURE 3: Left panel: This focal mass with truly nonsharp margins (BI-RAD 4 lesion) was diagnosed as a tubular carcinoma on stereotactic core biopsy. Right panel: A well-circumscribed lesion containing fat (BI-RAD 2 lesion), which is pathognomonic for a breast hamartoma (fibroadenolipoma). BI-RAD = Breast Imaging Reporting Data System.

FIGURE 4: Focal architectural distortion may be difficult to see, but, if confirmed, it has the highest positive predictive value for breast carcinoma. This BI-RAD 4 lesion proved to be an invasive lobular carcinoma, which often has a subtle mammographic appearance. BI-RAD = Breast Imaging Reporting Data System.

FIGURE 5: This breast ultrasonographic image demonstrates a hypoechoic, solid mass, which exhibits posterior shadowing and is taller than wide. This BI-RAD 4 lesion proved to be an invasive ductal carcinoma, not otherwise specified (NOS). BI-RAD = Breast Imaging Reporting Data System.

FIGURE 6: A 42-year-old woman presents with axillary adenopathy, which was positive on fine-needle aspiration. Results of a clinical breast exam, mammography, and ultrasonography were normal. A 7-mm enhancing cancer is clearly seen on this MRI of the breast.

TABLE 4: BI-RAD classification of mammographic lesions

BI-RAD class	Description	Probability of malignancy (%)	Follow-up
0	Needs additional evaluation		Diagnostic mammogram, ultra-sonographic image
1	Normal mammogram	0	Yearly screening
2	Benign lesion	0	Yearly screening
3	Probably benign lesion	< 2	Short interval follow-up
4[a]	Suspicious for malignancy	20	Biopsy
5	Highly suspicious for malignancy	90	Biopsy
6	Biopsy-proven malignancy	100	Treatment

BI-RAD = Breast Imaging Reporting Data System

[a] The American College of Radiology recommends that each site be divided into three subcategories: 4A, low suspicion; 4B, intermediate suspicion; and 4C, moderate concern but not classic for malignancy.

A recent study characterized the impact of family structure on the prevalence of *BRCA* gene mutations among 306 women with breast cancer before age 50 years and no first- or second-degree relatives with breast or ovarian cancer. Limited family structure was defined as fewer than two first- or second-degree female relatives surviving beyond age 45 years in either lineage. *BRCA* mutations were detected in 13.7% of women with limited versus 5.2% with adequate family structure. Thus, family structure appears to be a strong predictor of mutation status (odds ratio = 2.8; 95% confidence interval, 1.19–6.73; *P* = .019). Clinicians should know that family structure can affect the accuracy of mutation probability models. Genetic testing guidelines may need to be more inclusive for single cases of breast cancer when the family structure is limited *(Weitzel JN, Lagos VI, Cullinane CA, et al: JAMA 297:2587-2595, 2007).*

younger than age 50 who had a limited family structure. This observation was cited as a justification for testing in this scenario in the 2008 National Comprehensive Cancer Network (NCCN) practice guidelines for genetics/familial high-risk cancer screening which are updated annually and published at www.nccn.org.

Signs and symptoms

Mammographic findings Increasing numbers of breast malignancies are being discovered in asymptomatic patients through the use of screening mammography. Mammographic features suggestive of malignancy include asymmetry, microcalcifications, a mass, or an architectural distortion.

When these features are identified on a screening mammogram (see Figures 1–5), they should, in most cases, be further evaluated with a diagnostic mammogram (and, in some cases, with a breast ultrasonographic image or in highly selected cases with MRI [Figure 6]) prior to determining the need for a tissue diagnosis. Often, pseudolesions, such as those caused by a summation artifact, dust on the mammographic cassettes, and dermal calcifications, are correctly identified in this manner. All mammographic lesions (and the examinations themselves) must be unambiguously categorized according to one of the six Breast Imaging Reporting Data System (BI-RAD) classifications developed by the American College of Radiology (ACR, Table 4).

Breast lump When signs or symptoms are present, the most common presenting complaint is a lump within the breast. The incidence of this complaint can range from 65% to 76%, depending on the study. Inflammatory breast cancer is particularly aggressive, although relatively uncommon, accounting for about 5% of all breast cancers. On breast palpation, there often is no definite mass, but the breast appears to be engorged with erythema, skin edema (peau d'orange), and skin ridging. Ultrasonography may help to distinguish mastitis or abscess from inflammatory breast cancer. Antibiotics, which are prescribed for presumed mastitis, are not helpful for women with inflammatory carcinoma.

The Genetic Information Nondiscrimination Act of 2008 (GINA) was recently approved by the House of Representatives, by a vote of 414 to 1 and passed unanimously by the Senate, and signed by President Bush on May 21, 2008. This law bars employers from hiring or firing an employee based on genetic test results that indicate a predisposition to develop a disease. GINA would also prohibit insurance companies from denying or canceling coverage based on the information. This new law provides a Federal framework for protections based upon a genetic predisposition for a disease, instead of the patchwork of state laws throughout the country. As GINA further states, "genetic testing can allow individuals to take steps to reduce the likelihood that they will contract a particular disorder. New knowledge about genetics may allow for the development of better therapies that are more effective against disease or have fewer side effects than current treatments."

Paget's disease has been associated with intraductal carcinoma involving the terminal ducts of the breasts and may have an associated invasive component. It presents as an eczematoid change in the nipple, a breast mass, or bloody nipple discharge. Cytology may be helpful in establishing the diagnosis; however, negative cytologic results should not preclude a biopsy.

Other local symptoms Breast pain is the presenting symptom in ~5% of patients; breast enlargement, in 1%; skin or nipple retraction, in ~5%; nipple discharge, in ~2%; and nipple crusting or erosion, in 1%.

Screening and diagnosis

Screening

Breast self-examination The role of breast self-examination is controversial. The American Cancer Society (ACS) recommends that beginning in their 20s, women should be instructed in the technique and informed about both the benefits and limitations of this screening tool. Other groups have suggested that routine breast self-examination may lead to more false-positive results and therefore more benign biopsies. One meta-analysis of 12 studies involving a total of 8,118 patients with breast cancer correlated the performance of breast self-examination with tumor size and regional lymph node status. Women who performed breast self-examination were more likely to have smaller tumors and less likely to have axillary node metastases than those who did not. A recent multicenter study, from Memorial Sloan-Kettering Cancer Center and the University of Virginia, attempted to measure the benefits and costs of adding clinical breast exams to yearly screening mammography. These exams detected an additional 14 breast cancers, or 0.02% of the 60,027 exams performed, and the cost for each additional cancer detected was $122,598. Based on this report, the benefit of clinical breast exams appear to be marginal.

A major problem with breast self-examination as a screening technique is that it is rarely performed well. Only 2% to 3% of women do an ideal examination a year after instruction has been provided.

Clinical breast examination The ACS recommends that women begin clinical breast examination at the age of 20 and have an examination every 3 years between ages 20 and 39, and annually beginning at age 40. Beginning at age 40, the clinical breast examination should be timed to occur near or prior to screening mammography. If the clinician detects an abnormality, the patient should then undergo diagnostic imaging rather than screening. Clinical breast examination should be performed and a complete breast history obtained when a woman presents for routine health care. The clinical examination should include inspection and palpation of the breast and regional lymph nodes. Between 14% and 21% of breast cancers are detected by clinical breast examination.

Mammography Despite conflicting coverage in the lay press, the benefit of screening mammography is well established by the findings of an evidence-based clinical trial. The ACS, the ACR, and the American Medical Association have updated their guidelines since 1997 and recommend annual mammography beginning at age 40. The National Cancer Institute (NCI) also updated its guidelines in 1997, recommending that women undergo screening mammography every 1 to 2 years beginning in their 40s. The US Preventive Services Task Force updated its guidelines in 2002 and now recommends mammography every 1 to 2 years, alone or with clinical breast examination, for women aged 40 and older.

Screening mammography is performed in the asymptomatic patient to detect an occult breast cancer. This contrasts with diagnostic mammography, which is performed in a patient with a breast abnormality (palpable mass, bloody nipple discharge, or some other clinical finding) to further identify the etiology of the problem.

Physical examination and mammography are complementary. Mammography has a sensitivity of 85% to 90% and, thus, would miss 10% to 15% of clinically evident tumors while detecting the majority of cases an average of 2 years prior to any perceptible clinical signs or symptoms.

Screening recommendations for average-risk patients No upper age limit has been suggested, and the previous recommendation for a "baseline" mammogram between the ages of 35 and 40 has been withdrawn. Thus, both the ACS and the NCCN recommend annual mammography starting at age 40 for women at average risk of breast cancer.

Screening recommendations for high-risk patients Based on epidemiologic evidence that premenopausal familial breast cancer often presents at similar ages among affected family members, many breast imaging centers recommend that yearly screening for such high-risk individuals begin 5 to 10 years prior to the youngest age at which a first-degree relative was diagnosed with breast cancer. For example, according to this algorithm, a woman whose mother developed breast cancer at age 45 could begin yearly screening at age 35, in addition to biannual clinical breast examinations. Screening for women at genetic risk may begin at age 25. These commonly used screening algorithms are not based on formal studies but have arisen based on the natural history of the disease. They are, however, in keeping with the recommendations of the NCCN guidelines.

Digital mammography was approved by the US Food and Drug Administration (FDA) in 2000 and is rapidly being adopted by leading breast cancer centers worldwide. Initial trials indicate a comparable sensitivity to film-based mammography, with the benefit of a reduced risk of women called back from screening for additional work-up. The FDA also approved computer-aided detection systems for mammography beginning in 2001. Mammograms are scanned by a computer and possible lesions are marked for further review by a radiologist. A number of studies have shown a reduced risk of "missed cancers" when computer-aided diagnosis is thus employed. Although some physician are skeptical about the benefits of such computer-aided detection systems for mammography, many investigators in the field continue to support its use. For example, Lindfors et al published data showing that these systems increased the effectiveness of mammographic screening by 29%, with a comparable increase in screening cost.

Screening ultrasonography Sensitivity of mammography is diminished when the breast tissue is dense. There have been recent reports in the literature concerning the role of screening breast ultrasonography in women with dense breasts on mammography and normal mammography and clinical breast examination. The results from a multicenter trial of leading breast imagers (ACRIN 6666) showed that the addition of ultrasound to mammography increased detection of breast cancer compared to mammography alone among women at increased risk of breast cancer who also had dense breast tissue. However, there was also an increase in the number of benign biopsies. Furthermore, ultrasonography and MRI are used as adjunct studies and should not replace mammography. However, breast MRI appears to be an effective screening tool for high-risk women, particularly those with *BRCA1* and *BRCA2* mutations.

Breast MRI is a sensitive tool for detecting occult breast cancer foci. Due to its limited specificity and high cost, MRI is not likely to become a screening tool for avergage-risk women. However, the role of breast MRI for detecting breast cancers in high-risk women (ie, *BRCA* gene mutation carriers) continues to evolve. Although controversial, recent guidelines from the ACS called for consideration of breast MRI for women with at least a 20% lifetime risk for breast cancer.

Vitamin D is a regulator of cellular growth and differentiation. In a prospective Canadian study, vitamin D levels in women newly diagnosed with breast cancer (T1-3, N0-1, M0) more than 10 years ago were assessed in archived blood samples taken after surgery and prior to systemic therapy (N = 512). Vitamin D deficiency was associated with an increased risk of distant recurrence (independent of age, BMI, insulin level, and T and N stage, and not significantly modified by ER status, adjuvant chemotherapy or tamoxifen) and death, while patients with insufficient and sufficient Vitamin D levels had similar outcomes. These early findings raise the question of whether Vitamin D supplementation might improve breast cancer–specific survival (Goodwin PJ, Ennis M, Pritchard KI, et al: *J Clin Oncol* 26[suppl]:511, 2008).

Two major studies have demonstrated the increased sensitivity of MRI for detecting cancers in women with inherited susceptibility to breast cancer compared with clinical breast examination, mammography, or ultrasonography. The sensitivity of breast MRI is > 75%, in contrast to mammography and ultrasonography, which is approximately 30% each. The combined sensitivity of MRI plus mammography is about 95%, suggesting that it may be a viable strategy for screening young women at high risk for breast cancer.

Evaluation of a cystic mass

FNA When a dominant breast mass is present and the history and physical examination suggest that it is a cyst, the mass can simply be aspirated with a fine needle. Aspiration of a simple benign breast cyst should yield nonbloody fluid and result in complete resolution of the lesion.

Ultrasonography can also be used to determine whether a mass is solid or cystic and whether a cyst is simple, complicated, or complex. Simple cysts are anechoic and oval, with thin walls; if asymptomatic, a simple cyst may be treated as an incidental finding. Complicated cysts are similar, except that low-level echoes are present in the cyst lumen. In many instances, complicated cysts may be managed conservatively, unless a worrisome feature or history prompts aspiration. Complex cysts demonstrate an intracystic mass, or focally thickened walls or septa, and necessitate a percutaneous biopsy for diagnosis.

Biopsy A biopsy is indicated if the cyst fluid is bloody, the lesion does not resolve completely after aspiration, or the cyst recurs after repeated aspirations. Cytologic examination of the fluid is not routinely indicated, as the yield for positive cytology is so low. Cystic carcinoma accounts for < 1% of all breast cancers. However, an intraluminal solid mass is a worrisome sign suggesting (intra) cystic carcinoma and should be biopsied.

Evaluation of a solid mass

A solid, palpable mass can be evaluated in a variety of ways. The decision to observe a patient with a solid breast mass that appears to be benign should be made only after careful clinical and radiologic examinations. Either FNA for cytology or percutaneous core biopsy should also be performed.

Mammography is used to assess the radiologic characteristics of the mass and is important for the evaluation of the remainder of the ipsilateral breast as well as the contralateral breast.

FNA is a simple, easy-to-perform method for obtaining material for cytologic examination. The overall incidence of false-positive results ranges from 0% to 2.5% (0.7% when performed by experienced technicians), and the incidence of false-negative results varies from 3% to 27% (3% to 9% in experienced hands). Reasons for false-negative readings include less-than-optimal technique in preparing the cytologic material, a missed lesion on aspiration, tumor necrosis, and incorrect cytologic interpretation. FNA is limited in its ability to distinguish invasive from noninvasive cancers. For these reasons, the trend at leading breast centers has been to replace FNA with core biopsy.

Biopsy In the past, an excisional biopsy of a small breast mass or incisional biopsy of a larger breast mass was performed to establish a histologic diagnosis of breast cancer. In recent years, excisional biopsy is being performed less often, except for a presumably benign lesion. For a suspected malignancy, core biopsy has become the preferred diagnostic tool. With a core biopsy, the surgeon can plan for the cancer surgery, allowing for definitive surgical management in a single procedure. Core biopsy is also more advantageous than an FNA because architectural as well as cellular characteristics can be evaluated.

Image-guided core biopsies

When a palpable mass is extremely deep within the breast or a mass is relatively small, an ultrasonography-guided core biopsy can be performed to increase the diagnostic yield. When the procedure is performed with a large core needle (8 to 11 gauge) and vaccum assistance, a mass up to approximately 2 to 3 cm can be excised.

Ductal lavage

Ductal lavage is currently being developed and analyzed as a minimally invasive tool to identify cellular atypia within breast ducts in women who are already at high risk for developing breast cancer. Nipple aspiration is performed, and ducts that produce fluid should undergo lavage. The ductal orifice is cannulated and infused with 2 to 6 mL of saline. The ductal effluent is collected and evaluated by cytology. A careful record is maintained of each duct that has been lavaged by means of a nipple grid and photography.

The results of the cytologic evaluation may then be used to guide women in their decision-making process with respect to interventions to reduce their risk for breast cancer. For high-risk women who undergo ductal lavage and the cytology is benign, repeat lavage can be performed in 1 to 3 years, although the optimal time for repeat lavage is not currently known. When mild atypia is identified by ductal lavage, the location of the duct should be carefully recorded using a nipple grid and photography to ensure the accurate localization of the duct. A repeat lavage can then be performed in 6 to 12 months. Women who have benign cytology and mild atypia on ductal lavage should also consider tamoxifen or participation in a chemoprevention trial.

Severe atypia is seen in approximately 6% of women who undergo ductal lavage. Patients with severe atypia on ductal lavage should undergo a thorough evaluation, including a repeat lavage, to confirm this diagnosis and exclude malignancy. The evaluation could also include repeated mammography with ductography, breast MRI, and/or ductoscopy. If no suspicious lesions are found, patients should be carefully followed. Fewer than 1% of patients have had malignant cells identified on ductal lavage.

Lavage of the duct producing the malignant cells should be repeated to confirm the diagnosis. If the diagnosis is confirmed, patients should then undergo the same evaluation as patients with marked atypia. Any suspicious lesion should be biopsied. Patients without suspicious lesions can be offered duct excision after the ductal system has been injected with dye or after close follow-up. These patients should also consider tamoxifen.

<table>
<tr><td>

Low-fat intake has been hypothesized to reduce the risk for breast cancer. To assess the effects of undertaking a low-fat dietary pattern on breast cancer incidence, a randomized, controlled, primary prevention trial of 48,835 postmenopausal women, aged 50 to 79 years, without prior breast cancer, was conducted at 40 US clinical centers from 1993 to 2005. Women were randomly assigned to the dietary modification intervention group (n = 19,541) or the comparison group (n = 29,294). The intervention was designed to promote dietary change of reducing total fat to 20% and increasing daily consumption of vegetables and fruit to at least 5 servings and grains to at least 6 servings. Comparison group participants were not asked to make dietary changes. Overall, a low-fat dietary pattern did not result in a statistically significant reduction in invasive breast cancer risk over an 8.1-year average follow-up period. The number of women who developed invasive breast cancer (annualized incidence rate) was 655 (0.42%) in the intervention group and 1,072 (0.45%) in the comparison group (hazard ratio, 0.91; 95% confidence interval, 0.83-1.01). Secondary analyses suggest that among adherent women having a high-fat diet at baseline, a greater risk reduction might be achieved and that dietary effect varied by hormone receptor characteristics of the tumor (*Prentice RL, Caan B, Chlebowski RT, et al: JAMA 295:629-642, 2006*).

</td><td>

Evaluation of nonpalpable mammographic abnormalities

Excisional biopsy Prior to 1991, almost all nonpalpable mammographic lesions were excised using surgical excision. This technique has become less prevalent with the availability of image-guided percutaneous biopsy techniques.

Stereotactic and ultrasonography-guided core biopsies have revolutionized the management of nonpalpable breast lesions, and currently the majority of biopsies can be performed percutaneously, which is quicker, less invasive, and less expensive than excisional biopsy. Tissue acquisition is performed with automated core needles or directional vacuum-assisted biopsy probes. Guidance for percutaneous biopsy is usually provided by stereotaxis, ultrasonography, and, more recently, MRI.

Numerous studies comparing the sensitivity and specificity of stereotactic biopsy versus surgical biopsy have consistently found the two procedures to be statistically equivalent. The long-term false-negative rate for stereotactic biopsy is 1.4%, which equals best published results with surgical biopsy.

Up to 80% of patients with nonpalpable mammographic lesions are candidates for stereotactic core biopsy. Lesions near the chest wall or immediately behind the nipple often cannot be reached on the stereotactic table. Diffuse lesions, such as scattered calcifications or a large asymmetric density, are subject to undersampling with the percutaneous

</td></tr>
</table>

TABLE 5: Examples of eligible risk profiles used in the Breast Cancer Prevention Trial

Age (yr)	Risk profile
35	Two affected first-degree relatives plus personal history of biopsy
40	Two affected first-degree relatives plus no live births
45	Two affected first-degree relatives *or* one affected first-degree relative plus personal history of biopsy

approaches. Some patients are unable to lie prone on the stereotactic table for the duration of the examination. Finally, stereotactic units and trained personnel are not universally available.

Ultrasonography-guided core biopsies are another accurate percutaneous technique, useful for lesions best imaged by ultrasonography. Since the biopsy gun is handheld and guided in real time by the ultrasound imager, there is more vari-

TABLE 6: Number of events among Breast Cancer Prevention Trial participants

Type of event	Placebo	Tamoxifen	Total
Invasive breast cancer	154 (5)[a]	85 (3)[a]	239 (8)[a]
Noninvasive breast cancer	59	31	90
Hip fracture	20	9	29
Colles' fracture	12	7	19
Spinal fracture	39	31	70
Endometrial cancer	14	33	47
All other invasive cancers	88	85	173
Fatal stroke	3	4	7
Nonfatal stroke	21	30	51
Transient ischemic attack	21	18	39
Fatal pulmonary embolism	0	2	2
Nonfatal pulmonary embolism	6	15	21
Deep vein thrombosis requiring hospitalization	3	3	6
Deep vein thrombosis not requiring hospitalization	16	27	43
Total	456	380	836

[a] Numbers in parentheses indicate the number of deaths due to breast cancer.

TABLE 7: TNM staging system for breast cancer

Primary tumor (T)

Tx	Primary tumor cannot be assessed
T0	No evidence of primary tumor
Tis	(DCIS) Carcinoma in situ
Tis	(LCIS) Carcinoma in situ
Tis	Paget's disease of the nipple with no tumor
T1	Tumor $\leq$ 2 cm in greatest dimension
T1mic	Microinvasion $\leq$ 0.1 cm in greatest dimension
T1a	Tumor > 0.1 but not > 0.5 cm in greatest dimension
T1b	Tumor > 0.5 cm but not >1 cm in greatest dimension
T1c	Tumor > 1 cm but not > 2 cm in greatest dimension
T2	Tumor > 2 cm but not > 5 cm in greatest dimension
T3	Tumor > 5 cm in greatest dimension
T4	Tumor of any size, with direct extension to (a) the chest wall or (b) skin only, as described below
T4a	Extension to the chest wall, not including the pectoralis muscle
T4b	Edema (including peau d'orange) or ulceration of the skin of the breast or satellite skin nodules confined to the same breast
T4c	Both T4a and T4b
T4d	Inflammatory carcinoma

Note: Paget's disease associated with a tumor is classified according to the size of the tumor.

Regional lymph nodes (N)

Nx	Regional lymph nodes cannot be assessed (eg, previously removed)
N0	No regional lymph node metastasis
N1	Metastasis in movable ipsilateral axillary lymph node(s); pathologic involvement of one to three axillary lymph nodes
N2	Metastasis in ipsilateral axillary lymph node(s) fixed or matted, or in clinically apparent[a] ipsilateral internal mammary nodes in the *absence* of clinically evident axillary lymph node metastasis; pathologic involvement of four to nine axillary lymph nodes
N2a	Metastasis in ipsilateral axillary lymph nodes fixed to one another (matted) or to other structures
N2b	Metastasis only in clinically apparent[a] ipsilateral internal mammary nodes and in the *absence* of clinically evident axillary lymph node metastasis
N3	Metastasis in ipsilateral infraclavicular lymph node(s) with or without axillary lymph node involvement, or in clinically apparent[a] ipsilateral internal mammary lymph node(s) and in the presence of clinically evident axillary lymph node metastasis; or metastasis in ipsilateral supraclavicular lymph node(s) with or without axillary or internal mammary lymph node involvement; pathologic involvement of 10 or more axillary lymph nodes
N3a	Metastasis in ipsilateral infraclavicular lymph node(s) and axillary lymph node(s)
N3b	Metastasis in ipsilateral internal mammary lymph node(s) and axillary lymph node(s)
N3c	Metastasis in ipsilateral supraclavicular lymph node(s)

[a] "Clinically apparent" is defined as detected by imaging studies (excluding lymphoscintigraphy) or by clinical examination or grossly visible pathologically.

Pathologic classification (pN)

pNx   Regional lymph nodes cannot be assessed (eg, previously removed)

pN0   No regional lymph node metastasis

     pN0(I–)   No regional lymph node metastasis histologically; negative IHC

     pN0(I+)   No regional lymph node metastasis histologically; positive IHC; no IHC cluster > 0.2 mm

     pN0(mol–)   No regional lymph node metastasis histologically; negative molecular findings (RT-PCR)

     pN0(mol+)   No regional lymph node metastasis histologically; positive molecular findings (RT-PCR)

pN1   Metastasis in 1 to 3 axillary lymph nodes, and/or internal mammary nodes with microscopic disease detected by SLN dissection but not clinically apparent

     pN1mi   Micrometastasis (> 0.2 mm but ≤ 2.0 mm)

     pN1a   Metastasis in 1 to 3 axillary lymph nodes

     pN1b   Metastasis in internal mammary nodes with microscopic disease detected by SLN dissection but not clinically apparent

     pN1c   Metastasis in 1 to 3 axillary lymph nodes and in internal mammary lymph nodes with microscopic disease detected by SLN dissection but not clinically apparent

pN2   Metastasis in 4 to 9 axillary lymph nodes, or in clinically apparent internal mammary lymph nodes in the absence of axillary lymph node metastasis to ipsilateral axillary lymph node(s) fixed to each other or other structures

     pN2a   Metastasis in 4 to 9 axillary lymph nodes (at least 1 tumor deposit > 2.0 mm)

     pN2b   Metastasis in clinically apparent internal mammary lymph nodes in the absence of axillary lymph node metastasis

pN3   Metastasis in ≥ 10 axillary lymph nodes, or in infraclavicular lymph nodes, or in clinically apparent ipsilateral mammary lymph nodes(s) in the presence of 1 or more positive axillary lymph node(s); or, in > 3 axillary lymph nodes with clinically negative microscopic metastasis in internal mammary lymph nodes; or in ipsilateral supraclavicular lymph nodes

     pN3a   Metastasis in ≥ 10 axillary lymph nodes (at least 1 tumor deposit > 2.0 mm); or, metastasis to the infraclavicular lymph nodes

     pN3b   Metastasis in clinically apparent ipsilateral internal mammary lymph nodes in the presence of ≥ 1 positive axillary lymph node(s); or, in > 3 axillary lymph nodes and in internal mammary lymph nodes with microscopic disease detected by SLN dissection but not clinically apparent

     pN3c   Metastasis in ipsilateral supraclavicular lymph nodes

Distant metastasis (M)

Mx   Distant metastasis cannot be assessed

M0   No distant metastasis

M1   Distant metastasis   *continued on following page*

DCIS = ductal carcinoma in situ; IHC = immunohistochemistry; LCIS = lobular carcinoma in situ; RT-PCR = reverse transcriptase-polymerase chain reaction; SLN = sentinel lymph node

TABLE 7: TNM staging system for breast cancer *(continued)*

Stage grouping

Stage	T	N	M
Stage 0	Tis	N0	M0
Stage I	T1[b]	N0	M0
Stage IIA	T0	N1	M0
	T1[b]	N1	M0
	T2	N0	M0
Stage IIB	T2	N1	M0
	T3	N0	M0
Stage IIIA	T0	N2	M0
	T1[b]	N2	M0
	T2	N2	M0
	T3	N1-2	M0
Stage IIIB	T4	N0	M0
	T4	N1	M0
	T4	N2	M0
Stage IIIC	Any T	N3	M0
Stage IV	Any T	Any N	M1

[b] T1 includes T1mic

From: Greene FL, Page DL, Fleming ID, et al (eds): AJCC Cancer Staging Manual, 6th ed. New York, Springer-Verlag, 2002.

ability in performance, depending on the experience and skill of the practitioner. The overall reported accuracy rate of ultrasonography-guided biopsy is comparable to rates achieved with stereotactic and surgical biopsies.

Ultrasonography-guided or stereotactic FNA is another biopsy option. Although somewhat less invasive than core biopsy, FNA provides only cytologic (not histologic) pathology results. This technique can result in both false-positive and false-negative results, whereas a false-positive result has not been reported to date for core breast biopsies. FNA is most successful in centers that have an experienced cytopathologist, who, ideally, is available on site to review smears for adequacy during FNA procedures.

Breast MRI is currently used to search for an occult primary tumor in the setting of known metastasis, evaluate the extent of disease in a biopsy-proven breast carcinoma (useful if breast conservation is being considered), and assess lesions in implant-augmented breasts. It also is useful for screening high-risk women with dense breasts on mammography and nondiagnostic ultransonography or evaluating a borderline lesion when it is obscured by dense tissue. Breast MRI has a high sensitivity, and clinical developments have improved its specificity. Breast MRI examinations have recently been facilitated by the development of computer-aided detection software, which can help to streamline the interpretation of these images and produce a more uniform result.

Breast surgeons are increasingly utilizing breast MRI for surgical planning. In a study reported by Bedrosian et al (a retrospective review of 267 patients who had preoperative MRI prior to undergoing definitive surgery), preoperative breast MRI changed the planned surgical approach in 26% of cases, including 16.5% of cases of breast conservation switched to mastectomy. Imaging centers across the United States have a varying degree of expertise in performing, interpreting, and providing a standard reporting nomenclature for breast MRI. The ACR is currently developing an accreditation program in breast MRI to address this issue.

Ultrasonography Stavros et al have described ultrasonographic features of solid masses that suggest benign or malignant disease, such as sharp margins (benign) and taller-than-wide lesions (malignant). Although these features are useful for clinical decision-making, their utility in increasing the specificity of the breast lesion work-up has not been verified.

Sestamibi nuclear medicine scanning can help differentiate benign from malignant mammographic asymmetries and may play a role in evaluating palpable masses. Due to its limited spatial resolution and scatter, this technique is not reliable for lesions 1 cm or smaller. New gamma cameras designed specifically for breast scanning may overcome this limitation in the future.

Prevention

LIFESTYLE CHANGES ASSOCIATED WITH BREAST CANCER RISK REDUCTION

There is increasing evidence that lifestyle changes may alter an individual's breast cancer risk.

Physical activity has been associated with a reduction in breast cancer risk. The benefit was greatest in younger, premenopausal women. The activity can be related to leisure or work-time activities.

It has been suggested that women who exercise 3.5 to 4.0 times per week have a reduced incidence of breast cancer, compared with women who do not exercise. Exercise's protective effect may be associated with a reduction in the frequency of ovulatory cycles and circulating estrogen and progesterone levels.

Alcohol consumption Numerous studies on the effects of alcohol consumption on breast cancer risk and the results of a cohort study addressing this issue have been published. When compared with nondrinkers, women who consumed 2.3 to 4.5 bottles of beer per day, 2.5 to 5.6 glasses of wine per day, or 2 to 4 shots of liquor per day had a 41% higher risk of developing invasive breast cancer. Some reports indicate that the consumption of a moderate amount of alcohol (red wine) may decrease the risk of breast cancer, although these results are not conclusive. The biologic basis for the association between alcohol consumption and an increased risk of breast cancer is unclear. It has been proposed that there is a positive correlation between alcohol and estrogen levels.

Alterations in diet and tobacco use A reduced incidence of breast cancer has been observed in countries where the diet is typically low in fat. However, no reduction in breast cancer risk has been observed in the United States when women followed low-fat diets. An association between red meat consumption or tobacco use and breast cancer risk has not been demonstrated.

Lactation Although it has been suggested that lactation may protect against breast cancer, it is unclear whether lactation reduces breast cancer risk. A recent study failed to demonstrate any breast cancer risk reduction in women who breast-fed and showed no dose-response effect in women who breast-fed for longer periods.

CHEMOPREVENTION

Breast Cancer Prevention Trial

The NIH and NCI have publicized the results of the National Surgical Adjuvant Breast and Bowel Project (NSABP) Breast Cancer Prevention Trial (BCPT). Women who had a risk of developing breast cancer equivalent to that of women 60 years of age qualified as participants in this double-blind, randomized trial. (For representative eligibility profiles, see Table 5.) A total of 13,388 women were randomized to receive tamoxifen or placebo.

Benefits of therapy The summary results indicate that tamoxifen prevented about half of both invasive and noninvasive breast cancers in all age groups. A secondary benefit of tamoxifen appeared to be a reduction in the incidence of hip fracture (Table 6). At present, no survival advantage has been shown for participants in this trial.

Side effects Tamoxifen-treated women younger than age 50 had no apparent increase in side effects. However, women older than age 50 experienced serious side effects, including vascular events and endometrial cancer. Particularly worrisome was the increased incidence of endometrial cancer in the tamoxifen-treated patients (Table 6). In addition, a significant increase in pulmonary embolism and deep vein thrombosis was noted, especially in women older than age 50 (Table 6).

Current recommendations

Based on results of the BCPT, the FDA has approved tamoxifen for use in women at high risk (1.66% chance of getting breast cancer in the next 5 years, based on the Gail model) of breast cancer.

The NCI and NSABP are in the process of developing risk profiles based on age, number of affected first-degree relatives with breast cancer, number of prior breast biopsies, presence or absence of atypical hyperplasia or LCIS, age at menarche, and age at first live birth. These risk profiles may help guide women in making the decision as to whether or not to take tamoxifen.

An ASCO working group published an assessment of tamoxifen use in the setting of breast cancer risk reduction. All women older than 35 years of age with a Gail model risk of > 1.66% (or the risk equivalent to that of women 60 years of age) should be considered candidates for this treatment strategy. Comorbid conditions, such as a history of deep vein thrombosis, must be a part of the consent process and treatment decision.

Although the BCPT results establish tamoxifen as the standard of care for the primary chemoprevention of breast cancer in high-risk women, concern over the side effects of tamoxifen has prompted a continuing search for an agent that displays a more desirable efficacy/toxicity profile. Raloxifene (Evista), approved for the prevention of osteoporosis in postmenopausal women, displays antiestrogenic properties in the breast and endometrium and estrogenic effects in the bone, making it an attractive candidate for comparison with tamoxifen.

The Continuing Outcomes Relevant to Evista (CORE) trial, a 4-year follow-up to the Multiple Outcomes of Raloxifene (MORE) trial that examined the effect of long-term therapy with raloxifene in postmenopausal women with breast cancer, found that daily intake of the agent reduced the risk of invasive breast cancer by 59%. Compared with placebo, the incidence of invasive estrogen receptor-positive breast cancer was also reduced in the raloxifene arm ($P <$ .001). Women who took raloxifene were more likely to develop blood clots in their legs or lungs, but the increased risk was not statistically significant. However, long-term use of raloxifene did not increase the risk of uterine cancer, as does long-term use of tamoxifen.

The Study of Tamoxifen and Raloxifene (STAR or NSABP P-2) began in July 1999 at almost 400 centers in North America. A total of 19,747 postmenopausal women, or women $\geq$ 35 years old at increased risk of breast cancer by Gail criteria, were randomized to receive either tamoxifen (20 mg/d) or raloxifene (60 mg/d) for 5 years. Study endpoints included invasive and noninvasive breast cancers, cardiovascular disease, endometrial cancer, bone fractures, and vascular events.

There were 163 cases of invasive breast cancer in women assigned to tamoxifen and 168 of those assigned to raloxifene (incidence, 4.30 per 1,000 vs 4.41 per 1,000; risk ratio (RR), 1.02; 95% confidence interval (CI), 0.82–1.28). There were fewer cases of noninvasive breast cancer in the tamoxifen group (57 cases) than in the raloxifene group (80 cases); (incidence, 1.51 vs 2.11 per 1,000; RR, 1.40; 95% CI, 0.98–2.00). There were 36 cases of uterine cancer with tamoxifen and 23 with raloxifene (RR, 0.62; 95% CI, 0.35–1.08). The risk of other cancers, fractures, ischemic heart disease, and stroke is similar for both drugs. There was no difference in the total number of deaths (101 for tamoxifen vs 96 for raloxifene) or in causes of death. The authors concluded that raloxifene is as effective as tamoxifen in reducing the risk of invasive breast cancer and has a lower risk of thromboembolic events and cataracts but a nonstatistically significant higher risk of noninvasive breast cancer.

Staging and prognosis

Staging system The most widely used system to stage breast cancer is the American Joint Committee on Cancer (AJCC) classification, which is based on tumor size, the status of regional lymph nodes, and the presence of distant metastasis (Table 7).

Clinical staging is performed initially and is determined after the physical examination and appropriate radiologic studies have been performed.

Pathologic staging Pathologic stage is determined following surgery for operable breast cancer. Pathologic tumor size may differ from clinical tumor size. In addition, axillary nodal metastases that were not clinically evident may be detected after pathologic examination. With the advent of powerful molecular techniques, isolated tumor cells (ITCs) can be identified in histologically negative nodes. In the current AJCC staging, pathologic staging of nodes for detection of ITCs was included to obtain more information and hopefully gain insight into the biologic significance of these ITCs.

Prognostic factors Numerous prognostic factors for breast cancer have been identified.

Lymph node status Axillary nodal metastasis is the most important prognostic factor. Axillary nodal involvement and survival were evaluated in patients with breast cancer. Survival was examined relative to the number of nodes involved and the location of nodes that contained metastatic deposits. For any given number of positive nodes, survival was independent of the *level* of involvement but was directly related to the *number* of involved nodes.

Overall, patients who have node-negative disease have a 10-year survival rate of 70% and a 5-year recurrence rate of 19%. As the number of positive nodes increases, so does the likelihood of relapse. Patients with > 10 positive lymph nodes have a recurrence rate of 72% to 82%. The majority of patients who develop recurrence after initial curative treatment of early-stage breast cancer will have distant metastases.

Hormone-receptor status In general, hormone receptor-positive tumors have a more indolent course than do hormone receptor-negative tumors. However, the hormone receptor status of a tumor is a stronger predictive than prognostic factor; that is, hormone receptor-negative tumors are unlikely to respond to endocrine therapy in contrast to hormone receptor-positive tumors.

Other factors that have been utilized to predict outcome are histologic grade, lymphovascular permeation, S-phase fraction, and ploidy.

More recently, molecular prognostic factors have been evaluated to determine their utility in predicting outcome. They include the growth factor receptors (epidermal growth factor receptor and c-*erb*B-2/*neu*), tumor suppressor genes (*p53*), proteolytic enzymes that may be associated with invasion of disease and metastasis (cathepsin D), and metastasis suppressor genes (*nm23*).

Of these molecular markers, HER2/*neu* or c-*erb*B-1/*neu* is probably the most widely studied in breast cancer to date. HER2/*neu* amplification is often associated with a more aggressive behavior and thus a poorer outcome for patients with HER2/*neu*-positive tumors. Fortunately, targeted therapy with trastuzumab (Herceptin) has changed the course of treatment, providing longer survival when used in combination with chemotherapy for patients with metastatic disease.

SUGGESTED READING

ON RISK FACTORS AND GENETIC CANCER RISK ASSESSMENT

Daly M, National Comprehensive Cancer Network: Genetic/familial high-risk assessment: Breast and ovarian. Clinical Practice Guidelines in Oncology v.1.2008.

Metcalfe KA, Lynch HT, Ghadirian P, et al: The risk of ovarian cancer after breast cancer in BRCA1 and BRCA2 carriers. Gynecol Oncol 96:222–226, 2005.

Ravdin PM, Cronin KA, Howlader N, et al: The decrease in breast-cancer incidence in 2003 in the United States. N Engl J Med 356:1670–1674, 2007.

Walsh T, Casadei S, Coats KH, et al: Spectrum of mutations in BRCA1, BRCA2, CHEK2, and TP53 in families at high risk of breast cancer. JAMA 295:1379–1388, 2006.

Weitzel JN, Lagos VI, Cullinane CA, et al: Limited family structure and BRCA gene mutation status in single cases of breast cancer. JAMA 297:2587–2595, 2007.

ON PREVENTION

Anderson GL, Judd HL, Kaunitz AM, et al: Effects of estrogen plus progestin on gynecologic cancers and associated diagnostic procedures. The Women's Health Initiative Randomized Trial. JAMA 290:1739–1748, 2003.

Rebbeck TR, Friebel T, Lynch HT, et al: Bilateral prophylactic mastectomy reduces breast cancer risk in *BRCA1* and *BRCA2* mutation carriers: The PROSE Study Group. J Clin Oncol 22:1055–1062, 2004.

Vogel VG, Costantino JP, Wickerham DL, et al; National Surgical Adjuvant Breast and Bowel Project (NSABP): Effects of tamoxifen vs raloxifene on the risk of developing invasive breast cancer and other disease outcomes: The NSABP Study of Tamoxifen and Raloxifene (STAR) P-2 trial. JAMA 295:2727–2741, 2006.

Weitzel JN, Buys SS, Sherman WH, et al: Reduced mammographic density with use of a gonadotropin-releasing hormone agonist-based chemoprevention regimen in BRCA1 carriers. Clin Cancer Res 13:654–658, 2007.

ON SCREENING AND DIAGNOSIS

Feigin KN, Keating DM, Telford PM, et al: Clinical breast examination in a comprehensive breast cancer screening program: Contribution and cost. Radiology 240:650–655, 2006.

Kriege M, Biekelmans CTM, Boetes C, et al: Efficacy of MRI and mammography for breast cancer screening in women with a familial or genetic predisposition. N Engl J Med 351:427–437, 2004.

Lindfors KK, McGahan MC, Rosenquist CJ, et al: Computer-aided detection of breast cancer: A cost-effectiveness study. Radiology 239:710–717, 2006.

Schnall MD, Blume J, Bluemke DA, et al: MRI detection of distinct incidental cancer in women with primary breast cancer studied in IBMC 6883. J Surg Oncol 92:32–38, 2005.

CHAPTER 9

Stages 0 and I breast cancer

Lori Jardines, MD, Bruce G. Haffty, MD, and Melanie Royce, MD, PhD

This chapter focuses on the diagnosis and management of early-stage breast cancer, ie, stages 0 and I disease. This is an important area, since more noninvasive and small breast cancers are being diagnosed due to the increasing use of screening mammography. Treatment of these malignancies will continue to evolve as the results of clinical trials lead to further refinements in therapy.

STAGE 0 BREAST CANCER

Stage 0 breast cancer includes noninvasive breast cancer—lobular carcinoma in situ (LCIS) and ductal carcinoma in situ (DCIS)—as well as Paget's disease of the nipple when there is no associated invasive disease.

LOBULAR CARCINOMA IN SITU

LCIS is nonpalpable, produces no consistent mammographic changes, and is often an incidental finding after breast biopsy performed for another reason.

The biologic behavior of LCIS continues to be an issue of debate. Most clinicians agree that it is a marker for increased risk for all types of breast cancer (both noninvasive and invasive).

Epidemiology and etiology

The incidence of LCIS has doubled over the past 25 years and is now 2.8 per 100,000 women. In the past, the peak incidence of LCIS was in women in their 40s. Over the past 3 decades, the peak incidence has increased to the 50s. The incidence of LCIS decreases in women who are in their 60s to 80s. It has been suggested that the increase in the age of peak incidence of LCIS is related to the use of hormone replacement therapy (HRT). It is also possible that the use of HRT prevents the usual regression of LCIS normally seen at the time of menopause.

Signs and symptoms

LCIS is nonpalpable and has no consistent features on breast imaging. Most often, LCIS is found in association with a completely separate mammographic abnormality or palpable mass.

STAGES 0-I BREAST

Risk of invasive cancer

Approximately 20% to 25% of women with LCIS will develop invasive cancer within 15 years after the diagnosis of LCIS. More often, the invasive cancer is ductal in origin, and both breasts are at risk. At this point, there are no reliable molecular markers to determine which patients with LCIS will progress to invasive cancer.

Just as the incidence of LCIS has increased, there has also been an associated increase in the incidence of cases of infiltrating lobular carcinoma in post-menopausal women. The increase in invasive lobular carcinoma peaks in women in their 70s.

Pathology

LCIS appears to arise from the terminal duct-lobular apparatus, and the disease tends to be multifocal, multicentric, and bilateral. Subsequently, other types of LCIS have also been described and include pleomorphic LCIS. This entity tends to be associated with infiltrating lobular carcinoma, and the cytologic features are similar to those of intermediate- or high-grade DCIS. Pleomorphic LCIS may be more aggressive, with a higher likelihood of progression to invasion than classic LCIS.

Treatment options

The management of LCIS is continuing to evolve since the disease appears to be heterogeneous. Presently, treatment options include close follow-up, participation in a chemoprevention trial, tamoxifen, or bilateral prophylactic total mastectomy with or without reconstruction. At present, the decision for a given treatment will depend upon the patient's individual risk profile for DCIS or invasive breast cancer after careful counseling. In the future, treatment decisions may be based upon an analysis of a series of molecular markers, which can separate those patients with a low risk for invasion from those who are at high risk for disease progression.

DUCTAL CARCINOMA IN SITU

DCIS is being encountered more frequently with the expanded use of screening mammography. In some institutions, DCIS accounts for 25% to 50% of all breast cancers.

Long-term outcome results from a cohort of DCIS patients from two NSABP randomized trials were presented at the 2007 ASCO. A total of 2,615 women with primary DCIS from NSABP B-17 and B-24 trials, with a median follow-up of > 12 years, were analyzed for ipsilateral breast tumor recurrence (IBTR). IBTR was a first failure in 465 patients (243 invasive, 222 noninvasive). The 12-year cumulative incidence of all IBTRs was 32.9% for lumpectomy only (LO), 15.8% for lumpectomy with whole-breast irradiation (LRT), and 12.5% for LRT plus tamoxifen. Radiotherapy significantly reduced invasive IBTR. Tamoxifen conferred additional benefit on reducing invasive IBTR. Women with invasive IBTR had a two-fold greater mortality risk relative to those without invasive IBTR; the effect was greater for LRT patients than for LO patients. However, overall mortality was low. The investigators concluded that occurrence of an invasive IBTR after DCIS, particularly after RT, confers increased risk for subsequent mortality, as is seen after an invasive index tumor (Wapnir I, Dignam J, Julian TB, et al: J Clin Oncol 25[18s]:520, 2007).

Epidemiology

DCIS, like invasive ductal carcinoma, occurs more frequently in women, although it accounts for approximately 5% of all male breast cancers. The average age at diagnosis of DCIS is 54 to 56 years, which is approximately a decade later than the age at presentation for LCIS.

Signs and symptoms

The clinical signs and symptoms of DCIS include a mass, breast pain, or bloody nipple discharge. On mammography, the disease most often appears as microcalcifications. Because these microcalcifications are nonpalpable and are not always associated with a mass, DCIS is often discovered with mammography alone. Approximately 5% of patients who present with pathologic nipple discharge will have underlying breast cancer, and many of them will have DCIS alone.

Risk of invasive cancer

The risk of developing an invasive carcinoma following a biopsy-proven diagnosis of DCIS is between 25% and 50%. Virtually all invasive cancers that follow DCIS are ductal and ipsilateral and generally present in the same quadrant within 10 years of the diagnosis of DCIS. For these reasons, DCIS is considered a more ominous lesion than LCIS (which is considered a marker for risk) and appears to be a more direct precursor of invasive cancer.

Pathology

A variety of histologic patterns are seen with DCIS, including solid, cribriform, and papillary. Some researchers have divided DCIS into two subgroups: comedo and noncomedo types. As compared with the noncomedo subtypes, the comedo variant has a higher proliferative rate, overexpression of human epidermal growth factor receptor 2 (HER2/*neu*), and a higher incidence of local recurrence and microinvasion. DCIS is less likely to be bilateral and has approximately a 30% incidence of multicentricity.

Kuhl and colleagues investigated the detection rates of DCIS by mammography and breast MRI. During a 5-year study period, 193 women had a pathologic diagnosis of pure DCIS, without associated invasive breast cancer or microinvasion. Of them, 167 had undergone both imaging tests preoperatively; 93 of the 167 DCIS (56%) were diagnosed by mammography, and 153 (92%) were diagnosed by MRI ($P < .001$). With increasing nuclear grade, sensitivity of mammography decreased; it was highest in low-grade DCIS and lowest in high-grade DCIS. It even dropped further to 35% in high-grade DCIS without necroses. The sensitivity of MRI was superior to that of mammography across all DCIS subtypes. In addition, sensitivity increased with nuclear grade of DCIS; it was lowest in low-grade DCIS (80%) and highest in high-grade DCIS (98%), independent of presence or absence of necroses (Kuhl CK, Schrading S, Wardelmann E, et al. 30th SABCS, [abstract 44], December 13-16, 2007).

Treatment of noninvasive breast carcinoma

DUCTAL CARCINOMA IN SITU

Breast-conserving surgery

Breast-conserving surgery, followed by radiation therapy to the intact breast, is now considered the standard treatment of DCIS. Because the incidence of positive lymph nodes after axillary lymph node dissection for DCIS is ~ 1% to 2%, axillary dissection is not indicated in most instances.

The most important factor in determining local tumor control within the breast is margin status. A surgical margin of 1 mm has been associated with a 43% chance of having residual disease at the time of reexcision. When a surgical margin of 10 mm can be obtained, there is an extremely low rate of recurrence (4%). A 10-mm surgical margin may not be practical, however, when trying to provide a good cosmetic outcome. When breast-conserving therapy is used alone (without irradiation), a margin of at least 10 mm is required, and the tumor should be small (< 1 cm) and a noncomedo type. Although a wide margin is always desirable, narrower margins are acceptable for DCIS when radiation therapy is used after lumpectomy.

Sentinel node biopsy

The sentinel lymph node is the first node in the draining lymphatic basin that receives primary lymph flow. The technique of sampling the first draining lymph node was initially described in the management of patients with melanoma to determine who would benefit from regional lymph node dissection and was performed using a vital blue dye. This same technique has been used in patients with breast cancer, and sentinel lymph node biopsy represents a minimally invasive way to determine whether the axilla is involved with disease. The precise methods for identifying the sentinel lymph node (filtered vs unfiltered Tc-99m sulfur colloid and/or blue dye) and assessing the node (hematoxylin and eosin staining vs immunohistochemistry [IHC] vs polymerase chain reaction [PCR]) are being studied.

When blue dye is used, it can be injected into the breast parenchyma at the primary tumor or subareolar site. The radioactive tracer can be injected subdermally or intraparenchymally at the site of the primary tumor or in the subareolar location. The site and technique of injection will be based upon individual patient factors, including the type and location of the previous breast biopsy.

When lymphatic mapping and sentinel lymph node biopsy are performed, a blue vital dye and/or a radioactive tracer (generally technetium-labeled sulfur colloid) can be used. When a radiotracer is used, lymphoscintigraphy can also be performed to aid in locating the sentinel node. When a sentinel node biopsy is performed using blue dye, the axillary surgery should be performed carefully to avoid disrupting the blue-stained afferent lymphatic channels. When a radioisotope is used, a hand-held gamma counter is used to locate the sentinel node.

Axillary lymph node dissection is not routinely recommended for patients with DCIS. Recently, however, investigators have used sentinel lymph node biopsy to determine whether individuals with DCIS may harbor occult nodal metastases. Current studies have identified metastatic disease to the axillary nodes in up to 12% of patients who have undergone sentinel lymph node biopsy. Despite this relatively high percentage of positive sentinel nodes, recurrence in the nodal basins is rare (about 2%). Based on this and recent work, there is no indication for routine sentinel lymph node biopsy in patients with DCIS.

Factors associated with an increased risk of axillary metastasis with a diagnosis of DCIS are extensive DCIS requiring mastectomy, suspicion of microinvasion, DCIS associated with a palpable mass, and evidence of lymphovascular permeation or invasion seen on review of the slides. These factors likely are associated with a preoperatively nondiagnosed invasive component. However, for patients diagnosed with DCIS who are scheduled for mastectomy, sentinel lymph node sampling, prior to mastectomy, is a reasonable practice. In the event that an occult invasive cancer within the mastectomy is found, a negative sentinel node would be reassuring and perhaps would make it possible to avoid follow-up axillary dissection.

Patients whose sentinel node biopsy is negative do not require a complete node dissection, because the risk of an axillary recurrence is extremely low. Many institutions are using IHC in the evaluation of the sentinel node. When there is no evidence of metastatic disease by routine hematoxylin and eosin staining and the node is IHC-negative, the node is considered pN0(i–). When the routine staining is negative and isolated tumor cells are seen on IHC alone and no tumor cluster is greater than 0.2 mm, the node is staged as pN0(i+). The majority of the data suggest

Partial breast brachytherapy irradiation (PBBI) trial, using the MammoSite balloon delivery system in margin-negative lumpectomies, was reported by Streeter et al. Patients ≥ 45 years with unicentric pure DCIS, clinically node-negative, mammogram size ≤ 3 cm, gross tumor removed 5 cm or less in size, and all margins negative were eligible for the study. An iridium-192 high-dose rate brachytherapy source was guided through a central tube in the balloon to deliver a dose of 34 Gy in 10 fractions twice daily, prescribed to 1 cm from the balloon's surface. There have been 4 recurrences, all ipsilateral and noninvasive, in 100 patients treated. There has not been any recurrences to date in nuclear grade 1 or 2 patients without comedo necrosis. No serious adverse events were noted. The investigators concluded that this method is well tolerated, with a 98% good, to excellent cosmesis rate. (Streeter Jr OE, Benitez P, Vicini F, et al. 30th SABCS, [abstract 4079], December 13-16, 2007).

A study evaluated toxicity and cosmetic results in 43 selected patients ≥ 60 years of age with early-stage breast cancer receiving high-dose rate (HDR) brachytherapy using the MammoSite device as sole treatment in patients with T1 breast cancer. After a median follow-up of 13 months, there were no local recurrences and one contralateral lobular carcinoma. Seventeen (68%), 13 (52%), 7 (28%), 5 (20%), and 4 (16%) patients had erythema, seroma, inflammation, hematoma, and infection, respectively. At 3 months, breast erythema grade ≥ 2 was significantly correlated to cosmetic results. A trend of excellent cosmetic outcome was observed in patients with skin spacing ≥ 19 mm (50%) compared with patients with < 19 mm (11%; P = .087). At 1 year, the rate of "good-to-excellent" cosmetic results was 84% (Belkacemi Y, Chauvet MP, Giard S, et al: 30th SABCS, [abstract 4080], December 13-16, 2007).

that there is no effect on survival, the patient is considered node-negative, and a complete axillary node dissection is not warranted. Some authors suggest, however, that the presence of isolated tumor cells on sentinel node biopsy has been associated with the presence of additional disease within the remaining axillary nodes and a decreased survival when an axillary node dissection was not performed. Additional studies will be necessary to resolve this conflict. If the focus of metastatic disease is greater than 0.2 mm but less than 2 mm, the node is staged as pN1mi. In this instance, consideration should be given to a complete axillary node dissection or the administration of axillary radiation. The likelihood that additional nodal disease will be identified in the axilla increases with the size of the primary tumor.

Adjuvant radiation therapy

Retrospective series of patients with DCIS, as well as subsets of patients with early invasive cancer, have been treated with conservative surgery alone, omitting radiation therapy to the intact breast. In addition, several prospective, randomized trials have attempted to address this issue of omission of breast irradiation for both invasive cancer and DCIS. It is clear from all of these series that omission of breast irradiation results in a significantly higher ipsilateral breast tumor recurrence rate but has not, as yet, had an impact on overall survival.

Two large prospective randomized trials have demonstrated a significant reduction in local relapse with the use of postlumpectomy irradiation in treatment of DCIS. In the National Surgical Adjuvant Breast and Bowel Project (NSABP) B-17, the local recurrence rate at 8 years was reduced from 27% to 12% with postlumpectomy irradiation.

Similar results have been reported by a European cooperative group study of 1,010 women with DCIS randomly assigned to receive either 50 Gy of radiotherapy to the whole breast over 5 weeks or no further treatment. With a median follow-up of 4.25 years, the 4-year local relapse-free rate was 91% in the radiotherapy arm versus 84% in the observation arm. Hazard ratios with postexcision radiotherapy were 0.62 for all local relapses, 0.65 for DCIS recurrences, and 0.60 for noninvasive recurrences.

Both trials showed that radiotherapy reduces the risk of both noninvasive and invasive recurrences. Identification of a subgroup of patients who did not benefit from postlumpectomy irradiation has not as yet been clearly defined.

The Van Nuys Prognostic Index (VNPI), based on tumor size, grade, presence of necrosis, and width of the excision margin, is an algorithm commonly used to predict local recurrence after breast-conserving surgery for DCIS. In some series, VNPI lacked discriminatory power for guiding further patient management. In studies performed by this group, it appears that the width of the excision margin is the most important predictor of local recurrence after breast-conserving surgery for DCIS.

One study demonstrated acceptable local control in patients with DCIS treated by excision alone, provided that wide negative margins were obtained. In this retrospective series of 469 patients, radiation therapy did not lower the local recurrence rate in patients with wide ($\geq$ 10 mm) negative margins but did produce a significant benefit in patients with close ($\leq$ 1 mm) margins. The authors concluded that radiation therapy is unlikely to benefit patients with wide negative margins and small tumors. These findings need to be confirmed in prospective, randomized trials.

Although there may be some patients for whom wide excision alone is appropriate therapy, the available literature has not consistently identified the specific subgroup of patients. Clearly, the omission of radiation therapy in subsets of patients remains a controversial issue worthy of further investigation. It is hoped that ongoing randomized studies will help to resolve some of the conflicts generated by selective, retrospective studies.

Two trials have addressed the need for postlumpectomy radiation therapy (RT) in older women with breast cancer. Both studies randomized patients, following lumpectomy and adjuvant hormonal therapy, to receive RT or observation. Both studies confirmed statistically significant improvements in local control with RT, and local relapse rates were acceptable in carefully selected patients. The authors concluded that selected elderly patients may be treated with hormonal therapy alone (without RT) following breast-conserving therapy.

Adjuvant tamoxifen therapy

Adjuvant chemotherapy is not routinely employed for patients with DCIS. In NSABP B-24, 1,804 women with DCIS treated with lumpectomy and irradiation were randomly assigned to receive placebo or tamoxifen. At a median follow-up of 74 months, women in the tamoxifen group had fewer breast cancer events than those in the placebo group (8.2% vs 13.4%; $P = .0009$). Tamoxifen decreased the incidence of both ipsilateral and contralateral events. The risk of ipsilateral invasive cancers was reduced by tamoxifen, regardless of the presence or absence of comedo-necrosis or margin involvement.

In a more recent analysis of NSABP B-24, it was found that the benefit from tamoxifen is derived exclusively by patients with hormone receptor-positive disease. Based on these results, tamoxifen should be considered as adjuvant therapy for patients with hormone receptor-positive DCIS. The use of tamoxifen for the prevention of secondary breast cancers in women at high risk for breast cancer, which includes women previously diagnosed with DCIS, has led some clinicians to consider the use of tamoxifen in women diagnosed with DCIS.

STAGE I BREAST CANCER

Stage I breast cancer ranges from microinvasive tumors (≤ 0.1 cm) to tumors ≤ 2 cm without evidence of spread to the regional lymph nodes.

Pathology of invasive breast cancer

Ductal carcinoma Most cases of invasive carcinomas of the breast are ductal in origin. Of the different histologic subtypes of ductal carcinoma that have been described, tubular, medullary, mucinous (colloid), and papillary subtypes have been associated with a favorable outcome.

Lobular carcinoma Approximately 5% to 10% of invasive breast cancers are lobular in origin. This histology has been associated with synchronous and metachronous contralateral primary tumors in as many as 30% of cases.

Treatment

SURGICAL AND RADIATION TREATMENTS

Multiple studies have demonstrated that patients with stage I breast cancer who are treated with either breast-conserving therapy (lumpectomy and radiation therapy) or modified radical mastectomy have similar disease-free and overall survival rates.

Breast-conserving therapy

Extent of local surgery The optimal extent of local surgery has yet to be determined and, in the literature, has ranged from excisional biopsy to quadrantectomy. A consensus statement on breast-conserving therapy issued by the National Cancer Institute (NCI) recommended that the breast cancer be completely excised with negative surgical margins.

The extent of axillary surgery also continues to evolve. In recent years, patients with early-stage breast cancer who have clinically node-negative disease have the option to undergo sentinel lymph node biopsy rather than axillary node dissection. The present standard of care for patients with a positive sentinel node is complete nodal dissection. A study is under way to determine whether patients with a positive sentinel node require further axillary surgery.

Patient selection Specific guidelines must be followed when selecting patients for breast conservation. Patients may be considered unacceptable candidates for conservative surgery and radiation therapy either because the risk of breast recurrence following the conservative approach is significant enough to warrant mastectomy or the likelihood of an unacceptable cosmetic result is high. Some patients who are candidates for breast conservation can undergo breast MRI to identify sites of additional disease within the breast that may preclude breast-conserving treatment, although this is not a standard for evaluation. Contraindications to breast-conserving surgery are listed in Table 1.

Risk factors for ipsilateral recurrence For patients undergoing conservative surgery followed by radiation therapy to the intact breast, the risk of ipsilateral breast tumor recurrence has been reported to range from 0.5% to 2.0% per year, with long-term failure rates varying from 7% to 20%. Risk factors for ipsilateral breast tumor recurrence include, but are not limited to, young age (< 35 to 40 years), an extensive intraductal component, major lymphocytic stromal reaction, peritumoral invasion, presence of tumor necrosis, and positive resection margins. After a wide excision has been performed, the specimen should be oriented and inked; the pathologist may then ink each margin a different color. If a positive surgical margin is present, the color-coded system will guide the reexcision to obtain negative surgical margins with the removal of the least amount of breast tissue possible.

Earlier studies demonstrated that an extensive intraductal component was a risk factor for local relapse. However, in subsequent reports, when negative surgical margins are achieved, patients with an extensive intraductal component can be safely treated with breast conservation. Although it is desirable to achieve negative surgical margins, the available data do not preclude the use of conservative treatment, provided that adequate radiation doses (> 6,000 cGy) to the tumor bed are employed. The role of the remaining risk factors previously cited in predicting recurrence is unclear, and patients should not be denied breast conservation because of their presence.

Cosmetic considerations include primary tumor size and location, overall breast size, total body weight, and a history of preexisting collagen vascular disease.

Tumor size and breast size are important in determining whether the patient will have an acceptable cosmetic outcome after surgical resection. Patients with large tumors with respect to breast size may consider neoadjuvant chemotherapy to reduce the size of the primary tumor and allow breast preservation. (See chapter 11 for discussion of neoadjuvant chemotherapy.)

Obese women with large, pendulous breasts may experience marked fibrosis and retraction of the irradiated breast, making a good to excellent cosmetic outcome less likely. Techniques of brachytherapy may prove beneficial for these women. Women in this situation can undergo bilateral reduction mammo-

TABLE 1: Contraindications to breast conservation

Absolute contraindications	Relative contraindications
Multicentric disease[a]	Tumor size vs breast size
Diffuse malignant microcalcifications	Tumor location
Pregnancy	Collagen vascular disease (excluding rheumatoid arthritis)
Persistently positive surgical margins	
Previous breast or mantle irradiation	

[a] If a satisfactory cosmetic outcome is anticipated, multicentric disease is considered to be a relative contraindication.

plasty after the wide excision of the primary tumor site has been completed. The partial mastectomy specimen should be evaluated by the pathologist to ensure adequate resection margins. Radiopaque clips can be left to mark and identify the primary tumor site for the radiation oncologist. The follow-up mammograms will be more difficult to interpret due to scarring and radiotherapy effect.

Patients with collagen vascular disease may develop more severe reactions following radiation therapy. Although initial anecdotal reports demonstrated higher complication rates in patients with collagen vascular disease, a case-controlled study of patients with early-stage breast cancer showed higher complication rates only in those patients with scleroderma. Other case-controlled studies have also failed to demonstrate significantly higher complication rates in patients with collagen vascular disease undergoing radiation therapy. It appears that most patients without active significant collagen vascular diseases may be candidates for breast-conserving surgery and irradiation, although this approach remains controversial.

In some instances, it is necessary to excise skin to obtain a negative surgical margin. This does not necessarily preclude the patient from undergoing breast-conserving therapy and does not mean the patient should have a poor cosmetic outcome. When skin must be removed to obtain a negative surgical margin, complex skin closures, such as V-Y advancement flaps or Z-plasties, can be utilized to enhance cosmesis.

Patients with centrally located tumors Traditionally, patients who have centrally located tumors requiring excision of the nipple-areolar complex have not been offered the option of breast conservation. However, the cosmetic result achieved after local tumor excision that includes the nipple-areolar complex may not differ significantly from that obtained following mastectomy and reconstruction.

Furthermore, conservatively treated patients with subareolar lesions do not necessarily need to have the nipple-areolar complex sacrificed, as long as negative surgical margins can be achieved. However, if the complex is not removed, the remaining breast tissue and overlying skin remain sensate. Recent studies also indicate that the incidence of local recurrence is not increased when primary tumors in this location are treated conservatively.

Genetically predisposed breast cancer patients For women harboring germline mutations in *BRCA1* or *BRCA2*, there are limited data regarding long-term outcome. Studies, to date, have shown acceptable local control rates in the short term and increased but acceptable rates of acute, subacute, and chronic normal tissue reactions with lumpectomy followed by radiation therapy. Women with germline *BRCA1* and *BRCA2* mutations, however, are at high risk for second primary tumors in the contralateral breast.

A study from Yale University demonstrated high rates of second primary tumors in the ipsilateral breast. This study suggests that if breast-conserving therapy is chosen, some prophylactic measures, such as selective estrogen receptor modulators or oophorectomy, might be considered to reduce the risk of second primary tumors in the ipsilateral or contralateral breast. Other studies also indicate a trend toward higher rates of late local relapses in *BRCA* carriers. Further studies are clearly warranted to assess the long-term risks and benefits of breast-conserving strategies in women harboring mutations in *BRCA1* and *BRCA2*.

Role of axillary lymph node dissection The role of axillary lymph node dissection in the management of breast cancer has been questioned, particularly when a patient with a clinically negative axilla is undergoing breast-conserving therapy. In most instances, the breast surgery is performed with the patient under local anesthesia and sedation on an outpatient basis. When axillary lymph node dissection is added, the surgery is performed with the patient under general anesthesia.

It has also been suggested that if the status of the nodes will not alter therapy, the dissection is unnecessary and the axilla can be treated with irradiation. On the other hand, if axillary lymph node staging is not performed, the patient will not be accurately staged and important prognostic information will be unavailable.

Patients who may not be candidates for sentinel node biopsy are women who are pregnant or breast-feeding and women who have had prior irradiation. A prior excisional biopsy does not preclude the use of lymphatic mapping and sentinel node biopsy. It has been suggested that sentinel node biopsy accurately evaluates the axilla, even in patients with tumors > 5 cm and in those who have been treated with neoadjuvant chemotherapy.

Once the sentinel node(s) have been identified, they can be sent to pathology for frozen section or touch-prep analysis.

Sensitivity and specificity In breast cancer, lymphatic mapping has been performed using a vital blue dye and/or lymphoscintigraphy. Studies have suggested that the success rate for identifying the sentinel node can be increased when these techniques are used in combination. The ability to identify the sentinel node can reach as high as 97% when blue dye and Tc-99m sulfur colloid are used together. When blue dye is used alone, the success rate is 83%, and when Tc-99m sulfur colloid is used alone, the success rate is 94%.

Results from a multi-institution practice have demonstrated that sentinel lymph node biopsy using dual-agent injection provides optimal sensitivity. In the study, 806 patients were enrolled by 99 surgeons for sentinel

> **A** collaborative group of 10 institutions reported results of breast-conserving surgery with radiation in 160 *BRCA1/2* mutation carriers compared with 440 matched sporadic controls. There was no statistically significant difference in the 15-year risk of local relapse in the carriers compared with controls (24% vs 17%; $P = .19$). However, when carriers who had undergone oophorectomy were removed from analysis, there was a higher risk of in-breast recurrence associated with *BRCA1/2* mutations (hazard ratio = 1.99; $P = .04$). The study suggests that in *BRCA1/2* carriers treated with breast-conserving surgery and radiation therapy, prophylactic oophorectomy reduces the risk of an in-breast relapse to levels comparable to those in sporadic controls *(Pierce LJ, Levin AM, Rebbeck TR, et al: J Clin Oncol 24:2437-2443, 2006).*

lymph node biopsy by single-agent (blue dye alone or radioactive colloid alone) or dual-agent injection at the discretion of the surgeons. All patients underwent complete level I/II dissection following the sentinel procedure. There were no significant differences in the identification of a sentinel node among patients who underwent single- compared with dual-agent injection. However, the false-negative rate was 11.8% for single-agent versus 5.8% for dual-agent injections ($P = .05$).

The sensitivity and specificity of sentinel lymph node biopsy are high, and the likelihood of a false-negative result is extremely low. False-negative rates vary among series, ranging from 0% to 11%. In one series, in 18% of the cases where the frozen-section evaluation of the node was negative, the final pathologic evaluation revealed metastatic disease, and the patient ultimately required lymph node dissection. This potential result can be distressing to patients; however, they should be informed of this possibility at the time of the procedure.

Patients whose sentinel node biopsy is normal do not require a complete node dissection, because the risk of an axillary recurrence is extremely low. Many institutions are using IHC in the evaluation of the sentinel node. When there is no evidence of metastatic disease by routine hematoxylin and eosin staining and the node is IHC–, the node is considered pN0 (i–). When there are isolated tumor cells seen but no cluster is greater than 0.2 mm, the node is staged as pN0 (i+) and the patient does not require a complete node dissection. If the focus of metastatic disease in the node is greater than 0.2 mm but less than 2 mm, the node is staged as pN1mi. In this instance, consideration should be given to performing a complete axillary node dissection or axillary radiation therapy, unless the patient is participating in a clinical trial. The likelihood that nonsentinel lymph nodes will also contain metastatic disease increases as the size of the primary tumor increases.

The EORTC boost trial randomized 5,318 women with microscopically complete resections for early-stage breast cancer treated with whole-breast irradiation to receive a 16-Gy boost or no further radiation. With a median follow-up of 10.8 years, the 10 year risk of local relapse was 6.2% in the boost arm compared with 10.2% without a boost (hazard ratio = .59; P < .0001). In this recent update, although the absolute benefit was greater in younger women, the benefit to the boost was seen in all age groups. However, there was no difference in overall survival in this trial (Bartelink H, Horiot JC, Poortmans PM, et al: J Clin Oncol 25:3259-3265, 2007).

Radiation therapy after breast-conserving surgery

Based on the results of a number of retrospective single-institution experiences, as well as several prospective randomized clinical trials, breast-conserving surgery followed by radiation therapy to the intact breast is now considered a standard treatment for the majority of patients with stage I or II invasive breast cancer.

Radiation dose and protocol Radiation therapy after breast-conserving surgery should employ careful treatment planning techniques that minimize treatment of the underlying heart and lungs. To achieve the optimal cosmetic result, efforts should be made to obtain a homogeneous dose distribution throughout the breast. Doses of 180 to 200 cGy/d to the intact breast, to a total dose of 4,500 to 5,000 cGy, are considered standard.

Additional irradiation to the tumor bed is often administered. Although the necessity of a boost to the tumor bed has been questioned, at least two randomized clinical trials have demonstrated a small but statistically significant reduction in ipsilateral breast tumor relapses with the use of a radiation boost to the tumor bed following whole-breast irradiation of 50 Gy. In one of these trials, involving more than 5,000 women randomized to receive either a 16-Gy boost to the tumor bed or not, a 3% absolute reduction in local relapse was seen with the use of the radiation boost (4.3% vs 7.3%; $P < .0001$). This effect was particularly evident in patients younger than age 50. The boost is directed at the original tumor bed with either electron-beam irradiation or an interstitial implant, to bring the total dose to 50 to 66 Gy.

Regional nodal irradiation For patients who undergo axillary dissection and are found to have negative nodes, regional nodal irradiation is no longer routinely employed. For patients with positive nodes, radiation therapy to the supraclavicular fossa and/or internal mammary chain may be considered on an individualized basis (see chapter 10).

Partial breast irradiation There have been several reports demonstrating promising results with the use of partial breast irradiation, a potentially more convenient option for patients than the extended course of postoperartive radiotherapy.

Additional options are now available to shorten the radiotherapy treatment time to 1 to 5 days (accelerated) and to focus an increased dose of radiation on just the breast tissue around the excision cavity (partial breast). Current accelerated partial breast irradiation (APBI) approaches include interstitial brachytherapy, intracavitary (balloon) brachytherapy, and accelerated external beam (three-dimensional conformal) radiotherapy. Intraoperative radiotherapy is even shorter, with the entire treatment given as a single dose delivered immediately after surgery. Each approach has benefits and limitations.

Ongoing randomized trials will shape how APBI is utilized in routine clinical practice. Some of the more important outcomes from

Two meta-analyses evaluating patients treated with breast-conserving therapy confirm not only a substantial reduction in local relapse, but a small statistically significant decrease in breast cancer mortality with the use of radiation following breast-conserving surgery. Vinh-Hung demonstrated a three-fold reduction in local relapse and an 8.6% improvement in breast cancer mortality in a meta-analysis of over 8,000 patients in 13 trials. The Early Breast Cancer Trialists Collaborative Group meta-analysis included over 7,300 women from 10 trials treated with breast-conserving surgery and randomized to receive observation or radiation. As expected, they showed a highly significant three-fold reduction in local relapse with radiation, with a 5-year local relapse risk of 7% in those allocated to radiation compared with 26% in the non-irradiated cohorts. There was also a significant improvement in breast cancer mortality with the use of postlumpectomy radiation. The 15-year risk of death from breast cancer was 30.5% among those allocated to radiotherapy and 35.9% among those not *(Vinh-Hung V, Verschraegen C: J Natl Cancer Inst 21:115-121, 2004); (Clarke M, Collins R, Darby S, et al: Lancet 366:2087-2106, 2005).*

TABLE 2: Adjuvant chemotherapy regimens for node-negative breast cancer

Regimen	Dose and frequency
MF	
Methotrexate	100 mg/m^2 IV on days 1 and 8
5-FU	600 mg/m^2 IV on days 1 and 8 (1 h after methotrexate)
Folinic acid	10 mg/m^2 PO q6h × 6 doses (24 h after methotrexate)
Repeat every 4 weeks for 12 cycles.	
CMF (Bonadonna regimen)	
Cyclophosphamide	600 mg/m^2 IV on day 1
Methotrexate	40 mg/m^2 IV on day 1
5-FU	600 mg/m^2 IV on day 1
Repeat every 3 weeks for 9 cycles.	
or	
Cyclophosphamide	100 mg/m^2 IV on days 1-14
Methotrexate	40 mg/m^2 IV on days 1 and 8
5-FU	600 mg/m^2 IV on days 1 and 8
Repeat every 28 days for 6 cycles.	
CMFP	
Cyclophosphamide	100 mg/m^2 PO on days 1-14
Methotrexate	40 mg/m^2 IV on days 1 and 8
5-FU	600 mg/m^2 IV on days 1 and 8
Prednisone	40 mg/m^2 PO on days 1 and 14
Repeat every 4 weeks for 6 cycles.	
FAC	
5-FU	500 mg/m^2 IV on days 1 and 4 or 8
Adriamycin (doxorubicin)	50 mg/m^2 IV by continuous 72-h infusion on days 1-3 (or 50 mg/m^2 on day 1)
Cyclophosphamide	500 mg/m^2 IV on day 1
Repeat at 21-day intervals if hematologic recovery occurs for 6 cycles.	
CAF	
Cyclophosphamide	600 mg/m^2 IV on day 1
Adriamycin (doxorubicin)	60 mg/m^2 IV on day 1
5-FU	600 mg/m^2 IV on day 1
Repeat every 21-28 days.	
FEC	
5-FU	500 mg/m^2 IV on day 1
Epirubicin	100 mg/m^2 IV on day 1
Cyclophosphamide	500 mg/m^2 IV on day 1
Repeat every 21 days.	
AC	
Adriamycin (doxorubicin)	60 mg/m^2 IV on day 1
Cyclophosphamide	600 mg/m^2 IV on day 1
Repeat every 21-28 days depending on hematologic recovery for 4 cycles.	

these trials will be local toxicity, local and regional recurrence, and overall survival. If APBI is ultimately demonstrated to be as safe and effective as whole-breast radiotherapy, breast conservation may become an even more appealing choice, and the overall impact of treatment may be further reduced for certain women with newly diagnosed breast cancer.

Mastectomy options

Patients who are not candidates for breast conservation or who are not interested in breast conservation are offered mastectomy. For patients who desire immediate reconstruction at the time of mastectomy, a skin-sparing approach is recommended, provided it is oncologically safe. In most instances, the mastectomy can be performed through a circumareolar incision, where the nipple-areolar complex (NAC) is excised in continuity with the breast tissue. If a biopsy has been performed, this skin should also be excised with the mastectomy specimen. There have been reports in the literature in which the NAC has been spared during the course of a skin-sparing mastectomy. This concept awaits further study and is not considered standard of care.

MEDICAL TREATMENT

Medical management of local disease depends on clinical and pathologic staging. Systemic therapy is indicated only for invasive (infiltrating) breast cancers.

In the past, systemic therapy was not offered to patients with stage I disease (tumors up to 2.0 cm). However, adjuvant chemotherapy and hormonal therapy have been shown to improve disease-free and overall survival in selected patients with node-negative disease.

The sequence of systemic therapy and radiation therapy for patients treated with breast-conserving therapy has been the subject of considerable debate. Although concurrent CMF (cyclophosphamide, methotrexate, fluorouracil [5-FU]) and radiation therapy have been used with acetable toxicity, the concurrent use of chemoradiation therapy has fallen out of favor due to reports of enhanced toxicities. Delaying chemotherapy for 6 to 8 weeks of radiation therapy does not appear to negatively impact systemic disease or survival. Recent studies do not demonstrate a compromise in local con-

Interim results of a randomized, prospective, multicenter clinical trial to test the effect of a dietary intervention in women with resected, early-stage breast cancer receiving conventional cancer management (Women's Intervention Nutrition Study, WINS) showed that a lifestyle intervention reducing dietary fat intake, with modest influence on body weight, may improve relapse-free survival. A total of 2,437 women were randomly assigned in a ratio of 40:60 to dietary intervention (n = 975) or control (n = 1,462) groups. After a median follow-up of 60 months, dietary fat intake was lower in the intervention than in the control group (fat grams/day at 12 months, 33.3, vs 51.3 corresponding to a statistically significant (P = .005), 6-pound lower mean body weight in the intervention group. A total of 277 relapse events (local, regional, distant, or ipsilateral breast cancer recurrence or new contralateral breast cancer) have been reported in the dietary group (9.8%) and 181 women (12.4%) in the control group. The hazard ratio of relapse events in the intervention group compared with the control group was 0.76 (Chlebowski RT, Blackburn GL, Thomson CA, et al: *J Natl Cancer Inst.* 98:1767-1776, 2006).

trol if radiation is delayed until chemotherapy is complete. Currently, the majority of patients receiving chemotherapy and radiation therapy are treated with chemotherapy prior to radiation therapy.

For patients receiving tamoxifen or other hormonal agents, there had been considerable controversy regarding whether the hormonal agents should be administered during or after radiation therapy. Theoretically, tamoxifen may place cells in a resting state, making them less radiosensitive. Three retrospective studies, conducted independently but published together, all reached a similar conclusion: The timing of therapy had no impact on local relapse rates. Additionally, no significant difference was found in time to any event, metastasis, or death whether subsequent therapy was radiotherapy first or chemotherapy first among patients with breast conservation.

Treatment regimens

Multiagent therapy with CMF, CMF and prednisone (CMFP), sequential methotrexate and 5-FU (MF), and Adriamycin (doxorubicin) and cyclophosphamide (AC) has been used in patients with node-negative disease (Table 2). Hormonal therapy with tamoxifen (20 mg PO every day for 5 years) has been shown to be of value in women ≥ 50 years of age with estrogen- and/or progesterone receptor-positive tumors. (See chapter 10 for further discussion about tamoxifen and the ATAC trial [Arimidex and Tamoxifen Alone or in Combination] as well as for adjuvant chemotherapy regimens for node-positive breast cancer.)

Taxanes (ie, paclitaxel and docetaxel [Taxotere]) are now routinely used in the adjuvant therapy for node-positive breast cancer. The role of taxanes in node-negative disease is still evolving.

Node-negative tumors < 1.0 cm The reduction in the odds of recurrence and death with adjuvant therapy is similar in estrogen receptor-negative and [node]-negative patients. Therefore, patients who have the lowest risk of recurrence are least likely to benefit from systemic treatment when the attendant risks of treatment are considered. None of the reported trials in node-negative breast cancer included women with tumors < 1.0 cm, and because of the low risk of recurrence (≤ 10%) in this group, systemic adjuvant therapy is not used routinely. Recent results from the NSABP in this group of patients are provocative in suggesting a potential benefit from systemic therapy.

In this validation study, the likelihood of distant recurrence in tamoxifen-treated patients with node-negative, estrogen receptor-positive breast cancer was tested using a reverse transcriptase (RT)-PCR assay of 21 prospectively selected genes (16 cancer-related genes and 5 reference genes) in paraffin-embedded tumor tissue. The levels of expression of the 21 genes were used in a prospectively defined algorithm to calculate a recurrence score and to determine a risk group for each patient.

The proportions of patients categorized as having a low, intermediate, or high risk by the RT-PCR assay were 51%, 22%, and 27%, respectively. The Kaplan-Meier estimates of the rates of distant recurrence at 10 years in the low-, intermediate-, and high-risk groups were 6.8%, 14.3%, and 30.5%, respectively. The rate in the low-risk group was significantly lower than that in the high-risk group ($P < .001$). In a multivariate Cox model, the recurrence score provided significant predictive power that was independent of age and tumor size ($P < .001$). The recurrence score was also predictive of overall survival ($P < .001$) and could be used as a continuous function to predict distant recurrence in individual patients.

Node-negative tumors ≥ 1.0 cm The selection of a specific treatment program and the characteristics that predict risk of recurrence and death in women with node-negative breast cancer require further delineation and clarification in clinical trials. At present, women with tumors ≥ 1.0 cm who have poor histologic or nuclear differentiation, negative estrogen receptors, a high S-phase percentage, or high Ki-67 can be considered appropriate candidates for adjuvant systemic therapy.

An update of the NSABP B-20 trial indicated a significant advantage in the estrogen receptor-positive, node-negative population when chemotherapy with CMF or sequential MF is added to tamoxifen in the adjuvant setting. Patients receiving CMF plus tamoxifen appeared to derive the greatest benefit. Benefits with respect to both disease-free and overall survival have been reported for patients given chemotherapy and tamoxifen.

Chemotherapy and ovarian function suppression are both effective adjuvant therapies for patients with early-stage breast cancer. The efficacy of their sequential combination was investigated by the International Breast Cancer Study Group (IBCSG) Trial VIII. This study randomized more than 1,000 pre- and perimenopausal women with lymph node-negative breast cancer to receive either goserelin (Zoladex) for 24 months (n = 346), 6 courses of "classic" CMF chemotherapy (n = 360), or 6 courses of classic CMF followed by 18 months of goserelin (CMF then goserelin; n = 357). The primary outcome was disease-free survival.

In this study, patients with estrogen receptor-negative tumors achieved better 5-year disease-free survival rates if they received CMF (84% and 88% for CMF and CMF then goserelin, respectively) than if they received goserelin alone (73%). However, for patients with estrogen receptor-positive disease, chemotherapy alone and goserelin alone provided similar outcomes (81% 5-year disease-free survival rates for both treatment groups), whereas sequential therapy provided a statistically nonsignificant improvement compared with either modality alone.

Follow-up of long-term survivors

There is no consensus among oncologists as to the optimal follow-up routine for long-term breast cancer survivors. Based on guidelines from the National Comprehensive Cancer Network (NCCN), patients with stage 0 breast cancer should undergo a medical history and physical examination every 6 months for 5 years and then annually thereafter; mammography should be performed every year. Patients with stage I breast cancer should undergo a medical history and physical examination every 4 to 6 months for 5 years and then annually thereafter. In stage I patients, mammography should be performed every 6 months in the ipsilateral breast after radiation therapy following breast-conserving surgery and then annually thereafter, including the contralateral breast; if mastectomy was performed, mammography should be performed annually in the contralateral breast. Women receiving tamoxifen should undergo pelvic examination every 12 months if the uterus is present. All other follow-up evaluations are dictated by the development of symptoms.

SUGGESTED READING

Chlebowski RT, Blackburn GL, Thomson CA, et al: Dietary fat reduction and breast cancer outcome: Interim efficacy results from the Women's Intervention Nutrition Study. J Natl Cancer Inst 98:1767–1776, 2006.

Fyles AW, McCready DR, Manchul LA, et al: Tamoxifen with or without breast irradiation in women 50 years of age or older with early breast cancer. N Engl J Med 351:963–970, 2004.

Hughes KS, Schnaper LA, Berry D, et al: Cancer and Leukemia Group B; Radiation Therapy Oncology Group; Eastern Cooperative Oncology Group: Lumpectomy plus tamoxifen with or without irradiation in women 70 years of age or older with early breast cancer. N Engl J Med 351:971–977, 2004.

Kerlikowske K, Molinaro A, Cha I, et al: Characteristics associated with recurrence among women with ductal carcinoma in situ treated by lumpectomy. J Natl Cancer Inst 95:1692–1702, 2003.

King TA, Fey JV, Van Zee KJ, et al: A prospective analysis of the effect of blue-dye volume on sentinel lymph node mapping success and incidence of allergic reaction in patients with breast cancer. Ann Surg Oncol 11:535–541, 2004.

Paik S, Shak S, Tang G, et al: A multigene assay to predict recurrence of tamoxifen-treated, node-negative breast cancer. N Engl J Med 351:2817–2826, 2004.

Vinh-Hung V, Verschraegen C: Breast-conserving surgery with or without radiotherapy: Pooled-analysis for risks of ipsilateral breast tumor recurrence and mortality. J Natl Cancer Inst 96:115–121, 2004.

Voogd AC, Nielsen M, Peterse JL, et al: Differences in risk factors for local and distant recurrence after breast-conserving therapy or mastectomy for stage I and II breast cancer: Pooled results of two large European randomized trials. J Clin Oncol 19:1688–1697, 2001.

CHAPTER 10

Stage II breast cancer

Lori Jardines, MD, Bruce G. Haffty, MD, and Melanie Royce, MD, PhD

This chapter focuses on the treatment of stage II breast cancer, which encompasses primary tumors > 2 cm in greatest dimension that involve ipsilateral axillary lymph nodes as well as tumors up to 5 cm without nodal involvement.

Stage II breast cancer is further subdivided into stages IIA and IIB. Patients classified as having stage IIA breast cancer include those with T0-1, N1, and T2, N0 disease. Stage IIB breast cancer includes patients with T2, N1, and T3, N0 disease. Therefore, this patient population is more heterogeneous than the populations with stages 0 and I disease. The pretreatment evaluation and type of treatment offered to patients with stage II breast cancer are based on tumor size, nodal status, and estrogen receptor status.

Treatment

SURGICAL AND RADIATION TREATMENT

Multiple studies have demonstrated that patients with stage II breast cancer who are treated with either breast-conservation therapy (lumpectomy and radiation therapy) or modified radical mastectomy have similar disease-free and overall survival rates.

Breast-conservation therapy

The optimal extent of local surgery has yet to be determined and, in the literature, has ranged from excisional biopsy to quadrantectomy. A consensus statement issued by the National Cancer Institute (NCI) recommended that the breast cancer be completely excised with negative surgical margins and that a level I–II axillary lymph node dissection be performed. Patients should subsequently be treated with adjuvant breast irradiation.

Patients with tumors > 4 to 5 cm may not be optimal candidates for breast conservation due to the risk of significant residual tumor

A prospective study designed to determine the survival impact of micrometastases in sentinel nodes (SNs) of patients with invasive breast cancer included 790 patients who underwent sentinel node biopsy. The investigators found no significant difference in 8-yr disease-free survival or overall survival among patients with micrometastatic tumor deposits in the SN defined as pN0(i+) or pN1mic compared with SN-negative patients. The true significance of these micrometastatic deposits is still unclear but may help to eventually better define which patients should receive maximum adjuvant therapy, medical or surgical, and in which patients additional therapy could be avoided (Hansen NM, Grube BL, Ye C, et al: 30th Annual SABCS; December 13-17, 2007; San Antonio, TX [abstract 52]).

Factors affecting the rate of positive non-sentinel lymph node (NSN) and the necessity of axillary dissection (AD) following a positive sentinel lymph node resection (SNR) were evaluated in NSABP B-32. Women with operable invasive breast cancer and clinically negative nodes were randomized to undergo SNR with immediate conventional AD (group 1) or SNR without AD (group 2). Group 2 patients with positive sentinel nodes (SNs) underwent AD. Data from 1,166 patients with positive SNs were available for multivariate analysis (595 from group 1; 571 from group 2). Multivariate analysis indicated that a significantly higher percentage of group 2 patients had positive NSNs than did group 1 (41.5% vs 35.5%; *P* = .032). Clinical tumor size was a significant predictor for positive NSNs (*P* = .0010). Percentages of patients having positive NSNs were significantly increased by the number of positive SNs, and lymphovascular invasion was a significant predictor for positive NSNs. The percentages of patients with positive NSNs significantly decreased as the number of hot spots identified increased, and as the number of SNs removed increased. Therefore, although helpful in prognosis and treatment planning, completion AD after a positive SNB may not be required in patients with small tumors and in the absence of lymphovascular invasion (Julian TB, Anderson SJ, Fourchotte V, et al: 30th Annual SABCS; December 13-17, 2007; San Antonio, Texas [abstract 51]).

burden and the potential for a poor cosmetic result following lumpectomy (or partial mastectomy). Neoadjuvant chemotherapy, typically used for locally advanced breast cancer, is increasingly used in earlier stage, operable breast cancers to reduce the size of the primary tumor and allow conservative treatment.

In a study of more than 300 patients treated with neoadjuvant chemotherapy at the M. D. Anderson Cancer Center, promising results were reported. At a median follow-up of 60 months, the 5-year actuarial rates of intrabreast tumor recurrence-free and locoregional recurrence-free survival were 95% and 91%, respectively. The authors concluded that breast-conservation therapy after neoadjuvant chemotherapy results in acceptably low rates of recurrence-free survival in appropriately selected patients, even those with T3 or T4 disease. Advanced nodal involvement at diagnosis, residual tumor larger than 2 cm, multifocal residual disease, and lymphovascular space invasion predict higher rates of recurrence.

In some patients, preoperative chemotherapy results in sufficient reduction in tumor response that breast-conserving therapy becomes possible. The National Surgical Adjuvant Breast and Bowel Project (NSABP) B-18 trial showed that preoperative doxorubicin-based chemotherapy decreases tumor size by > 50% in approximately 90% of operable breast cancers, resulting in a greater frequency of lumpectomy.

In a subsequent trial, NSABP B-27, women with invasive breast cancer were randomized to receive 4 cycles of preoperative AC chemotherapy followed by surgery or 4 cycles of preoperative AC (Adriamycin [doxorubicin] and cyclophosphamide) followed by 4 cycles of docetaxel (Taxotere) followed by surgery, or 4 cycles of preoperative AC chemotherapy followed by surgery followed by 4 cycles of postoperative docetaxel. A higher rate of complete pathologic response was seen at surgery in patients treated with AC followed by docetaxel versus AC alone. There were no significant differences in disease-free and overall survival between the treatment groups. However, those who had a complete pathologic response in the breast had significant improvement in disease-free (hazard ratio [HR], 0.45; P < .0001) and overall survival (HR, 0.33; P < .0001) compared with those with residual disease after preoperative chemotherapy. Since preoperative chemotherapy does not have a negative impact on survival, the preoperative approach is a reasonable option and has gained favor among many patients.

Preoperative chemotherapy had an ability to convert patients requiring mastectomy to candidates for breast-conserving surgery. However, there was an increase in local recurrence in the "converted" group compared with those deemed eligibile initially for breast-conserving surgery.

The timing of sentinel node biopsy in patients undergoing preoperative chemotherapy is controversial. Preoperative chemotherapy can sterilize the axillary nodes and lead to errors in determination of nodal involvement. Formal studies are required to determine whether sentinel node biopsy can be safely performed after the patient has completed neoadjuvant chemotherapy.

Radiation therapy after breast-conserving surgery

For patients with stages I and II breast cancer, radiation therapy following lumpectomy remains an acceptable standard of care. Randomized trials as well as single-institution experiences have consistently demonstrated a significant reduction in local relapse rates for radiotherapy following breast-conserving surgery. Furthermore, small but significant differences in distant metastasis and disease-free survival have been observed in randomized trials comparing lumpectomy alone with lumpectomy and radiation therapy for patients with invasive breast cancer.

Based on the results of a number of retrospective single-institution experiences, as well as several prospective randomized clinical trials, breast-conserving surgery followed by radiation therapy to the intact breast is now considered standard treatment for the majority of patients with stage II invasive breast cancer.

Radiation dose and protocol Radiation dose to the intact breast follows the same guidelines as are used in patients with stages 0 and I disease, described in chapter 9.

Regional nodal irradiation For patients who undergo axillary lymph node dissection and are found to have negative lymph nodes, regional nodal irradiation is no longer em-

The Early Breast Cancer Trialists Collaborative Group meta-analysis included 8,500 women, primarily with node-positive disease, who were treated with mastectomy and axillary clearance. They were randomized to receive postmastectomy radiation versus no postmastectomy radiation. The 5-year risk of local relapse was significantly lower in the radiation group (6%) than in those randomized to no radiation (23%). Radiotherapy produced similar proportional reductions in local recurrence, regardless of patient age or tumor characteristics. The 15-year breast cancer mortality risk was also markedly lower in the radiation patients (54.7% vs 61.2%; P = .0002). The 5-year risk of local recurrence in patients with one to three positive nodes was 4%, compared with 16% in the controls, whereas in patients with four or more nodes the 5-year risk of local recurrence was 12% in the irradiated group compared with 26% in the control group *(Clarke M, Collins R, Darby S, et al: Lancet 366:2087-2106, 2005).*

For the first time, the type of taxane (paclitaxel vs docetaxel) and the schedule of therapy (every 3 weeks vs weekly) were compared in the adjuvant therapy of operable breast cancer. The E1199 trial accrued 4,950 eligible patients with lymph node-positive or high-risk (tumor $\geq$ 2 cm) node-negative breast cancer. All patients received 4 cycles of AC (doxorubicin 60 mg/m^2 and cyclophosphamide 600 mg/m^2) every 3 weeks, followed by either: (1) paclitaxel 175 mg/m^2 every 3 weeks $\times$ 4 (P3), (2) paclitaxel 80 mg/m^2 weekly $\times$ 12 (P1), (3) docetaxel 100 mg/m^2 every 3 weeks $\times$ 4 (D3), or (4) docetaxel 35 mg/m^2 weekly $\times$ 12 (D1). After a median follow-up of 60.2 months, there remains no significant difference in the hazard ratio (HR) for the taxane (1.02; P = 0.73) or schedule (1.07; P = 0.30) for the primary comparison. The incidence of worst grade toxicity (grade 3/4) was 24%/6% for arm P3, 24%/3% for arm P1, 21%/50% for arm D3, and 38%/6% for arm D1. In addition to concluding no differences in disease-free survival (DFS) when comparing taxane or schedule overall, investigators further concluded that DFS was significantly improved in the weekly paclitaxel and every-3-week docetaxel arms compared with the every-3-week paclitaxel arm *(Sparano JA, Wang M, Martino S, et al: J Clin Oncol 25[18S]:516, 2007).*

ployed routinely. For patients with positive lymph nodes, radiation therapy to the supra-clavicular fossa and/or internal mammary chain may be considered on an individualized basis.

Regional nodal irradiation should be administered using careful treatment planning techniques to minimize the dose delivered to the underlying heart and lungs. Prophylactic nodal irradiation to doses of 4,500 to 5,000 cGy results in a high rate of regional nodal control and may improve disease-free survival in subsets of patients.

Given the widespread use of systemic therapy for patients with both node-negative and node-positive disease, the role of axillary dissection has recently come into question. In patients with clinically negative axillae who do not undergo axillary dissection, radiation therapy to the supra-clavicular and axillary regions at the time of breast irradiation results in a high rate (> 95%) of regional nodal control with minimal morbidity.

Radiation therapy after mastectomy

Available data suggest that in patients with positive postmastectomy margins, primary tumors > 5 cm, or involvement of four or more lymph nodes at the time of mastectomy, the risk of locoregional failure remains significantly high enough to consider postmastectomy radiation therapy.

Several prospective randomized trials have evaluated the role of postmastectomy radiotherapy in addition to chemotherapy. Most of these trials have been limited to patients with pathologic stage II disease or patients with T3 or T4 primary lesions. All of these trials have shown an improvement in locoregional control with the addition of adjuvant irradiation, and several recent trials have demonstrated a disease-free and overall survival advantage in selected patients. Clinical practice guidelines developed by the American Society of Clinical Oncology (ASCO) support the routine use of postmastectomy radiation therapy for women with stage III or T3 disease or who have four or more involved axillary lymph nodes.

Most ongoing trials evaluating dose-intensive chemotherapy, with or without bone marrow or stem-cell transplantation, routinely include postmastectomy radiation therapy to the chest wall and/or regional lymph nodes to minimize locoregional recurrence.

Current recommendations There is no clearly defined role for postmastectomy irradiation in patients with small (T1 or T2) primary tumors and negative nodes.

For patients with four or more positive lymph nodes, with or without a large primary tumor, postmastectomy radiation therapy should be considered to lower the rate of local relapse and improve disease-free survival. For patients with T1 or T2 tumors and one to three positive nodes, postmastectomy radiation therapy may have a benefit with respect to disease-free and overall survival. However, controversies and uncertainties regarding this issue remain, and individualized decision-making, based on the patient's overall condition and specific risk factors, is reasonable.

Minimizing pulmonary and cardiac toxicities Early trials employing postmastectomy radiation therapy showed that the modest improvement in breast cancer mortality was offset by an excess risk of cardiovascular deaths, presumably due to the radiation treatment techniques used, which resulted in delivery of relatively high radiation doses to the heart. Recent trials employing more modern radiation therapy techniques have *not* demonstrated an excess of cardiac morbidity and, hence, have shown a slight improvement in overall survival due to a decrease in breast cancer deaths. Thus, in any patient being considered for postmastectomy radiation therapy, efforts should be made to treat the areas at risk while minimizing the dose to the underlying heart and lungs.

Radiation dose and protocol The available literature suggests that doses of 4,500 to 5,000 cGy should be sufficient to control subclinical microscopic disease in the postmastectomy setting. Electron-beam boosts to areas of positive margins and/or gross residual disease, to doses of ~6,000 cGy, may be considered.

In patients who have undergone axillary lymph node dissection, even in those with multiple positive nodes, treatment of the axillae does not appear to be necessary in the absence of gross residual disease. Treatment of the supraclavicular and/or internal mammary chain should employ techniques and field arrangements that minimize overlap between adjacent fields and decrease the dose to underlying cardiac and pulmonary structures.

MEDICAL TREATMENT

Medical management of local disease depends on clinical and pathologic staging. Systemic therapy is indicated only for invasive (infiltrating) breast cancers.

A discussion of the sequencing of chemotherapy and irradiation and hormonal therapy with irradiation is provided in chapter 9.

Treatment regimens

Systemic adjuvant therapy has been shown to decrease the risk of recurrence and in some cases also the risk of death. Systemic therapy may be divided into chemotherapy and endocrine (hormonal) therapy. Chemotherapy often involves use of combination regimens, given for 4 to 8 cycles. Chemotherapy is most often delivered after primary surgery for breast cancer and before radiation therapy for those who are candidates for irradiation.

Chemotherapy Multiagent therapy with cyclophosphamide, methotrexate, and fluorouracil (5-FU, CMF regimen); cyclophosphamide, methotrexate, 5-FU, and prednisone (CMFP); AC; and sequential methotrexate and 5-FU (MF) has been used in patients with node-negative disease (see Table 2 in Chapter 9).

For node-positive disease, systemic chemotherapy has changed over the past few years. Anthracycline-containing regimens are being used with greater frequency and have been shown to be of greater benefit than nonanthracycline-containing regimens (eg, CMF). Epirubicin (Ellence) was approved by the US Food and Drug Administration (FDA) for use in combination with cyclophosphamide and 5-FU (CEF regimen) for the adjuvant treatment of patients with node-positive breast cancer following resection of the primary tumor.

In a pivotal trial conducted by the NCI of Canada, premenopausal women with node-positive breast cancer were randomly allocated to receive either CEF or CMF, administered monthly for 6 months. With a median follow-up of 59 months, the 5-year relapse-free survival rates were 53% and 63% ($P = .009$), and 5-year survival rates were 70% and 77% for CEF and CMF, respectively ($P = .03$).

Several trials have also shown the benefit of incorporating taxanes (paclitaxel and docetaxel [Taxotere]) in the adjuvant treatment of node-positive breast cancer, and they are now routinely used in this setting. Taxanes can either be given in combination with an anthracycline or sequentially, either before or after an anthracycline.

The Breast Cancer International Research Group (BCIRG) compared Taxotere (docetaxel), Adriamycin (doxorubicin), and cylophosphamide (TAC regimen) with 5-FU, Adriamycin, and cyclophosphamide (FAC regimen) in 1,480 women with node-positive breast cancer (BCIRG 001/TAX 316). At a median follow-up of 55 months, the estimated 5-year disease-free survival rate was 75% for patients treated with TAC versus 68% for those treated with FAC. This represents a statistically significant reduction in the risk of relapse of 28% (P= .001). Furthermore, treatment with TAC resulted in a statistically significant reduction in the risk of death (30%; P= .008). Although there was more febrile neutropenia with TAC, it was ameliorated with growth factor support.

In another study by the Cancer and Leukemia Group B (CALGB 9344), 3,121 women with operable, node-positive breast cancer were randomly assigned to receive 3 doses of doxorubicin with a standard dose of cyclophosphamide followed by either no further therapy or 4 cycles of paclitaxel (175 mg/m^2). This study did not show any substantial benefit from dose escalation of doxorubicin. However, the addition of 4 cycles of paclitaxel improved disease-free and overall survival. At 5 years, the disease-free survival was 65% and 70%, and overall survival was 77% and 80% after AC versus AC plus paclitaxel, respectively. An unplanned subset analysis showed that the majority of the benefit was seen in those with estrogen receptor-negative tumors. Tamoxifen was given to 94% of patients with hormone receptor-positive tumors. Toxicity was modest with the addition of 4 cycles of paclitaxel.

In a similar study by the NSABP B-28, the addition of paclitaxel (225 mg/m^2) did not initially result in improvement of either disease-free or overall survival. However, with longer follow-up (median 67 months), improvement in disease-free survival in favor of AC followed by paclitaxel has emerged.

Dose-dense treatment CALGB 9741 tested two novel concepts: dose density and sequential therapy. A total of 2,005 women with operable, node-positive breast cancer were randomly assigned to receive one of the following regimens: (1) sequential Adriamycin (A) × 4 (doses) followed by Taxol (T) × 4 followed by cyclophosphamide (C) × 4, with doses every 3 weeks; (2) sequential A × 4 followed by T × 4 followed by C × 4, every 2 weeks with filgrastim (Neupogen); (3) concurrent AC × 4 followed by T × 4, every 3 weeks; or (4) concurrent AC × 4 followed by T × 4, every 2 weeks with filgrastim. At a median follow-up of 36 months, there was an improvement in disease-free (risk ratio = 0.74; P=.010) and overall survival (risk ratio = 0.69; P=.013) in favor of dose density. Four-year disease-free survival was 82% for the dose-dense regimens and 75% for the others. There was no difference in disease-free or overall survival between the concurrent (dose-dense) and sequential schedules.

The dosages, schedules, and frequencies of chemotherapy regimens used for node-positive breast cancer are detailed in Table 1. Other regimens also used in node-negative (Chapter 9) and/or metastatic disease (Chapter 11) are listed in their respective chapters.

Jones et al previously reported 5-year results of a randomized trial of 4 cycles of TC compared to 4 cycles of standard AC in women with node-negative (~50%) and node-positive early breast cancer, showing a significant improvement in disease-free survival with a disease-free survival rate of 86% for TC compared with 80% for AC (HR = 0.67; 95% confidence interval [CI], 0.50 to 0.94; P= .015). However, no difference in overall survival was observed, with overall

TABLE 1: Adjuvant chemotherapy regimens in node-positive breast cancer

Regimen	Dose and frequency
TAC	
Taxotere (docetaxel)	75 mg/m^2 IV on day 1
Adriamycin (doxorubicin)	50 mg/m^2 IV on day 1
Cyclophosphamide	500 mg/m^2 IV on day 1

Repeat every 21 days for 6 cycles.
Martin M, Pienkowski T, Mackey J, et al: Eur J Cancer 2(suppl):70, 2004.

AC → T (conventional regimen)

Adriamycin (doxorubicin)	60 mg/m^2 IV on day 1
Cyclophosphamide	600 mg/m^2 IV on day 1 × 4 cycles

followed by

Taxol (paclitaxel)	175 mg/m^2 IV by 3-h infusion every 3 weeks × 4 cycles

Dose-dense (concurrent regimen)

Adriamycin	60 mg/m^2 IV on day 1 every 2 weeks
Cyclophosphamide	600 mg/m^2 IV on day 1 every 2 weeks × 4 cycles

followed by

Paclitaxel	175 mg/m^2 IV by 3-h infusion every 2 weeks × 4 cycles

Dose-dense (sequential regimen)

Adriamycin	60 mg/m^2 IV on day 1 every 2 weeks × 4 cycles

followed by

Paclitaxel	175 mg/m^2 IV by 3-h infusion every 2 weeks × 4 cycles

followed by

Cyclophosphamide	600 mg/m^2 IV on day 1 every 2 weeks × 4 cycles

Citron M, Berry DA, Cirrincione C, et al: J Clin Oncol 21:1431–1439, 2003.

A-CMF

Adriamycin (doxorubicin)	75 mg/m^2 IV on day 1

Repeat every 3 weeks for 4 courses.

Cyclophosphamide	600 mg/m^2 IV on day 1
Methotrexate	40 mg/m^2 IV on days 1 and 8
Fluorouracil	600 mg/m^2 on day 1

Repeat every 3 weeks for 8 courses.

Buzzoni R, Bonadonna G, Valagussa P, et al: J Clin Oncol 9:2134–2140, 1991.

---

survival rates of 90% for TC versus 87% for AC (HR = 0.76; 95% CI, 0.52 to 1.1; P = .13). With longer follow-up, TC was associated with improved disease-free survival as well as overall survival compared with standard AC. With a

Regimen	Dose and frequency

AC → T + trastuzumab

Adriamycin (doxorubicin)	60 mg/m² IV on day 1
Cyclophosphamide	600 mg/m² IV over 30 minutes on day 1
Repeat every 21 days for 4 cycles.	

followed by

Taxol (paclitaxel)	175 mg/m² IV by 3-h infusion on day 1
Repeat every 21 days for 4 cycles.	

NOTE: All patients should receive dexamethasone (20 mg orally) 12 and 6 hours before paclitaxel, diphenhydramine (50 mg IV), and ranitidine (50 mg IV) 30 to 60 minutes before paclitaxel.

Or

Taxol (paclitaxel)	80 mg/m² IV over 1 hour weekly for 12 doses

NOTE: All patients should receive dexamethasone (20 mg orally) 12 and 6 hours before the first dose of paclitaxel. If no hypersensitivity reaction occurs, convert to dexamethasone (10 mg IV), completed 30 minutes before each subsequent paclitaxel administration (dexamethasone may be tapered during the 12 weeks of paclitaxel).

along with

Trastuzumab	4 mg/kg IV, loading dose over 90 minutes on day of the first paclitaxel cycle (On the weeks paclitaxel is given, trastuzumab will be given after paclitaxel.)
	2 mg/kg IV, maintenance dose over 30 minutes every week for 51 weeks starting on day 8

Romond E, Perez EA, Bryant J, et al: N Engl J Med 353:1673-1684, 2005.

median follow-up of now 6.9 years, the difference in overall survival between TC and AC is significant; in the TC group, there were 75 disease-free survival events (15%) and 57 deaths (11%); the AC group had 108 disease-free survival events (21%) and 83 deaths (16%).

The investigators also reported on the effect of treatment by age (using 65 years as the cutoff) on outcome and toxicity. In this trial, 16% (160 patients) were ≥ 65 years of age. Younger women in both the TC and AC groups had less febrile neutropenia (4.4% and 2.3%, respectively) than older women (7.7% and 3.7%, respectively). Toxicity, by treatment, was similar in both age groups to the groups as a whole. The investigators concluded that TC should now be a standard nonanthracycline combination for early breast cancer. In addition, TC was well tolerated in older women without excessive toxicity compared with their younger counterparts, and may be preferable due to its lack of cardiotoxicity.

Recommendations All patients with stage II breast cancer should be considered for systemic adjuvant therapy. Adjuvant chemotherapy in node-positive breast cancer improves disease-free and overall survival by 24% and 15%, respectively. Risk reductions for multiagent chemotherapy are proportionately the same in patients with node-negative and node-positive disease.

Chemotherapy for women 50 years of age and older is similar to that for younger women. However, multiagent chemotherapy affords the greatest benefit in women younger than age 50 with respect to reductions in the risk of recurrence and death from breast cancer. For instance, CMF or AC chemotherapy improves disease-free survival in women aged 50 to 69 by 18%, versus 33% for women younger than age 50. Limited data are available from randomized trials regarding women aged 70 and older. However, in the absence of comorbidity, such as heart, renal, or liver disease, systemic adjuvant therapy can be offered to women ≥ 70 years old.

During 1996 to 2005, ATLAS randomized 11,500 women (59% ER+, 41% untested) who had completed ~5 years of adjuvant tamoxifen to 5 more years of tamoxifen (10 years total tamoxifen) versus stopping. Less than 1% of patients had switched to any other adjuvant hormonal therapy in the trial treatment period. At a mean follow-up of 4.2 years, the annual recurrence rate in each of the two treatment groups was approximately constant during and after the 5-year trial treatment period. Approximately 1,500 recurrences have been reported. A total of ~1,300 occurred during years 5 to 9, but only ~200 occurred during years 10 to 14. Overall, the recurrence rate was significantly lower among those allocated to continue tamoxifen. There was no significant heterogeneity in the recurrence rate reduction with respect to ER status, time period, age, or nodal status at the time of diagnosis. Although breast cancer mortality and overall mortality were lower among those allocated to continue tamoxifen, these differences were not statistically significant. The investigators caution that further follow-up is needed to reliably assess the longer-term effects on recurrence and the net effects on mortality (Peto R, Davies C, on behalf of the ATLAS Collaboration. 30th Annual SABCS; December 13-17, 2007; San Antonio, Texas [abstract 48]).

Endocrine (hormonal) therapy

The Early Breast Cancer Trialists' Collaborative Group (EBCTCG) overview analyses demonstrated a significant advantage with the addition of tamoxifen (20 mg/d oral) for 5 years to the adjuvant therapy regimen of women with estrogen receptor-positive breast cancer regardless of age. Treatment with tamoxifen reduced the risk of death by 14% in women younger than age 50 and by 27% in those 50 years of age and older. Long-term follow-up from the NSABP conclusively demonstrates that there is no benefit to continuing tamoxifen therapy beyond 5 years. However, results from much larger studies have recently reported that a longer duration of tamoxifen may be more beneficial than 5 years of therapy.

Premenopausal women

Approximately 60% of premenopausal women with primary breast cancer have estrogen receptor-positive tumors. For this group of patients, the benefit of adjuvant endocrine therapy, either tamoxifen or ovarian ablation, was established in the EBCTCG overview. Endocrine therapy has comparable efficacy to that of chemotherapy. For premenopausal women, however, the long-term morbidity associated with permanent ovarian suppression may be significant. Ovarian suppression with luteinizing hormone-releasing hormone (LHRH) analogs offers an alternative to permanent ovarian ablation, which is potentially reversible on cessation of therapy.

The Zoladex Early Breast Cancer Research Association (ZEBRA) trial is a randomized trial directly comparing goserelin (Zoladex) monotherapy with CMF in premenopausal women 50 years of age and younger with node-positive, stage II breast cancer. The primary efficacy population included 1,614 patients: 797 randomized to receive goserelin and 817, CMF. Estrogen-receptor status was known for 92.5% of patients; 80% had estrogen receptor-positive tumors.

At a median follow-up of 6 years, the estrogen receptor-positive patients treated with goserelin fared comparably to those who received CMF in terms of disease-free survival (HR = 1.01; P = .94) and overall survival (HR = 0.99; P = .92). Not surprisingly, CMF was superior to goserelin in patients with estrogen receptor-negative tumors. The onset of amenorrhea occurred sooner with goserelin; by 6 months, more than 95% of patients on goserelin were amenorrheic, versus 59% for CMF recipients. Reversibility of amenorrhea was also greater for goserelin; 1 year after cessation of goserelin treatment, 23% remained amenorrheic, versus 77% for CMF recipients.

> In premenopausal women with early breast cancer, addition of zoledronic acid (Zometa) to adjuvant endocrine therapy significantly improved clinical outcomes beyond endocrine therapy alone. In ABCSG-12, a phase III randomized study of 1,800 premenopausal women with stage I-II disease undergoing ovarian suppression with goserelin (Zoladex), therapy with tamoxifen or anastrozole (Letrozole) plus zoledronic acid reduced the risk of disease-free survival (DFS) events by 36% and relapse-free survival by 35% vs endocrine therapy alone (P = .011 and .015, respectively). At 5-year follow-up, DFS was 94% and overall survival was 98.2%. Investigators concluded some premenopausal women with early breast cancer may achieve a strong treatment benefit without receiving chemotherapy (Gnant M, Mlineritsch B, Schippinger W, et al: J Clin Oncol 26:LBA4, 2008).

Several studies have compared adjuvant chemotherapy with combined endocrine therapies in premenopausal women, consisting of tamoxifen for 5 years and an LHRH agonist for 2 to 3 years. Overall, combination endocrine treatment yielded better results than chemotherapy alone. Whether a strategy of combined endocrine therapy is better than tamoxifen alone, either with or without chemotherapy, in premenopausal patients with hormone receptor-positive tumors is the subject of several ongoing clinical trials.

In the Suppression of Ovarian Function Trial (SOFT), following adjuvant chemotherapy, tamoxifen alone is being compared with tamoxifen plus ovarian function suppression/ablation versus ovarian function suppression plus an aromatase inhibitor (exemestane [Aromasin]). The role of ovarian suppression and aromatase inhibitors in this setting is being further investigated by the complementary Tamoxifen and Exemestane Trial (TEXT) comparing ovarian suppression with the LHRH analog triptorelin (Trelstar) plus tamoxifen versus triptorelin plus exemestane.

Currently, almost all premenopausal women with lymph node-positive, hormone receptor-positive breast cancer receive chemotherapy. Whether combined endocrine therapies alone may be sufficient to achieve excellent outcomes without chemotherapy is a question being investigated in the Premenopausal Endocrine Responsive Chemotherapy (PERCHE) trial. This trial is comparing ovarian function suppression with an LHRH agonist plus chemotherapy followed by tamoxifen or exemestane versus ovarian function suppression and tamoxifen or exemestane without chemotherapy for premenopausal patients with hormone receptor-positive tumors.

Postmenopausal women

For many years, tamoxifen has been the standard adjuvant endocrine therapy for postmenopausal women with hormone receptor-positive tumors. However, demonstrable benefits of aromatase inhibitors, as from several large, randomized clinical trials, have led to increasing use of these agents in the adjuvant treatment of postmenopausal women with hormone receptor-positive tumors.

The Arimidex, Tamoxifen, Alone or in Combination (ATAC) trial was the first large randomized trial demonstrating the superiority of an aromatase inhibitor over tamoxifen in the adjuvant treatment of postmenopausal women with hormone receptor-positive breast cancer. After the initial ATAC analyses, the combination arm was closed because of low efficacy. The ATAC trial was recently updated, with a median follow-up of 68 months.

ATAC has shown that anastrozole (Arimidex; n = 3,125) is significantly more effective than tamoxifen (n = 3,116) in preventing recurrences and is better tolerated but associated with a higher risk of fractures on treatment. After treatment completion, fractures and serious adverse events continued to be collected in a blinded fashion.

New data comparing tamoxifen at a median follow-up of 100 months have been presented. Significant improvements were seen for anastrozole compared with tamoxifen for disease-free survival, time to recurrence, time to distant recurrence and contralateral breast cancer. In the hormone receptor-positive population– the results follow: disease-free survival (hazard ratio (HR) 0.85; 95% CI, 0.76–0.94; P = .003), (HR 0.77; 95% CI, 0.67–0.88; P = .0001) TTDR (HR 0.84; 95% CI, 0.72–0.98; P = .027); and CLBC (odds ratio 0.6; 95% CI, 0.42–0.85; P = .004). Absolute differences for anastrozole and tamoxifen increased over time and hazard rates remained lower on anastrozole compared with tamoxifen after treatment completion. Breast cancer deaths were nonsignificantly fewer with anastrozle than tamoxifen (351 vs 380 intent-to-treat; 246 vs 268 hormone receptor-positive), but there was no difference in overall survival (HR = 0.97, hormone receptor-positive). After treatment completion, fracture rates for anastrozole and tamoxifen were similar, and safety benefits were maintained. Myocardial infarction rates on patients were identical to those on or off treatment, and endometrial cancer rates remained lower for anastrozole than tamoxifen off treatment. No new safety concerns were seen. These data confirm the long-term superior efficacy and safety of anastrozole over tamoxifen as initial adjuvant therapy for post-menopausal women with hormone-sensitive early breast cancer.

The use of an aromatase inhibitor as up-front adjuvant endocrine therapy for postmenopausal women with hormone receptor-positive breast cancer was confirmed in the BIG (Breast International Group) 1-98 trial. This study compared letrozole (Femara) with tamoxifen for 5 years as adjuvant endocrine therapy for this patient population. The study was later modified to include a crossover for both agents, but results from the crossover arms have not yet been reported. At a median follow-up time of 51 months for the monotherapy (non-crossover) arms, 352 disease-free survival events among 2,463 women receiving letrozole and 418 events among 2,459 women receiving tamoxifen were observed. This reflected an 18% reduction in the risk of an event (HR 0.82; 95% CI, 0.71 to 0.95; $P = .007$). No predefined subsets showed differential benefit. Adverse events were similar to previous reports, with patients on tamoxifen experiencing more thromboembolic events, endometrial pathology, hot flashes, night sweats, and vaginal bleeding, whereas patients on letrozole experienced more bone fractures, arthralgia, low-grade hypercholesterolemia, and cardiovascular events other than ischemia and cardiac failure. The present updated analysis yields results similar to those from the previous primary analysis but more directly comparable with results from other trials of continuous therapy using a single endocrine agent.

Other randomized trials have investigated the use of an aromatase inhibitor after tamoxifen. Two sequential strategies after tamoxifen were studied: (1) a switch to an aromatase inhibitor after 2 or 3 years of tamoxifen, to complete a 5-year course of endocrine therapy or (2) a switch to an aromatase inhibitor after 5 years of tamoxifen, to complete 10 years of endocrine therapy, also called extended adjuvant therapy. With either strategy, the use of an aromatase inhibitor after tamoxifen provided significant reduction in events (recurrence, contralateral breast cancer, or death).

In the Intergroup Exemestane Study (IES), 4,742 patients who had received 2 to 3 years of tamoxifen were randomized to receive either additional tamoxifen or a switch to exemestane, to complete a 5-year course of endocrine therapy. After a median follow-up of 55.7 months, 809 events contributing to the analysis of disease-free survival had been reported (354 exemestane, 455 tamoxifen); unadjusted HR of 0.76 (95% CI, 0.66–0.88; $P = .0001$) was in favor of exemestane, with an absolute benefit of 3.3% (95% CI, 1.6–4.9) by the end of treatment (ie, 2.5 years after randomization). A total of 222 deaths occurred in the exemestane group compared with 261 deaths in the tamoxifen group, with an unadjusted HR of 0.85 (95% CI, 0.71–1.02; $P = .08$) in the intent-to-treat group. When 122 patients with estrogen receptor-negative disease were excluded, the HR was 0.83 (0.69–1.00; $P = .05$). Results suggest that early improvements in DFS noted in patients who switch to exemestane after 2 to 3 years on tamoxifen persist after treatment, and translate into a modest improvement in overall survival.

Severe toxic events of exemestane were rare, and toxicity profiles were generally similar to those previously reported for aromatase inhibitors. Patients who received exemestane reported fewer venous thromboembolic events than did those on tamoxifen. No other statistically significant differences in reported cardiovascular events (excluding venous thromboembolic events) were noted either on treatment or including the post-treatment period. Myocardial infarctions were rare and occurred in 31 (1.3%) exemestane-treated patients compared with 19 (0.8%) tamoxifen-treated patients ($P = .08$). Any effect of treatment on the risk of myocardial infarction seemed largely restricted to patients with a history of hypertension. Musculoskeletal pain, carpal tunnel syndrome, joint stiffness, paraesthesia, and arthralgia were reported more frequently in patients who switched to exemestane than in those who remained on tamoxifen. These effects emerged during the on-treatment period. In total, fractures occurred in 277 patients, but hip, spine, and wrist fractures were few. Including on-treatment and post-treatment follow-up, other types of fractures were more common in patients who switched to exemestane than in those on tamoxifen. Fewer clinically serious gynecologic events were reported in patients who switched to exemestane than in those on tamoxifen in the on-treatment period and throughout follow-up. The number of endometrial cancers did not differ significantly between the groups.

Three other randomized trials showed a benefit to switching to anastrozole after 2 to 3 years of tamoxifen treatment versus continued tamoxifen for a total of 5 years. The ITA (Italian Tamoxifen Arimidex) trial, with 448 patients enrolled and a median follow-up of 36 months, showed significant benefits in event-free (HR = 0.35; 95% CI, 0.20–0.63; P = .0002) and recurrence-free survival (HR = 0.35; 95% CI, 0.18–0.68; P = .001) in the women switched to anastrozole. There were 19 total events in the tamoxifen group (n = 225) and 10 in the anastrozole group (n = 223). The 3-year difference in recurrence-free survival was 5.8% (95% CI, 5.2–6.4). Significantly longer locoregional recurrence-free survival (HR = 0.15; 95% CI, 0.03–0.65; P = .003) was noted for the anastrozole group. The difference in distant recurrence-free survival approached statistical significance (HR = 0.49; 95% CI, 0.22–1.05; P = .06).

A combined analysis of the ABCSG (Austrian Breast and Colorectal Cancer Study Group) Trial 8 and ARNO (Arimidex - Nolvadex) 95 Trial, with 3,224 patients and a median follow-up of 28 months, investigated a similar strategy. It showed that sequential endocrine therapy with tamoxifen for 2 years followed by anastrozole for 3 years was superior to 5 years of tamoxifen in terms of event-free (HR = 0.6; 95% CI, 0.44–0.81; P = .0009) and distant recurrence-free survival (HR = 0.61; 95% CI, 0.42–0.87; P = .0067). No statistically significant difference in overall survival has emerged at this point (P = .16). Updated results from the ARNO 95 trial have recently been reported, indicating that switching to anastrozole resulted in a significant reduction in the risk of disease recurrence (HR, 0.66; 95% CI, 0.44–1.00; P = .049) and improved overall survival (HR, 0.53; 95% CI, 0.28–0.99; P = .045) compared with continuing on tamoxifen. The overall safety profile for anastrozole was consistent with previous reports, and no new safety issues were identified.

In the MA-17 trial, 5,187 postmenopausal women who had taken tamoxifen for 5 years were randomly assigned to receive either letrozole or placebo for an additional 5 years. After the first interim analysis, the independent data and safety monitoring committee recommended termination of the trial since letrozole therapy after the completion of standard tamoxifen treatment significantly improved disease-free survival. With a median follow-up of approximately 27 months, the 4-year disease-free survival rates for letrozole and placebo were 93% and 87%, respectively (P < .001). No significant difference was noted in overall survival. However, in an updated analysis, an advantage in distant disease-free and overall survival was reported in the subset of women with node-positive disease. Toxicities associated with letrozole were similar to those seen with aromatase inhibitors in other trials.

Bone effects

The third-generation aromatase inhibitors have been shown to reduce bone mineral density (BMD) when compared with tamoxifen in the advanced, adjuvant and neoadjuvant settings in women with early breast cancer. Five-year results from the ATAC trial showed that patients treated with anastrozole had an annual decline in lumbar BMD of 2% during the first 2 years of treatment and ~ 1% in years 3 to 5.

The bone subprotocol of IBIS-II (International Breast Cancer Intervention Study-II) assessed changes in the BMD in postmenopausal women aged 40 to 70 years with a high risk of breast cancer receiving anastrozole versus placebo for 5 years. To date, of the 1,540 women in the prevention study, 613 women have taken part in the bone subprotocol of the study. Of the 250 women whose lumbar spine and femoral neck BMD has been assessed at baseline and 1 year by dual-energy x-ray absorptiometry (DEXA) scans, 162 with normal BMD received only monitoring without bisphosphonate treatment, 59 osteopenic women were further randomized to receive either risedronate (Actonel) or placebo, and 29 osteoporotic women received treatment with risedronate. Data from this trial confirm the BMD losses observed with third-generation aromatase inhibitors on breast cancer patients, but it is also reassuring that BMD loss can be controlled if women receive DEXA scans at baseline and bisphosphonate treatment as needed along with aromatase inhibitors.

ABCSG-12 is a randomized, open-label, phase III, four-arm trial comparing tamoxifen (20 mg/d orally) and goserelin (3.6 mg every 28 days subcutaneously) with or without zoledronic acid (Zometa; 4 mg intravenously every 6 months) versus anastrozole (1 mg/d orally) and goserelin with or without zoledronic acid for 3 years in premenopausal women with endocrine-responsive breast cancer. The median patient age at diagnosis was 44 years. In a BMD subprotocol, patients underwent serial BMD measurements at 0, 6, 12, 24, 36, and 60 months. Of 1,801 patients in the trial, 404 were prospectively included in a bone substudy. A total of 201 patients received adjuvant zoledronic acid together with their endocrine treatment, whereas 203 patients did not. After 3 years of treatment, patients who did not receive zoledronic acid showed a BMD loss of 11.3% as compared with baseline ($P < .0001$). Bone loss was more pronounced if anastrozole was used in combination with goserelin as compared with tamoxifen (−13.6% vs −9%). At 60 months of follow-up (ie, 2 years after the completion of treatment), patients without zoledronic acid still showed impaired BMD as compared to baseline (−6.8%; $P = .0005$). In contrast, patients who received zoledronic acid showed unchanged BMD at 36 months (+.3%; $P = .85$) and increased BMD at 60 months (+3.9%; $P = .02$).

The Z-FAST study evaluated the efficacy and safety of zoledronic acid in preventing aromatase inhibitors-associated bone loss in postmenopausal women with early breast cancer who are receiving adjuvant letrozole therapy. A total of 602 patients with estrogen receptor-positive and/or progesterone receptor-positive early breast cancer starting letrozole were randomized to up-front zoledronic acid versus delayed zoledronic acid. The delayed group received zoledronic acid when either the post-baseline T-score decreases to < −2 or a clinical fracture occurs. All patients are treated with calcium and vitamin D.

The Z-FAST trial showed that the overall difference in the percentage change in BMD between the up-front and delayed zoledronic acid treatment groups, at both lumbar spine and total hip, progressively increased from baseline through 36 months, demonstrating that zoledronic acid every 6 months for up to 36 months is effective in preventing bone loss associated with adjuvant aromatase inhibitor therapy in postmenopausal women with early breast cancer. At 36 months, the upfront zoledronic acid group (n = 189) showed a mean increase of 3.72% in lumbar spine BMD, whereas the delayed group (n = 188) showed a mean decrease of 2.95%, resulting in an absolute difference of 6.7% ($P <$ .001). The up-front group (n = 189) showed a mean increase of 1.66% in total hip BMD, whereas the delayed group (n = 187) showed a mean decrease of 3.51%, resulting in an absolute difference of 5.2% ($P < .001$). The study was not designed to detect a significant difference in the fracture rate between treatment arms. It was safe and well tolerated; no serious renal adverse events and no confirmed osteonecrosis of the jaw cases were reported.

Recommendations

Recent guidelines from ASCO and the National Comprehensive Cancer Network (NCCN) highlight the appropriate use of aromatase inhibitors in postmenopausal women with hormone receptor-positive breast cancer. Aromatase inhibitors have a significant role in reduction of recurrence in early-stage breast cancer and should be included as part of the adjuvant endocrine therapy for postmenopausal women with hormone receptor-positive disease. Using an aromatase inhibitor as up-front therapy or switching at some point after 2 to 3 years of tamoxifen is an acceptable strategy. Since the risk of breast cancer recurrence after completion of adjuvant endocrine therapy remains substantial, extended therapy with an aromatase inhibitor is another viable strategy for patients who are completing 5 years of tamoxifen.

Several questions on the optimal use of aromatase inhibitors remain, and we must await completion of ongoing trials and/or development of new trials for answers. For instance, neither the optimal timing nor the duration of aromatase inhibitor therapy has been established, and the role of biomarkers (such as HER2/*neu* status) in selecting optimal endocrine therapy remains controversial. Furthermore, long-term effects of aromatase therapy, including osteoporosis, have not yet been well characterized.

HER2-positive tumors

HER2/*neu*-expressing breast cancers have been shown to have a worse outcome than their HER2/*neu*-negative counterpart. Studies demonstrating significant benefit to the addition of trastuzumab (Herceptin) to chemotherapy in metastatic breast cancer have prompted several groups to test this agent in the adjuvant setting. These studies have completed accrual, and early results are astoundingly positive.

Three major trials of trastuzumab in the adjuvant setting have been published, and results of the fourth trial have been presented. The NSABP B-31 and the North Central Cancer Treatment Group (NCCTG) 9831 were jointly analyzed to include a total of 3,351 HER2-positive patients, with a median follow-up of 2.0 years (2.4 years in trial B-31 and 1.5 years in trial N9831). Both trials included two similar treatment arms: adjuvant chemotherapy with AC followed by paclitaxel with or without weekly trastuzumab for 1 year. Although there were differences between the two studies, including a third treatment arm in N9831 sequencing trastuzumab after paclitaxel that was not included in the joint analysis, the common question addressed was the effect of adding trastuzumab to AC followed by paclitaxel.

There were 261 events in the control group and 133 events in the trastuzumab group. The HR for a first event in the trastuzumab group, as compared with the control group, was 0.48 (95% CI, 0.39–0.59; $P < .0001$). The percentages of patients alive and disease-free at 3 years were 75.4% in the control group and 87.1% in the trastuzumab group (absolute difference, 11.8 percentage points; 95% CI, 8.1–15.4). At 4 years, the respective percentages were 67.1% and 85.3% (absolute difference, 18.2%; 95% CI, 12.7–23.7). Distant metastases were reported in 193 patients in the control group and 96 in the trastuzumab group. The HR for a first distant recurrence was 0.47 in the trastuzumab group as compared with the control group (95% CI, 0.37–0.61; $P < .0001$). At 3 years, 90.4% of women in the trastuzumab group were free of distant recurrence, as compared with 81.5% of women in the control group (absolute difference, 8.8%; 95% CI, 5.5–12.1); the respective rates at 4 years were 89.7% and 73.7% (absolute difference, 15.9%; 95% CI, 11.1–20.8). Both disease-free and distant disease-free survival were so highly statistically significant for trastuzumab, such results were unlikely to be due to chance alone.

Furthermore, there appears to be an early survival benefit to the addition of trastuzumab. There were 62 deaths in the trastuzumab group, as compared with 92 deaths in the control group (HR 0.67; 95% CI, 0.48–0.93; $P = .015$). The absolute survival rate at 3 years was 94.3% in the trastuzumab group and 91.7% in the control group (absolute difference, 2.5%; 95% CI, 0.1–5.0); at 4 years, the respective rates were 86.6% and 91.% (absolute difference, 4.8%; 95% CI, 0.6–9.0 percentage points). The principal adverse event associated with trastuzumab therapy among patients with prior exposure to anthracyclines is cardiac dysfunction.

In trial B-31, for patients initiated on trastuzumab therapy, the cumulative incidence of New York Heart Association (NYHA) class III or IV congestive heart failure or death from cardiac causes at 3 years was 0.8% in the control group (4 patients had congestive heart failure, and 1 died of cardiac causes) and 4.1% in the trastuzumab group (31 patients had congestive heart failure). Of the 31 women in the trastuzumab group who had congestive heart failure, 27 have been followed for at least 6 months after the onset of heart failure, and only 1 reported persistent symptoms of heart failure at the most recent follow-up visit.

In trial N9831, the 3-year cumulative incidence of NYHA class III or IV congestive heart failure or death from cardiac causes was 0% in the control group and 2.9% in the trastuzumab group (20 patients had congestive heart failure, 1 of whom died of cardiomyopathy).

During treatment with paclitaxel alone or with trastuzumab, there was little imbalance between treatment groups in the incidence of any toxicity except for a higher incidence of left ventricular dysfunction in the trastuzumab group. Since the dramatic results are changing the way breast cancer is treated and many clinicians have adopted the use of trastuzumab for similar groups of patients, the same monitoring used in these trials can be adopted in clinical practice to minimize cardiac toxicity. Additional toxicities were rare cases of interstitial pneumonitis, some of which appeared to be related to trastuzumab therapy. In trial B-31, four patients in the trastuzumab group had interstitial pneumonitis, one of whom died. In the N9831 trial, five patients in the trastuzumab group had grade 3+ pneumonitis or pulmonary infiltrates, one of whom died.

The international HERA (Herceptin Adjuvant) trial had a different design and assessed HER2-positive patients who received a variety of chemotherapeutic regimens, randomized to either observation versus 1 or 2 years of every-3-week trastuzumab. Results were reported for only the 1 year of trastuzumab versus the observation arm, which included 5,081 patients with 1-year medial follow-up. Similar to the previously mentioned joint analysis, reduction observed events (recurrence of breast cancer, contralateral breast cancer, second nonbreast malignant disease, or death) were noted for women who received trastuzumab. The unadjusted HR for an event in the trastuzumab group, as compared with the observation group, was 0.54 (95% CI, 0.43–0.67; $P < .0001$) in favor of trastuzumab. This represents an absolute benefit in terms of disease-free survival at 2 years of 8.4%. Overall survival in the two groups was not significantly different (29 deaths with trastuzumab vs 37 with observation). Severe cardiotoxicity developed in 0.5% of the women who were treated with trastuzumab.

The BCIRG 006 study evaluated the benefit of adjuvant trastuzumab (H) in 3,222 patients with HER2-positive breast cancer. Unique to this study was a nonanthracycline-containing regimen, which was expected to minimize the cardiotoxicity seen with trastuzumab following anthracycline-based chemotherapy. There were three treatment arms: 1) AC followed by T; 2) AC→TH (docetaxel + trastuzumab); or 3) TCH (docetaxel, carboplatin, trastuzumab).

For the second interim analysis, there were 192, 128, and 142 events in the 3 arms, respectively. HR for (AC→TH vs AC→T) disease-free survival was 0.61 (95% CI, 0.48–0.76; $P < .0001$), whereas for (TCH vs AC→T) was 0.67 (95% CI, 0.54–0.83; $P = .0003$). The absolute disease-free survival benefits (from years 2 to 4) were for AC→TH versus AC→T and TCH versus AC→T were 6% and 5%, respectively. There was no statistically significant difference in the disease-free survival between the two trastuzumab-containing arms. HR for (AC→TH vs AC→T) overall survival was 0.59 (95% CI, 0.42–0.85; $P = .004$), while HR for (TCH vs AC→T) was 0.66 (95% CI, 0.47–0.93; $P = .017$). There was a statistically significant higher incidence of cardiac events in the AC→TH

(20 grade 3/4 events) arm but not in the TCH (4 grade 3/4 events) arm when compared with AC→T (5 grade 3/4 events). There was also a statistically significant higher incidence of asymptomatic declines in left ventricular ejection fraction with AC→TH in comparison to AC→T or TCH. Furthermore, four leukemias were seen in the anthacycline-based arms versus 0 in the TCH arm. Thus, the investigators concluded, that in light of similar efficacy, global safety appears to favor the use of TCH.

There are unresolved questions about the adjuvant use of trastuzumab, including sequential versus concurrent use with chemotherapy, the optimal duration, and whether anthracyclines can be omitted. Furthermore, the long-term safety of trastuzumab in this setting remains to be determined.

High-dose chemotherapy Because of the higher rate of recurrence in patients with stage IIB breast cancer, high-dose chemotherapy can also be considered as part of a clinical trial. See chapter 11 for a discussion of the current status of this approach.

Toxic effects of medical therapy

Chemotherapy The most frequent acute toxicities are nausea/vomiting, alopecia, and hematologic side effects, such as leukopenia and thrombocytopenia. Neutropenia, with its attendant risk of infection, is a potentially life-threatening complication that requires prompt medical attention and broad-spectrum antibiotics until hematologic recovery occurs.

Other toxicities may include amenorrhea, cystitis, stomatitis, myocardial failure, and nail/skin changes. Amenorrhea is drug- and dose-related and is often permanent in women older than age 40. Recent evidence demonstrates that chemotherapy-induced ovarian failure in the adjuvant chemotherapy setting is associated with a high risk of rapid bone demineralization in the first 6 to 12 months after treatment. Thus, premenopausal women undergoing adjuvant chemotherapy must be closely evaluated to prevent the development of early osteoporosis. Cardiac failure, although rare, is potentially life-threatening and may be irreversible.

Endocrine therapy Toxicities with tamoxifen or aromatase inhibitors include hot flashes, menstrual irregularities, vaginal discharge, and weight gain. Thrombophlebitis and endometrial hyperplasia are more common with tamoxifen. Arthralgias, osteoporosis, and fractures are more common with aromatase inhibitors, although the incidence of hip fractures is low.

Follow-up of long-term survivors

There is no consensus among oncologists as to the appropriate and optimal follow-up routine for long-term breast cancer survivors. Recommendations for follow-up testing vary. The vast majority of relapses, both locoregional and distant, occur within the first 3 years. Surveillance is most intensive in the initial 5 years; thereafter, the frequency of follow-up visits and testing is reduced (Table 2).

TABLE 2: Follow-up recommendations for asymptomatic long-term breast cancer survivors as per NCCN guidelines

Intervention*	Year 1	Year 2	Years 3–5	Year 6+
History and physical exam	Every 4 mo	Every 4 mo	Every 6 mo	Annually
Mammography	Annually (or 6 mo after post BCS irradiation)	Annually	Annually	Annually
Chest x-ray	Annually?	NRR	NRR	NRR
Pelvic exam[a]	Annually	Annually	Annually	Annually
Bone density[b]	Every 1 to 2 yr	Every 1 to 2 yr	Every 1 to 2 yr	Every 1 to 2 yr

NCCN = National Comprehensive Cancer Network; NRR = not routinely recommended; BCS = breast-conserving surgery

[a] For patients with an intact uterus on tamoxifen
[b] For patients at risk for osteoporosis
* Bone scan, liver function tests, and tumor markers are not routinely recommended and are performed only if clinically indicated.

History and physical examination Surveillance methods include a detailed history and physical examination at each office visit. They are performed every 4 to 6 months for 5 years after completion of initial therapy, then annually thereafter. Patients at higher risk of recurrence or complications of treatment may require surveillance at shorter intervals. Patients who have been treated by mastectomy can be seen in the office annually after they have been disease-free for 5 years. Patients who were treated with breast-conserving surgery and radiotherapy can be followed at 6-month intervals until they have been disease-free for 6 to 8 years and then annually.

Approximately 71% of breast cancer recurrences are detected by the patients themselves, and they will report a change in their symptoms when questioned carefully. In patients who are asymptomatic, physical examination will detect a recurrence in another 15%. Therefore, a patient's complaint on history or a new finding on physical examination will lead to the detection of 86% of all recurrences.

Mammography should be performed annually in all patients who have been treated for breast cancer. For patients who have undergone breast-conserving surgery, the first follow-up mammogram should be performed approximately 6 months after completion of radiation therapy. The risk of developing contralateral breast cancer is approximately 0.5% to 1.0% per year. In addition, approximately one-third of ipsilateral breast tumor recurrences in patients who have been treated by conservation surgery and radiotherapy are detected by mammography alone. As the time interval between the initial therapy and follow-up mammography increases, so does the likelihood that local breast recurrence will develop elsewhere in the breast rather than at the site of the initial primary lesion.

Chest x-ray Routine chest radiographs detect between 2.3% and 19.5% of recurrences in asymptomatic patients and may be indicated on an annual basis.

Liver function tests detect recurrences in relatively few asymptomatic patients, and their routine use has been questioned. However, these tests are relatively inexpensive, and it may not be unreasonable to obtain them annually.

Tumor markers There is no evidence that tumor markers, such as carcinoembryonic assay (CEA), CA-15-3, and CA-57-29, provide an advantage in survival or palliation of recurrent disease in asymptomatic patients. Therefore, the use of tumor markers to follow long-term breast cancer survivors is not recommended.

Bone scans Postoperative bone scans are also not recommended in asymptomatic patients. In the NSABP B-09 trial, in which bone scans were regularly performed, occult disease was identified in only 0.4% of patients.

Liver and brain imaging Imaging studies of the liver and brain are not indicated in asymptomatic patients. PET scans are not routinely recommended. Their utility is primarily as an adjunct study, often to establish the extent of metastatic disease.

Pelvic examinations Women with intact uteri who are taking tamoxifen should have yearly pelvic examinations because of their risk of tamoxifen-associated endometrial carcinoma, especially among postmenopausal women. The vast majority of women with tamoxifen-associated uterine carcinoma have early vaginal spotting, and any vaginal spotting should prompt rapid evaluation. However, since neither endometrial biopsy nor ultrasonography has demonstrated utility as a screening test in any population of women, routine use of these tests in asymptomatic women is not recommended.

Bone density Premenopausal women who become permanently amenorrheic from adjuvant chemotherapy and postmenopausal women who are treated with an aromatase inhibitor are at increased risk for bone fracture from osteopenia/osteoporosis. These patients should undergo monitoring of bone health every 1 to 2 years.

SUGGESTED READING

Boccardo F, Rubagotti A, Puntoni M, et al: Switching to anastozole versus continued tamoxifen treatment of early breast cancer: Preliminary results of the Italian Tamoxifen Anastrozole Trial. J Clin Oncol 23:5138–5147, 2005.

Chen AM, Meric-Bernstam F, Hunt KK, et al: Breast conservation after neoadjuvant chemotherapy: The M. D. Anderson Cancer Center experience. J Clin Oncol 22:2303–2312, 2004.

Citron ML, Berry DA, Cirrincione C, et al: Randomized trial of dose-dense versus conventionally scheduled and sequential versus concurrent combination chemotherapy as postoperative adjuvant treatment of node-positive primary breast cancer: First report of Intergroup trial C9741/Cancer and Leukemia B trial 9741. J Clin Oncol 21:1431–1439, 2003.

Clarke M, Collins R, Darby S, et al: Effects of radiotherapy and of differences in the extent of surgery for early breast cancer on local recurrence and 15-year survival: An overview of the randomised trials. Lancet 366:2087–2106, 2005.

Coates AS, Keshaviah A, Thurlimann B, et al: Five years of letrozole compared with tamoxifen as initial adjuvant therapy for postmenopausal women with endocrine-responsive early breast cancer: Update of study BIG 1-98. J Clin Oncol 25:486–492, 2007.

Coombes RC, Hall E, Gibson LJ, et al: A randomized trial of exemestane after 2 to 3 years of tamoxifen therapy in postmenopausal women with primary breast cancer. N Engl J Med 350:1081–1092, 2004.

Coombes RC, Kilburn LS, Snowdon CF, et al: Survival and safety of exemestane versus tamoxifen after 2–3 years' tamoxifen treatment (Intergroup Exemestane Study): A randomised controlled trial. Lancet 369:559–570, 2007.

Goss PE, Ingle JN, Martino S, et al: A randomized trial of letrozole in postmenopausal women after 5 years of tamoxifen therapy for early-stage breast cancer. N Engl J Med 349:1793–1802, 2003.

Henderson IC, Berry DA, Demetri GD, et al: Improved outcomes from adding sequential paclitaxel but not from escalating doxorubicin dose in an adjuvant chemotherapy regimen for patients with node-positive primary breast cancer. J Clin Oncol 21:976–983, 2003.

Jakesz R, Kaufmann M, Gnant M, et al: Benefits of switching postmenopausal women with hormone-sensitive early breast cancer to anastrozole after 2 years of adjuvant tamoxifen: Combined results from 3,123 women enrolled in the ABCSG Trial 8 and the ARNO 95 Trial (abstract). Breast Cancer Res Treat 88(suppl 2):S7, 2004.

Jonat W, Kaufmann M, Sauerbrei W, et al: Goserelin versus cyclophosphamide, methotrexate, and fluorouracil as adjuvant therapy in premenopausal patients with node-positive breast cancer: The Zoladex Early Breast Cancer Research Association Study. J Clin Oncol 20:4628–4635, 2002.

Kaufmann M, Jonat W, Hilfrich J, et al: Improved overall survival in postmenopausal women with early breast cancer after anastrozole initiated after treatment with tamoxifen compared with continued tamoxifen: The ARNO 95 Study. J Clin Oncol 25:2664–2670, 2007.

Mamounas EP, Bryant J, Lembersky BC, et al: Paclitaxel (T) following doxorubicin/cyclophosphamide (AC) as adjuvant chemotherapy for node-positive breast cancer: Results from NSABP B-28 (abstract). Proc Am Soc Clin Oncol 22:4, 2003.

Martin M, Pienkowski T, Mackey J, et al; Breast Cancer International Research Group 001 Investigators: Adjuvant docetaxel for node-positive breast cancer. N Engl J Med 352:2302–2313, 2005.

Piccart-Gebhart MJ, Procter M, Leyland-Jones B, et al; Herceptin Adjuvant (HERA) Trial Study Team: Trastuzumab after adjuvant chemotherapy in HER2-positive breast cancer. N Engl J Med 353:1659–1672, 2005.

Pierce LJ, Hutchins LF, Green SR, et al: Sequencing of tamoxifen and radiotherapy after breast-conserving surgery in early-stage breast cancer. J Clin Oncol 23:24–29, 2005.

Romond EH, Perez EA, Bryant J, et al: Trastuzumab plus adjuvant chemotherapy for operable HER2-positive breast cancer. N Engl J Med 353:1673–1684, 2005.

Thurlimann BJ, Keshaviah A, Mouridsen H, et al: Randomized double-blind phase III study to evaluate letrozole (L) vs tamofixen (T) as adjuvant endocrine therapy for postmenopausal women with receptor-positive breast cancer (abstract). J Clin Oncol 23(suppl):6s, 2005.

Winer EP, Hudis C, Burstein HJ, et al: American Society of Clinical Oncology technology assessment on the use of aromatase inhibitors as adjuvant therapy for postmenopausal women with hormone receptor-positive breast cancer: Status report. J Clin Oncol 23:619–629, 2005.

CHAPTER 11

Stages III and IV breast cancer

Lori Jardines, MD, Bruce G. Haffty, MD, Melanie Royce, MD, PhD, and Ishmael Jaiyesimi, DO

This chapter addresses the diagnosis and management of locally advanced, locally recurrent, and metastatic breast cancer, ie, stages III and IV disease.

Approximately 20% to 25% of patients present with locally advanced breast cancer. Inflammatory breast cancer is a particularly aggressive form of breast cancer that falls under the heading of locally advanced disease and accounts for 1% to 3% of all breast cancers.

Locoregional recurrence of breast cancer remains a major clinical oncologic problem. Rates of locoregional recurrence may vary from < 10% to > 50%, depending on initial disease stage and treatment.

Metastatic disease is found at presentation in 5% to 10% of patients with breast cancer. The most common sites of distant metastasis are the lungs, liver, and bone.

The optimal therapy for stage III breast cancer continues to evolve. Recently, the use of neoadjuvant chemotherapy has been effective in downstaging locally advanced breast cancer prior to surgical intervention. The optimal neoadjuvant chemotherapeutic regimens continue to evolve, and studies are being performed to evaluate new agents and delivery methods.

Diagnosis

Locally advanced disease

Patients with locally advanced breast cancer do not have distant metastatic disease and are in this group based on tumor size and/or nodal status. Such patients often present with a large breast mass or axillary nodal disease, which is easily palpable on physical examination. In some instances, the breast is diffusely infiltrated with disease, and no dominant mass is evident.

Patients with inflammatory breast cancer often present with erythema and edema of the skin of the breast (peau d'orange) and may not have a discrete mass within the breast. These patients often are treated with antibiotics unsuccessfully for presumed mastitis.

Mammography is beneficial in determining the local extent of disease in the ipsilateral breast, as well as in studying the contralateral breast.

Fine-needle aspiration (FNA) or biopsy The diagnosis of breast cancer can be confirmed by either FNA cytology or core biopsy. Core biopsy is preferred to perform the wide variety of marker analyses.

Search for metastasis The presence of distant metastatic disease should be ruled out by physical examination, chest radiography, CT of the liver, bone scan, and CT of the chest. [18]Fluorodeoxyglucose-positron emission tomography (FDG-PET) has moderate accuracy for detecting axillary metastasis. It is highly predictive for nodal tumor involvement when multiple intense foci of tracer uptake are identified but fails to detect small nodal metastasis. The addition of FDG-PET to the standard workup of patients with locally advanced breast cancer may lead to the detection of unexpected distant metastases. Abnormal PET findings should be confirmed to prevent patients from being denied appropriate treatment.

Locoregional recurrence

Biopsy or FNA Locoregional recurrence of breast cancer can be diagnosed by surgical biopsy or FNA cytology. Whichever modality is appropriate, material should be sent for hormone-receptor studies, since there is only an 80% concordance in hormone-receptor status between the primary tumor and recurrent disease. When the suspected recurrent disease is not extensive, the biopsy procedure of choice is a negative margin excisional biopsy. For an extensive recurrence, an incisional biopsy can be used.

Search for distant metastasis Prior to beginning a treatment regimen for a patient with locoregional recurrence, an evaluation for distant metastasis should be instituted, since the findings may alter the treatment plan.

Distant metastasis from the breasts

Metastatic breast cancer may be manifested by bone pain, shortness of breath secondary to a pleural effusion, parenchymal or pulmonary nodules, or neurologic deficits secondary to spinal cord compression or brain metastases. In some instances, metastatic disease is identified after abnormalities are found on routine laboratory or radiologic studies.

Assessment of disease extent by radiography, CT, and radionuclide scanning is important. Organ functional impairment may be determined by blood tests (liver/renal/hematologic) or may require cardiac and pulmonary function testing. Biopsy may be required to confirm the diagnosis of metastasis; this is especially important when only a single distant lesion is identified.

Metastasis to the breasts

The most common source of metastatic disease to the breasts is a contralateral breast primary. Metastasis from a nonbreast primary is rare, representing < 1.5% of all breast malignancies. Some malignancies that could metastasize to the breast include non-Hodgkin lymphoma, leukemias, melanoma, lung cancer (particularly small-cell lung cancer), gynecologic cancers, soft-tissue sarcomas, and GI adenocarcinomas. Metastasis to the breasts from a nonbreast primary is more common in younger women. The average age at diagnosis ranges from the late 30s to 40s. Treatment depends on the status and location of the primary site.

Mammographic findings Mammography in patients with metastatic disease to the breasts most commonly reveals a single lesion or multiple masses with distinct or semidiscrete borders. Less common mammographic findings include skin thickening or axillary adenopathy.

FNA or biopsy FNA cytology has been extremely useful in establishing the diagnosis when the metastatic disease has cytologic features that are not consistent with a breast primary. When cytology is not helpful, core biopsy or even open biopsy may be necessary to distinguish primary breast cancer from metastatic disease.

Treatment

TREATMENT OF LOCALLY ADVANCED DISEASE

The optimal treatment for patients with locally advanced breast cancer has yet to be defined, due to the heterogeneity of this group. There are approximately 40 different substage possibilities with the different combinations of tumor size and nodal status. Between 66% and 90% of patients with stage III breast cancer will have positive lymph nodes at the time of dissection, and approximately 50% of patients will have four or more positive nodes.

Patients with locally advanced breast cancer have disease-free survival rates ranging from 0% to 60%, depending on the tumor characteristics and nodal status. In general, the most frequent type of treatment failure is due to distant metastases, and the majority of them appear within 2 years of diagnosis.

With the increased utilization of multimodality therapy, including chemotherapy, radiation therapy, and surgery, survival for this patient population has improved significantly.

Neoadjuvant systemic therapy

Neoadjuvant therapy with cytotoxic drugs permits in vivo chemosensitivity testing, can downstage locally advanced disease and render it operable, and may allow breast-conservation surgery to be performed. Preoperative chemotherapy requires a coordinated multidisciplinary approach to plan for surgical and radiation therapy. A multimodality treatment approach can provide improved control of locoregional and systemic disease. When neoadjuvant therapy is used, accurate pathologic staging is not possible. The majority of patients receiving neoadjuvant chemotherapy, treated with either breast conservation or mastectomy will require radiation therapy following surgery.

Active regimens Preoperative chemotherapy regimens reported to result in high response rates (partial and complete responses) include CAF (cyclo-

TABLE 1: Doses and schedules of chemotherapy agents commonly used in patients with metastatic breast cancer

Drug/combination	Dose and schedule
FAC	
5-FU	500 mg/m^2 IV on days 1 and 8
Adriamycin	50 mg/m^2 IV on day 1
Cyclophosphamide	500 mg/m^2 IV on day 1
Repeat cycle every 3-4 weeks.	
TAC	
Taxotere	75 mg/m^2 IV on day 1
Adriamycin	50 mg/m^2 IV on day 1
Cyclophosphamide	500 mg/m^2 IV on day 1
Repeat cycle every 21 days.	
FEC	
5-FU	500 mg/m^2 IV on day 1
Epirubicin	100 mg/m^2 IV on day 1
Cyclophosphamide	500 mg/m^2 IV on day 1
Repeat cycle every 21 days.	
Note: An absolute granulocyte count < 1,500/μL and/or platelet count <100,000/μL on day 21 will cause a treatment delay of at least 1 week. Treatment wil be terminated if hematology recovery takes more than 3 weeks.	
Paclitaxel	175 mg/m^2 by 3-h IV infusion every 3 weeks or 80-100 mg/m^2/week
Docetaxel	60-100 mg/m^2 by 1-h IV infusion every 3 weeks or 40 mg/m^2/week
Repeat if hematologic recovery has occurred (ie, absolute granulocyte count ≥ 1,500/μL and platelet count ≥ 100,000/μL).	
Capecitabine	2,000 to 2,500 mg/m^2 PO bid (divided dose, AM and PM) for 14 days, followed by 1-week rest
Repeat cycle every 21 days.	
Capecitabine + docetaxel	
Capecitabine	2,000 to 2,500 mg/m^2 PO bid (divided dose, AM and PM) for 14 days, followed by 1-week rest
Docetaxel	75 to 100 mg/m^2 IV infusion over 1 hour
Repeat cycle every 3 weeks.	
Vinorelbine + trastuzumab	
Vinorelbine	25 mg/m^2 IV on day 1 every week
Trastuzumab	4 mg/kg IV loading dose, then 2 mg/kg IV every week
Lapatinib and trastuzumab for HER-2 overexpressing metastatic breast cancer	
Lapatinib	1,000 mg orally daily
Trastuzumab	4 mg/kg IV loading dose, then 2 mg/kg IV every week
Lapatinib and pazopanib for HER-2 overexpressing metastatic breast cancer	
Lapatinib	1,000 mg orally daily
Pazopanib	400 mg orally daily

Drug/combination	Dose and schedule

Docetaxel or paclitaxel + carboplatin + trastuzumab (every-3-week dosing)

Docetaxel	75 mg/m^2 IV on day 1 every 21 days
	or
Paclitaxel	175 mg/m^2 IV on day 1 every 21 days
	plus
Carboplatin	AUC of 5 to 6 on day 1 every 21 days
	plus
Trastuzumab	4 mg/kg IV loading dose on day 1, followed by 2 mg/kg weekly

Note: Patients must be premedicated with dexamethasone prior to docetaxel.

Trastuzumab

	4 mg/kg IV loading dose, then 2 mg/kg weekly
	8 mg/kg IV loading dose, then 6 mg/kg every 3 weeks

Paclitaxel or docetaxel + carboplatin + trastuzumab (weekly dosing)

Paclitaxel	80 mg/m^2 IV on day 1 every week
	or
Docetaxel	35 mg/m^2 IV on day 1 every week
	plus
Carboplatin	AUC of 2 IV on day 1 every week
	plus
Trastuzumab	4 mg/kg IV loading dose, then 2 mg/kg every week

Gemcitabine + paclitaxel

Gemcitabine	1,250 mg/m^2 IV on days 1 and 8 (as a 30-minute infusion) every 21 days
Paclitaxel	175 mg/m^2 IV on day 1 (over 3 hours) every 21 days

Note: Standard paclitaxel premedications should be given.

Pegylated doxorubicin

Doxil	30 to 50 mg/m^2 IV on day 1 every 21 to 28 days

Nab-paclitaxel

	260 mg/m^2 IV on day 1 every 3 weeks

Ixabepilone plus capecitabine

Ixabepilone	40 mg IV over 3 hours on days 1 of 21-day cycle
Capecitabine	2,000 mg/m^2 orally (divided doses) on days 1 to 14 and one week off

Lapatinib plus capecitabine

Lapatinib	1,250 mg per day orally continuously
Capecitabine	2,000 mg/m^2/d orally (divided doses) days 1 through 14, followed by one week rest
Repeat cycle every 21 days	

Paclitaxel plus bevacizumab

Paclitaxel	IVPB 90 mg/m^2 on days 1, 8, and 15 of a 28-day schedule
Bevacizumab	10 mg/kg IVPB on day 1 and on day 15 of a 28-day schedule

AUC = area under the curve; IVPB = intravenous piggy back

phosphamide, doxorubicin [Adriamycin], and fluorouracil [5-FU]), FAC (5-FU, Adriamycin, and cyclophosphamide), CMF (cyclophosphamide, methotrexate, and 5-FU), and CMFVP (cyclophosphamide, methotrexate, 5-FU, vincristine, and prednisone). Combination chemotherapy with an anthracycline-based regimen—FAC or AC—is used most often. Recently published data suggest that the AT regimen of Adriamycin and docetaxel (Taxotere) given concomitantly may produce equivalently high response rates. Combination agents for metastastic breast cancer also include paclitaxel plus trastuzumab (Herceptin) with carboplatin, gemcitabine (Gemzar) and paclitaxel, and capecitabine (Xeloda) and docetaxel (Table 1). Although not yet definitive, recent data indicate that enhancing dose density may increase the pathologic complete response rate for women with locally advanced disease. The doses of these combination chemotherapy regimens are given in Table 1, chapter 10.

There seems to be no difference in survival in women with locally advanced disease who receive chemotherapy before or after surgery. Neoadjuvant chemotherapy results in complete response rates ranging from 20% to 53% and partial response rates (≥ 50% reduction in bidimensionally measurable disease) ranging from 37% to 50%, with total response rates ranging from 80% to 90%. Patients with large lesions are more likely to have partial responses. Pathologic complete responses (pCRs) do occur and are more likely to be seen in patients with smaller tumors. A pCR in the primary tumor is often predictive of a complete axillary lymph node response. Patients with locally advanced breast cancer who have a pCR in the breast and axillary nodes have a significantly improved disease-free survival rate compared with those who have less than a pCR. However, a pCR does not entirely eliminate the risk for recurrence.

Patients should be followed carefully while receiving neoadjuvant systemic therapy to determine treatment response. In addition to clinical examination, it may also be helpful to document photographically the response of ulcerated, erythematous, indurated skin lesions. Physical examination, mammography, and breast ultrasonography are best for assessing primary tumor response, whereas physical examination and ultrasonography are used to evaluate regional nodal involvement.

The role of MRI in evaluating response to preoperative chemotherapy is still evolving. Dynamic contrast-enhanced MRI performed at baseline, during chemotherapy, and before surgery has yielded more than 90% diagnostic accuracy in identifying tumors achieving a pCR and can potentially provide functional parameters that may help to optimize neoadjuvant chemotherapy strategies. However, despite its high sensitivity, a large number of patients still may have either false-negative or false-positive results on MRI scanning.

Multimodality approach

A multimodality treatment plan for locally advanced breast cancer (stages IIIA and IIIB, M1 supraclavicular nodes) is shown schematically in Figure 1. This approach has been shown to result in a 5-year survival rate of 84% in patients with stage IIIA disease and a 44% rate in those with stage IIIB disease. The most striking benefit has been seen in patients with inflammatory breast cancer,

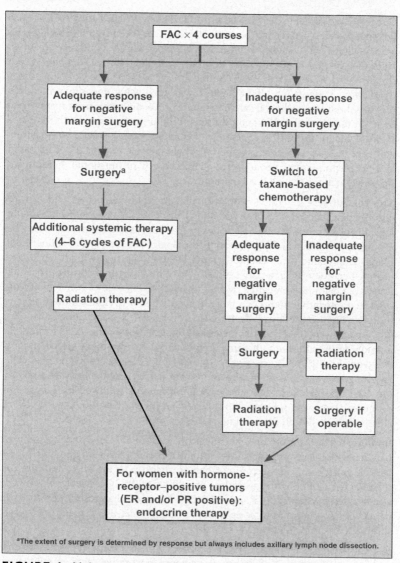

FIGURE 1: Multimodality approach to locally advanced breast cancer
FAC = 5-FU, Adriamycin, and cyclophosphamide

with 5-year survival rates of 35% to 50% reported for a multimodality treatment approach including primary chemotherapy followed by surgery and radiation therapy and additional adjuvant systemic therapy. The same chemotherapy drugs, doses, and schedules used for single-modality therapy are employed in the multimodality approach.

Surgery Traditionally, the surgical procedure of choice for patients with locally advanced breast cancer has been mastectomy. In recently published studies, some patients with locally advanced breast cancer who responded to treatment with neoadjuvant chemotherapy became candidates for breast-conservation therapy and were treated with limited breast surgery and adjuvant breast irradiation. Patients who have been downstaged using neoadjuvant chemotherapy should be evaluated carefully before proceeding with conservative treatment. It may be helpful to mark the site of the primary tumor with the placement of a clip during the course of percutaneous biopsy prior to beginning adjuvant therapy. There can sometimes be a complete clinical and/or radiographic response after neoadjuvant chemotherapy or hormonal therapy, and this may facilitate a wide local incision.

The role of sentinel node biopsy in the treatment of breast cancer after neoadjuvant chemotherapy has yet to be defined. Studies have shown that pathologically positive axillary lymph nodes can be sterilized when neoadjuvant chemotherapy is utilized. There are other biologic concerns with sentinel node biopsy after neoadjuvant chemotherapy. The lymphatics may undergo fibrosis or may become obstructed by cellular debris, making the mapping procedure unreliable, with false-negative rates of up to 25%. The rate of conversion from positive to negative nodes can be enhanced when 4 cycles of a doxorubicin-based regimen are followed by 4 cycles of docetaxel. Sentinel node biopsy will only be accurate then if all the metastatic deposits within the axilla respond in a similar fashion to chemotherapy. Preliminary data from the National Surgical Adjuvant Breast and Bowel Project (NSABP) B-27 trial demonstrated an 11% false-negative rate in women who underwent sentinel node biopsy after receiving 4 cycles of doxorubicin and cyclophosphamide followed by 4 cycles of docetaxel. However, patients with clinically positive nodes prior to neoadjuvant chemotherapy should have full node dissection.

Radiation therapy remains an integral component of the management of patients with locally advanced breast cancer. For patients with operable breast cancer undergoing mastectomy, radiation therapy to the chest wall and/or regional lymph nodes (to a total dose of 5,000–6,000 cGy) is usually employed, as discussed in chapter 10. Randomized trials suggest that postmastectomy patients with any number of positive nodes derive a disease-free and/or overall survival benefit from postmastectomy irradiation.

In a retrospective review of over 500 patients on six prospective trials treated with neoadjuvant chemotherapy, mastectomy, and radiation were compared with 134 patients treated with the same therapy, mastectomy, but without radiation. Despite the more unfavorable characteristics, the radiated patients had a lower rate of local-regional relapse than the unirradiated group (11% vs 22%). Patients who presented with clinically advanced stage III or IV disease but subsequently achieved a pathological complete response to neoadjuvant chemotherapy still had a high rate of locoregional response, which was significantly reduced with radiation (10-year rates: 33% vs 3%; $P = .006$). Radiation improved cause-specific survival (CSS) in the subsets of patients with stage IIIB disease, clinical T4 tumors, and four or more positive nodes. The authors conclude that radiation should be considered for these patients regardless of their response to initial chemotherapy.

Available data do not suggest a problem in delaying radiation therapy until the completion of systemic chemotherapy. Even in patients undergoing high-dose chemotherapy with autologous bone marrow or stem-cell transplantation, irradiation is generally indicated following mastectomy for patients with locally advanced disease (primary tumors ≥ 5 cm and/or ≥ four positive axillary nodes).

For patients whose disease is considered to be inoperable, radiation therapy may be integrated into the management plan prior to surgery.

High-dose chemotherapy The role of adjuvant high-dose chemotherapy (HDC) with autologous hematopoietic stem-cell transplantation for primary breast cancer at high risk of recurrence (at least four involved axillary lymph nodes) has not been well defined. Individually, the available trials have limited power to determine whether HDC has any benefit for this indication, or for any subgroup of patients. Based on a meta-analysis from 15 known randomized trials 6,210 patients (3,118 HDC, 3092 standard-dose chemotherapy [SDC]) were followed for a median of 6 years. Median age was 46 years. After adjusting for age and trial, HDC significantly prolonged disease-free survival but not breast cancer-specific survival (BCSS) or overall survival. After adjusting as well for hormone receptor status in the subset for which it was available, HDC significantly prolonged disease-free survival and had a modest and marginally significant benefit on BCSS and overall survival. For BCSS and overall survival, neither age nor hormone receptor status had a statistically significant interaction with treatment, yet there was a significant interaction between age and treatment for disease-free survival. The investigators caution that any benefits of HDC in the context of contemporary regimens such as taxanes and targeted therapies are unknown.

To date, the results of available clinical trials have not all shown improved disease-free and overall survival in patients treated with dose-intensive regimens. However, trial design, power, and strategy have all been questioned. Outside the context of a clinical trial, high-dose chemotherapy cannot be recommended for patients with primary or metastatic breast cancer.

TREATMENT OF LOCOREGIONAL RECURRENCE AFTER EARLY INVASIVE CANCER OR DCIS

When a patient develops a local failure after breast-conservation treatment for early invasive cancer or ductal carcinoma in situ (DCIS), it is generally in the region of the initial primary tumor. The risk of ipsilateral breast tumor recurrence after conservative treatment in patients with early invasive cancer ranges from 0.5% to 2.0% per year, with long-term local failure rates plateauing at about 15% to 20%. Local failure rates after wide excision alone for DCIS vary from 10% to 63%, as compared with rates between 7% and 21% after wide excision plus radiation therapy. Most patients whose disease recurs after conservative treatment for DCIS can be treated with salvage mastectomy. In one study, 14% of patients who developed local recurrence had synchronous distant metastatic disease.

The optimal treatment of a local or regional recurrence after mastectomy has yet to be defined. Locoregional recurrences are associated with initial nodal status and primary tumor size. Appropriate treatment may result in long-term control of locoregional disease. In many instances, these patients develop simultaneous distant metastasis, or distant disease develops some time after the locoregional recurrence manifests itself.

Recurrence of invasive cancer after breast conservation

Recurrence after wide excision and breast irradiation For patients with early invasive cancer who have undergone conservative surgery followed by irradiation and whose cancer recurs in the ipsilateral breast, salvage mastectomy is the most common treatment modality. The same is true for ipsilateral recurrence (of invasive or in situ disease) after conservative treatment for DCIS, when there is no evidence of distant metastatic disease.

Some studies with limited follow-up have reported acceptable results with repeated wide local excision for ipsilateral breast tumor relapses following conservative surgery and radiation therapy. Selection criteria for this approach are unclear, however, and use of this salvage procedure remains controversial. Although the use of limited-field reirradiation has been reported, selection criteria for this management option and long-term follow-up data are lacking.

Recurrence after wide excision alone In patients initially treated with wide local excision alone who sustain an ipsilateral breast tumor recurrence, small series with limited follow-up suggest that wide local excision followed by radiation therapy to the intact breast at the time of local recurrence may be a reasonable treatment alternative. In this situation, standard radiation doses would be employed.

Recurrent disease in the chest wall after mastectomy

In general, patients who develop minimal recurrent disease in the chest wall after a long disease-free interval may be treated by excision alone, although this approach is controversial and may not be ideal. Locoregional control obtained by radiation therapy alone is related to the volume of residual disease and may not be durable. When possible, disease recurring in the chest wall or axillary nodes should be resected and radiation therapy should be delivered to aid in local control.

Radiation treatment techniques are generally similar to those employed for patients treated with standard postmastectomy irradiation and consist of photon- and/or electron-beam arrangements directed at the chest wall and adjacent lymph node regions. Treatment planning should strive for homogeneous dose distributions to the target areas while minimizing the dose to the underlying cardiac and pulmonary structures.

Radiation dose and protocol Conventional fractionation of 180 to 200 cGy/d to the area of locoregional recurrence and immediately adjacent areas at risk, to a total dose of 4,500 to 5,000 cGy, is indicated. A boost to the area of recurrence or gross residual disease, to a dose of approximately 6,000 cGy, results in acceptable long-term locoregional control.

Radical chest wall resection A select group of patients with local chest wall recurrence secondary to breast cancer may be candidates for a radical chest wall resection, which may include resection of skin, soft tissue, and bone. Flap coverage or prosthetic chest wall reconstruction is required. Appropriate candidates would include patients who do not have distant metastases and who have persistent or recurrent chest wall disease after chest wall irradiation and patients who present with a chest wall recurrence after a long disease-free interval.

ADJUVANT SYSTEMIC THERAPY FOR LOCOREGIONAL RECURRENCE

Ipsilateral breast tumor recurrence

Limited data support the use of adjuvant systemic therapy at the time of ipsilateral breast tumor recurrence. Retrospective studies have suggested a 20% to 50% risk of systemic metastases in patients who sustain an ipsilateral breast tumor recurrence. A study conducted at Yale University found that ipsilateral breast tumor recurrence was a significant predictor of distant metastases, particularly among women who relapsed within 4 years of the original diagnosis; these women had a rate of distant metastasis of approximately 50%. Similar findings were noted by the NSABP investigators.

These data suggest that women whose tumors recur in the ipsilateral breast within the first few years following the original diagnosis may be considered for adjuvant systemic therapy. Given the lack of prospective, randomized data, specific treatment recommendations for these women remain highly individualized.

Regional nodal recurrence and postmastectomy recurrence of disease in the chest wall

Although there are limited data addressing the use of adjuvant systemic therapy at the time of locoregional relapse following mastectomy, given the high rate of systemic metastasis in this population, these patients may be considered for adjuvant systemic therapy. A randomized trial demonstrated a disease-free survival benefit with the use of adjuvant tamoxifen following radiation therapy at the time of postmastectomy recurrence of disease in the chest wall in patients with estrogen receptor-positive tumors. The 5-year disease-free survival rate was increased from 36% to 59%, and the median disease-free survival was prolonged by > 4.5 years.

Patients with estrogen receptor-negative tumors and aggressive locoregional recurrences may also be considered for systemic cytotoxic chemotherapy, given their relatively poor prognosis and the high rate of metastasis.

MEDICAL TREATMENT OF METASTATIC BREAST CANCER

Patients with metastatic cancer can be divided into two groups: those with stage IV disease at presentation and those who develop metastases after primary treatment. The management of stage IV disease depends on the site and extent of metastases, comorbid conditions, and clinical tumor characteristics.

Patients with delayed metastatic disease can be divided into two groups, ie, so-called low risk and intermediate or high risk, based on the biologic aggressiveness of the disease. As shown schematically in Figure 2, the management approach to these two groups differs.

Low-risk patients

The low-risk group includes patients who develop metastatic disease after a long disease-free interval (ie, a long disease-free interval from primary breast cancer diagnosis to presentation with metastasis), those whose tumors are positive for hormone receptors (estrogen and progesterone), those with bone-only disease, and those without extensive visceral organ involvement.

Hormone therapy Low-risk patients, whose tumor is hormone receptor-positive (ie, estrogen receptor-positive and/or progesterone receptor-positive), may be treated with a trial of hormone therapy.

First-line hormonal therapy consists of an aromatase inhibitor, with careful serial assessment of clinical and disease responses.

Hormone therapy may be associated with a "flare" response, a temporary worsening of signs and symptoms of disease within the first few weeks of treatment. This response generally means clinical benefit will follow.

If the tumor initially responds to first-line hormone therapy and then progresses, a second hormonal manipulation is warranted. Various hormonal agents are available (Table 3). They may be used sequentially and may provide disease palliation for prolonged periods in some patients.

Second-line hormonal agents The choice of second-line endocrine therapy depends on the front-line endocrine agent used. Typically, if tamoxifen was used, the second-line agent includes an aromatase inhibitor or fulvestrant (Faslodex) for postmenopausal women. For premenopausal women, the choice may be megestrol or induction of menopause with an LHRH (luteinizing hormone-releasing hormone) agonist with or without an aromatase inhibitor. If aromatase inhibitors were used as front-line agents for postmenopausal women, second-line options can be to change to another class of aromatase inhibitor, fulvestrant, or tamoxifen.

The Evaluation of Faslodex versus Exemestane Clinical Trial (EFECT) is a randomized, double-blind, placebo-controlled, multicenter, trial comparing the efficacy and tolerability of fulvestrant versus exemestane (Aromasin) in postmenopausal women with hormone receptor-positive advanced breast cancer following non-steroidal aromatase inhibitor therapy. A fulvestrant loading-dose regimen was utilized (via intramuscular injection): 500 mg on day 0, followed by 250 mg on days 14, 28, and every 28 ± 3 days, thereafter. Exemestane was given as a 25-mg capsule PO, once daily. Treatment was administered until disease progression or death, or withdrawal for any other reason. EFECT is the first phase III trial to specifically evaluate endocrine treatment options following disease progression/recurrence on a nonsteroidal aromatase inhibitor. This trial includes 693 women, ~60% of whom have received ≥ two prior endocrine therapies.

Low-risk hormone receptor-positive patients[a]

↓

Aromatase inhibitor or fulvestrant for postmenopausal women; tamoxifen, LHRH against +/- aromatase inhibitor for premenopausal women

↓

If partial or complete response, continue therapy until progressive disease

↓

Progressive disease

↓

Megestrol or tamoxifen

↓

If partial or complete response, continue therapy until progressive disease

↓

Progressive disease

↓

Trial of third-line hormone

↓

Hormone-refractory disease

Intermediate- or high-risk hormone receptor-negative patients[b]

↓

**No prior anthracycline: pegylated doxorubicin, FA/EC, CA/EF, A/ET
Prior anthracycline: taxane (paclitaxel or docetaxel) single agent or in combination (such as paclitaxel/gemcitabine or docetaxel/capecitabine)**

↓

If partial or complete response, continue 2 cycles past best response or until disease progression or unacceptable toxicity

↓

Progressive disease

↓

Trial of paclitaxel or docetaxel: if taxane-resistant, use single-agent vinorelbine or capecitabine

If partial or complete response, continue 2 cycles past best response or until disease progression or unacceptable toxicity

If no response, consider referral for investigational trial

Trastuzumab + taxane +/- platinum until partial response or complete response Maintain on trastuzumab until disease progression Change chemo (eg, vinorelbine, gemcitabine) +/- continue trastuzumab

If no response to two consecutive chemotherapy regimens + poor performance status, give symptomatic/supportive care

[a]Low-risk patients include those with a long disease-free interval, tumors that are positive for hormone receptors (estrogen and progesterone), or bone-only disease, as well as those without extensive visceral involvement.

[b]Intermediate- or high-risk patients include those with rapidly progressive disease, visceral involvement, hormone-refractory disease, or tumors that are negative for hormone receptors.

FIGURE 2: Treatment approach to metastatic breast cancer

In the primary analysis (median follow-up of 13 months), the median time to disease progression was 3.7 months in both the fulvestrant and exemestane groups (HR 0.963; 95% confidence interval [CI] 0.819–1.133; P = .06531). Objective response and clinical benefit rates were also similar between groups, although the median duration of response (n = 38; from randomization: 13.5 months vs 9.8 months) and clinical benefit (n = 172; 9.3 months vs 8.3 months) appeared slightly longer in patients receiving fulvestrant. Overall survival data were immature at the time of the primary analysis. However, in a recent update with a median follow-up of 20.9 months, 209 patients (59.5%) in the fulvestrant group and 197 patients (57.9%) in the exemestane group had died. Median overall survival was not significantly different between treatments (24.3 months vs 23.1 months in the fulvestrant and exemestane groups, respectively [HR 1.012; 95% CI, 0.833–1.229; P = .9072].

The most commonly used second-line hormonal agents had been progestational drugs, such as megestrol. Recent randomized trials have indicated that the aromatase inhibitors, such as anastrozole (Arimidex), letrozole (Femara), fulvestrant, and exemestane, are equally effective for palliation of metastatic disease, have less toxicity, and may provide a survival advantage compared with megestrol. Therefore, they are the drugs of choice for second-line therapy following tamoxifen administration. Tamoxifen may also be considered as second-line therapy for patients initially treated with an aromatase inhibitor.

Hormonal therapy continues until evidence of disease progression, or drug-related toxicity precludes further therapy with the same agent. If a partial or complete response to the first hormonal treatment is documented at the time of disease progression, a second hormonal agent may provide further palliation of symptoms and avoid the initiation of systemic chemotherapy. However, subsequent hormonal responses tend to be of shorter duration, and, ultimately, the disease will become refractory to hormonal treatment.

Cytotoxic agents Hormone-refractory disease can be treated with systemic cytotoxic therapy. FAC, paclitaxel, TAC (Taxotere [docetaxel], Adriamycin [doxorubicin], cyclophosphamide), or docetaxel may be used in this situation. (For a more detailed discussion of these agents, see section on "Intermediate- or high-risk patients." For doses, see Table 1.)

A prospective, multicenter study assessed the role of circulating tumor cells in predicting survival in 177 metastatic breast cancer patients before the start of a new treatment. Patients with levels of circulating tumor cells $\geq$ 5/7.5 mL of whole blood had a shorter median progression-free survival (2.7 vs 7.0 months; P < .001) and shorter overall survival (10.1 vs > 18 months; P < .001) than those with < 5/7.5 mL circulating tumor cells. Of all the variables in the statistical model, the levels of circulating tumor cells at baseline and at the first follow-up visit were the most significant predictors of progression-free and overall survival in this group of patients.

TABLE 2: Doses and schedules of hormonal agents commonly used in patients with metastatic breast cancer

Agent	Dose and schedule
Postmenopausal	
Tamoxifen	20 mg PO every day
or	
Toremifene	60 mg PO every day
Anastrozole	1 mg PO every day
or	
Letrozole	2.5 mg PO every day
or	
Exemestane	25 mg PO every day
Fulvestrant	250 mg IM every month
Megestrol	40 mg PO 4 times a day
Fluoxymesterone	10 mg PO 3 times a day
Aminoglutethimide	250 mg PO 4 times a day
Premenopausal	
Tamoxifen	20 mg PO every day
Luteinizing hormone-releasing hormone analogues (LHRH)	
Leuprolide	7.5 mg IM depot every 28 days
	22.5 mg IM every 3 months
	30 mg IM every 4 months
Goserelin	3.6 mg SC depot every 28 days
	10.8 mg SC every 3 months
Megestrol	40 mg PO 4 times a day
Fluoxymesterone	10 mg PO 3 times a day

Intermediate- or high-risk patients

Intermediate- or high-risk patients include those with rapidly progressive disease or visceral involvement, as well as those with disease shown to be refractory to hormonal manipulation by a prior therapeutic trial.

Anthracycline-containing combinations, such as FAC (see Table 1), are preferred for these patients. However, newer combinations of doxorubicin and a taxane are gaining favor for use in patients who have not received > 450 mg/m^2 of an anthracycline and whose relapse has occurred more than 12 months after the completion of adjuvant therapy.

Single agents Many single cytotoxic drugs have shown some activity in metastatic breast cancer (Table 1). They include vinblastine, mitomycin, thiotepa, capecitabine, vinorelbine, and gemcitabine.

Paclitaxel One of the most active agents is paclitaxel. It has demonstrated anti-tumor activity in patients with anthracycline-resistant disease, as well as in those who have received three or more prior chemotherapy regimens for metastatic disease.

High-dose paclitaxel (250 mg/m^2 over 3 hours) has not been shown to be superior to 175 mg/m^2 over 3 hours. The higher dose regimen is associated with greater hematologic and neurologic toxicities.

Docetaxel, approved by the US Food and Drug Administration (FDA) for anthracycline-resistant locally advanced or metastatic breast cancer, has demonstrated overall response rates of 41% in patients with doxorubicin-resistant disease. It has been shown to be superior to mitomycin/vinblastine in patients whose disease progressed after an anthracycline-based chemotherapy regimen.

The recommended starting dose of docetaxel—100 mg/m^2 as a 1-hour IV infusion—requires premedication with dexamethasone to avoid fluid retention and the capillary leak syndrome. The usual regimen of dexamethasone is 8 mg twice daily for a total of 3 days, beginning 24 hours prior to the administration of docetaxel.

Although 100 mg/m^2 is the dose of docetaxel approved by the FDA, many recent trials have demonstrated a high rate of grade 4 hematologic toxicity at this dose level; a dose of 60 to 70 mg/m^2 may achieve equivalent therapeutic benefit with improved safety. As with paclitaxel, the docetaxel dosage must be modified in patients who have hepatic impairment, manifested by elevated transaminase or alkaline phosphatase levels.

To determine whether weekly infusion of paclitaxel improves response rates versus the standard 3-hour infusion, 577 patients with metastatic breast cancer who had received one or two prior regimens were randomized to receive standard (175 mg/m^2) or weekly (80 mg/m^2) paclitaxel. Weekly paclitaxel was shown to be superior with respect to response rate (40% vs 28%; $P = .017$), time to disease progression (9 months vs 5 months; $P = .0008$), and overall survival (24 months vs 16 months). When trastuzumab became standard therapy for HER2-positive tumors, all patients with HER2-positive disease received trastuzumab, whereas patients with HER2-negative disease were randomized to receive either the addition of trastuzumab or not. The addition of trastuzumab did not improve any of these endpoints. Weekly paclitaxel caused more grade 3 sensory/motor neuropathy and less grade 3 granulocytopenia. The authors concluded that weekly is superior to standard paclitaxel in the management of metastatic breast cancer.

Capecitabine, an orally active fluorinated pyrimidine carbonate, has been shown to have a substantial antitumor effect in patients whose disease has recurred or progressed after prior anthracycline or taxane therapy. Prolonged survival, limited toxicity, and response in visceral as well as soft-tissue disease add to the benefit of capecitabine. Toxicities include diarrhea, stomatitis, and hand-foot syndrome.

New approaches Multiple new approaches to treating metastatic breast cancer are being explored. Weekly schedules of docetaxel and paclitaxel have been reported to produce high response rates and lower toxicity than 3-week schedules. Combinations of doxorubicin with paclitaxel or docetaxel have also shown substantial antitumor activity, as have combinations of capecitabine and docetaxel, carboplatin and paclitaxel, and gemcitabine and cisplatin. These newer combinations need to be compared with standard AC or FAC (CAF) regimens in phase III trials. Recent studies also suggest that sequential weekly chemotherapy may be as effective as more intensive combinations with respect to overall survival in patients with metastatic breast cancer.

Monoclonal antibody therapy and other targeted agents

Trastuzumab, a humanized monoclonal antibody to the HER2-*neu* protein, has been approved for use as a single agent in second- and third-line therapy for metastatic breast cancer and in combination with paclitaxel as first-line therapy in this setting. A randomized trial consisting of 469 women showed that the combination of trastuzumab with chemotherapy yielded a 45% overall response rate, as compared with a 29% rate with chemotherapy alone—a 55% increase. The addition of trastuzumab had the greatest impact on response when combined with paclitaxel. Among the study group as a whole, 79% of women treated with trastuzumab chemotherapy were alive at 1 year, as compared with 68% of those given chemotherapy alone.

An update of these data has shown a superior median overall survival with chemotherapy plus trastuzumab compared with chemotherapy alone (25.4 months vs 20.9 months). The survival advantage was seen with both AC plus trastuzumab and paclitaxel plus the monoclonal antibody.

In another single-arm trial involving 222 women who had not responded to prior chemotherapy, trastuzumab shrunk tumors by 50% in 14% of women, with a median duration of response of 9 months. Overall, trastuzumab was well tolerated in both trials. Due to an increased risk of cardiac dysfunction observed in women treated with trastuzumab plus an anthracycline, trastuzumab should not be used in combination with this drug class.

At ASCO 2008, researchers reported on the largest study to date of two targeted agents—lapatinib and trastuzumab—in HER2+ metastatic breast cancer. Women had been heavily pretreated with anthracyclines and taxanes (median of six prior chemotherapy regimens), and had progressed on prior trastuzumab. They were randomized to either lapatinib only (L; 1,500 mg daily dose) or to trastuzumab (T; 4 mg/kg loading dose then 2 mg/kg weekly) plus lapatinib (L + T; 1,000 mg daily dose of lapatinib). There were 148 patients in each group. Women could cross over to L + T if they progressed on L. The response rate with L was 6.9% and with L + T was 10.3%. Median progression-free survival was 8.1 weeks with L vs 12 weeks with L + T (HR 0.73, P = .008). Median overall survival was 39 weeks with L vs 52 weeks with L + T (P = .11). Both regimens were well tolerated; asymptomatic decline in LVEF (> 20% and below LLN) occurred in 2% of patients in the L arm and in 5% of patients in L+T arm. There was one death due to cardiac toxicity in the L + T arm. Investigators noted that the role of combined anti-HER2 therapy, in combination with chemotherapy, in less heavily pretreated patients with early-stage disease is ongoing in the ALTTO study (Adjuvant L and/or T Treatment Optimization) (O'Shaughnessy J, Blackwell KL, Burstein H, et al: J Clin Oncol [abstract 1015] 26[suppl 15S]:44s, 2008).

It is important to point out that trastuzumab also produces cardiac toxicity when administered by itself, particularly in patients who have had extensive prior exposure to an anthracycline. Finally, essentially all of the clinical benefit of trastuzumab (alone or in combination) is confined to patients whose breast cancer expresses high (3+) levels of the HER2-*neu* oncoprotein.

One study explored the relationship between circulating HER2 extracellular domain (ECD) and tissue HER2 status and examined its predictive value in a cohort of metastatic breast cancer patients treated with weekly trastuzumab and paclitaxel. Retrospective analysis of patients treated on a previous trial evaluated the associations between pretreatment serum HER2 ECD and tissue HER2 status and the change in serum HER2 ECD after 12 weeks of therapy and response. Stored serum samples were available for 55 of 95 patients (58%). A statistically significant association was found between HER2 status and baseline serum HER2 ECD level. Patients whose ECD normalized after 12 weeks of therapy had a higher response proportion thatn did those with persistently high ECD levels (68% vs 15%; $P = .005$). A relative decline of more than 55% from baseline HER2 ECD predicted response to trastuzumab-based therapy.

Lapatinib (Tykerb) Lapatinib is a tyrosine kinase inhibitor of HER2-*neu* and epidermal growth factor receptor (EGFR), and is active in combination with capecitabine in women with HER2-positive metastatic breast cancer. Women with HER2-positive, locally advanced or metastatic breast cancer that had progressed after treatment with regimens that included an anthracycline, a taxane, and trastuzumab were randomly assigned to receive either lapatinib (at a dose of 1,250 mg/d continuously) plus capecitabine (at a dose of 2,000 mg/m^2 of body surface area) on days 1 through 14 of a 21-day cycle or monotherapy with capecitabine alone (at a dose of 2,500 mg/m^2 on days 1 through 14 of a 21-day cycle).

The interim analysis of time to disease progression met specified criteria for early reporting on the basis of superiority in the combination-therapy group. The HR for the independently assessed time to disease progression was 0.49 (95% CI, 0.34–0.71; $P < .001$), with 49 events in the combination-therapy group and 72 events in the monotherapy group. The median time to disease progression was 8.4 months in the combination-therapy group, compared with 4.4 months in the monotherapy group. This improvement was achieved without an increase in serious toxic effects or symptomatic cardiac events. In March 2007, lapatinib in combination with capecitabine was approved by the FDA for treatment of women with HER2-positive advanced breast cancer that has progressed after treatment with trastuzumab.

Ixebepilone (Ixempra) has recently been approved for the treatment of advanced breast cancer after failure of an anthracycline and a taxane, either as monotherapy or in combination with capecitabine. Its approval was based on two pivotal trials. One is a phase II study evaluating the efficacy and safety of ixabepilone in patients with metastatic breast cancer resistant to anthracycline, taxane, and capecitabine. Patients were heavily pretreated: 88% of the 126 patients had received at least two lines of prior chemotherapy in the metastatic setting. Ixabepilone (40 mg/m²) was administered as a 3-hour intravenous infusion on day 1 of a 21-day cycle. The primary endpoint was objective response rate, assessed by an independent radiology facility (IRF). A total of 113 patients were assessable for response: IRF-assessed overall response rate was 11.5% (95% CI, 6.3%–18.9%). Fifty percent of patients achieved stable disease; 14.3% achieved stable disease ≥ 6 months. The median duration of response and progression-free survival were 5.7 and 3.1 months, respectively. The median overall survival was 8.6 months. Grade 3/4 treatment-related events included peripheral sensory neuropathy (14%), fatigue/asthenia (13%), myalgia (8%), and stomatitis/mucositis (6%). Resolution of grade 3/4 peripheral sensory neuropathy occurred after a median of 5.4 weeks.

The AVADO trial, in nearly 750 HER2-negative patients with locally recurrent or metastatic breast cancer, assessed first-line docetaxel (Taxotere) with or without bevacizumab (Avastin) at either its standard dose (15 mg/kg every 3 weeks) or at half the standard dose. Patient characteristics were similar between AVADO and E2100, the trial that led to FDA approval of Avastin as front-line treatment for metastatic disease in early 2008. In AVADO, patients did not have to receive chemotherapy until progression, and docetaxel could be discontinued after 6 or 9 cycles of chemotherapy while continuing treatment with bevacizumab (or placebo). Patients in both bevacizumab arms had a prolonged TTP vs those receiving chemotherapy alone (HR, 0.72-0.79; P < .05), but the improvements were modest vs E2100: Median TTP was increased from 8 months with docetaxel alone to 8.7 and 8.8 months with addition of the half-dose and standard dose of bevacizumab, respectively. Response rates with docetaxel alone vs half-dose and standard-dose bevacizumab were 44%, 55%, and 63%, respectively, and 1-year survival rates were 73%, 78%, and 83% (Miles D, Chan A, Romeiu G, et al: J Clin Oncol [abstract LBA101] 26 [suppl 15S]:2008).

The other study was a randomized phase III trial evaluating the efficacy and safety of ixebepilone in combination with capecitabine. This trial included 752 patients who were previously treated with anthracyclines and taxanes and whose tumors had demonstrated prior resistance to these therapies. Ixabepilone plus capecitabine prolonged progression-free survival relative to capecitabine (median, 5.8 months vs 4.2 months), with a 25% reduction in the estimated risk of disease progression (HR, 0.75; 95% CI, 0.64–0.88; P = .0003). Objective response rate was also increased (35% vs 14%; P < .0001). Grade 3/4 treatment-related sensory neuropathy (21% vs 0%), fatigue (9% vs 3%), and neutropenia (68% vs 11%) were more frequent with combination therapy, as was the rate of death as a result of toxicity (3% vs 1%, with patients with liver dysfunction [≥ grade 2 liver function tests] at greater risk). Capecitabine-related toxicities were similar for both treatment groups.

Bevacizumab (Avastin) is the first antiangiogenic agent to demonstrate benefit in women with breast cancer. The phase III Eastern Cooperative Oncology Group (ECOG) 2100 trial randomized patients to receive either standard doses of weekly paclitaxel or the same chemotherapy with bevacizumab as front-line treatment for metastatic disease. The overall response rate was significantly better with the combination (28.2% vs 14.2%; $P < .0001$). Noteworthy were the significant increases in progression-free and overall survival for patients treated with the combination, although the survival data are still immature. Toxicities associated with the bevacizumab combination included hypertension, proteinuria, and neuropathy. There was also a trend toward an increase in thrombosis and bleeding, but it was not statistically significant.

Capecitabine combined with bevacizumab in heavily pretreated metastatic breast cancer improved the response rate but not progression-free survival. In untreated metastatic breast cancer, the addition of bevacizumab to chemotherapy significantly improves progression-free survival which suggests that bevacizumab, is most effective in early disease. A single-arm, phase II study to evaluate progression-free survival in metastatic breast cancer patients receiving first-line treatment with capecitabine at $(1,000 \text{ mg/m}^2$ twice daily) on days 1 to 15 (28 doses) and bevacizumab (15 mg/kg) on day 1 repeated every 21 days until disease progression was recently reported. Results are based on 103 patients (intent-to-treat population), with 84 patients alive at this time. Tumor response, which is based on 91 patients evaluated, showed a 38.5% (35/91) patients have had a response: complete response, 5.5%; partial response, 33.0%. Stable disease was 42.9%, with a 81.4% clinical benefit. The planned dose received was 77.7% for capecitabine and 99.0% for bevacizumab. The majority of adverse events were mild or moderate. The most common grade 3 toxicities were hand-foot syndrome (13%) and pain (10%); grade 4 pulmonary embolism occurred in 2% in the first phase of the study.

High-dose chemotherapy

Patients who present with or subsequently develop distant metastasis may be candidates for high-dose intensive chemotherapy programs with autologous stem-cell support. Multiple feasibility and phase II studies of this approach have been undertaken. The majority of programs include the use of multiple alkylating agents. The role of high-dose chemotherapy in metastatic disease remains controversial, and analysis and observation of ongoing clinical trials continue to be important.

The results from multiple centers indicate an overall 5-year disease-free survival rate of 25% in patients with metastatic disease treated with high-dose chemotherapy. However, it must be remembered that these results were obtained in a select patient population—generally individuals < 60 years of age with good performance status; chemotherapy-sensitive disease; and normal cardiac, pulmonary, renal, and hepatic function. The use of intensive supportive outpatient care, such as colony-stimulating factors and antibiotics, has significantly reduced the morbidity and mortality associated with the high-dose chemotherapy approach.

In randomized trials of high-dose chemotherapy in patients with metastatic breast cancer (Table 3), it appears that most of the benefit occurs in women with low-bulk disease, especially those in complete clinical remission. A metaanalysis with longer follow-up also demonstrated a benefit for the addition of high-dose therapy to standard, anthracycline-containing chemotherapy for advanced disease in the setting of patients in complete clinical remission. This therapeutic modality remains investigational for patients with stage IV disease, however; women referred for high-dose therapy should be enrolled in a clinical trial.

Adjunctive bisphosphonate therapy

Multiple published reports have now confirmed the benefit of bisphosphonates as an adjunct to treatment of patients with bone metastasis. Use of these agents results in a significant reduction in skeleton-related events, including pathologic fracture, bone pain, and the need for radiation therapy to bone. Pamidronate and zoledronic acid (Zometa), both in IV formulations, are available in the United States. Oral bisphosphonates used for this indication, such ibandronate (Boniva) and clodronate, are not in the US market.

Patients with breast carcinoma who had all types of bone metastases (osteolytic, mixed, or osteoblastic) were randomized to receive treatment with either 4 or 8 mg of zoledronic acid as a 15-minute infusion or 90 mg of pamidronate as a 2-hour infusion every 3 to 4 weeks for 12 months. The proportion of patients who had a skeleton-related event (defined as a pathologic fracture, spinal cord compression, radiotherapy, or surgery to bone) was comparable between treatment groups (approximately 45%). However, among patients who had breast carcinoma with at least one osteolytic lesion, treatment with 4 mg of zoledronic acid was more effective than 90 mg of pamidronate in reducing skeletal complications.

The most commonly reported adverse events for both zoledronic acid and pamidronate were bone pain, nausea, fatigue, emesis, and fever. The 4-mg dose of zoledronic acid results in elevated serum creatinine levels in about 7.7% of patients, versus 6.0% with pamidronate. A larger proportion of patients had elevated serum creatinine levels with 8-mg of zoledronic acid; therefore, this dose is not recommended. Symptomatic hypocalcemia, although relatively rare, requires frequent monitoring of calcium and phosphate levels during treatment.

ROLE OF RADIATION THERAPY IN METASTATIC DISEASE

Irradiation remains an integral component of the management of metastatic breast carcinoma. Although bone metastases are the most commonly treated metastatic sites in patients with breast cancer, brain metastases, spinal cord compression, choroidal metastases, endobronchial lung metastases, and metastatic lesions in other visceral sites can be effectively palliated with irradiation.

Radiation dose and schedule Depending on the disease site and volume of the radiation field, fractionation schedules ranging from 20 Gy in 5 fractions to 30 Gy in 10 fractions are used most commonly. In some situations, more protracted courses using lower daily doses may be indicated.

Bone metastasis For patients with widespread bone metastasis, hemibody irradiation (6–7 Gy in one fraction to the upper body or 8 Gy to the lower

TABLE 3: Randomized studies of high-dose chemotherapy in metastatic breast cancer

| | | Median | Survival rate (%) | | |
Investigators	Number of patients	follow-up (yr)	High-dose treatment	Standard treatment	P value
Stadtmauer et al	553	3	32.0	38.0	NS
Lotz et al	61	5	29.8	18.5	NS

NS = not significant

body) has been shown to be effective. Strontium-89 chloride (Metastron) and other systemic radionuclides also provide effective palliation for widespread bone disease.

Consolidation after high-dose chemotherapy Since patients with metastatic disease treated with high-dose chemotherapy and autologous bone marrow or stem-cell transplantation often develop progressive disease in previously involved sites, studies have suggested the use of "consolidative radiation therapy" for patients undergoing high-dose chemotherapy. Although this approach appears to be well tolerated and preliminary data are encouraging, whether it will affect survival remains to be determined.

Brain metastasis Patients who develop metastasis to the brain generally have poor outcomes. Nonetheless, radiation therapy can often be helpful in palliating their symptoms and may help control disease for some time. In one randomized trial, patients with one to three newly diagnosed brain metastases (breast as well as other sites) were randomly allocated to receive either whole-brain radiation therapy (WBRT, 164 patients) or WBRT followed by a stereotactic radiosurgery boost (167 patients). Univariate analysis showed that there was a survival advantage in the WBRT and surgery group for patients with a single brain metastasis (median survival, 6.5 months vs 4.9 months; $P = .0393$). Patients in the stereotactic surgery group were more likely to have a stable or improved Karnofsky performance status score at 6 months' follow-up than were patients allocated to WBRT alone (43% vs 27%, respectively; $P = .03$.

ROLE OF SURGERY IN METASTATIC DISEASE

There are selected indications for surgical intervention in patients with metastatic breast cancer, and the role of surgery at this point is generally palliative. Most commonly, palliative surgery is offered to patients with brain metastases, spinal cord compression, fractures, or symptomatic pleural or pericardial effusions not controlled by other means. It is also used for GI complications stemming from metastatic deposits. The curative benefit of surgery in the treatment of metastatic disease to the lungs or liver is not proven, but, in highly selected cases, surgery may be beneficial.

Spinal cord compression Patients with spinal cord compression who have progressive symptoms during irradiation, disease recurrence after irradiation, or spinal instability or who require diagnosis are candidates for surgery.

Solitary brain metastasis Patients with a long disease-free interval and solitary brain metastasis may be candidates for resection. Evidence suggests an improved disease-free survival, overall survival, and quality of life in this subset of patients when treated with surgery combined with postoperative cranial irradiation, as compared with radiation therapy alone.

Gamma- and Cyber-knife radiosurgery is increasingly used to manage brain metastases. In some instances, these modalities have been used in patients who have multiple metastatic brain lesions or in patients who had previously received conventional treatment modalities for brain metastases, including whole-brain irradiation. No radiation-induced dementia and a remarkably low incidence of local failure were reported with these treatments. Although in the past, local control of brain metastasis was an issue, these treatment modalities are shifting the question of survival to that of systemic control.

Chest wall resection It is extremely rare for a patient with distant metastatic disease to be a candidate for chest wall resection; however, patients with symptomatic recurrence of disease in the chest wall who have limited distant disease and a life expectancy of > 12 months may be appropriate candidates.

Solitary liver metastatic disease Although rarely indicated, patients with single metastases or a prolonged disease-free or disease-stable interval may be candidates for resection.

Liver metastasis Patients with metastatic disease to the liver have a poor prognosis. In the past, patients with a single focus of disease in the liver who had no evidence of extrahepatic disease were offered liver resection as a means to control their disease and improve outcome. With advanced surgical techniques, the morbidity and mortality for liver resection have decreased. Hepatic resection was undertaken in patients with breast cancer metastases to the liver and not limited to patients whose disease was solely confined to the liver. A 5-year disease-free survival rate of 21% and an overall 5-year survival rate of 37% were observed. These results suggest an expanded role for hepatic resection in patients with breast cancer metastases to the liver.

Follow-up of long-term survivors

For recommendations on the type and timing of follow-up evaluations, see chapter 10.

SUGGESTED READING

Adam R, Aloia T, Krissat J, et al: Is liver resection justified for patients with hepatic metastases from breast cancer? Ann Surg 244:897–908, 2006.

Berry DA, Broadwater G, Klein JP, et al: High-dose versus standard chemotherapy in metastatic breast cancer: Comparison of Cancer and Leukemia Group B Trials with data from the Autologous Blood and Marrow Transplant Registry. J Clin Oncol 20:743–750, 2002.

Cristofanilli M, Budd GT, Ellis MJ, et al: Circulating tumor cells, disease progression, and survival in metastatic breast cancer. N Engl J Med 351:781–791, 2004.

Fornier MN, Seidman AD, Schwartz MK, et al: Serum HER2 extracellular domain in metastatic breast cancer patients treated with weekly trastuzumab and paclitaxel: Association with HER2 status by immunohistochemistry and fluorescence in situ hybridization and with response rate. Ann Oncol 16:234–239, 2005.

Geyer CE, Forster J, Lindquist D, et al: Lapatinib plus capecitabine for HER2-positive advanced breast cancer. N Engl J Med 355:2733–2743, 2006.

Geyer CE, Martin A, Newstat B, et al: Lapatinb (L) plus capecitabine (C) in HER2+ advanced breast cancer (ABC): Genomic and updated effiacy data. J Clin Oncol 25[18S]:1035, 2007.

Green MC, Buzdar AU, Smith T, et al: Weekly paclitaxel improves pathologic complete remission in operable breast cancer when compared with paclitaxel once every 3 weeks. J Clin Oncol 23:5983–5992, 2005.

Howell A, Robertson JF, Quaresma AJ, et al: Fulvestrant, formerly ICI 182,780, is as effective as anastrozole in postmenopausal women with advanced breast cancer progressing after prior endocrine treatment. J Clin Oncol 20:3396–3403, 2002.

Kuerer HM, Hunt K: The rationale for integration of lymphatic mapping and sentinel node biopsy in the management of breast cancer after neoadjuvant chemotherapy. Semin Breast Dis 5:80–87, 2002.

Loesch D, Robert N, Asmar L, et al: Phase II multicenter trial of a weekly paclitaxel and carboplatin regimen in patients with advanced breast cancer. J Clin Oncol 20:3857–3864, 2002.

Martincich L, Montemurro F, De Rosa G, et al: Monitoring response to primary chemotherapy in breast cancer using dynamic contrast-enhanced magnetic resonance imaging. Breast Cancer Res Treat 83:67–76, 2004.

O'Shaughnessy J, Miles D, Vukelja S, et al: Superior survival with capecitabine plus docetaxel combination therapy in anthracycline-pretreated patients with advanced breast cancer: Phase III trial results. J Clin Oncol 20:2812–2823, 2002.

Perez EA, Lerzo G, Pivot X, et al: Efficacy and safety of ixabepilone (BMS-247550) in a phase II study of patients with advanced breast cancer resistant to an anthracycline, a taxane, and capecitabine. J Clin Oncol 25:3407–3414, 2007.

Robertson JF, Osborne CK, Howell A, et al: Fulvestrant versus anastrozole for the treatment of advanced breast carcinoma in postmenopausal women: A prospective combined analysis of two multicenter trials. Cancer 98:229–238, 2003.

Rodenhuis S, Bontenbal M, Beex LV, et al: High-dose chemotherapy with hematopoietic stem-cell rescue for high-risk breast cancer. N Engl J Med 349:7–16, 2003.

Rosen LS, Gordon DH, Dugan W Jr, et al: Zoledronic acid is superior to pamidronate for the treatment of bone metastases in breast carcinoma patients with at least one osteolytic lesion. Cancer 100:36–43, 2004.

Sledge G, Miller K, Moisa C, et al: Safety and efficacy of capecitabine (C) plus bevacizumab (B) as first-line in metastatic breast cancer. J Clin Oncol 25:[18S]:1013, 2007.

Sledge GW, Neuberg D, Bernardo P, et al: Phase III trial of doxorubicin, paclitaxel, and the combination of doxorubicin and paclitaxel as front-line chemotherapy for metastatic breast cancer: An intergroup trial (E1193). J Clin Oncol 21:588–592, 2003.

Thomas ES, Gomez HL, Li RK, et al: Ixabepilone plus capecitabine for metastatic breast cancer progressing after anthracycline and taxane treatment. J Clin Oncol 25:5210–5217, 2007.

van der Hoeven JJ, Krak NC, Hoekstra OS, et al: 18F-2-fluoro-2-deoxy-d-glucose positron emission tomography in staging of locally advanced breast cancer. J Clin Oncol 22:1253–1259, 2004.

Wahl RL, Siegel BA, Coleman RE, et al: Prospective multicenter study of axillary nodal staging by positron emission tomography in breast cancer: A report of the staging breast cancer with PET study group. J Clin Oncol 22:277–285, 2004.

CHAPTER 12

Esophageal cancer

Jimmy J. Hwang, MD, Rajesh V. Iyer, MD, and Michael Mulligan, MD

Although still relatively uncommon in Western countries, esophageal cancer is fatal in the vast majority of cases. In the United States, an estimated 16,470 new cases will be diagnosed in the year 2008, and 14,280 deaths will result from the disease. This high percentage of deaths rivals that of pancreatic cancer and is more than four times that of rectal cancer.

The esophagus extends from the cricopharyngeal sphincter to the gastro-esophageal (GE) junction and is commonly divided into the cervical, upper to mid-thoracic, and thoracic portions. This can be important, as histology and optimal treatment approaches may vary considerably based on the site of the cancer. It may not be possible to determine the site of origin if the cancer involves the GE junction itself.

Epidemiology

Gender Esophageal cancer is seven times more common and slightly more lethal in men than in women.

Age Adenocarcinoma of the esophagus (now more common in the United States than the squamous cell type) has a median age at diagnosis of 69 years. The incidence of squamous cell cancer of the esophagus increases with age as well and peaks in the seventh decade of life.

Race The incidence of squamous cell esophageal cancer is three times higher in blacks than in whites, whereas adenocarcinomas are more common in white men.

Geography Evidence of an association between environment and diet and esophageal cancer comes from the profound differences in incidence observed in various parts of the world. Esophageal cancer occurs at a rate 20 to 30 times higher in China than in the United States. An esophageal "cancer belt" extends from northeast China to the Middle East.

Survival Although the overall outlook for patients diagnosed with esophageal cancer has improved in the past 30 years, most patients still present with advanced disease, and their survival remains poor. One-third to one-half of patients treated with either chemoradiation therapy or chemoradiation therapy plus surgery are alive at 2 years, without recurrence of esophageal cancer.

Disease site The rate of cancer of the distal esophagus is about equal to that of the more proximal two-thirds. In general, squamous cell carcinoma is found in the body of the esophagus, whereas adenocarcinoma predominates in lesions closer to the GE junction.

Etiology and risk factors

Cigarettes and alcohol Squamous cell carcinomas of the esophagus have been associated with cigarette smoking and/or excessive alcohol intake. Furthermore, cigarette smoking and alcohol appear to act synergistically, producing high relative risks in heavy users of tobacco and alcohol. Esophageal adenocarcinoma is increased twofold in smokers.

Diet High-fat, low-protein, and low-calorie diets have been shown to increase the risk of esophageal cancer. Exposure to nitrosamines has been proposed as a factor in the development of both squamous cell carcinoma and adenocarcinoma of the esophagus.

Barrett's esophagus and other factors Gastroesophageal reflux disease (GERD) and Barrett's esophagus (adenomatous metaplasia of the distal esophagus) have been linked to adenocarcinoma of the esophagus. Tylosis, Plummer-Vinson syndrome, history of head and neck cancer, and achalasia have also been associated with a higher-than-normal risk of developing squamous cell cancer of the esophagus.

Signs and symptoms

Because symptoms do not alert the patient until the disease is advanced, few esophageal cancers are diagnosed at an early stage.

Dysphagia The most common presenting complaint is dysphagia, which generally is not noted until the esophageal lumen is narrowed to one-half to one-third of normal, due to its elasticity.

Weight loss is common and has a significant role in prognosis (> 10% of total body weight as poor prognosis).

Cough that is induced by swallowing is suggestive of local extension into the trachea with resultant tracheoesophageal fistula.

Odynophagia and pain Pain with swallowing (odynophagia) is an ominous sign. Patients who describe pain radiating to the back may well have extra-esophageal spread. Supraclavicular or cervical nodal metastases may be appreciated on examination.

Hoarseness may be a sign of recurrent laryngeal nerve involvement due to extraesophageal spread.

Metastatic disease may present as malignant pleural effusion or ascites. Bone metastasis can be identified by pain involving the affected site or by associated hypercalcemia. The most common metastatic sites are retroperitoneal or celiac lymph nodes.

The American College of Surgeons conducted a study utilizing its national cancer database to assess the presentation, stage distribution, and treatment of patients diagnosed with esophageal cancer between 1994 and 1997 (n = 5,044). The most common presenting symptoms were dysphagia (74.0%), weight loss (57.3%), reflux (20.5%), odynophagia (16.6%), and dyspnea (12.1%). The American College of Surgeons Database finds 50% of patients present with tumors in the lower third of the esophagus; 42% have adenocarcinoma histology, and 52% have squamous histology. Barrett's esophagus was found in 39% of those patients with adenocarcinoma. Patients undergoing initial surgical resection had the following stage distribution: stage I (13.3%), II (34.7%), III (35.7%), and IV (12.3%).

Diagnosis

In Western countries, the diagnosis of esophageal cancer is generally made by endoscopic biopsy of the esophagus. In the Far East, cytologic evaluation is frequently utilized.

Endoscopic ultrasonography (EUS) is extremely accurate (> 90%) in establishing the depth of tumor invasion (T stage) but less accurate (70%–80%) in determining nodal involvement (N stage) unless combined with fine-needle aspiration (FNA) of the involved nodes (93% accuracy) when nodes greater than 5 mm are biopsied. The addition of FNA increases the sensitivity from 63% to 93% and the specificity from 81% to 100%. EUS is not reliable in determining the extent of response to neoadjuvant treatment.

Endoscopy and barium x-rays Endoscopy allows for direct visualization of abnormalities and directed biopsies. Barium x-rays are less invasive and provide a good assessment of the extent of esophageal disease.

Bronchoscopy should be performed to detect tracheal invasion in all cases of esophageal cancer except adenocarcinoma of the distal third of the esophagus.

CT scan Once a diagnosis has been established and careful physical examination and routine blood tests have been performed, a CT scan of the chest, abdomen, and pelvis should be obtained to help assess tumor extent, nodal involvement, and metastatic disease.

PET A prospective trial designed to evaluate the utility of PET versus CT and EUS was performed by obtaining these studies in 48 consecutive patients prior to esophagectomy. PET achieved a 57% sensitivity, 97% specificity, and 86% accuracy compared with CT, which was 99% sensitive, 18% specific, and 78% accurate. In terms of nodal staging, PET was correct in 83% of cases, as compared with 60% of cases for CT and 58% for EUS ($P = .006$). This analysis suggests the improved accuracy of PET in the staging work-up of patients with esophageal cancer.

Numerous studies report the accuracy of PET scanning in determining the presence of metastatic disease, with sensitivity approaching 90% and specificity over 90%.

As PET becomes more widely available, its use will probably become an important part of the preoperative evaluation of these patients. In a prospective trial of 39 patients with esophageal cancer, PET detected additional sites of metastatic disease at the initial evaluation when compared with conventional imaging. After induction therapy, PET did not add to the estimation of locoregional resectability and did not detect new distant metastases. However, this study suggested that changes in [^{18}fluorodeoxyglucose] FDG-PET following induction therapy may predict disease-free and overall survival after induction therapy and resection in patients with esophageal cancer. A large prospective national trial will evaluate the use of PET in the treatment of esophageal cancer.

Bone scan A bone scan should be obtained if the patient has bone pain or an elevated alkaline phosphatase level.

Thoracoscopy/laparoscopy Investigators have recently begun to examine the role of surgical staging prior to definitive therapy. These procedures are designed to allow pathologic review of regional lymph nodes and the accurate assessment of extraesophageal tumor spread by direct visualization. A multi-institution trial (Cancer and Leukemia Group B [CALGB] 9380) found these procedures to be feasible in over 70% of patients; they resulted in the upstaging of patients in 38% of cases reviewed. Further investigations need to be completed to determine the appropriate use of these tools in treatment algorithms for patients with esophageal cancer.

Warning Staging studies should be performed in a sequential manner. Invasive, lower yield, and less accurate studies and procedures should only be undertaken if management would change on the basis of specific findings.

Screening and surveillance

HIGH-RISK PATIENTS

Adenocarcinoma The role of screening patients with GERD and surveillance of patients with Barrett's esophagus by upper GI endoscopy remains under investigation. In 833 patients studied by endoscopy, there was a 13% incidence of intestinal metaplasia (Barrett's esophagus). Dysplasia or cancer was seen in 31% of patients with long-segment Barrett's esophagus, in 10% of short-segment Barrett's esophagus, and in 6% of GE-junction intestinal metaplasia.

Squamous cell carcinoma Mass screening in the high-risk areas of China and Japan is considered appropriate.

Pathology

Adenocarcinoma The incidence of esophageal adenocarcinoma involving the GE junction has risen 4% to 10% per year since 1976 in the United States and Europe. As a result, adenocarcinoma is now the predominant histologic subtype of esophageal cancer. The distal one-third of the esophagus is the site of origin of most adenocarcinomas.

Squamous cell carcinomas occur most often in the proximal two-thirds of the esophagus. Squamous cell carcinoma is still the most prevalent histologic subtype worldwide.

Other tumor types Other, less frequently seen histologic subtypes include mucoepidermoid carcinoma, small-cell carcinoma, sarcoma, adenoid cystic

TABLE I: 1983 and 2002 AJCC TNM staging systems for esophageal cancer

1983 Classification (clinical)				2002 Classification (pathologic)		
Primary tumor (T)						
Tis	Carcinoma in situ			Same		
T1	Tumor involves ≤ 5 cm of esophageal length, produces no obstruction, and has no circumferential involvement			Tumor invades lamina propria or submucosa		
T2	Tumor involves > 5 cm of esophageal length, causes obstruction, or involves the circumference of the esophagus			Tumor invades muscularis propria		
T3	Extraesophageal spread			Tumor invades adventitia		
T4	Not applicable			Tumor invades adjacent structures		
Regional lymph nodes (N)						
Nx	Regional nodes cannot be assessed			Same		
N0	No nodal metastases			No regional nodal metastases		
N1	Unilateral, mobile, regional nodal metastases (if clinically evaluable)			Regional nodal metastases		
N2	Bilateral, mobile, regional nodal metastases (if clinically evaluable)			Not applicable		
N3	Fixed nodes			Not applicable		
Distant metastases (M)						
M0	No distant metastases			Same		
M1	Distant metastases			Distant metastases		
				Tumors of lower thoracic esophagus:		
				M1a	Metastases in celiac lymph nodes	
				M1b	Other distant metastases	
				Tumors of mid-thoracic esophagus:		
				M1a	Not applicable	
				M1b	Nonregional lymph nodes and/or other distant metastases	
				Tumors of upper thoracic esophagus:		
				M1a	Metastases in cervical nodes	
				M1b	Other distant metastases	
Stage grouping						
Stage I	T1	N0 or NX	M0	T1	N0	M0
Stage II	T2	N0 or NX	M0			
Stage IIA				T2-3	N0	M0
Stage IIB				T1-2	N1	M0
Stage III	T3	Any N	M0	T3	N1	M0
				T4	Any N	M0
Stage IV	Any T	Any N	M1	Any T	Any N	M1
Stage IVA				Any T	Any N	M1a
Stage IVB				Any T	Any N	M1b

AJCC = American Joint Committee on Cancer

TABLE 2: Treatment options and survival by stage in esophageal cancer

Stage[a]		Standard treatment	5-Year survival rate (%)
Stage 0	(Tis N0 M0)	Surgery	> 90
Stage I	(TI N0 M0)	Surgery	> 70
Stage IIA	(T2-3 N0 M0)	Surgery, chemoradiation therapy, or combination	15-30
Stage IIB	(TI-2 NI M0)	Surgery, chemoradiation therapy, or combination	10-30
Stage III	(T3 NI M0 or T4 Any N M0)	Chemoradiation therapy Palliative resection of T3a tumors	< 10
Stage IV	(Any T Any N MI)	Radiation therapy ± intraluminal intubation and dilation ± chemotherapy	Rare

[a] According to the AJCC TNM system definitions (see Table I)

Note: Surgical results are based on the pathologic staging system, whereas patients treated with combined-modality therapy or neoadjuvant chemoradiation therapy are clinically staged.

leiomyosarcoma, and primary lymphoma of the esophagus. Occasionally, metastatic disease from another site may present as a mass in the esophagus or a mass pressing on the esophagus.

Metastatic spread The most common sites of metastatic disease are the regional lymph nodes, lungs, liver, bone, adrenal glands, and diaphragm. Adenocarcinoma can also metastasize to the brain.

Staging and prognosis

Based on data demonstrating that the depth of penetration has important prognostic significance, the American Joint Committee on Cancer (AJCC) TNM staging system for esophageal cancer was changed from a clinical one (1983) to a pathologic one in 2002. Both the clinical and pathologic staging systems are shown in Table 1, as patients may be cured without an operation. Although pathologic information obtained from an esophagectomy specimen is of prognostic importance, postoperative therapy to improve prognosis has not been rigorously tested. Moreover, recurrence rates for stage I (30%) and stage II (70%) cancers suggest early systemic spread undetected by current noninvasive staging.

Pathologic information obtained from an esophagectomy specimen is of significant prognostic importance. Immunohistochemical analysis of the initial biopsy specimen may also have prognostic relevance. Clinical staging has been shown to be of prognostic importance, particularly in patients managed with primary radiotherapy or chemoradiation therapy.

Histology and grade Neither histology nor grade has been shown to be of prognostic importance in esophageal carcinoma.

Other prognostic factors Patient age, performance status, and degree of weight loss are of prognostic importance. The prognostic implications of tumor-suppressor genes and oncogenes are an area of active investigation.

Treatment

Treatment options for the various disease stages are given in Table 2, along with 5-year survival rates.

TREATMENT OF LOCALIZED DISEASE

Only 40% to 60% of patients with esophageal cancer present with clinically localized disease. The National Comprehensive Cancer Network (NCCN) guidelines state that patients with clinically localized disease may be treated with resection or chemotherapy plus irradiation (Tables 3 and 4). The overall 5-year survival rates for either surgery alone or combined chemotherapy and irradiation appear equivalent.

Chemoradiation therapy as primary management of localized or locoregionally confined esophageal cancer has been shown to be superior to irradiation alone. A series of randomized trials have demonstrated that adjuvant postoperative chemoradiation therapy does not offer a survival advantage to patients with esophageal cancer. Adequate patient selection, tumor staging, and treatment standardization will be required before the optimal therapeutic modalities in these patients will be determined.

Surgery

Preoperative medical evaluation helps determine the patient's risk of developing postoperative complications and mortality. In addition to the staging and nutritional status, it should include an evaluation of the pulmonary, cardiac, renal, and hepatic functions.

Extent of surgical resection The extent of resection depends on the location of the primary tumor, histology of the tumor, and nature of the procedure (palliative vs curative). A retrospective study has reported that superficial mucosal lesions may be treated via endoscopic mucosal resection, but those patients with submucosal invasion require esophagectomy. For tumors of the intrathoracic esophagus (squamous cell carcinomas) and tumors with extensive Barrett's esophagus (adenocarcinomas), it is necessary to perform a total esophagectomy with cervical anastomosis to achieve a complete resection. For distal lesions of the abdominal esophagus (adenocarcinomas) and cardia, it is often possible to perform an intrathoracic esophageal anastomosis above the azygos vein, although many surgeons would prefer to perform a total esophagectomy.

The resected esophagus may be replaced with tubularized stomach in patients with tumors of the intrathoracic esophagus or with a colon interposition in

TABLE 3: Chemotherapy regimens for esophageal carcinoma

Drug/combination	Dose and schedule
Cisplatin/fluorouracil/radiation therapy	
Cisplatin	75 mg/m^2 IV on day 1 of weeks 1, 5, 8, and 11
Fluorouracil	1 g/m^2/d IV infused continuously on days 1-4 of weeks 1, 5, 8, and 11
Radiation therapy	200 cGy/d 5 days per week (total regional treatment, 3,000 cGy), followed by a 2,000-cGy boost field (total, 5,000 cGy) in 5 weeks

Give chemotherapy concurrently with radiation therapy.

Adapted from Herskovic A, Martz K, al-Sarraf M, et al: N Engl J Med 326:1593–1598, 1992.

FOLFOX4/radiation therapy	
Oxaliplatin	85 mg/m^2 IV on day 1
Leucovorin	200 mg/m^2 IVPB on day 1
Followed by	
Fluorouracil	400 mg/m^2 IV bolus and
Fluorouracil	600 mg/m^2, 22-hour continuous infusion on days 1 to 2

Repeat cycle every 2 weeks × 6 with radiation therapy.

Adenis A, Etienne P, Michel P, et al: 2007 Gastrointestinal Cancers Symposium [abstract 42].

Irinotecan /cisplatin	
Irinotecan	65 mg/m^2 IVPB every week × 4 weeks
Cisplatin	30 mg/m^2 IVPB every week × 4 weeks
Followed by 2 weeks rest and recycled every 6 weeks	

Ilson DH, Saltz L, Enzinger P, et al: J Clin Oncol 17:3270–3275, 1999.

IVPB = intravenous piggy back
Table prepared by Ishmael Jaiyesimi, DO

---

patients with tumors involving the proximal stomach, because such involvement makes this organ unsuitable for esophageal reconstruction. The esophageal replacement is usually brought up through the posterior mediastinum, although the retrosternal route is often used in palliative procedures.

Patient selection The indications for esophagectomy in esophageal cancer vary from center to center within the United States.

Clearly, patients with distant metastases, evidence of nodal metastases in more than one nodal basin, or tumor extension outside the esophagus (airway, mediastinum, vocal cord paralysis) are candidates for palliative therapy. Patients with disease limited to the esophagus and no evidence of nodal metastases (stages I and IIA) may be treated with esophagectomy, although these patients can also be considered for definitive treatment with chemoradiation therapy.

TABLE 4: Chemotherapy regimens for gastric esophageal cancer

Dose/combination	Dose and schedule
Adjuvant fluorouracil/leucovorin/radiation therapy for gastric and gastroesophageal junction adenocarcinoma	
Fluorouracil	425 mg/m² IV on days 1-5
Leucovorin	20 mg/m² IV on days 1-5 immediately before fluorouracil for 1 cycle then 3-4 weeks later
Followed by	
Radiation therapy	4,500 cGy (180 cGy a day) given concurrently with
Fluorouracil	400 mg/m² IV on days 1-4 and on the last 3 days of radiation therapy
Leucovorin	20 mg/m² IV on days 1-4 and on the last 3 days of radiation therapy
One month after completion of radiation therapy:	
Fluorouracil	425 mg/m² IV on days 1-5
Leucovorin	20 mg/m² IV on days 1-5 immediately before fluorouracil
Repeat cycle every 28 days for 2 cycles.	

Adapted from Macdonald JS, Smalley S, Benedetti J, et al: Proc Am Soc Clin Oncol 19:1, 2000.

Table prepared by Ishmael Jaiyesimi, DO

Method of resection Considerable controversy also exists among surgeons regarding the method of resection. To date, two randomized studies have compared transhiatal esophagectomy (without thoracotomy) with the Ivor-Lewis (transthoracic) esophagectomy (with thoracotomy). These studies failed to show differences between the two procedures with regard to operative morbidity and mortality. In a randomized trial of 220 patients treated with either a transthoracic or transhiatal esophageal resection, there was a trend toward an improvement in 5-year survival. A meta-analysis failed to show differences in 5-year survival rates. Over the past 5 years, successful attempts have been made to use minimally invasive approaches to esophageal cancer with thoracoscopy and laparoscopy. Although those studies have shown a decrease in morbidity and the minimally invasive approach appears to be oncologically sound from the point of view of resection margins, the number of nodes resected is still not comparable to that of the standard transthoracic approach.

The need for pyloric drainage (pyloroplasty) following esophagectomy is another area of debate. A meta-analysis of nine randomized trials that included 553 patients showed a trend favoring pyloric drainage in improving gastric emptying and nutritional status, whereas bile reflux was better in the nondrainage group. The gastric emptying time evaluated by scintigraphy was twice as long in the nondrainage group as in the pyloric drainage groups.

Lymphadenectomy Considerable controversy exists regarding the need for radical lymphadenectomy in esophageal disease. Much of the controversy is due to the fact that different diseases are being compared.

Japanese series include mostly patients with squamous cell carcinomas of the intrathoracic esophagus, with 80% of the tumors located in the proximal and middle sections of the esophagus. Americans report combined series, with at least 40% to 50% of patients with adenocarcinomas of the distal esophagus. Skinner and DeMeester favor en bloc esophagectomy with radical (mediastinal and abdominal) lymphadenectomy, based on 5-year survival rates of 40% to 50% in patients with stage II disease, as compared with rates of 14% to 22% in historic controls.

In a retrospective study, Akiyama found a 28% incidence of cervical node metastases in patients with squamous cell carcinomas located in the middle and distal portions of the esophagus, as opposed to 46% in those with tumors of the proximal third. Overall survival at 5 years was significantly better in patients who underwent extended lymphadenectomy (three fields) than in those who had conventional lymphadenectomy (two fields); this finding was true in patients with negative nodes (84% and 55%, respectively) and in those with positive nodes (43% and 28%, respectively). Extended lymphadenectomy afforded no survival advantage in patients with tumors in the distal third of the esophagus.

In a study of 1,000 patients with esophagogastric junction adenocarcinomas, the tumors were classified according to the location of the center of the tumor mass in adenocarcinomas of the distal esophagus, cardia, and subcardia. The tumors located in the cardia and subcardia regions spread primarily to the paragastric and left gastric vessel nodes and did not benefit from extended esophagectomy. Kato et al have studied the use of sentinel node mapping to improve the sensitivity of lymphadenectomy.

Preoperative chemotherapy

The frequency of metastatic disease as the cause of death in patients with esophageal cancer has resulted in exploration of the early application of systemic therapy for esophageal cancer. The first of the two large studies was intergroup study 113. A total of 440 patients were treated with surgical resection alone or preceded by 3 cycles of cisplatin and fluorouracil (5-FU). Objective responses were reported in only 19% of patients receiving chemotherapy. No difference in resectability, operative mortality, median survival (14.9 months with chemotherapy vs 16.1 months with surgery alone), or 2-year survival (35% vs 37%) was reported.

However, the Medical Research Council evaluated 802 patients with resectable esophageal cancer in a similar study. Patients randomized to receive chemotherapy were administered two cycles of cisplatin (80 mg/m^2) and 5-FU 1 g/m^2/d as a continuous infusion for 4 days). Microscopically complete resection was performed more frequently in patients receiving chemotherapy, with no difference found in postoperative complications or mortality. Moreover, patients receiving neoadjuvant chemotherapy had significantly longer median

(16.8 months vs 13.3 months) and 2-year survival (43% vs 34%) than patients treated with surgery alone. The reasons for the differences in the outcomes are unclear but may be related to the chemotherapy regimen and schedule employed in the intergroup study, patient population, or study design. As a result, the role of neoadjuvant chemotherapy remains in question but is promising, especially with the potentially more efficacious newer generation of chemotherapy agents.

Polee et al have evaluated a biweekly combination of cisplatin and paclitaxel in this setting in a phase II study, with promising results. Objective responses occurred in 59% of 49 patients. No patients had progressive disease. Although 71% of patients had severe neutropenia, it was often asymptomatic. Forty-seven patients underwent resection subsequently. Complete pathologic responses occurred in 14% of patients. The median survival of patients in this study was 20 months, but it was 32 months in patients who had disease responsive to chemotherapy. The 3-year survival rate was 32%.

Given the uncertainty about the efficacy of preoperative chemotherapy and chemoradiation therapy, some investigators have administered preoperative chemotherapy, followed by chemoradiation therapy, then surgery. The true utility of this approach will need to be defined by randomized studies, but clearly, it is feasible, without a significant increase in toxicity or operative morbidity. Interestingly, these reports have also demonstrated that most patients had significant improvement or resolution of dysphagia with the induction chemotherapy alone.

Adjuvant/postoperative chemotherapy

As the most common source of treatment failure in patients with esophageal cancer who have undergone surgical resection, postoperative chemotherapy has also undergone limited investigation. The Eastern Cooperative Oncology Group (ECOG) conducted a phase II study of 4 cycles of cisplatin (75 mg/m^2) and paclitaxel (175 mg/m^2 over 3 hours) every 3 weeks. Fifty-five eligible patients were treated. Therapy was well tolerated, with grade 3 or 4 neutropenia in 5% of patients, nausea/vomiting in 12% of patients, and neuropathy in 8% of patients. The 2-year survival rate was 60%, which exceeded the investigators' expectations. However, the predominant pattern of failure was distant, with the first site of disease recurrence being distant metastases alone in 76% of patients. Although this combination was not recommended for further investigation as adjuvant therapy, the promising results should encourage additional evaluation of this type of treatment.

Radiotherapy

Although radiotherapy alone is inferior to chemoradiation therapy in the management of locoregionally confined esophageal cancer, it may offer palliation to patients with advanced local disease too frail for chemotherapy.

Preoperative radiotherapy has been shown to be of little value in converting unresectable cancers into resectable ones or in improving survival. However, it decreases the incidence of locoregional tumor recurrence.

Stahl et al presented a randomized trial of preoperative chemotherapy alone versus preoperative chemoradiation therapy in 120 patients with T3-4 or N+ distal esophageal adenocarcinoma. Complete response at surgery was higher in the chemoradiation therapy arm (17% vs 2.5%). There was a trend for higher median (33 months vs 21 months) and 3 year overall survival (43% vs 27%) for preoperative chemoradiation therapy, despite higher mortality (5 patients vs 2 patients); (Stahl M, Walz MK, Stuschke M, et al: J Clin Oncol 25[18S]:4511, 2007).

Postoperative radiotherapy (usually to 50 or 60 Gy) can decrease locoregional failure following curative resection but has no effect on survival.

Brachytherapy Intraluminal isotope radiotherapy (intracavitary brachytherapy) allows high doses of radiation to be delivered to a small volume of tissue. Retrospective studies suggest that a brachytherapy boost may result in improved rates of local tumor control and survival over external-beam radiotherapy alone. This technique can be associated with a high rate of morbidity if not used carefully.

A multi-institution prospective trial was conducted by the Radiation Therapy Oncology Group (RTOG) to determine the feasibility and toxicity of chemotherapy, external-beam irradiation, and esophageal brachytherapy in potentially curable patients with esophageal cancer. Nearly 70% of patients were able to complete external-beam irradiation, brachytherapy, and at least 2 cycles of 5-FU/cisplatin. The median survival was 11 months, and the 1-year survival was 49%. Because of the 12% incidence of fistula formation, the investigators urged caution in the routine application of brachytherapy as part of a definitive treatment plan.

Chemoradiation therapy

Preoperative chemoradiation therapy Initial trials of preoperative chemoradiation therapy reported unacceptably high operative mortality (~26%). Subsequent trials reported operative mortality of 4% to 11%, median survival as long as 29 months, and 5-year survival rates as high as 34%. In general, 25% to 30% of patients have no residual tumor in the resected specimen, and this group tends to have a higher survival rate than those who have a residual tumor discovered by the pathologist.

The superiority of preoperative chemoradiation therapy over surgery alone in esophageal adenocarcinoma has been investigated in several prospective trials. The first trial included 113 patients with adenocarcinoma of the esophagus. These patients were randomized to receive either preoperative chemoradiation therapy (two courses of 5-FU and cisplatin given concurrently with 40 Gy of radiotherapy in 15 fractions) or surgery alone. Median survival was statistically superior in the combined-modality arm than in the surgery-alone arm (16 months vs 11 months). Rates of 3-year survival again statistically favored the combined-modality arm (32% vs 6%). Although toxicity was not severe, the short survival in the surgery control arm has minimized the impact of these results in the United States.

Another trial performed at the University of Michigan enrolled 100 patients and randomized them to undergo surgery alone or preoperative chemoradiation therapy (cisplatin, 20 mg/m^2/d), 5-FU (300 mg^2/d), and vinblastine (1 mg/m^2/d) and radiotherapy (45 Gy/1.5 Gy bid). With a median follow-up of 8.2 years, the 3-year survival was 16% (surgery alone) versus 30% (induction chemoradiation therapy). This difference did not reach statistical significance, as the study was designed to detect a relatively large increase in median survival from 1 to 2.2 years.

An Australian study of 257 patients by Burmeister et al also found no overall or progression-free survival advantage for those patients randomized to receive preoperative chemoradiation therapy versus surgery alone.

A meta-analysis of randomized trials comparing neoadjuvant chemoradiation therapy followed by surgery with surgery alone found that neoadjuvant concurrent chemoradiation therapy improved 3-year survival (odds ratio, 0.66) compared with surgery alone, with a nonsignificant trend toward increased mortality with neoadjuvant treatment.

Newer chemotherapy agents are active and may improve outcome over these older trials. A phase II trial of 129 patients employed paclitaxel/carboplatin/5-FU with 45 Gy of radiation therapy followed by esophagectomy. A pathologic complete response was seen in 38% of patients, with a median survival of 22 months and a 3-year survival of 41%.

Another phase II trial from the University of Michigan administered paclitaxel/cisplatin with 45 Gy of radiation therapy twice daily (1.5 Gy bid). In this study, 19% of patients exhibited a pathologic complete response, with a 24-month median survival and a 3-year survival of 34%. A phase II trial from Memorial Sloan-Kettering Cancer Center combined cisplatin and irinotecan with 50.4 Gy of radiation therapy followed by surgery. Twenty-five percent of patients had a pathologic complete response. Ongoing studies by the RTOG are employing these newer chemotherapy agents.

Primary chemoradiation therapy Patients with locally advanced esophageal cancer (T1-4 N0-1 M0) may be cured with definitive chemoradiation therapy. Randomized trials have demonstrated a survival advantage for chemoradiation therapy over radiotherapy alone in the treatment of esophageal cancer. In an RTOG randomized trial involving 129 patients with esophageal cancer, irradiation (50 Gy) with concurrent cisplatin and 5-FU provided a significant survival advantage (27% vs 0% at 5 years) and improved local tumor control over radiation therapy alone (64 Gy). Median survival also was significantly better in the combined-therapy arm than in the irradiation arm (14.1 vs 9.3 months).

A randomized trial of preoperative chemoradiation therapy followed by surgery versus chemoradiation therapy alone included 444 patients with T3N0-1 thoracic tumors, 88% with a squamous histology. A total of 259 patients responded to initial chemoradiation therapy and were randomized. After a median follow-up of 4 years, there was no statistical difference in median (17.7 months vs 19.3 months) or 2 year overall survival (34% vs 40%). Local tumor control and 3 month mortality were higher in the surgery arm. These results are similar to those in an earlier study by Stahl et al *(Bedenne L, Michel P, Bouche O, et al: J Clin Oncol 25:1160-1168, 2007).*

A randomized intergroup trial was designed to investigate the role of high-dose irradiation in conjunction with systemic therapy. This study compared doses of 50.4 Gy with 64.8 Gy. Both treatment arms of the study administered concurrent 5-FU and cisplatin. This trial was stopped after an interim analysis revealed no statistically significant difference in survival between the two groups. The authors concluded that higher dose radiation therapy did not offer any survival benefit over the 50.4-Gy dose.

Patient selection Patients with disease involving the mid to proximal esophagus are excellent candidates for definitive chemoradiation therapy because resection in this area can be associated with greater morbidity than resection of more distal tumors.

Most of the trials demonstrating the efficacy of chemoradiation therapy have had a high proportion of patients with squamous cell cancers. Chemoradiation therapy has thus become standard treatment of locoregionally confined squamous cell cancer of the esophagus. It is essential that chemotherapy be given concurrently with irradiation when this approach is chosen as primary treatment for esophageal cancer. A typical regimen is 50 to 60 Gy over 5 to 6 weeks, with cisplatin (75 mg/m^2) and 5-FU (1 g/m^2/24 h for 4 days) on weeks 1, 5, 8, and 11.

The literature also supports offering primary surgery, preoperative chemoradiation therapy, or primary chemoradiation therapy with surgical salvage if necessary to patients with adenocarcinoma. Entering these patients on protocols will allow us to further define standard treatment.

Sequential preoperative chemotherapy and radiation therapy Only modest benefits have been found with preoperative chemoradiation therapy to date, with systemic failure continuing to be an important problem. Thus, sequential therapy with chemotherapy followed by chemoradiation therapy has been explored.

Ajani et al reported a series of 43 patients who received 12 weeks of cisplatin and irinotecan followed by weekly paclitaxel with infusional 5-FU and concurrent radiation therapy (4,500 cGy) and then esophagectomy. Therapy was well tolerated, with no deaths from chemotherapy or chemoradiation therapy, and an operative mortality rate of 5%. Cisplatin and irinotecan induced responses in 37% of patients, and 91% of patients underwent complete resection. Pathologic complete responses occurred in 26% of patients, and some tumor shrinkage was noted in 63% of patients. With a median follow-up of more than 30 months, the median disease progression-free survival was 10.2 months, the median survival was 22.1 months, and the 2-year survival was 42%. The patients who had a pathologic response to therapy had significantly better outcomes than the rest of the study population. However, systemic recurrences remained a prominent cause of failure, with five patients experiencing recurrence first in the brain and an additional five patients, in the liver.

Esophagectomy following induction chemotherapy and chemoradiation therapy Controversy exists regarding the need for esophagectomy following chemoradiation therapy. Although previously described studies randomized patients to receive surgery with or without preoperative chemoradiation therapy,

Stahl et al randomized patients to receive chemoradiation therapy with or without surgery. Also, all 172 patients in the study underwent initial induction chemotherapy (bolus 5-FU, leucovorin, etoposide, and cisplatin for 3 cycles). Those randomized to receive preoperative chemoradiation therapy received cisplatin/etoposide with 40 Gy of radiation, followed by surgery 3 to 4 weeks later. Those randomized to receive definitive chemoradiation therapy received cisplatin/etoposide with 65 Gy of radiation.

After a 6-year median follow-up, the local progression-free survival favored the group undergoing surgery (64% vs 41%). However, the treatment-related mortality was higher in those patients undergoing surgery (13% vs 4%), and so overall survival was statistically equivalent (at 3 years, 31% vs 24%). Since induction chemotherapy was used in all patients, these results should not be extrapolated to indicate the value of esophagectomy following chemoradiotherapy alone.

The incidence of residual disease in patients who have a complete clinical response to chemoradiation therapy is 40% to 50%, and those patients who have a pathologic complete response to chemoradiation therapy have the best survival rates with surgery.

Treatment in elderly patients Since more patients are being diagnosed with esophageal cancer at older ages, research is ongoing as how to best treat elderly patients. Retrospective studies from Nallapareddy et al have found chemoradiaton therapy is tolerable in elderly patients, whereas Rice et al have found a trimodality approach of chemoradiation therapy followed by surgery is also tolerable in the elderly. Close monitoring for toxicities such as dehydration, nutritional concerns, anemia, and postoperative arrhythmia was recommended in these two studies.

TREATMENT OF ADVANCED DISEASE

The goal of esophageal cancer treatment is generally palliative for patients with bulky or extensive retroperitoneal lymph nodes or distant metastatic disease. Therapeutic approaches should temper treatment-related morbidity with the overall dismal outlook.

Local treatment In patients with a good performance status, the combination of 5-FU/mitomycin, or 5-FU/cisplatin, and radiotherapy (50 Gy) results in a median survival of 7 to 9 months. This regimen usually renders patients free of dysphagia until death.

Photodynamic therapy (PDT) Porfimer (Photofrin) and an argon-pumped dye laser can provide effective palliation of dysphagia in patients with esophageal cancer. A prospective, randomized multicenter trial comparing PDT with neodymium/yttrium-aluminum-garnet (Nd:YAG) laser therapy in 236 patients with advanced esophageal cancer found that improvement of dysphagia was equivalent with the two treatments.

A review of 119 patients treated with endoluminal palliation reported a significant improvement in dysphagia scores and an increased ability to relieve stenosis caused by tumor when PDT was used in conjunction with laser therapy and irradiation.

Other approaches include external-beam radiotherapy with or without intracavitary brachytherapy boost, simple dilatation, placement of stents, and laser recannulization of the esophageal lumen.

Palliative resection for esophageal cancer is rarely warranted, although it does provide relief from dysphagia in some patients.

Chemotherapy Phase I and II studies have demonstrated moderate response rates to taxanes in esophageal cancer. Taxanes in combination with platinum compounds and fluoropyrimidines are being tested in regimens with irradiation.

Although chemotherapy alone may produce an occasional long-term remission, there is no standard regimen for patients with metastatic cancer. Patients with advanced disease should be encouraged to participate in well-designed trials exploring novel agents and chemotherapy combinations.

CHEMOTHERAPY IN ADVANCED ESOPHAGEAL CANCER

In Britain, the ECF regimen, a combination of epirubicin (50 mg/m^2) and cisplatin (60 mg/m^2), both repeated every 21 days, with continuous infusion of 5-FU (200 mg/m^2/d), is considered to be a standard regimen for advanced esophagogastric cancers. Although the regimen has been fairly well tolerated, infusional 5-FU has rendered the combination unpopular in other countries. Several phase III studies have been performed and consistently demonstrated objective responses in about 40% of patients, with a median survival of 9 months and a 1-year survival of 36% to 40%. The main severe toxicities of this regimen are neutropenia, in about one-third of patients (32%–36%), lethargy (18%), and nausea and vomiting (11%–17%).

Attempts to improve the efficacy of this regimen, which is logistically difficult to administer, are ongoing. Given the accepted role of capecitabine (Xeloda), a 5-FU prodrug, in colorectal and breast cancers, as well as oxaliplatin, a study evaluating the potential roles of these drugs is being performed.

With the advent of many new chemotherapeutic agents (the taxoids, paclitaxel and docetaxel [Taxotere], irinotecan, and gemcitabine [Gemzar]) with varying mechanisms of activity, further studies have been conducted, and each of these drugs has demonstrated activity, with responses achieved in approximately 15% to 30% of patients.

However, the primary route of investigation for these new agents has been in combination with cisplatin and/or 5-FU. The results available to date

TABLE 5: Combination chemotherapy in advanced disease

Agents	Response rate (%)	Survival
Cisplatin/fluorouracil	19-40	Median = 7 months, 1 year = 27%
Cisplatin/paclitaxel	37-43	Median = 6-9 months
Cisplatin/gemcitabine	38-47	Median = 7-10 months
Cisplatin/irinotecan	30-57	Median = 9.6-14.6 months
Cisplatin/vinorelbine	33	Median = 6.8 months
Cisplatin/etoposide	45-48	Median = 8-10 months, 1 year = 26%-41%
Epirubicin/cisplatin/ fluorouracil	40-42	Median = 9 months, 1 year = 36%-40%
Cisplatin/fluorouracil/ paclitaxel	48	Median = 10.8 months, 1 year = 38%
Carboplatin/paclitaxel	45-50	Median = 9-11 months, 1 year = 43%-46%

suggest promising activity, with response rates often around 50% in phase II studies. Irinotecan (65 mg/m^2) and cisplatin (30 mg/m^2) administered weekly for 4 weeks every 6 weeks have also been active, with responses in 20 of 35 patients (57%) and an impressive median survival of 14.6 months. A Korean phase II study did not confirm these results but did suggest the combination was active, with a response rate of 31% of 32 patients, and a median survival of 9.6 months.

Following the example of the combination of irinotecan and 5-FU/leucovorin in colon cancer, the investigators have explored a modification of that schedule, with therapy administered for 2 weeks, with cycles repeated every 3 weeks. This simple modification has been investigated in 27 patients and was well tolerated, with severe neutropenia in 18% of patients and severe diarrhea in 11% of patients.

Paclitaxel (180 mg/m^2 over 3 hours) and cisplatin (60 mg/m^2 over 3 hours) administered every 14 days have been extensively evaluated in Europe and were reported to produce objective responses in 43% of 51 patients, including two complete responses, and 43% of patients were alive 1 year after initiation of therapy (Table 5).

Because of the toxic and logistic difficulties of using cisplatin, carboplatin has become a popular chemotherapeutic drug. Several studies of carboplatin with paclitaxel in esophageal cancer have been undertaken. El-Rayes et al administered carboplatin (area under the curve of 5) with paclitaxel (200 mg/m^2 over 3 hours) every 3 weeks in 33 chemotherapy-naive patients. Objective responses were reported in 45% of patients, with a median survival of 9 months and 1-year and 2-year survival rates of 43% and 17%.

Polee et al explored a weekly schedule of these drugs in a phase I study. With therapy administered for 3 consecutive weeks, followed by a 1-week break, a dose of carboplatin (area under the curve of 4) with paclitaxel (100 mg/m^2) was recommended for further investigation. Responses were noted in half of the 40 patients, with a median survival of 11 months and a 1-year survival of 46%. Both of these combinations were well tolerated, with the primary toxicity of myelosuppression.

Lorenzen et al treated 24 patients with esophageal and esophagogastric carcinomas and measurable disease with docetaxel (75 mg/m^2 IV) and capecitabine (1,000 mg/m^2 orally twice daily from days 1–14), with cycles repeated every 3 weeks. Only seven of the patients had adenocarcinomas, and eight had received prior chemotherapy. This combination had interesting antitumor activity, with objective responses in 11 patients (46%), including 56% of previously untreated patients and 2 of 8 patients who had received prior chemotherapy. Although patient numbers were small, there was no clear difference in response rates by histology. The therapy was reported to be fairly well tolerated overall, although dose reductions were necessary in 41% of patients. The main grade 3 and 4 toxicities were neutropenia (42% of patients, including two patients with neutropenic fever), diarrhea and neuropathy (13% of patients each), and hand-foot syndrome in 29% of patients.

The combination of docetaxel, cisplatin, and infusional 5-FU (DCF) has been approved by the U.S. Food and Drug Administration for the treatment of metastatic gastric and GE junction adenocarcinoma. The activity of this regimen in esophageal cancers is unclear. Chiarion-Sileni et al reported a study that provides some insight into the potential activity of this regimen. They studied a modification of the DCF regimen, with cisplatin (75 mg/m^2) and docetaxel (60 mg/m^2) given on day 1 and 5-FU (750 mg/m^2/d) given on days 2 to 5 every 21 days for 3 cycles in patients with locally advanced esophageal cancer. This regimen was followed by radiation therapy with concurrent carboplatin. The response rate to chemotherapy alone with this regimen was 48% in 37 patients, suggesting that this combination is active in esophageal cancers as well.

The antimetabolite gemcitabine has also been evaluated in combination with cisplatin in esophageal cancer. A Southwest Oncology Group Study reported by Urba et al combined 1,000 mg/m^2 of gemcitabine on days 1, 8, and 15 with 100 mg/m^2 of cisplatin on day 15 in 64 patients. Approximately one-quarter of these patients had received prior chemotherapy. Therapy was well tolerated, with severe neutropenia occurring in 31% of patients. The median survival of patients treated on this study was 7.3 months, and the 1-year survival rate was 20%. However, the heterogeneity of the patient population makes the efficacy of the therapy somewhat difficult to assess.

Oxaliplatin may also have a role in the treatment of esophageal cancer, both as a radiosensitizer and an agent in advanced disease. Mauer and colleagues reported the results of treatment with oxaliplatin, 5-FU, and leucovorin according to the FOLFOX4 schedule (oxaliplatin, 85 mg/m^2 on day 1; leucovorin, 500 mg/m^2 over 2 hours on days 1 and 2; and 5-FU, 400 mg/m^2 bolus, then 600 mg/m^2 over 22 hours on days 1 and 2, repeated every 14 days). Of 35 patients who were treated, objective responses were noted in 40%. The median survival rate was 7.1 months, 1-year survival rate was 31%, and 2-year survival was 11%. The median progression-free survival was 4.6 months. Although differences in patient populations were noted, these results are similar to those of other reported combinations.

The combination of oxaliplatin (130 mg/m² on day 1) with capecitabine (1,000 mg/m² twice daily on days 1 to 14) repeated every 21 days has also been studied in esophageal cancer. Thirty-eight percent of the 51 treated patients had objective responses, with a median survival of 8 months and a 1-year survival rate of 26%. This study was conducted in the Netherlands, and the tolerability and efficacy of this regimen in American patients remain to be determined.

The primary toxicity of these regimens is severe neutropenia, occurring in about 40% to 70% of patients. Severe diarrhea, nausea, and vomiting occur in ~10% to 15% of patients in many studies. Fatigue and asthenia also were significant side effects with both therapies.

With improving toxicity profiles and modest improvements in therapeutic outcomes, second-line therapy for advanced esophageal cancer is also increasingly being explored. Muro et al treated 28 Japanese patients with squamous cell carcinoma of the esophagus with docetaxel (70 mg/m²) every 3 weeks; these patients had previously received cisplatin and 5-FU. As expected, severe neutropenia was the dominant toxicity (88%, including nine episodes of febrile neutropenia), with severe anorexia, fatigue, and anemia also reported. Objective responses were noted in 16% of these patients.

In addition, Lordick et al determined that irinotecan (55 mg/m²) and docetaxel (25 mg/m²) given on days 1, 8, and 15, with cycles repeated every 28 days, were tolerable, with severe asthenia in 21% of 24 patients and severe diarrhea in 13%. However, only three partial responses (13%) and eight patients with stable disease were noted, with a resultant median survival of 26 weeks. Although these studies suggest the feasibility of second-line cytotoxic chemotherapy in esophageal cancer, the significant toxicity and limited objective response rate warrant its use only with caution and preferably on a clinical study.

Oral tyrosine kinase inhibitors of the epidermal growth factor receptor (EGFR) have also been investigated in esophageal cancer. Gefitinib (Iressa), at a daily dose of 500 mg, as second-line therapy in patients with esophageal adenocarcinomas was evaluated by Ferry et al. It produced partial responses in 11% of 27 patients, and an additional 7 patients had stable disease. In patients with esophageal cancer that had previously been treated with platinum-based chemotherapy, Janmaat et al treated 37 patients with the same regimen. They reported a confirmed response in only 1 patient, and stable disease in another 10, although 18% of patients were free of disease progression at 6 months, suggesting that some patients indeed experience disease control and benefit from this therapy. However, Radovich et al reported only 1 response in 23 patients treated with erlotinib (Tarceva; 150 mg daily). The toxicities were as expected, including rash, diarrhea, vomiting, and elevation in transaminase levels. As with lung and colon cancers, the optimal population for treatment with these targeted agents remains to be defined.

In addition to flavopiridol and the EGFR antagonists, it is anticipated that other targeted therapies, such as vascular endothelial growth factor antagonists, will be evaluated in this disease. Such avenues of exploration, in addition to early diagnosis and therapy for early-stage disease, are the most likely path toward significant improvements in therapy for esophageal cancer.

SUGGESTED READING

Ajani JA, Walsh G, Komaki R, et al: Preoperative induction of CPT-111 and cisplatin chemotherapy followed by chemoradiotherapy in patients with locoregional carcinoma of the esophagus or gastroesophageal junction. Cancer 100:2347–2354, 2004.

Armanios M, Xu R, Forastiere AA, et al; Eastern Cooperative Oncology Group: Adjuvant chemotherapy for resected adenocarcinoma of the esophagus, gastro-esophageal junction, and cardia: Phase II trial (E8296) of the Eastern Cooperative Oncology Group. J Clin Oncol 22:4495–4499, 2004.

Burmeister BH, Smithers BM, Gebski V, et al; Trans-Tasman Radiation Oncology Group; Australasian Gastro-Intestinal Trials Group: Surgery alone versus chemoradiotherapy followed by surgery for resectable cancer of the oesophagus: A randomised, controlled phase II trial. Lancet Oncol 6:659–668, 2005.

Chiarion-Sileni V, Corti L, Ruol A, et al: Phase II trial of docetaxel, cisplatin and fluorouracil followed by carboplatin and radiation in locally advanced oesophageal cancer. Br J Cancer 96:432–438, 2007.

Cunningham D, Rao S, Starling N, et al: Randomised multicentre phase III study comparing capecitabine with fluorouracil and oxaliplatin with cisplatin in patients with advanced esophagogastric (OG) cancer: The REAL 2 trial. J Clin Oncol 24[18S]:LBA 4017, 2006.

Downey RJ, Akhurst T, Ilson D, et al: Whole body 18FDG-PET and the response of esophageal cancer to induction therapy: Results of a prospective trial. J Clin Oncol 21:428–432, 2003.

Ferry DR, Anderson M, Beddard K, et al: A phase II study of gefitinib monotherapy in advanced esophageal adenocarcinoma: Evidence of gene expression, cellular, and clinical response. Clin Cancer Res 13:5869–5875, 2007.

Gerson LB, Triadafilopoulos G: Screening for esophageal adenocarcinomas: An evidence-based approach. Am J Med 113:499–505, 2002.

Hulscher JB, van Sandick JW, de Boer AG, et al: Extended transthoracic resection compared with limited transhiatal resection for adenocarcinoma of the esophagus. N Engl J Med 347:1662–1669, 2002.

Janmaat ML, Gallegos-Ruiz MI, Rodriguez JA, et al: Predictive factors for outcome in a phase II study of gefitinib in second-line treatment of advanced esophageal cancer patients. J Clin Oncol 24:1612–1619, 2006.

Kaklamanos IG, Walker GR, Ferry K, et al: Neoadjuvant treatment for resectable cancer of the esophagus and the gastroesophageal junction: A meta-analysis of randomized clinical trials. Ann Surg Oncol 10:754–761, 2003.

Kinkel K, Lu Y, Both M, et al: Detection of hepatic metastases from cancers of the gastrointestinal tract by using noninvasive imaging methods (US, CT, MR imaging, PET): A meta-analysis. Radiology 224:748–756, 2002.

Lee DH, Kim HT, Han JY, et al: A phase II trial of modified weekly irinotecan and cisplatin for chemotherapy-naive patients with metastatic or recurrent squamous cell carcinoma of the esophagus. Cancer Chemother Pharmacol 61:83–88, 2008.

Lorenzen S, Duyster J, Lersch C, et al: Capecitabine plus docetaxel every 3 weeks in first- and second-line metastastic oesophageal cancer: Final results of a phase II trial. Br J Cancer 92:2129–2133, 2005.

Mauer AM, Kraut EH, Krauss SA, et al: Phase II trial of oxaliplatin, leucovorin, and fluorouracil in patients with advanced carcincoma of the esophagus. Ann Oncol 16:1320–1325, 2005.

Medical Research Council Esophageal Cancer Working Group: Surgical resection with or without preoperative chemotherapy in esophageal cancer: A randomized controlled trial. Lancet 359:1727–1733, 2002.

Meluch AA, Greco FA, Gray JR, et al: Preoperative therapy with concurrent paclitaxel/carboplatin/infusional 5-FU and radiation therapy in locoregional esophageal cancer: Final results of a Minnie Pearl Cancer Research Network phase II trial. Cancer J 9:251–260, 2003.

Muro K, Hamaguchi T, Ohtsu A, et al: A phase II study of single-agent docetaxel in patients with metastatic esophageal cancer. Ann Oncol 15:955–959, 2004.

Nguyen NT, Roberts P, Follette DM, et al: Thoracoscopic and laparoscopic esophagectomy for benign and malignant disease: Lessons learned from 46 consecutive procedures. J Am Coll Surg 197:902–913, 2003.

Radovich D, Kelsen D, Shah M, et al: OSI-774 in advanced esophageal cancer: A phase II study (abstract). J Clin Oncol 22(suppl):14s, 2004.

Santharalingam M, Moughan J, Coia LR, et al: Outcome results of the 1996–1999 patterns of care survey of the national practice for patients receiving radiation therapy for carcinoma of the esophagus. J Clin Oncol 23:2325–2331, 2005.

Stahl M, Stuschke M, Lehmann N, et al: Chemoradiation with and without surgery in patients with locally advanced squamous cell carcinoma of the esophagus. J Clin Oncol 23:2310–2317, 2005.

Urschel JD, Blewett CJ, Young JE, et al: Pyloric drainage (pyloroplasty) or no drainage in gastric reconstruction after esophagectomy: A meta-analysis of randomized controlled trials. Dig Surg 19:160–164, 2002.

Urschel JD, Vasan H: A meta-analysis of randomized controlled trials that compared neoadjuvant chemoradiation and surgery to surgery alone for resectable esophageal cancer. Am J Surg 185:538–543, 2003.

Van Cutsem E, Moiseyenko VM, Tjulandin S, et al: Phase III study of docetaxel and cisplatin plus fluorouracil compared with cisplatin and fluorouracil as first-line therapy for advanced gastric cancer: A report of the V325 Study Group. J Clin Oncol 24:4991–4997, 2006.

van Meerten E, Eskens FA, van Gameren EC, et al: First-line treatment with oxaliplatin and capecitabine in patients with advanced or metastatic oesophageal cancer: A phase II study. Br J Cancer 96:1348–1352, 2007.

Visbal AL, Allen MS, Miller DL, et al: Ivor Lewis esophagogastrectomy for esophageal cancer. Ann Thorac Surg 71:1803–1808, 2001.

Walsh TN, Noonan N, Hollywood D, et al: A comparison of multinodal therapy and surgery for esophageal adenocarcinoma. N Engl J Med 335:462–467, 1996.

Jamie has non-small cell lung cancer, but it doesn't hold her back. She plays. She teaches. She conducts her life the way she likes to. With the help of TARCEVA, Jamie keeps living— one note at a time.

- TARCEVA significantly prolonged overall survival by 37% (HR=0.73; *P*<0.001).[1,2]
  - one-year survival rate increased by 45% vs placebo (31.2% vs 21.5%)[1]
  - median survival lengthened by 42.5% vs placebo (6.7 months vs 4.7 months)[1,2]

- Continue the support for the Playing For A Cure ensemble competition through LUNGevity Foundation by visiting www.lungevity.org/playingforacure.

- Encourage your patients to share their stories by calling 1-800-310-4700 or e-mailing shareyourstories@gene.com.

  Individual results may vary.

  Please see accompanying brief summary of full prescribing information.

Tarceva®
erlotinib
tablets

Proven to prolong survival

TARCEVA® (erlotinib) TABLETS BRIEF SUMMARY Please see the Tarceva package insert for full prescribing information.

INDICATIONS AND USAGE Non-Small Cell Lung Cancer (NSCLC) TARCEVA monotherapy is indicated for the treatment of patients with locally advanced or metastatic non-small cell lung cancer after failure of at least one prior chemotherapy regimen *[see Clinical Studies (14.1)]*. Results from two, multicenter, placebo-controlled, randomized, Phase 3 trials conducted in first-line patients with locally advanced or metastatic NSCLC showed no clinical benefit with the concurrent administration of TARCEVA with platinum-based chemotherapy [carboplatin and paclitaxel or gemcitabine and cisplatin] and its use is not recommended in that setting *[see Clinical Studies (14.3)]*. **Pancreatic Cancer** TARCEVA in combination with gemcitabine is indicated for the first-line treatment of patients with locally advanced, unresectable or metastatic pancreatic cancer *[see Clinical Studies (14.3)]*. **DOSAGE AND ADMINISTRATION Recommended Dose – NSCLC** The recommended daily dose of TARCEVA for non-small cell lung cancer is 150 mg taken at least one hour before or two hours after the ingestion of food. Treatment should continue until disease progression or unacceptable toxicity occurs. There is no evidence that treatment beyond progression is beneficial. **Recommended Dose – Pancreatic Cancer** The recommended daily dose of TARCEVA for pancreatic cancer is 100 mg taken at least one hour before or two hours after the ingestion of food, in combination with gemcitabine (see the gemcitabine package insert). Treatment should continue until disease progression or unacceptable toxicity occurs. **DOSAGE FORMS AND STRENGTHS 25 mg tablets** White film-coated tablets for daily oral administration. Round, biconvex face and straight sides, white film-coated, printed in orange with a "T" and "25" on one side and plain on the other side. **100 mg tablets** White film-coated tablets for daily oral administration. Round, biconvex face and straight sides, white film-coated, printed in gray with "T" and "100" on one side and plain on the other side. **150 mg tablets** White film-coated tablets for daily oral administration. Round, biconvex face and straight sides, white film-coated, printed in maroon with "T" and "150" on one side and plain on the other side. **CONTRAINDICATIONS None WARNINGS AND PRECAUTIONS Pulmonary Toxicity** There have been infrequent reports of serious Interstitial Lung Disease (ILD)-like events, including fatalities, in patients receiving TARCEVA for treatment of NSCLC, pancreatic cancer or other advanced solid tumors. In the randomized single-agent NSCLC study *[see Clinical Studies (14.1)]*, the incidence of ILD-like events (0.8%) was the same in both the placebo and TARCEVA groups. In the pancreatic cancer study -- in combination with gemcitabine – *[see Clinical Studies (14.3)]*, the incidence of ILD-like events was 2.5% in the TARCEVA plus gemcitabine group vs. 0.4% in the placebo plus gemcitabine group. The overall incidence of ILD-like events in approximately 4900 TARCEVA-treated patients from all studies (including uncontrolled studies and studies with concurrent chemotherapy) was approximately 0.7%. Reported diagnoses in patients suspected of having ILD-like events included pneumonitis, radiation pneumonitis, hypersensitivity pneumonitis, interstitial pneumonia, interstitial lung disease, obliterative bronchiolitis, pulmonary fibrosis, Acute Respiratory Distress Syndrome and lung infiltration. Symptoms started from 5 days to more than 9 months (median 39 days) after initiating TARCEVA therapy. In the lung cancer trials most of the cases were associated with confounding or contributing factors such as concomitant/prior chemotherapy, prior radiotherapy, pre-existing parenchymal lung disease, metastatic lung disease, or pulmonary infections. In the event of an acute onset of new or progressive unexplained pulmonary symptoms such as dyspnea, cough, and fever, TARCEVA therapy should be interrupted pending diagnostic evaluation. If ILD is diagnosed, TARCEVA should be discontinued and appropriate treatment instituted as needed *[see Dosage and Administration (2.3)]*. **Patients with Hepatic Impairment** In a pharmacokinetic study in patients with moderate hepatic impairment (Child-Pugh B) associated with significant liver tumor burden, 10 out of 15 patients died on treatment or within 30 days of the last TARCEVA dose. One patient died from hepatorenal syndrome, 1 patient died from rapidly progressing liver failure and the remaining 8 patients died from progressive disease. Six out of the 10 patients who died had baseline total bilirubin > 3 x ULN suggesting severe hepatic impairment. Treatment with TARCEVA should be used with extra caution in patients with total bilirubin > 3 x ULN. Patients with hepatic impairment (total bilirubin > ULN or Child-Pugh A, B and C) should be closely monitored during therapy with TARCEVA. TARCEVA dosing should be interrupted or discontinued if changes in liver function are severe such as doubling of total bilirubin and/or tripling of transaminases in the setting of pretreatment values outside normal range *[see Clinical Pharmacology (12.3) and Dosage and Administration (2.3)]*. **Hepatotoxicity** Cases of hepatic failure and hepatorenal syndrome (including fatalities) have been reported during use of TARCEVA, particularly in patients with baseline hepatic impairment. Therefore, periodic liver function testing (transaminases, bilirubin, and alkaline phosphatase) is recommended. In the setting of worsening liver function tests, dose interruption and/or dose reduction with frequent liver function test monitoring should be considered. TARCEVA dosing should be interrupted or discontinued if total bilirubin is > 3 x ULN and/or transaminases are > 5 x ULN in the setting of normal pretreatment values *[see Adverse Reactions (6.3) and Dosage and Administration (2.3)]*. **Renal Failure** Cases of hepatorenal syndrome, acute renal failure (including fatalities), and renal insufficiency have been reported. Some were secondary to baseline hepatic impairment while others were associated with severe dehydration due to diarrhea, vomiting, and/or anorexia or concurrent chemotherapy use. In the event of dehydration, particularly in patients with contributing risk factors for renal failure (eg, pre-existing renal disease, medical conditions or medications that may lead to renal disease, or other predisposing conditions including advanced age), TARCEVA therapy should be interrupted and appropriate measures should be taken to intensively rehydrate the patient. Periodic monitoring of renal function and serum electrolytes is recommended in patients at risk of dehydration *[see Adverse Reactions (6.3) and Dosage and Administration (2.3)]*. **Myocardial infarction/ischemia** In the pancreatic carcinoma study, six patients (incidence of 2.3%) in the TARCEVA/gemcitabine group developed myocardial infarction/ischemia. One of these patients died due to myocardial infarction. In comparison, 3 patients in the placebo/gemcitabine group developed myocardial infarction (incidence 1.2%) and one died due to myocardial infarction. **Cerebrovascular accident** In the pancreatic carcinoma study, six patients in the TARCEVA/gemcitabine group developed cerebrovascular accidents (incidence: 2.3%). One of these was hemorrhagic and was the only fatal event. In comparison, in the placebo/gemcitabine group there were no cerebrovascular accidents. **Microangiopathic Hemolytic Anemia with Thrombocytopenia** In the pancreatic carcinoma study, two patients in the TARCEVA/gemcitabine group developed microangiopathic hemolytic anemia with thrombocytopenia (incidence: 0.8%). Both patients received TARCEVA and gemcitabine concurrently. In comparison, in the placebo/ gemcitabine group there were no cases of microangiopathic hemolytic anemia with thrombocytopenia. **Use in Pregnancy Pregnancy Category D** Women of childbearing potential should avoid becoming pregnant while being treated with TARCEVA. Erlotinib administered to rabbits during organogenesis at doses that result in plasma drug concentrations of approximately 3 times those in humans (AUCs at 150 mg daily dose) was associated with embryo/fetal lethality and abortion. When erlotinib was administered to female rats prior to mating and through the first week of pregnancy, at doses 0.3 or 0.7 times the clinical dose of 150 mg, on a mg/m² basis, there was an increase in early resorptions that resulted in a decrease in the number of live fetuses. *[see Use in Specific Populations (8.1)]* **Elevated International Normalized Ratio and Potential Bleeding** International Normalized Ratio (INR) elevations and infrequent reports of bleeding events including gastrointestinal and non-gastrointestinal bleedings have been reported in clinical studies, some associated with concomitant warfarin administration. Patients taking warfarin or other coumarin-derivative anticoagulants should be monitored regularly for changes in prothrombin time or INR. *[see Adverse Reactions (6.3)]*. **ADVERSE REACTIONS Non-Small Cell Lung Cancer** Adverse reactions, regardless of causality, that occurred in at least 10% of patients treated with single-agent TARCEVA at 150 mg and at least 3% more often than in the placebo group in the randomized trial of patients with NSCLC are summarized by NCI-CTC (version 2.0) Grade in Table 1. The most common adverse reactions in patients receiving single-agent TARCEVA 150 mg were rash and diarrhea. Grade 3/4 rash and diarrhea occurred in 9% and 6%, respectively, in TARCEVA-treated patients. Rash and diarrhea each resulted in study discontinuation in 1% of TARCEVA-treated patients. Six percent and 1% of patients needed dose reduction for rash and diarrhea, respectively. The median time to onset of rash was 8 days, and the median time to onset of diarrhea was 12 days.

Table 1: Adverse Reactions Occurring More Frequently (≥ 3%) in the Single-agent TARCEVA Group than in the Placebo Group and in ≥ 10% of Patients in the TARCEVA Group.

NCI-CTC Grade MedDRA Preferred Term	TARCEVA 150 mg N = 485			Placebo N = 242		
	Any Grade	Grade 3	Grade 4	Any Grade	Grade 3	Grade 4
	%	%	%	%	%	%
Rash	75	8	< 1	17	0	0
Diarrhea	54	6	< 1	18	< 1	0
Anorexia	52	8	1	38	5	< 1
Fatigue	52	14	4	45	16	4
Dyspnea	41	17	11	35	15	11
Cough	33	4	0	29	2	0
Nausea	33	3	0	24	2	0
Infection	24	4	0	15	2	0
Vomiting	23	2	< 1	19	2	0
Stomatitis	17	< 1	0	3	0	0
Pruritus	13	< 1	0	5	0	0
Dry skin	12	0	0	4	0	0
Conjunctivitis	12	< 1	0	2	< 1	0
Keratoconjunctivitis sicca	12	0	0	3	0	0
Abdominal pain	11	2	< 1	7	1	< 1

Liver function test abnormalities (including elevated alanine aminotransferase (ALT), aspartate aminotransferase (AST) and bilirubin) were observed in patients receiving single-agent TARCEVA 150 mg. These elevations were mainly transient or associated with liver metastases. Grade 2 (> 2.5 – 5.0 x ULN) ALT elevations occurred in 4% and < 1% of TARCEVA and placebo treated patients, respectively. Grade 3 (> 5.0 – 20.0 x ULN) elevations were not observed in TARCEVA-treated patients. TARCEVA dosing should be interrupted or discontinued if changes in liver function are severe. *[see Dosage and Administration (2.3)]*. **Pancreatic Cancer** Adverse reactions, regardless of causality, that occurred in at least 10% of patients treated with TARCEVA 100 mg plus gemcitabine in the **Continued on next page**

Continued from previous page

randomized trial of patients with pancreatic cancer are summarized by NCI-CTC (version 2.0) Grade in Table 2. The most common adverse reactions in pancreatic cancer patients receiving TARCEVA 100 mg plus gemcitabine were fatigue, rash, nausea, anorexia and diarrhea. In the TARCEVA plus gemcitabine arm, Grade 3/4 rash and diarrhea were each reported in 5% of TARCEVA plus gemcitabine-treated patients. The median time to onset of rash and diarrhea was 10 days and 15 days, respectively. Rash and diarrhea each resulted in dose reductions in 2% of patients, and resulted in study discontinuation in up to 1% of patients receiving TARCEVA plus gemcitabine. The 150 mg cohort was associated with a higher rate of certain class-specific adverse reactions including rash and required more frequent dose reduction or interruption.

Table 2: Adverse Reactions Occurring in ≥ 10% of TARCEVA-treated Pancreatic Cancer Patients: 100 mg cohort

NCI-CTC Grade	TARCEVA + Gemcitabine 1000 mg/m² IV N = 259			Placebo + Gemcitabine 1000 mg/m² IV N = 256		
MedDRA Preferred Term	Any Grade	Grade 3	Grade 4	Any Grade	Grade 3	Grade 4
	%	%	%	%	%	%
Fatigue	73	14	2	70	13	2
Rash	69	5	0	30	1	0
Nausea	60	7	0	58	7	0
Anorexia	52	6	< 1	52	5	< 1
Diarrhea	48	5	< 1	36	2	0
Abdominal pain	46	9	< 1	45	12	< 1
Vomiting	42	7	< 1	41	4	< 1
Weight decreased	39	2	0	29	< 1	0
Infection*	39	13	3	30	9	2
Edema	37	3	< 1	36	2	< 1
Pyrexia	36	3	0	30	4	0
Constipation	31	3	1	34	5	1
Bone pain	25	4	< 1	23	2	0
Dyspnea	24	5	< 1	23	5	0
Stomatitis	22	< 1	0	13	1	0
Myalgia	21	1	0	20	< 1	0
Depression	19	2	0	14	< 1	0
Dyspepsia	17	< 1	0	13	< 1	0
Cough	16	0	0	11	0	0
Dizziness	15	< 1	0	13	0	< 1
Headache	15	< 1	0	10	0	0
Insomnia	15	< 1	0	16	< 1	0
Alopecia	14	0	0	11	0	0
Anxiety	13	1	0	11	< 1	0
Neuropathy	13	1	< 1	10	< 1	0
Flatulence	13	0	0	9	< 1	0
Rigors	12	0	0	9	0	0

*Includes all MedDRA preferred terms in the Infections and Infestations System Organ Class. In the pancreatic carcinoma trial, 10 patients in the TARCEVA/gemcitabine group developed deep venous thrombosis (incidence: 3.9%). In comparison, 3 patients in the placebo/gemcitabine group developed deep venous thrombosis (incidence 1.2%). The overall incidence of grade 3 or 4 thrombotic events, including deep venous thrombosis, was similar in the two treatment arms: 11% for TARCEVA plus gemcitabine and 9% for placebo plus gemcitabine. No differences in Grade 3 or Grade 4 hematological laboratory toxicities were detected between the TARCEVA plus gemcitabine group compared to the placebo plus gemcitabine group. Severe adverse reactions (≥ grade 3 NCI-CTC) in the TARCEVA plus gemcitabine group with incidences < 5% included syncope, arrhythmias, ileus, pancreatitis, hemolytic anemia including microangiopathic hemolytic anemia with thrombocytopenia, myocardial infarction/ischemia, cerebrovascular accidents including cerebral hemorrhage, and renal insufficiency [see Warnings and Precautions (5)]. Liver function test abnormalities (including elevated alanine aminotransferase (ALT), aspartate aminotransferase (AST) and bilirubin) have been observed following the administration of TARCEVA plus gemcitabine in patients with pancreatic cancer. Table 3 displays the most severe NCI-CTC grade of liver function abnormalities that developed. TARCEVA dosing should be interrupted or discontinued if changes in liver function are severe [see Dosage and Administration (2.3)].

Table 3: Liver Function Test Abnormalities (most severe NCI-CTC grade) in Pancreatic Cancer Patients: 100 mg Cohort

NCI-CTC Grade	TARCEVA + Gemcitabine 1000 mg/m² IV N = 259			Placebo + Gemcitabine 1000 mg/m² IV N = 256		
	Grade 2	Grade 3	Grade 4	Grade 2	Grade 3	Grade 4
Bilirubin	17%	10%	< 1%	11%	10%	3%
ALT	31%	13%	< 1%	22%	9%	0%
AST	24%	10%	< 1%	19%	9%	0%

NSCLC and Pancreatic Cancer Indications During the NSCLC and the combination pancreatic cancer trials, infrequent cases of gastrointestinal bleeding have been reported, some associated with concomitant warfarin or NSAID administration. [see Warnings and Precautions (5.9)]. These adverse reactions were reported as peptic ulcer bleeding (gastritis, gastroduodenal ulcers), hematemesis, hematochezia, melena and hemorrhage from possible colitis. Cases of acute renal failure or renal insufficiency, including fatalities, with or without hypokalemia have been reported. [see Warnings and Precautions (5.4)]. Cases of Grade 1 epistaxis were also reported in both the single-agent NSCLC and the pancreatic cancer clinical trials. NCI-CTC Grade 3 conjunctivitis and keratitis have been reported infrequently in patients receiving TARCEVA therapy in the NSCLC and pancreatic cancer clinical trials. Corneal ulcerations may also occur. [see Patient Counseling Information (17)]. Hair and nail disorders including alopecia, hirsutism, eyelash/eyebrow changes, paronychia and brittle and loose nails have been reported in clinical trials and during post-marketing use of TARCEVA. In patients who develop skin rash, the appearance of the rash is typically erythematous and maculopapular and it may resemble acne with follicular pustules, but is histopathologically different. This skin reaction commonly occurs on the face, upper chest and back, but may be more generalized or severe (NCI-CTC Grade 3 or 4) with desquamation. Associated symptoms may include itching, tenderness and/ or burning. Dry skin with or without digital skin fissures may occur. Hepatic failure has been reported in patients treated with single-agent TARCEVA or TARCEVA combined with chemotherapy in clinical studies and during post-marketing use of TARCEVA [see Warnings and Precautions (5.3)]; it is not possible to reliably estimate the frequency or establish a causal relationship to TARCEVA treatment. In general, no notable differences in the safety of TARCEVA monotherapy or in combination with gemcitabine could be discerned between females or males and between patients younger or older than the age of 65 years [see Use in Specific Populations (8.4)]. The safety of TARCEVA appears similar in Caucasian and Asian patients. **DRUG INTERACTIONS** Erlotinib is metabolized predominantly by CYP3A4, and inhibitors of CYP3A4 would be expected to increase exposure. Co-treatment with the potent CYP3A4 inhibitor ketoconazole increases erlotinib AUC by 2/3. When TARCEVA was co-administered with ciprofloxacin, an inhibitor of both CYP3A4 and CYP1A2, the erlotinib exposure [AUC] and maximum concentration [Cmax] increased by 39% and 17% respectively. Caution should be used when administering or taking TARCEVA with ketoconazole and other strong CYP3A4 inhibitors such as, but not limited to, atazanavir, clarithromycin, indinavir, itraconazole, nefazodone, nelfinavir, ritonavir, saquinavir, telithromycin, troleandomycin (TAO), voriconazole and grapefruit or grapefruit juice. [see Dosage and Administration (2.3)]. Pre-treatm ent with the CYP3A4 inducer rifampicin for 7 days prior to TARCEVA decreased erlotinib AUC by about 2/3 to 4/5, which is equivalent to a dose of about 30 to 50 mg in NSCLC patients. In a separate study, treatment with rifampicin for 11 days, with co-administration of a single 450 mg dose of TARCEVA on day 8 resulted in a mean erlotinib exposure (AUC) that was 57.6% of that observed following a single 150 mg TARCEVA dose in the absence of rifampicin treatment [see Dose Modifications (2.3)]. Use of alternative treatments lacking CYP3A4 inducing activity is strongly recommended. If an alternative treatment is unavailable, adjusting the starting dose should be considered. If the TARCEVA dose is adjusted upward, the dose will need to be reduced immediately to the indicated starting dose upon discontinuation of rifampicin or other inducers. Other CYP3A4 inducers include, but are not limited to, rifabutin, rifapentine, phenytoin, carbamazepine, phenobarbital and St. John's Wort [see Dosage and Administration (2.3)]. Cigarette smoking has been shown to reduce erlotinib AUC. Patients should be advised to stop smoking; however, if they continue to smoke, cautious increase in the dose of TARCEVA, not exceeding 300 mg may be considered, while monitoring the patient's safety. If the TARCEVA dose is adjusted upward, the dose should be reduced immediately to the indicated starting dose upon cessation of smoking. [see Dosage and Administration (2.3) and Clinical Pharmacology (12.3)]. Pretreatment and co-administration of TARCEVA decreased the AUC of CYP3A4 substrate, midazolam, by 24%. The mechanism is not clear. In a study, there were no significant effects of gemcitabine on the pharmacokinetics of erlotinib nor were there significant effects of erlotinib on the pharmacokinetics of gemcitabine. Drugs that alter the pH of the upper GI tract may alter the solubility of erlotinib and reduce its bioavailability. Co-administration of TARCEVA with omeprazole, a proton pump inhibitor, decreased the erlotinib AUC by 46%. Increasing the dose of TARCEVA when co-administered with such agents is not likely to compensate for the loss of exposure. Since proton pump inhibitors affect pH of the upper GI tract for an extended period, separation of doses may not eliminate the interaction. The concomitant use of proton pump inhibitors with TARCEVA should be avoided if possible. The use of antacids may be considered in place of histamine 2 receptor blockers (H₂ blockers) or proton pump inhibitors in patients receiving TARCEVA. However, no clinical study has been conducted to evaluate the effect of antacids on erlotinib pharmacokinetics. If an antacid is necessary, the antacid dose and the TARCEVA dose should be separated by several hours [see Clinical Pharmacology (12.3)]. **Manufactured for:** OSI Pharmaceuticals Inc., Melville, NY 11747 **Manufactured by:** Schwarz Pharma Manufacturing, Seymour, IN 47274 **Distributed by:** Genentech USA, Inc. 1 DNA Way, South San Francisco, CA 94080-4990. For further information please call 1-877-TARCEVA (1-877-827-2382) or visit www.tarceva.com.

℞ ONLY

Safety and effectiveness
have not been studied
in pediatric patients.

NSCLC efficacy overview

- Tarceva significantly prolonged overall survival by 37% (P<0.001).[1]
  - one-year survival rate increased by 45% vs placebo (31.2% vs 21.5%)[1]
  - median survival lengthened by 42.5% vs placebo (6.7 months vs 4.7 months)[1,2]

Indication

Tarceva monotherapy is indicated for the treatment of patients with locally advanced or metastatic Non-Small Cell Lung Cancer (NSCLC) after failure of at least one prior chemotherapy regimen.

Results from two multicenter, placebo-controlled, randomized, Phase III trials conducted in first-line patients with locally advanced or metastatic NSCLC showed no clinical benefit with the concurrent administration of Tarceva with platinum based chemotherapy, and its use is not recommended in that setting.

Important safety information

There have been infrequent reports of serious Interstitial Lung Disease (ILD)-like events, including fatalities, in patients receiving Tarceva for treatment of NSCLC, pancreatic cancer or other advanced solid tumors. In the event of an acute onset of new or progressive, unexplained pulmonary symptoms such as dyspnea, cough and fever, Tarceva therapy should be interrupted pending diagnostic evaluation. If ILD is diagnosed, Tarceva should be discontinued and appropriate treatment instituted as needed.

Cases of hepatic failure, hepatorenal syndrome, acute renal failure (all including fatalities), and renal insufficiency have been reported during use of Tarceva. Treatment with Tarceva should be used with extra caution in patients with total bilirubin > 3 x ULN. Tarceva dosing should be interrupted or discontinued if changes in liver function are severe. Patients should be closely monitored during therapy with Tarceva.

When receiving Tarceva therapy, women should be advised against becoming pregnant or breastfeeding. Tarceva is pregnancy category D.

The most common adverse reactions in patients with NSCLC receiving Tarceva monotherapy 150 mg were mild to moderate rash and diarrhea. Severe rash and diarrhea (9% & 6% NCI-CTC Grades 3–4, respectively) were reported. Rash and diarrhea each resulted in dose reductions (6% and 1%, respectively) and discontinuation in 1% of Tarceva-treated patients during the single-agent Phase III trial.

See accompanying brief summary of full prescribing information.

For further information, please call **1-877-TARCEVA (1-877-827-2382)** or visit our website at **www.tarceva.com**.

References: 1. Tarceva® (erlotinib) full prescribing information, OSI Pharmaceuticals, Inc., 2008. **2.** Data on file, OSI Pharmaceuticals, Inc.

Proven to prolong survival

CHAPTER 13

Gastric cancer

Charles D. Blanke, MD, Deborah Citrin, MD, and
Roderich E. Schwarz, MD, PhD

Gastric cancer is more common than esophageal cancer in Western countries but is less fatal. More than 21,000 new cases of gastric cancer will be diagnosed in the United States in the year 2008, with 10,880 deaths expected. Worldwide, gastric cancer represents approximately 930,000 new cases and accounts for more than 700,000 deaths. The incidence and mortality of gastric cancer have been declining in most developed countries, including the United States; the age-adjusted risk (world estimate) fell 5% from 1985-1990.

Gastric cancer is defined as any malignant tumor arising from the region extending between the gastroesophageal (GE) junction and the pylorus. It may not be possible to determine the site of origin if the cancer involves the GE junction itself, a situation that has become more common in recent years.

Epidemiology

Gender Gastric cancer occurs more frequently in men, with a male-to-female ratio of 2.3:1.0; mortality is approximately doubled in men.

Age The incidence of gastric cancer increases with age. In the United States, most cases occur between the ages of 65 and 74 years, with a median age of 70 for males and 74 for females.

Race Gastric cancer occurs 2.2 times more frequently in American blacks than whites; in black males, it tends to occur at a younger age (68 years).

Geography Evidence of an association between environment and diet and gastric cancer comes from the profound differences in incidence seen in various parts of the world. Almost 40% of cases occur in China, where it is the most common cancer, but age-adjusted incidence rates are highest in Korea.

Survival Most patients still present with advanced disease, and their survival remains poor. From 1989 to 1995, only 20% of patients with gastric cancer presented with localized disease. The relative 5-year survival rate for gastric cancer of all stages is 24%.

Incidence Significant increases in age-adjusted incidence rates for tumors arising in the gastric cardia have been seen in males. Rates for other gastric adenocarcinomas either have not significantly changed (black males) or have declined (white males). Overall, rates of gastric adenocarcinoma rose for white females between 1974 and 1994.

Etiology, risk factors, and prevention

Diet and environment Studies of immigrants have demonstrated that high-risk populations (eg, Koreans) have a dramatic decrease in the risk of gastric carcinoma when they migrate to the West and change their dietary habits. Low consumption of vegetables and fruits and high intake of salts, nitrates, and smoked or pickled foods have been associated with an increased risk of gastric carcinoma. Conversely, the increasing availability of refrigerated foods has contributed to the decline in incidence rates. Recent laboratory data from Japan suggest that oolong tea may contain a substance that can kill stomach cancer cells.

Occupational exposure in coal mining and processing of nickel, rubber, and timber has been reported to increase the risk of gastric carcinoma. Cigarette smoking may also increase the risk.

Intestinal metaplasia, a premalignant lesion, is common in locations where gastric cancer is common and is seen in 80% of resected gastric specimens in Japan.

Individuals with blood group A may have a greater risk of gastric carcinoma than individuals with other blood groups. The risk appears to be for the infiltrative type of gastric carcinoma (rather than the exophytic type).

Gastric resection Although reports have suggested that patients undergoing gastric resection for benign disease (usually peptic ulcer disease) are at increased risk of subsequently developing gastric cancer, this association has not been definitely proven. Gastric resection may result in increased gastric pH and subsequent intestinal metaplasia in affected patients.

Pernicious anemia Although it has been widely reported that pernicious anemia is associated with the subsequent development of gastric carcinoma, this relationship also has been questioned.

Hereditary diffuse gastric cancer (HDGC) occurs due to mutations in the E-cadherin (CDH1) gene, which has a penetrance of 70% to 80%. Lynch and colleagues recently studied 56 families with HDGC and found 46% of potential carrier individuals tested were CDH1 mutation positive. Prophylactic gastrectomies were performed in 50 individuals, and occult cancer was found in 80% of those for whom information was available. This report has profound implications regarding genetic testing and/or surgery in HDGC families (Lynch HT, Caldas C, Wirtzfeld D, et al: Proc Am Soc Clin Oncol 25[18S]:4500, 2007).

Genetic abnormalities The genetic abnormalities associated with gastric cancer are still poorly understood. Abnormalities of the tumor-suppressor gene TP53 (alias *p53*) are found in over 60% of gastric cancer patients and the adenomatous polyposis coli *(APC)* gene, in over 50%. The significance of these findings is not clear at present.

Overexpression, amplification, and/or mutations of oncogenes c-Ki-*ras*, HER-2/*neu (aka* c-*erb*-b2), and c-*myc* most likely play a role in the development of some gastric neoplasms. A high S-phase fraction has been associated with an increased risk of relapse as well.

E-cadherin has been linked to diffuse-type gastric cancer (see sidebar).

Family history Family members of a patient with gastric cancer have a two-fold to threefold higher risk of stomach cancer than the general population.

Prevention Recent studies strongly implicate cyclo-oxygenase 2 (COX-2) in the development of many human cancers, including gastric cancer. Potential mechanisms of oncogenesis include stimulation of tumor angiogenesis, inhibition of apoptosis, immune suppression, and enhancement of invasive potential. Furthermore, COX-2 inhibitors have been shown to decrease the size of gastric adenomas in mice. This information strongly suggests that COX-2 inhibitors may play a role in the prevention, and even treatment, of GI tumors. However, trials with COX-2 inhibitors in other advanced GI malignancies, such as colon cancer, have not been positive, so patients should not be treated with these agents outside the setting of a clinical trial.

Helicobacter pylori infection is associated with gastric lymphomas and adenocarcinomas. The overall risk of developing malignancy in the presence of infection is low; however, more than 40% to 50% of gastric cancers are linked with *H pylori*. The bacterium has been designated a class I carcinogen. Antibiotics alone can cure localized, node-negative MALT (mucosa-associated lymphoid tissue) lymphomas in about 50% of patients. With regard to gastric adenocarcinoma, *H pylori* infection is associated with a 2.8-fold increase in the relative risk of the disease compared with uninfected controls. Data from Japan and China suggest that *H pylori* infection can lead to chronic atrophic gastritis. This condition appears to be a major risk factor for gastric cancer. Eradication of *H pylori* should thus decrease the incidence of gastric cancer by preventing it.

Signs and symptoms

Most gastric cancers are diagnosed at an advanced stage. Presenting signs and symptoms are often nonspecific and typically include pain, weight loss, vomiting, and anorexia.

Hematemesis is present in 10% to 15% of patients.

Physical findings Peritoneal implants to the pelvis may be palpable on rectal examination (Blumer's shelf). Extension of disease to the liver may be appreciated as hepatomegaly on physical examination. Nodal metastases can be found in the supraclavicular fossa (Virchow's node), axilla, or umbilical region. Ascites can accompany advanced intraperitoneal spread of disease.

Screening and diagnosis

Routine screening for gastric cancer is generally not performed in Western countries because the disease is so uncommon. However, screening appears more effective in high-incidence areas. Mass screening, as has been practiced in Japan since the 1960s, has probably contributed to the 2.5-fold improvement in long-term survival compared with Western countries, though differences in biology may also play a role.

Endoscopy and barium x-rays The diagnosis of gastric cancer in a patient presenting with any constellation of the symptoms previously described revolves around the use of upper endoscopy or double-contrast barium x-rays. The advantage of endoscopy is that it allows for direct visualization of abnormalities and directed biopsies. Barium x-rays do not facilitate biopsies but are less invasive and may provide information regarding motility.

CT scan Once a diagnosis has been established and careful physical examination and routine blood tests have been performed, a CT scan of the chest, abdomen, and pelvis should be obtained to help assess tumor extent, nodal involvement, and metastatic disease. CT may demonstrate an intraluminal mass arising from the gastric wall or focal or diffuse gastric wall thickening. It is not useful in determining the depth of tumor penetration unless the carcinoma has extended through the entire gastric wall. Direct extension of the gastric tumor to the liver, spleen, or pancreas can be visualized on CT, as can metastatic involvement of celiac, retrocrural, retroperitoneal, and porta hepatis nodes. Ascites, intraperitoneal seeding, and distant metastases (liver, lungs, bone) can also be detected.

Endoscopic ultrasonography (EUS) is a staging technique that complements information gained by CT. Specifically, depth of tumor invasion, including invasion of nearby organs, can be assessed more accurately by EUS than by CT. Furthermore, perigastric regional nodes are more accurately evaluated by EUS, whereas regional nodes farther from the primary tumor are more accurately evaluated by CT. Specific ultrasonographic features may aid in the diagnosis and staging of patients with gastric lymphomas.

Capsule video endoscopy A capsule containing a tiny camera is swallowed by the patient. Two pictures per second are taken. Once clinical studies demonstrated that the procedure was safe and effective, the US Food and Drug Administration (FDA) cleared this device for clinical use in 2001. The capsule can be especially helpful in imaging the small intestine.

Laparoscopy Laparoscopy is particularly suited to detect small-volume visceral and peritoneal metastases missed on CT scan. It should be performed prior to curative-intent locoregional therapy or preoperative chemoradiation therapy.

Bone scan A bone scan should be obtained if the patient has bony pain or an elevated alkaline phosphatase level.

PET scan PET scanning may be used to show distant and metastatic disease and may also be helpful in assessing response to neoadjuvant therapy. In the latter setting, PET response correlates with better survival.

Pathology

Adenocarcinoma is the predominant form of gastric cancer, accounting for approximately 95% of cases. Histologically, adenocarcinomas are classified as intestinal or diffuse; mixed types occur but are rare. Intestinal-type cancers are characterized by cohesive cells that form glandlike structures and are often preceded by intestinal metaplasia. Diffuse-type cancers are composed of infiltrating gastric mucous cells that infrequently form masses or ulcers.

Primary lymphoma of the stomach is increasing in frequency and, occasionally, may be difficult to distinguish from adenocarcinoma.

Stromal tumors GI stromal tumors (GISTs) are mesenchymal tumors of the GI tract, most commonly arising from the stomach. These tumors share an ancestor with, or arise from, the interstitial cells of Cajal (the pacemaker cells of the gut). GISTs commonly express KIT (CD117), but this is not required for diagnosis. Most GISTs have mutations in either the C-KIT or PDGFR (platelet-derived growth factor receptor) genes.

Other histologic types Infrequently, other histologic types are found in the stomach, such as squamous cell carcinomas, small-cell carcinomas, and carcinoid tumors. Metastatic spread of disease from primaries in other organs (eg, breast cancer and malignant melanoma) is also seen occasionally.

Metastatic spread Gastric carcinomas spread by direct extension (lesser and greater omentum, liver and diaphragm, spleen, pancreas, transverse colon); regional and distant nodal metastases; hematogenous metastases (liver, lungs, bone, brain); and peritoneal metastases. Multicentricity characterizes up to 20% of gastric cancers.

Staging and prognosis

At present, epithelial gastric cancers are most commonly staged by the TNM system. Stromal tumors, lymphomas, carcinoids, and sarcomas are not covered by these TNM criteria. The most recent update of this staging system (Table 1) allows for a more precise nodal classification based on the number of lymph nodes involved.

A more detailed Japanese staging system has been shown to have prognostic importance in gastric cancer. However, these results have not yet been duplicated in the United States, and this system is not widely used around the world. Resected GISTs can be assigned a numeric risk of recurrence based on tumor size, mitotic rate, and location of the primary.

Prognostic factors Aneuploidy may predict a poor prognosis in patients with adenocarcinoma of the distal stomach. High plasma levels of vascular endothelial growth factor (VEGF) and the presence of carcinoembryonic antigen (CEA) in peritoneal washings predict poor survival in surgically resected patients. As with colorectal cancer, intratumoral levels of dihydropyrimidine dehydrogenase (DPD) may be prognostic of gastric cancer; low levels appear to predict better response to fluorouracil (5-FU)–based chemotherapy and longer survival. The prognostic implications of tumor-suppressor genes and oncogenes are an area of active investigation. Patients with cancers of the diffuse type fare worse than those with intestinal-type lesions.

TABLE 1: TNM staging system for gastric cancer

Primary tumor (T)

Tx	Primary tumor cannot be assessed
T0	No evidence of primary tumor
Tis	Carcinoma in situ: intraepithelial tumor without invasion of the lamina propria
T1	Tumor invades the lamina propria or submucosa
T2	Tumor invades the muscularis propria or subserosa[a]
T2a	Tumor invades the muscularis propria
T2b	Tumor invades the subserosa
T3	Tumor penetrates the serosa (the visceral peritoneum) without invasion of adjacent structures[b,c]
T4	Tumor invades adjacent structures[b,c]

Regional lymph nodes (N)

Nx	Regional lymph node(s) cannot be assessed
N0	No regional lymph node metastasis
N1	Metastasis in 1-6 regional lymph nodes
N2	Metastasis in 7-15 regional lymph nodes
N3	Metastasis in > 15 regional lymph nodes

Distant metastasis (M)

Mx	Distant metastasis cannot be assessed
M0	No distant metastasis
M1	Distant metastasis

Stage grouping

See Table 2

From Greene FL, Page DL, Fleming ID, et al (eds): AJCC Cancer Staging Manual, 6th ed. New York, Springer-Verlag, 2002.

[a] A tumor may penetrate the muscularis propria with extension into the gastrocolic or gastrohepatic ligaments, or into the greater or lesser omentum, without perforation of the visceral peritoneum covering these structures. In this case, the tumor is classified as T2. If there is perforation of the visceral peritoneum covering the gastric ligaments or the omentum, the tumor should be classified as T3.

[b] The adjacent structures of the stomach include the spleen, transverse colon, liver, diaphragm, pancreas, abdominal wall, adrenal gland, kidneys, small intestine, and retroperitoneum.

[c] Intramural extension of disease to the duodenum or esophagus is classified by the depth of greatest invasion in any of these sites, including the stomach.

Treatment

PRIMARY TREATMENT OF LOCALIZED DISEASE

Management of gastric cancer relies primarily on surgical resection of the involved stomach, with reconstruction to preserve intestinal continuity, as resection provides the only chance for cure. Radiotherapy and chemotherapy have potential roles as adjuncts to surgery and in patients with unresectable tumors. Preoperative chemo- and chemoradiation therapy are active areas of current investigation.

Surgery

The objectives of operative treatment for potentially curable gastric cancers are confirmation of resectability, performance of a complete resection, facilitation of appropriate pathologic staging, and reestablishment of GI continuity and function.

Confirmation of resectability

Laparoscopy has emerged as an excellent tool to assess the extent of disease and resectability before the surgeon performs an open laparotomy. Laparoscopy adds to the accuracy of preoperative imaging primarily in cases of peritoneal spread or small liver metastases. As a result, morbidity, hospital stay, and costs have been reduced significantly in patients with unresectable lesions. In addition, peritoneal washings can be obtained.

A thorough pathologic evaluation of resected lymph nodes is prognostic. Investigators from Italy reviewed pathologic data from 1,853 patients who underwent resection for gastric cancer. Patients with a higher percentage of lymph nodes involved were found to have worse outcomes, with the worst outcomes found in patients with more than 25% of resected lymph nodes involved with metastatic cancer. Outcomes were worse in patients with less than 15 resected lymph nodes, compared with patients with more than 15 lymph nodes resected, with a similar percentage of lymph nodes involved, which was attributed to understaging (Marchet A, Mocellin S, Ambrosi A, et al: Ann Surg 245:543-552, 2007).

The initial experience with laparoscopic ultrasonography has shown that its value lies in identifying lesions with a high risk of recurrence (T2b or >, N+), for which a preoperative chemotherapy protocol may be available.

Extent of resection The extent of gastric resection depends on the site and extent of the primary cancer. Subtotal gastrectomy is preferred over total gastrectomy, because it leads to comparable survival but lower morbidity. A 5-cm margin of normal stomach appears to be sufficient in proximal and distal resections. For lesions of the GE junction or the proximal third of the stomach, proximal subtotal gastrectomy can be performed. If total gastrectomy is necessary, transection of the distal esophagus and proximal duodenum is required, and omentectomy is performed. In Japan, there is a growing experience with more limited resections of early-stage gastric cancer. This trend includes endoscopic mucosal resection (EMR) of nonulcerated T1 N0 lesions and pylorus-preserving gastrectomy.

Newer chemotherapy regimens are being tested to improve disease outcomes and minimize toxicity. The Upper Gastrointestinal Clinical Studies Group of the National Cancer Research Institute of the United Kingdom compared triplet therapy with epirubicin and cisplatin plus either fluorouracil (ECF) or capecitabine (ECX) or triplet therapy with epirubicin and oxaliplatin plus either fluorouracil (EOF) or capecitabine (EOX) in patients with advanced esophagogastric cancer in a randomized trial (n = 1,002). Progression-free survival and response rates did not differ significantly between the regimens. Toxicity between capecitabine and fluorouracil were similar; however, oxaliplatin was associated with lower rates of grade 3 and 4 toxicity than cisplatin (Cunningham D, Starling N, Rao S, et al: N Engl J Med 358:36-46, 2008).

Laparoscopic resections are also being performed more frequently.

Extent of lymphadenectomy The extent of lymph node resection, including the number removed at the time of gastrectomy, continues to be controversial. Preferably, lymphadenectomy includes the lymphatic chains along the celiac, left gastric, splenic, and hepatic arteries, which allows for more precise lymph node staging. The exact level designation of lymph nodes varies with the site and intragastric location of the primary tumor. Based on the TNM staging criteria, 15 or more lymph nodes should be obtained and examined for an accurate N classification. Removal of lymph nodes immediately adjacent to the stomach (paracardial, paragastric at the lesser or greater curvature, parapyloric) has been termed D1 dissection. A more extensive D2 dissection would also remove retroperitoneal "second echelon" lymph nodes along the celiac trunk, left gastric artery, hepatic artery, splenic artery, and splenic hilus.

Improved long-term survival rates for Japanese patients had been attributed to the extended lymphadenectomies routinely performed in this country. Because the improvement in survival after gastrectomy during recent decades was usually associated with the performance of extended lymph node dissections (D2 dissections or greater), this practice appeared to be sensible if performed with acceptable complication rates. Retrospective data had shown that D2 lymphadenectomy is safe and does not increase morbidity.

On the other hand, two European randomized trials showed no significant differences in overall long-term survival between D1 and D2 dissection groups. Both studies found higher postoperative morbidity and mortality in the D2 (extended) group, largely due to a higher rate of splenectomy and/or partial pancreatectomy performed with those dissections. When a subset of patients with N2 disease were studied in long-term follow-up in the Dutch randomized trial, a survival advantage was shown with D2 dissection. Extended lymphadenectomy should primarily be performed in specialized centers by experienced surgeons, and splenectomy and pancreatectomy should be avoided; for adequate staging, at least 15 lymph nodes should be removed and analyzed.

TABLE 2: Treatment and survival by stage in patients with gastric carcinoma

Stage			Treatment	5-Year overall survival rate[a] (%)
Stage 0 (in situ)			Surgery	> 90%
Tis	N0	M0		
Stage IA			Surgery	60%-80%
T1	N0	M0		
Stage IB			Surgery ± CRT	50%-60%
T1	N1	M0		
T2a/b	N0	M0		
Stage II			Surgery + CRT	30%-50%
T1	N2	M0		
T2a/b	N1	M0		
T3	N0	M0		
Stage IIIA			Surgery + CRT	~20% (distal tumors)
T2a/b	N2	M0		
T3	N1	M0		
T4	N0	M0		
Stage IIIB			Same as for stage IIIA	~10%
T3	N2	M0	Consider preoperative CRT	
Stage IV			Palliative chemotherapy,	< 5%
T4	N1-2	M0	radiation therapy, and/or	
Any T	N3	M0	surgery, neoadjuvant	
Any T	Any N	M1	CRT	

Sources of data: American College of Surgeons Commission on Cancer and American Cancer Society

[a] Some American centers are reporting superior 5-year survival rates to those presented here. Confirmation of these results on a national level may be forthcoming.

CRT = chemoradiation therapy

Reconstruction methods After distal gastrectomy, Billroth I gastroduodenostomy or, more commonly, Billroth II gastrojejunostomy is an appropriate method for reconstruction. Reflux esophagitis is a common problem when the gastric reservoir is too small. After total or subtotal gastrectomy, a Roux-en-Y esophagojejunostomy is commonly performed.

Resection of extragastric organs may be required to control T4 disease. Such a resection can be associated with long-term survival. Splenectomy should be avoided unless it is indicated by direct tumor extension, because it significantly increases the rate of complications.

NEOADJUVANT THERAPY

Prompted by the promising results and acceptable toxicity of preoperative (neoadjuvant) chemoradiation therapy in other parts of the GI tract (eg, esophagus, rectum), there is growing interest in neoadjuvant therapy for gastric cancer. Neoadjuvant treatment may be performed in an attempt to convert an initially unresectable cancer to resectable status, or it may be used in advanced but resectable disease.

Most promising to date are the results from the European Medical Research Council Adjuvant Gastric Infusional Chemotherapy (MAGIC) trial using pre- and postoperative ECF (epirubicin, cisplatin, and 5-FU). Cunningham and associates randomized patients to receive preoperative and postoperative chemotherapy versus surgery alone. The 5-year survival rate for those offered systemic ECF therapy in addition to surgery was 36%, versus 23% for those who only underwent surgery. Chemotherapy also enhanced resectability. It remains to be seen whether these positive results, achieved with relatively uncommon (in the United States) chemotherapy and without irradiation, will lead to the adoption of this regimen in the United States.

ADJUVANT THERAPY

The 5-year survival rate after "curative resection" for gastric cancer is only between 30% and 40% (Table 2). Treatment failure stems from a combination of local or regional recurrence and distant metastases. Investigators have studied adjuvant therapy in the hope of improving treatment results. A North American Intergroup trial randomizing resected patients (stages IB–IV[M0]) to receive chemoradiation therapy or observation showed significant improvement in median disease-free (median 19 vs 30 months) and overall (26 vs 35 months) survival with adjuvant therapy, and the use of postoperative chemoradiation therapy, usually with continuous infusion of 5-FU, is the standard of care in the United States.

Radiotherapy

Radiotherapy can decrease the rate of locoregional failure but has not been shown to improve survival as a single postoperative modality. Postoperative radiotherapy may be appropriate in patients who are not candidates for chemotherapy.

Chemotherapy

Chemotherapy alone as a surgical adjunct does not have a defined role in the United States. Randomized trials of chemotherapy plus surgery versus resection alone have showed no definite survival advantage, with the possible exception of patients with widespread nodal involvement who may do better with chemotherapy. Interestingly, one meta-analysis included both Western and Asian studies; it showed a significant survival benefit with the use of chemotherapy in the Asian trials, but there was no benefit in the Western studies, possibly due to differences in biology or drug metabolism. No specific regimen could be recommended.

Chemoradiation therapy

Patients with T3–T4 any N M0 tumors are at highest risk of locoregional recurrence after potentially curative surgery (surgery in which all macroscopic tumor has been resected with no evidence of metastatic disease) for gastric cancer. Even patients with node-negative disease (T3 N0) have a gastric cancer-related mortality of about 50% within 5 years. Mortality is significantly worse in patients with node-positive disease or in those with incomplete (R1, R2) resection.

In the North American Intergroup trial mentioned in the section on "Adjuvant therapy," patients were randomized to receive chemoradiation therapy or observation following resection of stages IB–IV (M0) adenocarcinoma of the stomach. Chemoradiation therapy following resection of these high-risk patients significantly improved both disease-free and overall survival. Because of the apparent benefit of reducing locoregional recurrences, but not distant recurrences, it is possible that more routine use of D2 lymphadenectomy may modify this recommendation in the future. D2 lymphadenectomy was performed in only 10% of the patients in this trial. Subgroup analysis revealed that outcome did not differ based upon the type of lymphadenectomy ($P = .80$). Still, since only a small percentage of patients underwent the recommended D2 dissection, further research is necessary before firm conclusions can be made in this area.

Despite this trial, significant controversy regarding the need for adjuvant treatment persists and is perhaps growing. Many studies support the contention that aggressive, formal D2 resection may obviate the need for adjuvant treatment in many cases. Other studies and subgroup analyses support the recommendations for adjuvant treatment as concluded in the North American trial. These conflicting results, as well as distinct differences in results between Eastern and Western nations, suggest that this issue may take many years to resolve. In the interim, it is appropriate to recommend adjuvant chemoradiotherapy in the vast majority of cases in North America.

GISTs have a high risk of recurrence, even following complete resection. The American College of Surgical Oncologists performed a phase III trial of surgery alone versus surgery followed by 1 year of adjuvant imatinib (Gleevec) in patients with resected intermediate or high-risk gastrointestinal stromal tumors (GISTs). Accrual to the trial was halted early when it was apparent those given postoperative imatinib had a markedly lower 1-year relapse-free survival rate than did those treated with surgery alone (97% vs 83%; $P = .0000014$). Interestingly, there was no difference in overall survival, leaving open the question of whether patients should be treated immediately following surgery versus waiting for relapse and using imatinib in the salvage setting. Most North American GIST experts favor immediate imatinib.

Unresectable tumors

Patients with unresectable gastric cancers and no evidence of metastatic disease can be expected to survive approximately 6 months without any treatment.

Palliative resection Palliative resection, bypass, and/or stenting may be appropriate for some patients with obstructive lesions. Palliative resection may

TABLE 3: Chemotherapy regimens for gastric cancer

Drug/combination	Dose and schedule
ECF	
Epirubicin	50 mg/m^2 IV on day 1
Cisplatin	60 mg/m^2 IV on day 1
Repeat the cycle every 3 weeks to a maximum of 8 cycles.	
5-FU	200 mg/m^2/d as a continuous IV infusion for up to 6 months

Webb A, Cunningham D, Scarffe HJ, et al: J Clin Oncol 15:261–267, 1997.
Roth AD, Fazio N, Stupp R, et al: J Clin Oncol 25:3217–3223, 2007.

Drug/combination	Dose and schedule
Docetaxel plus cisplatin and 5-FU (DCF)	
Docetaxel	75 mg/m^2 IVPB on day 1
Cisplatin	75 mg/m^2 IVPB on day 1
5-FU	750 mg/m^2/d continuous IV infusion on days 1 to 5
Repeat the cycle every 3 weeks.	

Ajani JA, Moiseyenko VM, Tjulandin S, et al: J Clin Oncol 25:3210–3216, 2007.

IVPB = intravenous piggyback
Table prepared by Ishmael Jaiyesimi, DO

Survival remains poor in patients with advanced gastric cancer. Continuing chemotherapy may improve outcomes. Forty-one patients with advanced or recurrent gastric cancer were treated with sequential chemotherapy, which consisted of platinum plus 5-FU as first-line therapy, taxane-based chemotherapy as second-line therapy, and irinotecan plus 5-FU as third-line therapy. A median of 23 cycles was delivered with this regimen. The median time to disease progression was 6.4 (95% confidence interval (CI); 4.9–7.9) months in this series, and the median overall survival was 30 (95% CI, 19.5–40.5) months with no treatment-related mortality. These results compare favorably with historic survival data *(Lim J, Cho J, Paik Y, et al: 2008 Gastrointestinal Cancers Symposium [abstract 67]).*

also be suitable for patients with bleeding gastric cancers that are not resectable for cure. Generally, resection appears to offer better palliative results than bypass.

Radiotherapy Radiation therapy alone can provide palliation in patients with bleeding or obstruction who are not operative candidates. Radiotherapy may convert unresectable cancers to resectable tumors.

Chemoradiation therapy Patients with locally advanced disease may be appropriately treated with chemoradiation therapy. This approach can provide relatively long-lasting palliation and may render some unresectable cancers resectable. Older studies have shown that postoperative chemoradiation therapy can reduce relapse rates and prolong survival in patients with incompletely resected stomach cancer.

MEDICAL TREATMENT OF ADVANCED GASTRIC CANCER

When possible, all newly diagnosed patients with disseminated gastric cancer should be considered candidates for clinical trials, and those with good performance status should be offered systemic therapy. Even though cure is not expected with chemotherapy, such treatment may provide palliation in selected patients and sometimes durable remissions. At least four randomized chemotherapy trials have suggested improvement in survival and probably quality of life versus best supportive care alone.

Single-agent therapy

Several agents have established activity in gastric cancer: 5-FU, platinums (cisplatin, oxaliplatin [Eloxatin], and carboplatin, mitomycin, etoposide, some anthracyclines (doxorubicin and epirubicin), taxanes (paclitaxel and docetaxel [Taxotere]), irinotecan, antimetabolites (pemetrexed [Alimta], methotrexate, trimetrexate (Neutrexin), and oral fluoropyrimidines (uracil and tegafur [UFT], S-1, capecitabine [Xeloda]). 5-FU and cisplatin have been used most commonly. The responses seen with single-agent chemotherapy have been traditionally partial and mostly short-lived, with little, if any, impact on overall survival.

Novel agents recently tested in patients with advanced gastric cancer include the epidermal growth factor receptor inhibitor cetuximab (Erbitux) and the VEGF inhibitor bevacizumab (Avastin). Bevacizumab appears promising when given with chemotherapy.

Combination chemotherapy

Response rates are consistently higher when combination chemotherapy regimens are used in gastric cancer. Combination therapy has been generally preferred over single agents (Table 3).

In the 1980s, the combination of 5-FU, doxorubicin, and mitomycin (FAM) was considered the standard regimen in the treatment of advanced gastric cancer. However, the North Central Cancer Treatment Group (NCCTG) randomly compared this regimen with 5-FU plus doxorubicin and single-agent 5-FU and found no difference in survival among the patients treated with the three regimens.

Several different regimens, including FAMTX (5-FU, doxorubicin, and methotrexate) and ELF (etoposide, leucovorin, and 5-FU), have been tested. Most regimens show markedly better response rates and longer survival in early trials than in phase III studies. No combination has been confirmed as superior. However, ECF approaches standard of care in Canada and in some parts of Europe. This regimen has proved superior to FAMTX in terms of objective response rate and survival and superior to the mitomycin, cisplatin, 5-FU (MCF) regimen in terms of toxicity. A combination of docetaxel, cisplatin, and 5-FU was shown to offer superior survival rates versus cisplatin and 5-FU; however, grade 3/4 toxic events occurred in 81% of patients treated with triple therapy. The search for the optimal combination regimen continues, with the promising newer agents being introduced in combination regimens.

S-1 is a combination of the oral 5-fluorouracil (5-FU) pro-drug tegafur, gimeracil (an inhibitor of dihydropyrimidine dehydrogenase), and oteracil (an inhibitor of 5-FU phosphorylation in the gastrointestinal tract, which reduces the gastrointestinal toxicities of 5-FU). Combination studies with this drug were featured at the 2007 American Society of Clinical Oncology meeting. Narahara and associates performed a randomized phase III trial of S-1 plus cisplatin versus S-1 alone in patients with advanced gastric cancer (SPIRITS trial). Patients given combination therapy experienced improved survival (median 396 vs 336 days), and treatment was relatively well tolerated. Chin and colleagues randomized patients with advanced gastric cancer to S-1 alone versus S-1 with irinotecan. Patients given combination therapy had marked improvements in response rates (42% vs 27%; *P* = .035), and the combination was again reasonably well tolerated. Survival analysis is ongoing. It is likely S-1 may play a significant role in front-line combination therapy for patients with incurable gastric cancer *(Narahara H, Koizumi W, Hara T, et al: Proc Am Soc Clin Oncol 25[18S]:4514, 2007; Chin K, Iishi H, Imamura H, et al: Proc Am Soc Clin Oncol 25[18S]:4525, 2007).*

Newer agents with somewhat similar mechanisms of action to those of classic drugs have been tried in patients with advanced gastric cancer. S-1, alone or in combination, is particularly promising (see sidebar).

Gastric cancer patients should be encouraged to participate in well-designed clinical trials. Outside experimental regimens, the recommended therapy for patients with good performance status is a 5-FU– or cisplatin–based regimen.

Chemotherapy in the elderly

The benefits of chemotherapy for the general population with metastatic gastric cancer are well established. Until recently, however, there were few trials examining systemic treatment in the elderly.

Trumper and associates examined the results of 1,080 patients entered onto three randomized trials of chemotherapy and compared the outcomes between patients aged 70 and older and those younger than age 70. There were no significant differences in grade 3/4 hematologic or nonhematologic toxicities. Additionally, no significant differences were identified in response rates between the age groups. Multivariate analysis controlling for performance status, locally advanced disease status, and treatment showed no significant differences in overall or failure-free survival by age. The authors concluded that patients with gastric cancer aged 70 and older obtain the same benefit as younger patients from palliative chemotherapy with respect to symptomatic and standard responses and survival without increased toxicities.

SUGGESTED READING

Ajani JA, Moiseyenko VM, Tjulandin S, et al: Clinical benefit with docetaxel plus fluorouracil and cisplatin compared with cisplatin and fluorouracil in a phase III trial of advanced gastric or gastroesophageal cancer adenocarcinoma: The V-325 Study Group. J Clin Oncol 25:3205–3209, 2007.

Bennett JJ, Gonen M, D'Angelica M, et al: Is detection of asymptomatic recurrence after curative resection associated with improved survival in patients with gastric cancer? J Am Coll Surg 201:503–510, 2005.

Cunningham D, Allum WH, Stenning SP, et al: Perioperative chemotherapy versus surgery alone for resectable gastroesophageal cancer. N Engl J Med 355:11–20, 2006.

Cunningham D, Jost LM, Purkalne G, et al: ESMO Guidelines Task Force. ESMO Minimum Clinical Recommendations for diagnosis, treatment and follow-up of gastric cancer. Ann Oncol 16(suppl 1):i22–i23, 2005.

Cunningham D, Starling N, Rao S, et al: Capecitabine and oxaliplatin for advanced esophagogastric cancer. N Engl J Med 358:36–46, 2008.

DeMatteo R, Owzar K, Maki R, et al: Adjuvant imatinib mesylate increases recurrence free survival (RFS) in patients with completely resected localized primary gastrointestinal stromal tumors (GIST): North American Intergroup Phase III trial ACOSOG Z9001. Proc Am Soc Clin Oncol 25[18s]:10079, 2007.

Demetri GD, Benjamin RS, Blanke CD, et al: NCCN Task Force report: Management of patients with gastrointestinal stromal tumor (GIST)–Update of the NCCN clinical practice guidelines. J Natl Compr Canc Netw 59(suppl 2):S1–S29, 2007.

Di Bartolomeo M, Buzzoni R, Mariani L, et al: Feasibility of sequential therapy with FOLFIRI followed by docetaxel/cisplatin in patients with radically resected gastric adenocarcinoma: A randomized phase III trial. Oncology 71:341–346, 2006.

Hartgrink HH, van de Velde CJ, Putter H, et al: Extended lymph node dissection for gastric cancer: Who may benefit? Final results of the randomized Dutch gastric cancer group trial. J Clin Oncol 22:2069–2077, 2004.

Miettinen M, Lasota J: Gastrointestinal stromal tumors: Pathology and prognosis at different sites. Semin Diagn Pathol 23:70–83, 2006.

Miner TJ, Jaques DP, Karpeh MS, et al: Defining palliative surgery in patients receiving noncurative resections for gastric cancer. J Am Coll Surg 198:1013–1021, 2004.

Nakajima T, Kinoshita T, Nashimoto A, et al: Randomized controlled trial of adjuvant uracil-tegafur versus surgery alone for serosa-negative, locally advanced gastric cancer. Br J Surg 94:1468–1476, 2007.

Sakuramoto S, Sasako M, Yamaguchi T, et al: Adjuvant chemotherapy for gastric cancer with S-1, an oral fluoropyrimidine. N Engl J Med 357:1810–1820, 2007.

Sasako M, Sano T, Yamamoto S, et al: Left thoracoabdominal approach versus abdominal-transhiatal approach for gastric cancer of the cardia or subcardia: A randomised controlled trial. Lancet Oncol 7:644–651, 2006.

Smith DD, Schwarz RR, Schwarz RE: Impact of total lymph node count on staging and survival after gastrectomy for gastric cancer: Data from a large US-population database. J Clin Oncol 23:7114–7124, 2005.

Sumpter K, Harper-Wynne C, Cunningham D, et al: Report of two protocol planned interim analyses in a randomised multicentre phase III study comparing capecitabine with fluorouracil and oxaliplatin with cisplatin in patients with advanced oesophagogastric cancer receiving ECF. Br J Cancer 92:1976–1983, 2005.

CHAPTER 14

Pancreatic, neuroendocrine GI, and adrenal cancers

Al B. Benson III, MD, Robert J. Myerson, MD, PhD, and Aaron Sasson, MD

PANCREATIC CANCER

Pancreatic cancer is the fifth leading cause of cancer death in the United States. In the year 2008, an estimated 37,170 new cases are expected to be diagnosed, and 33,370 deaths are expected to occur.

Incidence and epidemiology

Gender The incidence of pancreatic cancer is slightly higher in males than in females. These gender differences are most prominent among younger individuals.

Age The peak incidence of pancreatic carcinoma occurs in the seventh decade of life. Two-thirds of new cases occur in people > 65 years old.

Race The incidence of pancreatic cancer is higher in the black population, with an excess risk of 40% to 50% over that in whites. Perhaps more importantly, black males probably have the highest risk of pancreatic cancer worldwide.

Survival Cancer of the pancreas is a highly lethal disease historically, with few reports of 5-year survivors. However, more recent series have shown a decrease in both operative mortality and overall morbidity. There has also been a significant increase in 5-year survival after curative resection (21%–25%). Factors that appear to be important in predicting long-term survival after resection include clear surgical margins, small tumor size (< 2 cm), negative lymph nodes, and reduced perioperative mortality.

Adenocarcinoma of the pancreas, the most common histologic type, has a median survival of 9 to 12 months and an overall 5-year survival rate of 3% for all stages. At the time of diagnosis, over 50% of patients with pancreatic adenocarcinoma have clinically apparent metastatic disease. Among patients whose disease is considered to be resectable, 50% will die of recurrent tumor within 2 years.

Etiology and risk factors

The specific risk factors for pancreatic cancer are not as striking as those for other GI malignancies, such as esophageal and gastric carcinomas. There does, however, appear to be a significant relationship between pancreatic cancer and environmental carcinogens.

Cigarette smoking Cigarette smoke is one of the carcinogens directly linked to the causation of pancreatic malignancies. Heavy cigarette smokers have at least a twofold greater risk of developing pancreatic carcinoma than nonsmokers. In Japan, cigarette smoking carries an even greater risk, which can be as much as 10-fold in men smoking one to two packs of cigarettes daily.

N-nitroso compounds, found particularly in processed meat products, reliably induce pancreatic cancer in a variety of laboratory animals. No study has directly linked dietary carcinogens to pancreatic cancers in humans.

Caffeine The contribution of caffeine consumption to the development of pancreatic carcinoma is controversial. A case-controlled study showed a correlation between caffeine consumption and pancreatic cancer. However, other studies have been unable to confirm this relationship.

Alcohol A clear-cut relationship between alcohol use and pancreatic carcinoma has not been shown.

Diabetes does not seem to be a risk factor for pancreatic cancer. However, 10% of all patients with pancreatic carcinoma present with new-onset diabetes.

Genetic factors Cancer of the pancreas is a genetic disease. To date, more than 80% of resected pancreatic cancers have been found to harbor activating point mutations in K-*ras*. In addition, the tumor-suppressor genes *p16, p53,* and *DPC4* are all frequently inactivated in this cancer.

Research is also focusing on aberrantly methylated genes in pancreatic cancer using methylation-specific polymerase chain reaction (PCR) and the identification of microRNAs as targets for detection strategies.

Familial pancreatic carcinoma has been associated with the following genetic syndromes: hereditary pancreatitis, ataxia-telangiectasia, hereditary nonpolyposis colorectal cancer (HNPCC), familial atypical mole melanoma (FAMM) syndrome, Peutz-Jeghers syndrome, and familial breast cancer. Families with *p16* germline mutations may be at higher risk of developing pancreatic cancer than those without these mutations.

Signs and symptoms

The initial clinical features of pancreatic carcinoma include anorexia, weight loss, abdominal discomfort or pain, and new-onset diabetes mellitus or thrombophlebitis. The vague nature of these complaints may delay diagnosis for several months.

Pain Specific symptoms usually relate to localized invasion of peripancreatic structures. The most common symptom is back pain, which stems from tumor invasion of the splanchnic plexus and retroperitoneum or pancreatitis. This pain is described as severe, gnawing, and radiating to the middle of the back. Pain can also be epigastric or in the right upper quadrant if bile duct obstruction is present.

Jaundice In a majority of cases, patients with pancreatic cancer present with epigastric or back pain and/or jaundice. Painless or sometimes painful jaundice occurs when lesions involve the intrapancreatic bile duct.

GI symptoms Tumor invasion of the duodenum or gastric outlet may give rise to nausea or vomiting as a presenting symptom. This symptom is rare early in the course of the disease. Changes in bowel habits related to pancreatic insufficiency may also be present, along with associated steatorrhea.

Glucose intolerance Recent onset of glucose intolerance in an elderly patient associated with GI symptoms should alert physicians to the possibility of pancreatic carcinoma.

A palpable gallbladder occurring in the absence of cholecystitis or cholangitis suggests malignant obstruction of the common bile duct until proven otherwise. This so-called Courvoisier's sign is present in about 25% of all patients with pancreatic cancer.

Other physical findings include Trousseau's syndrome (migratory superficial phlebitis), ascites, Virchow's node (left supraclavicular lymph node), or a periumbilical mass (Sister Mary Joseph's node).

Screening and diagnosis

Early diagnosis of pancreatic carcinoma is difficult but essential if surgical resection and cure are to be improved. Defining early lesions at a resectable stage remains a diagnostic challenge. To date, leading medical organizations have not recommended routine screening of asymptomatic individuals for pancreatic cancer.

Serum markers The use of serologic tumor markers for pancreatic carcinoma, such as CA19-9, was originally thought to be appropriate as a screening tool. However, since the prevalence of pancreatic carcinoma in the general population is extremely low (0.01%), many false-positive screening results are generated. Also, the sensitivity of CA19-9 is not high (20%) in stage I cancers. Nevertheless, CA19-9 may be a useful marker for diagnosing patients at high risk with the appropriate symptoms, such as smokers, recent-onset diabetics, those with familial pancreatic cancer, or those with unexplained weight loss or diarrhea. This marker correlates with tumor burden and is useful in following disease and in assessing the adequacy of resection or therapy. CA19-9 should be interpreted with caution in patients, who have jaundice, as it is falsely elevated in such patients. Furthermore, 5% to 15% of the population are unable to synthesize CA19-9, and in such patients, it would be falsely low, even in the presence of extensive tumor burden.

No currently available serum marker is sufficiently accurate to be considered reliable for screening asymptomatic patients.

Laparoscopy is useful for staging patients with pancreatic carcinoma and for formulating treatment plans. Approximately 10% to 15% of patients thought to have resectable disease are found to have distant metastases at laparoscopy. The false-negative rate of laparoscopy is < 10%. The strongest indications for laparoscopy are locally advanced disease and tumors of the body and tail of the pancreas.

Peritoneal cytology also is being explored for the diagnosis of pancreatic carcinoma. Cytology is positive in 5% to 10% of patients who are thought to have localized disease. There are anecdotal cases of long-term survival after resection where positive cytology of peritoneal washings was noted. However, the clinical/prognostic value of this test is not yet known. However, there is increasing evidence that the presence of positive peritoneal cytology is a marker of advanced disease, and curative resection is extremely unlikely.

Imaging techniques

Imaging for pancreatic carcinoma is best performed with conventional ultrasonography and CT.

Ultrasonography The limit of sonographic resolution for early pancreatic carcinoma is a diameter of 1.0 to 1.5 cm. A mass located in the pancreatic head will produce dilatation of the common bile duct and pancreatic duct. The actual sensitivity of ultrasonography in the diagnosis of pancreatic carcinoma is ~70%.

CT provides better definition of the tumor and surrounding structures than does ultrasonography and is operator-independent. CT correctly predicts unresectable tumors in 85% of patients and resectable tumors in 70% of patients. Findings of tumor unresectability on CT scanning include distant lymphadenopathy, encasement or occlusion of the superior mesenteric artery (SMA) or celiac artery, occlusion of the portal vein or superior mesenteric vein (SMV), and distant metastases. Spiral CT increases the accuracy of detecting pancreatic carcinoma in general and vessel encasement in particular. This technique permits rapid data acquisition and computer-generated three-dimensional (3D) images of the mesenteric arterial and venous tributaries in any plane. Spiral CT is quicker and less expensive and uses less contrast medium than angiography.

PET The use of positron emission tomography with [18]fluorodeoxyglucose (FDG-PET) in the evaluation of patients with pancreatic cancer is expanding. A recent study of 126 patients with focal, malignant, or benign pancreatic lesions showed high sensitivity of FDG-PET for detection of small pancreatic neoplasms. Lack of focal glucose uptake excludes pancreatic neoplasms (sensitivity 85.4%, specificity 60.9%).

MRI At present, MRI is not as accurate as CT in diagnosing and staging pancreatic carcinoma. MRI may be as useful as CT in staging and can provide magnetic resonance angiography and magnetic resonance cholangiopancreatography (MRC) images if needed. As yet, MRC is not a standard test for the diagnosis of pancreatic carcinoma, but it may become helpful in the future.

Endoscopic ultrasonography (EUS) is a newer modality for the diagnosis of pancreatic carcinoma, with an overall diagnostic accuracy rate of approximately 85% to 90%. For the assessment of regional lymph node metastases, the accuracy of EUS is 50% to 70%. This technique is also important in the evaluation of portal vein/SMV involvement by tumor. In addition, EUS-guided fine-needle cytology of periampullary tumors may yield new information with respect to the diagnosis of pancreatic cancer and may be less risky in spreading cells by needle tracking than by percutaneous biopsies.

In a comparison of EUS and spiral CT, both techniques showed comparable efficacy in detecting tumor involvement of lymph nodes and the SMVs and portal veins. However, EUS is less helpful in the evaluation of the SMA.

Endoscopic retrograde cholangiopancreatography (ERCP) may someday be supplanted as a diagnostic tool by EUS, although, at present, ERCP is used in many clinics. Also, if a patient presents with jaundice and the CT scan reveals dilatation of the common bile duct without an obvious mass, ERCP may be complementary to spiral CT. ERCP findings of pancreatic cancer include an abrupt or tapered cutoff of either or both the main pancreatic and common bile ducts.

Pathology

Adenocarcinoma arising from the exocrine gland ductal system is the most common type of pancreatic cancer, accounting for 95% of all cases. Two-thirds of these cancers originate in the pancreatic head, and the remainder arise in the body or tail. Most ductal carcinomas are mucin-producing tumors and usually are associated with a dense desmoplastic reaction.

Although most pancreatic adenocarcinomas arise from the ductal epithelium, pancreatic acinar carcinomas and cancers arising from mucinous cystic neoplasms are also found.

Multicentricity, which is usually microscopic, is not unusual.

Metastatic spread Perineural invasion occurs in the majority of patients with pancreatic carcinoma. In addition, pancreatitis distal to and surrounding the tumor is usually present. Most patients present with lymph node metastases in the region of the pancreaticoduodenal drainage basins. The subpyloric and inferior pancreatic head, SMA, and para-aortic lymph node groups also may be involved. Distant metastatic spread most commonly involves the liver and peritoneal surfaces.

Staging and prognosis

Pancreatic adenocarcinoma is staged according to local spread of disease, nodal status, and distant metastatic involvement using the American Joint Committee on Cancer (AJCC) TNM system (Table 1). The T staging of the primary tumor includes an analysis of direct extension of disease to the duodenum, bile duct, or peripancreatic tissues. A T4 advanced cancer may extend directly to the SMA or celiac axis, meaning that the cancer is unresectable.

TABLE 1: TNM staging of pancreatic tumors

Primary tumor (T)

Tx	Primary tumor cannot be assessed
T0	No evidence of a primary tumor
Tis	Carcinoma in situ
T1	Tumor limited to the pancreas, ≤ 2 cm in diameter
T2	Tumor limited to the pancreas, > 2 cm in diameter
T3	Tumor extends beyond the pancreas but without involvement of the celiac axis or the superior mesenteric artery
T4	Tumor involves the celiac axis or the superior mesenteric artery (unresectable primary tumor)

Regional lymph nodes (N)

N0	No involved regional lymph nodes
N1	Any involved regional lymph nodes

Distant metastases (M)

Mx	Presence of distant metastases cannot be assessed
M0	No distant metastases
M1	Distant metastases

Stage grouping

Stage 0	Tis	N0	M0
Stage IA	T1	N0	M0
Stage IB	T2	N0	M0
Stage IIA	T3	N0	M0
Stage IIB	T1-3	N1	M0
Stage III	T4	Any N	M0
Stage IV	Any T	Any N	M1

From Fleming ID, Cooper JS, Henson DE, et al (eds): AJCC Cancer Staging Manual, 6th ed. New York, Springer-Verlag, 2002.

Independent prognostic factors Lymph node metastases and tumor size and differentiation have independent prognostic value in patients with pancreatic carcinoma. Significantly improved survival is seen in patients with smaller lesions, lymph node-negative tumors, and tumors in which the surgical margins are not involved.

Lymph node and margin status Prior to the age of adjuvant therapy, lymph node status was the most dominant prognostic factor (Figure 1). It is now rivaled by surgical margin status in series where surgical margins have been meticulously examined.

Treatment

SURGICAL TREATMENT OF RESECTABLE DISEASE

The rate of resection for curative intent ranges from 10% to > 75%, with the higher percentage resulting from both a more aggressive approach and better

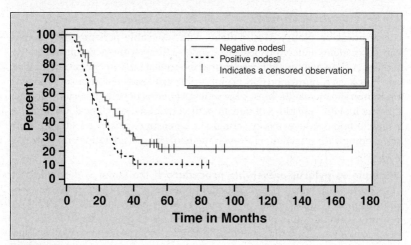

FIGURE 1: Actuarial survival as a function of regional lymph node status in patients with pancreatic cancer.

preoperative staging for resectability. Also, there is growing evidence that patients with potentially resectable pancreatic cancer have a shorter hospital stay, reduced surgical mortality, and an overall better outcome if the surgery is performed at "high-volume" medical centers staffed by experienced surgeons (approximately 16 operable cases per year).

Extended resections may include portal or superior mesenteric vessels, colon, adrenal glands, or stomach. If resection of adjacent organs or tissues results in the conversion of a positive to a negative resection margin, it is of great potential benefit to the patient. With regard to the extent of lymph node dissection, several recent prospective randomized studies have shown an increase in postoperative morbidity, but with no improvement in overall survival in patients undergoing an extended lymph node dissection.

Determination of resectability

The initial approach to surgery for pancreatic carcinoma includes a determination of resectability. This determination should be first made preoperatively with high-quality CT or MRI and perhaps EUS. Operative determination of resectability includes careful examination of the liver, porta hepatis, and portal and superior mesenteric vessels. The head of the pancreas and uncinate process are mobilized by an extensive Kocher maneuver to evaluate the head of the pancreas. The SMA is palpated, and its relationship to the tumor is assessed. The hepatic artery and celiac trunk are examined to make certain there is no vascular encasement.

Criteria for unresectability include distant metastases and involvement of the SMA and celiac axis.

Operative intervention

Intraoperative biopsy Most patients with resectable periampullary tumors can successfully undergo pancreaticoduodenectomy without an intraoperative biopsy. A time-consuming frozen section interpretation may not be informative, and histologic confirmation may be impossible with small lesions associated with peritumoral pancreatitis. Most large series of pancreaticoduodenectomy for carcinoma include resections of benign pathology based on clinical judgment. A negative fine-needle cytology should not deter an experienced surgeon from proceeding with resection. However, medicolegal considerations may prompt a biopsy.

Whipple vs pylorus-preserving procedure If the tumor is deemed to be resectable, a standard pancreaticoduodenectomy (Whipple procedure) or pylorus-preserving Whipple procedure (PPW) is performed. The PPW theoretically eliminates the nutritional problems caused by a reduced gastric reservoir and gastric dumping, but this finding has not been shown to alter long-term nutritional status. If there is any doubt about cancer proximity or blood supply to the pylorus, an antrectomy should be performed. If the tumor approaches the pylorus or involves the subpyloric nodes, classic antrectomy is preferred. Recent prospective randomized studies have shown there to be no significant difference between pylorus-preserving and standard Whipple resection.

Reconstruction technique The most common reconstruction technique after a Whipple resection requires a single retrocolic jejunal loop to complete the pancreaticojejunostomy, which is followed by a cholangiojejunostomy and gastrojejunostomy. A duct-mucosal anastomosis is preferred to the pancreaticojejunostomy. Pancreaticogastrostomy is also an effective and safe means of creating the anastomosis.

Postoperative complications Operative mortality of pancreaticoduodenectomy is currently < 6% in major surgical centers. The leading causes of postoperative mortality include postoperative sepsis, hemorrhage, and cardiovascular events. Most of the septic complications arise from pancreaticojejunostomy leaks.

In many series, early delayed gastric emptying is the leading cause of morbidity for pylorus-preserving procedures. The number-two cause of morbidity, seen in 5% to 15% of all patients, is a leak or fistula from the pancreatic anastomosis. Today, with appropriate drainage and nutritional support, more than 95% of pancreatic fistulas will heal using conservative measures.

An analysis of 200 patients who underwent resection of pancreatic adenocarcinoma in the era prior to adjuvant therapy found that the most important factors influencing long-term survival were the diameter of the primary tumor, status of the resected lymph nodes, and status of the resected margins. Patients with tumors < 3 cm in diameter had significantly longer median survival and 5-year survival rates (21 months and 28%, respectively) than those with tumors ≥ 3 cm (11.5 months and 15%). Patients with no lymph node involvement had a 5-year survival rate of 36%, as compared with < 5% for those with positive nodes. Patients who underwent resections with negative margins had a 5-year survival rate of 26%, versus 8% for those with positive margins. The type of resection (pylorus-preserving vs standard Whipple procedure) did not influence survival.

Body and tail tumors Tumors in the body and tail of the pancreas are typically larger than tumors in the head of the pancreas and are often metastatic upon presentation. For those patients who are surgical candidates, resection employs a distal pancreatectomy with concomitant splenectomy. Due to their large size, removal may require resection of adjacent organs. Of note, the rate of pancreatic leaks following distal pancreatectomy is approximately 30% to 40%, although with appropriate treatment they resolve, using conservative measures.

SURGICAL PALLIATION

Surgical palliation is also considered in patients undergoing exploration with curative intent. Jaundice, gastric obstruction, and pain may be alleviated by surgical palliation.

Biliary tract obstruction Either a choledochojejunostomy or cholecystojejunostomy can be used to bypass the biliary obstruction. Recurrent jaundice and cholangitis are less likely to develop when the common duct is used for decompression.

Duodenal obstruction Although duodenal obstruction is rare as a presenting symptom, duodenal involvement may occur eventually in 25% of patients. Some authors believe that prophylactic bypasses are safe and should be performed in all patients. One phase III trial supports prophylactic bypass, but the subject remains controversial.

Pain relief Severe back pain may be an incapacitating symptom. Pain relief may be achieved by chemoablation of the celiac plexus or by alcohol injection, which may be performed intraoperatively, percutaneously, or endoscopically. An intraoperative injection of 25 mL of ethanol (95%) on both sides of the celiac axis will ablate tumor pain. (For further discussion of these techniques, see chapter 37 on "Pain Management.")

A Radiation Therapy Oncology Group (RTOG)/Southwest Oncology Group (SWOG)/ Eastern Cooperative Oncology Group (ECOG) intergroup trial, the largest of its kind, compared infusional 5-FU with gemcitabine (Gemzar), both agents given before and after chemoradiation therapy, in patients with resected pancreatic cancer. Radiation therapy was administered without a treatment break and was given with continuous-infusion 5-FU in both arms. The study accrued 451 patients and demonstrated a survival advantage for patients with pancreatic head adenocarcinoma who received gemcitabine vs those treated with 5-FU (median overall survival 20.5 vs 16.9 months; P = .033); *(Regine WF, Winter KA, Abrams RA, et al: JAMA 299:1019-1026, 2008).* The study also included a rigorous review of radiation therapy delivery. Patient outcome was strongly associated with adherence to radiotherapy guidelines, on both arms of the study, with a significant trend toward impaired survival with radiotherapy deviations (P = .09 of the 5-FU arm and .023 on the gemcitabine arm). This underscores the importance of careful attention to how radiation therapy is delivered, which was not done in the European trials *(RA Abrams, K Winter, W Regine, et al: Int J Radiat Onc Biol Phys 66[suppl]:522, 2006).*

NEOADJUVANT AND ADJUVANT THERAPIES

Radiation therapy

Even with apparently adequate surgical resection, pancreatic cancer has a high risk of locoregional recurrence. Moreover, most lesions are unresectable, even when there is no apparent distant metastatic disease. Thus, there is a theoretical rationale for the adjunctive use of radiation therapy, either before or after surgery, in almost all patients. Preoperative (neoadjuvant) radiation therapy may help render locally advanced lesions resectable with negative margins (R0 resection). Postoperative (adjuvant) radiation therapy may help eliminate suspected residual microscopic disease in the tumor bed and/or regional lymphatics. Alternative radiation techniques, including intensity-modulated radiotherapy (IMRT) and 3D conformal radiation therapy, are being explored.

With an effective chemotherapeutic agent, there is greater potential for adequate locoregional cytotoxicity—as well as control of subclinical distant disease—than could be obtained with limited doses of adjuvant radiation therapy alone.

Preoperative chemoradiation therapy Several single-institution studies have evaluated the role of preoperative irradiation in conjunction with fluorouracil (5-FU)- and gemcitabine (Gemzar)-based chemotherapy. In these studies, 60% to 80% of the lesions were completely resected 1.0 to 1.5 months after the completion of chemoradiotherapy. Median survival has ranged from 16 to 36 months, but no phase III trials have been conducted to evaluate preoperative therapy versus postoperative sequencing.

Preoperative radiation therapy, to 4,500 to 5,000 cGy, in conjunction with chemotherapy should be considered for patients with pancreatic adenocarcinoma who are medically fit but who have marginally resectable disease. There are research initiatives to further address the role of neoadjuvant chemotherapy. For example, phase II studies explore high-dose gemcitabine and high-dose gemcitabine and cisplatin with short-term radiation therapy for locally advanced cancer. Other neoadjuvant strategies include the addition of oxaliplatin (Eloxatin), bevacizumab (Avastin), cetuximab (Erbitux), or erlotinib (Tarceva) to gemcitabine/irradiation combinations.

Postoperative chemoradiation therapy A total of 541 patients were enrolled in a trial conducted by the European Study Group for Pancreatic Cancer (ESPAC). This study evaluated the benefits of adjuvant therapy. The design was complex, attempting to assess several options. It included no further therapy after surgery, chemoradiation therapy (bolus 5-FU with split-course radiotherapy), chemotherapy (5-FU with leucovorin), and chemoradiation therapy followed by chemotherapy.

Interpretation of the results is confounded by the fact that some institutions opted for a full 2×2 randomization (all four options), whereas others allowed only two options (no further therapy vs chemotherapy or no further therapy vs chemoradiation therapy). Patients receiving these two options could also have therapy other than that prescribed in the randomization. Furthermore, no data were collected regarding time to disease recurrence or whether treatment was given after recurrence. Curiously, the median survival of those in the control group was more than 17 months, much longer than those of the control groups from the Gastrointestinal Tumor Study Group (GITSG) and European Organisation for Research and Treatment of Cancer (EORTC) trials.

Only the 5-FU–with-leucovorin arm would be considered a state-of-the-art approach, and it was demonstrated to improve survival significantly ($P = .0005$). This finding would suggest a strong benefit to postoperative chemotherapy. If radiation therapy is included, it would probably best be given after 1 to 2 months of full-dose chemotherapy. Most practitioners would recommend continuous-course radiation therapy rather than split-course treatment.

> A German randomized phase III trial including 368 patients with resected pancreatic cancer compared postoperative gemcitabine (Gemzar) given for 6 months observation. Disease-free survival was significantly superior for patients receiving postoperative gemcitabine (13.4 months vs 6.9 months; $P < .001$), including patients with either R0 or R1 resection. Overall survival, however, was not significantly different between the gemcitabine and control groups (22.1 months vs 20.2 months; $P = .06$). (Oettle H, Post S, Neuhaus P, et al: JAMA 297:267-277, 2007).

The ESPAC is now conducting a postoperative trial comparing gemcitabine and 5-FU. In the United States, the findings of several phase II trials of postoperative regimens as well as a phase III trial will be available soon. In addition, the GI Intergroup is conducting a randomized phase II trial to explore new combinations incorporating the monoclonal antibodies bevacizumab and cetuximab, each given with gemcitabine; irradiation is given with oral capecitabine (Xeloda).

Locally advanced but potentially resectable lesions

These lesions comprise 10% to 15% of cases presenting to physicians. Data from phase II preoperative chemoradiotherapy trials indicate that trimodality therapy is crucial for margin-free resection and long-term survival. A meta-analysis from the ESPAC1 trial showed that chemotherapy alone is ineffective for patients having had an R1 (residual microscopic disease at a margin) resection, thus adding further support to both chemotherapy and radiation therapy for these borderline resectable patients. ACOSOG (American College of Surgeons Oncology Group) will be mounting a trial with preoperative capecitabine, bevacizumab, and radiation therapy for these patients within the next year.

> A systematic review of 11 trials including 794 patients with locally advanced pancreatic cancer using radiation/combined-modality therapy showed a survival benefit for chemoradiation over irradiation alone, but there was not a significant advantage for chemoradiation followed by chemotherapy compared with chemotherapy alone (Sultana A, Tudur Smith C, Cunningham D, et al: Br J Cancer 96:1183-1190, 2007).

TREATMENT OF UNRESECTABLE DISEASE

Irradiation can prolong and/or improve quality of life in some patients with unresectable adenocarcinoma of the pancreas. It is better combined with chemotherapy. Long-term survival is, unfortunately, highly unusual.

Chemoradiation therapy The addition of chemotherapy to radiation therapy has been shown to improve the survival of patients with unresectable pancreatic adenocarcinoma, with moderate doses of radiation only slightly less effective than higher doses. In a GITSG trial of unresectable disease, moderate-dose radiation (4,000 cGy) with 5-FU chemotherapy significantly improved survival, as compared with higher doses of radiation (6,000 cGy) and no chemotherapy (median survival, 9.6 vs 5.2 months). The GITSG has also compared chemotherapy plus irradiation with chemotherapy alone and demonstrated a significant improvement with combined-modality therapy (median survival, 42 vs 32 weeks).

Based on these data, except in a protocol setting, the palliative management of a patient with unresectable pancreatic adenocarcinoma who has significant local symptoms should probably consist of moderate doses of radiation (4,000–5,000 cGy) in conjunction with 5-FU–based chemotherapy. As in adjuvant treatment, carefully shaped portals approximately 12 × 12 cm should be used.

Approaches under investigation At present, numerous trials are exploring a variety of chemoradiation therapy approaches, including single-agent or combination therapy with oral or infusional 5-FU, paclitaxel, cisplatin, gemcitabine, docetaxel (Taxotere), and oxaliplatin. The radiosensitizing properties of the biologic agents, including cetuximab, bevacizumab, and erlotinib, are being explored in radiation therapy clinical trials in combination with chemotherapy. Trials with combined gemcitabine and irradiation are of particular interest due to the activity of this drug in pancreatic cancer and the fact that it is a potent radiosensitizer. The benefit of irradiation for patients with locally advanced disease, however, remains a research question because of toxicity concerns and the relatively brief survival rates. Therefore, an Eastern Cooperative Oncology Group (ECOG) trial evaluated gemcitabine alone versus gemcitabine and irradiation for this group of patients. Low accrual resulted in early trial closure; however, an analysis will be available later in 2008.

If gemcitabine is given either before or after a course of radiation therapy, full doses of 1,000 mg/m² are possible. If irradiation and gemcitabine are given concurrently, doses of either modality must be sharply reduced. A phase II trial is combining "full-dose" gemcitabine (1,000 mg/m²) with radiation therapy directed at the primary tumor alone (36 Gy). It was reported that 17 of 20 patients thought to have resectable disease before treatment underwent pancreatic resection. Of them, 41% are alive without recurrence at 18 months. In addition, a Radiation Therapy Oncology Group (RTOG) randomized trial evaluated radiation therapy (50.4 Gy) and weekly gemcitabine and paclitaxel with or without the farnesyl transferase inhibitor R115777 (tipifarnib, Zarnestra) for locally advanced pancreatic cancer. In that trial, the gemcitabine dose was 75 mg/m²/wk and the paclitaxel dose was 40 mg/m²/wk. Radiation was conventionally fractionated to a dose of 50.4 Gy. Both these trials are now completed and being analyzed.

TABLE 2: Chemotherapy regimens for pancreatic cancer

Drug/combination	Dose and schedule
Fluorouracil (5-FU)/radiation therapy (GITSG regimen)	
Fluorouracil	500 mg/m^2/d IV bolus for 3 consecutive days once every 4 weeks during radiation therapy
Radiation therapy	Two courses of 2,000 cGy each, separated by 2 weeks (total dose, 4,000 cGy)

Gastrointestinal Tumor Study Group: Cancer 59:2006–2010, 1987.

Infusional 5-FU with radiation therapy	
Concurrent radiation therapy and chemotherapy phase:	
Fluorouracil	150-250 mg/m^2/d, 24 hours/d during radiation therapy
Radiation therapy	Median dose of 4,500 cGy/25 fractions (range 4,000 cGy/ 20 fractions to 5,040 cGy/28 fractions)

Fisher B, Perera F, Kocha W, et al: Int J Radiat Oncol Biol Phys 45:291–295, 1999.

Single-agent regimen	
Gemcitabine	1,000 mg/m^2 IV infused over 30 minutes once a week for 7 weeks, followed by a 1-week rest period

Subsequent cycles once a week for 3 consecutive weeks of every 4 weeks

Burris HA, Moore MJ, Andersen J, et al: J Clin Oncol 15:2403–2413, 1997.

Erlotinib plus gemcitabine	
Erlotinib	100 mg oral daily
Gemcitabine	1,000 mg/m^2 IV infused over 30 minutes once a week for 7 weeks, followed by a 1-week rest period

Subsequent cycles once a week for 3 consecutive weeks of every 4 weeks

Moore MJ, Goldstein D, Hamm J, et al: J Clin Oncol 23(suppl):16s, 2005. Abstract 1.

Gemcitabine adjuvantly in resected pancreatic carcinoma	
Gemcitabine	1,000 mg/m^2 IV over 30 minutes on days 1, 8, and 15 every 4 weeks for 6 cycles

Neuhaus P, Riess H, Post S, et al: J Clin Oncol 26: 2008. Abstract LBA4504.

Table prepared by Ishmael Jaiyesimi, DO

The dose of gemcitabine that can be given concurrently with irradiation depends on the volume and dose of radiation. If full doses of gemcitabine (1,000 mg/m^2/wk) are given concurrently with irradiation, the dose of radiation must be markedly reduced to avoid unacceptable GI toxicity.

TREATMENT OF METASTATIC ADENOCARCINOMA

Pancreatic adenocarcinoma is still one of the most frustrating, resistant solid neoplasms to treat, and therapy for metastatic disease remains palliative. Few agents have demonstrated activity of > 10%. Moreover, most of the reported series have been small, and not all encouraging results have been duplicated.

Chemotherapy

As metastatic pancreatic carcinoma is incurable, the anticipated risks of chemotherapy, which are often substantial, must be balanced against the gains that may be achieved; unfortunately, they are few. Patients who are debilitated due to their underlying or comorbid disease should not be offered chemotherapy, as their likelihood of deriving any benefit is exceedingly slim. However, patients who desire therapy and who, while symptomatic, still have a good performance status may be offered "standard" chemotherapy (Table 2) or, if possible, should be encouraged to participate in a clinical trial.

5-FU Historically, single-agent 5-FU has been associated with a response rate of 25% in pancreatic cancer. FAM (5-FU, Adriamycin [doxorubicin], and mitomycin) and 5-FU plus doxorubicin offer no advantage over 5-FU alone. 5-FU plus leucovorin appears to be ineffective.

Gemcitabine is indicated for the treatment of locally advanced or metastatic pancreatic adenocarcinoma. Gemcitabine was compared with 5-FU in a group of 126 previously untreated patients and showed a small, but statistically significant, improvement in response rate. Median survival in the gemcitabine group was 5.7 months, with 18% of patients alive at 12 months, as compared with a median survival of 4.4 months in the group receiving 5-FU, with 2% of patients alive at 12 months. Perhaps more important, clinical benefit response (a composite measurement of pain, performance status, and weight) occurred in 23.8% of the gemcitabine-treated group, as compared with 4.8% of the 5-FU–treated group. Due to its palliative potential, gemcitabine has become the standard of care for patients with unresectable pancreatic adenocarcinoma.

A recent randomized, phase II trial of dose-intense gemcitabine administered by standard infusion versus a fixed-dose rate (10 mg/m^2/min) suggested an improved 1-year survival with the fixed-dose rate.

Combination therapy There have been a number of attempts to improve the therapeutic outcome for patients with metastatic pancreatic cancer by comparing promising combinations of agents in randomized clinical trials. Unfortunately, the results have been disappointing. The ECOG compared gemcitabine with or without 5-FU, demonstrating a median survival of 5.4 months for gemcitabine versus 6.7 months for the combination; however, this difference was not statistically significant. Another trial explored the addition of irinotecan to gemcitabine.

A European randomized trial for 319 patients with advanced pancreatic cancer compared capecitabine (Xeloda)/gemcitabine (Gemzar) versus gemcitabine and showed no difference in overall survival (8.4 vs 7.2 months; $P = .234$). The combination showed improved median overall survival in good performance status patients (10.1 vs 7.4 months; $P = .014$); *(Herrmann R, Bodoky G, Ruhstaller T, et al: J Clin Oncol 25:2212-2217, 2007).*

There was no survival benefit when this regimen was compared with gemcitabine alone, although the combination did increase the tumor response rate (16.1% vs 4.4%; $P < .001$).

A meta-analysis of 15 randomized trials showed a significant survival benefit for patients with advanced pancreatic cancer and a good performance status who received gemcitabine either with a platinum analog (hazard ratio [HR] = 0.85; $P = .01$) or a fluoropyrimidine (HR = 0.9; $P = .03$).

Preliminary results from a randomized phase II trial comparing FOLFIRINOX (5-FU/leucovorin, irinotecan, oxaliplatin) versus gemcitabine for 88 patients with metastatic pancreatic cancer showed response rates of 38.7% versus 11.7%, respectively, with a median duration of response of 6.3 months versus 4.6 months, respectively. The trial will continue as a phase III study.

A phase III study of 565 patients compared gemcitabine with the combination of gemcitabine plus the multitargeted antifolate pemetrexed (Alimta) and demonstrated a significant response benefit with the combination (14.8% vs 7.1%; $P = .004$). However, overall and disease progression-free survival rates were comparable. There was increased hematologic toxicity with the combination.

Agents with marginal activity include mitomycin, doxorubicin, ifosfamide, streptozocin (Zanosar), and docetaxel. To date, monoclonal antibody therapy and hormonal manipulation have been ineffective. A phase II study of the anti–epidermal growth factor receptor (EGFR)–antibody cetuximab combined with gemcitabine has shown a 12% partial response rate and 39% stable disease in advanced pancreatic cancer. Side effects included rash/folliculitis and fatigue. A phase III trial of the combination is accruing patients.

The ECOG is also exploring EGFR-directed therapy in pancreatic cancer with a new randomized phase II trial comparing docetaxel and irinotecan with or without cetuximab. The trial will correlate EGFR expression with outcome after therapy. Other "targeted" therapies are under investigation.

Novel approaches A progressively better understanding of the molecular biology of pancreatic cancer has revealed numerous new therapeutic targets. Areas of active current research include attempts to replace tumor-suppressor genes (ie, *p53*) and to inhibit K-*ras* protein function.

PANCREATIC ENDOCRINE TUMORS

Pancreatic endocrine tumors (PETs) cover a spectrum of neoplasms. Many, although not all, originate from the pancreatic islets of Langerhans.

PETs are not rare. Autopsy studies have documented an incidence as high as 1.5%. Most of these lesions are clinically silent.

Approximately 20% of patients with Zollinger-Ellison syndrome develop the syndrome in the setting of the MEN-1 (multiple endocrine neoplasia type 1) syndrome. MEN-1 is inherited as an autosomal-dominant trait and is characterized by tumors of multiple endocrine organs, including the pituitary, pancreas, and parathyroid. The gene for MEN-1, which has been localized to the long arm of chromosome 11, has been identified and named *MENIN*.

The normal islet contains α, β, γ cells and enterochromaffin cells, which primarily secrete glucagon, insulin, somatostatin, and serotonin, respectively. All of these hormones may be secreted in excess by PETs. Other hormones that may be secreted by these tumors include vasoactive intestinal peptide (VIP), gastrin, pancreatic polypeptide (PP), and calcitonin. The aggressiveness of a PET in terms of its metastatic potential appears to be due to the cell of origin.

Types of tumors

Insulinomas are β-cell tumors of the pancreatic islets that produce insulin. Four-fifths of insulinomas occur as a solitary lesion, and < 10% of these tumors demonstrate malignant potential (in terms of invasiveness or the development of metastases). In patients with the MEN-1 syndrome, insulinomas are multicentric (10% of patients). In addition, a small group of insulinomas are associated with diffuse islet-cell hyperplasia or nesidioblastosis.

Gastrinomas are gastrin-secreting tumors associated with the Zollinger-Ellison syndrome (ZES). These tumors can be either sporadic or familial. Sporadic gastrinomas do not have associated endocrinopathies, whereas hereditary gastrinomas occur in patients with MEN-1 syndrome. Patients with the sporadic form of ZES may have single or multiple gastrinomas. This finding contrasts with patients with hereditary MEN-1 PETs, who generally have a more diffuse tumor process within the pancreas.

It is known that 80% to 90% of gastrinomas are located within the "gastrinoma triangle," defined as the junction of (1) the cystic and common duct, (2) the second and third portions of the duodenum, and (3) the neck and body of the pancreas. Although tumors most characteristically are located within the pancreas, a significant percentage of patients with ZES demonstrate primary tumors of the duodenal wall. Extrapancreatic and extraintestinal locations occur in approximately 10% of patients.

More than 90% of gastrinomas are malignant. The spectrum of clinical disease progression includes localized tumors, regional lymph node metastases, and widespread metastatic disease.

Other types Approximately three-quarters of VIPomas and approximately half of all glucagonomas and somatostatinomas are malignant.

'Nonfunctional' tumors Although many PETs cause considerable morbidity due to the inappropriately elevated levels of the hormones that they secrete, even "nonfunctional" PETs, ie, those without an associated demonstrable hormone-related syndrome (such as PPomas, neurotensinomas, and nonsecretory PETs), may be aggressive. Nonfunctional tumors account for up to 30% of all PETs. Two-thirds of these nonfunctional tumors will demonstrate metastatic lesions at some point during the patient's lifetime.

Signs and symptoms

The symptom complex that is observed depends on which hormone or hormones are secreted in excess.

Insulinomas are associated with symptoms of recurrent hypoglycemia. Diagnosis of these tumors is made by the demonstration of inappropriately elevated levels of insulin, proinsulin, and C peptide at the time of hypoglycemia and an elevated insulin-glucose ratio (> 0.3).

Gastrinomas Symptoms of gastrinoma-ZES are due to the effect of elevated levels of circulating gastrin. Ulceration of the upper GI tract is seen in > 90% of patients. Diarrhea is the second most common symptom. Approximately 25% of gastrinomas occur in the context of MEN-1 and are associated with parathyroid hyperplasia and hypercalcemia.

The diagnosis of ZES is established by the demonstration of hypergastrinemia (fasting serum gastrin concentration > 1,000 pg/mL) and gastric acid hypersecretion in a patient with ulcerative disease.

VIPomas An excess of VIP causes a profuse, watery diarrhea, hypokalemia, hypophosphatemia, and hypochlorhydria (WDHA syndrome).

Glucagonomas are associated with a rash (described as a necrotizing migratory erythema), glossitis, cheilosis, constipation and ileus, venous thrombosis, and hyperglycemia. Not all of these manifestations are secondary to elevated glucagon levels alone. The etiology of these signs and symptoms remains unknown, but some patients respond to supplemental zinc and amino acid infusions.

Somatostatinomas, which are rare, are associated with elevated blood glucose levels, achlorhydria, cholelithiasis, and diarrhea.

Tumor localization

Insulinomas Ultrasonography, CT, MRI, and selective arteriography with portal vein sampling have been utilized for the preoperative localization of insulinomas. The sensitivity of these preoperative imaging tests ranges from approximately 30% to 60%. This is because 40% of insulinomas are ≤ 1 cm and two-thirds of these tumors are < 1.5 cm.

Because the success of preoperative localization tests is disappointing and 90% of these tumors will be found and successfully resected by an experienced endocrine surgeon, there is a general trend toward performing fewer tests. Some centers utilize preoperative ultrasonography if the patient has not undergone prior pancreatic surgery. Other centers still routinely employ portal vein catheterization and angiography. Most centers with EUS availability use the modality as a standard diagnostic tool for these tumors.

More recently, intraoperative sonography has been shown to aid the surgeon. In one series, 84% of tumors not localized preoperatively were correctly located by surgical exploration and intraoperative sonography. Many lesions not discovered by surgical palpation may be found by this technique. At present, there is much less reliance on blind distal resection than was previously advocated. Obviously, the technique of intraoperative ultrasonography may not be as helpful in the MEN-1 syndrome, in which multiple small insulinomas may be found.

Gastrinomas CT, ultrasonography, selective abdominal angiography, selective venous sampling of gastrin, intraoperative ultrasonography, EUS, and intraoperative endoscopy have all been reported to be useful in localizing gastrinomas. More recently, somatostatin receptor scintigraphy (SRS) has become a valuable tool for PET localization; several studies have suggested greater sensitivity and specificity with SRS than with other diagnostic tests.

Treatment

Surgery for insulinomas

For larger insulinomas in the body or tail of the pancreas, a distal pancreatectomy may be preferable to enucleation. For tumors in the head of the pancreas, enucleation of the tumor is usually possible. Patients with MEN-1 or islet-cell hyperplasia may benefit from an 80% distal pancreatectomy. If the insulinoma is not found at surgery, a blind pancreatectomy is not warranted. Further imaging and venous sampling studies may reveal the exact location of the tumor.

A surgical cure results in normal values on subsequent provocative testing, during which blood insulin and glucose concentrations are measured simultaneously. Some insulinoma recurrences actually represent persistent disease after incomplete tumor excisions or overlooked secondary multiple tumors.

Surgery for gastrinoma-ZES

The ideal treatment of gastrinoma-ZES is surgical excision of the gastrinoma. However, this approach is possible in only 20% of patients, most of whom have a sporadic tumor. With the development of effective antisecretory agents and preoperative localization with octreotide scanning, the majority of patients demonstrating widespread metastatic disease can be identified and spared surgical exploration. In addition, some series report that patients with nonmetastatic sporadic gastrinoma may have a higher incidence of extrapancreatic sites than was previously thought. One series has reported that two-thirds of gastrinomas are extrapancreatic.

Patients with sporadic gastrinoma All patients with sporadic gastrinoma should undergo localization studies and be considered for exploratory laparotomy, with the goal of potential cure of ZES. Recent evidence suggests that resection of primary gastrinoma decreases the incidence of liver metastases and ZES. Overall, surgery produces complete remission in approximately 60% of patients with sporadic ZES, and subsequent survival is excellent.

Patients with ZES and MEN-1 Some experts believe that surgery should not be used in the management of patients with MEN-1 and ZES. Instead, they recommend treatment with antisecretory medications. This approach is somewhat controversial, as some authors believe that all patients without demonstrated liver metastases should undergo surgery to remove duodenal and pancreatic gastrinomas.

Moreover, since many patients with ZES and MEN-1 die of metastatic gastrinoma at a young age, a surgical approach may be warranted. Surgery should be performed only if imaging studies localize the tumor. Although radical surgery may not provide a cure, removal of large tumors may decrease metastatic potential and increase survival.

Surgical procedure During surgery, the entire pancreas should be mobilized and scanned ultrasonographically to permit a thorough examination of the pancreatic head, duodenum, stomach, mesentery, liver, and splenic hilum. Intraoperative endoscopy with transillumination of the bowel wall may also be useful in identifying duodenal lesions. In general, enucleation is the treatment of choice, except for lesions within the duodenal wall, which may require pancreaticoduodenectomy. If no tumor is found, blind distal pancreatectomy should be avoided, since 90% of gastrinomas are located within the gastrinoma triangle. (This triangle is formed by the angles at the junction between the cystic and common bile ducts, the junction between the second and third parts of the duodenum, and the junction between the head and neck of the pancreas.)

Surgical resection of liver metastases is controversial. However, several authors have demonstrated meaningful survival in patients with small, isolated lesions. The use of ablative procedures, with open, laparoscopic, or percutaneous techniques, can reduce the neurohormonal tumor burden.

Radiation therapy for PETs

Adjuvant therapy The role of adjuvant radiation therapy for PETs of the pancreas is unclear. Because of the rarity of these lesions and their often indolent behavior, the role of this therapy will probably never be demonstrated. However, postoperative irradiation can be considered for patients with positive nodes or microscopically close margins. Concurrent chemotherapy with such agents as 5-FU and/or streptozocin also can be considered. Radiation doses are the same as are used in adjuvant treatment of pancreatic cancer.

Palliative therapy Anecdotal reports indicate that pancreatic PETs may respond to palliative doses of irradiation. Long-term control of unresectable disease has been reported.

Chemotherapy for PETs

PETs are more sensitive to chemotherapy than are carcinoid tumors.

Single agents Agents that have demonstrated antitumor activity include recombinant human interferon alfa-2a and alfa-2b (Roferon-A, Intron A, respectively), 5-FU, doxorubicin, dacarbazine, and streptozocin.

Combination regimens Combination chemotherapy is often more effective than monotherapy. For example, in an ECOG study, the combination of 5-FU and streptozocin demonstrated a higher response rate than streptozocin alone (63% vs 36%) in PETs, as well as a better complete response rate (33% vs 12%) and median survival duration (26.0 vs 16.5 months). Therapy with doxorubicin plus streptozocin was superior to therapy with both 5-FU plus streptozocin and single-agent chlorozotocin in terms of response and survival and is the combination most widely used in the United States. Etoposide combined with cisplatin is active in poorly differentiated neuroendocrine malignancies but is marginally effective in well-differentiated lesions.

New agents Antiangiogenic approaches and the recognition of other potential biologic targets have contributed to the development of a number of early-phase clinical trials incorporating bevacizumab with temozolomide (Temodar) and with FOLFOX (5-FU, leucovorin, and oxaliplatin) chemotherapy, sunitinib (Sutent), sorafenib (Nexavar), vatalanib, imatinib (Gleevec), thalidomide (Thalomid), temsirolimus (Torisel), and everolimus. Phase III trials are planned or ongoing to further evaluate sunitinib and everolimus.

TREATMENT OF SYMPTOMS

Octreotide

Octreotide (Sandostatin) is often successful in palliating symptoms in patients with PETs, although this success depends somewhat on the cell type. For example, insulinomas are marginally responsive to octreotide, whereas gastrinomas and VIPomas often respond. However, compared with carcinoid tumors, the median duration of response of PETs to octreotide is significantly shorter (~ 10 weeks).

Recent Surveillance, Epidemiology, and End Results (SEER) data between 1973 and 1999 suggest an increasing median survival of patients with metastatic carinoid tumors since the era of octreotide treatment.

As discussed more fully in the section on carcinoid tumors below, a promising experimental approach for patients whose tumors express somatostatin receptors is the use of octreotide conjugated to a therapeutic radioisotope.

Other agents

Omeprazole (Prilosec), an inhibitor of the function of the parietal cell hydrogen pump, is more effective than H_2-receptor antagonists in blocking gastric acid production and is useful in the symptomatic management of gastrinomas.

Other agents available for symptomatic treatment of insulinomas include diazoxide (Hyperstat), an insulin-release inhibitor, and, more recently, glucagon, by continuous infusion through a portable pump. Both of these agents are used in conjunction with frequent high-carbohydrate meals.

Patients with the glucagonoma syndrome are treated symptomatically with insulin, high-protein meals, supplemental zinc, amino acid infusions, and anticoagulants.

Hepatic arterial embolization

Hepatic arterial embolization, with or without chemotherapy (chemoembolization), is an alternative palliative therapy for patients with either carcinoid tumors or a PET who have predominant liver metastases or who are symptomatic. Embolization is best reserved for patients with < 75% tumor involvement of the liver, bilirubin level < 2 mg/dL, and an ECOG performance status of ≤ 2. In addition, a patent portal vein is required for this procedure.

Other liver-directed therapeutic strategies include radiofrequency ablation (RFA) for select patients and clinical trials investigating the role of yttrium-90 microspheres.

CARCINOID TUMORS OF THE GI TRACT

Carcinoid tumors typically arise from components derived from the primitive gut, lungs, and, rarely, the gonads. Approximately 85% of all carcinoids originate from the gut, predominantly the appendix, followed by the small bowel and rectum.

These tumors have the propensity to cause considerable morbidity by virtue of creating a syndrome of hormonal excess. For example, although the majority of carcinoids are hormonally inert, these neoplasms may produce excessive amounts of serotonin (from dietary tryptophan), prostaglandins, kinins (secondary to kallikrein release), and a variety of other hormones, which may account for the "carcinoid syndrome." Recent SEER data suggest an increase in the incidence of carcinoid tumors between 1973 and 1990.

Signs and symptoms

Flushing The most common sign of the carcinoid syndrome is flushing, which is often triggered by alcohol, catecholamines, or emotional stress. It ranges in severity from a minor annoyance to profound vasodilatation with near syncope and hypotension.

Diarrhea is also common and is due to GI hypermotility. It usually occurs after meals and is rarely voluminous, bulky, or foul-smelling.

Abdominal cramps Diarrhea may be associated with crampy pain, although other etiologies for the pain must be considered, including bowel obstruction due to tumor or mesenteric fibrosis.

Bronchospasm Patients may also develop bronchospasm, which may be mediated by histamine. This problem is often associated with (although less common than) flushing.

Valvular heart disease A late finding is right-sided valvular heart disease, although left-sided lesions may be noted occasionally. The fibrous deposits may lead to tricuspid insufficiency and/or pulmonary stenosis. Valve replacement is rarely necessary, however.

Symptom triad If there is sufficient shunting of dietary tryptophan from niacin to serotonin synthesis, patients may develop diarrhea, dermatitis, and dementia, although this symptom triad is rare if patients maintain adequate intake of a balanced diet.

Diagnosis

Diagnostic studies include CT/MRI of the abdomen and a 24-hour urine test for 5-hydroxyindoleacetic acid (5-HIAA). Some radiologists prefer to obtain a triple-phase CT scan of the liver to detect these highly vascular liver metastases.

Octreotide scanning Indium-111 octreotide scintigraphy (OctreoScan) has been shown to have a higher sensitivity for detecting pancreatic tumors and is superior to CT or MRI for detecting metastatic disease, particularly extrahepatic disease. One study suggests that indium-111 octreotide scintigraphy can reduce costs by avoiding unnecessary surgeries. Also, a positive scan may predict which patients may benefit from treatment with somatostatin analogs (eg, octreotide). Initial studies with a new peptide tracer, indium-111 DOTA-lanreotide, suggest high tumor uptake and a more favorable dosimetry than is seen with indium-111 DTPA-D-Phel-octreotide.

Prognosis

Site and size of tumor The site of tumor origin is potentially prognostic, as most appendiceal carcinoids (75%) are < 1 cm when found and are usually cured by resection. Similarly, rectal carcinoids are usually small and completely resectable for cure.

In contrast, small bowel carcinoids tend to present at a more advanced stage, and approximately one-third have multicentric primary lesions. However, if the disease is completely resectable, patients have a 20-year survival rate of 80%; patients with unresectable intra-abdominal or hepatic metastases have median survival durations of 5 and 3 years, respectively.

Treatment

The management of carcinoid tumors focuses not only on treating bulky disease, in common with other solid malignancies, but also on treating the complications of hormonal excess.

TREATMENT OF BULKY DISEASE

Surgery

Appendiceal carcinoids For tumors that are found incidentally in the appendix and that are probably between 1 and 2 cm, appendectomy is the treatment of choice. For tumors > 2 cm, a right hemicolectomy and lymph node dissection are appropriate.

Small intestines and rectal carcinoids should be resected with a wedge lymphadenectomy to evaluate nodal disease. Small distal rectal tumors (< 2 cm) can undergo local excision via transanal techniques. Duodenal lesions should be locally excised if small (< 2 cm), with radical resection reserved for larger tumors.

Tumor debulking Liver resection or ablation of liver metastases with cryotherapy or radiofrequency techniques is useful in patients with limited extrahepatic disease and/or symptomatic carcinoid syndrome. Tumor debulking can protect liver functional reserve and improve quality of life.

Liver transplantation may be of benefit in selected patients without extrahepatic disease whose cancer progresses after other therapeutic interventions.

Radiation therapy

Carcinoid tumors are responsive to radiation therapy and frequently are well palliated with this modality. Overall, treatment with higher radiation doses (29 to 52 Gy) has been associated with higher response rates (40% to 50%) than treatment with lower doses (10%).

Chemotherapy

Since carcinoid tumors tend to be resistant to most chemotherapeutic agents, there are no standard regimens for the treatment of unresectable tumors.

Single agents Agents that have reported activity include 5-FU, doxorubicin, and recombinant human interferon alfa-2a and alfa-2b. However, the response rate with these agents is in the range of 10% to 20%, the response duration is < 6 months, and complete remission is rare.

Combination regimens Combination chemotherapy regimens represent little improvement over single-agent therapy, with response rates ranging from 25% to 35%, response durations < 9 months, and rare complete remissions.

New agents Antiangiogenic approaches and the recognition of other potential biologic targets have contributed to the development of a number of early-phase clinical trials incorporating bevacizumab with temozolomide and with FOLFOX chemotherapy, sunitinib, sorafenib, vatalanib, imatinib, thalidomide, temsirolimus, and everolimus. Phase III trials are planned or ongoing to further evaluate sunitinib and everolimus. The Southwest Oncology Group (SWOG) is currently coordinating an intergroup randomized phase III trial comparing depot octreotide (Sandostatin LAR) plus interferon alfa-2b versus depot octreotide plus bevacizumab in advanced, poor-prognosis carcinoid patients.

TREATMENT OF SYMPTOMS

Somatostatin analogs

Octreotide The most active agent is the somatostatin analog octreotide. Even though native somatostatin is effective in controlling many symptoms, due to its short half-life (< 2 minutes), this agent would have to be administered via continuous infusion to be clinically useful. However, octreotide may be administered subcutaneously every 8 to 12 hours, facilitating outpatient therapy. The initial dose of octreotide is 100 to 600 µg/d in two to four divided doses, although the effective dose varies between patients and must be titrated to the individual patient's symptoms.

Octreotide not only is useful in managing the chronic problems of the carcinoid syndrome but also is effective in treating carcinoid crisis (volume-resistant hypotension), which may be precipitated by surgery or effective antitumor treatment.

Octreotide is well tolerated, although chronic treatment may be associated with cholelithiasis, increased fecal fat excretion, fluid retention, nausea, and glucose intolerance. Occasional objective antitumor responses have been observed in patients who have received octreotide; the median duration of symptomatic improvement is 1 year. One report evaluating the cost-effectiveness of octreotide suggested that it may double survival time. Other somatostatin analogs, including lanreotide and vapreotide, are under investigation.

SMS 201-995 pa LAR is a long-acting somatostatin analog that allows for monthly dosing, avoiding the need for three daily injections. This relatively new agent improves quality of life while apparently maintaining the same activity seen with daily octreotide. The usual monthly dose is 20 or 30 mg.

Patients who demonstrate disease resistance with somatostatin analog treatment alone may benefit from combination therapy with interferon-α and this somatostatin analog.

Radiolabeled somatostatin analogs A promising experimental treatment approach involves the use of octreotide or other somatostatin analogs conjugated to radioisotopes (eg, indium-111 or yttrium-90) in patients whose tumors express somatostatin receptors (eg, those with a positive OctreoScan result). This approach allows targeted in situ radiotherapy by taking advantage of internalization of the radioligand into the cell to produce DNA damage and cell death, with little effect on normal tissue. Initial reports have shown favorable results with this technique.

Other agents

Other agents that have been used for symptomatic management include H_1- and H_2-receptor antagonists, methoxamine (Vasoxyl), cyproheptadine, and diphenoxylate with atropine. The symptom complex of diarrhea, dermatitis, and dementia may be prevented or treated with supplemental niacin.

Hepatic arterial embolization

Hepatic arterial embolization with such agents as Ivalon or Gelfoam, with or without chemotherapy (chemoembolization), is an option for patients with either a carcinoid tumor or an islet-cell carcinoma who have predominant liver metastases or who are symptomatic. These lesions often are hypervascular, and, thus, peripheral hepatic embolization may provide symptomatic relief in some patients. It is unclear whether this therapy has any effect on patient survival.

Other liver-directed therapeutic strategies include RFA for select patients and clinical trials investigating the role of yttrium-90 microspheres.

ADRENOCORTICAL CARCINOMA

Adrenocortical carcinoma is a rare, highly malignant neoplasm that accounts for about 0.2% of cancer deaths. Long-term survival is dismal overall; the survival rate is 23% at 5 years and 10% at 10 years.

Etiology

The etiology of adrenocortical cancer is unknown, but some cases have occurred in families with a hereditary cancer syndrome.

Signs and symptoms

Approximately half of adrenocortical neoplasms produce hormonal and metabolic syndromes of hormone hypersecretion (such as Cushing's syndrome, virilizing or feminizing syndromes, and hyperaldosteronism). In children, Cushing's syndrome is rare but is often due to adrenal carcinoma. Mixed syndromes, such as Cushing's syndrome and virilization, strongly suggest adrenal carcinoma. The combination of hirsutism, acne, amenorrhea, and rapidly progressing Cushing's syndrome in a young female is a typical presentation. In men, estrogen-secreting tumors are associated with gynecomastia, breast tenderness, testicular atrophy, impotence, and decreased libido.

Often the diagnosis of adrenocortical carcinoma is not evident until the discovery of metastases or until the primary tumor becomes large enough to produce abdominal symptoms. Smaller tumors may be discovered incidentally, when unrelated abdominal complaints are investigated radiographically.

Treatment

Surgery

Complete surgical resection is the treatment of choice in patients with localized disease, as it offers the best chance of extending the disease-free interval and survival.

Medical therapy

Mitotane (Lysodren) is one of only a few effective agents; it exerts a specific cytolytic effect on adrenocortical cells and has been used to treat unresectable or metastatic adrenocortical carcinoma. Only 15% to 30% of patients experience objective tumor regression, with a median duration of about 7 months. Mitotane is given at a dose of 4–8 g/d as tolerated, although the dose is variable.

Chemotherapy Doxorubicin has been of benefit in a limited number of patients, and combination chemotherapy is under investigation.

Suramin, a sulfonated drug that is cytotoxic to human adrenocortical carcinoma cell lines, has been evaluated but has not proven useful in inoperable adrenocortical cancer. Innovative chemotherapy programs are clearly needed for this disease.

Controlling hormone hypersecretion Hormone hypersecretion can be controlled medically in most cases. Agents that are effective in reducing steroid production and in palliating associated clinical syndromes include the antifungal drug ketoconazole, 800 mg/d; aminoglutethimide (Cytadren), 1–2 g/d; and metyrapone (Metopirone), 1–4 g/d or higher as needed to control cortisol levels. These agents may be used alone or with mitotane.

PHEOCHROMOCYTOMA

Pheochromocytomas are catecholamine-secreting tumors that arise from chromaffin cells in the adrenal medulla or extra-adrenal sympathetic ganglia. These tumors constitute a surgically correctable cause of hypertension in 0.1% to 1.0% of hypertensive persons.

Only about 10% of pheochromocytomas are considered to be malignant. The vast majority (90%) of pheochromocytomas are found in the adrenal medulla, and 97% are located below the diaphragm. Approximately 10% each of pheochromocytomas are bilateral, malignant, multifocal, extra-adrenal, found in children, or associated with a familial syndrome.

Pheochromocytomas in patients with familial syndromes, such as MEN-2 and von Hippel-Lindau syndrome (VHL), are less likely to be malignant than other adrenal lesions. In contrast, pheochromocytomas in patients with a family history of malignant pheochromocytoma are more apt to be malignant.

Epidemiology and etiology

Pheochromocytomas occur in all age groups, but the incidence peaks in the third to fifth decades of life. Most pheochromocytomas (90%) are sporadic. Approximately 10% of cases are inherited as an autosomal-dominant trait, either independently or as a part of the MEN-2 syndrome; bilateral tumors are more common in this setting.

Both MEN-2A and MEN-2B include medullary thyroid carcinoma and pheochromocytoma. MEN-2A includes hyperparathyroidism, whereas MEN-2B includes ganglioneuromas and marfanoid habitus. In MEN-2 families, pheochromocytoma occurs in 5.5% to 100% (mean, 40%), depending on the kindred studied. Bilateral medullary hyperplasia is almost always present. Pheochromocytomas are bilateral in 70% of cases and usually multicentric, but they are rarely extra-adrenal or malignant.

Signs and symptoms

Patients can present with various symptoms, ranging from mild labile hypertension to hypertensive crisis, myocardial infarction, or cerebral vascular accident, all of which can result in sudden death. The classic pattern of paroxysmal hypertension occurs in 30% to 50% of cases; sustained hypertension may also occur and resembles essential hypertension. A characteristic presentation includes "spells" of paroxysmal headaches, pallor or flushing, tremors, apprehension, palpitations, hypertension, and diaphoresis.

Diagnosis

The diagnosis of pheochromocytoma relies on an appropriate history and documentation of excessive catecholamine production.

Catecholamine measurements Measurement of 24-hour urinary catecholamines and their metabolites, vanillylmandelic acid and metanephrine, is commonly used; the metanephrine level is considered to be the most specific single test. Serum catecholamine measurements are more susceptible to false elevations due to stress-related physiologic fluctuations. The evaluation of serum catecholamines after clonidine suppression, however, provides a useful diagnostic tool that is more convenient than urine collection. Dynamic provocative tests are rarely indicated. Recently, the measurement of plasma-free metanephrines has been shown to be an excellent test for excluding or confirming pheochromocytoma.

Radiologic studies Almost all pheochromocytomas are localized in the abdomen, mostly in the adrenal medulla; other locations include the posterior mediastinum or any distribution of the sympathetic ganglia. After the diagnosis is established biochemically, radiologic methods may be needed for preoperative localization of the lesion; CT and MRI are most widely used. Iodine methyl-iodobenzyl guanidine (MIBG) and SRS provide a "functional" image; they are most helpful in the detection of occult contralateral or extra-adrenal lesions.

Differentiating benign from malignant tumors The histologic differentiation between benign and malignant lesions is extremely difficult and often impossible to make; this distinction may require the development of lymph node, hepatic, bone, or other distant metastases. Recurrent symptoms of pheochromocytoma, often emerging many years after the original diagnosis, are suggestive of malignancy. Biochemical confirmation of recurrent catecholamine hypersecretion and localization of metastatic lesion(s) with iodine-131–MIBG scan constitute diagnostic proof.

Treatment

PREOPERATIVE MEDICAL MANAGEMENT

Phenoxybenzamine (Dibenzyline), an oral, long-acting, noncompetitive α-adrenoceptor blocker, is a widely used, very helpful first drug; it is given at a dose of 10–40 mg/d. Propranolol, a β-blocker (20–80 mg/d), is usually added after a few days to prevent tachycardia or arrhythmia. The use of β-blockers alone is hazardous because they may precipitate a paradoxical rise in blood pressure. The tyrosine hydroxylase inhibitor metyrosine (Demser) may be added in patients whose blood pressure is not well controlled with the combination of an α- and a β-blocker.

SURGERY

The principles of pheochromocytoma resection are complete tumor resection, avoidance of tumor seeding, and minimal tumor manipulation. Adrenalectomy can be performed by means of an open anterior transabdominal, open posterior retroperitoneal, laparoscopic lateral transabdominal, or laparoscopic posterior retroperitoneal approach. In the past, an open anterior approach was the standard because it allowed for complete exploration and inspection for potential tumor foci. However, with the improved accuracy of preoperative imaging and increased experience with laparoscopic procedures, there is little need for exploration in areas in which a tumor has not been identified.

Except in tumors < 6 cm, the laparoscopic approach to pheochromocytoma is probably the technique of choice. In the absence of obvious local tumor invasion or metastatic disease, a laparoscopic procedure is acceptable to many experienced endocrine surgeons.

The most critical intraoperative aspect of surgery is control of blood pressure immediately after removal of the tumor, when all agonistic effects are abolished and the effects of α- and β-blockers are still present. Close cooperation with the anesthesiologist to expand fluid volume and prepare the appropriate infusions of agonists to support vascular stability is critical.

TREATMENT OF METASTATIC MALIGNANT PHEOCHROMOCYTOMA

The treatment of choice for metastatic malignant pheochromocytoma remains problematic.

Medical and radiation therapy

Medical therapy with α- or β-blockers, as well as metyrosine, is almost always required to maintain hemodynamic stability. Chemotherapy utilizing streptozocin-based regimens or the combination of cyclophosphamide, vincristine, and dacarbazine has yielded promising responses. Treatment with iodine-131–MIBG or (in Europe) with radiolabeled somatostatin has met with only limited success. In most cases, uncontrolled catecholamine hypersecretion eventually escapes biochemical blockade, and fatal hypertensive crisis ensues.

Surgery

In those cases in which limited and resectable lesions can be identified, surgery can effect complete and lasting remission of the disease.

SUGGESTED READING

ON PANCREATIC CANCER

Bilimoria KY, Bentrem DJ, Ko CY, et al: Multimodality therapy for pancreatic cancer in the US: Utilization, outcomes, and the effect of hospital volume. Cancer 110:1227–1234, 2007.

Chua YJ, Cunningham D: Adjuvant treatment for resectable pancreatic cancer. J Clin Oncol 23:4532–4537, 2005.

Crane CH, Varadhachary G, Pisters PW, et al: Future chemoradiation strategies in pancreatic cancer. Semin Oncol 34:335–346, 2007.

Goggins M: Molecular markers of early pancreatic cancer. J Clin Oncol 23:4524–4531, 2005.

Heinemann V, Hinke A, Bock S, et al: Gemcitabine-based combinations (gem+x) vs gemcitabine (gem) alone in the treatment of advanced pancreatic cancer: A meta-analysis of sixteen randomized trials. J Clin Oncol 25(18S):2007. Abstract 4515.

Herrmann R, Bodoky G, Ruhstaller T, et al: Gemcitabine plus capecitabine compared with gemcitabine alone in advanced pancreatic cancer: A randomized, multicenter, phase III trial of the Swiss Group for Clinical Cancer Research and the Central European Cooperative Oncology Group. J Clin Oncol 25:2212–2217, 2007.

Moore MJ, Goldstein D, Hamm J, et al: Erlotinib plus gemcitabine compared with gemcitabine alone in patients with advanced pancreatic cancer: A phase III trial of the National Cancer Institute of Canada Clinical Trials Group. J Clin Oncol 25:1960–1966, 2007.

Mulcahy MF: Adjuvant therapy for pancreas cancer: Advances and controversies. Semin Oncol 34:321–326, 2007.

Neoptolemos JP, Stocken DD, Friess H, et al; European Study Group for Pancreatic Cancer: A randomized trial of chemoradiotherapy and chemotherapy after resection of pancreatic cancer. N Engl J Med 350:1200–1210, 2004. Erratum in: N Engl J Med 351:726, 2004.

Oettle H, Post S, Neuhaus P, et al: Adjuvant chemotherapy with gemcitabine vs observation in patients undergoing curative-intent resection of pancreatic cancer: A randomized controlled trial. JAMA 297:267–277, 2007.

O'Reilly EM, Abou-Alfa GK: Cytotoxic therapy for advanced pancreatic adenocarcinoma. Semin Oncol 34:347–353, 2007.

Russo S, Butler J, Ove R, et al: Locally advanced pancreatic cancer: A review. Semin Oncol 34:327–334, 2007.

Stocken DD, Buchler MW, Dervenis C, et al: Meta-analysis of randomised adjuvant therapy trials for pancreatic cancer. Br J Cancer 92:1372–1381, 2005.

Teh SH, Deveney C, Sheppard BC: Aggressive pancreatic resection for primary pancreatic neuroendocrine tumor: Is it justifiable? Am J Surg 193:610–613, 2007.

Ujiki MB, Talamonti MS: Guidelines for the surgical management of pancreatic adenocarcinoma. Semin Oncol 34:311–320, 2007.

Willett CG, Czito BG, Bendell JJ, et al: Locally advanced pancreatic cancer. J Clin Oncol 23:4538–4544, 2005.

Wong GY, Schroeder DR, Carns PE, et al: Effect of neurolytic celiac plexus block on pain relief, quality of life, and survival in patients with unresectable pancreatic cancer: A randomized controlled trial. JAMA 3:1092–1099, 2004.

Ychou M, Desseigne F, Guimbaud R, et al: Randomized phase II trial comparing folfirinox (5FU/leucovorin [LV], irinotecan [I] and oxaliplatin [O]) vs gemcitabine (G) as first-line treatment for metastatic pancreatic adenocarcinoma (MPA): First results of the ACCORD 11 trial. J Clin Oncol 25(18S):2007. Abstract 4516.

ON NEUROENDOCRINE GI TUMORS

Durán I, Salazar R, Casanovas O, et al: New drug development in digestive neuroendocrine tumors. Ann Oncol 18:1307–1313, 2007.

Faiss S, Pape UF, Bohmig M, et al: Prospective, randomized, multicenter trial on the antiproliferative effect of lanreotide, interferon alfa, and their combination for therapy of metastatic neuroendocrine gastroenteropancreatic tumors. The International Lanreotide and Interferon Alfa Study Group. J Clin Oncol 15:2689–2696, 2003.

Fazio N, Oberg K: Prospective, randomized, multicenter trial on the antiproliferative effect of lanreotide, interferon alfa, and their combination for therapy of metastatic neuroendocrine gastroenteropancreatic tumors. J Clin Oncol 22:573–574, 2004.

Ho AS, Picus J, Darcy MD, et al: Long-term outcome after chemoembolization and embolization of hepatic metastatic lesions from neuroendocrine tumors. AJR Am J Roentgenol 188:1201–1207, 2007.

Kvols LK, Krenning EP, Pauwels S, et al: Phase I study of 90Y-SMT487 (Octreother) in patients with somatostatin receptor (SS-R) positive neuroendocrine (NE) tumors (abstract). Proc Am Soc Clin Oncol 19:207, 2000.

Kwekkeboom DJ, Teunissen JJ, Bakker WH, et al: Radiolabeled somatostatin analog [177Lu-DOTA0,Tyr3]octreotate in patients with endocrine gastroenteropancreatic tumors. J Clin Oncol 23:2754–2762, 2005.

Mazzaglia PJ, Berber E, Milas M, et al: Laparoscopic radiofrequency ablation of neuroendocrine liver metastases: A 10-year experience evaluating predictors of survival. Surgery 142:10–19, 2007.

Musunuru S, Chen H, Rajpal S, et al: Metastatic neuroendocrine hepatic tumors: Resection improves survival. Arch Surg 141:1000–1004, 2006.

Oberg K, Kvols L, Caplin M, et al: Consensus report on the use of somatostatin analogs for the management of neuroendocrine tumors of the gastroenteropancreatic system. Ann Oncol 15:966–973, 2004.

Yao JC, Hoff PM: Molecular targeted therapy for neuroendocrine tumors. Hematol Oncol Clin North Am 21:575–581, 2007.

ON ADRENAL NEOPLASMS

Jossart GH, Burpee SE, Gagner M: Surgery of the adrenal glands. Endocrinol Metab Clin North Am 29:57–68, 2000.

Kendrick ML, Lloyd R, Erickson L, et al: Adrenocortical carcinoma: Surgical progress or status quo? Arch Surg 136:543–549, 2001.

Libè R, Fratticci A, Bertherat J: Adrenocortical cancer: Pathophysiology and clinical management. Endocr Relat Cancer 14:13–28, 2007.

Terzolo M, Angeli A, Fassnacht M, et al: Adjuvant mitotane treatment for adrenocortical carcinoma. N Engl J Med 356:2372–2380, 2007.

Vassilopoulou-Sellin R, Schultz PN: Adrenocortical carcinoma: Clinical outcome at the end of the 20th century. Cancer 92:1113–1121, 2001.

Wajchenberg BL, Albergaria Pereira MA, Medonca BB, et al: Adrenocortical carcinoma: Clinical and laboratory observations. Cancer 88:711–736, 2000.

ON CARCINOIDS

Anthony LB, Kang T, Shyr T: Malignant carcinoid syndrome: Survival in the octreotide era (abstract 4084). J Clin Oncol 23(suppl):328s, 2005.

Goede AC, Winslet MC: Surgery for carcinoid tumours of the lower gastrointestinal tract. Colorectal Dis 5:123–128, 2003.

Kolby L, Persson G, Franzen S, et al: Randomized clinical trial of the effect of interferon alpha on survival in patients with disseminated midgut carcinoid tumours. Br J Surg 90:687–693, 2003.

Krenning EP, de Jong M: Therapeutic use of radiolabelled peptides. Ann Oncol 11(suppl 3):267–271, 2000.

Modlin IM, Lye KD, Kidd M: A 5-decade analysis of 13,715 carcinoid tumors. Cancer 97:934–959, 2003.

Moller JE, Connolly HM, Rubin J, et al: Factors associated with progression of carcinoid heart disease. N Engl J Med 348:1005–1015, 2003.

Schell SR, Camp ER, Caridi JG, et al: Hepatic artery embolization for control of symptoms, octreotide requirements, and tumor progression in metastatic carcinoid tumors. J Gastrointest Surg 6:664–670, 2002.

van der Horst-Schrivers AN, Wymenga AN, de Vries EG: Carcinoid heart disease. N Engl J Med 348:2359–2361, 2003.

ON PHEOCHROMOCYTOMAS

Baghai M, Thompson GB, Young WF Jr, et al: Pheochromocytomas and paragangliomas in von Hippel-Lindau disease: A role for laparoscopic and cortical-sparing surgery. Arch Surg 137:682–689, 2002.

Goldstein RE, O'Neill JA Jr, Holcomb GW III, et al: Clinical experience over 48 years with pheochromocytoma. Ann Surg 229:755–764, 1999.

Lenders JW, Eisenhofer G, Mannelli M, et al: Phaeochromocytoma. Lancet 366:665–675, 2005.

Rose B, Matthay KK, Price D, et al: High-dose 131I-metaiodobenzylguanidine therapy for 12 patients with malignant pheochromocytoma. Cancer 98:239–248, 2003.

Safford SD, Coleman RE, Gockerman JP, et al: Iodine-131 metaiodobenzylguanidine is an effective treatment for malignant pheochromocytoma and paraganglioma. Surgery 134:956–962, 2003; discussion 962–963.

Scholz T, Eisenhofer G, Pacak K, et al: Clinical review: Current treatment of malignant pheochromocytoma. J Clin Endocrinol Metab 92:1217–1225, 2007.

Vaughan ED Jr: Diseases of the adrenal gland. Med Clin North Am 88:443–466, 2004.

Zendron L, Fehrenbach J, Taverna C, et al: Pitfalls in the diagnosis of phaeochromocytoma. Br Med J 13:629–630, 2004.

CHAPTER 15

Liver, gallbladder, and biliary tract cancers

Lawrence D. Wagman, MD, John M. Robertson, MD, and Bert O'Neil, MD

HEPATOCELLULAR CANCER

Hepatocellular carcinoma is one of the most common malignancies in the world, with approximately 1 million new cases recorded annually.

Epidemiology

Gender Hepatocellular carcinoma is the most common tumor in males worldwide, with a male-to-female ratio of 5:1 in Asia and 2:1 in the United States.

Geography Tumor incidence varies significantly, depending on geographic location. In the United States, hepatocellular carcinoma represents < 2% of all tumors, whereas in the Far East and sub-Saharan Africa, this neoplasm occurs at an incidence of 150 per 100,000 population and comprises almost 50% of all diagnosed tumors. A study analyzing SEER (Surveillance, Epidemiology, and End Results) data has shown that the incidence of hepatocellular carcinoma is rising in both white and black populations in the United States, with a current incidence of about 3.4 cases per 100,000 in whites and 5.6 per 100,000 in blacks. Modeling of the spread of hepatitis C virus (HCV) suggests that this number may continue to increase dramatically.

Age The incidence of hepatocellular cancer increases with age. The mean age at diagnosis is 53 years in Asia and 67 years in the United States.

Race The incidence of hepatocellular tumors is higher in Asian immigrants and blacks than in whites.

Survival In patients who undergo curative resection, the 5-year survival rate is approximately 20%–90% depending on initial stage and functional liver status. Recurrence is common, with metastases arising in the remaining liver, lungs, bone, kidneys, and heart. Most patients present with unresectable disease. Patients with unimpaired liver function who can undergo resection may experience significantly longer survival than those whose disease is not resected.

HEPATOBILIARY

Etiology and risk factors

Hepatitis B The close geographic relationship between hepatitis B incidence and hepatocellular carcinoma rates is well recognized. In endemic areas of hepatitis B, approximately 90% of all patients with hepatocellular carcinoma are positive for hepatitis B surface antigen (HBsAg). The presence of the hepatitis B "e" antigen has been found to increase risk ninefold. The most compelling epidemiologic evidence of a causal relationship between hepatitis B infection and hepatocellular carcinoma is the observation of a significant decline in the incidence of childhood hepatocellular carcinoma after the introduction of a national immunization program in Taiwan. The hepatitis B "x" gene, which can interact with *p53*, has been a focus of study on the pathogenesis of hepatocellular carcinoma.

Hepatitis C has also been implicated in hepatocellular carcinoma development. The molecular mechanisms of HCV infection and carcinogenesis are poorly understood. Unlike patients with hepatitis B infection, patients with hepatocellular carcinoma infected with hepatitis C usually have cirrhotic livers at diagnosis; this finding suggests an extended period of infection (or hepatic damage) before malignancy develops.

Alcohol Patients with alcoholic cirrhosis are at risk for hepatocellular carcinoma, but the addition of HCV infection increases that risk dramatically.

Other possible etiologies include aflatoxin, hemochromatosis, hepatic venous obstruction, thorotrast (a contrast agent no longer used for radiologic procedures), androgens, estrogens, and α_1-antitrypsin deficiency.

Prevention A large 5-year randomized study performed in China has confirmed that treatment of chronic hepatitis B infection with the antiviral lamivudine not only decreases the risk of progression to cirrhosis of the liver but also decreases the rate of progression to hepatocellular cancer. Treated patients had a 3.9% risk of hepatocellular cancer over 5 years, compared with 7.4% for those in the placebo group (hazard ratio: 0.49; $P = 0.047$.

Signs and symptoms

Nonspecific symptoms Patients usually present with abdominal pain and other vague symptoms, including malaise, fever, chills, anorexia, weight loss, and jaundice.

Physical findings An abdominal mass is noted on physical examination in one-third of patients. Less common findings include splenomegaly, ascites, abdominal tenderness, muscle wasting, and spider nevi. Up to 10% of patients may present with an acute abdomen due to a ruptured tumor.

Screening and diagnosis

Presently, no organization recommends routine screening of average-risk, asymptomatic adults for liver, gallbladder, and biliary tract cancers.

α-Fetoprotein is produced by 70% of hepatocellular carcinomas. The normal range for this serum marker is 0–20 ng/mL, and a level > 200 ng/mL is essentially diagnostic for hepatocellular cancer in the absence of chronic, active hepatitis B infection. In the presence of active hepatitis B infection, the diagnostic cutoff is considered to be at least 1,000 ng/mL. In the setting of hepatitis C infection, the cutoff for diagnosis of hepatocellular carcinoma has not been well studied. In hepatitis C, values > 200 ng/mL appear to be highly predictive of hepatocellular carcinoma. False-positive results may be due to acute or chronic hepatitis, germ-cell tumors, or pregnancy. In its guidelines for diagnosis of hepatic masses suspicious for hepatocellular carcinomas, the National Comprehensive Cancer Network (NCCN) does not recommend biopsy for patients with an α-fetoprotein level > 400 ng/mL, except in the presence of HBsAg positivity. In that situation, a cutoff value of 4,000 ng/mL is recommended for biopsy.

Hepatitis B and C Given the association between hepatitis B and C and hepatocellular cancer, blood should be sent for hepatitis B and C antigen and antibody determinations.

Imaging The initial diagnostic test in the symptomatic patient may be ultrasonography, as it is noninvasive and can detect lesions as small as 1 cm. Ultrasound findings should be followed up with more specific imaging.

Triple-phase, high-resolution CT and contrast-enhanced MRI are the primary imaging modalities used to diagnose and stage hepatocellular carcinoma. Recent reports have documented a high number of false-positive results with CT angioportography (CTAP) and CT hepatic angiography (CTHA). CT scan predicts resectability in only 40%–50% of cases and does not accurately determine the functional extent of cirrhosis. Major difficulties arise when the liver parenchyma is not homogeneous and the lesions are smaller than 1 cm.

Laparoscopy is useful for the evaluation of small tumors, the extent of cirrhosis, peritoneal seeding, and the volume of noninvolved liver and therefore may be used prior to open laparotomy for resection. Laparoscopic or intraoperative ultrasonography should be used to confirm preoperative imaging tests. The laparoscopic results may change surgical management in up to one-third of selected patients.

High-risk patients should be screened for hepatocellular carcinoma using ultrasonography and serum α-fetoprotein levels. At present, however, there is no standard screening interval, and screening has not been shown to affect survival. Data suggest that, for screened patients, there is an increase in the proportion of cancers that are resectable. A study comparing 6-month and 12-month survival intervals in a cohort of HCV-infected patients with hemophilia showed no substantial benefit to more frequent screening.

TABLE 1: TNM staging of liver and intrahepatic bile duct tumors

Primary tumor (T)

Tx	Primary tumor cannot be assessed
T0	No evidence of primary tumor
TI	Solitary tumor without vascular invasion
T2	Solitary tumor with vascular invasion or multiple tumors (none > 5 cm)
T3	Multiple tumors > 5 cm or tumor involving a major branch of the portal or hepatic vein(s)
T4	Tumor(s) with direct invasion of adjacent organs other than the gallbladder or perforation of the visceral peritoneum

Regional lymph nodes (N)

Nx	Regional lymph nodes cannot be assessed
N0	No regional lymph node metastasis
NI	Regional lymph node metastasis

Distant metastasis (M)

Mx	Distant metastasis cannot be assessed
M0	No distant metastasis
MI	Distant metastasis

Stage grouping

Stage I	TI	N0	M0
Stage II	T2	N0	M0
Stage IIIA	T3	N0	M0
Stage IIIB	T4	N0	M0
Stage IIIC	Any T	NI	M0
Stage IV	Any T	Any N	MI

From Greene FL, Page DL, Fleming ID, et al (eds): AJCC Cancer Staging Manual, 6th ed. New York, Springer-Verlag, 2002.

Pathology

Three morphologic patterns of hepatocellular carcinoma have been described: nodular, diffuse, and massive. Diffuse and massive types account for > 90% of cases. The nodular type usually has multiple lesions in both lobes.

Histologic arrangements Several histologic arrangements have been identified: trabecular, compact, pseudoglandular or acinar, clear cell, and a fibrolamellar variant, which is associated with a relatively favorable prognosis.

Staging and prognosis

The staging system for hepatocellular cancer is based on the number and size of lesions and the presence or absence of vascular invasion (Table 1). The Okuda staging system accounts for the degree of liver dysfunction and may better predict prognosis than the TNM stage. However, the Okuda staging system does not adequately predict resectability. Because of the limited value of standard staging, the most important factors determining survival are technical resectability of lesions and degree of dysfunction of the normal liver. Groups in Spain, Italy, and China have created prognostic indices that may prove useful for making treatment decisions.

Of the 5%–30% of patients who can undergo resection, factors associated with improved survival include curative resection, small tumor size, well-differentiated tumors, and normal performance status. Cirrhosis, nodal metastases, and an elevated prothrombin time are indicative of a poor prognosis, as are male sex, age > 50 years, poor performance status, duration of symptoms < 3 months, tumor rupture, aneuploidy, high DNA synthesis rate, hypocalcemia, vascular invasion, and a high serum α-fetoprotein level.

Treatment

SURGERY

Surgery is the form of treatment that offers the greatest potential for cure, even though only a small minority of patients will actually be cured. Unfortunately, many patients whose disease is thought to be resectable are clinically understaged preoperatively.

Only stage I or II tumors have a significant likelihood of being resectable for cure. However, a large tumor may still be potentially resectable for cure. Moreover, contiguous involvement of large vessels (including the portal vein and inferior vena cava) or bile ducts does not automatically mitigate against a resection, especially in patients with a fibrolamellar histology, although such resections are considerably more difficult.

Bilobar disease may be addressed with formal resection, tumor ablation techniques (eg, cryoablation, radiofrequency ablation, and ethanol injection ablation), or a combination of the two modalities.

Contraindications to resection include imminent clinical hepatic failure (jaundice in the absence of biliary obstruction), hypoalbuminemia, ascites, renal insufficiency, hypoglycemia, prolongation of the prothrombin and partial thromboplastin times, main portal vein involvement, extrahepatic metastatic disease, or other comorbid diseases that would preclude surgery of any kind.

Noncirrhotic vs cirrhotic patients Resection should be performed in all noncirrhotic patients when feasible. Resection of hepatocellular carcinoma in the presence of cirrhosis is more controversial due to its increased morbidity in this setting. Cirrhosis has been a major deterrent to resection in western nations. Resectability rates vary from 0%–43% for cirrhotic patients, whereas up to 60% of patients without cirrhosis undergo resection. Use of the modified Child-Pugh classification of liver reserve may guide the surgeon in preoperative assessment of liver function status and may aid in the selection of operable patients.

When resection is performed in the presence of cirrhosis, Child class A patients fare better than Child class B or C patients. Survival rates at 5 years following resection range from 4% to 36%, with noncirrhotic patients living longer than cirrhotic patients.

Transplantation Owing to the risk of hepatic failure following resection in cirrhotic patients, transplantation has become an option for patients with hepatocellular cancer and cirrhosis. In a study of 181 patients with hepatocellular carcinoma, Starzl and Iwatsuki found similar overall 5-year survival rates in patients treated with transplantation vs resection (36% vs 33%). Survival rates were similar in the two groups when tumors were compared for TNM stage. However, survival was significantly improved in patients with concomitant cirrhosis if they were treated with transplantation. Tumor recurrence rates for stages II and III tumors were significantly lower after transplantation than after resection, but no differences were seen for stage IV tumors.

Patients with cirrhosis and single tumors < 5 cm or multiple tumors (up to 3 with none > 3 cm) can be considered for transplantation. Larger tumors may be treated with resection when feasible. Chemoembolization followed by transplantation may be considered in selected patients. The use of transplantation is significantly limited by the scarcity and lack of immediate availability of donor organs. Recently, changes in the organ allocation system have decreased waiting times for patients with documented hepatocellular cancer.

NON-RESECTIONAL THERAPIES

Given the high risk of recurrence after resection, the multifocal nature of hepatocellular carcinoma, and its association with chronic liver disease, nonresectional therapies can play an important role in management. A number of prognostic factors have been identified for patients with unresectable hepatocellular carcinoma. These factors, taken alone, can have a great effect on survival rates, making cross-treatment comparisons more difficult because considerable selection bias may be present in any nonrandomized trial. Additionally, comparisons are difficult, as there are few randomized trials among the large number of non-resectional, liver-directed therapies currently available.

Radiation therapy

Adjuvant treatment Intrahepatic recurrence has been observed in up to two-thirds of patients treated with partial hepatectomy for hepatocellular carcinoma. Such a recurrence may represent growth at the resected edge, metastatic disease, or a new primary tumor. There is no evidence, however, that adjuvant radiation therapy can reduce this risk.

Unresectable disease Whole-liver radiation therapy can provide palliation in pa-

> A phase I trial of stereotactic radiation therapy in 82 patients with intrahepatic tumors found that doses as high as 60 Gy in 6 fractions could be given successfully. The 32 patients with hepatocellular carcinoma had an in-field response rate of 67% and a median survival of 11 months (Dawson LA, Tse R, Kim J, et al: J Clin Oncol 25[18S]:4590, 2007).

tients with unresectable tumors but is limited to a total dose of ≤ 30 Gy due to the risk of radiation-induced liver disease. Whole-liver irradiation has been combined with chemotherapy and transcatheter arterial chemoembolization, with objective response rates of approximately 40%–50% and median survival rates of about 18 months. Patients with tumor regrowth after chemoembolization may respond to radiotherapy.

Radiation therapy has also been delivered using yttrium-90 microspheres infused via the hepatic artery. This approach has encouraging response rates and a low toxicity profile and may be complementary with other forms of therapy.

Three-dimensional conformal radiation therapy treatment planning can allow patients with nondiffuse disease to be safely irradiated to doses well above the whole-liver tolerance dose, with doses up to 90 Gy given safely to selected patients and a response rate of 40%, with a median survival of 15 months.

Multiple institutions have reported response rates as high as 90% with acceptable toxicity when conformal radiation therapy was combined with transcatheter arterial chemoembolization (TACE). Good response and local control rates have also been reported for proton, carbon ion, and stereotactic radiotherapy.

Hepatic TACE

Normal hepatocytes receive most of their blood supply from the portal vein, whereas tumors create new blood vessels from branches of the hepatic arterial system. This target is exploited by embolization of the hepatic artery with any number of substances, resulting in radiographic response rates in about 50% of patients and evidence of tumor liquefaction in over two-thirds of patients. Embolization is accomplished by advancing a catheter within the tumor-feeding branch of the hepatic artery. Materials injected have included Gelfoam powder, polyvinyl alcohol, iodized oil (Lipiodol), collagen, and autologous blood clot. Chemoembolization should be reserved for symptomatic tumors, reducing tumor size for resection or ablation, or as a bridge while awaiting transplant.

Methodologies for delivering TACE (transcatheter arterial chemoembolization) are numerous. A recent innovation in chemotherapy delivery during TACE is the drug-eluting bead (DEB). These perforated beads allow for slow, localized release of chemotherapy after embolization. In a study by Varela et al, 27 patients with Child-Pugh A liver disease and unresectable hepatocellular cancer underwent DEB-TACE. PK samples were analyzed for doxorubicin, demonstrating lower systemic drug exposure than expected with conventional TACE. Two patients had abscesses, but the radiographic response rate was a promising 75%. Studies of this technology are now being planned and conducted at multiple sites *(Varela M, Real MI, Burrel M, et al: J Hepatol 46:474-481, 2007).*

The effect of TACE on survival remains controversial, with randomized studies returning mixed results. A randomized, controlled trial in Spain was stopped early due to a survival benefit. Meta-analysis of studies does indicate a positive impact on overall survival.

Intratumoral ethanol injection

The direct injection of 95% ethanol into a neoplastic lesion causes cellular dehydration and coagulation necrosis. Intratumoral ethanol ablation is employed via a percutaneous route under ultrasonographic guidance. Percutaneous intratumoral ethanol injection is best suited for use in patients with few lesions, each < 5 cm, although larger lesions may be injected multiple times.

Although intratumoral ethanol injection appears to be an effective palliative modality in certain patients, its effect on patient survival is unclear.

CRYOTHERAPY AND RADIOFREQUENCY ABLATION

Similar to ethanol ablation, cryotherapy and radiofrequency ablation (RFA) techniques are suitable for treatment of localized disease. Cryotherapy has been used intraoperatively to ablate small solitary tumors outside a planned resection (ie, in patients with bilobar disease). Cryotherapy must be performed using laparotomy, which limits its use in the palliative setting. RFA can be performed either via laparotomy or percutaneously and has limitations similar to those of ethanol ablation. As with ethanol ablation, there are no data about a survival advantage with these therapies, which may prove to be most useful for temporary tumor control in patients awaiting liver transplants. A randomized trial comparing RFA with ethanol injection found a significant benefit to RFA for local recurrence-free survival (96% vs 62% at 2 years) but not for overall survival (98% vs 88%).

A cautionary note regarding percutaneous RFA has been raised by publication of a report from Barcelona, citing 4 of 32 patients in a series who developed needle-track tumor seeding relating to subcapsular tumor location and poorly differentiated tumors.

Chemotherapy

Systemically administered chemotherapy has, for the most part, been disappointing in patients with hepatocellular carcinoma. This fact relates to both low rates of response to available agents and to difficulty with toxicity for modestly active agents because of liver dysfunction. Agents with partial response rates near or above 10% include doxorubicin, fluorouracil (5-FU), and cisplatin. Two newer agents, oxaliplatin (Eloxatin) and gemcitabine (Gemzar), which do not require liver metabolism or excretion, have garnered some interest. Both agents appear to be more active when partnered with a second agent, but results from phase II combination studies are mixed.

Hepatic arterial infusion (HAI) Use of HAI, principally floxuridine (fluorodeoxyuridine [FUDR]), has good biologic rationale but is hampered by high rates of biliary complications and the requirement for surgical pump placement in patients who are generally poor surgical candidates. A meta-analysis concluded that HAI after curative liver resection improved survival significantly at both 2 (23% benefit) and 3 (28% benefit) years.

Biologic therapy Interferon-alpha (IFN-α) has been shown to have potential beneficial effects in prevention of hepatocellular carcinoma; however, recent randomized studies have failed to show a benefit in patients with pre-existing cirrhosis and advanced cancers. Adjuvant interferon, however, was associated with a reduction in recurrence in two small randomized trials. This finding needs to be confirmed in a much larger trial. Moderate-to-high doses of interferon are poorly tolerated by patients with frankly cirrhotic livers.

Biochemotherapy Results of combination biochemotherapy in a study of 154 patients by Leung et al were encouraging. Using a combination of cisplatin, interferon-α-2a (Roferon-A), doxorubicin, and 5-FU for 4 days out of 28 days, resulted in a response rate of around 20%. Moreover, 10% of patients whose tumors were initially thought to be unresectable subsequently underwent complete resection. Eight of these patients had documented pathologic complete re-

Based on promising phase II data from the SHARP study, a trial comparing sorafenib (Nexavar: 400 mg PO bid) versus placebo in patients with advanced or metastatic hepatocellular cancer was presented at the 2007 ASCO meeting. Patients enrolled in this study were required to have Child-Pugh A liver disease. About one-third of the patients had undergone embolization and the disease progressed. A total of 70% of patients had portal vein thrombosis, metastatic disease, or both. In spite of a low radiographic response rate (only 2% of tumors responded by radiographic criteria), median survival for the 300 patients who received sorafenib was significantly better than that for the placebo group (10.7 vs 7.9 months). This is the first well-powered trial to convincingly demonstrate a survival benefit associated with a systemic agent for this disease *(Llovet J, Ricci S, Mazzaferro V, et al: J Clin Oncol 25 [18S]:LBA1, 2007).*

Due to the extensive vascularity of many hepatocellular cancers (HCCs), bevacizumab (Avastin) has seemed a perfect drug candidate for study in this disease. Two small single-agent studies of bevacizumab demonstrated apparent activity with tumor responses by RECIST criteria. HCC also expresses significant amounts of epidermal growth factor receptor. Single-agent erlotinib (Tarceva) produced few responses but promising survival in one (but not another) single-agent trial. At ASCO 2007, data were presented for a combination of bevacizumab and erlotinib, which resulted in an interesting 20% radiographic response rate and preliminary overall survival of 19 months (almost certain to be less with further follow-up, but promising nonetheless). A phase III study of this combination against sorafenib (Nexavar) is planned *(Thomas MB, Chadha R, Iwasaki M, et al: J Clin Oncol 25[18S]:4567, 2007).*

. missions. A phase III study of PIAF (cisplatin [Platinol]/interferon-α-2b/doxorubicin[Adriamycin]/5-FU) versus single-agent doxorubicin has confirmed a higher response rate for PIAF, but survival was not significantly better than with doxorubicin. Of note, all patients in this series had hepatitis B-associated hepatocellular carcinoma. Patt et al have studied a less-toxic regimen of continuous 5-FU with interferon-α-2b, demonstrating a median survival of 15.5 months.

Targeted therapies

A group led by Philip at Karmanos Cancer Institute has reported results of a phase II trial of the epidermal growth factor receptor (EGFR)-targeting agent erlotinib (Tarceva) in HCC and biliary tumors. Erlotinib was administered orally, 150 mg daily, to 35 patients with HCC. The response rate was only 9%, but OS for the group was an encouraging 13 months.

Sorafenib (Nexavar), an inhibitor of RAF and VEGF kinases, was recently demonstrated to be the first systemic agent to convinicingly improve survival in a placebo-controlled randomized study. This now represents standard of care for patients with advanced disease that is not amenable to locoregional therapy such as embolization. Studies in conjunction with embolization are already underway. The drug is the first approved for this indication by the FDA.

BILIARY TRACT CANCERS

Gallbladder carcinoma is diagnosed approximately 5,000 times a year in the United States, making it the most common biliary tract tumor and the fifth most common GI tract cancer. Approximately 4,500 cases of bile duct tumors occur each year in the United States.

Epidemiology

GALLBLADDER CANCER

Gender Women are more commonly afflicted with gallbladder cancer than are men, with a female-to-male ratio of 1.7:1.

Age The median age at presentation of gallbladder cancer is 73 years.

Race An incidence five to six times that of the general population is seen in southwestern Native Americans, Hispanics, and Alaskans.

BILE DUCT CANCER

Gender Bile duct tumors are found in an equal number of men and women.

Age Extrahepatic bile duct tumors occur primarily in older individuals; the median age at diagnosis is 70 years.

Etiology and risk factors

GALLBLADDER CANCER

The risk of developing gallbladder cancer is higher in patients with cholelithiasis or calcified gallbladders and in typhoid carriers.

BILE DUCT CANCER

Ulcerative colitis is a clear risk factor for bile duct tumors. Patients with ulcerative colitis have an incidence of bile duct cancer that is 9-21 times higher than that of the general population. This risk does not decline after total colectomy for ulcerative colitis.

Other risk factors Primary sclerosing cholangitis, congenital anomalies of the pancreaticobiliary tree, and parasitic infections are also associated with bile duct tumors. No association of bile duct cancer with calculi, infection, or chronic obstruction has been found.

Signs and symptoms

GALLBLADDER CANCER

Early disease In the early stages, gallbladder cancer is usually asymptomatic.

Late disease Later, symptoms similar to those of benign gallbladder disease arise; they include right upper quadrant pain, nausea, vomiting, fatty food intolerance, anorexia, jaundice, and weight loss. This nonspecificity of symptoms delays presentation for medical attention and contributes to the low curability of gallbladder cancer.

Physical findings may include tenderness, an abdominal mass, hepatomegaly, jaundice, fever, and ascites.

BILE DUCT CANCER

Jaundice is the most frequent symptom found in patients with high bile duct tumors; it is present in up to 98% of such patients.

Nonspecific signs and symptoms Patients who do not present with jaundice have vague complaints, including abdominal pain, weight loss, pruritus, fever, and an abdominal mass.

Diagnosis

GALLBLADDER CANCER

Gallbladder carcinomas are often diagnosed at an advanced stage, such that by the time symptoms have developed, most tumors are unresectable.

Laboratory values in patients with gallbladder carcinoma are nonspecific but may include anemia, leukocytosis, and an elevated bilirubin level.

TABLE 2: TNM staging of gallbladder cancer

Primary tumor (T)

Tx		Primary tumor cannot be assessed
T0		No evidence of primary tumor
Tis		Carcinoma in situ
TI		Tumor invades the lamina propria or muscle layer
	TIa	Tumor invades the lamina propria
	TIb	Tumor invades the muscle layer
T2		Tumor invades perimuscular connective tissue; no extension beyond the serosa or into the liver
T3		Tumor perforates the serosa (visceral peritoneum) and/or directly invades the liver and/or one other adjacent organ or structure, such as the stomach, duodenum, colon, pancreas, omentum, or extrahepatic bile ducts
T4		Tumor invades the main portal vein or hepatic artery or invades two or more extrahepatic organs or structures

Regional lymph nodes (N)

Nx	Regional lymph nodes cannot be assessed
N0	No regional lymph node metastasis
NI	Regional lymph node metastasis

Distant metastasis (M)

Mx	Distant metastasis cannot be assessed
M0	No distant metastasis
MI	Distant metastasis

Stage grouping

Stage 0	Tis	N0	M0
Stage IA	TI	N0	M0
Stage IB	T2	N0	M0
Stage IIA	T3	N0	M0
Stage IIB	TI	NI	M0
	T2	NI	M0
	T3	NI	M0
Stage III	T4	Any N	M0
Stage IV	Any T	Any N	MI

From Greene FL, Page DL, Fleming ID, et al (eds): AJCC Cancer Staging Manual, 6th ed. New York, Springer-Verlag, 2002.

Ultrasonography is useful for defining a thickened gallbladder wall and may show tumor extension into the liver.

CT is more helpful than ultrasonography in assessing adenopathy and spread of disease into the liver, porta hepatis, or adjacent structures. MRI may be used to evaluate intrahepatic spread.

Endoscopic retrograde cholangiopancreatography (ERCP) or transhepatic cholangiography (THC) may be useful in the presence of

TABLE 3: Staging of bile duct tumors

Primary tumor (T)

Tx	Primary tumor cannot be assessed
T0	No evidence of primary tumor
T1	Tumor confined to the bile duct histologically
T2	Tumor invades beyond the wall of the bile duct
T3	Tumor invades the liver, gallbladder, pancreas, and/or ipsilateral branches of the portal vein (right or left) or hepatic artery (right or left)
T4	Tumor invades any of the following sites: main portal vein or its branches bilaterally; common hepatic artery; or other adjacent structures, such as the colon, stomach, duodenum, or abdominal wall

Regional lymph nodes (N)

Nx	Regional lymph nodes cannot be assessed
N0	No regional lymph node metastasis
N1	Regional lymph node metastasis

Distant metastasis (M)

Mx	Distant metastasis cannot be assessed
M0	No distant metastasis
M1	Distant metastasis

Stage grouping

Stage 0	Tis	N0	M0
Stage IA	T1	N0	M0
Stage IB	T2	N0	M0
Stage IIA	T3	N0	M0
Stage IIB	T1	N1	M0
	T2	N1	M0
	T3	N1	M0
Stage III	T4	Any N	M0
Stage IV	Any T	Any N	M1

From Greene FL, Page DL, Fleming ID, et al (eds): AJCC Cancer Staging Manual, 6th ed. New York, Springer-Verlag, 2002.

jaundice to determine the location of biliary obstruction and involvement of the liver.

BILE DUCT CANCER

Cholangiocarcinoma may present earlier than gallbladder cancer by virtue of the development of biliary obstruction with jaundice, which may be painless. Tissue confirmation of suspected bile duct cancer can be difficult. The goals of the diagnostic evaluation include the determination of the level and extent of obstruction, the extent of local invasion of disease, and the identification of metastases.

Many patients with cholangiocarcinoma are thought to have metastatic adenocarcinoma of an unknown primary, although occasionally the metastatic lesion may produce biliary dilatation without the primary lesion itself being radiographically visualized.

Ultrasonography It is generally accepted that ultrasonography should be the first imaging procedure in the evaluation of the jaundiced patient.

CT is a complementary test to ultrasonography, but both tests are accurate for staging in only 50% of patients and for determining resectability in < 45% of patients.

Cholangiography is essential to determine the location and nature of the obstruction. Percutaneous THC is used for proximal lesions, and ERCP is used for distal lesions. Magnetic resonance cholangiopancreatography (MRCP) may replace invasive studies in the near future. Histologic confirmation of tumor can be made in 45%–85% of patients with the use of exfoliative or brush cytology during cholangiography.

Pathology

GALLBLADDER CANCER

Histologic types Over 85% of gallbladder neoplasms are adenocarcinomas and the remaining 15% are squamous cell or mixed tumors.

Route of spread The initial route of spread of gallbladder cancer is locoregional rather than distant. For patients undergoing resection for presumed high-risk gallbladder masses or preoperatively defined disease limited to the gallbladder, 25% of patients will have lymphatic involvement and 70% will have direct extension of disease into the liver defined at operation.

BILE DUCT CANCER

Adenocarcinoma Morphologically, more than 90% of bile duct tumors are adenocarcinomas. Three macroscopic appearances have been identified: The papillary and nodular types occur more frequently in the distal bile duct, whereas the sclerosing type is found in the proximal bile duct. Patients with papillary lesions have the best prognosis.

Other histologic types Unusual malignant diseases of the biliary tract include adenosquamous carcinoma, leiomyosarcoma, and mucoepidermoid carcinoma.

Route of spread Most bile duct tumors grow slowly, spreading frequently by local extension and rarely by the hematogenous route. Nodal metastases are found in up to one-third of patients.

Staging and prognosis

GALLBLADDER CANCER

Gallbladder cancer is staged primarily at the time of surgery, and staging is determined by lymphatic involvement and extension of disease into adjacent structures (Table 2).

Stage Survival of gallbladder carcinoma is directly related to disease stage. The 5-year survival rate is 83% for tumors that are confined to the gallbladder mucosa; this rate decreases to 33% if the tumor extends through the gallbladder. For patients who have involvement of the lymph nodes or metastatic disease, 5-year survival rates range from 0%–15%.

Type of therapy Median survival is also improved in patients who have undergone curative resection, as compared with those who have had palliative procedures or no surgery (17 months vs 6 and 3 months, respectively).

BILE DUCT CANCER

Over 70% of patients with cholangiocarcinoma present with local extension, lymph node involvement, or distant spread of disease. The AJCC (American Joint Committee on Cancer) staging system for extrahepatic tumors is shown in Table 3.

Stage Survival for these patients is poor and is directly related to disease stage. Median survival is 12–20 months for patients with disease limited to the bile ducts and ≤ 8 months when the disease has spread.

Tumor location Survival is also related to tumor location, with patients with distal lesions doing better than those with mid or proximal tumors.

Success of therapy Curative resection and negative margins result in improved survival.

Treatment

In the absence of polyps identified ultrasonographically and confirmed by CT during the work-up of suspected cholelithiasas, relatively few patients with gallbladder cancer are diagnosed prior to surgery. Only 1%–2% of cholecystectomy specimens are found to contain malignancy.

SURGERY FOR GALLBLADDER CANCER

Surgical management of gallbladder carcinoma is based on the local extension of the tumor.

Early-stage disease Tumors that invade the mucosa, those that do not penetrate the muscularis, and those that penetrate full thickness but do not abut the liver or muscularis require cholecystectomy alone. Laparoscopic cholecystectomy may be adequate for T1 tumors. If there is direct extension of disease to or through the serosa, the resection should include the gallbladder bed (segments IVb and V) and a porta hepatis lymphadenectomy. Disease that involves the gallbladder node is particularly curable and should be resected. Nodal disease beyond the pericholedochal (porta hepatis) nodes defines the surgically incurable patient.

SURGERY FOR BILE DUCT CANCER

The rate of resectability is 15%–20% for high bile duct tumors and up to 70% for distal lesions.

Assessing resectability Higher resolution CT or MRI with biliary reconstruction may be supplemented with hepatic arteriography, portal venography, or duplex imaging preoperatively to assess resectability.

Preoperative treatments Three randomized trials have shown no benefit to preoperative decompression of the biliary tree in patients with obstructive jaundice. Some authors advocate the preoperative placement of biliary stents to facilitate dissection of the hilus. This procedure should be performed close to the planned resection to reduce the risk of cholangitis and maintain the duct at its maximally dilated size.

Proximal tumors Local excision is often possible for proximal lesions. Hepatic resection is indicated for high bile duct tumors. Resection is not indicated in situations in which a clear surgical margin cannot be obtained.

Mid-ductal and distal tumors Mid-ductal lesions can often be removed by resection of the bile duct with associated portal lymphadenectomy. Distal or mid-ductal lesions that cannot be locally excised should be removed by pancreaticoduodenectomy.

Reconstruction techniques Biliary-enteric continuity is usually reconstructed with a Roux-en-Y anastomosis to the hilum for high lesions and in a standard drainage pattern following pancreaticoduodenectomy.

Liver transplantation has been attempted for unresectable tumors, but early recurrence and poor survival have prevented the widespread application of this approach.

Surgical bypass For patients found to have unresectable disease at surgical exploration, operative biliary bypass may be performed using a variety of techniques. Bypass results in excellent palliation and obviates the need for further intervention.

ADJUVANT RADIATION THERAPY FOR BILIARY TRACT CANCER

A review of the patterns of initial disease recurrence after resection of gallbladder cancer (80 patients, in whom disease recurred in 53) and hilar cholangiocarcinoma (76 patients, in whom disease recurred in 52) found a distinct difference with regard to total locoregional failure versus total distant failure. Hilar cholangiocarcinomas were much more likely to include locoregional failure alone or as a component (65% of all failures), compared with gallbladder cancer (28% of all failures). Distant failure was found alone or as a component in 72% of all recurrences of gallbladder cancer but only in 36% of hilar cholangiocarcinomas.

ADJUVANT CHEMOTHERAPY

A randomized trial performed in Japan showed that treatment with 5-FU and mitomycin (Mutamycin) produced a survival benefit in patients with resected gallbladder cancers. These data came from a planned subset of a larger trial in which 112 patients with gallbladder cancer were randomized. At 5 years, 26% of chemotherapy-treated patients were alive, compared with 14% of those treated with surgery and observation alone. Based on these data, consideration of chemotherapy for these patients is warranted, but definitive conclusions would require a larger randomized trial.

TREATMENT OF UNRESECTABLE DISEASE

Like pancreatic adenocarcinoma, unresectable biliary tract carcinoma has a poor prognosis.

Stenting

Many patients with unresectable disease, particularly those with pain, nausea, or pruritus, will benefit from nonsurgical percutaneous or endoscopic stenting.

Radiation therapy

There are few data on radiation therapy for unresectable gallbladder cancer, other than reports of intraoperative radiation therapy. External-beam radiation therapy would be anticipated to provide a palliative benefit.

There is considerable experience using brachytherapy alone or combined with external-beam radiation therapy for unresectable bile duct tumors. Median survival ranges from 10–24 months, and 5-year survival rates are approximately 10% with these approaches. Cholangitis, however, may occur more frequently in people treated with brachytherapy. A randomized trial of stenting alone versus with photodynamic therapy (PDT) found a significantly longer median survival and improved quality of life in the PDT group. Although it is unlikely that all of the tumor was treated with PDT, this study did show the importance of local control and its association with quality of life. Radiation therapy may also ultimately play a role in the promotion of viral replication for gene therapy.

Chemotherapy

Because biliary tract malignancies are uncommon cancers, the number of clinical trials and the number of patients in those trials are limited. Generally speaking, responses to chemotherapy are infrequent and brief. However, newer drugs and drug combinations are better tolerated and stand to improve on past results.

5-FU has historically been the most active single agent, with single-agent response rates in the 10%–20% range.

Capecitabine (Xeloda), a prodrug of 5-FU (see chapter 16), produced responses in 4 of 8 gallbladder cancers but in only 1 of 18 cholangiocarcinomas in a phase II study presented by Hassan et al from M. D. Anderson Cancer Center.

The role of adjuvant radiation therapy for biliary disease has not been studied in a randomized trial; however, there is some evidence that a role may be present. A review of 3,187 cases of gallbladder cancer recorded in the Surveillance, Epidemiology, and End Results survey from the National Cancer Institute found that, despite a higher stage, patients treated with adjuvant radiation therapy demonstrated a longer median survival than those who were treated with resection only (14 vs 8 months; *P* < .0001). On subgroup analysis, this benefit was most evident for patients with involved regional lymph nodes or liver invasion *(Mojica P, Smith D, Ellenhorn J: J Surg Oncol 96:8-13, 2007)*. A Cox proportional hazards survival analysis was applied to 75 consecutive patients with hilar cholangiocarcinoma treated surgically with curative intent. It found that the most powerful predictors of outcome (in descending order) were resection type, adjuvant radiation therapy, regional lymph node involvement, and preoperative maximum serum total bilirubin *(Cheng Q, Luo X, Zhang B, et al: Eur J Surg Oncol 33:202-207, 2007)*.

Gemcitabine Multiple studies have documented gemcitabine as an active agent, particularly in gallbladder cancer. Cisplatin and gemcitabine may be a synergistic doublet, with reported response rates for gallbladder cancer in the range of 30%–50%.

Combination chemotherapy with both 5-FU and gemcitabine (Gemzar) have modest activity in biliary malignancies. A group in Toronto published results of combination therapy with capecitabine (Xeloda) and gemcitabine. The mix of cholangiocarcinoma and gallbladder cancer in the 45 patients studied was nearly 50:50. The overall response rate was 31%, and the median survival was a promising 14 months. This regimen is a reasonable alternative to gemcitabine and cisplatin for biliary tract neoplasms.

Hepatic arterial chemotherapy There is limited experience with hepatic arterial chemotherapy for biliary tract neoplasms, but there are case reports of responses to floxuridine in the literature.

Treatment recommendations In the absence of a clinical trial, patients should be offered gemcitabine and/or 5-FU (or capecitabine), with or without leucovorin. Other agents, such as doxorubicin or cisplatin, may be added, but, as noted, there is no unequivocal evidence that combination chemotherapy produces any substantial benefits in improving quality of life or survival.

SUGGESTED READING

ON HEPATOCELLULAR CARCINOMA

Ben-Josef E, Normolle D, Ensminger WD, et al: Phase II trial of high-dose conformal radiation therapy with concurrent hepatic artery floxuridine for unresectable intrahepatic malignancies. J Clin Oncol 23:8739–8747, 2005.

Gupta S, Bent S, Kohlwes J: Test characteristics of alpha-fetoprotein for detecting hepatocellular carcinoma in patients with hepatitis C: A systematic review and critical analysis. Ann Intern Med 139:46–50, 2003.

Hashimoto T, Tokuuye K, Fukumitsu N, et al: Repeated proton beam therapy for hepatocellular carcinoma. Int J Radiat Oncol Biol Phys 65:196–202, 2006.

Llovet J, Bruix J: Systematic review of randomized trials for unresectable hepatocellular carcinoma: Chemoembolization improves survival. Hepatology 37:429–442, 2003.

Mathurin P, Raynard B, Dharancy S, et al: Meta-analysis: Evaluation of adjuvant therapy after curative liver resection for hepatocellular carcinoma. Aliment Pharmacol Ther 17:1247–1261, 2003.

Mok TS, Yeo W, Yu S, et al: An intensive surveillance program detected a high incidence of hepatocellular carcinoma among hepatitis B virus carriers with abnormal alpha-fetoprotein levels or abdominal ultrasonography results. J Clin Oncol 23:8041–8047, 2005.

Yao FY, Bass NM, Ascher NL, et al: Liver transplantation for hepatocellular carcinoma: Lessons from the first year under the Model of End-Stage Liver Disease (MELD) organ allocation policy. Liver Transpl 10:621–630, 2004.

Yeo W, Mok TS, Zee B, et al: A randomized phase III study of doxorubicin versus cisplatin/interferon alpha-2b/doxorubicin/fluorouracil (PIAF) combination chemotherapy for unresectable heaptocellular carcinoma. J Natl Cancer Inst 97:1532–1538, 2005.

ON GALLBLADDER TUMORS

Doval DC, Sekhon JS, Gupta SK, et al: A phase II study of gemcitabine and cisplatin in chemotherapy-naive, unresectable gall bladder cancer. Br J Cancer 90:1516–1520, 2004.

Jarnagin WR, Ruo L, Little SA, et al: Patterns of initial disease recurrence after resection of gallbladder carcinoma and hilar cholangiocarcinoma: Implications of adjuvant therapeutic strategies. Cancer 98:1689–1700, 2003.

Mojica P, Smith D, Ellenhorn J: Adjuvant radiation therapy is associated with improved survival for gallbladder carcinoma with regional metastatic disease. J Surg Oncol 96:8–13, 2007.

Patt YZ, Hassan MM, Aguayo A, et al: Oral capecitabine for the treatment of hepatocellular carcinoma, cholangiocarcinoma, and gallbladder carcinoma. Cancer 101:578–586, 2004.

Takada T, Amano H, Yasuda H, et al: Is postoperative adjuvant chemotherapy useful for gallbladder carcinoma? A phase III multicenter prospective randomized controlled trial in patients with resected pancreaticobiliary carcinoma. Cancer 95:1685–1695, 2002.

ON BILE DUCT TUMORS

Alberts SR, Al-Khatib H, Mahoney MR, et al: Gemcitabine, 5-fluorouracil, and leucovorin in advanced biliary tract and gallbladder carcinoma: A North Central Cancer Treatment Group phase II trial. Cancer 103:111–118, 2005.

Ben-David MA, Griffith KA, Abu-Isa E, et al: External-beam radiotherapy for localized extrahepatic cholangiocarcinoma. Int J Radiat Oncol Biol Phys 66:772–779, 2006.

Cheng Q, Luo X, Zhang B, et al: Predictive factors for prognosis of hilar cholangiocarcinoma: Postresection radiotherapy improves survival. Eur J Surg Oncol 33:202–207, 2007.

Knox JJ, Hedley D, Oza A, et al: Combining gemcitabine and capecitabine in patients with advanced biliary cancer: A phase II trial. J Clin Oncol 23:2332–2338, 2005.

Rea DJ, Heimbach JK, Rosen CB, et al: Liver transplantation with neoadjuvant chemoradiation is more effective than resection for hilar cholangiocarcinoma. Ann Surg 242:451–461, 2005.

For previously untreated diffuse large B-cell, CD20-positive NHL in combination with CHOP or other anthracycline-based chemotherapy regimens

When planning a treatment course for DLBCL

Take the essential path toward improved survival

RITUXAN+CHOP is proven to prolong survival in DLBCL

47% INCREASE
in 7-year OS in GELA* trial[1,2]

R-CHOP (n=202)
CHOP† (n=197)
p=0.0004

Cumulative Proportion Surviving
Years

- At 7 years, 8 cycles of RITUXAN+ CHOP increased overall survival (OS) from 36% to 53% compared with CHOP alone[1]

- At 5 years, 8 cycles of RITUXAN+ CHOP increased OS from 46% to 58% compared with CHOP alone[5]

RITUXAN® (Rituximab) Brief summary—Please consult full prescribing information.

> **WARNING: FATAL INFUSION REACTIONS, TUMOR LYSIS SYNDROME (TLS), SEVERE MUCOCUTANEOUS REACTIONS, and PROGRESSIVE MULTIFOCAL LEUKOENCEPHALOPATHY (PML)**
> **Infusion Reactions:** Rituxan administration can result in serious, including fatal infusion reactions. Deaths within 24 hours of Rituxan infusion have occurred. Approximately 80% of fatal infusion reactions occurred in association with the first infusion. Carefully monitor patients during infusions. Discontinue Rituxan infusion and provide medical treatment for Grade 3 or 4 infusion reactions [*see Warnings and Precautions, Adverse Reactions*].
> **Tumor Lysis Syndrome (TLS):** Acute renal failure requiring dialysis with instances of fatal outcome can occur in the setting of TLS following treatment of non-Hodgkin's lymphoma (NHL) patients with Rituxan [*see Warnings and Precautions, Adverse Reactions*].
> **Severe Mucocutaneous Reactions:** Severe, including fatal, mucocutaneous reactions can occur in patients receiving Rituxan [*see Warnings and Precautions, Adverse Reactions*]. Progressive Multifocal Leukoencephalopathy (PML): JC virus infection resulting in PML and death can occur in patients receiving Rituxan [*see Warnings and Precautions, Adverse Reactions*].

INDICATIONS AND USAGE Non-Hodgkin's Lymphoma (NHL) Rituxan® (rituximab) is indicated for the treatment of patients with: Relapsed or refractory, low-grade or follicular, CD20-positive, B-cell NHL as a single agent; Previously untreated follicular, CD20-positive, B-cell NHL in combination with CVP chemotherapy; Non-progressing (including stable disease), low-grade, CD20-positive B-cell NHL, as a single agent, after first-line CVP chemotherapy; Previously untreated diffuse large B-cell, CD20-positive NHL in combination with CHOP or other anthracycline-based chemotherapy regimens. **WARNINGS AND PRECAUTIONS Infusion Reactions** Rituxan can cause severe, including fatal, infusion reactions. Severe reactions typically occurred during the first infusion with time to onset of 30–120 minutes. Rituxan-induced infusion reactions and sequelae include urticaria, hypotension, angioedema, hypoxia, bronchospasm, pulmonary infiltrates, acute respiratory distress syndrome, myocardial infarction, ventricular fibrillation, cardiogenic shock, or anaphylactoid events. Premedicate patients with an antihistamine and acetaminophen prior to dosing. Institute medical management (e.g., glucocorticoids, epinephrine, bronchodilators, or oxygen) for infusion reactions as needed. Depending on the severity of the infusion reaction and the required interventions, consider resumption of the infusion at a minimum 50% reduction in rate after symptoms have resolved. Closely monitor the following patients: those with preexisting cardiac or pulmonary conditions, those who experienced prior cardiopulmonary adverse reactions, and those with high numbers of circulating malignant cells (≥25,000/mm³). [*See Boxed Warning, Warnings and Precautions, Adverse Reactions.*] **Tumor Lysis Syndrome (TLS)** Rapid reduction in tumor volume followed by acute renal failure, hyperkalemia, hypocalcemia, hyperuricemia, or hyperphosphatemia, can occur within 12–24 hours after the first infusion. Fatal TLS cases have occurred after administration of Rituxan. A high number of circulating malignant cells (≥25,000/mm³) or high tumor burden confers a greater risk of TLS after rituximab. Consider prophylaxis for TLS in patients at high risk. Correct electrolyte abnormalities, monitor renal function and fluid balance, and administer supportive care, including dialysis as indicated. [*See Boxed Warning.*] **Severe Mucocutaneous Reactions** Mucocutaneous reactions, some with fatal outcome, can occur in patients treated with Rituxan. These reactions include paraneoplastic pemphigus, Stevens-Johnson syndrome, lichenoid dermatitis, vesiculobullous dermatitis, and toxic epidermal necrolysis. The onset of these reactions has varied from 1–13 weeks following Rituxan exposure. Discontinue Rituxan in patients who experience a severe mucocutaneous reaction. The safety of readministration of Rituxan to patients with severe mucocutaneous reactions has not been determined. [*See Boxed Warning, Adverse Reactions.*] **Progressive Multifocal Leukoencephalopathy (PML)** JC virus infection resulting in PML and death can occur in Rituxan-treated patients with hematologic malignancies or with autoimmune diseases. The majority of patients with hematologic malignancies diagnosed with PML received Rituxan in combination with chemotherapy or as part of a hematopoietic stem cell transplant. The patients with autoimmune diseases had prior or concurrent immunosuppressive therapy. Most cases of PML were diagnosed within 12 months of their last infusion of Rituxan. Consider the diagnosis of PML in any patient presenting with new-onset neurologic manifestations. Discontinue Rituxan and consider discontinuation or reduction of any concomitant chemotherapy or immunosuppressive therapy in patients who develop PML. [*See Boxed Warning, Adverse Reactions.*] **Hepatitis B Virus (HBV) Reactivation** Hepatitis B Virus (HBV) reactivation with fulminant hepatitis, hepatic failure, and death can occur in patients with hematologic malignancies treated with Rituxan. The median time to the diagnosis of hepatitis was approximately 4 months after the initiation of Rituxan and approximately one month after the last dose. Screen patients at high risk of HBV infection before initiation of Rituxan. Closely monitor carriers of hepatitis B for clinical and laboratory signs of active HBV infection for several months following Rituxan therapy. Discontinue Rituxan and any concomitant chemotherapy in patients who develop viral hepatitis, and institute appropriate treatment including antiviral therapy. Insufficient data exist regarding the safety of resuming Rituxan in patients who develop hepatitis subsequent to HBV reactivation. [*See Adverse Reactions.*] **Other Viral Infections** The following additional serious viral infections, either new, reactivated, or exacerbated, have been identified in clinical studies or postmarketing reports. The majority of patients received Rituxan in combination with chemotherapy or as part of a hematopoietic stem cell transplant. These viral infections included cytomegalovirus, herpes simplex virus, parvovirus B19, varicella zoster virus, West Nile virus, and hepatitis C. In some cases, the viral infections occurred as late as one year following discontinuation of Rituxan and have resulted in death. [*See Adverse Reactions.*] **Cardiovascular** Discontinue infusions for serious or life-threatening cardiac arrhythmias. Perform cardiac monitoring during and after all infusions of Rituxan for patients who develop clinically significant arrhythmias or who have a history of arrhythmia or angina. [*See Adverse Reactions.*] **Renal** Severe, including fatal, renal toxicity can occur after Rituxan administration in patients with hematologic malignancies. Renal toxicity has occurred in patients with high numbers of circulating malignant cells (≥25,000/mm³) or high tumor burden who experience tumor lysis syndrome and in patients with NHL administered concomitant cisplatin therapy during clinical trials. The combination of cisplatin and Rituxan is not an approved treatment regimen. Use extreme caution if this non-approved combination is used in clinical trials and monitor closely for signs of renal failure. Consider discontinuation of Rituxan for patients with a rising serum creatinine or oliguria. **Bowel Obstruction and Perforation** Abdominal pain, bowel obstruction and perforation, in some cases leading to death, can occur in patients receiving Rituxan in combination with chemotherapy. In postmarketing reports, the mean time to documented gastrointestinal perforation was 6 (range 1–77) days in patients with NHL. Perform a thorough diagnostic evaluation and institute appropriate treatment for complaints of abdominal pain, especially early in the course of Rituxan therapy. [*See Adverse Reactions.*] **Immunization** The safety of immunization with live viral vaccines following Rituxan therapy has not been studied and vaccination with live virus vaccines is not recommended. For NHL patients, the benefits of primary or booster vaccinations should be weighted against the risks of delay in initiation of Rituxan therapy. **Laboratory Monitoring** Because Rituxan binds to all CD20-positive B lymphocytes (malignant and non-malignant), obtain complete blood counts (CBC) and platelet counts at regular intervals during Rituxan therapy and more frequently in patients who develop cytopenias [*see Adverse Reactions*]. The duration of cytopenias caused by Rituxan can extend months beyond the treatment period. **ADVERSE REACTIONS** The most common adverse reactions of Rituxan (incidence ≥25%) observed in patients with NHL are infusion reactions, fever, chills, infection, asthenia, and lymphopenia. The most important serious adverse reactions of Rituxan are infusion reactions, tumor lysis syndrome, mucocutaneous toxicities, hepatitis B reactivation with fulminant hepatitis, PML, other viral infections, cardiac arrhythmias, renal toxicity, and bowel obstruction and perforation. **Clinical Trials Experience Non-Hodgkin's Lymphoma** Because clinical trials are conducted under widely varying conditions, adverse reaction rates observed in the clinical trials of a drug cannot be directly compared to rates in the clinical trials of another drug and may not reflect the rates observed in practice. The data described below reflect exposure to Rituxan in 1606 patients, with exposures ranging from a single infusion up to 6–8 months. Rituxan was studied in both single-agent and active-controlled trials (n = 356 and n = 1250). These data were obtained in adults with low-grade, follicular, or DLBCL NHL. Most patients received Rituxan as an infusion of 375 mg/m² per infusion, given as a single agent weekly for up to 8 doses, in combination with chemotherapy for up to 8 doses, or following chemotherapy for up to 16 doses. **Infusion Reactions** In the majority of patients with NHL, infusion reactions consisting of fever, chills/rigors, nausea, pruritus, angioedema, hypotension, headache, bronchospasm, urticaria, rash, vomiting, myalgia, dizziness, or hypertension occurred during the first Rituxan infusion. Infusion reactions typically occurred within 30 to 120 minutes of beginning the first infusion and resolved with slowing or interruption of the Rituxan infusion and with supportive care (diphenhydramine, acetaminophen, and intravenous saline). The incidence of infusion reactions was highest during the first infusion (77%) and decreased with each subsequent infusion. [*See Boxed Warning, Warnings and Precautions.*] **Infections** Serious infections (NCI CTCAE Grade 3 or 4), including sepsis, occurred in less than 5% of patients with NHL in the single-arm studies. The overall incidence of infections was 31% (bacterial 19%, viral 10%, unknown 6%, and fungal 1%). [*See Warnings and Precautions.*] In randomized, controlled studies where Rituxan was administered following chemotherapy for the treatment of follicular or low-grade NHL, the rate of infection was higher among patients who received Rituxan. In diffuse large B-cell lymphoma patients, viral infections occurred more frequently in those who received Rituxan. **Cytopenias and hypogammaglobulinemia** In patients with NHL receiving rituximab monotherapy, NCI-CTC Grade 3 and 4 cytopenias were reported in 48% of patients. These included lymphopenia (40%), neutropenia (6%), leukopenia (4%), anemia (3%), and thrombocytopenia (2%). The median duration of lymphopenia was 14 days (range, 1–588 days) and of neutropenia was 13 days (range, 2–116 days). A single occurrence of transient aplastic anemia (pure red cell aplasia) and two occurrences of hemolytic anemia following Rituxan therapy occurred during the single-arm studies. In studies of monotherapy, Rituxan-induced B-cell depletion occurred in 70% to 80% of patients with NHL. Decreased IgM and IgG serum levels occurred in 14% of these patients. **Single-Agent Rituxan** Adverse reactions in Table 1 occurred in 356 patients with relapsed or refractory, low-grade or follicular, CD20-positive, B-cell NHL treated in single-arm studies of Rituxan administered as a single agent. Most patients received Rituxan 375 mg/m² weekly for 4 doses.

Table 1
Incidence of Adverse Events in ≥5% of Patients with Relapsed or Refractory, Low-Grade or Follicular NHL, Receiving Single-agent Rituxan (N = 356)[a,b]

	All Grades (%)	Grade 3 and 4 (%)		All Grades (%)	Grade 3 and 4 (%)
Any Adverse Events	99	57	Respiratory System	38	4
Body as a Whole	86	10	Increased Cough	13	1
Fever	53	1	Rhinitis	12	1
Chills	33	3	Bronchospasm	8	1
Infection	31	4	Dyspnea	7	1
Asthenia	26	1	Sinusitis	6	0
Headache	19	1	Metabolic and Nutritional		
Abdominal Pain	14	1	Disorders	38	3
Pain	12	1	Angioedema	11	1
Back Pain	10	1	Hyperglycemia	9	1
Throat Irritation	9	0	Peripheral Edema	8	0
Flushing	5	0	LDH Increase	7	0
Heme and Lymphatic System	67	48	Digestive System	37	2
Lymphopenia	48	40	Nausea	23	1
Leukopenia	14	4	Diarrhea	10	1
Neutropenia	14	6	Vomiting	10	1
Thrombocytopenia	12	2	Nervous System	32	1
Anemia	8	3	Dizziness	10	1
Skin and Appendages	44	2	Anxiety	5	1
Night Sweats	15	1	Musculoskeletal System	26	3
Rash	15	1	Myalgia	10	1
Pruritus	14	1	Arthralgia	10	1
Urticaria	8	1	Cardiovascular System	25	3
			Hypotension	10	1
			Hypertension	6	1

[a]Adverse reactions observed up to 12 months following Rituxan. [b]Adverse reactions graded for severity by NCI-CTC criteria.

In these single-arm Rituxan studies, bronchiolitis obliterans occurred during and up to 6 months after Rituxan infusion. **Rituxan in Combination With Chemotherapy** Adverse reactions information below is based on 1250 patients who received Rituxan in combination with chemotherapy or following chemotherapy. **Rituxan in Combination With Chemotherapy for Low-Grade NHL** In Study 4, patients in the R-CVP arm experienced a higher incidence of infusional toxicity and neutropenia compared to patients in the CVP arm. The following adverse reactions occurred more frequently (≥5%) in patients receiving R-CVP compared to CVP alone: rash (17% vs. 5%), cough (15% vs. 6%), flushing (14% vs. 3%), rigors (10% vs. 2%), pruritus (10% vs. 1%), neutropenia (8% vs. 3%), and chest tightness (7% vs. 1%). In Study 5, the following adverse reactions were reported more frequently (≥5%) in patients receiving Rituxan following CVP compared to patients who received no further therapy: fatigue (39% vs. 14%), anemia (35% vs. 20%), peripheral sensory neuropathy (30% vs. 18%), infections (19% vs. 9%), pulmonary toxicity (18% vs. 10%), hepato-biliary toxicity (17% vs. 7%), rash and/or pruritus (17% vs. 5%), arthralgia (12% vs. 3%), and weight gain (11% vs. 4%). Neutropenia was the only Grade 3 or 4 adverse reaction that occurred more frequently (≥2%) in the Rituxan arm compared with those who received no further therapy (4% vs. 1%). **Rituxan in Combination With Chemotherapy for DLBCL** In Studies 6 and 7, the following adverse reactions, regardless of severity, were reported more frequently (≥5%) in patients age ≥60 years receiving R-CHOP as compared to CHOP alone: pyrexia (56% vs. 46%), lung disorder (31% vs. 24%), cardiac disorder (29% vs. 21%), and chills (13% vs. 4%). Detailed safety data collection in these studies was primarily limited to Grade 3 and 4 adverse reactions and serious adverse reactions. In Study 7, a review of cardiac toxicity determined that supraventricular arrhythmias or tachycardia accounted for most of the difference in cardiac disorders (4.5% for R-CHOP vs. 1.0% for CHOP). The following Grade 3 or 4 adverse reactions occurred more frequently among patients in the R-CHOP arm compared with those in the CHOP arm: thrombocytopenia (9% vs. 7%) and lung disorder (6% vs. 3%). Other Grade 3 or 4 adverse reactions occurring more frequently among patients receiving R-CHOP were viral infection (Study 7), neutropenia (Studies 7 and 8), and anemia (Study 8). **Immunogenicity** As with all therapeutic proteins, there is a potential for immunogenicity. The observed incidence of antibody (including neutralizing antibody) positivity in an assay is highly dependent on several factors including assay sensitivity and specificity, assay methodology, sample handling, timing of sample collection, concomitant medications, and underlying disease. For these reasons, comparison of the incidence of antibodies to Rituxan with the incidence of antibodies to other products may be misleading. Using an ELISA assay, anti-human anti-chimeric antibody (HACA) was detected in 4 of 356 (1.1%) patients with low-grade or follicular NHL receiving single-agent Rituxan. Three of the four patients had an objective clinical response. The clinical relevance of HACA

formation in rituximab treated patients is unclear. **Postmarketing Experience** The following adverse reactions have been identified during postapproval use of Rituxan in hematologic malignancies. Because these reactions are reported voluntarily from a population of uncertain size, it is not always possible to reliably estimate their frequency or establish a causal relationship to drug exposure. Decisions to include these reactions in labeling are typically based on one or more of the following factors: (1) seriousness of the reaction, (2) frequency of reporting, or (3) strength of causal connection to Rituxan. *Hematologic:* prolonged pancytopenia, marrow hypoplasia, and late-onset neutropenia, hyperviscosity syndrome in Waldenstrom's macroglobulinemia. *Cardiac:* fatal cardiac failure. *Immune/Autoimmune Events:* uveitis, optic neuritis, systemic vasculitis, pleuritis, lupus-like syndrome, serum sickness, polyarticular arthritis, and vasculitis with rash. *Infection:* viral infections, including progressive multifocal leukoencephalopathy (PML), increase in fatal infections in HIV-associated lymphoma, and a reported increased incidence of Grade 3 and 4 infections in patients with previously treated lymphoma without known HIV infection. *Neoplasia:* disease progression of Kaposi's sarcoma. *Skin:* severe mucocutaneous reactions. *Gastrointestinal:* bowel obstruction and perforation. *Pulmonary:* fatal bronchiolitis obliterans and pneumonitis (including interstitial pneumonitis). **DRUG INTERACTIONS** Formal drug interaction studies have not been performed with Rituxan. **USE IN SPECIFIC POPULATIONS Pregnancy Category C:** There are no adequate and well-controlled studies of rituximab in pregnant women. Postmarketing data indicate that B-cell lymphocytopenia generally lasting less than six months can occur in infants exposed to rituximab in-utero. Rituximab was detected postnatally in the serum of infants exposed in-utero. Non-Hodgkin's lymphoma is a serious condition that requires treatment. Rituximab should be used during pregnancy only if the potential benefit to the mother justifies the potential risk to the fetus. Reproduction studies in cynomolgus monkeys at maternal exposures similar to human therapeutic exposures showed no evidence of teratogenic effects. However, B-cell lymphoid tissue was reduced in the offspring of treated dams. The B-cell counts returned to normal levels, and immunologic function was restored within 6 months of birth. **Nursing Mothers** It is not known whether Rituxan is secreted into human milk. However, Rituxan is secreted in the milk of lactating cynomolgus monkeys, and IgG is excreted in human milk. Published data suggest that antibodies in breast milk do not enter the neonatal and infant circulations in substantial amounts. The unknown risks to the infant from oral ingestion of Rituxan should be weighed against the known benefits of breastfeeding. **Pediatric Use** The safety and effectiveness of Rituxan in pediatric patients have not been established. **Geriatric Use** *Diffuse Large B-Cell NHL* Among patients with DLBCL evaluated in three randomized, active-controlled trials, 927 patients received Rituxan in combination with chemotherapy. Of these, 396 (43%) were age 65 or greater and 123 (13%) were age 75 or greater. No overall differences in effectiveness were observed between these patients and younger patients. Cardiac adverse reactions, mostly supraventricular arrhythmias, occurred more frequently among elderly patients. Serious pulmonary adverse reactions were also more common among the elderly, including pneumonia and pneumonitis. *Low-Grade or Follicular Non-Hodgkin's Lymphoma* Clinical studies of Rituxan in low-grade or follicular, CD20-positive, B-cell NHL did not include sufficient numbers of patients aged 65 and over to determine whether they respond differently from younger subjects. **OVERDOSAGE** There has been no experience with overdosage in human clinical trials. Single doses of up to 500 mg/m² have been given in dose-escalation clinical trials. **NONCLINICAL TOXICOLOGY Carcinogenesis, Mutagenesis, Impairment of Fertility** No long term animal studies have been performed to establish the carcinogenic or mutagenic potential of Rituxan or to determine potential effects on fertility in males or females. **PATIENT COUNSELING INFORMATION** Patients should be provided the Rituxan Medication Guide and provided an opportunity to read prior to each treatment session. Because caution should be exercised in administering Rituxan to patients with active infections, it is important that the patient's overall health be assessed at each visit and any questions resulting from the patient's reading of the Medication Guide be discussed. Rituxan is detectable in serum for up to six months following completion of therapy. Individuals of childbearing potential should use effective contraception during treatment and for 12 months after Rituxan therapy.

Revised 9/2008 (4835505)

Jointly Marketed by:
Biogen Idec Inc. 5200 Research Place San Diego, CA 92122
Genentech USA, Inc. 1 DNA Way South San Francisco, CA 94080-4990

Genentech
BIO●NCOLOGY™   biogen idec

CHAPTER 16

Colon, rectal, and anal cancers

Joshua D. I. Ellenhorn, MD, Carey A. Cullinane, MD,
Steven R. Alberts, MD, and Deborah Citrin, MD

COLORECTAL CANCER

Despite the existence of excellent screening and preventive strategies, colorectal carcinoma (CRC) remains a major public health problem in Western countries. The American Cancer Society (ACS) estimated that in 2008, 148,810 people will be diagnosed with CRC, and 49,960 will die of the disease. CRC is the third most common type of cancer in both sexes (after prostate and lung cancers in men and lung and breast cancers in women) and the second most common cause of cancer death in the United States.

About 72% of new CRCs arise in the colon, and the remaining 28% arise in the rectum. Rectal cancer is defined as cancer arising below the peritoneal reflection, up to approximately 12 to15 cm from the anal verge.

The lifetime risk of being diagnosed with CRC in the United States is estimated to be 5.9% for men and 5.5% for women.

Epidemiology

Gender Overall, the incidence of CRC and mortality rates are higher in men than in women; tumors of the colon are slightly more frequent in women than in men (1.2:1), whereas rectal carcinomas are more common in men than in women (1.7:1).

Age The vast majority, 90%, of all new CRC cases occur in individuals older than age 50. In the United States, the median age at presentation is 72 years.

Race The incidence and mortality rates of CRC are highest among African-American men and women compared with white men and women (15% higher and 40% higher, respectively). The incidence rates among Asian Americans, Hispanics/Latinos, and American Indians/Alaskan natives are lower than those among whites.

Geography The incidence of CRC is higher in industrialized regions (the United States, Canada, the Scandinavian countries, northern and western Europe, New Zealand, Australia) and lower in Asia, Africa (among blacks), and South America (except Argentina and Uruguay).

TABLE 1: Five-year relative survival rates in colorectal cancer[a] by stage at diagnosis (1995–2000)

Time of detection	5-year survival rate (%)
All stages	64
In early, localized stage	90
After spread to adjacent organs or lymph nodes	67
After spread to distant sites	10
Unstaged	35

[a] Source: Cancer Facts & Figures—2005. Atlanta: American Cancer Society; 2005. Surveillance, Epidemiology, and End Results (SEER) Program.

Survival Five-year survival rates (Table 1) for patients with CRC have improved in recent years. This fact may be due to wider surgical resections, modern anesthetic techniques, and improved supportive care. In addition, better pathologic examination of resected specimens, preoperative staging, and abdominal exploration reveal clinically occult disease and allow treatment to be delivered more accurately. Survival also has improved through the use of adjuvant chemotherapy for colon cancer and adjuvant chemoradiation therapy for rectal cancer. Mortality from colorectal cancer is decreasing, likely from earlier diagnosis and screening as well as improvements in treatment modalities.

Etiology and risk factors

The specific causes of CRC are unknown, but environmental, nutritional, genetic, and familial factors, as well as preexisting diseases, have been found to be associated with this cancer. A summary of selected risk factors for CRC is shown in Table 2.

Environment Asians, Africans, and South Americans who emigrate from low-risk areas assume the colon cancer risk for their adopted country, suggesting the importance of environmental factors in CRC. Smoking and alcohol intake (four or more drinks per week) increase the risk of CRC.

Diet Diets rich in fat and cholesterol have been linked to an increased risk of colorectal tumors. Dietary fat causes endogenous production of secondary bile acids and neutral steroids and increases bacterial degradation and excretion of these acids and steroids, thereby promoting colonic carcinogenesis. Historically, diets rich in cereal fiber or bran and yellow and green vegetables are said to have protective effects, although recent studies have failed to prove a risk reduction with increasing dietary fiber intake. A protective role also has been ascribed to calcium salts and calcium-rich foods, because they decrease colon-cell turnover and reduce the cancer-promoting effects of bile acid and fatty acids.

TABLE 2: Selected risk factors for colorectal cancer

Risk factor	Relative risk
Family and medical histories	
Family history (first-degree relative)	1.8
Inflammatory bowel disease (diagnosed ≥ 10 years)	1.5
Modifiable factors that increase risk	
Obesity (body mass index ≥ 30)	1.5–2.0
Red meat (≥ 7 servings/week vs 1 serving/month)	1.5
Cigarette use (current vs never)	1.5
Alcohol (≥ 4 drinks/week vs none)	1.4
Modifiable factors that decrease risk	
Physical activity (more than 3 hours/week vs none)	0.6
Vegetable and fruit consumption (≥ 5 vs < 3 servings/day)	0.7

Source: Colorectal Cancer Facts & Figures–2005. Atlanta: American Cancer Society; 2005.

Physical activity Several studies have reported a lower risk of CRC in individuals who participate in regular physical activity. High levels of physical activity may decrease the risk by as much as 50%. Being overweight or obese has been consistently associated with a higher risk of CRC.

Inflammatory bowel disease Patients with inflammatory bowel disease (ulcerative colitis, Crohn's disease) have a higher incidence of CRC. The risk of CRC in patients with ulcerative colitis is associated with the duration of active disease, extent of colitis, development of mucosal dysplasia, and duration of symptoms.

The risk of CRC increases exponentially with the duration of colitis, from approximately 3% in the first decade to 20% in the second decade to > 30% in the third decade. CRC risk also is increased in patients with Crohn's disease, although to a lesser extent.

Adenomatous polyps Colorectal tumors develop more often in patients with adenomatous polyps than in those without polyps. There is approximately a 5% probability that carcinoma will be present in an adenoma; the risk correlates with the histology and size of the polyp. The potential for malignant transformation is higher for villous and tubulovillous adenomas than for tubular adenomas. Adenomatous polyps < 1 cm have a slightly greater than 1% chance of being malignant, in comparison with adenomas > 2 cm, which have up to a 40% likelihood of malignant transformation.

Cancer history Patients with a history of CRC are at increased risk of a second primary colon cancer or other malignancy. The risk of a second CRC is higher if the first diagnosis was made prior to age 60.

Prior surgery Following ureterosigmoidostomy, an increased incidence of colon cancer at or near the suture line has been reported. Cholecystectomy also has been associated with colon cancer in some studies but not in others.

Family history and genetic factors Individuals with a first-degree relative with the disease have an increased risk of developing CRC. Those with two or more relatives with the disease make up about 20% of all people with CRC. The risk of developing CRC is significantly increased in several forms of inherited susceptibility (Table 3). About 5% to 10% of all patients with CRC have an inherited susceptibility to the disease. The risks of developing CRC in the subgroups of familial or hereditary CRC vary from 15% in relatives of patients with CRC diagnosed before 45 years of age, through 20% for family members with two first-degree relatives with CRC, to approximately 70% to 95% in patients with familial adenomatous polyposis and hereditary nonpolyposis CRC (HNPCC).

Familial adenomatous polyposis (FAP) is inherited as an autosomal-dominant trait with variable penetrance. Patients characteristically develop pancolonic and rectal adenomatous polyps. Approximately 50% of patients with FAP will develop adenomas by 15 years of age and 95% by age 35. Left untreated, 100% of patients with FAP will develop CRC, with an average age at diagnosis ranging from 34 to 43 years. Total colectomy, usually performed on patients in their mid-to-late teens, is the preventive treatment of choice in this group of patients. The familial adenomatous polyposis coli *(APC)* gene has been localized to chromosome 5q21. Currently, it is possible to detect mutations in the *APC* gene in up to 82% of families with FAP. Mutations in the *APC* gene combined with mutational activation of proto-oncogenes, especially K-*ras*, occur sequentially in the neoplastic transformation of bowel epithelium in patients with FAP. Use of cyclo-oxygenase-2 (COX-2) inhibitors such as celecoxib (Celebrex) has been shown to reduce the number of polyps in patients with FAP.

HNPCC is transmitted as an autosomal-dominant trait. It is associated with germline mutations in one of five DNA mismatch repair genes (*MSH2, MLH1, PMS1, PMS2,* and *MSH6).* The incidence of a mutated mismatch repair gene is approximately 1 in 1,000 people. The Amsterdam criteria were proposed in 1991 as a way to help identify patients at risk of HNPCC. In 1999, they were revised (Amsterdam II) to recognize extracolonic manifestations as part of the family history. The criteria include the following factors:

- three or more relatives with a histologically verified HNPCC-associated cancer (colorectal, endometrial, small bowel, ureter, or renal pelvis), one of whom is a first-degree relative of the other two (FAP should be excluded)
- CRC involving at least two generations
- one or more CRCs diagnosed before the age of 50.

The Bethesda criteria were developed based upon an analysis of high-risk patients who did not meet the Amsterdam criteria but still demonstrated germline mutations in either the *MSH2* or *MLH1* gene. These criteria are much less restrictive than the Amsterdam criteria and serve to help identify those individual patients at risk of HNPCC who might benefit from further evaluation. They include the following:

- individuals with cancer in families who meet the Amsterdam criteria

TABLE 3: Hereditary polyposis syndromes

Adenomatous polyposis

Familial adenomatous polyposis (FAP)

Characterized by hundreds or thousands of sessile or pedunculated polyps throughout the large intestine; histologic examination reveals microscopic adenomas; average age at onset of polyps, 25 years; at onset of symptoms, 33 years; at diagnosis, 36 years; at diagnosis of colon cancer, 42 years; extracolonic features include mandibular osteomas, upper GI polyps, and congenital hypertrophy of the retinal pigment epithelium. An attenuated form of FAP that is clinically characterized by the presence of tens or hundreds of polyps exists.

Gardner's syndrome

Same colonic manifestations as FAP; extracolonic features more evident and varied, including osteomas of the skull, mandible, and long bones; desmoid tumors; dental abnormalities; neoplasms of the thyroid, adrenal glands, biliary tree, and liver; upper GI polyps; and congenital hypertrophy of the retinal pigment epithelium; fibromatosis of the mesentery is a potentially fatal complication (occurring in 8% to 13% of patients).

Turcot's syndrome

This rare syndrome is characterized by malignant colon and brain tumors. Two different types of Turcot's have been identified: one characterized by an adenomatous polyposis coli (APC) mutation resulting in colon cancer and malignant glioblastoma; the second characterized by a mismatch repair gene mutation resulting in colon cancer and astrocytoma.

Hamartomatous polyposis

Peutz-Jeghers syndrome

In infancy and childhood, melanin deposits manifest as greenish-black to brown mucocutaneous pigmentation (which may fade at puberty) around the nose, lips, buccal mucosa, hands, and feet; polyps (most frequent in the small intestines; also found in the stomach and colon) are unique hamartomas with branching bands of smooth muscle surrounded by glandular epithelium; may produce acute and chronic GI bleeding, intestinal obstruction, or intussusception; 50% of patients develop cancer (median age at diagnosis, 50 years); ovarian cysts and unique ovarian sex-cord tumors reported (5% to 12% of female patients).

Juvenile polyposis

Three forms: familial juvenile polyposis coli (polyps limited to the colon), familial juvenile polyposis of the stomach, and generalized juvenile polyposis (polyps distributed throughout the GI tract); polyps are hamartomas covered by normal glandular epithelium, found mostly in the rectum in children and sometimes in adults; may produce GI bleeding, obstruction, or intussusception; mixed juvenile/adenomatous polyps or synchronous adenomatous polyps may lead to cancer, but gastric cancer has not been reported in patients with familial juvenile polyposis of the stomach.

Cowden's disease (multiple hamartoma syndrome)

Multiple hamartomatous tumors of ectodermal, mesodermal, and endodermal origin; mucocutaneous lesions are prominent and distinctive; also reported: breast lesions ranging from fibrocystic disease to cancer (50% of patients), thyroid abnormalities (10% to 15%), cutaneous lipomas, ovarian cysts, uterine leiomyomas, skeletal and developmental anomalies, and GI polyps; no associated risk of cancer in GI polyps; probably does not warrant clinical surveillance.

- individuals with two HNPCC-related cancers, including synchronous and metachronous CRCs or associated extracolonic cancers; endometrial, ovarian, gastric, hepatobiliary, small bowel, or transitional cell carcinoma of the renal pelvis or ureter

- individuals with CRC and a first-degree relative with CRC and/or HNPCC-related extracolonic cancer and/or a colorectal adenoma; one of the cancers diagnosed at age younger than 45 years; and the adenoma diagnosed at age younger than 40 years

- individuals with CRC or endometrial cancer diagnosed at age < 45 years

- individuals with right-sided CRC with an undifferentiated pattern (solid/cribriform) on histology diagnosed at age < 45 years

- individuals with signet ring-cell–type CRC diagnosed at age < 45 years

- individuals with colorectal adenomas diagnosed at age < 40 years.

Mutations in the DNA mismatch repair genes *MLH1* or *MSH2* can be found in approximately 40% of individuals who meet these criteria. Genetic evaluation for HNPCC should be considered in families that meet the Amsterdam criteria, in affected individuals who meet the Bethesda criteria, and in first-degree relatives of those individuals with known mutations. For situations in which HNPCC is suspected but the first three Bethesda criteria are not met, microsatellite instability (MSI) testing may be considered. Over 90% of HNPCCs will demonstrate MSI, compared with 15% to 20% of sporadic CRC, and thus a normal result in the absence of compelling clinical criteria usually excludes the diagnosis of HNPCC. Alternatively, *MSH6* may be involved in a substantial proportion of patients in whom HNPCC is suspected and should be considered in those with tumors that are low in MSI.

Chemoprevention

Chemoprevention aims to block the action of carcinogens on cells before the development of cancer.

Antioxidants and calcium Controlled trials of vitamins C and E and calcium have produced mixed results. Clinical trials have shown that calcium supplementation modestly decreases the risk of colorectal adenomas.

Nonsteroidal anti-inflammatory drugs inhibit colorectal carcinogenesis, possibly by reducing endogenous prostaglandin production through COX inhibition. Sulindac (Clinoril) has induced regression of large bowel polyps in patients with FAP. Controlled studies have shown a reduction in the incidence of colorectal polyps with regular, long-term use of aspirin. HMG-CoA (hydroxymethyl glutaryl coenzyme A) reductase inhibitors may reduce the risk of CRC after extended treatment.

Postmenopausal hormones Women who use postmenopausal hormones appear to have a lower rate of CRC than do those who do not. Postmenopausal hormones may increase the risk of other types of cancer, however.

Signs and symptoms

Early stage During the early stages of CRC, patients may be asymptomatic or complain of vague abdominal pain and flatulence, which may be attributed to gallbladder or peptic ulcer disease. Minor changes in bowel movements, with or without rectal bleeding, are also seen; they are frequently ignored and/or attributed to hemorrhoids or other benign disorders.

Left side of the colon Cancers occurring in the left side of the colon generally cause constipation alternating with diarrhea; abdominal pain; and obstructive symptoms, such as nausea and vomiting.

Right side of the colon Right-sided colon lesions produce vague, abdominal aching, unlike the colicky pain seen with obstructive left-sided lesions. Anemia resulting from chronic blood loss, weakness, weight loss, and/or an abdominal mass may also accompany carcinoma of the right side of the colon.

Rectum Patients with cancer of the rectum may present with a change in bowel movements; rectal fullness, urgency, or bleeding; and tenesmus.

Pelvic pain is seen at later stages of the disease and usually indicates local extension of the tumor to the pelvic nerves.

Screening and diagnosis

Screening

Fecal occult blood testing (FOBT) or fecal immunochemical test (FIT) guaiac-based fecal occult blood tests are, in themselves, inexpensive but have been associated with many false-positive and false-negative results. Almost all colonic polyps and > 50% of all CRCs go undetected because they are not bleeding at the time of the test. The newer FOBTs, including a guaiac-based product called Hemoccult SENSA and immunochemical tests for hemoglobin (HemeSelect), appear to have better sensitivity than the older tests without sacrificing specificity.

Three large randomized controlled clinical trials have demonstrated decreased CRC mortality associated with detection of earlier-stage cancer and adenomas by FOBT. Recently, results from a large trial also showed a decreased incidence of CRC associated with FOBT, largely because of increased use of polypectomy resulting from diagnostic endoscopy following positive tests.

Digital rectal examination is simple to perform and can detect lesions up to 7 cm from the anal verge.

Sigmoidoscopy Flexible proctosigmoidoscopy is safe and more comfortable than examination using a rigid proctoscope. Almost 50% of all colorectal neoplasms are within the reach of a 60-cm sigmoidoscope. Even though flexible sigmoidoscopy visualizes only the distal portion of the colorectum, the identification of adenomas can lead to colonoscopy. When we add the percentage of colorectal neoplasms in the distal 60 cm of the colorectum to the percentage of patients with distal polyps leading to complete colonoscopy, 80% of those individuals with a significant neoplasm anywhere in the colorectum can be identified.

Colonoscopy (optical) provides information on the mucosa of the entire colon, and its sensitivity in detecting tumors is extremely high. Most physicians consider colonoscopy to be the best screening modality for CRC. Colonoscopy can be used to obtain biopsy specimens of adenomas and carcinomas and permits the excision of adenomatous polyps. For this reason, colonoscopy is the only screening modality ever shown to reduce the incidence of cancer in screened individuals. Colonoscopy is the best follow-up strategy for evaluating patients with positive guaiac-based FOBTs and the best screening modality for high-risk patients.

Limitations of colonoscopy include its inability to detect some polyps and small lesions because of blind corners and mucosal folds and the fact that sometimes the cecum cannot be reached. A supplementary double-contrast barium enema may be needed if a colonoscopic exam fails to reach the cecum.

Colonoscopy (CT virtual) Some recent studies have suggested that CT virtual colonoscopy may have sensitivity and specificity for detecting neoplastic polyps that approach those of optical colonoscopy. Unfortunately, other studies have demonstrated clear superiority of optical colonoscopy. Until additional confirmatory studies are available, virtual CT colonoscopy should not replace routine optical colonoscopic screening.

Barium enemas can accurately detect CRC; however, the false-negative rate associated with double-contrast barium enemas ranges from 2% to 61% because of misinterpretation, poor preparation, and difficulties in detecting smaller lesions. A supplementary colonoscopy may be needed if a double-contrast barium enema does not adequately visualize the entire colon or to obtain histopathology or perform polypectomy in the event of abnormal findings.

Recommendations for average-risk individuals Adults at average risk should begin CRC screening at age 50. The ACS guidelines on screening and surveillance for the early detection of colorectal adenomatous polyps and cancer provide several options for screening average-risk individuals (Table 4).

For those individuals who elect FOBT/FIT alone, or in combination with flexible sigmoidoscopy, a single test of a stool sample in the clinical setting (as, for instance, is often performed with the stool sample collected on the fingertip during a digital rectal examination) is not an adequate substitute for a full set of samples using the take-home card system. Because combining flexible sigmoidoscopy with FOBT/FIT can substantially increase the benefits of either test alone, the ACS regards annual FOBT/FIT accompanied by flexible sigmoidoscopy every 5 years as a better choice than either FOBT/FIT or flexible sigmoidoscopy alone.

The choice of colonoscopy or double-contrast barium enema for screening may depend on factors such as personal preference, cost, and the local availability of trained clinicians to perform a high-quality examination. For those who elect either colonoscopy or double-contrast barium enema for screening, there is no need for annual FOBT/FIT. Digital rectal examination should be performed at the time of the sigmoidoscopy or colonoscopy.

TABLE 4: American Cancer Society guidelines on screening and surveillance for the early detection of colorectal adenomas and cancer—Average risk

Test	Interval (beginning at age 50)	Comment
FOBT or FIT and flexible sigmoidoscopy	FOBT annually and flexible sigmoidoscopy every 5 years	Flexible sigmoidoscopy together with FOBT is preferred over FOBT or flexible sigmoidoscopy alone. All positive test results should be followed up with colonoscopy.[a]
Flexible sigmoidoscopy	Every 5 years	All positive test results should be followed up with colonoscopy.[a]
FOBT	Annually	The recommended take-home multiple sample method should be used. All positive test results should be followed up with colonoscopy.[a,b]
Colonoscopy	Every 10 years	Colonoscopy provides an opportunity to visualize, sample, and/or remove significant lesions.
Double-contrast barium enema	Every 5 years	All positive test results should be followed up with colonoscopy.

[a] If colonoscopy is unavailable, not feasible, or not desired by the patient, double-contrast barium enema (DCBE) alone or the combination of flexible sigmoidoscopy and DCBE is an acceptable alternative. Adding flexible sigmoidoscopy to DCBE may provide a more comprehensive diagnostic evaluation than DCBE alone in finding significant lesions. A supplementary DCBE may be needed if a colonoscopic exam fails to reach the cecum, and a supplementary colonoscopy may be needed if a DCBE identifies a possible lesion or does not adequately visualize the entire colorectum.

[b] There is no justification for repeating FOBT in response to an initial positive finding.

FOBT = fecal occult blood test; FIT = fecal immunochemical test

Adapted with permission from Smith RA, von Eschenbach AC, Wender R, et al: CA Cancer J Clin 53:27–43, 2003.

Recommendations for screening increased-risk and high-risk individuals

Risk of CRC is even higher among individuals with hereditary syndromes or a history of inflammatory bowel disease of significant duration.

Those individuals who have been diagnosed as having adenomatous polyps or a personal history of curative-intent resection of CRC should undergo a colonoscopy to remove all polyps from the colorectum, after which a colonoscopic exam should be repeated at an interval to be determined on the basis of the size, multiplicity, and histologic appearance of the adenoma(s) (Table 5). If colonoscopy is not available, or not feasible, flexible sigmoidoscopy followed by double-contrast barium enema may be used for surveillance.

TABLE 5: American Cancer Society guidelines on screening and surveillance for the early detection of colorectal adenomas and cancer—Increased or high risk

Risk category	Age to begin	Practice
Increased risk		
A single, small (< I cm) adenoma	3-6 years after initial polypectomy	Colonoscopy[a]
If the exam is normal, the patient can thereafter be screened as per average-risk guidelines.		
A large (> I cm) adenoma, multiple adenomas, or adenomas with high-grade dysplasia or villous change	Within 3 years after the initial polypectomy	Colonoscopy[a]
If the exam is normal, repeat examination in 3 years; if the exam is normal then, the patient can thereafter be screened as per average-risk guidelines.		
Personal history of curative-intent resection of colorectal cancer	Within I year after cancer resection	Colonoscopy[a]
If the exam is normal, repeat examination in 3 years; if the exam is normal then, repeat examination every 5 years.		
Either colorectal cancer or adenomatous polyps in any first-degree relative before age 60 or in two or more first-degree relatives at any age (if not a hereditary syndrome)	Age 40, or 5-10 years before the youngest case in the immediate family	Colonoscopy[a]
Every 5-10 years. Colorectal cancer in relatives more distant than first-degree relatives does not increase risk substantially above the average-risk group.		
High risk		
Family history of familial adenomatous polyposis (FAP)	12 years	Early surveillance with endoscopy and counseling to consider genetic testing
If the genetic test result is positive, colectomy may be indicated. These patients are best referred to a center with experience in the management of FAP.		
Family history of hereditary nonpolyposis colorectal cancer (HNPCC)	Age 21	Colonoscopy and counseling to consider genetic testing
If the genetic test result is positive or the patient has not undergone genetic testing, every 1-2 years until age 40, then annually. These patients are best referred to a center with experience in the management of HNPCC.		
Inflammatory bowel disease, chronic ulcerative colitis, Crohn's disease	Cancer risk begins to be significant 8 years after the onset of pancolitis or 12-15 years after the onset of left-sided colitis	Colonoscopy with biopsies for dysplasia
Every 1-2 years. These patients are best referred to a center with experience in the surveillance and management of inflammatory bowel disease.		

[a] If colonoscopy is unavailable, not feasible, or not desired by the patient, double-contrast barium enema (DCBE) alone or the combination of flexible sigmoidoscopy and DCBE is an acceptable alternative. Adding flexible sigmoidoscopy to DCBE may provide a more comprehensive diagnostic evaluation than DCBE alone in finding significant lesions. A supplementary DCBE may be needed if a colonoscopic exam fails to reach the cecum, and a supplementary colonoscopy may be needed if a DCBE identifies a possible lesion or does not adequately visualize the entire colorectum.

Adapted with permission from Smith RA, von Eschenbach AC, Wender R, et al: CA Cancer J Clin 53:27–43, 2003.

Treatment of endoscopically removed polyps Adenomatous colon polyps should be completely removed endoscopically to prevent progression to malignancy. Colon polyps with dysplasia or carcinoma in situ can also be managed with colonoscopic polypectomy as long as the entire polyp is removed. A malignant polyp is defined as one with cancer invading through the muscularis mucosa and into the submucosa (pT1). Management of malignant polyps removed by colonoscopy is somewhat controversial. In general, malignant polyps can be removed colonoscopically as long as they can be removed with a confirmed negative margin and do not invade the submucosa beneath the polyp stalk. Sessile polyps with submucosal invasion should probably be removed by colon resection.

Diagnosis

Initial work-up An initial diagnostic work-up for patients suspected of having colorectal tumors should include:

- digital rectal examination and FOBT
- colonoscopy
- biopsy of any detected lesions.

Adequate staging prior to surgical intervention requires:

- chest x-ray
- CT scan of the abdomen and pelvis
- CBC with platelet count
- liver and renal function tests
- urinalysis
- measurement of carcinoembryonic antigen (CEA) level. If CEA levels are elevated preoperatively, postoperative CEA levels should be monitored every 3 months for 3 years in patients with stage II or III CRC and every 6 to 12 months thereafter.

In monitoring response to therapy for metastatic cancer, CEA levels should be measured every 1 to 8 months during active treatment.

FDG-PET scanning FDG ([18]fluorodeoxyglucose)-PET scanning has emerged as a highly sensitive study for the evaluation of patients who have metastatic disease. Although not usually recommended in the evaluation of early-stage primary disease, this modality can aid in the staging of recurrence.

Pathology

Adenocarcinomas constitute 90% to 95% of all large bowel neoplasms. These tumors consist of cuboidal or columnar epithelium with multiple degrees of differentiation and variable amounts of mucin.

Mucinous adenocarcinoma is a histologic variant characterized by huge amounts of extracellular mucus in the tumor and the tendency to spread within the

TABLE 6: TNM staging of colorectal cancer

TNM stage	Primary tumor[a]	Lymph node metastasis[b]	Distant metastasis[c]	Modified Astler-Coller
Stage 0	Tis	N0	M0	–
Stage I	T1	N0	M0	A
	T2	N0	M0	B1
Stage IIA	T3	N0	M0	B2
IIB	T4	N0	M0	B3
Stage IIIA	T1-2	N1	M0	C1[d]
IIIB	T3-4	N1	M0	C2-3[d]
IIIC	Any T	N2	M0	C1-3[d]
Stage IV	Any T	Any N	M1	D

[a] Tis = carcinoma in situ; T1 = tumor invades submucosa; T2 = tumor invades muscularis propria; T3 = tumor invades through the muscularis propria into the subserosa or into nonperitoneal pericolic or perirectal tissues; T4 = tumor perforates the visceral peritoneum or directly invades other organs or structures

[b] N0 = no regional lymph node metastasis; N1 = metastases in one to three pericolic or perirectal lymph nodes; N2 = metastases in four or more pericolic or perirectal lymph nodes

[c] M0 = no distant metastasis; M1 = distant metastasis

[d] C1 = T2 N1, T2 N2   C2 = T3 N1, T3 N2   C3 = T4 N1, T4 N2

From Greene FL, Page DL, Fleming ID, et al (eds): AJCC Cancer Staging Manual, 6th Ed. New York, Springer-Verlag, 2002.

peritoneum. Approximately 10% of colorectal adenocarcinomas are mucinous. It is more commonly seen in younger patients.

Signet-ring–cell carcinoma is an uncommon variant, comprising 1% of colorectal adenocarcinomas. These tumors contain large quantities of intracellular mucinous elements (causing the cytoplasm to displace the nucleus) and tend to involve the submucosa, making their detection difficult with conventional imaging techniques.

Other tumor types Squamous cell carcinomas, small-cell carcinomas, carcinoid tumors, and adenosquamous and undifferentiated carcinomas also have been found in the colon and rectum. Nonepithelial tumors, such as sarcomas and lymphomas, are exceedingly rare.

Metastatic spread CRC has a tendency toward local invasion by circumferential growth and for lymphatic, hematogenous, transperitoneal, and perineural spread. Longitudinal spread is usually not extensive, with microscopic spread averaging only 1 to 2 cm from gross disease, but radial spread is common and depends on anatomic location.

The most common site of extralymphatic involvement is the liver, with the lungs the most frequently affected extra-abdominal organ. Other sites of hematogenous spread include the bones, kidneys, adrenal glands, and brain.

Staging and prognosis

The TNM staging classification, which is based on the depth of tumor invasion in the intestinal wall, the number of regional lymph nodes involved, and the presence or absence of distant metastases, has largely replaced the older Dukes' classification scheme (Table 6).

Pathologic stage is the single most important prognostic factor following surgical resection of colorectal tumors. The prognosis for early stages (I and II) is favorable overall, in contrast to the prognosis for advanced stages (III and IV). However, there appears to be superior survival for patients with stage III disease whose disease is confined to the bowel wall (ie, ≤ T2, N+).

Histologic grade may be correlated with survival. Five-year survival rates of 56% to 100%, 33% to 80%, and 11% to 58% have been reported for grades 1, 2, and 3 colorectal tumors, respectively.

Other prognostic factors (such as age at diagnosis, presurgical CEA level, gender, presence and duration of symptoms, site of disease, histologic features, obstruction or perforation, perineural invasion, venous or lymphatic invasion, ploidy status, and S-phase fraction) have not consistently been correlated with overall disease recurrence and survival. Furthermore, the size of the primary lesion has had no influence on survival. Elevated expression of thymidylate synthase and allelic loss of chromosome 18 have been correlated with a poor prognosis.

Treatment

PRIMARY TREATMENT OF LOCALIZED DISEASE

Management of CRC relies primarily on resection of the bowel with the adjacent draining lymph nodes. The need for adjuvant systemic or local chemotherapy or immunotherapy, with or without concurrent irradiation, depends on tumor location (colon vs rectum) and stage of disease.

Surgery

Colon The primary therapy for adenocarcinoma of the colon is surgical extirpation of the bowel segment containing the tumor, the adjacent mesentery, and draining lymph nodes. Based on studies that correlated the number of lymph nodes removed and survival, it is recommended that at least 12 lymph nodes be available for examination by a pathologist to confirm. Surgical resection can be performed by open or laparoscopic approach. The type of resection depends on the anatomic location of the tumor. Right, left, or transverse colectomy is the surgical treatment of choice in patients with right, left, or transverse colonic tumors, respectively. Tumors in the sigmoid colon may be treated with wide sigmoid resection. The length of colon resected depends largely on the requirement for wide mesenteric nodal clearance.

Rectum For rectal carcinoma, the distal surgical margin should be at least 2 cm, although some investigators have suggested that a smaller but still negative margin may be adequate. The resection should include the node-bearing

In a large multicenter prospective trial, 413 patients with colon cancer and 381 patients with rectal cancer were randomized to undergo laparoscopic versus open surgical resection. No differences were seen in the overall survival rates or rates of local recurrence, despite a statistically significant increase in the positive margin rate with laparoscopic rectal resections (Jayne DG, Guillou PJ, Thorpe H, et al: J Clin Oncol 25:3061-3068, 2007). The results of this study are in concordance with two other multicenter randomized trials in colon cancer and in one other study in rectal cancer. All of the studies to date demonstrate the oncologic safety of minimally invasive surgery for colorectal cancer.

mesorectum surrounding the rectum. This procedure, which is termed total mesorectal excision (TME), is accomplished using a sharp dissection technique (see Figure 1). Posteriorly, the mesorectal dissection is carried out along the presacral fascia. Anteriorly, the dissection follows the posterior vaginal wall in females or Denonvilliers' fascia in males, either of which may be resected in the presence of an anterior wall rectal cancer. The use of TME has been associated with a significant reduction in local recurrence rates for patients with rectal cancer.

Reported rates of local recurrence following TME for rectal cancer have generally been < 10%, compared with rates of recurrence up to 30% prior to the advent of TME. Selective use of radiation therapy can improve upon the results of TME alone.

Sphincter-sparing approaches Technologies (eg, circular stapling devices) and the application of surgical techniques, such as coloanal anastomosis and creation of intestinal pouches, are employed to maintain anal sphincter function for tumors in the lower one-third of the rectum. If the tumor is located proximally between 6 and 15 cm from the anal verge, a low anterior resection with end-to-end anastomosis may be performed.

Abdominoperineal resection, removing the anus and sphincter muscle with permanent colostomy, may be necessary if the tumor is located in the distal rectum and other characteristics of the tumor (eg, bulky size, proximity to the sphincter musculature) preclude an oncologically adequate sphincter-sparing approach. An alternative procedure for tumors 2 to 5 cm from the anal verge is to resect the entire rectum, sparing the anoderm and anal sphincter musculature, and to perform a coloanal anastomosis. Either procedure can be performed with autonomic nerve preservation, minimizing bladder and sexual function morbidity.

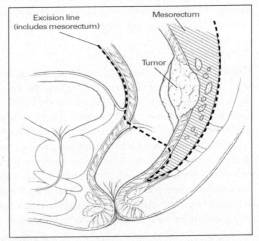

FIGURE 1: Mesorectal excision

Local excision alone may be indicated for selected patients who have small (< 3 to 4 cm), T1, well to moderately differentiated rectal cancers without histologic evidence of lymphovascular involvement, provided that a full-thickness negative margin can be achieved. In some series, transanal excision for these good histology T1 lesions results in excellent long-term control. However, some large studies with long-term follow-up demonstrated significant local recurrence rates, even with T1 lesions. For T2 or T3 tumors, the standard therapy remains a transabdominal resection because of the risk of mesorectal nodal spread. Preoperative transrectal ultrasonography is useful in defining lesions that can be resected by local excision alone. A trial sponsored by the CALGB (Cancer and Leukemia Group B) demonstrated reasonable results for patients with T2 rectal cancer undergoing negative margin local excision followed by fluorouracil (5-FU) and external-beam radiation therapy. The locoregional recurrence rate at 6 years was only 14%. Good results with local excision alone following chemoradiotherapy for rectal cancer have been reported. The role of local excision alone in this clinical scenario awaits confirmatory studies.

Laparoscopic colonic resection Multiple large randomized trials have established laparoscopic colonic resection as an oncologically acceptable method of treating cancer of the colon. Resection of rectal cancer using laparoscopic approaches has also been evaluated in a number of randomized trials. Laparoscopy for rectal resection still requires confirmation as an oncologically equivalent procedure to open surgery. The potential advantages include a shorter hospital stay, reduced postoperative ileus, decreased time away from work, fewer adhesive complications, and a lower risk of hernia formation. The potential disadvantages compared with open transabdominal resection include longer operative time, higher operative costs, and technical considerations related to operative skill. Large randomized trials with long-term follow-up are still needed.

Patterns of failure

The natural history and patterns of failure following "curative" resection are different for colon and rectal carcinomas. Locoregional failure as the only or major site of recurrence is common in rectal cancer, whereas colon cancer tends to recur in the peritoneum, liver, and other distant sites, with a lower rate of local failure. As a result, local therapy, such as irradiation, may play a significant role in the treatment of rectal tumors but is not used routinely for colon cancers.

ADJUVANT THERAPY FOR COLON CANCER

Approximately 75% of all patients with colorectal carcinoma will present at a stage when all gross carcinoma can be surgically resected. Nevertheless, despite the high resectability rate, almost half of all patients with colorectal adenocarcinoma die of metastatic disease, primarily because of residual disease that is not apparent at the time of surgery. These individuals are candidates for adjuvant local or systemic therapies.

Systemic chemotherapy

Systemic combined chemotherapy is the principal adjuvant therapy for colon cancer (Table 7). The current standard for resected stage III colon cancer is a combination of 5-FU, leucovorin, and oxaliplatin (Eloxatin; FOLFOX, FLOX). For patients in which the use of oxaliplatin is thought to be contraindicated (eg, in the presence of a peripheral neuropathy), alternatives for adjuvant therapy include capecitabine (Xeloda) or 5-FU and leucovorin. The development of 5-FU–containing regimens is described in the section on treatment of advanced and metastatic CRC.

The use of chemotherapy for resected stage II colon cancer is of uncertain survival benefit. When determining the benefit of adjuvant therapy for this group of patients, several factors should be taken into consideration, including the number of lymph nodes analyzed after surgery, the prognostic features (T4 lesion, perforation, peritumoral lymphovascular invasion, poorly differentiated histology, microsatellite stable), anticipated life expectancy, and comorbid conditions.

FOLFOX, FLOX Oxaliplatin has been approved by the U.S. Food and Drug Administration (FDA) for adjuvant therapy for resected stage III CRC. In a phase III trial for resected stages II and III colon cancer from Europe (MOSAIC), the use of FOLFOX4 compared with the same infusional regimen without oxaliplatin led to a higher 3-year disease-free survival rate (78% vs 73%) in those receiving FOLFOX. In a subgroup analysis, a significant disease-free survival benefit was seen for patients with stage III colon cancer and for patients with high-risk stage II colon cancer. A significant overall survival advantage was also seen for patients with stage III disease.

In a separate randomized phase III trial, conducted by the National Surgical Adjuvant Breast and Bowel Project (NSABP), for patients with resected stage II or III colon cancer, FLOX was compared with a weekly bolus of 5-FU and leucovorin. The 3-year disease-free survival benefit from FLOX was similar to that seen with FOLFOX4. Stages II and III disease were not evaluated separately.

A randomized trial (NSABP C-07) compared infusional 5-FU, oxaliplatin, and leucovorin (FLOX) with the same regimen without oxaliplatin in resected stages II and III colon cancer. Four-years disease-free survival was 67% versus 73% favoring the oxaliplatin-containing regimen. Grade 3 neurosensory toxicity and hospitalization for diarrhea were more common with the oxaliplatin-containing regimen (Kuebler JP, Wieand HS, O'Connell MJ, et al: J Clin Oncol 25:2198-2204, 2007).

Capecitabine is an oral fluorinated pyrimidine recently approved by the FDA for adjuvant therapy for patients with stage III colon cancer who have undergone complete resection of the primary tumor when treatment with fluoropyrimidine therapy alone is preferred. Capecitabine was not inferior to bolus 5-FU and low-dose leucovorin for disease-free survival, with a hazard ratio in the capecitabine group of 0.87 (95% confidence interval, 0.75–1.00). Capecitabine is an alternative for patients who are unlikely to tolerate 5-FU, leucovorin, and oxaliplatin.

5-FU plus leucovorin Studies have demonstrated the benefits of 5-FU plus leucovorin in the adjuvant treatment of colon car-

TABLE 7: Adjuvant chemotherapy regimens for colorectal adenocarcinoma (nonmetastatic)

Drug/combination	Dose and schedule
Oxaliplatin/fluorouracil/leucovorin (FOLFOX4)	
Oxaliplatin	85 mg/m^2 IV piggyback over 2 hours on day 1 only
Leucovorin	200 mg/m^2/d over 2 hours on day 1 given simultaneously with oxaliplatin
Fluorouracil	400 mg/m^2 IV bolus over 2 to 4 minutes on days 1 and 2
Fluorouracil	600 mg/m^2 continuous infusion over 22 hours on days 1 and 2 every 14 days for 12 cycles
Andre T, Boni C, Mounedji-Boudiaf L, et al: N Engl J Med 350:2343–2351, 2004.	
FLOX	
Fluorouracil	500 mg/m^2 IV bolus weekly for 6 weeks
Leucovorin	500 mg/m^2 IV weekly for 6 weeks each 8-week cycle x 3
Oxaliplatin	85 mg/m^2 IV administered on weeks 1, 3, and 5 of each 8-week cycle x 3
Kuebler JP, Weiand HS, O'Connell MJ, et al: J Clin Oncol 25:2198–2204, 2007.	
Capecitabine	
Capecitabine	1,250 mg/m^2 twice daily on days 1–14 every 3 weeks for 24 weeks
Twelves C, Wong A, Nowacki MP, et al: N Engl J Med 352:2696–2704, 2005.	

cinomas. Acceptable adjuvant regimens of 5-FU plus leucovorin for colon cancer include both low-dose leucovorin and high-dose leucovorin regimens (Table 7).

Irinotecan (CPT-11; Camptosar) Two phase III trials of FOLFIRI (5-FU, irinotecan, leucovorin) compared the same infusional regimen without irinotecan in either patients with resected stages II and III colon cancer (PETACC3) or high-risk stage III disease (ACCORD-2) did not show a benefit to the use of irinotecan in the adjuvant setting. Given the results of these two studies, the use of irinotecan currently is not considered a primary option for patients with resected stage II or III colon cancer.

Radiation therapy

Postoperative irradiation to the tumor bed should be considered in patients with T3 node-positive and T4 (B3 or C3) tumors located in retroperitoneal portions of the colon because more than 30% of these patients develop a local recurrence. Retrospective studies suggest improved local control with irradiation, particularly in patients with positive resection margins. If available, intraoperative radiotherapy may be considered for patients with T4 or recurrent cancers as an additional boost.

Patients with stage II disease may have a low recurrence rate after complete resection and may have less benefit from chemotherapy. The QUASAR trial evaluated the role of observation compared with chemotherapy with 5-FU and folinic acid in patients with colon or rectal cancer after curative resection. At a median follow-up of 5.5 years, the relative risk of death with chemotherapy versus observation was .82 (95% confidence interval [CI], .70–.95; P = .008). A second randomized trial of observation vs weekly 5-FU and leucovorin in 500 patients with stage II colon cancer found no significant difference in overall survival or risk of relapse for patients on the surveillance arm (hazard ratio, .69; 95% CI; .45–1.06; P = .09); (Quasar Collaborative Group: Gray R, Barnwell J, McConkey C: Lancet 370:2020-2029, 2007; Schippinger W, Samonigg H, Schaberl-Moser R, et al: Br J Cancer 97:1021-1027, 2007).

ADJUVANT THERAPY FOR RECTAL CANCER

Local recurrence alone or in combination with distant metastases occurs in up to 50% of patients with rectal carcinoma. Nodal metastases and deep bowel wall penetration are significant risk factors for locoregional failure.

In the absence of nodal metastases, the rate of local recurrence may be as low as 5% to 10% for stage I rectal cancer and 15% to 30% for stage II tumors. In stage III disease, the incidence of pelvic failure increases to 50% or more. The use of TME significantly reduces this risk of local recurrence; however, local recurrence remains a concern in patients with stages II and III disease.

Local recurrence in the pelvis is complicated by involvement of contiguous organs, soft and bony tissues, and deep nodal disease. Presenting symptoms vary from vague pelvic fullness to sciatica related to mass effect in the fixed space of the bony pelvis and invasion of the sciatic nerve.

Because local recurrence in the absence of metastatic disease is more common in rectal cancer than in colon cancer, aggressive resections, such as pelvic exenteration (anterior and posterior), sacral resection, and wide soft-tissue and pelvic floor resection, have been employed to treat these recurrences. Modern techniques of pelvic floor reconstruction, creation of continent urinary diversion, and vaginal reconstruction may be required for functional recovery.

The findings of the NSABP R-02 trial indicated postoperative adjuvant chemotherapy resulted in similar survival rates as those of postoperative chemoradiation therapy but was associated with a significantly higher rate of locoregional failure.

Pre- or postoperative radiation therapy

Radiation therapy has been used to reduce the locoregional recurrence rate of rectal tumors. Preoperative radiation therapy has been demonstrated to reduce local tumor recurrence, even in patients undergoing TME surgery. However, with the exception of one recent study, preoperative therapy has not affected overall survival in patients with stage II or III rectal cancer. An improvement in local control also has been observed with postoperative irradiation, but again with no benefit with regard to disease-free or overall survival. Preoperative radiation therapy reduced local recurrence rates when combined with total mesorectal resection (8% vs 2%; P < .001) in a Dutch phase III trial. In a French study of 762 patients, preoperative chemoradiation therapy compared with preoperative radiotherapy reduced local failure rates in patients with T3–T4 rectal cancers from 16.5% to 8%.

Chemoradiation therapy

Postoperative chemoradiation therapy Clinical trials of surgical adjuvant treatment indicate that postoperative radiation therapy with concurrent chemotherapy (chemoradiation therapy) is superior to postoperative radiation therapy alone or surgery alone. Postoperative chemoradiation therapy is a standard of care for patients with stage II or III rectal cancer based largely on the findings of the North Central Cancer Treatment Group (NCCTG) and Gastrointestinal Tumor Study Group (GITSG) trials. A summary of the 5-year survival results of the Patterns of Care Study (PCS) of the American College of Radiology and the results of the National Cancer Data Base (NCDB), both of which are representative of American national averages, is shown in Table 8.

The most effective combination of drugs, optimal mode of administration, and sequence of irradiation and chemotherapy still need to be determined. Radiation doses of 45 to 55 Gy are recommended in combination with 5-FU–based chemotherapy. Postoperative bolus 5-FU administration with irradiation is inferior to protracted venous infusion, resulting in lower 3-year rates of both overall survival (68% vs 76%) and disease-free survival (56% vs 67%).

An adjuvant treatment combining chemotherapy and pelvic irradiation in patients with stage II or III rectal cancer used the following regimen: 5-FU, 500 mg/m^2/d administered as a rapid IV infusion on days 1 to 5 and 450 mg/m^2/d on days 134 to 138 and days 169 to 173. Patients received a protracted IV infusion of 5-FU, 225 mg/m^2/d, by portable ambulatory infusion pump during the entire period of pelvic irradiation. Pelvic radiation therapy began on day 64 with a multiple-field technique to the tumor bed and nodal groups. A total of 4,500 cGy in 180-cGy fractions was administered over a 5-week period. Patients received a minimal boost dose of 540 cGy to the entire tumor bed, adjacent nodes, and 2 cm of adjacent tissue. A second boost dose of 360 cGy was allowed in selected patients with excellent displacement of the small bowel.

Neoadjuvant therapy For rectal cancers approaching the anal sphincter, preoperative (neoadjuvant) irradiation or the combination of chemotherapy and irradiation will significantly reduce the size of the majority of tumors. This approach allows for sphincter-preserving surgery in many patients. In addition, the long-term morbidity of radiation therapy for rectal cancer may be reduced if it is administered prior to surgery. The use of preoperative chemotherapy and radiation therapy is particularly important for patients presenting with locally advanced, unresectable rectal cancer, as the disease of the majority will be rendered resectable following neoadjuvant therapy. One additional role of neoadjuvant therapy may be in facilitating transanal excision of T2 and T3 rectal cancers in poor surgical risk patients. A number of investigators have reported good results with transanal excision of T2 and T3 tumors following a complete response to neoadjuvant therapy. However, this approach cannot be considered the current standard of care.

TABLE 8: Five-year overall survival in Patterns of Care Study (PCS) vs the National Cancer Data Base (NCDB), Gastro-intestinal Tumor Study Group (GITSG), and Mayo/North Central Cancer Treatment Group (Mayo/NCCTG) studies

Study	5-year survival	
Bimodality vs trimodality	**S + RT**	**S + RT + CT**
Stage II		
PCS	61%	81%
NCDB	55%	62%
Stage III		
PCS	33%	65%
NCDB	39%	42%
Postop CRT vs postop RT	**Postop RT**	**Postop CRT**
GITSG (7175)	52%	59%
Mayo/NCCTG (7945)	48%	57%
PCS	50%	69%

S = surgery; RT = radiation therapy; CT = chemotherapy; CRT = concurrent radiation therapy and chemotherapy

Adapted from Coia LR, Gunderson LL, Haller D, et al: Cancer 86:1952–1958, 1999.

Preoperative vs postoperative chemoradiation therapy Preoperative chemoradiation therapy may be preferred to postoperative adjuvant treatment, particularly in patients with T3 or T4 lesions. Such treatment may enhance resectability and may be associated with a lower frequency of complications compared with postoperative treatment. In a report of a randomized trial conducted by the German Rectal Cancer Study, Sauer et al found that compared with postoperative chemoradiotherapy, preoperative chemoradiotherapy significantly decreased local failure (7% vs 11%; $P = .02$) and sphincter preservation in low-lying tumors (39% vs 19%; $P < .004$). In addition, the incidence of chronic anastomotic recurrence was also lowest in the preoperative chemoradiotherapy group (2.7% vs 8.5%; $P = .001$).

TREATMENT OF ADVANCED AND METASTATIC COLON CANCERS

Local recurrences from colon cancers usually occur at the site of anastomosis, in the resection bed, or in the contiguous and retroperitoneal (para-aortic, para-caval) lymph nodes. Anastomotic recurrences heralded by symptoms are the most curable, followed by local soft-tissue recurrences. Regional and retroperitoneal lymph node recurrences portend a poor prognosis and systemic disease.

Chemotherapy

The development of chemotherapy for advanced CRC has become a very active field (Table 9). After decades of 5-FU–based treatment, and of little clinical gains, the arrival of new, effective agents has significantly changed the way this cancer is treated. Although 5-FU remains the backbone of most regimens, the new agents irinotecan and oxaliplatin have become an important part of front-line treatment of this disease in the United States and abroad. The recent development of molecular targeted agents has provided additional improvements in both response and survival for patients with CRC.

5-FU remains an important agent in the treatment of advanced CRC. Mainly in the past, 5-FU was administered as a bolus injection either weekly or daily for 5 days, every 4 to 5 weeks (Table 9). With these regimens, response rates have been approximately 10% to 15%. The development of permanent venous access devices and portable infusion pumps has permitted the prolonged infusion of 5-FU on an outpatient basis. The pattern of 5-FU toxicity differs depending on whether it is administered as a bolus or a prolonged infusion than by other methods. Bolus administration has pronounced myelotoxic effects, whereas the dose-limiting toxic effects of prolonged infusion 5-FU are mucositis and diarrhea. Palmar-plantar erythrodysesthesia (hand-foot syndrome) has been reported with prolonged infusions. Infusional 5-FU is now an important component of therapy when combined with either irinotecan or oxaliplatin.

Biochemical modulation of 5-FU Interest in the biochemical modulation of 5-FU by leucovorin is based on preclinical studies demonstrating that leucovorin raises the level of N5,N10-methylenetetrahydrofolate and, thus, forms a stable tertiary complex of thymidylate synthase (TS), the folate coenzyme, and 5-FU (in the form of 5-fluorodeoxyuridine). The use of 5-FU with leucovorin results in higher response rates than 5-FU alone and may prolong survival.

Although there is no agreement as to the optimal dose of leucovorin, historically two dosing schedules (as shown in Table 7) have been used with either low-dose or high-dose leucovorin.

FOLFOX was approved by the FDA in 2004 as first-line therapy. Initial evidence of activity was demonstrated in patients with pretreated, 5-FU–resistant CRC (45% response rate). In subsequent trials, patients with untreated metastatic CRC receiving FOLFOX had response rates of over 50%. In addition, patients receiving oxaliplatin, infusional 5-FU, and leucovorin have achieved overall survival rates of > 20 months in several reported trials. However, many of these patients have received second- and even third-line therapies at the time of disease progression, reducing the validity of survival evaluation. Currently, there are several accepted FOLFOX regimens in use, including FOLFOX4, FOLFOX6, modified FOLFOX6, and FOLFOX 7.

Oxaliplatin's toxicity profile includes nausea/vomiting and cumulative, reversible peripheral neuropathy. Patients may also develop a reversible, cold-induced, acute pharyngolaryngeal neuropathy. The OPTIMOX trials (OPTIMOX1 and OPTIMOX2) demonstrated that patients with either stable or responding metastatic CRC may benefit from an oxaliplatin-free interval

TABLE 9: Chemotherapy for advanced or metastatic disease

Drug/combination	Dose and schedule
Oxaliplatin/fluorouracil/leucovorin (FOLFOX6)	
Leucovorin	400 mg/m^2 IV infused over 2 hours on day 1
Oxaliplatin	100 mg/m^2 IV infused over 2 hours on day 1*
Fluorouracil	400 mg/m^2 IV bolus on day 1 then 1,200 mg/m^2/d for 2 days (total 2,400 mg/m^2 over 46-48 hours) continuous infusion

Cycle repeated every 2 weeks.
* Modified FOLFOX6 uses 85 mg/m^2

Maindrault-Goebel F, Louvet C, Andre T, et al: Eur J Cancer 35:1338–1342, 1999.

Capecitabine/oxaliplatin (CAPOX)	
Oxaliplatin	130 mg/m^2 IV infused on day 1 only followed by
Capecitabine to the morning of day 15	1,000 mg/m^2 orally twice daily in the evening on day 1

Cycle repeated every 3 weeks.

Cassidy J, Tabernero J, Twelves C, et al: J Clin Oncol 22:2084-2091, 2004.

Fluorouracil as an irradiation enhancer—bolus	
Leucovorin	20 mg/m^2 IV bolus on days 1-5, 29-33 immediately before fluorouracil
Fluorouracil	325 mg/m^2/d IV bolus on days 1-5, 29-33

Hyams DM, Mamounas EP, Petrelli N, et al: Dis Colon Rectum 40:131–139, 1997.

Fluorouracil as an irradiation enhancer—continuous infusion	
Fluorouracil	225 mg/m^2/d IV continuous infusion during irradiation

O'Connell MJ, Martenson JA, Wieand HS, et al: N Engl J Med 331:502–507, 1994.

Capecitabine as an irradiation enhancer	
Capecitabine	825 mg/m^2 twice daily during radiation

Dupuis O, Vie B, Lledo G, et al: Oncology 73:169–176, 2007.

with either no therapy or maintenance 5-FU and leucovorin followed by reintroduction of FOLFOX at the time of disease progression. The use of maintenance therapy compared with continued FOLFOX provided a comparable overall period of disease control. Maintenance therapy lessened the amount of oxaliplatin-induced neuropathy.

Irinotecan has significant clinical activity in patients with metastatic CRC whose disease has recurred or spread after standard chemotherapy. Its FDA approval was based on two phase III trials showing that irinotecan (350 mg/m^2 once every 3 weeks) significantly increased survival, compared with best supportive care and infusional 5-FU, respectively, in patients with recurrent or progressive cancer following first-line 5-FU therapy. Irinotecan increased the median

Irinotecan/fluorouracil/leucovorin (FOLFIRI)

Leucovorin	400 mg/m^2 IV infused over 2 hours prior to 5-FU on days 1 and 2
Irinotecan	180 mg/m^2 IV infused over 90 minutes on day 1
Fluorouracil	400 mg/m^2 IV bolus on day 1, then 600 mg/m^2 IV over 22 hours continuous infusion on days 1 and 2

Repeat cycle every 2 weeks.

Andre T, Louvet C, Maindrault-Goebel F, et al: Eur J Cancer 35:1343–1347, 1999.

Fluorouracil and leucovorin plus bevacizumab

Leucovorin	500 mg/m^2 IV infused over 2 hours once a week for 6 weeks, then a 2-week rest period
Fluorouracil	500 mg/m^2 IV bolus slow push 1 hour after leucovorin infusion once a week for 6 weeks, then a 2-week rest period
Bevacizumab	5 mg/kg IV continuous infusion over 90 minutes every 2 weeks

Kabbinavar F, Hurwitz H, Fehrenbacher I, et al: J Clin Oncol 21:60–65, 2003.

FOLFIRI with cetuximab in wild type KRAS

Irinotecan	180 mg/m^2 IV on day 1
Folinic acid	400 mg/m^2 on day 1
Fluorouracil	400 mg/m^2 bolus IV on day 1
Fluorouracil infusion	2.4 g/m^2 over 46 hours IV continuous infusion every 2 weeks
Cetuximab	400 mg/m^2 on day 1, then 250 mg/m^2/week 4

Van Cutsem E, Lang I, D'haens G, et al: J Clin Oncol 26(18S, part II):1006s [abstract 2], 2008.

FOLFOX with cetuximab in wild type KRAS

Oxaliplatin	85 mg/m^2 IV over 2 hours on day 1
Fluorouracil bolus	400 mg/m^2 IV bolus over 2 to 4 minutes
Leucovorin	400 mg/m^2 IV on day 1
Fluorouracil	2,400 to 3,000 mg/m^2 IV continuous infusion over 46 hours

Cycle repeated every 2 weeks.

Cetuximab	400 mg/m^2 IV on day 1, then 250 mg/m^2 IV once a week

Bokeymeyer C, Bondarenko I, Hartmann JT, et al: J Clin Oncol 26(18S, part I):178s [abstract 4000], 2008.

---

survival by 27% and 41%, respectively, in the two trials. Irinotecan is active in patients whose disease progressed while receiving 5-FU. Reproducible 15% to 20% response rates in this patient population led to the approval of irinotecan for use in patients with 5-FU–refractory disease. The dosage schedules most commonly used are 125 mg/m^2 weekly for 4 weeks, followed by a 2-week rest period (United States) and 350 mg/m^2 every 3 weeks (Europe). The primary toxicities of irinotecan are diarrhea and neutropenia. Intensive loperamide is important in the management of the former complication. An initial 4-mg loading dose is given at the first sign of diarrhea, followed by 2-mg doses every 2 hours until diarrhea abates for at least a 12-hour period.

Recent studies have shown that variation in the metabolism of irinotecan is associated with the pattern of allelic inheritance with the gene UGT 1A1. Although it is recommended that UGT 1A1 testing be performed prior to the use of irinotecan, dose-modification recommendations, based on the pattern of alleles inherited, are not currently available. However, it is recommended that patients with the UGT 1A1*28 pattern of inheritance should receive a reduced dose of irinotecan.

FOLFIRI Several randomized trials have shown improved response rates and overall survival when irinotecan is added to an infusional regimen of 5-FU and leucovorin compared with 5-FU and leucovorin alone. A bolus combination of irinotecan, 5-FU, and leucovorin (IFL) had also shown better response rates and overall survival but proved to be much more toxic. The use of IFL is no longer recommended.

In a phase III trial comparing the sequence of FOLFIRI followed by FOLFOX or the reverse sequence for patients with metastatic CRC, no difference in median survival was seen. Grade 3 or 4 mucositis, nausea, and vomiting occurred more frequently with FOLFIRI, whereas grade 3 or 4 neutropenia and neurosensory toxicity were more frequent with FOLFOX. Response rates were similar between the two groups. The results of this clinical trial and others stress the importance of using all available agents in the treatment of metastatic CRC, and the sequence of their use appears to be less important.

Capecitabine In a phase III trial of previously untreated patients with metastatic colon cancer, capecitabine produced higher response rates than did 5-FU and leucovorin. Overall survival and time to disease progression were similar (noninferior) to those with 5-FU and leucovorin. As established in European trials, the recommended dose of capecitabine is 2,500 mg/m^2 each day, given as a twice-daily dose, for 14 days followed by a 1-week rest period. However, most North American patients will not tolerate this dose of capecitabine and should instead receive 2,000 mg/m^2 each day, given as a twice-daily dose, for 14 days followed by a 1-week rest period. The side effects of capecitabine tend to be similar to those seen with prolonged infusion of 5-FU, with hand-foot syndrome being the most common.

Capecitabine and oxaliplatin may also provide significant benefit. Results of completed clinical trials with capecitabine and oxaliplatin are similar to those obtained with FOLFOX. This combination avoids the need for a central venous catheter.

Capecitabine and irinotecan may also be of benefit. This combination should be used with caution. Although some clinical trials have shown this combination to be tolerable and active, other trials of capecitabine and irinotecan have shown significant toxicity.

Molecular targeted agents

A variety of monoclonal antibodies and small molecules are being evaluated in clinical trials and preclinical studies. Three of these agents (bevacizumab [Avastin], cetuximab [Erbitux], and panitumumab [Vectibix]) have been approved by the FDA for use in CRC.

Bevacizumab is a humanized monoclonal antibody that binds circulating vascular endothelial growth factor (VEGF). When given with a 5-FU–containing regimen in several different trials as first-line therapy in patients with metastatic CRC, bevacizumab led to an improved outcome. The addition of bevacizumab to 5-FU and leucovorin resulted in significant improvement in disease progression-free survival. Even better results were seen with IFL, when the addition of bevacizumab to IFL resulted in significant improvement in overall survival and response rates. These studies led to approval by the FDA of bevacizumab. It is indicated for use in first-line therapy for metastatic CRC when combined with 5-FU–based chemotherapy, such as FOLFOX.

Cetuximab is a human/mouse chimeric antibody directed against the epithelial growth factor receptor (EGFR). In a randomized trial of patients with CRC refractory to irinotecan, patients were randomized to receive either cetuximab and irinotecan or cetuximab alone. The addition of cetuximab to irinotecan led to a significantly higher response rate compared with cetuximab alone. The median survival for those receiving cetuximab and irinotecan was also longer, though not significantly. Based on the results of this study, cetuximab has been approved by the FDA for use in patients whose disease is refractory to irinotecan with tumors expressing EGFR. Recent data from a phase III trial in which cetuximab was evaluated in addition to FOLFIRI compared to FOLFIRI alone suggests that patients with tumors harboring a

The CRYSTAL trial evaluated patients with first-line metastatic colon cancer treated with FOLFIRI vs FOLFIRI with cetuximab (Erbitux). The initial presentation of data from the Crystal trial presented at ASCO 2007 indicated a statistically significant improvement in progression-free survival (PFS) of approximately 1 month for the cetuximab arm. A second presentation of the data made at ASCO 2008 focused on the impact of KRAS on the outcome of this trial.

Eric Van Cutsem, MD, PhD, and colleagues used available archival tumor samples from 540 of the 1,198 patients and reported that when clinical responses were re-evaluated based on whether tumors showed normal or mutant KRAS expression, progression-free survival (PFS) and overall objective responses were better for patients with tumors that expressed normal KRAS (1 yr PFS 25% and 43% for patients with normal KRAS receiving FOLFIRI and the combination of FOLFIRI and cetuximab, respectively). Median progression-free survival also improved for patients receiving cetuximab and FOLFIRI in the presence of normal KRAS tumors (8.7 vs. 9.9 months; hazard ratio [HR] 0.68; $P = .017$). When clinical responses were re-evaluated for the 192 patients whose tumors harbored the KRAS mutation, OR and PFS rates were similar whether patients received FOLFIRI or FOLFIRI plus cetuximab. Adding cetuximab to FOLFIRI did not improve clinical responses in patients with KRAS mutation (Van Cutsem E, Lang I, D'haens G, et al: J Clin Oncol 26[abstract 2]: 2008).

mutant KRAS derived no benefit from the addition of cetuximab. A benefit in progression-free survival and response rates were seen with the addition of cetuximab in patients with wild type KRAS.

Panitumumab is a monoclonal antibody that targets EGFR. In a pivotal phase III trial, 463 patients with metastatic CRC who had failed to respond to previous standard therapy were randomized between panitumumab (6 mg/kg every 2 weeks) plus best supportive care (BSC) versus BSC alone. Patients in the panitumumab arm achieved a significantly improved time to disease progression (96 days vs 60 days) and objective response rate (8% vs 0%). On the basis of the results of this trial, the FDA approved panitumumab for the treatment of patients with CRC that has metastasized following standard chemotherapy.

Chemotherapy and surgery for stage IV CRC

Previously untreated patients with stage IV disease and limited organ involvement, such as liver-only metastases, in whom surgery is thought possible, consideration should be given to neoadjuvant chemotherapy followed by synchronous or staged partial colectomy and metastasectomy. The appropriate chemotherapy in this setting is uncertain. However, the use of FOLFOX or FOLFIRI is reasonable. The addition of bevacizumab may enhance response. However, because of the potential risk for bleeding or other surgical complications, bevacizumab should be discontinued 6 to 8 weeks before surgery. In addition, because of liver-associated changes with oxaliplatin or irinotecan, it is preferable to proceed with surgery after approximately 3 months of chemotherapy. Additional chemotherapy can be given after recovery from surgery. Patients with the development of limited metastatic disease after surgery and adjuvant therapy for stages I to III disease may also obtain long-term benefit from further chemotherapy and surgery.

Metastasectomy

Metastases to the liver and lungs account for most cases of non-nodal systemic disease in CRC. Resection of metastases, or metastasectomy, has gained recognition as a viable treatment. Resection of liver metastases results in cure rates of 5% to 60%, depending on the number of metastases and the stage of disease. Resection of solitary metastases in patients with stage I or II disease results in a 5-year survival rate of ~40% to 60%.

Metastasectomy for liver metastases should only be considered when complete resection is feasible on the basis of anatomic grounds and when adequate hepatic function can be maintained. Debulking resections are generally not recommended. Patients who are initially unresectable can be considered for resection after neoadjuvant chemotherapy as long as all disease, including the primary tumor can be resected. Hepatic resection is the treatment of choice for resectable liver metastases from colorectal cancer. Ablative techniques can be considered in amenable lesions where surgical resection is not feasible.

Adjuvant therapy after resection of hepatic metastases has been assessed in several randomized trials. Intra-arterial administration of floxuridine, using a hepatic artery catheter, alternating with systemic 5-FU and leucovorin, improves

TABLE 10: NCCN recommendations for post-treatment surveillance/monitoring*

- History and physical examination every 3 months for 2 years, then every 6 months for a total of 5 years
- CEA level evaluation every 3 months for 2 years, then every 6 months or years 2 to 5 for T2 or greater lesions
- Colonoscopy in 1 year, repeat in 1 year if results are abnormal or at least every 2 to 3 years if results are negative for polyps. If no preoperative colonoscopy has been performed due to an obstructing lesion, colonoscopy in 3 to 6 months
- Abdominal/pelvic CT scan in addition to chest x-ray or chest CT for patients with resected stage IV disease only: Every 6 months for 2 years, then every 6 to 12 months for a total of 5 years

* http://www.nccn.org

CEA = carcinoembryonic antigen; NCCN = National Comprehensive Cancer Network

overall survival and reduces the risk of recurrence within the liver.

Metastasectomy for lung metastases can be considered for highly selected patients where complete resection is feasible with maintenance of adequate pulmonary function. Resectable extrapulmonary metastases, particularly liver metastases, do not preclude resection.

TREATMENT OF ADVANCED RECTAL CANCER

Radiation therapy

Radiation therapy is moderately effective in palliating the symptoms of advanced rectal cancer. Pain is decreased in 80% of irradiated patients, although only 20% report complete relief. Bleeding can be controlled in more than 70% of patients. Obstruction cannot be reliably relieved by irradiation, and diverting colostomy is recommended. Only 15% of patients with recurrent rectal cancers achieve local disease control with irradiation, and median survival is < 2 years.

Chemoradiation therapy may be useful to convert fixed unresectable lesions into resectable lesions. These regimens have generally used protracted infusions of 5-FU (200 to 250 mg/m^2/d) delivered via a portable infusion pump during pelvic radiation therapy (450 cGy over 5 weeks).

Intraoperative radiotherapy (localized irradiation given to the tumor or tumor bed at the time of resection) is under active investigation in advanced and locoregionally recurrent rectal cancers.

Laser photoablation

Laser photoablation is occasionally employed for temporary relief of obstructive rectal cancer in patients who are not surgical candidates because of the presence of distant metastases, surgical comorbidity, or extensive intra-abdominal disease.

Follow-up of long-term survivors

Patients who have completed therapy for CRC require monitoring for potential treatment-related complications, recurrent disease, and new metachronous cancers. Specific follow-up recommendations for these patients are controversial. Guidelines for post-treatment surveillance/monitoring adopted by the National Comprehensive Cancer Network (NCCN), a consortium of American cancer centers, are shown in Table 10.

ANAL CANAL CARCINOMA

Epidemiology, etiology, and risk factors

In the United States, about 4,650 new cases of anal canal carcinoma are diagnosed each year. Overall, it is slightly more common in women than men. More than 80% of anal canal tumors occur in individuals > 60 years of age. Recent epidemiologic studies suggest that receptive anal intercourse is strongly related to anal cancer.

The incidence rate of anal cancer for single men is reported to be six times that for married men. In people < 35 years old, anal carcinoma is more common in men than women. A history of genital warts has been observed, suggesting that papillomavirus may be an etiologic factor.

Signs and symptoms

The diagnosis of anal canal carcinoma is usually delayed because the symptoms (bleeding, pain, and sensation of mass) are so often attributed to benign anorectal disorders, such as hemorrhoids or anal fissures.

Diagnosis

Evaluation should include a careful rectal examination, endoscopic examination with description of lesion size, and assessment of whether there is invasion of disease into adjacent organs (vagina, urethra, or bladder). Reexamination under general anesthesia may be necessary. A diagnostic incisional biopsy is required.

Pelvic CT is suggested to evaluate pelvic nodes. Although distant metastases are uncommon at diagnosis, a chest x-ray and liver function tests are recommended. Suspicious inguinal nodes discovered on physical examination must be assessed pathologically. The incidence of inguinal nodal metastases at diagnosis varies from 13% to 25%. The presence of perirectal, inguinal, and pelvic lymph node involvement correlates with tumor size and is unusual for tumors < 2 cm in diameter. Formal groin dissection is not advised; needle aspiration should be performed, with limited surgical biopsy if results of aspiration are inconclusive.

Pathology

Squamous cell carcinomas Most anal canal malignancies are squamous cell carcinomas. They have been classified as cloacogenic carcinomas, basaloid carcinomas, transitional cell carcinomas, or mucoepidermoid carcinomas. However, there is little difference in the natural history of these various types.

Unusual tumors arising in the anal canal include small-cell carcinomas, anal melanomas, and adenocarcinomas.

Small-cell carcinomas of the anal canal are aggressive neoplasms similar in natural history to bronchogenic small-cell carcinomas. If such a histology is identified, the clinician should be alerted to the possibility of early distant metastases, and treatment should include chemotherapeutic regimens used in bronchogenic small-cell carcinomas.

Anal melanomas Although advanced anal melanomas generally are associated with a dismal survival, prognosis may be related to the depth of disease penetration. Early anal melanomas < 2.0 mm in depth can be cured with wide excision. More advanced disease can be treated with local excision and external-beam irradiation with excellent local control. Abdominoperineal resection is indicated only rarely in the management of anal melanoma, because lesions large enough to require radical surgery are almost always associated with distant spread of disease.

Adenocarcinomas are uncommon cancers associated with a poor prognosis. Treatment should be aggressive and based on a multimodality approach. The rarity of this tumor precludes the development of specific clinical trials.

Staging

Size of the primary tumor is the most important clinical predictor of survival for patients with anal carcinomas. Both the International Union Against Cancer (UICC) and the American Joint Committee on Cancer (AJCC) have agreed on a unified staging system (Table 11). The TNM classification distinguishes between anal canal carcinoma and anal margin tumors, because the latter exhibit biologic behavior similar to that of other skin cancers and are staged as skin cancers.

Treatment

Surgery

In selected individuals with small superficial T1 tumors, local excision has achieved adequate local control and survival. However, most studies of local excision have been retrospective, with small numbers of patients. Prior to the advent of primary radiotherapy and combined-modality treatment (see later

> **A** retrospective review of patients undergoing salvage abdominoperineal resection for persistent or recurrent epidermoid carcinoma of the anal canal following chemoradiation therapy revealed a 5-year survival rate of 64%. Patients who received an initial radiation dose of less than 55 Gy, and those with positive lymph nodes at presentation had a significantly worse survival rate *(Mullen JT, Rodriguez-Bigas MA, Chang GJ, et al: Ann Surg Oncol 14:478-483, 2007).*

TABLE 11: TNM classification of anal canal tumors

Primary tumor (T)

Tx	Primary tumor cannot be assessed
T0	No evidence of primary tumor
Tis	Carcinoma in situ
T1	Tumor ≤ 2 cm in greatest dimension
T2	Tumor > 2 cm but not > 5 cm in greatest dimension
T3	Tumor > 5 cm in greatest dimension
T4	Tumor of any size that invades adjacent organs (eg, vagina, bladder, urethra, bladder)[a]

Regional lymph nodes (N)

Nx	Regional lymph nodes cannot be assessed
N0	No regional lymph node metastasis
N1	Metastasis in perirectal lymph node(s)
N2	Metastasis in unilateral internal iliac and/or inguinal lymph node(s)
N3	Metastasis in perirectal and inguinal lymph nodes and/or bilateral internal iliac and/or inguinal lymph nodes

Distant metastasis (M)

Mx	Distant metastasis cannot be assessed
M0	No distant metastasis
M1	Distant metastasis

Grade (G)

Gx	Grade of differentiation cannot be assessed
G1	Well differentiated
G2	Moderately differentiated
G3	Poorly differentiated
G4	Undifferentiated

Stage groupings

Stage 0	Tis	N0	M0
Stage I	T1	N0	M0
Stage II	T2	N0	M0
	T3	N0	M0
Stage IIIA	T1-3	N1	M0
	T4	N0	M0
Stage IIIB	T4	N1	M0
	Any T	N2-3	M0
Stage IV	Any T	Any N	M1

[a] Direct invasion of the rectal wall, perirectal skin, subcutaneous tissue, or the sphincter muscle(s) is not classified as T4.

From Greene FL, Page DL, Fleming ID, et al (eds): AJCC Cancer Staging Manual, 6th Ed. New York, Springer-Verlag, 2002.

TABLE 12: Chemotherapy regimens for anal canal cancer

Drug/combination	Dose and schedule
Fluorouracil/mitomycin/radiation therapy	
Fluorouracil	1 g/m^2/d IV infused continuously on days 1-4 and 29-32
Mitomycin	15 mg/m^2 IV on day 1
Irradiation	200 cGy/d for 5 days per week (total dose, 3,000 cGy)
Give chemotherapy concurrently with irradiation; start both modalities on the same day.	
Leichman L, Nigro ND, Vaitkevicius VK, et al: Am J Med 78:211–215, 1985.	
Fluorouracil/cisplatin/radiation therapy	
Fluorouracil	1 g/m^2/d IV infused continuously for 4 days
Cisplatin	25 mg/m^2/d IV on days 2-5 following standard hydration
Irradiation	200 cGy/d for 5 days per week (total dose, 3,000 cGy)
Give chemotherapy concurrently with irradiation, except in elderly or frail patients.	
Wagner JP, Mahe MA, Romestaing P, et al: Int J Radiat Oncol Biol Phys 29:17–23, 1994.	

Table prepared by Ishmael Jaiyesimi, DO

in this chapter), abdominoperineal resection was considered to be the conventional treatment for patients with invasive anal canal cancer. Unfortunately, even with radical surgical procedures, local recurrences are frequent. Currently, radical extirpative surgery is indicated only after the failure of combined-modality treatment.

Radiation therapy

Trials of primary external-beam radiotherapy in patients with anal canal carcinomas have used doses varying between 4,500 and 7,550 cGy. Local control rates of 60% to 90%, with 5-year survival rates of 32% to 90%, are similar to the results of surgical series when the trials are controlled for tumor size.

Interstitial radiation therapy alone has been used primarily in Europe for early-stage lesions. A relatively high radiation dose is delivered to a small volume. This modality carries a high potential for radiation necrosis and fails to incorporate treatment of the inguinal nodes.

Combined-modality treatment

Chemotherapy given concurrently with irradiation is the preferred therapy for most patients with anal canal cancer (Table 12). Investigators from Wayne State University pioneered the use of simultaneous pelvic irradiation and chemotherapy in the treatment of patients with anal canal carcinomas. They demonstrated that the majority of such patients could be treated with this combination, obviating the need for an abdominoperineal resection. The original study design used 3,000 cGy over 3 weeks with 5-FU (1,000 mg/m^2/d) as a continu-

The Intergroup RTOG 98-11 trial randomized 682 patients with anal carcinoma to receive 5-FU (1,000 mg/m^2) on days 1-4 and 29-32) plus mitomycin (10 mg/m^2 on days 1 and 29) and radiation (45 to 59 Gy) or 5-FU (1,000 mg/m^2 on days 1-4, 29-32, 57-60, and 85-88) plus cisplatin (75 mg/m^2 on days 1, 29, 57, and 85) and radiation (45 to 59 Gy). Early results indicate no significant difference in 5-year disease-free survival (56% vs 48%; P = .28) and 5-year overall survival (69% for both arms; P = .24). Hematologic toxicity was higher in the mitomycin-containing regimen (Ajani JA, Winter KA, Gunderson LL, et al: JAMA 299:1914-1921, 2008).

ous infusion on days 1 to 4 and then repeated on days 29 to 32. Mitomycin, 15 mg/m^2, was administered as an IV bolus on day 1. A total of 4 to 6 weeks after the completion of therapy, patients had a deep muscle biopsy of the anal canal scar.

An updated analysis of this experience demonstrated that 38 of 45 patients (84%) were rendered disease free after chemotherapy and irradiation. Individuals who had positive results on biopsy underwent an abdominoperineal resection.

Because of the success of this experience, other investigators have attempted to implement infusional 5-FU and mitomycin with irradiation as definitive therapy. Most studies have used similar schedules of 5-FU and mitomycin but have used higher doses of pelvic irradiation (4,500 to 5,700 cGy). Five-year survival rates > 70% have been reported.

A randomized trial from the Radiation Therapy Oncology Group (RTOG) showed that the use of mitomycin with irradiation and 5-FU increased complete tumor regression and improved colostomy-free survival over irradiation and 5-FU alone. At 4 years, the colostomy-free survival rate was higher in the mitomycin arm than in the 5-FU–alone arm (71% vs 59%), as was the disease-free survival rate (73% vs 51%). Current studies are examining the role of cisplatin versus mitomycin along with radiation therapy and 5-FU.

Several investigators have compared the results of irradiation alone versus irradiation plus chemotherapy. Cummings et al found that with identical irradiation doses and techniques, the local control rate for cancers > 2 cm rose from 49% with radiation therapy alone to 85% when 5-FU and mitomycin were combined with irradiation. Papillon and Montbarbon found an increase in the rate of local control with a combined-modality approach compared with pelvic irradiation alone (81% vs 66%). Two recent randomized studies have shown improved local control with chemoradiation therapy over irradiation.

A complete response to combined chemotherapy and radiation therapy is expected in 80% to 90% of patients with anal cancer. It is important to evaluate the response of therapy with a careful examination of the anal canal after treatment. Anal canal cancers can continue to regress for up to 3 or more months after completion of treatment. For this reason, it is recommended that a biopsy be performed no sooner than 3 months after the completion of treatment, unless there is evidence of disease progression or other evidence to suggest early recurrence. If pathologic evidence of recurrence is diagnosed, abdominoperineal resection is expected to yield long-term disease control and survival in 40% to 60% of patients.

Chemotherapy

Reports of other chemotherapeutic agents in anal cancer have been relatively anecdotal, with limited phase II studies. Because of the activity of cisplatin in other squamous cell carcinomas, this agent has been employed as a single agent or combined with infusional 5-FU in advanced disease.

SUGGESTED READING

ON COLORECTAL CARCINOMA

Bentrem DJ, Okabe S, Wong WD, et al: T1 adenocarcinoma of the rectum: Transanal excision or radical surgery? Ann Surg 242:472–477, 2005.

Bosset JF, Collette L, Calais G, et al: Chemotherapy with preoperative radiotherapy in rectal cancer. N Engl J Med 355:1114–1123, 2006.

Cunningham D, Humblet Y, Siena S, et al: Cetuximab monotherapy and cetuximab plus irinotecan in irinotecan-refractory metastatic colorectal cancer. N Engl J Med 351:337–345, 2005.

Fazio VW, Zutshi M, Remzi FH, et al: A randomized multicenter trial to compare long-term functional outcome, quality of life, and complications of surgical procedures for low rectal cancers. Ann Surg 246:481–488, 2007.

Jayne DG, Guillou PJ, Thorpe H, et al: Randomized trial of laparoscopic-assisted resection of colorectal carcinoma: 3-year results of the UK MRC CLASICC Trial Group. J Clin Oncol 25:3061–3068, 2007.

Kuebler JP, Wieand HS, O'Connell MJ, et al: Oxaliplatin combined with weekly bolus fluorouracil and leucovorin as surgical adjuvant chemotherapy for stage II and III colon cancer: Results from NSABP C-07. J Clin Oncol 25:2198–2204, 2007.

Lembersky BC, Wieand HS, Petrelli NJ, et al: Oral uracil and tegafur plus leucovorin compared with intravenous fluorouracil and leucovorin in stage II and III carcinoma of the colon: Results from National Surgical Adjuvant Breast and Bowel Project Protocol C-06. J Clin Oncol 24:2059–2064, 2006.

Leung KL, Kwok SP, Lam SC, et al: Laparoscopic resection of rectosigmoid carcinoma: Prospective randomised trial. Lancet 363:1187–1192, 2004.

Peeters KC, Marijnen CA, Nagtegaal ID, et al: The TME trial after a median follow-up of 6 years: Increased local control but no survival benefit in irradiated patients with resectable rectal carcinoma. Ann Surg 246:693–701, 2007.

Poynter JN, Gruber SB, Higgins PD, et al: Statins and the risk of colorectal cancer. N Engl J Med 352:2184–2192, 2005.

Toxicity from combined radiotherapy (CRT) and chemotherapy for anal carcinoma is significant. Two recently completed trials have addressed the use of 3D-CRT and intensity-modulated radiotherapy (IMRT) to reduce these toxicities. A comparison of 60 patients treated with conventional radiotherapy to 62 patients treated with 3D CRT found improvements in 5-year local control (85.1% and 61.1%; $P = .0056$) and overall survival (80.7% and 53.9%; $P = .0171$) with 3D CRT. All patients received 5-FU and mitomycin or 5-FU and cisplatin concurrently with radiotherapy. A second series evaluated IMRT for the treatment of anal carcinoma with standard doses and chemotherapy regimens. Toxicity compared favorably with historic rates as did disease outcomes, suggesting that IMRT may be effective and reduce toxicity (*Vuong T, Kopek N, Ducruet T, et al: Int J Radiat Oncol Biol Phys 67:1394-1400, 2007; Salama JK, Mell LK, Schomas DA, et al: J Clin Oncol 25:4581-4586, 2007*).

Quasar Collaborative Group, Gray R, Barnwell J, McConkey C, et al: Adjuvant chemotherapy versus observation in patients with colorectal cancer: A randomised study. Lancet 370:2020–2029, 2007.

Saltz LB, Niedzwiecki D, Hollis D, et al: Irinotecan fluorouracil plus leucovorin is not superior to fluorouracil plus leucovorin alone as adjuvant treatment for stage III colon cancer: Results of CALGB 89803. J Clin Oncol 25:3456–3461, 2007.

Schippinger W, Samonigg H, Schaberl-Moser R, et al: A prospective randomised phase III trial of adjuvant chemotherapy with 5-fluorouracil and leucovorin in patients with stage II colon cancer. Br J Cancer 97:1021–1027, 2007.

Van Cutsem E, Peeters M, Siena S, et al: Open-label phase III trial of panitumumab plus best supportive care compared with best supportive care alone in patients with chemotherapy-refractory metastatic colorectal cancer. J Clin Oncol 25:1658–1664, 2007.

ON ANAL CANAL CARCINOMA

Das P, Bhatia S, Eng C, et al: Predictors and patterns of recurrence after definitive chemoradiation for anal cancer. Int J Radiat Oncol Biol Phys 68:794–800, 2007.

Ghouti L, Houvenaeghel G, Moutardier V, et al: Salvage abdominoperineal resection after failure of conservative treatment in anal epidermoid cancer. Dis Colon Rectum 48:16–22, 2005.

Mullen JT, Rodriguez-Bigas MA, Chang GJ, et al: Results of surgical salvage after failed chemoradiation therapy for epidermoid carcinoma of the anal canal. Ann Surg Oncol 14:478–483, 2007.

Podnos YD, Tsai NC, Smith D, et al: Factors affecting survival in patients with anal melanoma. Am Surg 72:917–920, 2006.

Salama JK, Mell LK, Schomas DA, et al: Concurrent chemotherapy and intensity-modulated radiation therapy for anal canal cancer patients: A multicenter experience. J Clin Oncol 25:4581–4586, 2007.

Vuong T, Kopek N, Ducruet T, et al: Conformal therapy improves the therapeutic index of patients with anal canal cancer treated with combined chemotherapy and external beam radiotherapy. Int J Radiat Oncol Biol Phys 67:1394–1400, 2007.

CHAPTER 17

Prostate cancer

Judd W. Moul, MD, FACS, Andrew J. Armstrong, MD, SCM,
Brent K. Hollenbeck, MD, MS, Joseph Lattanzi, MD,
Deborah Bradley, MD, and Maha Hussain, MD

Prostate cancer is the most common non-skin cancer and the second leading cause of cancer mortality in American men. Despite the fact that this cancer will be diagnosed in an estimated 186,320 American men in the year 2008 and will lead to the death of approximately 28,660 men, there is no universally agreed-upon strategic plan for its diagnosis and management.

Epidemiology

Age The risk of developing prostate cancer begins to increase at age 50 years in white men who have no family history of the disease and at age 40 years in black men and those who have a first-degree relative (father, brother) with prostate cancer. Risk increases with age, but, unlike other cancers, prostate cancer has no "peak" age or modal distribution. There has been a downward "age migration" in the PSA (prostate-specific antigen) era such that the median age at diagnosis is now approximately 60 years old.

Race The highest incidence of prostate cancer in the world is found in American black men, who have approximately a 9.8% lifetime risk of developing this cancer. This rate is slightly higher than the 8% lifetime risk for American white men. Black men have an incidence of prostate cancer that is 1.6 times that of white men.

The Japanese and mainland Chinese populations have the lowest rates of prostate cancer. Interestingly, although Japanese immigrants to the United States have a higher incidence of prostate cancer than Japanese people living in Japan, their rate is still about half that of American whites.

Socioeconomic status appears to be unrelated to the risk of prostate cancer, and the explanation for racial variability is unknown. However, an interplay of diet, hormonal factors, and genetics likely accounts for the variability.

Geography The incidence of prostate cancer is highest in Scandinavian countries (22 cases per 100,000 population) and lowest in Asia (5 per 100,000). Risk may be inversely related to ultraviolet light exposure, as the incidence increases the farther one lives from the equator. However, recent studies show extremely high rates in populations of African heritage, such as Jamaicans.

Etiology and risk factors

Family history Men who have a first-degree relative with prostate cancer have approximately a twofold increased risk of developing prostate cancer during their lifetime. An individual who has two first-degree relatives with prostate cancer has a ninefold increase in lifetime risk.

True hereditary prostate cancer occurs in a small number of men and tends to develop at an early age (< 55 years old).

Dietary fat Studies have suggested that dietary fat may increase the risk of prostate cancer. However, no definitive proof of its role has yet been found.

These studies indicate that progression of prostate cancer, which is likely to be more clinically relevant, has different risk factors than those associated with its initiation/incidence and that some of these risk factors are likely modifiable. Recent findings from the Health Professionals Follow-up study have, however, demonstrated different dietary risk factors for the incidence compared with progression of prostate cancer. For example, African-American race, a positive family history, low consumption of tomato products, and high consumption of alpha-linolenic acid have been associated with higher risks of incident prostate cancer. However, height, body mass index, low physical activity, smoking, low consumption of tomato sauce, high calcium and alpha-linolenic acid intake, African-American race, and positive family history have all been associated with fatal cancer.

In addition, recent findings suggest that cruciferous or brassica family vegetables may reduce the risk of advanced prostate cancer. This family includes broccoli, cauliflower, cole slaw, and sauerkraut. Interestingly, the intake of brussels sprouts, spinach, and mustard greens did not appear to be protective, and the consumption of fruit was not associated with the incidence or progression of prostate cancer.

Vasectomy Several large epidemiologic studies suggest that vasectomy may increase the relative risk of prostate cancer by as much as 1.85. However, these same studies do not report an increased risk of dying from prostate cancer associated with vasectomy but do indicate a statistically increased risk of dying from lung cancer. These findings argue against an association between vasectomy and prostate cancer. Currently, this association is unproven and does not constitute grounds for fundamental changes in the use of vasectomy.

Sexual activity/sexually transmitted disease A large prospective study of more than 29,000 men demonstrated an association between high ejaculatory frequency (more than 21 ejaculations/month) and a decreased risk of prostate cancer, with a lifetime relative risk of 0.67. However, there may be several confounding factors associated with high sexual activity, such as differences in prostate cancer screening or lifestyle. There was no associated increased risk for men in the lowest ejaculatory frequency category.

Inflammation may underlie the findings associated with a relatively higher risk of prostate cancer in men seen in STD (sexually transmitted disease) clinics, but it may also be related to screening bias. Several cohort studies and one meta-analysis have demonstrated a protective role for the daily intake of aspirin and the risk of prostate cancer. In addition, the lipid-lowering and anti-inflammatory statin compounds have been associated with a reduction in the risk of high-grade tumors. These findings require prospective validation in randomized trials.

Prevention Active research on the chemoprevention of prostate cancer is ongoing. The only prospective randomized trial to demonstrate an effect was the Prostate Cancer Prevention Trial (PCPT), which showed a 24.8% reduction in the risk of prostate cancer among men randomized to receive finasteride (Proscar) daily versus those men on the placebo arm. Finasteride as a chemopreventive agent has not been universally accepted, however, because patients in the treatment arm were possibly more likely to exhibit higher-grade prostate cancer. Recent follow-up studies of the PCPT suggest that finasteride probably does not induce high-grade disease, and the observation may be a detection artifact. Other agents under study include vitamin E and selenium, both of which have been associated with a decreased risk of prostate cancer. A large prospective randomized trial to evaluate the effects of these agents in healthy men is currently under way.

> **D**espite data from the Prostate Cancer Prevention Trial demonstrating the ability of finasteride to reduce the risk of prostate cancer, the adoption of this preventive measure may be hindered by concerns over the induction of high-grade disease in the treatment arm. Recent evidence from two different studies suggest that the ascertainment of more high-grade disease in the finasteride arm was due to sampling density bias and the impact of the treatment on prostate volume *(Cohen YC, Liu KS, Heyden NL, et al: J Natl Cancer Inst 99:1366-1374, 2007; Lucia MS, Epstein JI, Goodman PJ, et al: J Natl Cancer Inst 99:1375-1383, 2007).*

Signs and symptoms

Early-stage disease Men with organ-confined prostate cancer often are completely asymptomatic. Men with a large component of benign prostatic hyperplasia often present with bladder outlet obstruction unrelated to prostate cancer.

Locally advanced disease Bladder outlet obstruction is the most common sign of locally advanced prostate cancer. A few men with locally advanced disease present with hematuria, urinary tract infections, and irritative voiding symptoms secondary to bladder outlet obstruction.

Advanced disease Rarely, men with bulky lymph node metastasis may present with bilateral lower-extremity edema. Men with bony metastasis often present with bone pain and, uncommonly, with lower-extremity weakness or paralysis from spinal cord compression.

Screening and diagnosis

Prostate cancer screening with PSA and digital rectal examination (DRE) has resulted in not only an increase in prostate cancer detection but also a stage shift. More cancers are now being detected at earlier stages, when they are potentially curable. Prior to screening efforts, most prostate cancers were detected when they produced local symptoms or distant metastases, at which point treatment for cure often was impossible.

Digital rectal examination Prostate biopsy prompted by abnormal findings on DRE, such as nodularity or induration of the prostate, leads to a diagnosis of prostate cancer in only 15% to 25% of cases. This rate compares with a prostate cancer prevalence of < 5% among men of similar age without an abnormal DRE. Although neither accurate nor sensitive for prostate cancer detection, abnormal DRE is associated with a fivefold increased risk of cancer present at the time of screening.

PSA is a serine protease produced by the prostatic epithelium and secreted in the seminal fluid in large quantities. The level of PSA in serum is increased by inflammation of the prostate, urinary retention, prostatic infection, benign prostatic hyperplasia, prostate cancer, and prostatic manipulation. The optimal threshold to recommend prostatic biopsy has come under increasing scrutiny. The overall sensitivity for PSA levels is approximately 50% to 70% depending on the threshold used, but it is not as specific and does not allow for differentiation between indolent and aggressive disease. For example, by using a threshold of 4.1 ng/mL, the majority of cancers in men < age 60 would potentially be missed. However, a PSA cutoff of 4.1 ng/mL only has a positive predictive value of approximately 30%, meaning two out of three men would undergo biopsy for benign disease.

A more worthwhile approach for PSA screening may be to use the rate of rise in PSA (PSA velocity) in combination with the absolute PSA value. This approach has been shown to be useful recently in the form of age-adjusted PSA velocity, but accepted guidelines are still controversial.

Another commonly employed test for patients with a PSA level < 10 ng/mL is the percent-free PSA level. There is an inverse relationship between the percent-free PSA level and the risk of a cancer diagnosis. Most urologists utilize a cutoff of 10% to prompt a recommendation for biopsy. In men who have never had a prostate biopsy but who have a total PSA level > 4.0 ng/mL, a percent-free PSA less than 25% may suggest a 50% to 60% probability of prostate cancer.

In men who have had a prior negative biopsy but who have a persistently elevated PSA level > 4.0 ng/mL, a percent-free PSA < 10% should prompt a repeat biopsy.

Current screening recommendations The American Cancer Society and the American Urological Association (AUA) recommend that the PSA test and the DRE should be offered annually beginning at age 50 to men who have a life expectancy of at least 10 years. In high-risk men (African Americans and those with a first-degree relative diagnosed with prostate cancer), screening should be offered at an earlier age (40–45 years old). Prior to testing, physicians should discuss with their patients the potential benefits of early prostate cancer detection and its implications in the need for subsequent treatment so that patients can make an informed decision about undergoing screening.

> Using administrative data, Welch and colleagues found that 32% of Medicare recipients who underwent prostate biopsy were diagnosed with prostate cancer. This is among the first population-based studies to empirically demonstrate detection rates in the PSA era. Further, the incidence rose with age (to 41% among those 80 and older) and with repetitive biopsies *(Welch HG, Fisher ES, Gottlieb DJ, et al: J Natl Cancer Inst 99:1395-1400, 2007).*

There are currently two ongoing major prostate cancer screening trials: The Prostate, Lung, Colorectal, and Ovarian (PLCO) trial in the United States funded by the National Cancer Institute and the European Organisation for Research and Treatment of Cancer (EORTC) trial. The National Comprehensive Cancer Network (NCCN) has recently published aggressive screening guidelines on its website (www.nccn.org). These new controversial guidelines call for baseline PSA levels at a younger age (generally age 40) and suggest that any young man with a PSA level > 0.7 ng/mL (median in men aged 40–49) be tested annually.

Biopsy When indicated, prostate biopsy is usually performed as an office procedure by transrectal ultrasonographic guidance using an automated 18-gauge biopsy gun. The procedure is performed with, at most, local anesthesia and carries a risk of significant infection of only 1 in 200 cases. Additional side effects of hematuria and hematochezia are common for 2 to 3 days following the biopsy. Hematospermia may last for up to 4 to 6 weeks. Since about the year 2000, prostate biopsy includes laterally directed extended core protocols employing 8 to 12 biopsy cores per procedure. Multiple studies have demonstrated that the addition of the lateral cores improves the accuracy of biopsy.

If the biopsy result is negative, these men are typically followed conservatively with serial PSA levels and DRE repeated annually. Repeat biopsy is performed only when PSA levels rise at abnormal rates (> 0.8 ng/mL/yr) or if DRE findings show new nodularity or induration. Men in whom high-grade prostatic intraepithelial neoplasia is found on biopsy usually should undergo repeat biopsy, since one-third to one-half will be found to have prostate cancer.

Recently, a new test, the UPM-3 urine test, has become more widely available. This test, performed on voided urine after an "attentive" DRE, is based on reverse transcriptase–polymerase chain reaction assay for a PSA product (DD3).

TABLE 1: TNM staging system of prostate cancer

Localized disease

T1a Tumor incidental histologic finding in ≤ 5% of resected tissue; not palpable

T1b Tumor incidental histologic finding in > 5% of resected tissue

T1c Tumor identified by needle biopsy (eg, because of elevated PSA level)

T2a Tumor involves one-half of one lobe or less

T2b Tumor involves more than one-half of one lobe but not both lobes

T2c Tumor involves both lobes

Local extension

T3a Extracapsular extension (unilateral or bilateral)

T3b Tumor invades seminal vesicle(s)

T4   Bladder invasion, fixed to pelvic side wall, or invasion of adjacent structures

Metastatic disease

N1   Positive regional lymph nodes

M1   Distant metastasis

PSA = prostate-specific antigen
Adapted from Greene FI, Page DL, Fleming ID, et al (eds): AJCC Cancer Staging Manual, 6th ed. New York, Springer-Verlag, 2002.

It is becoming useful not as a primary screening test, but to dictate the need for repeat prostate biopsy in men with persistently elevated PSA levels.

In addition, researchers at Johns Hopkins University have developed a blood-based test called EPCA-2, which detects a nuclear matrix protein linked to prostate cancer. Elevated levels of EPCA-2 were found to be more sensitive and specific for prostate cancer, even in men with normal PSA levels and benign prostatic hypertrophy, and predicted extracapsular disease as well. Currently, this test is being further optimized and validated in a large series of patients. Additional future studies will investigate the role of a novel fusion protein (TMPRSS2-ETS) commonly found in prostate tumors, both as a diagnostic and prognostic marker. This fusion gene is androgen regulated and directs oncogenic signals and has been found in over 50% of localized prostate cancer.

Pathology

Adenocarcinomas make up the vast majority of prostate carcinomas. A total of 70% of prostate adenocarcinomas occur in the peripheral zone, 20% in the transitional zone, and approximately 10% in the central zone.

Other tumor types are relatively rare and include ductal adenocarcinoma, which occurs in the major ducts and often projects into the urethra; and mucinous adenocarcinoma, which secretes abundant mucin and does not arise

TABLE 2: D'Amico et al risk stratification for clinically localized prostate cancer

Low risk	Diagnostic PSA < 10.0 ng/mL *and* highest biopsy Gleason score ≤ 6 *and* clinical stage T1c or T2a
Intermediate risk	Diagnostic PSA > 10 but < 20 ng/mL *or* highest biopsy Gleason score = 7 *or* clinical stage T2b
High risk	Diagnostic PSA > 20 ng/mL *or* highest biopsy Gleason score ≤ 8 *or* clinical stage T2c/T3

PSA = prostate-specific antigen

from the major ducts. Transitional carcinoma of the prostate occurs within the ducts and, to a lesser extent, in the prostatic acini. Typically, primary transitional carcinomas are aggressive cancers that have a poor prognosis. Similarly, neuroendocrine (small-cell) tumors are rare and aggressive, have a poor prognosis, and typically require aggressive surgical management. Other rare types include foamy carcinoma, mucinous adenocarcinoma, large cell neuroendocrine tumors, and signet ring tumors.

Histologic grade The grading system developed by Gleason from data accumulated by the Veterans Administration Cooperative Urologic Research Group appears to provide the best prognostic information in addition to clinical stage and is the predominant grading system in widespread use.

Metastatic spread Adenocarcinoma of the prostate may spread locally through direct extension into periprostatic fat or via the ejaculatory ducts into seminal vesicles; lymphatically to regional lymph nodes, including the hypogastric and obturator lymph nodes; and hematogenously to bone. The most common sites of bony metastases are the lumbosacral spine (probably related to venous drainage of the prostate through Baston's plexus) and the axial skeleton, but any bone, including the skull and ribs, can be involved. Rare sites of metastatic spread include the liver and lungs.

Prevention

Until 2004, there was no intervention known to prevent prostate cancer. The primary objective of the PCPT was to describe the prevalence of histologically proven prostate cancer among men randomized to receive daily finasteride (a 5-alpha-reductase inhibitor that decreases prostate size and serum/prostate dihydrotestosterone levels) or placebo. The authors described a 24.8% reduction in the prevalence of prostate cancer among men taking finasteride, suggesting that it either prevents or delays the appearance of prostate cancer. The

TABLE 3: Risk of dying of clinically localized prostate cancer without definitive locoregional therapy

Gleason score	Age			
	55-59	60-64	65-69	70-74
2-4	4%	5%	6%	7%
5	6%	8%	10%	11%
6	18%	23%	27%	30%
7	70%	62%	53%	42%
8-10	87%	81%	72%	60%

Adapted from Albertsen PC, Hanley JA, Fine J: JAMA 293:2095–2101, 2005.

caveat of their findings, however, was that these cancers that developed in the treatment arm were of a higher grade.

Prognosis and natural history

Staging systems The most widely used and universally accepted staging system for prostate cancer is the TNM system (Table 1). In the TNM system, T1 and T2 tumors are confined to the gland, whereas T3 and T4 tumors have local extension.

Risk-adapted staging The development of the "Partin Tables" in 1993 ushered in a new era of combining clinical stage, Gleason score, and PSA level to predict pathologic stage after radical prostatectomy. More recently, this has led to the D'Amico et al risk groupings for newly diagnosed men with clinically localized disease (Table 2). Patients are divided into three risk groups (low, intermediate, or high) of occult micrometastases and relapse after initial local therapy. Although not perfect, this system is currently in widespread use and allows a framework for multimodal and multidisciplinary treatment strategies based on risk grouping. Finally, Kattan et al have developed preoperative and postoperative nomograms as clinical tools to predict the risk of recurrence after radical prostatectomy. Although these nomograms are imperfect, they may be useful for estimating risk and planning therapy as well as for stratifying and selecting patients for clinical trials.

Indicators of the quality of life of prostate cancer care have been developed. However, in a multi-institutional study using the National Cancer Database, Miller and colleagues noted that compliance with the indicators was highly variable and generally more common among those undergoing radiation therapy opposed to those undergoing surgery (Miller DC, Spencer BA, Ritchey J, et al: Med Care 45:401-409, 2007).

Prognosis The optimal management of patients with prostate cancer varies widely and is highly dependent upon a patient's age, overall health, and tumor risk assessment. The natural history of the disease process can be heterogeneous, ranging from an incidental finding unlikely to result in cancer-specific mortality, to very aggressive, resulting in early widespread metastatic disease and death. Therefore, treating physicians should carefully consider the value of curative therapy with potential toxicity in the context of a patient's comorbidities and life expectancy.

Volume outcome relationships are evident for a variety of surgeries. Multi-institutional data suggest that the learning curve for radical prostatectomy is steep and does not begin to plateau until at least 250 cases *(Vickers AJ, Ulmert D, Serio AM, et al: J Natl Cancer Inst 99:1171-1177, 2007).*

Among patients with clinically localized prostate cancer treated conservatively (observation or hormonal therapy alone), those with a low Gleason score (2–4) have a small risk of dying of their cancer within 15 years (4%–7%). However, those with poorly differentiated tumors (Gleason score 8–10) have a greater risk of dying of prostate cancer than of any other cause, even when the cancer is diagnosed in the eighth decade of life. Indeed, a man diagnosed before the age of 60 with a clinically localized, Gleason score 8 to 10 prostate cancer has an 87% risk of dying of the disease within 15 years if untreated (Table 3).

D'Amico et al combined a number of national datasets to report 10-year cancer-specific mortality rates for men undergoing radical prostatectomy or external-beam radiotherapy (EBRT) by this risk grouping and age at diagnosis. These 10-year mortality graphs are useful to counsel contemporary-era men contemplating surgery or radiation therapy. Given recent advances in the treatment of metastatic disease, identifying men at high risk for metastatic disease following local therapy is important, as these agents are incorporated earlier in the disease course.

Treatment of localized prostate cancer

There are several treatment options for localized prostate cancer, including radical prostatectomy, EBRT, and brachytherapy (interstitial radiation/seeds). Multiple treatment series with each modality have documented the validity of the risk-stratification model based on clinical palpation stage, Gleason score, and serum PSA level. More recently, it has been suggested that biopsy quantification may also be an important factor. Specifically, counting the number of involved needle biopsy cores or the percentage of each core involved by cancer may be prognostic. Low-risk patients experience a favorable 85% to 90% freedom from recurrence, compared with approximately 75% and 35% to 50% for the intermediate- and high-risk patients, respec-

Recent evidence using SEER-Medicare data suggests that older men (those aged 65-80) with low- and intermediate-risk prostate cancer may benefit from aggressive therapy (surgery or irradiation). However, this study did not control for unobserved heterogeneity between patients, which may result in considerable selection bias *(Wong YN, Mitra N, Hudes G, et al: JAMA 296:2683-2693, 2006).*

tively. Although no randomized studies have been performed, contemporary series, which stratify patients by the risk model, demonstrate remarkably similar outcomes independent of the treatment modality. For this reason, treatment recommendations should be individualized based on patient preference, life expectancy, and discussion of potential toxicities.

TREATMENT OF CLINICALLY LOCALIZED DISEASE (T1, T2)

Radical prostatectomy

Radical prostatectomy can be performed retropubically through a lower midline incision—an approach that may include pelvic lymph node dissection. Alternatively, some urologists prefer the perineal approach. With the latter approach, a separate incision is required if lymph node removal is desired.

Although the morbidity of radical prostatectomy was a major concern in the past, improvements were made during the 1980s. Among the various treatment options for prostate cancer, only radical prostatectomy has been demonstrated to confer a survival advantage over no treatment. Bill-Axelson and colleagues found a 44%, 40%, and 67% decrease in the risk of prostate cancer mortality, distant metastases, and disease progression, respectively, among those undergoing radical prostatectomy compared with those treated expectantly. The hazards of anesthesia, risk of blood loss, and hospital stay have all been minimized. Nationwide, Medicare data suggest that surgical outcomes are significantly better at those centers performing > 40 prostatectomies per year than at other hospitals with a lower surgical volume.

Transfusion is usually unnecessary, and treatment-related mortality is < 0.05% at leading prostate cancer centers. The average hospital stay of a man undergoing radical prostatectomy is now approximately 1 to 3 days at leading referral centers in the United States; several institutions routinely discharge patients within 24 hours. Although urinary incontinence is common in the first few months after prostatectomy, most men recover urinary control; at some leading centers, 90% to 98% of men report few or no long-term urinary problems.

Nerve-sparing radical prostatectomy is appropriate for men with small-volume disease. It offers those men with good potency prior to surgery the probability of recovering that function following the operation. By permitting better visualization of Santorini's dorsal venous plexus, the apical prostate, the urethra, and the striated urethral sphincter, the nerve-sparing technique also reduces blood loss and improves recovery of urinary continence. In appropriately selected individuals, a nerve-sparing procedure confers no greater risk of prostate cancer recurrence after considering other relevant clinical information (PSA level, Gleason score, margin status, seminal vesicle involvement, and the presence of extraprostatic spread).

Referral centers have reported that 50% to 90% of patients who are fully potent prior to surgery recover erections following a nerve-sparing procedure, but the quality (rigidity and duration) of these recovered erections may be compromised compared with preoperative erections. Erection recovery rates can be higher than 80% in patients < 60 years of age and lower in older men. Potency may return anywhere from 2 to 24 months following surgery. Regardless of potency, sensation of the penis is not changed after this procedure, and men still experience orgasm. Nerve-sparing radical prostatectomy has not compromised cancer control outcomes in well-selected men with early-stage disease. Also, a recent study has suggested that early postoperative use of sildenafil (Viagra) may facilitate the return of natural erections more quickly. Generally speaking, recovery of erectile function after radical prostatectomy is mediated by age (the younger, the better), pretreatment erectile function (the stronger, the better), and a nerve-sparing approach (bilateral is better than unilateral, which is better than none, which is better than wide dissection).

Robotic radical prostatectomy

Laparoscopic prostatectomy was initially described by Schuessler in 1997 but was abandoned because of its technical difficulty and long operative time with little apparent benefit over the conventional technique. A resurgence in the technique was prompted by improved instrumentation and refinements in the procedure itself, although the laparoscopically naive urologist must endure a substantial learning curve (with attendant perioperative morbidity) prior to meeting the outcome standards set by the open technique.

The robotic-assisted prostatectomy was developed to overcome some of the difficulties of the standard laparoscopic prostatectomy (eg, intracorporeal suturing). The robotic technique allows for three-dimensional (3D) visualization of the operative field and provides for a significantly wider range of movements intracorporeally than do standard laparoscopic instruments. This advance has prompted the assimilation of the technique into the armamentarium of many urologists.

Current evidence suggests that in experienced hands, the laparoscopic and robotic techniques have similar oncologic efficacy to that of the open procedure. However, the length of follow-up (usually < 12 months) in these studies is limited, suggesting that a measure of caution be taken when interpreting the results. Furthermore, recent studies suggest the learning curve is prolonged, with 200 to 250 cases necessary before results can be compared with those of experienced surgeons. Long-term effects of these modalities on sexual and urinary health (as measured by a psychometrically valid survey) have not been reported, and such data are critical in the context of the prostatectomy patient when evaluating technical results. Though it is a promising advance in the treatment of prostate cancer, published data suggest further research in this area is warranted.

Pelvic lymph node dissection Studies now indicate that regional pelvic lymph node dissection may not be necessary for patients with stage T1c disease if the total Gleason score is < 7 and the PSA level is < 10.0 ng/mL, ie, low-risk individuals. Selected intermediate-risk men may also not require this staging procedure, but in high-risk men, it is still considered imperative.

Neoadjuvant hormonal therapy

Approximately 15% to 35% of men who undergo radical prostatectomy for clinical stage T2 prostate cancer will be found to have pathologic T3 disease following surgery. This finding led some investigators to evaluate the efficacy of neoadjuvant androgen deprivation therapy in prospective clinical trials. Early data from these trials suggested that neoadjuvant hormonal therapy led to a reduction in positive surgical margins. However, these findings need to be considered in a technical context: Androgen deprivation therapy causes artifactual changes in prostate morphology that cause difficulties for the pathologic identification of prostate cancer foci.

Indeed, more recent data from prospective studies have shown no benefit of neoadjuvant therapy with regard to disease progression-free survival. At present, therefore, it appears that neoadjuvant hormonal therapy does not improve the curative potential of radical prostatectomy but instead is associated with morphologic alterations that complicate the prognostic utility of standard pathology. Consequently, neoadjuvant hormonal therapy should be reserved for evaluation as an experimental modality in the context of clinical trials.

Adjuvant therapy postprostatectomy

The potential indications for adjuvant therapy following radical prostatectomy in patients with clinical T1 or T2 malignancy include pathologic evidence of T3 disease, positive nodes, a rising PSA level, and positive surgical margins, among others. Possible adjuvant treatments include radiation therapy and androgen deprivation either alone or in combination. Best available evidence suggests that early salvage radiotherapy (eg, postprostatectomy PSA level < 1.0 ng/mL) affords the best results in terms of subsequent biochemical recurrence.

Radiation therapy Men with positive margins or pathologic T3 disease following radical prostatectomy are potential candidates for adjuvant EBRT. Some controversy exists as to the efficacy of early postoperative therapy versus intervention once a biochemical failure has been documented.

In a multi-institutional study, 425 men were randomized to receive either external beam radiation or observation following a prostatectomy for pathologic T3 disease. Treatment patients received 60 to 64 Gy delivered to the prostatic fossa. With a median follow-up of 10 years, the overall survival difference was not statistically significant. However, patients in the treatment group demonstrated a significant improvement in PSA relapse-free survival (10.3 vs 3.1 years) and in median recurrence-free survival (13.8 vs 9.9 years); *(Thompson IM, Tangen CM, Paradelo J, et al: JAMA 296:2329-2335, 2006).*

Valicenti et al demonstrated that the 5-year PSA control rate with immediate postoperative radiation therapy for patients with pathologic T3 disease was 89%, compared with 55% for a matched-pair analysis of surgery alone. Additionally, they demonstrated a favorable dose response in patients receiving EBRT doses above 64.8 Gy.

More recently, Bolla et al reported the results of a randomized, controlled study of observation versus EBRT in 500 patients with pathologic T3 disease following radical prostatectomy. Although to date there are no data demonstrating an overall survival difference, with a median follow-up of 5 years, the progression-free survival was significantly improved with treatment (74% vs 53%). A subsequent update suggested the benefit might be limited to patients with positive margins.

Less controversy exists regarding the role of salvage radiation therapy for PSA recurrence. Approximately 60% to 70% of patients with favorable disease after surgical failure (PSA level < 2.0 ng/mL, a slow PSA doubling time, and a long interval to failure after surgery) will experience durable disease-free survival after adjuvant radiotherapy, presumably due to a smaller tumor burden and a lower likelihood of occult metastatic disease.

Stephenson et al evaluated a large number of patients with persistent or increasing PSA levels after surgery from five American academic institutions. Forty-five percent of patients were free of disease at 4 years. Patients with no adverse risk features achieved a 4-year progression-free probability of 77%. The authors subsequently developed a nomogram based on established risk factors to more accurately identify patient-specific risks to assist in clinical decision-making. Patients who experience PSA failure after radical prostatectomy should be restaged with pelvic CT, bone scan, and DRE. Patients with no evidence of metastatic disease should be evaluated for adjuvant radiotherapy.

Hormonal therapy Significant controversy exists within the academic community as to the timing of initiating androgen deprivation following radical prostatectomy. Clinical trials have documented a benefit only for those patients with nodal involvement.

Treatment recommendations for postprostatectomy recurrence

Following radical prostatectomy, it is expected that serial PSA levels will become undetectable. Any detectable PSA level (> 0.2 ng/mL) following surgery indicates possible recurrent disease and the need for restaging and possible salvage therapies, including radiation or hormonal therapy, experimental protocols, or observation. However, some patients can develop low levels of detectable PSA after prostatectomy without cancer recurrence, presumably due to small foci of benign prostate tissue in situ. Although there is concern for recurrence when the PSA level is > 0.2 ng/mL, most clinicians will wait until a PSA threshold > 0.4 ng/mL is reached to assume that the rise in PSA level represents real recurrence.

Recent findings have suggested that tumor grade, time to PSA recurrence after surgery, and PSA doubling time predict the 5-, 10-, and 15-year risks of prostate cancer mortality and can help to guide the timing and need for androgen ablation. Although these findings do not prove that early androgen ablation is more beneficial than delayed androgen ablation based on a PSA threshold or development of metastatic disease, it does help to risk-stratify patients into those most likely to derive benefit from androgen ablation early. Moreover, men with a PSA doubling time of less than 15 months may be more likely to die of prostate cancer than of other competing causes, suggesting that these men should be evaluated in controlled trials of hormonal or novel therapeutic agents.

Definitive radiation therapy

EBRT EBRT utilizes high-energy photons to destroy cancer cells by damaging cellular DNA. Traditional EBRT utilized bony landmarks and standard beam arrangements to deliver dose to the pelvic region. Technologic advances in treatment planning, driven by improved computing power and the incorporation of individualized patient anatomy, have led to dramatic improvements in treatment delivery. (For a more complete discussion of radiation therapy techniques, see chapter 1.)

3D conformal EBRT creates 3D representations of target structures (ie, the prostate) and designs highly tailored treatment portals utilizing various angles to create a volume of high radiation dose that conforms to the target shape. The anatomic information used to define the target is generally derived from CT images obtained while the patient is placed in an immobilization device in the precise treatment position. With the selective delivery of dose to the target and avoidance of the surrounding normal tissue, the therapeutic ratio is improved. This approach has permitted the use of doses far higher than tolerable with traditional therapy, with fewer bowel and bladder complications.

Treatment volumes in patients with low-risk disease are designed to encompass the prostate plus a margin for daily variations. Patients with a high risk for periprostatic extension and/or regional lymph node metastasis receive initial pelvic treatment of 45 to 50 Gy, followed by a coned-down boost to the prostate.

RTOG (Radiation Therapy Oncology Group) 9413 was designed to test the addition of whole pelvic radiation and the timing of androgen deprivation in the treatment of high-risk patients (lymph node–positive potential > 15% or locally advanced [Gleason score ≥ 6 and > cT2c] cancers). At a median follow-up of 59.5 months, Roach et al noted an improved 4-year disease progression-free survival (60%) among those receiving whole pelvic radiotherapy in conjunction with neoadjuvant androgen deprivation, compared with other treatment arms (44%–50%). An update at 7 years confirmed improved progression-free survival for larger fields in this group.

EBRT dose The previous standard radiation dose with conventional therapy was 70 Gy given over 7 weeks; however, much recent work has suggested a positive dose response, particularly in the intermediate- and high-risk patient populations. Multiple single-institution experiences have demonstrated that 3D conformal EBRT techniques with doses of 75 Gy and higher can be delivered with minimal toxicities.

A randomized trial from the M. D. Anderson Cancer Center compared 70 Gy given conventionally with 78 Gy delivered with a conformal boost. With a median follow-up of 8.7 years, it showed an advantage in freedom from failure for the higher-dose arm in patients with a PSA level > 10 ng/mL (78% vs 39%). Kupelian et al presented pooled data for nearly 5,000 patients from 9 institutions over a narrow time range (1994–1995) to remove treatment technique, stage migration, and lead-time bias. They demonstrated favorable biochemical control outcomes for doses higher than 72 Gy in all risk groups.

The RTOG has completed a dose-escalation trial to assess toxicity with 3D conformal EBRT. In this multi-institutional trial, 78 Gy (prescribed as a minimum to the tumor volume in 2-Gy fractions) was well tolerated, with only 3% of patients experiencing significant (grade 3+) acute gastrointestinal/genitourinary (GI/GU) morbidity and a 6% rate of significant late toxicity. A comparison trial is being conducted by the RTOG (P0126); it will accrue 1,520 cases and provide information regarding any beneficial effect on mortality with higher radiation doses. Although no standard exists, doses ≥ 75 Gy with 3D conformal EBRT techniques appear to be well tolerated and improve biochemical response rates.

Intensity-modulated radiation therapy (IMRT) is becoming a widely used treatment for prostate cancer. This refinement of conformal therapy employs high nonuniform beam intensity profiles and dynamic multileaf collimation to create even more conformal dose distributions. Further improving the therapeutic index compared with 3D conformal EBRT, IMRT is associated with reduced toxicity, permitting further dose escalations previously unattainable.

IMRT was pioneered in several major centers, and Memorial Sloan-Kettering Cancer Center has reported a series of 772 patients treated with doses between 81 and 86.4 Gy. With a median follow-up of 24 months, the side-effect profile was improved, despite these higher doses, with less than 1% of patients experiencing late grade 3+ GI/GU toxicity. The early PSA relapse-free survival rates for favorable, intermediate, and unfavorable risk groups were 92%, 86%, and 81%, respectively. Although IMRT is quickly becoming the standard of care at most institutions, some caution should be exercised. The precision of dose delivery and the complexity of treatment planning demand a strong commitment by both physicians and physics personnel to ensure high-quality IMRT.

Proton therapy Technically a form of EBRT, proton therapy has been utilized in clinical practice for more than 10 years. It offers a potential advantage over photon-based IMRT by exploiting superior dose distributions of the Bragg peak effect. The routine implementation of this technology has been hampered by the staggering costs of building and maintaining a facility. The largest experience involving 1,277 patients at the Loma Linda proton facility was reported in 2004 and demonstrated "comparable control rates with minimal toxicity" compared with other local therapies. Although there are theoretical benefits and ongoing trials evaluating the possibility of further safe dose escalation with protons, to date there is little clinical evidence to support a significant benefit over IMRT. With several new centers now under construction, and a published economic evaluation questioning its cost-effectiveness, the future of eventual widespread application of proton therapy remains unclear.

Androgen ablation with EBRT Two potential benefits of the use of transient androgen ablation prior to EBRT have been identified. First, there may be some synergy between the apoptotic response induced by androgen deprivation and radiotherapy that may increase local control.

Second, androgen deprivation results in an average 20% decrease in prostate volume. This volume reduction not only may reduce the number of target cells, and thereby improve tumor control, but also may shrink the prostate and, thus, diminish the volume of rectum and bladder irradiated during conformal therapy. Complete androgen blockade can be achieved with luteinizing hormone-releasing hormone (LHRH) agonists plus an oral antiandrogen.

The survival benefits of androgen suppression therapy (AST) for patients with intermediate-risk disease have been uncertain. A recent single-institution prospective trial by D'Amico et al randomized patients with a PSA level > 10 ng/ mL, a Gleason score ≥ 7, or radiographic evidence of extraprostatic disease to receive EBRT (70 Gy) alone or the same EBRT with 6 months of AST. After a median follow-up of 4.5 years, patients treated with combined EBRT and AST were found to have improved disease progression-free, prostate cancer–specific, and overall survival ($P = .04$). Although hormone therapy for 3 years has been shown to be beneficial in locally advanced cases, this trial in men with more localized disease showed a benefit to shorter duration of hormone therapy. However, it is not known whether high-dose radiotherapy will obviate the need for AST in this group of patients. The survival benefit in this study was largely confined to those men with few cardiovascular comorbidities, illustrating the importance of patient selection for AST.

Recent secondary findings from a large randomized study (RTOG 9202) suggest that men with high-grade tumors (Gleason score 8–10) and high-risk (T2c–T4) localized disease benefit from long-term androgen ablation (2 years) compared with short-term androgen ablation (4 months), based on improved prostate cancer–specific and overall survival. A caveat to these findings has been the increased incidence or acceleration of incident cardiovascular death in men older than 65 years of age starting androgen ablation compared with those men who did not receive androgen ablation. These findings suggest that cardiac evaluation should be considered in those men older than age 65 with cardiovascular risk factors prior to undergoing androgen ablation.

Interstitial radiotherapy In the 1970s, the use of permanently placed radioactive iodine implants produced initial results as good as those obtained with other available radiotherapy techniques and posed a small risk of impotence and other morbidity when compared with conventional EBRT and radical prostatectomy. However, ultimate control rates were unacceptable. The technique used (freehand placement of seeds during laparotomy) was found to distribute the radioactive seeds unevenly throughout the gland; cold regions may have contributed to the relatively poor outcome.

The advent of improved imaging and seed placement techniques coupled with better patient selection has resulted in vast improvements in cancer control. The perception of fewer side effects in a single outpatient treatment has also contributed to a recent surge in this treatment modality. Transrectal ultrasonography is now utilized to guide seed placement from a transperineal approach, which has corrected the problem of poor seed placement in experienced hands. Two radioactive seed isotopes have been used: iodine (I-125), with a half-life of 60 days, and palladium (Pd-103), with a shorter half-life (17 days) and subsequent higher dose rate. The advantage of the brachytherapy technique is that substantial dose can be delivered to the prostate with minimal effect on the surrounding tissue.

Although concentrating dose with brachytherapy represents a potential advantage over EBRT, it also highlights the need for appropriate patient selection. Significant dose falloff 2 to 3 mm beyond placement of the seeds within the gland limits the application of seed monotherapy in patients with potential periprostatic or regional disease extension. Large studies from several leading institutions have now matured and confirm the long-term effectiveness and safety of this approach in low-risk populations. Favorable results have also been reported in selected intermediate-risk patients. Typical monotherapy doses of 145 Gy for I-131 and 125 Gy for Pd-103 are utilized. To date, the data do not support the use of either isotope over the other.

In addition to disease risk factors, certain patient selection factors are important in considering implants. A large prostate size (> 60 cc) may make the procedure more challenging, both from the perspective of increased prostate gland swelling due to the increased number of needles and the difficulty of the pubic bone obstructing needle placement. Patients with outlet obstruction symptoms (American Urological Society score > 15) have an increased risk of requiring catheterization following implantation. Patients who have undergone prior transurethral resection of prostate (TURP) have been reported to have an increased risk of incontinence; recognizing this risk and placing seeds farther from the defect may help to minimize this risk. Therefore, with proper counseling, patients with small TURP defects may still be considered implant candidates.

For patients with intermediate- or high-risk disease, implants may be combined with EBRT. There is sound logic in combining high-dose therapy to the prostate with an implant and moderate doses of EBRT to the regional tissues to sterilize micrometastatic disease. In this situation, an implant (110 Gy of I-131 or 100 Gy of Pd-104) usually either precedes or follows 20 to 45 Gy delivered to the pelvis. Some reports have suggested an increase in rectal toxicity with this approach; however, this is likely due to the poor quality of the implant. At least one study from a leading implant center suggested no significant increase in severe early or late GI/GU morbidity with combination therapy. The value of supplemental EBRT needs to be evaluated in comparison to full-dose EBRT in terms of long-term morbidity and cancer control.

High-dose–rate (HDR) devices Besides permanent implants, which deliver low-dose–rate (LDR) radiotherapy, brachytherapy for prostate cancer has been delivered using temporary high-dose–rate devices, usually in patients with locally advanced disease. In this technique, a high dose (minimum, approximately 5 Gy) is delivered to the prostate over ≤ 1 hour by remotely inserting a highly radioactive source into catheters placed into the prostate under ultrasonographic guidance while the patient is under anesthesia. Several treatments are given on separate occasions, and EBRT is used for approximately 5 weeks as well.

More reports are accumulating on the application of HDR brachytherapy to prostate cancer. Various dose-fractionation combinations of HDR with or without combined pelvic EBRT have been employed, with a dose-response relationship apparent in biochemical control. Although the follow-up is short and no prospective randomized trials evaluating this approach have yet been published, it appears that HDR prostate brachytherapy in combination with pelvic

EBRT may be effective. The long-term consequences for normal tissue of delivering large doses per fraction using this technique are unclear.

Medications and devices to manage impotence after prostatectomy, EBRT, or brachytherapy

Treatment for postprostatectomy impotence includes the phosphodiesterase inhibitors sildenafil, vardenafil (Levitra), and tadalafil (Cialis); prostaglandin E_1, administered as a urethral suppository (Muse); intercavernosal injection (Caverject, Edex); or vacuum-pump erection aids that are useful for improving erections in men who have poor erectile function after prostatectomy, radiation therapy, or brachytherapy. These therapies are effective in 15% to 40% of men with postprostatectomy impotence and in 50% to 75% of men with postradiotherapy erectile dysfunction. Insertion of a penile prosthesis is typically offered to patients only after unsuccessful trials with the previously mentioned less invasive interventions.

DETECTION AND TREATMENT OF RECURRENCE

Significance and definition of a rising PSA level postirradiation

The use of PSA levels following definitive therapy (either radiotherapy or radical prostatectomy) can detect early recurrences that may be amenable to salvage treatment. A rising PSA profile following radiotherapy is unequivocal evidence of the presence of a residual prostatic neoplasm. However, the definition of a rising PSA level after radiation therapy varies in the literature. A 1996 consensus conference recommended that PSA failure be considered to have occurred after three consecutive PSA level rises, with the rate of failure defined as halfway between the first rise and the previous PSA level.

Moreover, patients with a rising PSA level after irradiation may be a heterogeneous group, including patients with truly localized failure as well as those with metastatic disease. Also, certain patients will have a slowly rising PSA level after irradiation and may not require additional treatment. In patients who do not receive androgen ablation, the 5-year actuarial risk of distant metastasis from the time that the PSA level begins to rise is ~50%. A rapidly emerging key concept in rising PSA levels is PSA velocity, or more specifically PSA doubling time. Multiple recent studies have found that a PSA doubling time < 10 to 12 months predicts early clinical relapse if biochemical recurrence is untreated.

Treatment recommendations for recurrence postirradiation

In general, men who have clear evidence of a rising PSA level 2 years after definitive radiotherapy for localized prostate cancer should be advised about the options of hormonal therapy (see section on "Treatment of locally advanced disease [T3, T4]"), salvage surgery, salvage cryotherapy, observation, or experimental therapy.

If patients have minimal comorbidity, good life expectancy, and only local evidence of disease recurrence, salvage surgery is an option but should be preceded by a bone scan, CT scan, cystoscopy, and extensive counseling because urinary difficulties after salvage prostatectomy are substantial and highly prevalent. Factors that determine success of salvage surgery after radiation therapy include low (< 4–10 ng/mL) preoperative PSA level, low pathologic stage (T3a or less), and prior type of radiation therapy (brachytherapy, IMRT being favorable). However, no randomized trials have been conducted in this setting to provide level I evidence favoring surgery over other modes of treatment.

TREATMENT OF LOCALLY ADVANCED DISEASE (T3, T4)

The treatment of patients with locally advanced prostate cancer is centered on a multimodality and multidisciplinary approach, including radiation therapy (EBRT with or without HDR interstitial therapy), androgen ablation plus EBRT, or radical prostatectomy with or without androgen deprivation.

EBRT with and without HDR interstitial therapy

For patients with locally extensive prostate cancer, local failure remains a potential problem after EBRT. This problem has prompted investigations into alternative means to intensify therapy.

One strategy has been to deliver large fractions of radiotherapy using HDR interstitial techniques in combination with EBRT. The large interstitial fractions, which may be on the order of 5 Gy, deliver a high dose to the prostate but spare normal tissues, due to the rapid dose falloff outside the implanted volume. Early experience with this strategy is encouraging, but long-term data on outcome, particularly in patients with locally extensive disease, and on morbidity are awaited.

Patients with locally advanced prostate cancer probably are not good candidates for permanent prostate implants. Patients with stage T3/T4 tumors are at high risk of gross extraprostatic involvement, and this localized therapy may not offer adequate dosimetric coverage of extraprostatic disease.

As mentioned in the previous section, there may be a synergistic effect between hormonal therapy given in conjunction with radiation therapy. In addition to enhancing apoptosis and producing local cytoreduction, the use of early androgen deprivation may possibly delay or even prevent the development of metastatic disease.

The current body of evidence from two large randomized trials (RTOG 85-10 and EORTC 22863) suggests that immediate long-term androgen deprivation in conjunction with EBRT improves outcomes among men with locally advanced or high-risk (Gleason score ≥ 8) prostate cancer compared with radiation therapy alone. An analysis of RTOG 85-31 by Horwitz et al, which employed early indefinite androgen deprivation, demonstrated that patients with locally advanced disease (T3N0) had improved cause-specific failure and distant metastatic failure compared with EBRT alone. Furthermore, a comparison to RTOG 86-10, which studied similar patients treated with only 4 months of hormonal therapy, favored the long-term approach. The EORTC trial randomized 415 patients and demonstrated a 15% overall survival benefit to 3

TABLE 4: Hormonal approaches to the treatment of advanced prostate cancer

Method	Mechanism of action	Side effects
Surgical castration	Removal of testicular androgens	Hot flashes (50%), psychological effects
Diethylstilbestrol (DES)	Inhibition of gonadotropin secretion	Gynecomastia, cardiovascular risks at high doses
LHRH analogs (goserelin, leuprolide)	Inhibition of gonadotropin secretion	Hot flashes (50%), less gynecomastia than with DES, fatigue
Antiandrogens (bicalutamide, flutamide, nilutamide)	Blockade of binding of dihydrotestosterone to its receptor	Abnormal liver function studies, diarrhea (10%)

LHRH = luteinizing hormone-releasing hormone

years of combined therapy versus radiation therapy alone.

Radical prostatectomy with or without adjuvant therapy

Surgical monotherapy can be considered a reasonable option for patients with locally advanced prostate cancer. Stage T3 disease can be successfully treated with low morbidity and significant reductions in risk of local recurrence, with clinical overstaging (up to 26%) reported by Yamada et al. Well- and moderately differentiated cancers have cancer-specific survival rates of 76% at 10 years, comparable to those of other treatment modalities.

The Mayo Clinic has one of the largest radical prostatectomy series for T3 disease, consisting of more than 1,000 patients. In this population, of whom 34% received adjuvant therapy, 15-year cancer-specific survival and local recurrence rates were 77% and 21%, respectively. Ninety-eight men who were found to have nodal metastases following radical prostatectomy and pelvic lymphadenectomy were randomized to receive immediate androgen deprivation or be followed until clinical disease progression. At a median follow-up of 7 years, 18 of 51 men in the observation group had died, compared with only 4 of 47 in the treatment group ($P = .02$).

Positive margins are not uncommon after radical prostatectomy (37% in this study by Simon et al). Despite these strikingly high rates, approximately only one in five will recur, suggesting that adjuvant therapy is not always necessary (Simon MA, Kim S, Soloway MS: J Urol 175:140-145, 2006).

Treatment of node-positive disease

Whether any local treatment adds to the overall survival duration in patients with known nodal involvement is debatable. Until recently, the standard of care had been to perform frozen-section pathologic analysis on pelvic lymph nodes at the time of radical prostatectomy, prior to removal of the prostate. If this analysis revealed micrometastases, radical prostatectomy was thought to be contraindicated. Although retrospective in nature, recent data from several American centers, including one large study from the Mayo Clinic, have reported a survival benefit in men who undergo radical prostatectomy despite the presence of micrometastases to regional pelvic lymph nodes. These men tend to do better and survive longer when started on early hormonal therapy, either with orchiectomy or an LHRH agonist.

> Patients with positive lymph nodes at the time of radical prostatectomy who receive immediate androgen deprivation have a survival advantage over those who receive deferred therapy (deferred vs early hazard ratio, 1.84; 95% confidence interval, 1.01-3.35) *(Messing EM, Manola J, Yao J, et al: Lancet Oncol 7:472-479, 2006).*

Radiation therapy There are also compelling data that long-term survival is achievable in these patients with combination radiation and hormonal therapy. Data from the M. D. Anderson Cancer Center indicate a benefit to pelvic/prostate radiation therapy plus immediate hormonal manipulation compared with hormones alone. A subset analysis of patients with node-positive disease from RTOG 85-31 revealed immediate hormonal therapy plus radiation therapy resulted in 5- and 9-year cause-specific survival rates of 84% and 76%, respectively. Therefore, aggressive locoregional therapy appears to be effective in this cohort of unfavorable patients.

TREATMENT OF ADVANCED SYSTEMIC DISEASE

Defining advanced disease

Metastatic prostate cancer This is a heterogeneous group of patients that ranges from those with pathologically detected locoregional nodal metastases at the time of radical prostatectomy to those with widespread systemic disease. The most common sites of metastatic disease are the bone and pelvic and abdominal lymph nodes. Other, less common sites include the liver and lungs. Complications of metastatic prostate cancer include pain, fatigue, skeletal fractures, spinal cord compression, urinary outlet obstruction, and failure to thrive. First-line hormonal therapy for men with metastatic prostate cancer delays these complications.

Rising PSA level A large series of more than 2,000 patients treated with radical prostatectomy at Johns Hopkins University demonstrated that approximately 17% of cases recurred, with only 5.8% being local disease. In the remaining patients, disease recurred initially with either a rise in PSA level alone (9.7%) or evidence of clinical metastases (1.7%).

Outcomes for men with only a rising PSA level can vary greatly. Time to PSA recurrence (< vs > 2 years), PSA doubling time (< vs > 9 months), and Gleason score (8–10 vs 5–7) are among the important factors for predicting the development of metastatic disease and survival. The major developments for hormonal therapy in advanced prostate cancer were achieved prior to routine PSA testing and were often complicated by problematic study design. There are no prospective data that confirm a benefit to early hormonal therapy for men with a rising PSA alone. However, for patients with a rising PSA level who are at high risk for the development of metastases, some physicians agree that early hormonal therapy is likely to benefit this group of patients as well as those with radiologic evidence of metastatic disease.

First-line therapies for advanced disease

The standard first-line treatment of advanced prostate cancer, regardless of whether local treatment has been applied, is to ablate the action of androgens by medical or surgical means. For the majority of patients, androgen ablation can result in a decline in PSA level, palliation of disease-related symptoms, and regression of metastatic disease on imaging.

Bilateral orchiectomy The advantages of orchiectomy over other means of castration include an immediate decline in testosterone levels and ease of compliance for patients. Given these advantages, however, many men still opt for medical castration, with the potential advantage of intermittent hormonal therapy. In addition, the psychological impact of orchiectomy can be significant. Nonetheless, bilateral orchiectomy may be appropriate and cost-effective for a select group of patients.

LHRH analogs LHRH agonists, such as leuprolide (Lupron, Eligard) and goserelin (Zoladex), interfere with the normal pulsatile secretion of LH from the pituitary gland, resulting in an eventual decline in serum testosterone levels. The effect is reversible with cessation of therapy. Because LH is initially increased with LHRH agonists, testosterone levels may actually increase initially as well. This finding can result in a transient rise in PSA levels and potential growth of metastatic sites. Because of this initial "flare response" with LHRH agonists, consideration should be given to the administration of an antiandrogen prior to the LHRH, especially in patients who are at risk for complications from the disease (such as spinal cord compression, worsening pain, or urinary outlet obstruction; Table 4).

A pure LHRH antagonist (abarelix [Plenaxis]) has been approved by the US Food and Drug Administration (FDA). Its main advantage is the lack of an LHRH surge or flare, and it is indicated in men with impending spinal cord compression or other now uncommon clinical scenarios where a flare could be harmful. However, this drug must be administered every 2 weeks in the first month and monthly thereafter. Also, it can rarely be associated with an anaphylactic reaction.

The American Society of Clinical Oncology recently published guidelines for the initial management of androgen-sensitive (recurrent, metastatic) prostate cancer. Based on the literature, immediate androgen deprivation was associated with a moderate decrease in prostate cancer mortality and a moderate increase in other causes of mortality. Currently, there is no definitive evidence favoring the early initiation of androgen deprivation in this population *(Loblaw DA, Virgo KS, Nam R, et al: J Clin Oncol 25:1596-1605, 2007).*

Antiandrogens Antiandrogens function to block the binding of dihydro-testosterone (DHT) to the androgen receptor, blocking the translocation of the DHT-androgen receptor complex into the nuclei of cells. There are two general classes: steroidal and nonsteroidal. Steroidal antiandrogens include cyproterone and megestrol. The most commonly

TABLE 5: The incidence of complications from advanced prostate cancer with immediate vs deferred androgen deprivation

Complication	Immediate	Deferred
Pathologic fracture	2.3%	4.5%
Spinal cord compression	2.0%	5.0%
Ureteric obstruction	7.0%	11.8%
Extraskeletal metastases	7.9%	11.8%

used antiandrogens include the nonsteroidal agents flutamide, bicalutamide (Casodex), and nilutamide (Nilandron). These agents differ slightly in their affinity for the androgen receptor and their side-effect profiles.

Typically, antiandrogens are used in combination with surgical or medical castration. Some trials comparing antiandrogens alone with LHRH analogs have shown similar efficacy, but more recent trials suggest that monotherapy with antiandrogens may be inferior in terms of time to disease progression and possibly survival. For example, a randomized trial of monotherapy with high-dose bicalutamide (150 mg daily) compared with flutamide plus goserelin demonstrated that patients treated with bicalutamide monotherapy had fewer side effects, such as loss of libido or erectile dysfunction, and trended toward improved quality of life. However, in patients with radiographic evidence of metastases, bicalutamide monotherapy was associated with a small 6-week decrease in survival (hazard ratio, 1.3). Despite this finding, for men who are intolerant to the side effects of LHRH analogs, monotherapy with antiandrogens can be considered after careful discussion with patients.

Antiandrogen monotherapy with flutamide or bicalutamide is also sometimes used to treat PSA recurrence. Used alone or in combination with a 5-alpha reductase inhibitor (finasteride or dutasteride), this approach is associated with fewer side effects than traditional androgen suppression therapy, but the approches have not been approved by the FDA. A significant downside is nipple tenderness or gynecomastia, but this "peripheral blockade" approach may preserve potency and libido. Prophylactic breast irradiation may prevent this complication.

Combined androgen blockade Combined androgen blockade (CAB) refers to the elimination of testicular androgens in combination with blockade of adrenal androgens, generally with an LHRH analog and an antiandrogen agent. The use of CAB is somewhat controversial. Several randomized trials comparing LHRH antagonists alone versus CAB have demonstrated a survival benefit with CAB. However, in one of the largest trials conducted by the United States Intergroup, more than 1,300 men were randomized to undergo orchiectomy versus orchiectomy plus flutamide. There was no significant advantage to CAB in terms of time to disease progression or overall survival. Some investigators believe that bicalutamide, a more potent agent, may be associated with greater survival when used as part of CAB.

Many investigators believe that the advantages observed in trials that include an LHRH antagonist exist because of the "flare phenomenon," which occurs with LHRH antagonists alone and may be lost with a short period of treatment with antiandrogens during the expected flare period.

Diethylstilbestrol (DES) Estrogen administration, in the form of DES, also produces chemical castration. DES inhibits prostate growth, primarily through the inhibition of the hypothalamic-pituitary-gonadal axis, which blocks testicular synthesis of testosterone and thus lowers plasma testosterone levels. Since doses higher than 3 mg/d cause significant cardiovascular mortality, DES has fallen out of favor as a first-line therapy to induce castration.

Ketoconazole (Nizoral) Ketoconazole is an antifungal agent that can inhibit adrenal and testicular steroid synthesis at higher doses, leading to a decline in adrenal and testicular androgens. It has the benefit of a rapid decline in testosterone, which can be useful for patients who present emergently with a complication of newly diagnosed advanced disease. Ketoconazole is started at a dose of 200 mg three times daily and is increased to a total dose of 400 mg three times daily. Ketoconazole is associated with significant side effects (such as fatigue, nausea, and vomiting) and drug interactions, however, and must be given with supplemental hydrocortisone to avoid symptoms of adrenal insufficiency. Because of the side effects, its use is more common in the second-line setting, where responses can be expected in 20% to 40% of patients following disease progression with CAB.

Early versus late treatment Whether to treat patients early with hormonal therapy or wait until patients become symptomatic has been tested in a large European trial conducted by the Medical Research Council. Men were randomized to receive immediate hormonal therapy (orchiectomy or an LHRH analog) versus delayed therapy, which was initiated with symptomatic disease progression. Men who were treated with early therapy were less likely to experience urinary obstructive symptoms requiring intervention, pathologic fractures, and spinal cord compression than those treated in the delayed arm (Table 5). The survival benefit was less clear, however, because many of the men in the delayed arm died before they received any hormonal therapy. This study was also complicated by the initiation of PSA monitoring during the study period. Many patients and physicians currently are not comfortable delaying therapy until the onset of symptoms while the PSA level is rising; this fact limits the applicability of its findings in the modern era.

Other smaller trials have examined this issue as well. A Cochrane Database review was conducted in 2002; it demonstrated an increase in progression-free survival and a small, but significant, improvement in survival with early hormonal therapy.

One setting in which early adjuvant hormonal therapy has been associated with a survival benefit is in the postprostatectomy setting in men found to have pathologic lymph node–positive disease. Messing and colleagues published an adjuvant study that evaluated immediate hormonal therapy versus delayed treatment upon detection of distant metastases or symptomatic recurrence in men who had undergone radical prostatectomy and lymph node dissection and were found to have nodal metastases. At a median follow-up of 11.9 years (range, 9.7–14.5 for surviving patients), men assigned immediate androgen deprivation therapy had a significant improvement in overall survival, prostate cancer–specific survival, and progression-free survival.

Intermittent androgen deprivation Androgen deprivation is associated with several short-term and long-term adverse effects. These side effects make treatment breaks provided by intermittent androgen deprivation an attractive option. Additionally, results from preclinical studies suggest that hormonal resistance may be delayed with intermittent androgen deprivation. These potential advantages have led to significant interest among patients and caregivers in intermittent androgen deprivation.

Over the past decade, several phase II studies of intermittent androgen deprivation have demonstrated feasibility and safety with suggestion of improved quality of life without negative effects on time to disease progression or survival. More recently, a phase III trial was reported at the 2006 ASCO meeting. In this trial, patients randomized to the intermittent therapy arm were off therapy for a median of 52 weeks with no significant difference in time to disease progression or overall survival. The results of several ongoing phase III trials in metastatic disease and PSA-only relapse will better define the role of intermittent androgen deprivation. With the currently available information, intermittent androgen deprivation may be considered in select patient settings.

Treatment recommendations Just as for localized disease, initial treatment for advanced prostate cancer must be individualized. A patient who presents with a rising PSA level only after local treatment and a slow PSA doubling time, a prolonged time to PSA recurrence, and a low initial Gleason score may not require immediate therapy, especially if there are other more significant comorbidities. However, a patient with multiple metastatic sites will need immediate treatment, generally with orchiectomy or CAB initially followed by monotherapy with an LHRH analog, to prevent the sequelae of metastatic disease, such as fracture, spinal cord compression, and ureteral obstruction. Ketoconazole may be considered as the initial systemic therapy for patients presenting with spinal cord compression as the first presentation of prostate cancer. Given the overall limitations of hormone therapy, all appropriate patients should be offered access to clinical trials.

Several phase III trials evaluating the role of intermittent androgen deprivation are ongoing. Interim results from the South European Urological Group were presented at the 2006 ASCO meeting. Fifty percent of patients randomized to the intermittent arm were off therapy for a median of 52 weeks after their initial treatment period. For patients whose PSA level declined to < 2 ng/mL, the median time off therapy was 74 weeks. There was no significant difference in time to disease progression or overall survival. Main differences in quality of life were confined to sexual function, with sexual activity significantly greater in the intermittent arm (*P* < .1). Mature results of this trial are awaited. The results from two other large intergroup studies (S9346, INT-0162 and NCI Canada's JPR7) yet to be reported will help to more clearly define the role of intermittent hormonal therapy (*Calais Da Silva FM, Calais Da Silva F, Bono A, et al: J Clin Oncol 24[18s]:4513, 2006*).

For patients with a rising PSA level who are at high risk for the development of metastases, a discussion regarding the potential advantages to early treatment and an explanation of the lack of randomized prospective data are warranted. Some investigators favor early treatment for these patients based on the data from the Medical Research Council trial and the Cochrane Database review, understanding that this information is extrapolated from data obtained prior to PSA testing and from patients with clinical and radiographic metastases.

Second-line hormonal therapies

Outcomes with initial androgen ablation can vary from responses that last from months to years; they also vary as a function of the Gleason grade, pretreatment PSA velocity, and extent of disease at the time of initiating treatment. Once PSA levels begin to rise with androgen ablation, the disease is often referred to as "hormone refractory." This term is actually a misnomer, because preclinical data suggest that tumors may become hypersensitive to androgens, resulting in worsened disease if androgen ablation is removed entirely. Moreover, many patients have disease that remains sensitive to further hormonal manipulations, such as second-line antiandrogens, steroids, or ketoconazole.

An example of this sensitivity to hormonal manipulation is exemplified in the antiandrogen withdrawal response. Up to one-third of patients with a rising PSA level while receiving treatment with an antiandrogen will have a decline in PSA level and or clinical regression with antiandrogen withdrawal. The mechanism of this response has not been fully elucidated but supports the hypothesis that the androgen receptor remains important in progressive disease.

Although second-line hormonal therapy has demonstrated benefit in terms of PSA levels and response, there are no data to demonstrate a survival advantage with second-line hormonal therapy. Its role has further come into question with data that support the use of docetaxel (Taxotere) chemotherapy for men with metastatic androgen-independent prostate cancer to improve survival. The survival advantage of docetaxel is not limited by number of prior hormonal therapies.

For patients with a rising PSA level only, timing of chemotherapy is even less clear. The Eastern Cooperative Oncology Group attempted a trial comparing ketoconazole/hydrocortisone with docetaxel in patients with a rising PSA level but no evidence of metastatic disease after hormonal therapy, but the trial was closed early due to lack of accrual. Until prospective data are available, physicians will need to counsel patients carefully on the different options and timing of those options available at the time of disease progression, including second-line hormonal manipulation, chemotherapy, and especially clinical trials.

Chemotherapy for castration-resistant disease

Docetaxel The role of chemotherapy has changed significantly over the past several years, with the results of two large randomized trials demonstrating a survival benefit for men with castration-resistant metastatic prostate cancer treated with docetaxel-based chemotherapy (Table 6). Investigators from the Southwest Oncology Group randomized patients to receive mitoxantrone

TABLE 6: Standard chemotherapy regimens for prostate cancer

Drug/combination	Dose and schedule
Mitoxantrone/prednisone	
Mitoxantrone	12 mg/m^2 IV every 3 weeks
Prednisone	5 mg orally twice daily started on day 1
Repeat cycle every 21 days.	

Tannock IF, Osoba D, Stockler MR, et al: J Clin Oncol 14:1756–1764, 1996.

Docetaxel/prednisone	
Docetaxel	75 mg/m^2 IV every 3 weeks
Prednisone	5 mg orally twice daily started on day 1

Note: Standard docetaxel premedication should be given prior to the administration of docetaxel

Tannock IF, de Wit R, Berry WR, et al: N Engl J Med 351:1502–1512, 2004.

Table prepared by Ishmael Jaiyesimi, DO

(Novantrone) plus prednisone versus docetaxel (60 mg/m^2) plus estramustine (Emcyt) and dexamethasone every 3 weeks. Patients in the docetaxel arm had a significant improvement in survival by 2 to 3 months. Currently, estramustine is no longer being utilized in the front-line setting due to the 7% to 10% risk of arterial and venous thromboembolic events and the equivalent survival benefits seen with docetaxel alone compared with mitoxantrone.

A second trial by Tannock et al showed a similar survival benefit of 3 months with docetaxel (75 mg/m^2) plus prednisone given every 3 weeks compared with mitoxantrone and prednisone. These trials were the first to demonstrate a survival benefit with chemotherapy in advanced prostate cancer and have sparked numerous studies involving docetaxel in combination with newer agents. Toxicities of docetaxel include myelosuppression and neuropathy, both of which can be dose-limiting.

A recent 5-year update of this study has confirmed a 3-month survival advantage to every-3-week docetaxel in the overall study population. In addition, nearly 18% of men experienced normalized PSA levels with every-3-week docetaxel, as opposed to 8% of men treated with mitoxantrone. Men with normalized PSA levels lived on average 33 months, compared with 16 months among men without normalized PSA levels, nearly a two-fold difference. Current studies indicate that a 30% or greater decline in the serum PSA level within 3 months of treatment initiation is the best predictor of disease outcome of all current surrogate markers in this disease and may be used to assist in prognostication after treatment initiation.

Mitoxantrone plus prednisone Mitoxantrone (12 mg/m^2) plus prednisone has been approved for use in advanced prostate cancer based on improvement in

Satraplatin is a novel, orally bioavailable platinum compound. Preliminary results of the Satraplatin and Prednisone Against Refractory Cancer (SPARC) trial were presented at the 2007 ASCO meeting. In this phase III investigation, satraplatin plus prednisone was compared with placebo plus prednisone as second-line therapy for men with metastatic hormone-refractory prostate cancer. A 33% improvement in progression-free survival was demonstrated (11.1 vs 9.7 weeks; hazard ratio [HR] = 0.67; 95% confidence interval [CI] = 0.57–0.77; P = .0000003). All other prespecified endpoints (pain response, tumor response by RECIST criteria, and PSA response) were statistically significant in favor of satraplatin (Sternberg CN, Petrylak D, Witjes F, et al: J Clin Oncol 25[18S]:5019, 2007). According to data presented at the 2008 ASCO meeting, the SPARC trial failed to show an overall survival benefit for satraplatin in the general intent-to-treat population (61.3 vs 61.4 weeks). However, in a docetaxel (Taxotere)-pretreated intent-to-treat subgroup, a positive overall survival effect was observed (66.1 vs 62.9 weeks, HR = 0.78; 95% CI = 0.61–0.99), when adjusting for prespecified prognostic factors (Sartor AO, Petrylak DP, Witjes JA, et al: J Clin Oncol 26[15S]:5003, 2008).

palliation of pain and quality of life over prednisone alone despite no improvement in overall survival.

Bisphosphonates Bone metastases from prostate cancer are associated with increased bone formation around tumor deposits, resulting in characteristic osteoblastic metastases. However, concomitant with the osteoblastic activity is a marked increase in bone resorption and osteolysis, which can be inhibited by bisphosphonates.

Studies of bisphosphonates in prostate cancer have demonstrated mixed results. A combined analysis of two multicentered randomized controlled trials comparing pamidronate with placebo in men with androgen-independent progressive prostate cancer demonstrated no benefit in terms of skeleton-related events or palliation of symptoms. A phase III trial with an oral bisphosphonate, clodronate, demonstrated no difference in either symptomatic bone metastases or prostate cancer-related deaths when compared with placebo.

A phase III trial demonstrated a reduction in skeleton-related events for men with castration-resistant metastatic prostate cancer with a more potent bisphosphonate, zoledronic acid (Zometa). However, it is important to note that this trial did not show an improvement in quality of life with zoledronic acid, nor did it demonstrate a reduction in the development of new metastases.

At this time, the recommendation for zoledronic acid in prostate cancer is limited to men with androgen-independent prostate cancer. It is important to recognize the limitations of this therapy and to understand that there is no defined role for its use in men with androgen-dependent prostate cancer. Although these men are at higher risk for osteoporosis, less potent oral bisphosphonates may be a more reasonable approach, given the long-term side effects associated with zoledronic acid (renal insufficiency and osteonecrosis of the mandible).

TABLE 7: Phase III trials in hormone-refractory prostate cancer

Trial	Experimental agent	Type of therapy	Phase
Docetaxel/prednisone +/- bevacizumab	Bevacizumab	Antiangiogenesis	III
Docetaxel/prednisone +/- atrasentan	Atrasentan	ET-A receptor antagonist	III
Docetaxel/prednisone vs GVAX	GVAX	Vaccine	III
Docetaxel/prednisone vs docetaxel/GVAX	GVAX	Vaccine	III
Provenge vs placebo	Provenge	Vaccine	III
Abiraterone acetate and prednisone vs prednisone alone	Abiraterone	Androgen synthesis inhibitor	III
VEGF Trap (Aflibercept) and docetaxel vs docetaxel alone	VEGF Trap	Antiangiogenesis	III

Newer therapies

Several new therapies for men with prostate cancer (some as single agents and some with chemotherapy) are under investigation, with promising early results. They include the endothelin receptor antagonist atrasentan, vitamin D_3 (calcitriol), immunotherapies (Provenge and GVAX as autologous and allogeneic vaccination strategies), the vascular epidermal growth factor inhibitors bevacizumab (Avastin) and sunitinib (Sutent), a new class of antimicrotubule agents (the epothilones), and novel agents targeting the androgen receptor. There are ample preclinical and early clinical data to suggest that all of these agents may have activity against prostate cancer, but no definitive trials to establish their role have yet been completed. These agents are still considered investigational. Several trials are evaluating the combinations of docetaxel and bevacizumab, docetaxel and atrasentan, and docetaxel and a vaccine.

In addition, current trials are investigating the use of these systemic agents, including chemotherapeutic regimens such as docetaxel, in locally advanced disease, either prior to or adjuvant following surgery or radiation therapy (Table 7). Accrual to these trials (TAX3501, RTOG 0521, VA 553, and CALGB 90203) is a priority, as they are investigating the role of systemic therapy to prevent disease recurrence, similar to the widely accepted use of systemic therapy for other tumor types such as breast and colorectal cancers.

Radiation therapy for palliating bone metastasis

Radiotherapy is effective in controlling local pain associated with skeletal prostate metastasis. In general, a treatment regimen of 30 Gy over 10 treatments results in rapid and durable local symptom control and a reduced dependence on analgesics. Single-dose palliative XRT may provide equal palliation as well.

For patients with more extensive bone involvement causing pain that may be difficult to address with localized EBRT, alternatives include wide-field irradiation (ie, hemibody irradiation) or systemic administration of radioactive bone-seeking isotopes that can deliver therapeutic doses to skeletal metastatic disease. Radioactive isotopes used in this fashion include strontium-89 chloride (Metastron) and samarium SM 153 lexidronam (Quadramet). A more detailed discussion of these approaches can be found in chapter 37.

SUGGESTED READING

Albertsen PC, Hanley JA, Fine J, et al: 20-year outcomes following conservative management of clinically localized prostate cancer. JAMA 293:2095–2101, 2005.

Armstrong AJ, Garrett-Mayer E, Ou Yang YC, et al: Prostate-specific antigen and pain surrogacy analysis in metastatic hormone-refractory prostate cancer. J Clin Oncol 25:3965–3970, 2007.

Bill-Axelson A, Holmberg L, Ruutu M, et al: Radical prostatectomy versus watchful waiting in early prostate cancer. N Engl J Med 352:1977–1984, 2005.

D'Amico AV, Chen MH, Roehl KA, et al: Preoperative PSA velocity and the risk of death from prostate cancer after radical prostatectomy. N Engl J Med 351:125–135, 2004.

D'Amico AV, Denham JW, Crook J, et al: Influence of androgen suppression therapy for prostate cancer on the frequency and timing of fatal myocardial infarctions. J Clin Oncol 25:2420–2425, 2007.

D'Amico AV, Renshaw AA, Sussman B, et al: Pretreatment PSA velocity and risk of death from prostate cancer following external beam radiation therapy. JAMA 294:440–447, 2005.

Freedland SJ, Humphreys EB, Mangold LA, et al: Death in patients with recurrent prostate cancer after radical prostatectomy: Prostate-specific antigen doubling time subgroups and their associated contributions to all-cause mortality. J Clin Oncol 25:1765–1771, 2007.

Freedland SJ, Humphreys EB, Mangold LA, et al: Risk of prostate cancer-specific mortality following biochemical recurrence after radical prostatectomy. JAMA 294:433–439, 2005.

Giovannucci E, Liu Y, Platz EA, et al: Risk factors for prostate cancer incidence and progression in the health professionals follow-up study. Int J Cancer 121:1571–1578, 2007.

Kirsh VA, Peters U, Mayne ST, et al: Prospective study of fruit and vegetable intake and risk of prostate cancer. J Natl Cancer Inst 99:1200–1209, 2007.

Lawton CA, Winter K, Grignon D, et al: Androgen suppression plus radiation versus radiation alone for patients with stage D1/pathologic node-positive adenocarcinoma of the prostate: Updated results based on national prospective randomized trial Radiation Therapy Oncology Group 85-31. J Clin Oncol 23:800–807, 2005.

Loblaw DA, Virgo KS, Nam R, et al: Initial hormonal management of androgen-sensitive metastatic, recurrent, or progressive prostate cancer: 2006 update of an American Society of Clinical Oncology practice guideline. J Clin Oncol 25:1596–1605, 2007.

Messing EM, Manola J, Sarosdy M, et al: Immediate hormonal therapy compared with observation after radical prostatectomy and pelvic lymphadenectomy in men with node-positive prostate cancer. N Engl J Med 341:1781–1788, 1999.

Messing EM, Manola J, Yao J, et al: Immediate versus deferred androgen deprivation treatment in patients with node-positive prostate cancer after radical prostatectomy and pelvic lymphadenectomy. Lancet Oncol 7:472–479, 2006.

Moul JW, Wu H, Sun L, et al: Early versus delayed hormonal therapy for prostate specific antigen only recurrence of prostate cancer after radical prostatectomy. J Urol 171:1141–1147, 2004.

Petrylak DP, Tangen CM, Hussain MH, et al: Docetaxel and estramustine compared with mitoxantrone and prednisone for advanced refractory prostate cancer. N Engl J Med 351:1513–1520, 2004.

Sharifi N, Gulley JL, Dahut WL: Androgen deprivation therapy for prostate cancer. JAMA 294:238–244, 2005.

Smith MR, Kabbinavar F, Saad F, et al: Natural history of rising serum prostate-specific antigen in men with castrate nonmetastatic prostate cancer. J Clin Oncol 23:2918–2925, 2005.

Stephenson AJ, Shariat SF, Zelefsky MJ, et al: Salvage radiotherapy for recurrent prostate cancer after radical prostatectomy. JAMA 291:1325–1332, 2004.

Tannock IF, de Wit R, Berry WR, et al: Docetaxel plus prednisone or mitoxantrone plus prednisone for advanced prostate cancer. N Engl J Med 351:1502–1512, 2004.

Tannock IF, Osoba D, Stockler MR, et al: Chemotherapy with mitoxantrone plus prednisone or prednisone alone for symptomatic hormone-resistant prostate cancer: A Canadian randomized trial with palliative end points. J Clin Oncol 14:1756–1764, 1996.

Thompson IM, Ankerst DP, Chi C, et al: Assessing prostate cancer risk: Results from the Prostate Cancer Prevention Trial. J Natl Cancer Inst 98:529–534, 2006.

Thompson IM, Ankerst DP, Chi C, et al: Operating characteristics of prostate-specific antigen in men with an initial PSA level of 3.0 ng/ml or lower. JAMA 294:66–70, 2005.

Thompson IM, Pauler DK, Goodman PJ, et al: Prevalence of prostate cancer among men with a prostate-specific antigen level < or = 4.0 ng per milliliter. N Engl J Med 350:2239–2246, 2004.

Wong YN, Mitra N, Hudes G, et al: Survival associated with treatment vs observation of localized prostate cancer in elderly men. JAMA 296:2683–2693, 2006.

CHAPTER 18

Testicular cancer

Patrick J. Loehrer, MD, Thomas E. Ahlering, MD,
Mark K. Buyyounouski, MD, MS, and Douglas Skarecky, BS

Testicular cancer, although an uncommon malignancy, is the most frequently occurring cancer in young men. In the year 2008, an estimated 8,090 cases of testicular cancer will be diagnosed in the United States. For unknown reasons, the incidence of this cancer has increased since the turn of the century, from 2 cases per 100,000 population in the 1930s, to 3.7 cases per 100,000 population from 1969 to 1971, to 5.4 cases per 100,000 population from 1995 to 1999. The greatest rise has been observed in Puerto Rico (1973 to 1997: 220%). This trend seems greatest for the development of seminoma.

Most testicular tumors are of germ-cell origin. These cancers are uniquely sensitive to chemotherapy and are considered the model for the treatment of solid tumors. Perhaps the most controversial area in the management of germ-cell tumors is the proper approach to early-stage disease (ie, surveillance vs primary lymphadenectomy [for nonseminoma germ-cell tumors] or radiation therapy [for seminomas]). In advanced disease, chemotherapy plays an essential role, but novel treatment regimens are currently being evaluated through multi-institution clinical trials.

Epidemiology

Age Testicular cancer can occur at any age but is most common between the ages of 15 and 35 years. There is a secondary peak in incidence after age 60. Seminoma is the most common histology in the older population but is rare in those younger than age 10. There is a slight increased prevalence of testicular cancer among fathers and brothers of testicular cancer patients.

Race Although testicular cancer is rare in African-Americans (1.6/100,000 population), these men present with higher grade disease and have significantly worse survival at 5 and 10 years. The incidence of this cancer has increased in whites during the 20th century but has remained flat in African Americans. Non-Hispanic white patients typically present with disease at early stages compared with

Surveillance, Epidemiology, and End Results (SEER) data show the incidence of testicular cancer in the United States continues to increase, albeit at an overall slower rate. Over the past 3 decades, the ratio of seminoma to nonseminoma increased from 50/50 to 60/40 in whites and from 60/40 to 70/30 in African Americans. National estimates of annual medical expenditures placed the total cost of treatment at $21.8 million in 2000, representing an increase of 10% over the total in 1994 *(Sokoloff MH, Joyce GF, Wise M, et al: J Urol 177:2030-2041, 2007).*

TESTICULAR

TABLE I: Anticipated cure rates in patients with germ-cell tumors, according to disease stage

Stage	Incidence at presentation (%)	Cure rate (%)
I (testis alone)	40	100
II (extension to retroperitoneal lymph nodes)	40	98
III (disseminated disease)	20	80

African Americans, Native Americans, Hawaiians, and Hispanic patients.

Geography Denmark has the highest incidence of testicular cancer; the Far East has the lowest.

Primary site Germ-cell tumors present most commonly in the testes (90%) and only infrequently in extragonadal sites (10%). The most common extragonadal sites (in decreasing order of frequency) are the retroperitoneum, mediastinum, and pineal gland. Many patients presumed to have a primary retroperitoneal germ-cell tumor may have an occult germ-cell tumor of the testicle. This possibility should be evaluated with testicular ultrasonography, especially when the retroperitoneal tumor is predominantly one-sided.

Survival The 5-year survival rate for all patients with testicular cancer is ~95%. Cure rates are highest for early-stage disease, which is treated primarily with surgery or radiation therapy (early seminoma), and lower for advanced disease, for which chemotherapy is the primary therapy (Table 1).

Etiology and risk factors

The specific cause of germ-cell tumors is unknown, but various factors have been associated with an increased risk of this malignancy.

Prior testicular cancer Perhaps the strongest risk factor for germ-cell tumors is a history of testicular cancer. Approximately 1% to 2% of patients with testicular cancer will develop a second primary in the contralateral testis over time. This represents a 500-fold increase in incidence over that in the normal male population.

The risk of contralateral testicular cancer was studied in a large population-based cohort of men diagnosed with testicular cancer before the age of 55. For 29,515 cases reported from 1973 through 2001 to the National Cancer Institute's Surveillance, Epidemiology, and End Results Program, the 15-year cumulative risk of developing metachronous contralateral testicular cancer was 1.9%, reaffirming the practice of not performing a biopsy on the contralateral testis at initial presentation.

Cryptorchidism Patients with cryptorchidism have a four- to eight-fold increased risk of developing germ-cell tumors compared with their normal counterparts. Orchiopexy, even at an early age, appears to reduce the incidence of germ-cell tumor only slightly (if at all). For an undescended testis, the most common malignant histology is seminoma. For those undergoing early orchiopexy, the most common malignancy is non-seminoma. Of note, in ~10% of patients with cryptorchidism who develop germ-cell tumors, the cancer is found in the normally descended testis. Biopsies of nonenlarged cryptorchid testes demonstrate an increased incidence of intratubal germ-cell neoplasm, a presumed precursor lesion.

Genetics Klinefelter's syndrome (47XXY) is associated with a higher incidence of germ-cell tumors, particularly primary mediastinal germ-cell tumors. For first-degree relatives of individuals affected with 47XXY, approximately a 6- to 10-fold increased risk for germ-cell tumors has been observed. In addition, patients with Down's syndrome have been reported to be at increased risk for germ-cell tumors. Also thought to be at greater risk are patients with testicular feminization, true hermaphrodites, persistent müllerian syndrome, and cutaneous ichthyosis.

> An undescended testis is a risk factor for testicular cancer and was studied in 16,983 men who were surgically treated. A cohort of men who underwent orchiopexy in Sweden between 1965 and 2000 was studied. Fifty-six cases of testicular cancer were identified. The relative risk of testicular cancer among those who underwent orchiopexy before reaching 13 years of age was 2.23 (95% confidence interval [CI], 1.58–3.06) compared with the Swedish general population. For those treated at 13 years of age or older, the relative risk was 5.4 (95% CI, 3.2–8.53); (Pettersson A, Richiardi L, Nordenskjold A, et al: N Engl J Med 356:1835-1841, 2007).

Family history Although familial testicular cancer has been observed, the incidence among first-degree relatives remains low. One investigator, however, reported a sixfold increased risk among male offspring of a patient with testicular cancer.

Environment Numerous industrial occupations and drug exposures have been implicated in the development of testicular cancer. Although exposure to diethylstilbestrol (DES) in utero is associated with cryptorchidism, a direct association between DES and germ-cell neoplasm is weak at best.

Reports have suggested an increased risk of testicular cancer among individuals exposed to exogenous toxins, such as Agent Orange and solvents used to clean jets. One author has suggested that based on epidemiologic evidence, ochratoxin A correlated with incidence data for testicular cancer.

Prior trauma, elevated scrotal temperature (secondary to the use of thermal underwear, jockey shorts, and electric blankets), and recurrent activities such as horseback riding and motorcycle riding, do not appear to be related to the development of testicular cancer.

No supporting findings substantiate a viral etiology.

Fertility An increased risk of infertility exists for men with unilateral testicular cancer successfully treated with orchiectomy. For example, 40% of patients have subnormal sperm counts, and by 1 year, 25% continue to have subnormal sperm counts.

Signs and symptoms

Local disease

Scrotal mass The most common complaint of patients on presentation is a painless scrotal mass that, on physical examination, cannot be separated from the testis. This finding distinguishes the mass from epididymitis. Not infrequently, the mass may be painful and thus may mimic epididymitis or testicular torsion.

Hydrocele Approximately 20% of patients with germ-cell tumors have an associated hydrocele.

Inguinal adenopathy Patients generally do not have inguinal adenopathy in the absence of prior scrotal violation.

Other symptoms include low back pain (from retroperitoneal adenopathy) and gynecomastia (usually bilateral). In cases of massive retroperitoneal lymphadenopathy, abdominal pain, nausea, vomiting, and constipation may be reported.

Disseminated disease

Patients with disseminated germ-cell tumors usually present with symptoms from lymphatic or hematogenous dissemination. Mediastinal adenopathy may be associated with chest pain or cough. Supraclavicular lymphadenopathy may also be present.

The cumulative 10-year risk of developing metachronous testicular cancer for patients with extragonadal germ-cell tumors is 10.3%. Patients with extragonadal tumors of the retroperitoneum and nonseminomatous cell type have a 14.3% 10-year risk for the development of metachronous testicular cancer. Some, however, may have previously undiagnosed occult testicular primary tumors.

Hematogenous spread to the lungs may be associated with dyspnea, cough, or hemoptysis. Infrequently, patients with extensive disease may present with signs and symptoms of CNS metastases or bone pain from osseous metastases (most common in patients with seminoma).

Metastases to the liver are not uncommon and may manifest as fullness in the upper abdomen or vague abdominal discomfort. More likely, they will be identified on CT scan in an otherwise asymptomatic patient.

Virtually all adult patients with germ-cell tumors have increased copies of isochromosome 12p, usually as i(12p). This is a useful marker in patients with undifferentiated tumors who fit the clinical profile of patients with germ-cell malignancy. Kit mutations have also been observed in seminoma, especially of primary mediastinal origin. The clinical significance of this observation is unknown at present.

Primary mediastinal germ-cell tumors

Primary mediastinal germ-cell tumors are associated with several unique syndromes, including Klinefelter's syndrome and acute megakaryocytic leukemia. In addition, mediastinal tumors have a great propensity for the development of non–germ-cell malignant histology as a major component of the tumor (eg, embryonal rhabdomyosarcoma, adenocarcinoma, and peripheral neuroectodermal tumor).

Screening and diagnosis

Screening

Self-examination Testicular self-examination is both simple to learn and safe to perform. The rarity of this disease, however, calls into question the value of routine aggressive screening procedures.

Testicular biopsy Testicular biopsy of a suspicious lesion is not recommended. Approximately 95% of patients with a mass within the testicle have a malignancy. Orchiectomy is the preferred treatment for patients with a testicular mass.

Carcinoma in situ (CIS) appears to be the precursor lesion for most testicular germ-cell tumors, except spermatocytic seminoma. Most patients harboring CIS can be expected to develop testicular cancer but with a latency period of a decade or more. The incidence of CIS in infertile men is about 0.6%. In patients with prior testicular cancer, biopsy will reveal CIS in the contralateral testis at a rate of ~5% to 6%. Men with a history of cryptorchidism and presumed extragonadal germ-cell tumor are at greater risk for CIS. Some investigators suggest routine biopsy of the contralateral testis in men with CIS.

Diagnosis

Ultrasonography can reliably identify masses within the testis. In virtually all patients, ultrasonography can distinguish a testicular from an extratesticular mass and may detect lesions that are not palpable on physical examination. Ultrasonographic findings cannot consistently differentiate benign from malignant tumors of the testis (95% of such masses are malignant). Most patients with testicular cancer, especially seminoma, have hypoechoic lesions compared to adjacent tissue. Nonseminomatous tumors, however, may have mixed signals, including hyperechoic masses, which are commonly seen with teratoma.

Serum markers Serum levels of β-subunit human chorionic gonadotropin (β-hCG) and α-fetoprotein (AFP) are elevated in ~80% to 85% of patients with extensive germ-cell tumors. Patients with pure seminoma may have elevated levels of β-hCG but not AFP (a significantly elevated AFP level usually indicates the presence of nonseminomatous germ-cell elements). False-positive β-hCG levels can be seen in patients who have hypogonadism (cross-reactivity with luteinizing hormone) or who pursue the use of marijuana; AFP levels may be elevated in patients with liver dysfunction or hepatitis.

Inguinal orchiectomy When a testicular mass is discovered, the patient should undergo an orchiectomy through an inguinal incision.

Trans-scrotal incisions or biopsies should not be performed, as they ultimately lead to aberrant lymphatic drainage from the tumor.

Staging evaluation

The principal objective of the staging evaluation is to ascertain whether the patient has early-stage disease (which is amenable to local therapy, such as retroperitoneal lymphadenectomy [for nonseminoma] or radiation therapy [for seminoma]) or disseminated disease (which requires chemotherapy).

Chest x-ray A chest x-ray can determine whether or not a patient has gross supradiaphragmatic metastases, which would mandate initial chemotherapy.

Chest CT In patients with a normal chest x-ray, chest CT is recommended in both patients with seminoma and those with nonseminoma when abdominal adenopathy is found, to rule out occult metastases within the lungs or mediastinum. If such metastases are present, the patient should be treated with primary chemotherapy.

Abdominopelvic CT provides important information about the retroperitoneal lymph nodes. Usually, periaortic adenopathy is noted on the ipsilateral side of the primary tumor. Patients with primary retroperitoneal germ-cell tumors often show an enlarged retroperitoneal mass in the midline. Although hepatic metastases are infrequent, at present, CT is the most viable method of determining these metastatic lesions.

PET [18]Fluorodeoxyglucose (FDG)-PET is emerging as a significant adjunct in staging and follow-up. Seminomas are FDG-avid. In some cases, nodal and extranodal metastases not appreciated on CT scans may be noted with FDG-PET. The optimal use of FDG-PET is in patients with residual masses following systemic therapy for pure seminoma. In such cases, the scans should be performed at least 3 to 4 weeks beyond the last course of chemotherapy. As teratoma is not PET-avid, its usefulness in nonseminomatous germ-cell tumors (NSGCT) is limited.

Other scans In the absence of symptoms or signs, a CT scan (or MRI) of the head and radionuclide bone scan are unnecessary. A lymphangiogram is rarely used today to identify microscopic nodal involvement in patients with stage I disease who choose to undergo surveillance. PET scans may be useful in patients with residual disease following chemotherapy for seminoma. If a PET scan is positive in such patients, surgical resection of the residual mass is indicated. Otherwise, the residual mass can be simply followed with periodic radiographic evaluation.

Pathology

Germ-cell tumors are classified into two broad histologic categories: seminoma and NSGCT. Patients with seminoma who have increased AFP levels or any focus of NSGCT components (including teratoma) are considered to have an NSGCT.

Seminoma

Seminoma is the most common single histology, accounting for ~30% of all germ-cell tumors. Up to 10% of seminomas have focal syncytiotrophoblastic cells, thought to be the source of β-hCG in some cases. Elevated AFP levels connote NSGCT.

Spermatocytic seminoma, a rare subset of germ-cell tumors, often grows to large size, occurs almost exclusively in men older than age 50, and rarely, if ever, metastasizes.

Nonseminoma

Embryonal carcinoma is composed of large pleomorphic cells with different architectural patterns. This tumor may be associated with an elevation in the serum levels of β-hCG and/or AFP.

Endodermal sinus tumor (yolk sac carcinoma) is the most common testicular tumor seen in infants and young children. Like embryonal carcinoma, yolk sac tumor has a variety of architectural patterns. This tumor is associated with an elevated serum level of AFP.

Choriocarcinoma, as a pure entity, is one of the least common germ-cell tumors. These tumors have a great propensity for hematogenous spread, often skipping the retroperitoneum. Choriocarcinoma is associated with an increased serum level of β-hCG.

Teratoma is a generally benign tumor with elements from each of the germ layers (ectoderm, mesoderm, and endoderm). Teratoma is uncommonly seen as the sole histology in primary tumors, but it is frequently associated with other histologic elements, including those previously mentioned. Of patients with residual disease following chemotherapy for NSGCT, ~45% have teratoma in resected specimens.

A subset of patients with immature teratoma that contains non–germ-cell histologies (eg, sarcoma, adenocarcinoma) has been reported. In contrast to most teratomas, these tumors may grow locally and can be lethal. In addition, late recurrences of both teratoma and carcinoma have been reported in patients with teratoma. Serum markers are normal in patients with pure teratoma.

Pattern of spread

Testicular cancer spreads in a fairly predictable fashion: from the testicle to the retroperitoneal lymph nodes and later hematogenously to the lungs or other visceral sites. Only 10% of patients present with hematogenous metastases (usually in the lungs) in the absence of discernible retroperitoneal adenopathy.

Staging systems

Clinical staging systems (Royal Marsden and TNM systems) for testicular cancer are outlined in Table 2. These staging systems help define the population for appropriate primary therapy.

Good- and poor-risk subgroups For patients with nonseminomas who are candidates for chemotherapy, other staging systems (such as those by Indiana University and Memorial Sloan-Kettering Cancer Center) were developed to segregate patients into good- and poor-risk categories. More recently, the International Germ-Cell Collaborative Group Consensus Conference formulated a classification that more clearly defines good- and poor-risk disease (Table 3), and it is currently being used to stratify patients in ongoing trials.

Treatment

SURGICAL TREATMENT OF STAGE I OR II DISEASE

Initial intervention for testicular cancer is radical inguinal orchiectomy. Orchiectomy may be deferred temporarily in patients with advanced-stage disease in whom the diagnosis of NSGCT can be made on clinical grounds (elevated markers). In such patients, an orchiectomy must be performed sooner or later, as there is incomplete penetration of chemotherapy into the testes.

Further therapy hinges on the pathologic diagnosis. In general, most clinical stage I tumors are typically followed with surveillance. Patients with pure seminomas (normal AFP level with or without an elevated β-hCG level) are treated with radiotherapy or chemotherapy, whereas most nonseminomas are treated with surgery and/or chemotherapy.

Inguinal orchiectomy

In addition to removal of the testis, the spermatic cord is dissected high into the retroperitoneum. The vas deferens is isolated from the testicular vessels and ligated separately with a permanent suture. Also, the testicular vessels are freed from the peritoneum and carefully ligated with a permanent suture.

TABLE 2: Staging systems for testicular cancer

Royal Marsden system	TNM system	Description
I	Tx, N0, M0	Disease confined to the testis and peritesticular tissue
II	Tx, N1 or N2a, M0	Fewer than six positive lymph nodes without extension into retroperitoneal fat; no node > 2 cm (infradiaphragmatic)

A < 2 cm
  B 2-5 cm
  C > 5-10 cm
  D > 10 cm		

	Tx, N2b, M0	Six or more positive lymph nodes, well-encapsulated and/or retroperitoneal fat extension; any node > 2 cm
	Tx, N3, M0	Any node > 5 cm
III	Tx, Nx, M1	Supradiaphragmatic and infradiaphragmatic adenopathy (no extralymphatic metastasis)
IV		Disseminated disease (lungs, liver, bone)

Retroperitoneal lymphadenectomy (nonseminomas)

For patients with nonseminomatous testicular cancer and either no evidence or a small volume of disease on CT (stage I [N0] or stage II [N1, N2a, N2b] disease), retroperitoneal lymphadenectomy (RLND) is generally indicated because it (1) accurately and definitively defines the presence or absence of retroperitoneal metastases and (2) removes the retroperitoneum as a site of recurrence, thus obviating the need for surveillance with CT.

RLND can be accomplished transperitoneally or retroperitoneally through a thoracoabdominal approach. The thoracoabdominal approach is more technically difficult but eliminates the risk of postoperative small bowel obstruction and usually requires a shorter hospital stay.

Nerve-sparing surgery Regardless of the approach, urologic oncologists recommend a unilateral, nerve-sparing procedure. For right-sided tumors, the medial border of the template is the midpoint of the aorta, and for left-sided

TABLE 3: International Germ-Cell Collaborative Group Consensus Conference criteria for good- and poor-risk testicular cancer patients treated with chemotherapy

NONSEMINOMA

Good prognosis

All of the following:

- AFP < 1,000 ng/mL, β-hCG < 5,000 IU/L, and LDH < 1.5 × upper limit of normal
- Nonmediastinal primary
- No nonpulmonary visceral metastasis

Intermediate prognosis

All of the following:

- AFP = 1,000-10,000 ng/mL, β-hCG = 5,000-50,000 IU/L, or LDH = 1.5-10 × normal
- Nonmediastinal primary site
- No nonpulmonary visceral metastasis

Poor prognosis

Any of the following:

- AFP > 10,000 ng/mL, β-hCG > 50,000 IU/L, or LDH > 10 × normal
- Mediastinal primary site
- Nonpulmonary visceral metastasis

SEMINOMA

Good prognosis

- No nonpulmonary visceral metastasis

Intermediate prognosis

- Nonpulmonary visceral metastasis

AFP = α-fetoprotein; hCG = human chorionic gonadotropin; LDH = lactate dehydrogenase

TABLE 4: Chemotherapy regimens for testicular cancer

Drug/combination	Dose and schedule
BEP	
Bleomycin	30 IU IV bolus on days 2, 9, and 16
Etoposide	100 mg/m^2 IV infused over 30 minutes on days 1-5
Platinol (cisplatin)	20 mg/m^2 IV infused over 15-30 minutes on days 1-5

Repeat cycle every 21 days for 3 or 4 cycles.

NOTE: Treat patients every 21 days on schedule, regardless of the granulocyte count. Reduce etoposide dose by 20% in patients who previously received radiotherapy or had granulocytopenia with fever/sepsis during the previous cycle. Patients receiving 4 cycles of BEP should undergo pulmonary function tests at baseline and at 9 weeks.

Williams SD, Birch R, Einhorn LH, et al: N Engl J Med 316:1435–1440, 1987

EP	
Etoposide	100 mg/m^2 IV infused over 30 minutes on days 1-5
Platinol (cisplatin)	20 mg/m^2 IV infused over 15-30 minutes on days 1-5

Repeat cycle every 21 days for 4 cycles.

NOTE: Treat patients every 21 days on schedule, regardless of the granulocyte count. Reduce etoposide dose by 20% in patients who previously received radiotherapy or had granulocytopenia with fever/sepsis during the previous cycle.

de Wit R, Roberts JT, Wilkinson PM, et al: J Clin Oncol 19:1629–1640, 2001

VIP	
VePesid (etoposide)	75 mg/m^2/d IV on days 1-5
Ifosfamide	1.2 g/m^2/d IV on days 1-5
Platinol (cisplatin)	20 mg/m^2/d IV on days 1-5
Mesna	400 mg IV bolus prior to the first ifosfamide dose, then 1.2 g/m^2/d IV infused continuously on days 1-5

Repeat cycle every 21 days for 4 cycles.

Loehrer PJ, Lauer R, Roth BJ, et al: Ann Intern Med 109:540–546, 1988

TIP (salvage therapy)

Taxol (pacliaxel)	175 mg/m^2 on day 1
Ifosfamide	1 g/m^2 on days 1-5
Platinol (cisplatin)	20 mg/m^2 on days 1-5
Mesna	400 mg IV bolus prior to the first ifosfamide dose, then 1.2 g/m^2/d IV infused continuously on days 1-5

Repeat cycle every 21 days for 4 cycles.

Kon Dagunta GV, Bacik J, Donadio A, et al: J Clin Oncol 23:6549–6555, 2005
Mead GM, Cullen MH, Huddart R, et al: Br J Cancer 93:178–184, 2005

VeIP (salvage therapy)

Vinblastine	0.11 mg/kg/d on days 1 and 2
Ifosfamide	1.2 g/m^2/d IV on days 1-5
Platinol (cisplatin)	20 mg/m^2/d IV on days 1-5
Mesna	400 mg/m^2 IV bolus prior to first ifosfamide dose, then 1.2 g/m^2/d IV infused continuously for 5 days

Repeat cycle every 21 days for 4 cycles.

Loehrer PJ, Lauer R, Roth BJ, et al: Ann Intern Med 109:540–546, 1988
Miller KD, Loehrer PJ, Gonin R, et al: J Clin Oncol 15:1427–1431, 1997

Table prepared by Ishmael Jaiyesimi, DO

tumors, the medial border is the midpoint of the inferior vena cava (IVC). The sympathetic trunks responsible for normal bladder neck closure during ejaculation course lateral to the aorta on the left side and behind the IVC on the right side. Below the inferior mesenteric artery, both sympathetic trunks send branches to the region anterior to the aorta. The branches coalesce and then pass to the bladder neck.

Critical aspects of nerve-sparing surgery include preservation of the ipsilateral sympathetic nerve trunk and bilateral preservation

> Surveillance guidelines for stage I seminoma were reported by investigators from Princess Margaret Hospital based on a systematic review of 17 prospective studies with a total of 5,561 patients. Follow-up with abdominopelvic CT scan and chest x-ray was recommended three times for years 1 and 2, twice a year for years 3 and 4, and then annually until year 10 *(Martin JM, Panzarella T, Zwahlen DR, et al: Cancer 109:2248-2256, 2007).*

of branches below the level of the inferior mesenteric artery. In our experience and that of other authors, it is possible to maintain normal ejaculatory function in virtually all patients using this technique.

SURVEILLANCE (NONSEMINOMAS)

In patients with clinical stage I disease (normal serum markers and normal CT scans of the chest and abdomen), surveillance is a reasonable option. In unselected patients with clinical stage I NSGCTs, the risk of recurrence is approximately 25%. Thus, close follow-up with chest x-ray, serum markers (β-hCG and AFP), and physical exam should be performed.

When followed up in this way, most patients will be detected with low-volume disease. If recurrence occurs, such cases should be curable with 3 cycles of BEP (bleomycin, 30 IU/wk × 9/wk; etoposide, 100 mg/m²/d; and Platinol [cisplatin], 20 mg/m²/d) or 4 cycles of EP (etoposide plus cisplatin at the same doses; see Table 4). If patients recur with higher volume disease (ie, intermediate or poor prognosis), up to 50% may not be cured. Thus, diligent follow-up is crucial.

RADIATION THERAPY FOR STAGE I OR II SEMINOMAS

Seminomas of the testes are exquisitely sensitive to irradiation. This characteristic, combined with their predictable lymphatic spread, makes these cancers amenable to radiotherapy. Since low radiation doses are used, acute and late side effects are few.

Radiation fields and doses The radiotherapy portals have traditionally included the para-aortic lymph nodes from T10 to L5 and the ipsilateral hemipelvis, including the inguinal scar. However, recent studies that reduced the size of para-aortic fields and omitted hemipelvis irradiation in selected patients (eg, those who have not undergone prior orchiopexy or other pelvic, inguinal, or scrotal surgery) are encouraging. A study by Fossa and colleagues randomized 478 men with stage I seminomas to receive irradiation of the para-aortics (T11 to L5) and ipsilateral hemipelvis versus irradiation of the para-aortics only. The actuarial rate of 3-year freedom from relapse was about 96% for both groups, although there were more pelvic relapses in patients given para-aortic radiation therapy only. Pelvic and/or inguinal failures occurred in

TABLE 5: Follow-up Schedule for Germ-Cell Tumor

Surveillance	Chest X-ray	βhCG/AFP	Chest CT	ABD/ Pelvic CT
Clinical stage I seminoma	q4mo, years 1-2	q4mo, years 1-2	—	q4mo, years 1-2
	q6mo, years 3-5	q6mo, years 3-5	—	q6mo, years 3-5
	After 5 years, annually	After 5 years, annually	—	As indicated
Clinical stage I NSGCT	q2mo, year 1	q2mo, year 1	—	q4mo, years 1-2
	q4mo, year 2	q4mo, year 2	—	q6mo, years 3-5
	q6mo, years 3-5	q6mo, years 3-5,	—	As indicated
	After 5 years, annually	After 5 years, annually	—	As indicated
Following chemotherapy complete remission ± surgical RPLND	q2mo, year 1 q4mo, year 2 q6mo, years 3-5 After year 5, annually	q2mo, year 1 q4mo, year 2 q6mo, years 3-5 After year 5, annually	— — — —	q4mo, years 1 & 2[a] q6mo, years 3-5[a] As indicated
Following treatment for mediastinal or other GCT salvage	q2mo, year 1 q4mo, year 2 q6mo, years 3-5	q2mo, year 1 q4mo, year 22 q6mo, years 3-5	q4mo, years 1-2[a] q6mo, years 3-5[a] —	As indicated As indicated —
	After year 5, annually	After year 5, annually	—	As indicated

[a] For patients with resected teratoma only.

< 5% of these patients. The few failures observed following radiotherapy most often occurred in the next echelon of lymph node drainage sites, such as the mediastinum or left supraclavicular fossa.

The smaller treatment volume reduces the dose to the remaining testicle and probably the risk of secondary malignancy. The ipsilateral hemipelvis is treated only when there is a history of ipsilateral inguinal surgery. Violation of the inguinal region can alter the testicular lymphatic drainage pathway to the para-aortic region. The hemiscrotum is often treated if the tumor penetrated the tunica albuginea, a trans-scrotal incision was performed, or orchiopexy was performed for cryptorchidism. However, this practice has been questioned, since the incidence of scrotal failure is low, even in the presence of these risk factors. In fact, some surgeons advocate the use of trans-scrotal exploration in order to rule out benign lesions.

Side effects The acute side effects of radiotherapy are limited to nausea, vomiting, and infrequently diarrhea, all of which usually can be readily controlled with medication. Long-term complications recently reported at M. D. Anderson Cancer Center demonstrated increased mortality ratios for overall, cardiac-specific, and secondary cancer deaths for men treated with radiation therapy for seminoma between 1951 and 1999. No difference in mortality risk was noted in the first 15 years following treatment; however, over the entire period, the all-cause mortality risk was 1.59. The cardiac-specific mortality rate after 15 years was 1.61, and the secondary cancer mortality rate was 1.91.

Permanent infertility from scattered irradiation to the contralateral testis is uncommon, whereas prolonged aspermia for more than 1 year may occur, especially with irradiation of the hemiscrotum. Nevertheless, sperm banking is recommended for patients concerned about childbearing.

Stage I disease

Prophylactic radiotherapy vs surveillance vs chemotherapy Primary lymphatic drainage of the testes is to the para-aortic lymph nodes from the level of the renal vessels to the bifurcation of the aorta. Although ipsilateral pelvic nodal failures and, to a much lesser extent, inguinal failures occur following tumor resection by inguinal orchiectomy in patients with stage I disease, these sites are at a much lower risk of failure than the para-aortic region. Based on surveillance data, the overall incidence of disease failure without radiotherapy is 15% to 27% (median, 20%), whereas only 2% to 5% (median, 3%) of patients who are treated with radiotherapy relapse. Relapse rates with surveillance appear to be lower in patients with < 4 cm primary tumors and no evidence of rete testis involvement.

The identification of prognostic factors makes surveillance an attractive alternative to the more conventional approach of radiotherapy in selected patients. Follow-up in patients undergoing surveillance is rigorous because disease progression usually is not associated with symptoms until the tumor burden is large. Surveillance requires abdominopelvic CT scans and chest x-rays at 3- to 4-month intervals for about 3 years and then at 6-month intervals for at least an additional 2 years. Late failures beyond 5 years have been observed. Salvage rates reported in patients who relapse while undergoing surveillance are approximately 90% initially, with ultimate salvage rates after relapse of approximately 95%. Those patients who do develop recurrence usually receive 4 cycles of EP.

Thus, in summary, various options exist for the primary treatment of clinical stage I seminoma, including radiation therapy and observation with monitoring of serum markers and computed tomography. Primary chemotherapy has decreased risk of recurrence comparable to radiation therapy, but still requires abdominal CT imaging for follow-up. Risk-adapted therapy has not yet defined the optimal population for primary chemotherapy.

CHEMOTHERAPY FOR STAGE I SEMINOMAS

Several studies have evaluated the role of primary chemotherapy, typically carboplatin as adjuvant therapy, for clinical stage I seminoma. Single-cycle carboplatin has been studied as an alternative to adjuvant radiotherapy in a randomized trial conducted by the UK Medical Research Council/European Organisation for Research and Treatment of Cancer (UKMRC/EORTC). At a median follow-up of 4 years, 3-year relapse-free survival rates were similar among the 1,477 randomized patients. However, first-echelon para-aortic nodal recurrences were more common in the chemotherapy group (74% vs 9%), raising concern regarding the efficacy of single-cycle carboplatin. Para-aortic nodal recurrences following radiotherapy are typically marginal misses at the edge of the treatment field.

Further questioning the role of single-cycle carboplatin in stage I disease, a pooled analysis of two randomized trials in advanced-stage disease demonstrated that single-agent carboplatin is inferior to cisplatin-based combination therapy. Phase II results evaluating two cycles of carboplatin (400 mg/m^2) for prophylactic treatment of stage I seminomas are more promising. However, acute toxicity (ie, the degree of lethargy and time missed from work) is unlikely to be less than that of a 2-week course of radiotherapy. A risk-adjusted method has also been evaluated, but thus far, these chemotherapy options do not preclude the necessity for continued surveillance with computerized tomography. In summary, observation, radiation therapy and chemotherapy can be considered options after careful, informed decision-making.

Stage II disease

The majority of patients with infradia-phragmatic para-aortic and/or pelvic adenopathy < 5 cm are treated with radiotherapy alone. Those with larger lymph node metastases are typically treated with platinum-based chemotherapy. Among patients who are candidates for radiotherapy, it is essential that renal function be preserved in case chemotherapy is necessary for salvage treatment. Recent preliminary evidence indicates that the 5-year freedom-from-failure rates may be improved to 97% by administration of neoadjuvant carboplatin combined with reduced-field radiotherapy. Alternatively, systemic therapy alone (BEP × 3 vs EP × 4) may be used in lieu of radiation therapy.

Radiation fields The radiotherapy fields are similar to those used for stage I disease except that they are widened to include any para-aortic or pelvic adenopathy with a 2- to 3-cm margin. In the past, mediastinal and supraclavicular treatment was standard in patients with stage II disease. However, data from several series revealed only a 3% rate of mediastinal/supraclavicular relapse. In addition, late cardiac toxicity has been reported. Although treatment to supradiaphragmatic sites has largely been abandoned in these cases, one report indicates that the rate of failure in the left supraclavicular fossa is higher than was previously believed. An analysis from another group indicates the opposite, however, that supradiaphragmatic radiotherapy for stage IIA-B seminoma is unnecessary. The overall actuarial rate of freedom from disease at 5 years for patients with para-aortic adenopathy < 2 cm (IIA) is 95%, 2 to 5 cm (IIB) is 90%, and > 5 and < 10 cm (IIC) is 85%.

Treatment-specific risks of second malignancies and cardiovascular disease in 5-year survivors of testicular cancer was reported from investigators from the Netherlands. Seminomas and nonseminomas were equally common in the cohort of 2,707 patients (median follow-up 17.5 years). The majority of seminoma patients (83%) received radiotherapy, whereas most nonseminoma patients received chemotherapy (45%) or surgery alone (28%). Subdiaphragmatic radiotherapy and chemotherapy increased the risk of developing second malignancy or cardiovascular disease to a similar extent as smoking (1.7-fold). Radiotherapy strongly increased the risk of second malignancy (2.6-fold), whereas chemotherapy increased the risks of both second malignancy (2.1-fold) and cardiovascular disease (1.7-fold) (van den Belt-Dusebout AW, de Wit R, Gietema JA, et al: J Clin Oncol 25:4370-4378, 2007).

Radiation doses The involved areas are usually treated with 30 to 35 Gy and the uninvolved areas, with 20 to 25 Gy. There is no evidence of a dose-response effect above 20 Gy for uninvolved areas and above 30 Gy for involved areas. Failures within the irradiated volume are anecdotal.

TREATMENT OF STAGE II NONSEMINOMAS

Over the past several years, the threshold for primary surgery in patients with stage II disease on CT scans has changed. At present, masses > 3 cm in greatest cross-sectional diameter or those with more extensive longitudinal lymphatic spread are generally handled primarily with chemotherapy. For patients with tumor sizes ≤ 3 cm, primary RLND is considered the standard approach. It should be noted that up to 25% of patients with enlarged lymph nodes on CT scans will be found to have pathologic stage I (false-positive) disease by RLND.

Adjuvant chemotherapy for nonseminomas

The risk of systemic recurrence is 5% to 10% in patients with pathologic stage I nonseminomas, 15% to 30% in those with completely resected stage IIA (N2a) disease, and 30% to 50% in those with stage IIB (N2b) disease. Recurrence usually occurs in the lungs within the first 24 months after surgery. The risk of retroperitoneal recurrence in patients with stage I, IIA, or IIB disease is < 1% after a properly performed RLND. Following RLND, patients with complete resection of stage II disease can be considered candidates for adjuvant chemotherapy.

The decision of whether or not to prescribe adjuvant therapy following lymph node dissection is somewhat arbitrary and often depends on the patient's social circumstances and likelihood of adhering to close follow-up. A patient with completely resected carcinoma who undergoes RLND has a 70% chance of cure; thus, the majority of patients will never need chemotherapy. However, these patients must be monitored carefully with chest x-rays and serum marker determinations every month for 1 year, every 2 months for an additional year, and then every 6 months for the next 3 years. (CT scanning is not performed routinely unless clinically indicated.) The 30% of patients followed in such a manner who do develop recurrence will present with a tumor of low volume (eg, small pulmonary metastases or elevated serum markers); nearly 100% of these patients should be cured with appropriate systemic therapy.

However, some patients with resected stage II disease elect to receive adjuvant chemotherapy to minimize the risk of cancer recurrence. For such therapy, two cycles of BEP (bleomycin, 30 IU/wk × 8; etoposide, 100 mg/m^2 on days 1 to 5 and 29 to 34; and cisplatin, 20 mg/m^2 on days 1 to 5 and 29 to 34) are recommended (Table 4). It should be emphasized that in a patient who agrees to close follow-up, the chance of dying of cancer should be negligible in either scenario. For patients who have persistently elevated or increasing serum markers following RLND or who have undergone incomplete lymph node dissection, 3 cycles of BEP are indicated.

In a study of 75 patients with stage I NSGCTs, compliance with clinical examinations was 61.5% in year 1 and 35.5% in year 2, whereas compliance with abdominal/pelvic CT was only 25.0% and 11.8% in years 1 and 2, respectively. Careful selection of highly motivated patients for surveillance is indicated.

TREATMENT OF STAGE III DISEASE

Seminomas

Chemotherapy is the treatment of choice for patients with stage III seminomas (see Table 4). The management of patients with bulky disease after chemotherapy (residual mass > 3 cm) is somewhat controversial. Investigators at Memorial Sloan-Kettering Cancer Center suggest that such patients require consolidation with radiotherapy or surgical removal of radiographically evident disease. More recent data from the Royal Marsden Hospital and the Centre Léon Bérard report a relapse rate of 10% to 15% in patients with residual masses with or without postchemotherapy surgery or radiotherapy, supporting the practice of observation in patients with residual masses following chemotherapy. FDG-PET may be helpful in the decision to treat residual masses > 3 cm but should be performed 4 to 6 weeks after the last course of chemotherapy.

Nonseminomas

As mentioned previously, patients with nonseminomas being treated with chemotherapy can be classified as having good- or poor-risk disease (see Table 3).

Good-risk nonseminomas In patients with good-risk nonseminomas, 3 cycles of BEP given every 3 weeks or, alternatively, 4 cycles of EP at the same dosages appear to yield equivalent results. More than 90% of good-risk patients should be cured with these therapies.

Two prospective randomized trials comparing cisplatin with carboplatin in good-risk patients with disseminated germ-cell tumors have demonstrated inferior results for carboplatin-containing regimens.

Postchemotherapy resection If a patient has persistent radiographic disease with normal serum markers 4 to 6 weeks following chemotherapy for an NSGCT, surgical resection should be performed when possible. In patients with a seminoma, a residual mass > 3 cm, and an abnormal PET scan, resection is also recommended.

Postresection chemotherapy Histologic examination of residual disease will reveal necrotic fibrous tissue in ~45% of such cases, benign teratoma in ~45%, and persistent carcinoma in ~10% to 15%. If persistent carcinoma is detected in the resected specimen, 2 additional cycles of EP should be administered. For patients with complete resection of mature and immature teratoma or necrosis, no additional therapy is needed.

Poor-risk nonseminomas A cohort of patients with disseminated germ-cell tumors presents with advanced or poor-risk disease. "Poor risk" has been variously defined (see Table 3) but represents a patient population with a cure rate of ≤ 50% with standard cisplatin-based combination chemotherapy. Irradiation is useful in the treatment of metastatic nonseminomas to the brain.

Chemotherapy During the past few years, several trials have evaluated a variety of combination regimens in patients with poor-risk disease (Table 4). They include the use of high-dose therapy, sequential therapy, and VIP (VePesid [etoposide], ifosfamide, and Platinol). VIP appears to be therapeutically equivalent to BEP; however, for most patients with advanced disease, BEP is the preferred regimen because it produces less myelosuppression. In patients with underlying pulmonary dysfunction, VIP is preferred.

In a study by Bhatia et al, 65 patients with recurrent testicular cancer were treated with tandem cycles of high-dose etoposide plus carboplatin followed by peripheral stem-cell transplantation as initial salvage therapy. With a median follow-up of 39 months, 37 patients (57%) remain continuously disease-free, with 3 additional patients (5%) disease-free with subsequent surgery. There was no treatment-related mortality.

A prospective Intergroup trial evaluating high-dose chemotherapy and stem cell transplantation (SCT) was recently published. This trial comparing 4 cycles of BEP with 2 cycles of BEP followed by 2 tandem courses of high-dose chemotherapy plus SCT in previously untreated patients with poor-risk disease was recently completed.

Postchemotherapy resection The ultimate goal of combination chemotherapy in these patients is the resolution of all radiographically visible disease and the normalization of tumor markers. If residual radiographic abnormalities persist in the lungs and/or abdomen, surgical resection of residual disease is indicated.

Postchemotherapy RLND must clear the region of residual disease. In general, postchemotherapy resections are extremely difficult, and incomplete resections are unacceptable. After the retroperitoneum is cleared of persistent radiographic disease, persistent pulmonary lesions are resected. In cases with residual disease in the retroperitoneum and thorax, RLND should be performed first. If necrosis is found, the disease within the chest can be observed. If teratoma or cancer is noted, the supradiaphragmatic disease should be resected.

Complicating factors associated with postchemotherapy resection include the risk of oxygen toxicity secondary to bleomycin as well as intense fibrosis and adherence of residual disease to the aorta and other vital retroperitoneal organs. Inspired oxygen levels must remain below 35% to prevent bleomycin-related acute respiratory distress syndrome, which has a fatality rate $\geq 50\%$.

After successful resection, the only visible structures remaining should include the back muscles, nerves, anterior spinous ligament, aorta, IVC, renal vessels, kidneys, and ureters. Up to 20% of patients with advanced abdominal disease may require resection of a kidney or even the IVC. Operative mortality in centers with experience performing resection of these advanced-stage tumors should be < 2%.

Postresection chemotherapy As mentioned, 2 additional cycles of chemotherapy are indicated for patients with persistent viable carcinoma in the resected specimen. For patients with resected teratoma of nonviable necrotic tissue, no additional chemotherapy is warranted.

Salvage chemotherapy

Approximately 20% to 30% of patients with disseminated germ-cell tumors do not attain complete remission with induction chemotherapy or relapse after such therapy. These patients may be candidates for salvage chemotherapy. It should be noted that occasional patients may be erroneously classified as having recurrent disease based on false-positive markers or abnormal radiographic findings. Some of these false-positive results may be due to a growing teratoma; pseudonodules from bleomycin-induced pulmonary disease; or elevated markers from other causes, such as an elevated β-hCG level from marijuana usage, cross-reactivity with luteinizing hormone, or an elevated AFP level associated with hepatitis or liver dysfunction. Another cause of persistently elevated markers is a tumor sanctuary site (eg, in the testes or brain). Assuming that false disease progression has been ruled out, several approaches to salvage therapy can be used. When possible, autologous BMT is preferred. It can achieve slightly more durable response rates than other options.

VeIP Ifosfamide is one of a few drugs (including etoposide, gemcitabine [Gemzar], and paclitaxel) that has clinical activity in patients with cisplatin-refractory disease. As second-line therapy, VeIP (vinblastine, 0.11 mg/kg on days 1 and 2, total dose = .22 mg/kg; plus ifosfamide, 1.2 g/m^2 [plus mesna (Mesnex)]; plus Platinol, 20 mg/m^2, both on days 1 to 5) produces durable complete remissions in ~30% of non-seminoma germ cell tumor (NSGCT) patients and 50% of seminoma patients previously treated with BEP chemotherapy (Table 4). Toxicity is primarily hematologic, which can be minimized with the use of a colony-stimulating growth factor.

Seminoma Patients with recurrent seminoma appear to be more sensitive to salvage therapy. In a study by Miller et al, 24 patients with seminoma were treated with VeIP as second-line therapy (following relapse after cisplatin-etoposide combination therapy). Of the 24 patients, 20 patients (83%) achieved a complete response, and 13 patients (54%) are long-term survivors, including 4 of 6 with extragonadal primary sites. Thus, initial salvage therapy in these patients should be VeIP (Table 4) rather than high-dose chemotherapy with bone marrow rescue.

High-dose chemotherapy with stem-cell rescue High-dose chemotherapy with tandem courses of carboplatin and etoposide plus autologous stem-cell rescue produces durable complete remission in 5% to 10% of patients whose disease is overtly refractory to cisplatin. When this approach is used in patients with recurrent, but not cisplatin-refractory, disease, improved response rates are observed; over 60% of all patients with recurrence of testicular cancer (excluding extragonadal recurrence) will be cured. Approximately 70% of patients treated with second-line therapy are curable with this approach.

Surgery Some patients with recurrent disease appear to have localized or minimally metastatic disease. In such cases, "desperation" surgery may achieve a durable complete remission. A 25% cure rate was seen in a select group of patients with elevated serum markers who underwent such surgery at Indiana University. These patients had completely resected viable carcinoma without chemotherapy following surgery.

Other agents Few drugs besides etoposide and ifosfamide have activity in patients with cisplatin-refractory disease. Oral etoposide given in a chronic schedule (50 mg/m^2/d for 21 days) has produced objective responses in ~20% of patients who were previously treated with IV etoposide. Paclitaxel has a similar response rate in minimally pretreated patients (< 6 cycles). Gemcitabine produces a response rate of ~15% in patients with cisplatin-refractory disease.

The Eastern Cooperative Oncology Group conducted a phase II trial of gemcitabine (1,000 mg/m^2) plus paclitaxel (110 mg/m^2) every week × 3 given every 4 weeks in patients with recurrent germ-cell tumor not thought to be curable with standard chemotherapy or surgery. Of 28 evaluable patients, 6 responded, including 3 complete responses (2 of whom were free of disease at 15+ and 25+ months).

In a group of patients not considered to be curable with standard salvage chemotherapy, cisplatin plus epirubicin produced durable complete remissions in 7 of 30 patients.

Survivorship issues

Delayed toxicity from systemic therapy

Delayed toxicity from systemic therapy for germ-cell tumors has been well characterized. In the absence of signs and symptoms, specific monitoring for these late effects is not generally warranted. A number of late effects have been observed.

Fertility problems and fetal malformation Fertility problems, manifested by azoospermia or oligospermia at or beyond 2 years, occur in 45% to 55% of treated patients. No increased risk of fetal malformation has been observed in the offspring of men previously treated with chemotherapy for testicular cancer.

Cardiovascular disease The risk of hypertension or other cardiovascular disease may be increased in patients with testicular cancer who received chemotherapy, but this theory is controversial. The only exception is Raynaud's phenomenon, which occurs at a rate directly proportional to the number of cycles of cisplatin-based chemotherapy.

Renal and pulmonary toxicities Although renal and pulmonary dysfunction can occur acutely during therapy, long-term consequences from therapy are uncommon.

Secondary malignancies

Perhaps of greatest concern is the development of secondary malignancies.

Late recurrence A similar percentage of patients may suffer late recurrence of the primary tumor. These late recurrences typically occur beyond 5 years (longest 32+ years) from primary therapy, frequently present with an elevated serum level of AFP, and are particularly resistant to salvage chemotherapy. Thus, surgical resection of disease is the primary treatment strategy.

Testicular cancer Approximately 1% to 2% of patients may develop a second primary testicular cancer.

Other cancers In a large series of 40,000 men by Travis et al, the relative risk for developing secondary tumors was 1.9 for 10-year survivors of testicular cancer and remained 1.7 for 35-year survivors. The greatest elevated risk was for cancers of the pleura, pancreas, bladder, and stomach. In another large retrospective analysis of 635 patients with extragonadal germ-cell tumors treated from 1975 to 1996, only an increased number of hematologic and skin malignancies were observed.

The contribution of chemotherapy and/or radiation therapy to the development of these other malignancies, as opposed to a natural propensity toward their development, is unknown. However, in several series, etoposide has been shown to pose an increased risk for the development of secondary leukemia (dose-related). At higher dosages (> 2 g/m^2 cumulative), etoposide has been associated with a greater incidence of acute leukemia. Very high dosages of etoposide with stem-cell rescue do not appear to be linked to a higher risk than standard-dose chemotherapy. In one paper by Travis and colleagues, both increased dosages of radiation therapy and cisplatin were associated with an increased risk for acute leukemia. Although these risks are real, they still are low compared with the risk of death caused by testicular cancer. Nonetheless, indiscriminate use of chemotherapy for early-stage (stage I) disease should be tempered by the recognition of the long-term hazards of therapy.

Follow-up for relapse

Because the relapse rate for testicular cancer is low, patients with pathologically confirmed stage I NSGCTs require no further therapy, and follow-up can be accomplished easily with chest x-ray, tumor markers, and physical examination. Similarly, for patients who have stage II disease and receive adjuvant chemotherapy, the risk of relapse is low. For patients with either of these two clinical scenarios, follow-up tests (chest x-ray, serum markers) should be performed every 2 months for 1 year, every 4 months for the second year, every 6 months for years 3 through 5, and annually thereafter.

In patients with resected stage II NSGCTs who do not receive adjuvant chemotherapy, the follow-up tests are the same as those listed above. However, in these patients, follow-up tests are performed every month for 1 year, every 2 months for 2 years, every 6 months for years 3 through 5, and then annually.

SUGGESTED READING

Albqami N, Janetschek G: Laparoscopic retroperitoneal lymph-node dissection in the management of clinical stage I and II testicular cancer. J Endourol 19:683–692, 2005.

Aparicio J, Germa JR, Garcia del Muro X, et al: Risk-adapted management for patients with clinical stage I seminoma: The Second Spanish Germ Cell Cancer Cooperative Group study. J Clin Oncol 23:8717–8723, 2005.

Beck SD, Foster RS, Bihrle R, et al: Does the histology of nodal metastasis predict systemic relapse after retroperitoneal lymph node dissection in pathological stage B1 germ cell tumors? J Urol 174:1287–1290, 2005.

Beck SD, Foster RS, Bihrle R, et al: Impact of the number of positive lymph nodes on disease-free survival in patients with pathological stage B1 nonseminomatous germ cell tumor. J Urol 174:143–145, 2005.

Bedano PM, Brames MJ, Williams SD, et al: Phase II study of cisplatin plus epirubicin salvage chemotherapy in refractory germ cell tumors. J Clin Oncol 24:5403–5407, 2006.

Chung PW, Warde PR, Panzarella T, et al: Appropriate radiation volume for stage IIA/B testicular seminoma. Int J Radiat Oncol Biol Phys 56:746–748, 2003.

Classen J, Schmidberger H, Meisner C, et al: Radiotherapy for stages IIA/B testicular seminoma: Final report of a prospective multicenter clinical trial. J Clin Oncol 21:1101–1106, 2003.

Classen J, Schmidberger H, Meisner C, et al: Para-aortic irradiation for stage I testicular seminoma: Results of a prospective study in 675 patients. A trial of the German testicular cancer study group (GTCSG). Br J Cancer 90:2305–2311, 2004.

Corvin S, Sturm W, Schlatter E, et al: Laparoscopic retroperitoneal lymph-node dissection with the waterjet is technically feasible and safe in testis-cancer patients. J Endourol 19:823–826, 2005.

Daugaard G, Petersen PM, Rorth M: Surveillance in stage I testicular cancer. APMIS 111:76–83, 2003.

DeSantis M, Becherer A, Bokemeyer C, et al: 2-18Fluoro-deoxy-*D*-glucose positron emission tomography is a reliable predictor for viable tumor in postchemotherapy seminoma: An update of the prospective multicentric SEMPET trial. J Clin Oncol 22:1034–1039, 2004.

Einhorn LH: Curing metastatic testicular cancer. Proc Natl Acad Sci U S A 99:4592–4595, 2002.

Einhorn LH, Williams SD, Chamness A, et al: High-dose chemotherapy and stem-cell rescue for metastatic germ-cell tumors. N Engl J Med 357:340–348, 2007.

Hinton S, Catalano PJ, Einhorn LH, et al: Cisplatin, etoposide and either bleomycin or ifosfamide in the treatment of disseminated germ cell tumors. Cancer 97:1869–1875, 2003.

Holm M, Hoei-Hansen CE, Rajpert-DeMeyts E, et al: Increased risk of carcinoma in situ in patients with testicular germ cell cancer with ultrasonic microlithiasis in the contralateral testicle. J Urol 170:1163–1167, 2003.

Houck W, Abonour R, Vance G, et al: Secondary leukemias in refractory germ cell tumor patients undergoing autologous stem-cell transplantation using high-dose etoposide. J Clin Oncol 22:2155–2158, 2004.

Huyghe E, Matsuda T, Thonneau P: Increasing incidence of testicular cancer worldwide: A review. J Urol 170:5–11, 2003.

Jones WG, Fossa SD, Mead GM, et al: Randomized trial of 30 versus 20 Gy in the adjuvant treatment of stage I testicular seminoma: A report on Medical Research Council Trial TE18, European Organisation for the Research and Treatment of Cancer Trial 30942 (ISRCTN 18525328). J Clin Oncol 23:1200–1208, 2005.

Loehrer PJ, Bosl GJ: Carboplatin for stage I seminoma and the sword of Damocles. J Clin Oncol 23:8566–8569, 2005.

McGlynn KA, Devesa SS, Sigurdson AJ, et al: Trends in the incidence of testicular germ cell tumors in the United States. Cancer 97:63–70, 2003.

Melchior D, Mulle SC, Albers P: Extensive surgery in metastatic testicular cancer. Aktuelle Urol 34:214–222, 2003.

Oliver RT, Mason MD, Mead GM, et al: Radiotherapy versus single-dose carboplatin in adjuvant treatment of stage I seminoma: A randomised trial. Lancet 366:293–300, 2005.

Rick O, Bokemeyer C, Weinknecht T, et al: Residual tumor resection after high-dose chemotherapy in patients with relapsed or refractory germ cell cancer. J Clin Oncol 22:3713–3719, 2004.

Travis LB, Fossa SD, Schonfeld SJ, et al: Second cancers among 40,576 testicular cancer patients: Focus on long-term survivors. J Natl Cancer Inst 97:1354–1365, 2005.

Zagars GK, Ballo MT, Lee AK, et al: Mortality after cure of testicular seminoma. J Clin Oncol 22:640–647, 2004.

CHAPTER 19

Urothelial and kidney cancers

Mark Hurwitz, MD, Philippe E. Spiess, MD, Brian Rini, MD,
Louis L. Pisters, MD, and Bruce G. Redman, DO

UROTHELIAL CANCER

In the year 2008, an estimated 68,810 new cases of bladder cancer will be diagnosed in the United States, and approximately 14,100 patients will die of this disease.

Urothelial cancers encompass carcinomas of the bladder, ureters, and renal pelvis; these cancers occur at a ratio of 50:3:1, respectively. Cancer of the urothelium is a multifocal process. Patients with cancer of the upper urinary tract have a 30% to 50% chance of developing cancer of the bladder at some time in their lives. On the other hand, patients with bladder cancer have a 2% to 3% chance of developing cancer of the upper urinary tract. The incidence of renal pelvis tumors is decreasing.

Epidemiology

Gender Urothelial cancers occur more commonly in men than in women (3:1) and have a peak incidence in the seventh decade of life.

Race Cancers of the urothelial tract are also more common in whites than in blacks (2:1).

Etiology and risk factors

Cigarette smoking The major cause of urothelial cancer is cigarette smoking. A strong correlation exists between the duration and amount of cigarette smoking and cancers at all levels of the urothelial tract. This association holds for both transitional cell and squamous cell carcinomas.

Analgesic abuse Abuse of compound analgesics, especially those containing phenacetin, has been associated with an increased risk of cancers of the urothelial tract. This risk appears to be greatest for the renal pelvis, and cancer at this site is usually preceded by renal papillary necrosis. The risk associated with analgesic abuse is seen after the consumption of excessive amounts (5 kg).

Chronic urinary tract inflammation also has been associated with urothelial cancers. Upper urinary tract stones are associated with renal pelvis cancers. Chronic bladder infections can predispose patients to cancer of the bladder, usually squamous cell cancer.

Occupational exposure has been associated with an increased risk of urothelial cancers. Workers exposed to arylamines in the organic chemical, rubber, and paint and dye industries have an increased risk of urothelial cancer similar to that originally reported for aniline dye workers.

Balkan nephropathy An increased risk of cancer of the renal pelvis and ureters occurs in patients with Balkan nephropathy. This disorder is a familial nephropathy of unknown cause that results in progressive inflammation of the renal parenchyma, leading to renal failure and multifocal, superficial, low-grade cancers of the renal pelvis and ureters.

Genetic factors There are reports of families with a higher risk of transitional cell cancers of the urothelium, but the genetic basis for this familial clustering remains undefined.

Signs and symptoms

Hematuria is the most common symptom in patients presenting with urothelial tract cancer. It is most often painless, unless obstruction due to a clot or tumor and/or deeper levels of tumor invasion have already occurred.

Urinary voiding symptoms of urgency, frequency, and/or dysuria are also seen in patients with cancers of the bladder or ureters but are uncommon in patients with cancers of the renal pelvis.

Vesical irritation without hematuria can be seen, especially in patients with carcinoma in situ of the urinary bladder.

Symptoms of advanced disease Pain is usually a symptom of more advanced disease, as is edema of the lower extremities secondary to lymphatic obstruction.

Diagnosis

Initial work-up The initial evaluation of a patient suspected of having urothelial cancer consists of excretory urography, followed by cystoscopy. In patients with upper tract lesions, retrograde pyelography can better define the exact location of lesions. Definitive urethroscopic examination and biopsy can be accomplished utilizing rigid or flexible instrumentation.

At the time of cystoscopy, urine is obtained from both ureters for cytology, and brush biopsy is obtained from suspicious lesions of the ureter. Brush biopsies significantly increase the diagnostic yield over urine cytology alone. Also, at the time of cystoscopy, a bimanual examination is performed to determine whether a palpable mass is present and whether the bladder is mobile or fixed.

Evaluation of a primary bladder tumor In addition to biopsy of suspicious lesions, evaluation of a bladder primary tumor includes biopsy of selected mucosal sites to detect possible concomitant carcinoma in situ. Biopsies of the primary lesion must include bladder wall muscle to determine whether there is invasion of muscle by the overlying carcinoma.

CT For urothelial cancers of the upper tract or muscle invasive bladder cancers, a CT scan of the abdomen/pelvis is performed to detect local extension of the cancer and involvement of the abdominal lymph nodes.

Bone scan For patients with bone pain or an elevated alkaline phosphatase level, a radioisotope bone scan is performed.

A chest x-ray completes the staging evaluation.

Pathology

Transitional cell carcinomas constitute 90% to 95% of urothelial tract cancers.

Squamous cell cancers account for 3% to 7% of urothelial carcinomas and are more common in the renal pelvis and ureters.

Adenocarcinomas account for a small percentage (< 3%) of bladder malignancies and are predominantly located in the trigone region. Adenocarcinomas of the bladder that arise from the dome are thought to be urachal in origin.

Carcinoma in situ In approximately 30% of newly diagnosed bladder cancers, there are multiple sites of bladder involvement, most commonly with carcinoma in situ. Although carcinoma in situ can occur without macroscopic cancer, it most commonly accompanies higher disease stages.

When carcinoma in situ is associated with superficial tumors, rates of recurrence and disease progression (development of muscle invasion) are higher (50%–80%) than when no such association is present (10%). Carcinoma in situ involving the bladder diffusely without an associated superficial tumor is also considered an aggressive disease. Most patients with this type of cancer will develop invasive cancers of the bladder.

Staging and prognosis

Staging system Urothelial tract cancers are staged according to the American Joint Committee on Cancer (AJCC) TNM classification system (Table 1). Superficial bladder cancer includes papillary tumors that involve only the mucosa (Ta) or submucosa (T1) and flat carcinoma in situ (Tis). The natural history of superficial bladder cancer is unpredictable, and recurrences are common. Most tumors recur within 6 to 12 months and are of the same stage and grade, but 10% to 15% of patients with superficial cancer will develop invasive or metastatic disease.

Prognostic factors For carcinomas confined to the bladder, ureters, or renal pelvis, the most important prognostic factors are T stage and differentiation

TABLE 1: TNM staging of urothelial tract cancers

Primary tumor (T)

Tx		Primary tumor cannot be assessed
T0		No evidence of primary tumor
Ta		Noninvasive papillary tumor
Tis		Carcinoma in situ: "flat tumor"
T1		Tumor invades subepithelial connective tissue
T2		Tumor invades muscle
	pT2a	Tumor invades superficial muscle (inner half)
	pT2b	Tumor invades deep muscle (outer half)
T3		Tumor invades perivesical tissue
	pT3a	Microscopically
	pT3b	Macroscopically (extravesical mass)
T4		Tumor invades any of the following: prostate, uterus, vagina, pelvic wall, abdominal wall
	T4a	Tumor invades prostate, uterus, vagina
	T4b	Tumor invades pelvic wall, abdominal wall

Regional lymph nodes (N)

Nx	Regional lymph nodes cannot be assessed
N0	No regional node involvement
N1	Metastasis in a single node, ≤ 2 cm in greatest dimension
N2	Metastasis in a single node, > 2 cm but ≤ 5 cm in greatest dimension; or multiple lymph nodes, none > 5 cm in greatest dimension
N3	Metastasis in a lymph node, > 5 cm in greatest dimension

Distant metastasis (M)

Mx	Distant metastasis cannot be assessed
M0	No distant metastasis
M1	Distant metastasis

Stage grouping

Stage 0a	Ta	N0	M0
Stage 0is	Tis	N0	M0
Stage I	T1	N0	M0
Stage II	T2a	N0	M0
	T2b	N0	M0
Stage III	T3a	N0	M0
	T3b	N0	M0
	T4a	N0	M0
Stage IV	T4b	N0	M0
	Any T	N1-N3	M0
	Any T	Any N	M1

From Greene FL, Page DL, Fleming ID, et al (eds): AJCC Cancer Staging Manual, 6th ed. New York, Springer-Verlag, 2002.

pattern. The impact of associated carcinoma in situ on Ta and T1 lesions is discussed previously (see section on "Pathology"). Less-differentiated Ta–T1 lesions also are associated with higher recurrence and disease progression rates. Patients with well-differentiated Ta lesions without carcinoma in situ have a 95% survival rate, whereas those with high-grade T1 lesions have a 10-year survival rate of 50%. The presence of lymphovascular invasion within the surgical specimen appears to be independently associated with overall survival, cause-specific survival, as well as local and distant recurrence in patients with node-negative bladder cancer at the time of cystectomy. As such, the presence of lymphovascular invasion should be included in the pathologic assessment of bladder cancer.

Muscle invasive carcinoma carries a 5-year survival rate of 20% to 50%. When regional lymph nodes are involved, the 5-year survival rate is 0% to 20%.

Treatment

TREATMENT OF LOCALIZED DISEASE

Surgical approaches to superficial bladder cancer

Transurethral resection Most patients with superficial bladder cancer can be treated adequately with transurethral resection (TUR). Such procedures preserve bladder function, entail minimal morbidity, and can be performed repeatedly. Survival rates > 70% at 5 years are expected. Although TUR removes existing tumors, it does not prevent the development of new lesions. Patients should be followed closely.

Laser The neodymium:yttrium-aluminum-garnet (Nd:YAG) laser has achieved good local tumor control when used in the treatment of superficial bladder tumors. However, it has not been adopted for general use because of its limitations in obtaining material for staging and grading of tumors.

Partial cystectomy is an infrequently utilized treatment option for patients whose tumors are not accessible or amenable to TUR.

Radical cystectomy is generally not used for the treatment of superficial bladder tumors. The indications for radical cystectomy include:

- Unusually large tumors that are not amenable to complete TUR, even on repeated occasions
- Some high-grade tumors
- Multiple tumors or frequent recurrences that make TUR impractical
- Symptomatic diffuse carcinoma in situ (Tis) that proves unresponsive to intravesical therapy
- Prostatic stromal involvement.

Intravesical therapy The indications for intravesical therapy include:

- Stage T1 tumors, especially if multiple

- Multifocal papillary Ta lesions, especially grade 2 or 3
- Diffuse Tis
- Rapidly recurring Ta, T1, or Tis disease.

In the United States, four intravesical agents are commonly used: thiotepa, an alkylating agent; bacillus Calmette-Guérin (BCG), an immune modulator/stimulator; and mitomycin and doxorubicin, both antibiotic chemotherapeutic agents. The dose of BCG varies with the strain (50 mg [Tice] or 60 mg [Connaught]). Mitomycin doses range from 20 to 40 mg. Although all four agents reduce the tumor recurrence rate, BCG is the most effective. For the treatment of papillary Ta and T1 lesions, BCG and mitomycin have the greatest efficacy (complete response rate, approximately 50%). For the treatment of Tis, BCG is extremely effective.

In a recent meta-analysis, comparing intravesical BCG and chemotherapy (mitomycin, epirubicin, doxorubicin, or sequential mitomycin/doxorubicin), intravesical BCG was shown to be superior in reducing the risk of short- and long-term treatment failure for Tis. Therefore, intravesical BCG appears to be the agent of choice for Tis.

Surgical approaches to invasive bladder cancer

Radical cystectomy Invasive bladder cancer (stage II or higher) is best treated by radical cystectomy. Candidates for radical cystectomy include:

- Patients with muscle-invasive tumor (depth of invasion is not important, merely its presence), regardless of grade
- Patients with high-grade, invasive, lamina propria tumors with evidence of lymphovascular invasion, with or without Tis
- Patients with diffuse Tis or recurrent superficial cancer who do not respond to intravesical therapy.

In men, radical cystectomy includes en bloc pelvic lymph node dissection and removal of the bladder, seminal vesicles, and prostate. In women, radical cystectomy entails en bloc pelvic lymph node dissection and anterior exenteration, including both ovaries, fallopian tubes, uterus, cervix, anterior vaginal wall, bladder, and urethra.

Partial cystectomy is an infrequently utilized treatment option and should only be considered when there is a solitary lesion in the dome of the bladder and when random biopsy results from remote areas of the bladder and prostatic urethra are negative.

Urethrectomy is routinely included in the anterior exenteration performed in female patients. Urethrectomy in male patients is performed if the tumor grossly involves the prostatic urethra or if prior TUR biopsy results of the prostatic stroma are positive. Delayed urethrectomy for positive urethral cytology or biopsy is required in about 10% of male patients.

Urinary reconstruction may involve any one of the following: intestinal conduits (eg, ileal, jejunal, or colonic), continent cutaneous diversion (eg, Indiana or Kock pouch), or orthotopic reconstruction (in both male and female patients).

Surgical approaches to ureteral and renal pelvic tumors

Optimal surgical management of urothelial malignancies of the ureter and renal pelvis consists of nephroureterectomy with excision of a bladder cuff. Some tumors may respond well to local resection, and tumor specifics may allow for a more conservative intervention.

Upper ureteral and renal pelvic tumors (because of similar tumor behavior and anatomic aspects) may be considered as a group, whereas lower ureteral tumors may be considered as a separate group.

Upper ureteral and renal pelvic tumors are best treated with nephroureterectomy. Solitary, low-grade upper tract tumors may be considered for segmental excision or ureteroscopic surgery if close surveillance is feasible. Care should be exercised, however, as multicentricity is more probable and the risk of recurrence is greater than for lower ureteral lesions.

Lower ureteral lesions may be managed by nephroureterectomy, segmental resection, and neovesical reimplantation or by endoscopic resection. A 15% recurrence rate is seen after segmental resection or endoscopic excision. Careful follow-up is mandatory. Disease progression, the development of a ureteral stricture precluding periodic surveillance, and poor patient compliance are indications to abandon conservative management and perform nephroureterectomy.

ROLE OF RADIATION THERAPY

Radiation therapy for bladder cancer

Primary radiation or chemoradiation therapy Radiation therapy, either alone or in conjunction with chemotherapy, is the modality of choice for patients whose clinical condition precludes surgery, either because of extensive disease or poor overall status. Trials have shown that patients treated with irra-

TABLE 2: Chemotherapy regimens for bladder carcinoma

Drug/combination	Dose and schedule

M-VAC

Methotrexate	30 mg/m^2 IV on days 1, 15, and 22
Vinblastine	3 mg/m^2 IV on days 2, 15, and 22
Doxorubicin	30 mg/m^2 IV on day 2
Cisplatin	70 mg/m^2 IV on day 2

NOTE: Reduce doxorubicin dose to 15 mg/m^2 in patients who have received prior pelvic irradiation. On days 15 and 22, methotrexate (30 mg/m^2) and vinblastine (3 mg/m^2) are given only if the white blood cell count is > 2,500 cells/μL and the platelet count is > 100,000 cells/μL.

Repeat cycles every 28-32 days even if the interim dose is withheld due to myelosuppression or mucositis. Doxorubicin dose is reduced to 15 mg/m^2 in patients treated with prior pelvic radiation.

von der Maase H, Hansen SW, Roberts JT, et al: J Clin Oncol 18:3068–3077, 2000.

Paclitaxel/carboplatin

Paclitaxel	200 mg/m^2 IV infused over 3 hours
Carboplatin	Dose calculated by the Calvert formula to an area under the curve (AUC) of 5 mg/mL/min IV infused over 15 minutes after paclitaxel

Repeat cycle every 21 days

PREMEDICATIONS: Dexamethasone, 20 mg PO, 12 and 6 hours prior to paclitaxel; as well as ranitidine, 50 mg IV, and diphenhydramine, 50 mg IV, both 30-60 minutes prior to paclitaxel.

Redman B, Smith D, Flaherty L, et al: J Clin Oncol 16:1844-1848, 1998.

Gemcitabine/docetaxel

Gemcitabine	800 mg/m^2 IV on days 1, 8, and 15
Docetaxel	60 mg/m^2 IV on day 1

Repeat cycle every 28 days.

Gitlitz BJ, Baker C, Chapman Y, et al: Cancer 98:1863–1869, 2003.

Gemcitabine/cisplatin

Gemcitabine	1,000 mg/m^2 IV on days 1, 8, and 15
Cisplatin	70 mg/m^2 IV on day 2

Repeat cycle every 28 days.

von der Maase H, Hansen SW, Roberts JT, et al: J Clin Oncol 18:3068–3077, 2000.

---

diation and cisplatin with or without fluorouracil (5-FU) have improved local control, as compared with patients treated with irradiation alone.

The most frequently utilized systemic chemotherapy regimens for urothelial carcinoma are shown in Table 2. Other studies suggest that TUR followed by radiation therapy combined with cisplatin or 5-FU chemotherapy, with cystectomy reserved for salvage, provides a survival equivalent to that achieved with initial radical cystectomy while allowing for bladder preservation in many patients. The extent of TUR and the absence of hydronephrosis are important prognostic factors in studies of bladder-conserving treatment. Updates from

Drug/combination	Dose and schedule

PCG

Paclitaxel	200 mg/m^2 IV infused over 3 hours on day 1
Carboplatin	Dose calculated on AUC of 5 mg/mL/min, 15-minute IV infusion on day 1
Gemcitabine	800 mg/m^2 30-minute IV on days 1 and 8

Repeat cycle every 21 days.

PREMEDICATIONS: Dexamethasone, 20 mg PO, 12 and 6 hours prior to paclitaxel; diphenhydramine, 50 mg IV, 30 minutes prior to paclitaxel; and either cimetidine, 300 mg IV, or ranitidine, 50 mg IV, 30 minutes prior to paclitaxel.

Hussain M, Vaishampayan U, Du W, et al: J Clin Oncol 19:2527–2533, 2001.

Paclitaxel/cisplatin

Paclitaxel	135 mg/m^2 IV infused over 3 hours
Cisplatin	70 mg/m^2 IV infused over 2 hours

Repeat cycle every 3 weeks until disease progression or for a maximum of 6 cycles.

PREMEDICATIONS: Dexamethasone, 20 mg PO, 12 and 6 hours prior to paclitaxel; as well as ranitidine, 50 mg IV, or cimetidine, 300 mg IV, prior to paclitaxel, and diphenhydramine, 50 mg IV, 30 minutes prior to paclitaxel.

Burch PA, Richardson RI, Cha SS, et al: Proc Am Soc Clin Oncol 18:1266a, 1999.

TCG

Taxol (paclitaxel)	80 mg/m^2 IV infused over 1 hour on days 1 and 8
Cisplatin	70 mg/m^2 on day 1
Gemcitabine	1 g/m^2 IV on days 1 and 8

Repeat cycle every 21 days.

PREMEDICATIONS: Dexamethasone, 20 mg PO, 12 and 6 hours prior to paclitaxel; as well as diphenhydramine, 50 mg IV, 30 minutes prior to paclitaxel, and either cimetidine, 300 mg IV, or ranitidine, 50 mg IV, 30 minutes prior to paclitaxel.

Vaishampayan U, Smith D, Redman B, et al: Proc Am Soc Clin Oncol 18:333a (abstract 1282), 1999.

Table prepared by Ishmael Jaiyesimi, DO

---

institutions in Europe and the United States on over 600 patients with long-term follow-up support the durability of outcomes previously reported.

A randomized phase III study of bladder preservation with or without neoadjuvant chemotherapy following TUR, conducted by the Radiation Treatment Oncology Group (RTOG), revealed no advantage to the use of MCV (methotrexate, cisplatin, and vinblastine) before radiation therapy and concurrent cisplatin. The favorable outcome without neoadjuvant chemotherapy may make bladder preservation a more acceptable option for a wider range of patients.

Preoperative irradiation may improve survival in patients undergoing radical cystectomy. Its use is limited due to concern over complications occurring with the urinary diversions currently utilized.

Radiation dose and technique Initially, a pelvic field is treated to approximately 4,500 cGy utilizing a multifield box technique, with 180 cGy delivered daily. The bladder tumor is then boosted to a total dose of 6,480 cGy utilizing multifield techniques, with 180 cGy delivered daily. Alternatively, twice daily treatment may be considered.

Radiation therapy for renal pelvic and ureteral cancers

In patients with renal pelvic and ureteral lesions who have undergone nephroureterectomy, postoperative local-field irradiation is offered if there is periureteral, perirenal, or peripelvic extension or lymph node involvement. A dose of approximately 4,500 to 5,040 cGy is delivered utilizing multifield techniques.

Palliative irradiation

Palliative radiation therapy is effective in controlling pain from local and metastatic disease and in providing hemostatic control. A randomized study comparing 3,500 cGy in 10 fractions and 2,100 cGy in 3 hypofractionated treatments revealed high rates of relief of hematuria, frequency, dysuria, and nocturia with either regimen. In selected cases of bladder cancer, aggressive palliation to approximately 6,000 cGy may be warranted to provide long-term local tumor control. Concurrent chemotherapy should be considered.

NEOADJUVANT/ADJUVANT CHEMOTHERAPY

Perioperative chemotherapy to reduce the risk of recurrence before or after cystectomy is a debated topic. Multiple randomized trials of different designs have given various chemotherapy regimens before and/or after cystectomy. Many of these trials had inadequate power or methodologic flaws that limit interpretation. In general, there is likely a small (5% to 10%) reduction in the risk of recurrence for perioperative chemotherapy given to high-risk (T3 and/or N+) patients, with an uncertain effect on overall survival.

CHEMOTHERAPY FOR ADVANCED DISEASE

Treatment of advanced metastatic urothelial cancer is generally considered palliative. Response rates are high with cisplatin-containing regimens (50% to 60%), but the duration of response is short, and median survival is 12 to 14 months. A small subset of patients (5% to 10%; usually with only lymph node metastases) can have a complete response to chemotherapy. A randomized trial showed an advantage for a regimen of M-VAC (methotrexate, vinblastine, Adriamycin [doxorubicin], and cisplatin) over cisplatin alone with regard to disease progression-free and overall survival. In another randomized trial, the combination of gemcitabine (Gemzar) and cisplatin exhibited equivalent survival to M-VAC in metastatic bladder cancer but was clinically better tolerated. Thus, cisplatin plus gemcitabine is the standard of care. Carboplatin can be substituted if a contraindication to cisplatin exists (eg, neuropathy, poor renal function). The role of combination chemotherapy in the adjuvant treatment of resected urothelial cancer remains undetermined and an area of clinical research. A randomized trial of neoadjuvant M-VAC in locally advanced resectable bladder cancer showed a trend in survival favoring M-VAC over surgery alone, but it was not statistically significant.

KIDNEY CANCER

Approximately 54,390 new cases of renal cell carcinoma will be diagnosed in the year 2008 in the United States, with an associated 13,010 deaths. There has been a steady increase in the incidence of renal cell carcinoma that is not explained by the increased use of diagnostic imaging procedures. Mortality rates have also shown a steady increase over the past 2 decades.

Epidemiology

Gender and age This malignancy is twice as common in men as in women. Most cases of renal cell carcinoma are diagnosed in the fourth to sixth decades of life, but the disease has been reported in all age groups.

Ethnicity Renal cell carcinoma is more common in persons of northern European ancestry than in those of African or Asian descent.

Etiology and risk factors

Renal cell carcinoma occurs most commonly as a sporadic form and rarely as a familial form. The exact etiology of sporadic renal cell carcinoma has not been determined. However, smoking, obesity, and renal dialysis have been associated with an increased incidence of the disease.

Genetic factors More recently, a genetic basis has been sought for this disease.

von Hippel-Lindau disease (VHL), an autosomal-dominant disease, is associated with retinal angiomas, CNS hemangioblastomas, and renal cell carcinoma.

Chromosomal abnormalities Deletions of the short arm of chromosome 3 (3p) occur commonly in renal cell carcinoma associated with VHL disease. In the rare familial forms of renal cell carcinoma, translocations affecting chromosome 3p can be present. Sporadic renal cell carcinoma of the nonpapillary type is also associated with VHL-gene silencing.

Associated malignancy Two studies from large patient databases have reported a higher-than-expected incidence of both renal cell cancer and lymphoma. No explanation for this association has been found.

Signs and symptoms

Renal cell carcinoma has been associated with a wide array of signs and symptoms. The classic triad of hematuria, flank mass, and flank pain occurs in only 10% of patients and is usually associated with a poor prognosis. With the routine use of CT scanning for various diagnostic reasons, renal cell carcinoma is being diagnosed more frequently as an incidental finding.

Hematuria More than half of patients with renal cell carcinoma present with hematuria, either gross or microscopic.

Other common signs/symptoms Other commonly associated signs and symptoms of renal cell carcinoma include normocytic/normochromic anemia, fever, and weight loss.

Less common signs/symptoms Less frequently occurring, but often described, signs and symptoms include polycythemia, hepatic dysfunction not associated with hepatic metastasis, and hypercalcemia. Although not a common finding at the time of diagnosis of renal cell carcinoma, hypercalcemia ultimately occurs in up to 25% of patients with metastatic disease.

Diagnosis

Contrast-enhanced CT scanning has virtually replaced excretory urography and renal ultrasonography in the evaluation of suspected renal cell carcinoma. In most cases, CT imaging can differentiate cystic from solid masses and also supplies information about lymph nodes and renal vein/inferior vena cava (IVC) involvement.

Ultrasonography is useful in evaluating questionable cystic renal lesions if CT imaging is inconclusive.

Venography and MRI When IVC involvement by tumor is suspected, either IVC venography or MRI is needed to evaluate its extent. MRI is currently the preferred imaging technique for assessing IVC involvement at most centers.

Renal arteriography is not used as frequently now as it was in the past in the evaluation of suspected renal cell carcinoma. In patients with small, indeterminate lesions, arteriography may be helpful. It is also used by the surgeon as part of the preoperative evaluation of a large renal neoplasm.

Percutaneous cyst puncture is used in the evaluation of cystic renal lesions that are thought to be potentially malignant on the basis of ultrasonography or CT imaging. Percutaneous cyst puncture permits the collection of cyst fluid for analysis, as well as the evaluation of cyst structure via instillation of contrast medium after fluid removal. Benign cyst fluid is usually clear to straw-colored and low in protein, fat, and lactic dehydrogenase (LDH) content, whereas malignant fluid is usually bloody with high protein, fat, and LDH content.

Evaluation of extra-abdominal disease sites includes a chest x-ray or CT imaging of the chest. A bone scan is required if a patient has symptoms suggestive of bone metastasis and/or an elevated alkaline phosphatase level.

TABLE 3: TNM staging of renal cell carcinoma

Primary tumor (T)

Tx		Primary tumor cannot be assessed
T0		No evidence of primary tumor
T1		Tumor ≤ 7 cm in greatest dimension, limited to the kidneys
	T1a	Tumor ≤ 4 cm in greatest dimension, limited to the kidneys
	T1b	Tumor > 4 cm but not > 7 cm in greatest dimension, limited to the kidneys
T2		Tumor > 7 cm in greatest dimension, limited to the kidneys
T3		Tumor extends into major veins or invades adrenal gland or perinephric tissues but not beyond Gerota's fascia
	T3a	Tumor directly invades adrenal gland or perirenal and/or renal sinus fat but not beyond Gerota's fascia
	T3b	Tumor grossly extends into renal vein or its segmental (muscle-containing) branches or vena cava below the diaphragm
	T3c	Tumor grossly extends into the vena cava above the diaphragm or invades the wall of the vena cava
T4		Tumor invades beyond Gerota's fascia

Regional lymph nodes (N)

Nx	Regional lymph nodes cannot be assessed
N0	No regional lymph node metastasis
N1	Metastasis in a single regional lymph node
N2	Metastasis in more than one regional lymph node

Distant metastasis (M)

Mx	Distant metastasis cannot be assessed
M0	No distant metastasis
M1	Distant metastasis

Stage grouping

Stage I	T1	N0	M0
Stage II	T2	N0	M0
Stage III	T1	N1	M0
	T2	N1	M0
	T3a	N0-N1	M0
	T3b	N0-N1	M0
	T3c	N0-N1	M0
Stage IV	T4	N0-N1	M0
	Any T	N2	M0
	Any T	Any N	M1

From Greene FL, Page DL, Fleming ID, et al (eds): AJCC Cancer Staging Manual, 6th ed. New York, Springer-Verlag, 2002.

TABLE 4: Therapeutic regimens for renal cell carcinoma

Dose and schedule

High-dose IL-2

IL-2: 600,000 or 720,000 IU/kg IV infused over 15 minutes every 8 hours until toxicity develops; or 14 consecutive doses for 5 days

After a 5- to 9-day rest period, an additional 14 doses of IL-2 are administered over a 5-day period. If patients show evidence of tumor regression or stable disease, 1-2 more courses of treatment may be given.

Fyfe G, Fisher RI, Rosenberg SA, et al: J Clin Oncol 13:688–696, 1995.

Low-dose IL-2

IL-2: 72,000 IU/kg by IV bolus every 8 hours to a maximum of 15 doses every 7-10 days for 2 cycles

NOTE: The cycles represent one course of therapy. Patients who are stable or responding after one course of therapy receive a second course. Third and fourth courses are given only if patients demonstrate further tumor regression.

Yang JC, Topalian SL, Parkinson D, et al: J Clin Oncol 12:1572–1576, 1998.

Sunitinib

50 mg PO daily for 4 weeks. Repeat every 6 weeks (4 weeks on, 2 weeks off)

Motzer RJ, Hutson TE, Tomczak P, et al: N Engl J Med 356:115–124, 2007.

Sorafenib

400 mg PO bid daily continuously until disease progression

Escudier B, Eisen T, Stadler WM, et al: N Engl J Med 356:125–134, 2007.

Temsirolimus

25 mg IVPB every week

Hudes G, Carducci M, Tomczak P, et al: N Engl J Med 356:2271–2281, 2007.

IVPB = intravenous piggy back
Table prepared by Ishmael Jaiyesimi, DO

Pathology

Renal cell carcinoma arises from the proximal renal tubular epithelium. Histologically, renal cell carcinoma can be of various cellular types: clear cell (70% to 80%), papillary (10% to 15%), and chromophobe (5%). Oncocytoma is a benign renal tumor. Approximately 10% to 20% of renal cell carcinomas have sarcomatoid features (spindled cells that can occur in any subtype), which is a more aggressive malignancy with a worse prognosis.

Staging and prognosis

Staging system The preferred staging system for renal cell carcinoma is the TNM classification (Table 3).

Prognostic factors The natural history of renal cell carcinoma is highly variable. However, approximately 30% of patients present with metastatic disease at diagnosis, and one-third of the remainder will develop metastasis during follow-up.

Five-year survival rates after nephrectomy for tumors confined to the renal parenchyma (T1/2) are > 80%. Renal vein involvement without nodal involvement does not affect survival. Lymph node involvement and/or extracapsular spread is associated with a 5-year survival of 10% to 25%. Patients with metastatic disease have a median survival of 1 year and a 5-year survival of 0% to 20%.

Several prognostic schemes have been developed for both localized and metastatic renal cell carcinomas. In general, factors such as tumor stage and grade, performance status, hemoglobin value, calcium, LDH level, and time interval to development of metastatic disease are important.

Treatment

Surgery

Radical nephrectomy is the established therapy for localized renal cell carcinoma. At surgery, the kidneys, adrenal gland, and perirenal fat (structures bound by Gerota's fascia) are removed. Also, limited regional lymph node dissection is often performed for staging purposes. Partial nephrectomy is standard in patients with smaller tumors (eg, < 4 cm) or in whom radical nephrectomy would unacceptably compromise overall renal function.

Because complete resection is the only known cure for renal cell carcinoma, even in locally advanced disease, surgery is considered if the involved structures can be safely removed. In patients with metastatic renal cell carcinoma, two randomized, controlled trials have shown a survival benefit of 6 months (combined analysis) with a debulking nephrectomy prior to interferon-alpha immunotherapy, as compared with immunotherapy alone. However, patients must be carefully selected prior to the nephrectomy and should have a performance status of 0 to 1 according to the World Health Organization criteria. The performance status of a patient prior to treatment is an important determinant of disease-related outcome and should be considered in making treatment decisions.

Radiation therapy for renal cell carcinoma

Primary radiation therapy Radiation therapy may be considered for palliation as the primary therapy for renal cell carcinoma in patients whose clinical condition precludes surgery, either because of extensive disease or poor overall condition. A dose of 4,500 cGy is delivered, with consideration of a boost up to 5,500 cGy.

Postoperative radiation therapy has not been shown to prevent recurrence.

Palliation Radiation therapy is commonly used for palliation for metastatic and local disease.

Systemic therapy for advanced disease

Metastatic renal cell carcinoma is resistant to chemotherapeutic agents. An extensive review of currently available agents concluded that the overall response rate to chemotherapy is 6%.

Interleukin-2 The first US Food and Drug Administration (FDA)-approved treatment for metastatic renal cell carcinoma was high-dose interleukin-2 (IL-2, aldesleukin [Proleukin]; Table 4).

High-dose regimen High-dose IL-2 (720,000 IU/kg IV piggy back every 8 hours for 14 doses, repeated once after a 9-day rest) results in a 15% remission rate (7% complete responses, 8% partial responses). The majority of responses to IL-2 are durable, with a median response duration of 54 months.

The major toxicity of high-dose IL-2 is a sepsis-like syndrome, which includes a progressive decrease in systemic vascular resistance and an associated decrease in intravascular volume due to a "capillary leak." Management includes judicious use of fluids and vasopressor support to maintain blood pressure and intravascular volume and at the same time to avoid pulmonary toxicity due to noncardiogenic pulmonary edema from the capillary leak. This syndrome is totally reversible.

Other doses and schedules Because of the toxicity of high-dose IL-2, other doses and schedules have been and are being evaluated. Several trials of low-dose IL-2 (3–18 × 10^6 IU/d), either alone or combined with interferon-alpha, have reported outcomes similar to those achieved with high-dose IL-2.

Multikinase inhibitors Three oral multikinase inhibitors have been approved by the FDA for the treatment of advanced kidney cancer.

Sorafenib (Nexavar) targets several serine/threonine and receptor tyrosine kinases thought to be integral to the biology of renal cell carcinoma, especially vascular endothelial growth factor (VEGF). A phase III placebo-controlled trial was conducted in 769 patients with advanced renal cell carcinoma who had received prior systemic treatment. The recommended oral dose of sorafenib (400 mg twice daily) was used. The median progression-free survival was 5.5 months in the sorafenib group versus 2.8 months in the placebo group. Toxic effects associated with sorafenib included reversible skin rashes in 40% and hand-foot skin reactions in 30% of patients. Notably, the incidence of treatment-emergent cardiac ischemia/infarction events was higher with sorafenib (2.9% vs 0.4%).

Sunitinib (Sutent) targets several receptor tyrosine kinases. In a single-arm, multicenter phase II trial of patients with metastatic renal cell disease, the overall response rate with sunitinib was nearly 40% (all partial responses), with a median time to disease progression of 8.7 months. Diarrhea, skin dis-

> Preliminary results using axitinib (AG-013736), a potent inhibitor of several VEGF receptors (1, 2, and 3) have shown substantial antitumor activity (partial response, 14%; stable disease, 36%) in patients with sorafenib (Nexavar) refractory metastatic renal cell carcinoma. The toxicity profile of this agent is typical of tyrosine kinase inhibitors, which are generally manageable (Rini BI, Wilding GT, Hudes G, et al: J Clin Oncol 25:[18S]:5032, 2007).

coloration, and mucositis/stomatitis were the most common adverse events occurring more frequently with sunitinib. Decreases in left ventricular ejection fraction were noted with sunitinib, and dose reductions and/or antihypertensive or diuretic medications may be required.

Temsirolimus (Torisel) and bevacizumab (Avastin) were added to the NCCN Kidney Cancer Guidelines as options for first-line treatment of relapsed or medically unresectable stage IV renal cancer (RCC) with predominant clear cell histology and in the case of temsirolimus, non-clear cell histology. The recommendations were based on the results of large randomized trials. Temsirolimus significantly prolonged median overall survival in a phase III trial in 626 patients ($P = .0078$) and received FDA approval for first-line as well subsequent treatment (clear cell histology only) of advanced RCC. In the AVOREN trial, bevacizumab significantly increased progression-free survival (10.2 months vs 5.4 months; $P = .0001$) of patients with metastatic RCC when administered in combination with interferon-a2a.

RAD001 (everolimus) is an oral inhibitor of mTOR kinase that has shown activity in metastatic RCC in phase II studies. Motzer and colleagues recently presented results of a planned interim analysis of a phase III study assessing the clinical benefit of RAD001 in patients who had progressive metastatic RCC after receiving sunitinib, sorafenib, or both. The primary endpoint was progression-free survival. A total of 410 patients were randomized to receive RAD001, 10 mg, or placebo in a 2:1 ratio. Prior bevacizumab and/or cytokine treatment was allowed. The results showed a significant improvement in progression-free survival for RAD001 vs placebo (PFS = 4.0 months for RAD001 vs 1.9 months for placebo, $P < .001$). *(Motzer RJ, Escudier B, Oudard S, et al: J Clin Oncol 26:[abstract LBA5026], 2008).*

As always, patients should be encouraged to participate in ongoing clinical trials of metastatic renal cell cancer.

SUGGESTED READING

ON UROTHELIAL CANCER

Barton Grossman H, Natale RB, Tangen CM, et al: Neoadjuvant chemotherapy plus cystectomy compared with cystectomy alone for locally advanced bladder cancer. N Engl J Med 349:859–866, 2003.

Duchesne GM, Bolger JJ, Griffiths GD, et al: A randomized trial of hypofractionated schedules of palliative radiotherapy in the management of bladder carcinoma: Results of Medical Research Council Trial BA09. Int J Radiat Oncol Biol Phys 47:379–388, 2000.

Hudson MA, Herr HW: Carcinoma in situ of the bladder. J Urol 153:564–572, 1995.

Hussain MH, Glass TR, Forman J, et al: Combination cisplatin, 5-fluorouracil, and radiation therapy for locally advanced unresectable or medically unfit bladder cancer cases: A Southwest Oncology Group study. J Urol 165:56–60, 2001.

Lotan Y, Gupta A, Shariat SF, et al: Lymphovascular invasion is independently associated with overall survival, cause-specific survival, and local and distant recurrence in patients with negative lymph nodes at radical cystectomy. J Clin Oncol 23:6533–6539, 2005.

Milosevic M, Gospodarowicz M, Zietman A, et al: Radiotherapy for bladder cancer. Urology 69:80–92, 2007.

Sylvester RJ, van der Meijden AP, Witjes JA, et al: Bacillus calmette-guerin versus chemotherapy for the intravesical treatment of patients with carcinoma in situ of the bladder: A meta-analysis of the published results of randomized clinical trials. J Urol 174:86–92, 2005.

Von der Maase H, Hansen SW, Roberts JT, et al: Gemcitabine and cisplatin versus methotrexate, vinblastine, doxorubicin, and cisplatin in advanced or metastatic bladder cancer: Results of a large, randomized, multinational, multicenter, phase III study. J Clin Oncol 17:3068–3077, 2000.

ON KIDNEY CANCER

Dutcher JP, Szczylik C, Tannir N, et al: Correlation of survival with tumor histology, age, and prognostic risk group for previously untreated patients with advanced renal cell carcinoma (adv RCC) receiving temsirolimus (TEMSR) or interferon-alpha (IFN). J Clin Oncol 25:5033, 2007.

Escudier B, Eisen T, Stadler WM, et al: Sorafenib in advanced clear-cell renal-cell carcinoma. N Engl J Med 356:125–134, 2007.

Escudier B, Koralewski P, Pluzanska A, et al: A randomized, controlled, double-blind phase III study (AVOREN) of bevacizumab/interferon-α2a vs placebo/interferon-α2a as first-line therapy in metastatic renal cell carcinoma. J Clin Oncol 25:3, 2007.

Flanigan RC, Salmon SE, Blumenstein BA, et al: Nephrectomy followed by interferon alfa-2b compared with interferon alfa-2b alone for metastatic renal cell cancer. N Engl J Med 345:1655–1659, 2001.

Hudes G, Carducci M, Tomczak P, et al: Temsirolimus, interferon alfa, or both for advanced renal-cell carcinoma. N Engl J Med 356:2271–2281, 2007.

Mickisch GH, Garin A, van Poppel H, et al: Radical nephrectomy plus interferon-alfa-based immunotherapy compared with interferon alone in metastatic renal-cell carcinoma: A randomized trial. Lancet 358:966–970, 2001.

Motzer RJ, Hutson TE, Tomczak P, et al: Sunitinib versus interferon alfa in metastatic renal-cell carcinoma. N Engl J Med 356:115–124, 2007.

Parkinson DR, Sznol M: High-dose interleukin-2 in the therapy of metastatic renal cell carcinoma. Semin Oncol 22:61–66, 1995.

Rabinovitch RA, Zelefsky MJ, Gaynor JJ, et al: Patterns of failure following surgical resection of renal cell carcinoma: Implications for adjuvant local and systemic therapy. J Clin Oncol 12:206–212, 1994.

Stodlen WM, Vogelzang NJ: Low-dose interleukin-2 in the treatment of metastatic renal cell carcinoma. Semin Oncol 22:67–73, 1995.

Zisman A, Pantuck AJ, Dorey F, et al: Improved prognostication of renal cell carcinoma using an integrated staging system. J Clin Oncol 19:1649–1657, 2001.

In the **adjuvant** treatment of HER2+ breast cancer

With Herceptin, proven results are within her reach

NOW APPROVED (the first non-AC Herceptin regimen) TCH and AC-TH[§]

- Herceptin, in combination with paclitaxel following AC* therapy, reduced the risk of recurrence by **52%** vs chemotherapy alone (HR=0.48, CI: 0.39-0.59; P<0.0001)[†]
  - Benefit was similar regardless of age, hormone-receptor status, or tumor size[1]
- Herceptin, as a single agent following completion of surgery and chemotherapy with or without radiotherapy, reduced the risk of recurrence by **46%** (HR=0.54, CI: 0.44-0.67; P<0.0001).[†] The benefit was seen:
  - Regardless of nodal involvement[1]
  - Using a q3w dosing schedule
  - With a variety of anthracycline-based chemotherapy regimens used prior to Herceptin[1]

Adjuvant indications

Herceptin is indicated for adjuvant treatment of HER2-overexpressing node-positive or node-negative (ER/PR-negative or with one high-risk feature)[‡] breast cancer:

- As part of a treatment regimen containing doxorubicin, cyclophosphamide, and either paclitaxel or docetaxel
- With docetaxel and carboplatin
- As a single agent following multi-modality anthracycline-based therapy

52 weeks of Herceptin significantly **reduced**

the risk of breast cancer recurrence

*AC=anthracycline-based.
[†]HR=hazard ratio; CI=95% confidence interval.
[‡]High-risk features for patients with ER/PR+ breast cancer include: tumor size >2 cm, age <35 years, and histologic and/or nuclear grade 2/3.
[§]AC-TH is now approved with docetaxel, and for q3w dosing of Herceptin.

Boxed WARNINGS and Additional Important Safety Information

Herceptin administration can result in sub-clinical and clinical cardiac failure manifesting as congestive heart failure (CHF) and decreased left ventricular ejection fraction (LVEF). The incidence and severity of left ventricular cardiac dysfunction was highest in patients who received Herceptin concurrently with anthracycline-containing chemotherapy regimens. Discontinue Herceptin treatment in patients receiving adjuvant therapy and strongly consider discontinuation of Herceptin in patients with metastatic breast cancer who develop a clinically significant decrease in left ventricular function.

Patients should undergo monitoring for decreased left ventricular function before Herceptin treatment, and frequently during and after Herceptin treatment. More frequent monitoring should be employed if Herceptin is withheld in patients who develop significant left ventricular cardiac dysfunction. In one adjuvant clinical trial, cardiac ischemia or infarction occurred in the Herceptin-containing regimens.

Serious infusion reactions and pulmonary toxicity have occurred; fatal infusion reactions have been reported. In most cases, symptoms occurred during or within 24 hours of administration of Herceptin. Herceptin infusion should be interrupted for patients experiencing dyspnea or clinically significant hypotension. Patients should be monitored until signs and symptoms completely resolve. Discontinue Herceptin for infusion reactions manifesting as anaphylaxis, angioedema, interstitial pneumonitis, or acute respiratory distress syndrome.

Exacerbation of chemotherapy-induced neutropenia has also occurred.

Herceptin can cause oligohydramnios and fetal harm when administered to a pregnant woman.

The most common adverse reactions associated with Herceptin use were fever, nausea, vomiting, infusion reactions, diarrhea, infections, increased cough, headache, fatigue, dyspnea, rash, neutropenia, anemia, and myalgia.

Please see brief summary of full Prescribing Information, including **Boxed WARNINGS** and additional important safety information, on the following pages.

Reference: 1. Data on file. Genentech, Inc.

www.herceptin.com

Herceptin®
t r a s t u z u m a b
Targeted on HER2, Focused on Living

HERCEPTIN® (trastuzumab)

Brief Summary For full Prescribing Information, see package insert.

WARNING: CARDIOMYOPATHY, INFUSION REACTIONS, and PULMONARY TOXICITY

Cardiomyopathy

Herceptin can result in sub-clinical and clinical cardiac failure manifesting as CHF and decreased LVEF. The incidence and severity of left ventricular cardiac dysfunction was highest in patients who received Herceptin concurrently with anthracycline-containing chemotherapy regimens.

Evaluate left ventricular function in all patients prior to and during treatment with Herceptin. Discontinue Herceptin treatment in patients receiving adjuvant therapy and strongly consider discontinuation of Herceptin treatment in patients with metastatic breast cancer for clinically significant decrease in left ventricular function. [*see Warnings and Precautions and Dosage and Administration*]

Infusion Reactions; Pulmonary Toxicity

Herceptin administration can result in serious infusion reactions and pulmonary toxicity. Fatal infusion reactions have been reported. In most cases, symptoms occurred during or within 24 hours of administration of Herceptin. Herceptin infusion should be interrupted for patients experiencing dyspnea or clinically significant hypotension. Patients should be monitored until signs and symptoms completely resolve. Discontinue Herceptin for infusion reactions manifesting as anaphylaxis, angioedema, interstitial pneumonitis, or acute respiratory distress syndrome. [*see Warnings and Precautions*]

INDICATIONS AND USAGE **Adjuvant Breast Cancer** Herceptin is indicated for adjuvant treatment of HER2 overexpressing node positive or node negative (ER/PR negative or with one high risk feature [*see Clinical Studies*]) breast cancer • As part of a treatment regimen consisting of doxorubicin, Cyclophosphamide, and either paclitaxel or docetaxel • With docetaxel and carboplatin • As a single agent following multi-modality anthracycline based therapy. **Metastatic Breast Cancer** Herceptin is indicated: • In combination with paclitaxel for first-line treatment of HER2-overexpressing metastatic breast cancer • As a single agent for treatment of HER2-overexpressing breast cancer in patients who have received one or more chemotherapy regimens for metastatic disease. **CONTRAINDICATIONS** None. **WARNINGS AND PRECAUTIONS Cardiomyopathy** Herceptin can cause left ventricular cardiac dysfunction, arrhythmias, hypertension, disabling cardiac failure, cardiomyopathy, and cardiac death [*see Boxed Warning: Cardiomyopathy*]. Herceptin can also cause asymptomatic decline in left ventricular ejection fraction (LVEF). There is a 4–6 fold increase in the incidence of symptomatic myocardial dysfunction among patients receiving Herceptin as a single agent or in combination therapy compared with those not receiving Herceptin. The highest absolute incidence occurs when Herceptin is administered with an anthracycline. Withhold Herceptin for ≥16% absolute decrease in LVEF from pre-treatment values or an LVEF value below institutional limits of normal and ≥10% absolute decrease in LVEF from pre-treatment values. [*see Dosage and Administration*] The safety of continuation or resumption of Herceptin in patients with Herceptin-induced left ventricular cardiac dysfunction has not been studied. *Cardiac Monitoring* Conduct thorough cardiac assessment, including history, physical examination, and determination of LVEF by echocardiogram or MUGA scan. The following schedule is recommended: • Baseline LVEF measurement immediately prior to initiation of Herceptin • LVEF measurements every 3 months during and upon completion of Herceptin • Repeat LVEF measurement at 4 week intervals if Herceptin is withheld for significant left ventricular cardiac dysfunction [*see Dosage and Administration*] • LVEF measurements every 6 months for at least 2 years following completion of Herceptin as a component of adjuvant therapy. In Study 1, 16% (136/844) of patients discontinued Herceptin due to clinical evidence of myocardial dysfunction or significant decline in LVEF. In Study 3, the number of patients who discontinued Herceptin due to cardiac toxicity was 2.6% (44/1678). In Study 4, a total of 2.9% (31/1056) patients in the TCH arm (1.5% during the chemotherapy phase and 1.4% during the monotherapy phase) and 5.7% (61/1068) patients in the AC-TH arm (1.5% during the chemotherapy phase and 4.2% during the monotherapy phase) discontinued Herceptin due to cardiac toxicity. Among 32 patients receiving adjuvant chemotherapy (Studies 1 and 2) who developed congestive heart failure, one patient died of cardiomyopathy and all other patients were receiving cardiac medication at last follow-up. Approximately half of the surviving patients had recovery to a normal LVEF (defined as ≥50%) on continuing medical management at the time of last follow-up. Incidence of congestive heart failure is presented in Table 1. The safety of continuation or resumption of Herceptin in patients with Herceptin-induced left ventricular cardiac dysfunction has not been studied.

Table 1 Incidence of Congestive Heart Failure in Adjuvant Breast Cancer Studies

Study	Regimen	Incidence of CHF	
		Herceptin	Control
1 & 2[a]	AC[b]→Paclitaxel+Herceptin	2% (32/1677)	0.4% (7/1600)
3	Chemo→Herceptin monotherapy	2% (30/1678)	0.3% (5/1708)
4	AC[b]→Docetaxel+Herceptin	2% (20/1068)	0.3% (3/1050)
4	Docetaxel+Carbo+Herceptin	0.4% (4/1056)	0.3% (3/1050))

[a] Includes 1 patient with fatal cardiomyopathy.
[b] Anthracycline (doxorubicin) and cyclophosphamide.

Table 2 Incidence of Cardiac Dysfunction[a] in Metastatic Breast Cancer Studies

Study	Event	Incidence			
		NYHA I-IV		NYHA III-IV	
		Herceptin	Control	Herceptin	Control
5 (AC)[b]	Cardiac Dysfunction	28%	7%	19%	3%
5 (paclitaxel)	Cardiac Dysfunction	11%	1%	4%	1%
6	Cardiac Dysfunction[c]	7%	N/A	5%	N/A

[a]Congestive heart failure or significant asymptomatic decrease in LVEF. [b]Anthracycline (doxorubicin or epirubicin) and cyclophosphamide. [c]Includes 1 patient with fatal cardiomyopathy.

Infusion Reactions Infusion reactions consist of a symptom complex characterized by fever and chills, and on occasion included nausea, vomiting, pain (in some cases at tumor sites), headache, dizziness, dyspnea, hypotension, rash, and asthenia. [see Adverse Reactions]. In postmarketing reports, serious and fatal infusion reactions have been reported. Severe reactions which include bronchospasm, anaphylaxis, angioedema, hypoxia, and severe hypotension, were usually reported during or immediately following the initial infusion. However, the onset and clinical course were variable including progressive worsening, initial improvement followed by clinical deterioration, or delayed post-infusion events with rapid clinical deterioration. For fatal events, death occurred within hours to days following a serious infusion reaction. Interrupt Herceptin infusion in all patients experiencing dyspnea, clinically significant hypotension, and intervention of medical therapy administered, which may include: epinephrine, corticosteroids, diphenhydramine, bronchodilators, and oxygen. Patients should be evaluated and carefully monitored until complete resolution of signs and symptoms. Permanent discontinuation should be strongly considered in all patients with severe infusion reactions. There are no data regarding the most appropriate method of identification of patients who may safely be retreated with Herceptin after experiencing a severe infusion reaction. Prior to resumption of Herceptin infusion, the majority of patients who experienced a severe infusion reaction were pre-medicated with antihistamines and/or corticosteroids. While some patients tolerated Herceptin infusions, others had recurrent severe infusion reactions despite pre-medications. **Exacerbation of Chemotherapy-Induced Neutropenia** In randomized, controlled clinical trials in women with metastatic breast cancer, the per-patient incidences of NCI CTC Grade 3-4 neutropenia and of febrile neutropenia were higher in patients receiving Herceptin in combination with myelosuppressive chemotherapy as compared to those who received chemotherapy alone. The incidence of septic death was not significantly increased. [see Adverse Reactions]. **Pulmonary Toxicity** Herceptin use can result in serious and fatal pulmonary toxicity. Pulmonary toxicity includes dyspnea, interstitial pneumonitis, pulmonary infiltrates, pleural effusions, non-cardiogenic pulmonary edema, pulmonary insufficiency and hypoxia, acute respiratory distress syndrome, and pulmonary fibrosis. Such events can occur as sequelae of infusion reactions [see Warnings and Precautions]. Patients with symptomatic intrinsic lung disease or with extensive tumor involvement of the lungs, resulting in dyspnea at rest, appear to have more severe toxicity. **HER2 Testing** Detection of HER2 protein overexpression is necessary for selection of patients appropriate for Herceptin therapy because these are the only patients studied and for whom benefit has been shown. Assessment for HER2 overexpression and of HER2 gene amplification should be performed by laboratories with demonstrated proficiency in the specific technology being utilized. Improper assay performance, including use of suboptimally fixed tissue, failure to utilize specified reagents, deviation from specific assay instructions, and failure to include appropriate controls for assay validation, can lead to unreliable results. Several FDA-approved commercial assays are available to aid in the selection of patients for Herceptin therapy. These include HercepTest™ and Pathway® HER-2/neu (IHC assays) and PathVysion® and HER2 FISH pharmDx™ (FISH assays). Users should refer to the package inserts of specific assay kits for information on the validation and performance of each assay. Limitations in assay precision (particularly for the IHC method) and in the direct linkage between assay result and overexpression of the Herceptin target (for the FISH method) make it inadvisable to rely on a single method to rule out potential Herceptin benefit. A negative FISH result does not rule out HER2 overexpression and potential benefit from Herceptin. Treatment outcomes for metastatic breast cancer (Study 5) as a function of IHC and FISH testing are provided in Table 9. Treatment outcomes for adjuvant breast cancer (Studies 2 and 3) as a function of IHC and FISH testing are provided in Table 7. *HER2 Protein Overexpression Detection Methods* HER2 protein overexpression can be established by measuring HER2 protein using an IHC method. HercepTest®, one test approved for this use, was assessed for concordance with the Clinical Trial Assay (CTA), using tumor specimens collected and stored independently from those obtained in Herceptin clinical studies in women with metastatic breast cancer. Data are provided in the package insert for HercepTest®. *HER2 Gene Amplification Detection Method* The presence of HER2 protein overexpression and gene amplification are highly correlated, therefore the use of FISH to detect gene amplification may be employed for selection of patients appropriate for Herceptin therapy. PathVysion®, one test approved for this use, was evaluated in an exploratory, retrospective assessment of available CTA 2+ or 3+ tumor specimens collected as part of patient screening for clinical studies in metastatic breast cancer (Studies 5 and 6). Data are provided in the package insert for PathVysion®. **Embryo-Fetal Toxicity (Pregnancy Category D)** Herceptin can cause fetal harm when administered to a pregnant woman. Post-marketing case reports suggest that Herceptin use during pregnancy increases the risk of oligohydramnios during the second and third trimesters. If Herceptin is used during pregnancy or if a woman becomes pregnant while taking Herceptin, she should be apprised of the potential hazard to a fetus. [see Use in Specific Populations]. **ADVERSE REACTIONS** The following adverse reactions are discussed in greater detail in other sections of the label: • Cardiomyopathy [see Warnings and Precautions] • Infusion reactions [see Warnings and Precautions] • Exacerbation of chemotherapy-induced neutropenia [see Warnings and Precautions] • Pulmonary toxicity [see Warnings and Precautions] The most common adverse reactions in patients receiving Herceptin are fever, nausea, vomiting, infusion reactions, diarrhea, infections, increased cough, headache, fatigue, dyspnea, rash, neutropenia, anemia, and myalgia. Adverse reactions requiring interruption or discontinuation of Herceptin treatment include CHF, significant decline in left ventricular cardiac function, severe infusion reactions, and pulmonary toxicity [see Dosage and Administration]. **Clinical Trials Experience** Because clinical trials are conducted under widely varying conditions, adverse reaction rates observed in the clinical trials of a drug cannot be directly compared to rates in the clinical trials of another drug and may not reflect the rates observed in practice. *Adjuvant Breast Cancer Studies* The data below reflect exposure to Herceptin across three randomized, open-label studies, Studies 1, 2, and 3, with (n= 3355) or without (n= 3308) trastuzumab in the adjuvant treatment of breast cancer. The data summarized in Table 3 below, from Study 3, reflect exposure to Herceptin in 1678 patients; the median treatment duration was 51 weeks and median number of infusions was 18. Among the 3386 patients enrolled in Study 3, the median age was 49 years (range: 21 to 80 years), 83% of patients were Caucasian, and 13% were Asian.

Table 3 Adverse Reactions for Study 3, All Grades[a]:

MedDRA (v. 7.1) Adverse Event Preferred Term	1 Year Herceptin (n= 1678)	Observation (n= 1708)
Cardiac		
Hypertension	64 (4%)	35 (2%)
Dizziness	60 (4%)	29 (2%)
Ejection Fraction Decreased	58 (3.5%)	11 (0.6%)
Palpitations	48 (3%)	12 (0.7%)
Cardiac Arrhythmias[b]	40 (3%)	17 (1%)
Cardiac Failure Congestive	30 (2%)	5 (0.3%)
Cardiac Failure	9 (0.5%)	4 (0.2%)
Cardiac Disorder	5 (0.3%)	0 (0%)
Ventricular Dysfunction	4 (0.2%)	0 (0%)
Respiratory Thoracic Mediastinal Disorders		
Nasopharyngitis	135 (8%)	43 (3%)
Cough	81 (5%)	34 (2%)
Influenza	70 (4%)	9 (0.5%)
Dyspnea	57 (3%)	26 (2%)
URI	46 (3%)	20 (1%)
Rhinitis	36 (2%)	6 (0.4%)
Pharyngolaryngeal Pain	32 (2%)	8 (0.5%)
Sinusitis	26 (2%)	5 (0.3%)
Epistaxis	25 (2%)	1 (0.06%)
Pulmonary Hypertension	4 (0.2%)	0 (0%)
Interstitial Pneumonitis	4 (0.2%)	0 (0%)
Gastrointestinal Disorders		
Diarrhea	123 (7%)	16 (1%)
Nausea	108 (6%)	19 (1%)
Vomiting	58 (3.5%)	10 (0.6%)
Constipation	33 (2%)	17 (1%)
Dyspepsia	30 (2%)	9 (0.5%)
Upper Abdominal Pain	29 (2%)	15 (1%)
Musculoskeletal & Connective Tissue Disorders		
Arthralgia	137 (8%)	98 (6%)
Back Pain	91 (5%)	58 (3%)
Myalgia	63 (4%)	17 (1%)
Bone Pain	49 (3%)	26 (2%)
Muscle Spasm	46 (3%)	3 (0.2%)
Nervous System Disorders		
Headache	162 (10%)	49 (3%)
Paraesthesia	29 (2%)	11 (0.6%)
Skin & Subcutaneous Tissue Disorders		
Rash	70 (4%)	10 (0.6%)
Nail Disorders	43 (2%)	0 (0%)
Pruritus	40 (2%)	10 (0.6%)
General Disorders		
Pyrexia	100 (6%)	6 (0.4%)
Edema Peripheral	79 (5%)	37 (2%)
Chills	85 (5%)	0 (0%)
Asthenia	75 (4.5%)	30 (2%)
Influenza-like Illness	40 (2%)	3 (0.2%)
Sudden Death	1 (0.06%)	0 (0%)
Infections		
Nasopharyngitis	135 (8%)	43 (3%)
UTI	39 (3%)	13 (0.8%)
Immune System Disorders		
Hypersensitivity	10 (0.6%)	1 (0.06%)
Autoimmune Thyroiditis	4 (0.3%)	0 (0%)

[a]The incidence of Grade 3/4 adverse reactions was <1% in both arms for each listed term. [b]Higher level grouping term.

The data from Studies 1 and 2 were obtained from 3206 patients enrolled, of which 1635 patients received Herceptin; the median treatment duration was 50 weeks. The median age was 49.0 years (range: 24-80); 84% of patients were White, and 7% were Black, 4% were Hispanic, and 4% were Asian. In Study 1, only Grade 3–5 adverse events, treatment-related Grade 2 events, and Grade 2–5 dyspnea were collected during and for up to 3 months following protocol-specified treatment. The following non-cardiac adverse reactions of Grade 2-5 occurred at an incidence of at least 2% greater among patients randomized to Herceptin plus chemotherapy as compared to chemotherapy alone: arthralgia (31% vs. 28%), fatigue (28% vs. 22%), infection (22% vs. 14%), hot flashes (17% vs. 15%), anemia (13% vs. 7%), dyspnea (12% vs. 4%), rash/desquamation (11% vs. 7%), neutropenia (7% vs. 5%), headache (6% vs. 4%), and insomnia (3.7% vs. 1.5%). The majority of these events were Grade 2 in severity. In Study 2, data collection was limited to the following investigator-attributed treatment-related adverse reactions: NCI-CTC Grade 4 and 5 hematologic toxicities, Grade 3–5 non-hematologic toxicities, selected Grade 2–5 toxicities associated with taxanes (myalgia, arthralgia, nail changes, motor neuropathy, sensory neuropathy) and Grade 1–5 cardiac toxicities occurring during chemotherapy and/or Herceptin treatment. The following non-cardiac adverse reactions of Grade 2–5 occurred at an incidence of at least 2% greater among patients randomized to Herceptin plus chemotherapy as compared to chemotherapy alone: arthralgia (11% vs. 8.4%), myalgia (10% vs. 8%), nail changes (9% vs. 7%), and dyspnea (2.5% vs. 0.1%). The majority of these events were Grade 2 in severity. Safety data from Study 4 reflect exposure to Herceptin as part of an adjuvant treatment regimen from 2124 patients receiving at least one dose of study treatment [AC-TH: n = 1068; TCH: n = 1056]. The overall median treatment duration was 54 weeks in both the AC-TH and TCH arms. The median number of infusions was 26 in the AC-TH arm and 30 in the TCH arm, including weekly infusions during the chemotherapy phase and every three week dosing in the monotherapy period. Among these patients, the median age was 49 years (range 22 to 74 years). In Study 4, the toxicity profile was similar to that reported in Studies 1, 2, and 3 with the exception of a low incidence of CHF in the TCH arm. *Metastatic Breast Cancer Studies* The data below reflect exposure to Herceptin in one randomized, open-label study, Study 5, of chemotherapy with (n=235) or without (n=234) trastuzumab in patients with metastatic breast cancer, and one single-arm study (Study 6; n=222) in patients with metastatic breast cancer. Data in Table 5 are based on Studies 5 and 6. Among the 464 patients treated in Study 5, the median age was 52 years (range: 25–77 years). Eighty-nine percent were White, 5% Black, 1% Asian and 5% other racial/ethnic groups. All patients received 4 mg/kg initial dose of Herceptin followed by 2 mg/kg weekly. The percentages of patients who received Herceptin treatment for ≥6 months and ≥12 months were 58% and 9%, respectively. Among the 352 patients treated in single agent studies (213 patients from Study 6), the median age was 50 years (range 28–86 years), 100% had breast cancer, 86% were White, 3% were Black, 3% were Asian, and 8% in other racial/ethnic groups. Most of the patients received 4 mg/kg initial dose of Herceptin followed by 2 mg/kg weekly. The percentages of patients who received Herceptin treatment for ≥6 months and ≥12 months were 31% and 16%, respectively.

Table 4 Per-Patient Incidence of Adverse Reactions Occurring in ≥5% of Patients in Uncontrolled Studies or at Increased Incidence in the Herceptin Arm (Studies 5 and 6) (Percent of Patients)

	Single Agent[a] n = 352	Herceptin + Paclitaxel n = 91	Paclitaxel Alone n = 95	Herceptin + AC[b] n = 143	AC[b] Alone n = 135
Body as a Whole					
Pain	47	61	62	57	42
Asthenia	42	62	57	54	55
Fever	36	49	23	56	34
Chills	32	41	4	35	11
Headache	26	36	28	44	31
Abdominal pain	22	34	22	23	18
Back pain	22	34	30	27	15
Infection	20	47	27	47	31
Flu syndrome	10	12	5	12	6
Accidental injury	6	13	3	9	4
Allergic reaction	3	8	2	4	2
Cardiovascular					
Tachycardia	5	12	4	10	5
Congestive heart failure	7	11	1	28	7
Digestive					
Nausea	33	51	9	76	77
Diarrhea	25	45	29	45	26
Vomiting	23	37	28	53	49
Nausea and vomiting	8	14	11	18	9
Anorexia	14	24	16	31	26
Heme & Lymphatic					
Anemia	4	14	9	36	26
Leukopenia	3	24	17	52	34
Metabolic					
Peripheral edema	10	22	20	20	17
Edema	8	10	8	11	5
Musculoskeletal					
Bone pain	7	24	18	7	7
Arthralgia	6	37	21	8	9
Nervous					
Insomnia	14	25	13	29	15
Dizziness	13	22	24	24	18
Paresthesia	9	48	39	17	11
Depression	6	12	13	20	12
Peripheral neuritis	2	23	16	2	2
Neuropathy	1	13	5	4	4
Respiratory					
Cough increased	26	41	22	43	29
Dyspnea	22	27	26	42	25
Rhinitis	14	22	5	22	16
Pharyngitis	12	22	14	30	18
Sinusitis	9	21	7	13	6
Skin					
Rash	18	38	18	27	17
Herpes simplex	2	12	3	7	9
Acne	2	11	3	3	<1
Urogenital					
Urinary tract infection	5	18	14	13	7

[a] Data for Herceptin single agent were from 4 studies, including 213 patients from Study 6. [b] Anthracycline (doxorubicin or epirubicin) and cyclophosphamide.

The following subsections provide additional detail regarding adverse reactions observed in clinical trials of adjuvant breast, metastatic breast cancer, or post-marketing experience. *Cardiomyopathy* Serial measurement of cardiac function (LVEF) was obtained in clinical trials in the adjuvant treatment of breast cancer. In Study 3, the median duration of follow-up was 12.6 months (12.4 months in the observation arm; 12.6 months in the 1-year Herceptin arm); and in Studies 1 and 2, 23 months in the AC-T arm, 24 months in the AC-TH arm. In Studies 1 and 2, 6% of patients were not permitted to initiate Herceptin following completion of AC chemotherapy due to cardiac dysfunction (LVEF < 50% or ≥15 point decline in LVEF from baseline to end of AC). Following initiation of Herceptin therapy, the incidence of new-onset dose-limiting myocardial dysfunction was higher among patients receiving Herceptin and paclitaxel as compared to those receiving paclitaxel alone in Studies 1 and 2, and in patients receiving Herceptin monotherapy compared to observation in Study 3 (see Table 5, Figures 1 and 2).

Table 5[a] Per-patient Incidence of New Onset Myocardial Dysfunction (by LVEF) Studies 1, 2, 3 and 4

	LVEF <50% and Absolute Decrease from Baseline			Absolute LVEF Decrease	
	LVEF <50%	≥10% decrease	≥16% decrease	<20% and ≥10%	≥20%
Studies 1 & 2[b]					
AC→TH (n=1606)	22.8% (366)	18.3% (294)	11.7% (188)	33.4% (536)	9.2% (148)
AC→T (n=1488)	9.1% (136)	5.4% (81)	2.2% (33)	18.3% (272)	2.4% (36)
Study 3					
Herceptin (n=1678)	8.6% (144)	7.0% (118)	3.8% (64)	22.4% (376)	3.5% (59)
Observation (n=1708)	2.7% (46)	2.0% (35)	1.2% (20)	11.9% (204)	1.2% (21)
Study 4[c]					
TCH (n=1056)	8.5% (90)	5.9% (62)	3.3% (35)	34.5% (364)	6.3% (67)
AC→TH (n=1068)	17% (182)	13.3% (142)	9.8% (105)	44.3% (473)	13.2% (141)
AC→T (n=1050)	9.5% (100)	6.6% (69)	3.3% (35)	34% (357)	5.5% (58)

[a] For Studies 1, 2 and 3, events are counted from the beginning of Herceptin treatment. For Study 4, events are counted from the date of randomization. [b] Studies 1 and 2 regimens: doxorubicin and cyclophosphamide followed by paclitaxel (AC→T) or paclitaxel plus Herceptin (AC→TH). [c] Study 4 regimens: doxorubicin and cyclophosphamide followed by docetaxel (AC→T) or docetaxel plus Herceptin (AC→TH); docetaxel and carboplatin plus Herceptin (TCH).

Figure 1 Studies 1 and 2: Cumulative Incidence of Time to First LVEF Decline of ≥10 Percentage Points from Baseline and to Below 50% with Death as a Competing Risk Event

Time 0 is initiation of paclitaxel or Herceptin + paclitaxel therapy.

Figure 2 Study 3: Cumulative Incidence of Time to First LVEF Decline of ≥10 Percentage Points from Baseline and to Below 50% with Death as a Competing Risk Event

Time 0 is the date of randomization.

Figure 3 Study 4: Cumulative Incidence of Time to First LVEF Decline of ≥ 10 Percentage Points from Baseline and to Below 50% with Death as a Competing Risk Event

Time 0 is the date of randomization.

The incidence of treatment emergent congestive heart failure among patients in the metastatic breast cancer trials was classified for severity using the New York Heart Association classification system (I–IV, where IV is the most severe level of cardiac failure) (see Table 2). In the metastatic breast cancer trials the probability of cardiac dysfunction was highest in patients who received Herceptin concurrently with anthracyclines. *Infusion Reactions* During the first infusion with Herceptin, the symptoms most commonly reported were chills and fever, occurring in approximately 40% of patients in clinical trials. Symptoms were treated with acetaminophen, diphenhydramine, and meperidine (with or without reduction in the rate of Herceptin infusion); permanent discontinuation of Herceptin for infusional toxicity was required in <1% of patients. Other signs and/or symptoms may include nausea, vomiting, pain (in some cases at tumor sites), rigors, headache, dizziness, dyspnea, hypotension, elevated blood pressure, rash, and asthenia. Infusional toxicity occurred in 21% and 35% of patients, and was severe in 1.4% and 9% of patients, on second or subsequent Herceptin infusions administered as monotherapy or in combination with chemotherapy, respectively. In the post-marketing setting, severe infusion reactions, including hypersensitivity, anaphylaxis, and angioedema have been reported. *Anemia* In randomized controlled clinical trials, the overall incidence of anemia (30% vs. 21% [Study 5]), of selected NCI-CTC Grade 2–5 anemia (12.5% vs. 6.6% [Study 1]), and of anemia requiring transfusions (0.1% vs. 0 patients [Study 2]) were increased in patients receiving Herceptin and chemotherapy compared with those receiving chemotherapy alone. Following the administration of Herceptin as a single agent (Study 6), the incidence of NCI-CTC Grade 3 anemia was <1%. *Neutropenia* In randomized controlled clinical trials in the adjuvant setting, the incidence of selected NCI-CTC

Grade 4–5 neutropenia (2% vs. 0.7% [Study 2]) and of selected Grade 2–5 neutropenia (7.1% vs. 4.5 % [Study 1]) were increased in patients receiving Herceptin and chemotherapy compared with those receiving chemotherapy alone. In a randomized, controlled trial in patients with metastatic breast cancer, the incidences of NCI-CTC Grade 3/4 neutropenia (32% vs. 22%) and of febrile neutropenia (23% vs. 17%) were also increased in patients randomized to Herceptin in combination with myelosuppressive chemotherapy as compared to chemotherapy alone. *Infection* The overall incidences of infection (46% vs. 30% [Study 5]), of selected NCI-CTC Grade 2–5 infection/febrile neutropenia (22% vs. 14% [Study 1]) and of selected Grade 3–5 infection/febrile neutropenia (3.3% vs. 1.4%) [Study 2]), were higher in patients receiving Herceptin and chemotherapy compared with those receiving chemotherapy alone. The most common site of infections in the adjuvant setting involved the upper respiratory tract, skin, and urinary tract. In Study 4, the overall incidence of infection was higher with the addition of Herceptin to AC-T but not to TCH [44% (AC-TH), 37% (TCH), 38% (AC-T)]. The incidences of NCI-CTC grade 3-4 infection were similar [25% (AC-TH), 21% (TCH), 23% (AC-T)] across the three arms. In a randomized, controlled trial in treatment of metastatic breast cancer, the reported incidence of febrile neutropenia was higher (23% vs. 17%) in patients receiving Herceptin in combination with myelosuppressive chemotherapy as compared to chemotherapy alone. *Pulmonary Toxicity* Adjuvant Breast Cancer: Among women receiving adjuvant therapy for breast cancer, the incidence of selected NCI-CTC Grade 2–5 pulmonary toxicity (14% vs. 5% [Study 1]) and of selected NCI-CTC Grade 3–5 pulmonary toxicity and of spontaneous reported Grade 2 dyspnea (3.4% vs. 1% [Study 2]) was higher in patients receiving Herceptin and chemotherapy compared with chemotherapy alone. The most common pulmonary toxicity was dyspnea (NCI CTC Grade 2–5: 12% vs. 4% [Study 1]; NCI-CTC Grade 2–5: 2.5% vs. 0.1% [Study 2]). Pneumonitis/pulmonary infiltrates occurred in 0.7% of patients receiving Herceptin compared with 0.3% of those receiving chemotherapy alone. Fatal respiratory failure occurred in 3 patients receiving Herceptin, one as a component of multi-organ system failure, as compared to 1 patient receiving chemotherapy alone. In Study 3, there were 4 cases of interstitial pneumonitis in Herceptin-treated patients compared to none in the control arm. Metastatic Breast Cancer: Among women receiving Herceptin for treatment of metastatic breast cancer, the incidence of pulmonary toxicity was also increased. Pulmonary adverse events have been reported in the post-marketing experience as part of the symptom complex of infusion reactions. Pulmonary events include bronchospasm, hypoxia, dyspnea, pulmonary infiltrates, pleural effusions, non-cardiogenic pulmonary edema, and acute respiratory distress syndrome. For a detailed description, see *Warnings and Precautions*. *Thrombosis/ Embolism* In 4 randomized, controlled clinical trials, the incidence of thrombotic adverse events was higher in patients receiving Herceptin and chemotherapy compared to chemotherapy alone in three studies (3.0% vs. 1.3% [Study 1], 2.5% and 3.7% vs. 2.2% [Study 4] and 2.1% vs. 0% [Study 5]). *Diarrhea* Among women receiving adjuvant therapy for breast cancer, the incidence of NCI-CTC Grade 2–5 diarrhea (6.2% vs. 4.8% [Study 1]) and of NCI-CTC Grade 3–5 diarrhea (1.6% vs. 0% [Study 2]), and of Grade 1–4 diarrhea (7% vs. 1% [Study 3]) were higher in patients receiving Herceptin as compared to controls. In Study 4, the incidence of Grade 3–4 diarrhea was higher [5.7% AC-TH, 5.5% TCH vs. 3.0% AC-T] and of Grade 1–4 was higher [51%

AC-TH, 63% TCH vs. 43% AC-T] among women receiving Herceptin. Of patients receiving Herceptin as a single agent for the treatment of metastatic breast cancer, 25% experienced diarrhea. An increased incidence of diarrhea was observed in patients receiving Herceptin in combination with chemotherapy for treatment of metastatic breast cancer. *Glomerulopathy* In the post-marketing setting, rare cases of nephrotic syndrome with pathologic evidence of glomerulopathy have been reported. The time to onset ranged from 4 months to approximately 18 months from initiation of Herceptin therapy. Pathologic findings included membranous glomerulonephritis, focal glomerulosclerosis, and fibrillary glomerulonephritis. Complications included volume overload and congestive heart failure. **Immunogenicity** As with all therapeutic proteins, there is a potential for immunogenicity. Among 903 women with metastatic breast cancer, human anti-human antibody (HAHA) to Herceptin was detected in one patient using an enzyme-linked immunosorbent assay (ELISA). This patient did not experience an allergic reaction. Samples for assessment of HAHA were not collected in studies of adjuvant breast cancer. The incidence of antibody formation is highly dependent on the sensitivity and the specificity of the assay. Additionally, the observed incidence of antibody (including neutralizing antibody) positivity in an assay may be influenced by several factors including assay methodology, sample handling, timing of sample collection, concomitant medications, and underlying disease. For these reasons, comparison of the incidence of antibodies to Herceptin with the incidence of antibodies to other products may be misleading. **USE IN SPECIFIC POPULATIONS Pregnancy Teratogenic Effects: Category D [*see Warnings and Precautions*]** Herceptin can cause fetal harm when administered to a pregnant woman. Post-marketing case reports suggest that Herceptin use during pregnancy increases the risk for oligohydramnios during the second and third trimester. If Herceptin is used during pregnancy or if a woman becomes pregnant while taking Herceptin, she should be apprised of the potential hazard to a fetus. In the post-marketing setting, oligohydramnios was reported in women who received Herceptin during pregnancy, either alone or in combination with chemotherapy. In half of these women, amniotic fluid index increased after Herceptin was stopped. In one case, Herceptin was resumed after the amniotic fluid index improved, and oligohydramnios recurred. Women using Herceptin during pregnancy should be monitored for oligohydramnios. If oligohydramnios occurs, fetal testing should be done that is appropriate for gestational age and consistent with community standards of care. Additional intravenous (IV) hydration has been helpful when oligohydramnios has occurred following administration of other chemotherapy agents; however, the effects of additional IV hydration with Herceptin treatment are not known. Reproduction studies in cynomolgus monkeys at doses up to 25 times the recommended weekly human dose of 2 mg/kg trastuzumab have revealed no evidence of harm to the fetus. However, HER2 protein expression is high in many embryonic tissues including cardiac and neural tissues; in mutant mice lacking HER2, embryos died in early gestation. Placental transfer of trastuzumab during the early (Days 20-50 of gestation) and late (Days 120-150 of gestation) fetal development period was observed in monkeys. [*See Nonclinical Toxicology*] Because animal reproduction studies are not always predictive of human response, Herceptin should be used during pregnancy only if the potential benefit to the mother justifies the potential risk to the fetus. **Nursing Mothers** It is not known whether Herceptin is excreted in human milk, but human IgG is excreted in human milk. Published data suggest that breast milk antibodies do not enter the neonatal and infant circulation in substantial amounts. Trastuzumab was present in the breast milk of lactating cynomolgus monkeys given 12.5 times the recommended weekly human dose of 2 mg/kg of Herceptin. Infant monkeys with detectable serum levels of trastuzumab did not have any adverse effects on growth or development from birth to 3 months of age; however, trastuzumab levels in animal breast milk may not accurately reflect human breast milk levels. Because many drugs are secreted in human milk and because of the potential for serious adverse reactions in nursing infants from Herceptin, a decision should be made whether to discontinue nursing, or discontinue drug, taking into account the elimination half-life of trastuzumab and the importance of the drug to the mother. **Pediatric Use** The safety and effectiveness of Herceptin in pediatric patients has not been established. **Geriatric Use** Herceptin has been administered to 386 patients who were 65 years of age or over (253 in the adjuvant treatment and 133 in metastatic breast cancer treatment settings). The risk of cardiac dysfunction was increased in geriatric patients as compared to younger patients in both those receiving treatment for metastatic disease in Studies 5 and 6, or adjuvant therapy in Studies 1 and 2. Limitations in data collection and differences in study design of the 4 studies of Herceptin in adjuvant treatment of breast cancer preclude a determination of whether the toxicity profile of Herceptin in older patients is different from younger patients. The reported clinical experience is not adequate to determine whether the efficacy improvements (ORR, TTP, OS, DFS) of Herceptin treatment in older patients is different from that observed in patients <65 years of age for metastatic disease and adjuvant treatment. **OVERDOSAGE** There is no experience with overdosage in human clinical trials. Single doses higher than 8 mg/kg have not been tested. **PATIENT COUNSELING INFORMATION** • Advise patients to contact a health care professional immediately for any of the following: new onset or worsening shortness of breath, cough, swelling of the ankles/legs, swelling of the face, palpitations, weight gain of more than 5 pounds in 24 hours, dizziness or loss of consciousness [*see Boxed Warning: Cardiomyopathy*]. • Advise women with reproductive potential to use effective contraceptive methods during treatment and for a minimum of six months following Herceptin [*see Pregnancy*]. • Encourage pregnant women who are using Herceptin to enroll in the Cancer and Childbirth Registry [*see Pregnancy*].

HERCEPTIN® [trastuzumab]
Manufactured by: 4839802
Genentech, Inc.   Initial US Approval: Sept. 1998
1 DNA Way   Revision Date: May 2008
South San Francisco, CA   LK0726 9395300
94080-4990   ©2008 Genentech USA, Inc.

CHAPTER 20

Cervical cancer

Dennis S. Chi, MD, Carlos A. Perez, MD, and John Kavanagh, MD

The overall incidence of invasive cervical carcinoma has declined steadily since the mid-1940s. Of the predominant gynecologic cancers, cancer of the uterine cervix is the least common, with only 11,070 new cases anticipated in the United States in 2008. Nevertheless, approximately 3,670 women die of cancer of the uterine cervix annually in the United States.

Epidemiology

Age The peak age of developing cervical cancer is 47 years. Approximately 47% of women with invasive cervical cancer are < 35 years old at diagnosis. Older women (> 65 years) account for another 10% of patients with cervical cancer. Although these older patients represent only 10% of all cases, they are more likely to die of the disease due to their more advanced stage at diagnosis.

Socioeconomic class Carcinoma of the uterine cervix primarily affects women from the lower socioeconomic class and those with poor access to routine medical care.

Geography Although invasive cervical carcinoma is relatively uncommon in the United States compared with the more common cancers in women (breast, endometrial, and ovarian cancers), it remains a significant health problem for women worldwide. In many developing countries, not only is cervical carcinoma the most frequently occurring cancer among middle-aged women, but also it is a leading cause of death. This is due, in part, to poor access to medical care and the unavailability of routine screening in many of these countries.

Etiology and risk factors

Sexual activity Invasive cervical carcinoma can be viewed as a sexually transmitted disease. If a woman is never sexually active, she will never develop this cancer. Conversely, any woman who has been sexually active is at risk for invasive cervical carcinoma.

Human papillomavirus Molecular and epidemiologic evidence clearly indicates that certain types of human papillomavirus (HPV), which is sexually transmitted, are the principal causes of invasive cervical cancer and cervical intraepithelial neoplasia (CIN). More than 100 HPV types have been identified, and about 40

CERVICAL

Gardasil, a quadrivalent vaccine to prevent cervical cancer, has been approved by the US FDA to be used in girls and women aged 9 to 26. The vaccine uses virus-like particles to induce immunity to human papillomavirus (HPV) types 16 and 18, which cause approximately 70% of cervical cancers and more than 50% of precancerous lesions of the cervix, vulva, and vagina. It is also reported to be protective against HPV types 6 and 11, which cause more than 90% of genital wart cases. Overall, more than 50,000 women have participated in the phase III trials worldwide. With follow-up ranging from 1 to 4 years, the vaccine has been reported to be 90%–100% effective in preventing infection and precancerous lesions (*Prescribing information, US FDA. Issued June 2006. No. 9682300*). Cervarix, a bivalent vaccine that targets HPV 16/18, is currently undergoing phase III clinical trials involving more than 30,000 women worldwide.

infect the genital tract. HPV-16 and HPV-18 are the types most commonly linked with cancer, present in 70% of cervical cancers and high-grade CINs. A vaccine to prevent cervical cancer was approved by the US Food and Drug Administration (FDA) and became available in 2006.

Age of onset of sexual activity Population studies of women with invasive cervical carcinoma have demonstrated that early age of onset of sexual activity also plays a role in the later development of the cancer. It is postulated that during the time of menarche in early reproductive life, the transformation zone of the cervix is more susceptible to oncogenic agents, such as HPV. Women who begin sexual activity before 16 years of age or who are sexually active within 1 year of beginning menses are at particularly high risk of developing invasive cervical carcinoma.

Other risk factors include multiple sexual partners, a history of genital warts, and multiparity.

Cigarette smoking has been identified as a significant risk factor for cervical carcinoma. It is thought to increase risk by two-fold to five fold. The mechanism may be related to diminished immune function secondary to a systemic effect of cigarette smoke and its by-products or a local effect of tobacco-specific carcinogens.

Oral contraceptives may also play a role in the development of invasive cervical carcinoma, although this theory is controversial. Given that most women who use oral contraceptives are more sexually active than women who do not, this may represent a confounding factor rather than a true independent risk factor. The exception may be adenocarcinoma of the cervix; this relatively uncommon histologic subtype may be related to previous oral contraceptive use.

Immune system alterations In recent years, alterations in the immune system have been associated with an increased risk of invasive cervical carcinoma, as exemplified by the fact that patients who are infected with the human immunodeficiency virus (HIV) have increased rates of both preinvasive and invasive cervical carcinomas. These patients also are at risk for other types of carcinoma, including Kaposi's sarcoma, lymphomas, and other squamous cell carcinomas of the head and neck and the anogenital region. (For further discussion of AIDS-related malignancies, see chapter 27.)

CERVICAL

Data suggest that patients who are immunocompromised due to immuno-suppressive medications also are at risk for both preinvasive and invasive cervical carcinomas. This association is probably due to the suppression of the normal immune response to HPV, which makes patients more susceptible to malignant transformation. An exciting recent development in the prevention of carcinoma of the cervix is the increasing use of HPV vaccines; if used on a timely basis in young women (ideally before they are exposed to the HPV virus, they can decrease this infection and eventually the incidence of cervical cancer.

Signs and symptoms

Common symptoms A symptom of advanced cervical carcinoma is inter-menstrual bleeding in a premenopausal patient. Other commonly reported symptoms include heavier menstrual flow, metrorrhagia, and/or postcoital bleeding. With effective screening, cervical cancer is generally asymptomatic.

Less common presentations Less frequently, patients with advanced cancer will present with signs of advanced disease, such as bowel obstruction and renal failure due to urinary tract obstruction. Only rarely are asymptomatic patients with a normal screening Pap smear found to have a lesion on the cervix as their only sign or symptom of cervical cancer. Foul-smelling vaginal discharge, pelvic pain, or both are occasionally observed.

Screening and diagnosis

Screening

Pap smear The paradigm for a cost-effective, easy-to-use, reliable screening test is the cervical cytology screen, or Pap smear. In every population studied, the introduction of the Pap smear has resulted in a significant reduction in the incidence of invasive cervical carcinoma, as well as a shift toward earlier stage disease at the time of diagnosis. The success of cervical cytology, as measured by the lowered incidence of cervical cancer, ironically has led to some controversy regarding the most effective application of this screening tool. With the marked reduction in the incidence of cervical carcinoma, more patients are screened and greater costs incurred to detect each additional case of cervical carcinoma.

Current screening recommendations The current recommendation of the American College of Obstetricians and Gynecologists (ACOG) is that all women who are 18 years of age or older and are sexually active be screened. If the patient has three consecutive annual cervical cytology smears that are normal, she may be safely screened at a less frequent interval of perhaps 2–3 years. There are no data to support screening patients on a less frequent basis. Any patient who has a history of cervical dysplasia should be screened at least on a yearly basis.

The current American Cancer Society (ACS) revised guidelines for cervical cancer screening follow: Cervical cancer screening should begin ~3 years after the onset of vaginal intercourse but no later than age 21. Cervical screening should be performed every year with conventional cervical cytology smears, or every 2 years using liquid-based cytology until age 30. After age 30, as an alternative to annual routine cytology, HPV DNA testing may be added to cervical cytology for screening. After this initial dual testing, women whose results are negative by both HPV DNA testing and cytology should not be rescreened before 3 years. Women whose results are negative by cytology but who are high-risk HPV DNA (type 16, 18, most commonly) positive are at a relatively low risk of having high-grade cervical neoplasia, and colposcopy should not be performed routinely in this setting. Instead, HPV DNA testing along with cervical cytology should be repeated in these women at 6 or 12 months. If test results of either modality are positive, colposcopy should then be performed.

Women who are > 70 years old with an intact cervix and who have had three or more documented, consecutive, technically satisfactory normal cervical cytology tests and no abnormal cytology tests within the 10-year period prior to age 70 may elect to cease cervical cancer screening. Women with a history of cervical cancer, in utero exposure to diethylstilbestrol (DES), and/or who are immunocompromised (including HIV+) should continue cervical cancer screening for as long as they are in reasonably good health and do not have a life-limiting chronic condition. Women > 70 years old should discuss their need for cervical cancer screening with a health care professional and make an informed decision about continuing screening based on its potential benefits, harms, and limitations.

Women who have had a supracervical hysterectomy should continue cervical cancer screening as per current guidelines. Cervical cancer screening following total hysterectomy (with removal of the cervix) for benign gynecologic disease is not indicated. Women with a history of CIN2/3 or for whom it is not possible to document the absence of CIN2/3 prior to or as the indication for hysterectomy should be screened until three documented, consecutive, technically satisfactory normal cervical cytology tests and no abnormal cytology tests (within a 10-year period) are achieved. Women with a history of in utero DES exposure and a history of cervical carcinoma should continue screening after hysterectomy for as long as they are in reasonably good health and do not have a life-limiting chronic condition.

Techniques designed to improve the sensitivity of the Pap smear have been approved by the FDA. Liquid-based cytologies such as thin prep and SurePath are commercially available techniques. Computer-based analysis of these techniques has been developed but is still under evaluation.

Diagnosis

The diagnosis of invasive cervical carcinoma can be suggested by either an abnormal Pap smear or an abnormal physical finding.

Colposcopy In the patient who has an abnormal Pap smear but normal physical findings, colposcopy is indicated. Colposcopic findings consistent with invasive cervical carcinoma include dense white epithelium covering the ectocervix, punctation, mosaicism, and especially, an atypical blood vessel pattern.

Biopsy If the colposcopic findings are suggestive of invasion, biopsies are obtained from the ectocervix and endocervix. If these biopsies demonstrate only precancerous changes but not an invasive carcinoma, the patient should undergo an excisional biopsy of the cervix. In most current clinical settings, the loop electrosurgical excision procedure (LEEP) is the most expedient method for performing an excisional biopsy. This can be easily accomplished in the office with the patient under local anesthesia and provides adequate tissue for diagnosis. Once the diagnosis of either microinvasive or invasive carcinoma has been established, the patient can be triaged accordingly.

Patient with signs/symptoms of advanced disease The patient with signs/symptoms of advanced invasive cervical carcinoma requires a cervical biopsy for diagnosis and treatment planning. In this setting, a Pap smear is superfluous and may be misleading.

Pathology

Squamous cell carcinoma The most common histology associated with invasive cervical carcinoma is squamous cell carcinoma, which accounts for approximately 80% of all carcinomas of the uterine cervix. For the most part, the decline in the annual incidence of invasive cervical carcinoma has been seen primarily among patients with this subtype.

Adenocarcinoma In the past, adenocarcinoma was relatively uncommon as a primary histology of cervical cancer. As a result of the decrease in the overall incidence of invasive squamous cell cancer and, probably, an increase in the baseline incidence of adenocarcinoma of the uterine cervix, this histology now accounts for approximately 20% of all cervical cancers.

There is controversy over whether patients with adenocarcinoma of the cervix have a worse prognosis than those with the more common squamous cell histology. The poorer prognosis associated with adenocarcinoma may be due to the relatively higher frequency of late stage at the time of diagnosis among patients with this histologic type. In several series in which patients were stratified by stage and tumor size, the outcome of cervical adenocarcinoma appeared to be similar to that of squamous lesions of the cervix.

Aggressive subtypes Among the various subtypes of adenocarcinoma, certain types are particularly aggressive and are associated with a poor prognosis. Among them are the small cell or neuroendocrine tumors, which have a poor prognosis even when diagnosed at an early stage.

Rare tumor types More rare lesions of the cervix include lymphoma, sarcoma, and melanoma. These histologic subtypes account for < 1% of all cervical cancers.

TABLE 1: AJCC and FIGO staging for carcinoma of the uterine cervix

AJCC	FIGO	
Primary tumor (T)		
Tx		Primary tumor cannot be assessed
T0		No evidence of primary tumor
Tis		Carcinoma in situ
T1	I	Cervical carcinoma confined to the uterus (extension to the corpus should be disregarded)
T1a	IA	Preclinical invasive carcinoma, diagnosed by microscopy only
T1a1	IA1	Minimal microscopic stromal invasion ($\leq$ 3 mm stromal invasion (in depth), $\leq$ 7 mm in horizontal spread)
T1a2	IA2	Tumor with an invasive component more than 3 mm and not more than 5 mm and 7 mm or less in horizontal spread
T1b	IB	Clinical lesions confined to the cervix or preclinical lesions greater than stage IA
	IB1	Clinical lesions no greater than 4 cm
	IB2	Clinical lesions greater than 4 cm
T2	II	Cervical carcinoma invades beyond the uterus but not to the pelvic wall or to the lower third of the vagina
T2a	IIA	Tumor without parametrial invasion
T2b	IIB	Tumor with parametrial invasion
T3	III	Cervical carcinoma extends to the pelvic wall and/or involves the lower third of the vagina and/or causes hydronephrosis or nonfunctioning of the kidneys
T3a	IIIA	Tumor involves the lower third of the vagina, with no exension to the pelvic wall
T3b	IIIB	Tumor extends to the pelvic wall and/or causes hydronephrosis or nonfunctioning of the kidneys
T4[a]	IVA	Tumor invades the mucosa of the bladder or rectum and/or extends beyond the true pelvis
Regional lymph nodes[b] (N)		
Nx		Regional lymph nodes cannot be assessed
N0		No regional lymph node metastasis
N1		Regional lymph node metastasis
Distant metastasis (M)		
Mx		Presence of distant metastasis cannot be assessed
M0		No distant metastasis
M1	IVB	Distant metastasis

AJCC = American Joint Committee on Cancer; FIGO = International Federation of Gynecology and Obstetrics

[a] *Note:* The presence of bullous edema is not sufficient evidence to classify a tumor as T4.

[b] Regional lymph nodes include paracervical, parametrial, hypogastric (obturator), common, internal and external iliac, presacral, and sacral.

Modified from Greene FL, Page DL, Fleming ID, et al: AJCC Cancer Staging Manual, ed 6. N Y, Springer, 2002; Perez CA, Kavanagh BD: Uterine cervix. In: Perez CA, Brady LW, Halperin EC, eds: Principles and Practice of Radiation Oncology, ed 4, pp 1800–1915. Philadelphia, Lippincott Williams & Wilkins, 2004.

Staging and prognosis

Clinical staging: suspected early disease

When a diagnosis of invasive cervical cancer has been established histologically, an evaluation of all pelvic organs should be performed to determine whether the tumor is confined to the cervix or has extended to the adjacent vagina, parametrium, endometrial cavity, bladder, ureters, or rectum. According to the International Federation of Gynecology and Obstetrics (FIGO) guidelines for clinical staging (Table 1), diagnostic studies may include intravenous urography (IVU), cystoscopic examination of the bladder and urethra, a proctosigmoidoscopic study, a barium enema (BE), and in the case of early-stage disease, a colposcopic study of the vagina and the vaginal fornices. Colposcopic findings may be used for assigning a stage to the tumor (for instance, FIGO stage IIA), but the results must be confirmed by biopsy.

A pelvic examination must be performed as part of the staging process, and the procedure is best done with the patient completely relaxed by general anesthesia. In up to 20% of patients, the initial clinical classification of the disease has proved to be incorrect at the time of pelvic examination. Such an examination can reveal a more advanced stage of the disease than was originally found; additional biopsies (if indicated) or fractional curettage can be performed as well as colposcopy, cystoscopy, and proctosigmoidoscopy.

Clinical staging: suspected advanced disease

When studies detect ureteral obstruction, a tumor is classified as a stage IIIB lesion, regardless of the size of the primary lesion. Ureteral obstruction, either hydronephrosis or nonfunction of the kidneys, is well established as an indicator of poor prognosis, as recognized in the FIGO classification.

In women with bulky or advanced-stage tumors, the bladder mucosa also should be inspected cystoscopically for possible bullous edema, which indicates lymphatic obstruction within the bladder wall. Evidence of tumor in the bladder must be confirmed by biopsy before the lesion can be classified as stage IVA. Rectal mucosal lesions also require a biopsy via proctosigmoidoscopy, because they can be related to an inflammatory process rather than to the cervical tumor.

Surgical experience from pelvic lymphadenectomy has confirmed an error rate of 15%–25% in the clinical staging of patients with stage IB or II lesions. In 10%–30% of cases with stage II/III tumors, in addition to positive findings of occult pelvic lymph nodes, other metastases may be found in the para-aortic nodes. Unfortunately, pelvic examinations and clinical staging as defined by FIGO cannot detect such metastases.

Consequently, there is a growing body of literature showing the superiority of cross-sectional imaging (CT and MRI) over clinical staging in delineating the extent of disease in patients with cervical cancer. As stated previously, official FIGO guidelines do not incorporate the use of either CT or MRI findings into the staging of cervical cancer. However, as knowledge of prognostic factors and the value of cross-sectional imaging has accumulated, its use in treatment planning has increased without changing the official FIGO clinical staging guidelines. Similarly, although the benefits of laparoscopic extraperitoneal surgical staging have also been reported in this setting, this approach has not been incorporated into the FIGO staging system.

The value of CT scanning in the pretreatment evaluation of patients with cervical cancer is in the assessment of advanced disease (stage IIB and greater) and in the detection and biopsy of suspected lymph node metastasis. The treatment plan for patients with locally advanced disease must be modified if upper abdominal tumor masses and/or distant metastasis is discovered. The soft-tissue contrast resolution of CT scanning does not allow for consistent tumor visualization at the primary cervical site, and, therefore, neither tumor size nor early parametrial invasion can be evaluated reliably. However, T2-weighted MRI allows consistent tumor visualization and has been reported to be over 90% accurate in determining tumor size to within 5 mm of measurements of surgical specimens. Nevertheless, a recent ACRIN study in 208 patients with invasive cervical cancer evaluated with CT scans or MRI before radical hysterectomy showed that MRI was superior to CT and clinical exam in evaluating uterine body involvement and in measuring tumor size, but neither method was accurate in evaluating the cervical stromal depth of tumor invasion.

Recent reports show the value of positron emission tomography (PET) scanning in the pretreatment evaluation, treatment planning, and post-therapy assessment of response in patients with higher risk invasive carcinoma of the cervix.

Noteworthy, in 60 patients with stage IA2 to IIA cervical cancer up to 4 cm with MRI-negative nodes, preoperative FDG-PET (fluorodeoxyglucose PET) scanning detected 1 para-aortic node metastasis, but only 1 of 10 pelvic node metastasis, which led to the conclusion that PET scanning is of little value in evaluating patients with stage IA2 to IIA cervical cancer up to 4 cm.

Surgical staging

Clinical staging of cervical carcinoma, although widely utilized, is not without controversy. When compared with surgical staging performed by large cooperative groups, clinical staging is frequently inaccurate in predicting locoregional tumor spread. For many cooperative groups, including the Gynecologic Oncology Group (GOG), surgical staging may be required for patients who are entering prospective, randomized clinical protocols. However, because of the controversy of risk and benefit, the GOG considers surgical staging optional.

The most common method used to stage patients with advanced disease is extraperitoneal sampling of the pelvic and para-aortic lymph nodes. This approach minimizes the risk of subsequent radiation injury to the small bowel due to surgical adhesions and, in patients with advanced disease, allows for individualized treatment planning.

Work-up for advanced disease The standard work-up of a patient with advanced cervical carcinoma who is not considered a candidate for radical surgery includes an abdominopelvic CT scan with both intravenous and GI oral contrast. If there is evidence of para-aortic lymph node metastases, the patient should undergo fine-needle aspiration (FNA) of these enlarged lymph nodes. If FNA confirms that there is para-aortic lymph node metastasis, treatment should be individualized, and extended-field irradiation should be considered part of the primary treatment regimen.

Loft et al reported the diagnostic value of PET/CT scanning in 120 patients with newly diagnosed cervical cancer FIGO stage ≥ IB. Regarding the para-aortic lymph nodes, the positive predictive value (PPV) was 94%, negative predictive value (NPV) was 100%, sensitivity was 100%, and specificity was 99%. Regarding the distant metastases, the PPV was 63%, NPV was 100%, sensitivity was 100% and specificity was 94% *(Loft A, Berthelsen AK, Roed H, et al: Gynecol Oncol 106:29-34, 2007).*

If the scalene lymph nodes are negative on clinical examination and the patient is known to have positive metastatic disease to the para-aortic lymph nodes, consideration can be given to performing a scalene lymph node biopsy; the incidence of positive scalene nodes when para-aortic lymph nodes are known to be positive ranges from 0% to 17%. The rationale for biopsying the scalene nodes is that if there is disease outside the radiation therapy field, chemotherapy may be appropriate.

If the result of FNA is negative, or if the abdominopelvic CT scan does not demonstrate enlarged para-aortic lymph nodes, the patient can be considered for surgical staging.

Recent data reported the comparison of accuracy between PET and PET/CT for detecting lymph node metastasis in cervical cancer. In a series of 86 patients with stage IB–IVA cervical cancer, a total of 688 lymph node regions were evaluated. PET/CT was more sensitive than PET for detecting small (< 5 mm) lymph node metastasis (ASCO 2007).

Pros and cons of surgical staging The advantage of surgical staging is that patients with microscopic disease in the para-aortic lymph nodes can be treated with extended-field radiation therapy and, possibly, chemotherapy and potentially benefit in terms of long-term survival. The controversy regarding surgical staging stems from the fact that a small number of patients will actually benefit from the procedure; the majority of patients who undergo it will be found not to have metastatic disease and will receive the same treatment as planned prior to surgical staging; if they are found to have metastatic disease, they will be unlikely to benefit from extended-field radiation therapy. Because of this controversy, GOG considers surgical staging to be *optional* for patients with advanced-stage cervical cancer.

Laparoscopic surgery In more recent years, the introduction of minimal-access surgery has allowed surgeons to accurately stage patients via the laparoscope prior to initiation of radiation therapy. However, the safety and efficacy of laparoscopic surgical staging are areas of ongoing investigation.

Work-up for early-stage disease For patients who have early-stage disease for which surgery is contemplated, only a minimal diagnostic work-up is indicated prior to surgery. At most institutions, this would include a two-view chest x-ray. Patients who have stage IA cervical carcinoma (microinvasive carcinoma) do not require preoperative CT scanning prior to hysterectomy. For patients with a small stage IB carcinoma of the cervix, a CT scan of the abdomen and pelvis has a low yield and is unlikely to change the treatment plan.

Prognostic factors

Clinical stage The most important determinant of prognosis remains clinical stage, which is defined by tumor volume and extent of disease spread. The overall 5-year survival rate ranges from 95% to 100% for patients with stage IA cancer and from 75% to 90% for those with stage IB disease. Patients with stage IV disease have a $\leq 5\%$ chance of surviving 5 years after diagnosis.

Patients with early disease For patients with early invasive carcinoma (stage IB), the size of the lesion, percentage of cervical stromal invasion, histology, tumor grade, and lymphovascular space involvement are important local factors that predict prognosis. In general, good prognostic signs are lesions that are ≤ 2 cm in diameter, superficially invasive, and well differentiated with no lymphovascular space involvement. In a study of 1,067 patients treated with surgery, HPV-16 was detected in 63.8% and HPV-18 in 16.5% of samples. With a median follow-up of 77 months, HPV was not found to be a significant prognostic factor.

For patients who have undergone radical hysterectomy for early cervical carcinoma, poor prognostic factors, in addition to the local factors previously mentioned, include positive vaginal or parametrial margins and metastasis to the pelvic lymph nodes. For patients with stage IB disease and positive pelvic nodes, the 5-year survival rate drops from approximately 75%–85% to 50%.

Patients with advanced disease For patients with advanced-stage disease (stages IIB through IV), the primary determinants of prognosis are histology and size of the primary lesion. Survival is significantly longer for patients with small stage IIB cervical carcinomas and minimal parametrial involvement than for patients with large bulky tumors and bilateral parametrial involvement. Disease extension beyond the pelvis to the para-aortic nodes is associated with a significant decrease in overall survival rate. With regard to histology, a better prognosis is associated with a large-cell nonkeratinizing squamous cell cancer of the cervix, as opposed to a poorly differentiated adenocarcinoma.

Other prognostic factors Other factors that may predict outcome include the patient's general medical and nutritional status. Patients who are anemic may respond poorly to radiation therapy, as compared with those with normal hemoglobin levels. Patients with significant alterations in their immune system may not respond as well; this result is becoming increasingly apparent with regard to patients who are HIV-seropositive.

A retrospective review of 605 patients from seven institutions in Canada treated with irradiation for cervical cancer described average weekly nadir hemoglobin levels as significant prognostic factors for survival, second only in importance to tumor stage. Interestingly, Winter et al reported that hemoglobin levels during treatment were independent predictors of treatment outcome through a recent retrospective study of 494 patients from two consecutive prospective GOG trials. The pretreatment level was not a significant predictor of outcome in the multivariate regression model. Levels in the last part of treatment were the most predictive of disease recurrence and survival. However, erythropoietin should not be given outside a clinical trial, as thrombosis is a significant complication and cause/effect has not been proven.

> Meta-analysis shows that all conservative procedures to treat cervical intraepithelial neoplasia and microinvasive cervical cancer present similar pregnancy-related morbidities without apparent neonatal morbidities. Caution should be recommended in the treatment of young women with mild cervical abnormalities (*Kyrgiou M, Koliopoulos G, Martin-Hirsch P, et al: Lancet 367:489-498, 2006*).

PET scanning is being used to determine response and outcome after therapy. In 152 patients with cervical cancer treated with irradiation alone or in combination with chemotherapy, Grigsby et al reported cause-specific survival of 80% in 114 patients without post-therapy PET abnormalities, 32% in 20 patients with persistent abnormal scans, and no survivors in 18 patients who developed new sites of abnormal uptake.

Treatment

SURGICAL TREATMENT OF EARLY-STAGE DISEASE

The standard management of patients with early cervical carcinoma is surgical removal of the cervix. The extent of resection of surrounding tissue depends on the size of the lesion and the depth of tumor invasion.

Stage IA1 disease

Simple hysterectomy Patients who have a microinvasive squamous carcinoma of the cervix with ≤ 3 mm of tumor invasion, ≤ 7 mm of lateral extent, and no lymphovascular space involvement (stage IA1) can be treated with a simple hysterectomy. Vaginal, abdominal, and laparoscopic hysterectomies are equally effective.

Cone biopsy Although simple hysterectomy is considered the standard therapy for patients with microinvasive cervical carcinoma, there are some patients in whom preservation of future fertility is a strong consideration. A cone biopsy entails removal of the cervical transformation zone. Provided that the biopsy margins are free of dysplasia and microinvasive carcinoma, cone biopsy is probably a safe treatment for such patients who meet the criteria of having superficial invasion < 3 mm, minimal lateral extension, and no lymphovascular space involvement.

Since there is a small risk of recurrence among this population of patients treated by cone biopsy alone, they should be followed closely. Follow-up includes a Pap smear every 3 months for 2 years and then twice a year. An abnormal Pap smear is an indication for a repeat colposcopy. If such patients are successful in achieving pregnancy and have no evidence of recurrent squamous cell carcinoma, there is no need to proceed with hysterectomy at the completion of planned childbearing.

Stages IA2, IB1, and nonbulky IIA disease

Radical hysterectomy A standard treatment for patients with small cervical carcinomas (≤ 4 cm) confined to the uterine cervix or with minimal involvement of the vagina (stage IIA) is radical hysterectomy (removal of the uterus, cervix, and parametrial tissue), pelvic lymphadenectomy, and para-aortic lymph node sampling. The overall success of this treatment is similar to that of radiation therapy, and for patients with early lesions, radical hysterectomy may provide an improved quality of life. The benefits of surgical excision include rapid treatment, less time away from normal activities, and preservation of normal ovarian and vaginal function.

A randomized trial for patients with early-stage cervical cancer reported no difference in survival between radical hysterectomy and definitive radiation therapy. Because a significant percentage of patients following radical hysterectomy required postoperative pelvic radiotherapy, the morbidity was increased in the surgery arm. Therefore, patients selected for radical hysterectomy should have small-volume disease so adjuvant pelvic radiation therapy is unnecessary.

Currently, there are no specific contraindications to radical hysterectomy. Several studies have demonstrated that patients ≥ 65 years old tolerate this procedure well, and age alone should not be considered a contraindication. Obesity also is not a contraindication to radical hysterectomy.

Alternatives to radical hysterectomy Reports have described laparoscopically assisted radical vaginal hysterectomy and laparoscopic abdominal radical hysterectomy as less invasive alternatives to traditional radical hysterectomy. Although these procedures are not performed in all centers, the results from centers that have the surgical expertise are promising. The use of fertility-preserving surgery by means of pelvic lymphadenectomy combined with radical vaginal trachelectomy (removal of the uterine cervix) has also been evaluated

> In a prospective study, the rate of recurrence, fertility, and complications was evaluated in 118 women with stages IA2 and IB1 cervical cancer who had undergone radical vaginal trachelectomy (RVT) and pelvic lymphadenectomy. Six patients received chemoradiotherapy after surgery. The average follow-up was 45 months. There were 5 recurrences and 32 complications (6 intraoperative and 26 postoperative). The 5-year pregnancy rate among women trying to conceive was 52.8%. All but two women were delivered by cesarean section, and seven babies (25%) were born prematurely. Therefore, for selected women with early-stage cervical cancer, RVT and pelvic lymphadenectomy are fertility-sparing options (Shepherd JH, Spencer C, Herod J, et al: Br J Oncol Gynaecol 113:719-724, 2006).

in selected women with early cervical cancer (see box). Successful pregnancies after this procedure have been reported. However, further data are needed to assess the safety and efficacy of fertility-preserving surgery. There is a lack of long-term follow-up data and survival rates between conservative and radical treatment. These techniques should be performed by fully trained surgeons. The role of laparoscopic sentinel lymph node dissection is an area of active investigation.

Complications Due to improved surgical techniques, as well as the use of prophylactic antibiotics and prophylaxis against deep vein thrombosis, the morbidity and mortality associated with radical hysterectomy have declined significantly over the past several decades. The currently accepted complication rate for radical hysterectomy includes approximately a 0.5%–1.0% incidence of urinary tract injury, a 0.5%–1.0% incidence of deep vein thrombosis, and an overall mortality of < 1.0%.

The increased awareness of the risks associated with blood transfusion is reflected in the fact that, in many cases, no transfusions are administered. The need for heterologous blood transfusion also can be decreased by encouraging autologous blood donation prior to radical hysterectomy or by using intraoperative hemodilution.

The average hospital stay for patients undergoing radical hysterectomy is between 4 and 7 days. Follow-up should include a vaginal Pap smear every 3 months for 2 years, twice a year for 3 years, and yearly thereafter.

Stages IB2 and bulky IIA disease

Numerous studies have demonstrated that patients with early-stage "bulky" lesions (> 4 cm) have a worse prognosis than those with nonbulky tumors. Therefore, patients who have undergone radical hysterectomy and pelvic lymphadenectomy for early-stage bulky cervical cancer have traditionally received postoperative adjuvant pelvic radiation therapy. However, a randomized trial from Italy demonstrated that radical hysterectomy plus radiotherapy does not improve overall or disease-free survival in patients with early-stage bulky tumors, as compared with radiation therapy alone, but does significantly increase morbidity.

Furthermore, a recent GOG trial (GOG 123) demonstrated the benefit of the addition of cisplatin chemotherapy to pelvic radiation therapy followed by extrafascial hysterectomy in this group of patients (Figure 1). Therefore, many experts believe that patients with stage IB2 and bulky IIA cervical cancer should be treated initially with chemoradiation therapy instead of radical hysterectomy. Others argue that treatment decisions should not be based on tumor size alone, because some studies have demonstrated that significant independent predictors of disease-free survival are lymphovascular space involvement and outer two-thirds depth of invasion. GOG attempted to compare chemoradiation therapy with radical hysterectomy followed by chemoradiation therapy for bulky stage IB2 cervical cancer, but unfortunately, the trial closed prematurely due to poor accrual.

FIGURE 1: Relative risk estimate of survival from five phase III randomized, controlled clinical trials of chemoradiation therapy in women with cervical cancer. A relative risk of 1 indicates no difference in outcome between the treatment arms. A relative risk of < 1 indicates a benefit for the experimental treatment. A relative risk of 0.6, for example, indicates that the treatment has reduced the risk of death by 40%. The relative risks of survival for all five trials, with 90% confidence intervals shown, range from 0.70–0.50, indicating that the concurrent chemoradiation therapy decreased the risk of death by 30%–50% (Rose PG, Bundy BN: J Clin Oncol 20:891–893, 2002).

CHEMORADIATION THERAPY FOR LOCALLY ADVANCED DISEASE

The role of curative surgery diminishes once cervical cancer has spread beyond the confines of the cervix and vaginal fornices. Intracavitary irradiation for central pelvic disease and external-beam radiation therapy for lateral parametrial and pelvic nodal disease are typically combined to encompass the known patterns of disease spread with an appropriate radiation dose while sparing the bladder and rectum from receiving full doses. The addition of intracavitary irradiation to external-beam irradiation is associated with improved pelvic control and survival over external irradiation alone, as the combination can achieve high central doses of radiation.

Radiation techniques

Intracavitary brachytherapy Radioactive isotopes, such as cesium-137, can be introduced directly into the uterine cavity and vaginal fornices with special applicators. The most commonly used applicator is the Fletcher-Suit intrauterine tandem and vaginal ovoids.

Calculating dose rates With the advent of computerized dosimetry, the dose rate to a number of points from a particular source arrangement can be calculated. Adjustments in the strength or positioning of the sources can then be made to yield a selected dose rate to one or more points.

Quantification of acceptable implant geometry has been described by Katz and Eifel after review of 808 implants performed in 396 patients with cervical cancer treated with irradiation at M. D. Anderson Cancer Center. These guidelines set the standard for high-quality tandem and ovoid insertions.

Points of interest usually include the maximal rectal and bladder dose, as well as the dose to three standard pelvic points: A, B, and P (see Figure 2). Point A is located 2 cm cephalad from the cervical os and 2 cm lateral to the uterine canal. Anatomically, it represents the medial parametrium/lateral cervix, the approximate point at which the ureter and uterine artery cross. Point B is 5 cm lateral to the center of the pelvis at the same level as point A and approximates the region of the obturator nodes or lateral parametrium. Point P is located along the bony pelvic sidewall at its most lateral point and represents the minimal dose to the external iliac lymph nodes. Recent publications have advocated the use of imaging (CT or MRI) to delineate tumor/target volumes and to specify more precisely the doses of brachytherapy administered to patients with carcinoma of the cervix (Potter et al).

LDR vs HDR brachytherapy Standard dose rates at point A are typically 50–70 cGy/h; this level is considered low-dose-rate (LDR) brachytherapy. The applicator is placed into the uterus while the patient is under anesthesia in the operating room, and the patient must stay in the hospital for 2–3 days during the procedure. One or two implants are usually placed. Despite the fact that two insertions may allow time for regression of disease between placements, there are no data indicating that two insertions improve pelvic control or survival rates over one insertion.

Whereas LDR brachytherapy has been used successfully for decades in the treatment of carcinoma of the cervix, the use of high-dose-rate (HDR) brachytherapy has been increasing in the United States over the past decade. Dose rates are typically 200–300 cGy/min, with short treatment times allowing for stable position of the applicator.

The major benefit of HDR brachytherapy is that the procedure can be performed on an outpatient basis with less radiation exposure to personnel. The major disadvantage is biologic: large single fractions of radiation (5–10 Gy) are used with 3–10 insertions per patient, which may increase the rate of late complications.

Several series have cited comparable disease control and complication rates with HDR and LDR brachytherapy. A total of 237 patients with previously untreated invasive cervical cancer were enrolled into one randomized study to compare the clinical outcome between HDR and LDR intracavitary brachytherapy. The median follow-up for LDR and HDR groups was 40.2 and 37.2 months, respectively. The 3-year overall and relapse-free survival rates for all patients were 69.6% and 70.0%. There was no significant difference in the

FIGURE 2: Gynecologic Oncology Group (GOG) definitions of points A, B, and P.

following clinical parameters between LDR and HDR groups: the 3-year overall survival rate was 70.9% and 68.4% ($P = .75$), the 3-year pelvic control rate was 89.1% and 86.4% ($P = .51$), and the 3-year relapse-free survival rate in both groups was 69.9% ($P = .35$). Considering patient convenience, the small number of medical personnel needed, and the decreased radiation exposure to health care workers, HDR intracavitary brachytherapy is an alternative to conventional LDR brachytherapy. HDR brachytherapy is an alternative to LDR brachytherapy in current GOG and Radiation Therapy Oncology Group (RTOG) advanced cervical cancer trials.

Guidelines have been published for HDR brachytherapy for cervical cancer by the American Brachytherapy Society (see Suggested Reading).

External-beam pelvic radiation therapy is used in conjunction with intracavitary radiotherapy for stage IA2 disease and above when the risk of pelvic lymph node involvement is significant. The amount of external-beam irradiation delivered and the timing of its administration relative to intracavitary radiation

TABLE 2: Relationship between tumor size and outcome in patients with tumors ≥ 5 cm treated with irradiation alone[a]

Tumor size (cm)	Number of patients	Central pelvic control rate (%)	Total pelvic control rate (%)	DSS (%)
5-5.9	200	93	85	69
6-6.9	99	92	79	69
7-7.9	55	90	81	58
≥ 8	48	69	57	40

[a]Excludes patients who underwent adjuvant hysterectomy   DSS = disease-specific survival

are individualized. For example, the presence of a large exophytic cancer that distorts the cervix would initially preclude successful placement of intracavitary brachytherapy. External-beam radiotherapy would be administered first, and after significant regression of disease, it could be followed by intracavitary radiotherapy.

Various techniques have been developed to optimize external-beam irradiation, including CT simulation, conformal blocking, and, more recently, intensity-modulated radiation therapy (IMRT). These techniques reduce the volume of normal tissue having full-dose irradiation while coverage of the target is not compromised.

Several preliminary reports have been published describing highly conformal dose distributions for patients with carcinoma of the cervix in IMRT. Tumor control has been about 80% for various stages, and no patient has developed > grade 2 GI or genitourinary toxicity.

Advanced tumors require relatively more external irradiation due to the inability of central radioisotope sources to effectively irradiate disease in the lateral parametrium. Typically, external pelvic doses of 4,000–5,000 cGy are followed by 4,000–5,000 cGy to point A with intracavitary LDR brachytherapy, for a total dose of 8,000–9,000 cGy to point A. A parametrial boost completes treatment to the lateral pelvis, for a total dose to point B or P of 6,000 cGy from external-beam irradiation and brachytherapy, depending on the extent of disease.

With HDR brachytherapy, equivalent doses are prescribed using the linear quadratic equation. The HDR/LDR dose ratio ranges from .5 to .8 depending on the number of HDR fractions.

External-beam para-aortic radiation therapy may be used in addition to external-beam pelvic irradiation when para-aortic disease is confirmed or suspected. An RTOG trial found that external-beam para-aortic irradiation conferred a survival benefit in patients with advanced cervical cancer (stage IB > 4 cm, stage IIA, and stage IIB) over external-beam pelvic therapy alone. Although external-beam radiation therapy can successfully sterilize microscopic disease,

FIGURE 3: Top – Kaplan-Meier estimates of overall survival for patients who received extended-field radiotherapy (EFRT) or concurrent chemotherapy and radiotherapy (CT-RT; *P* < .0001). **Bottom** – Kaplan-Meier estimates of overall survival for patients who received EFRT or CT-RT in subgroups stratified by International Federation of Gynecology and Obstetrics stage (*P* < .0001).

its value in the treatment of gross para-aortic disease is limited, as the tolerance of surrounding organs (bowel, kidneys, spinal cord) precludes the delivery of sufficiently high doses to the para-aortic region.

In multivariate analysis, treatment factors associated with improved pelvic control for cervical cancer include the use of intracavitary brachytherapy, total point A dose > 8,500 cGy (stage III only), and overall treatment time < 8 weeks.

Definitive radiation therapy

CIS, stage IA disease Carcinoma in situ (CIS) and microinvasive cervical cancer (stage IA) are not associated with lymph node metastases. Therefore, intracavitary LDR brachytherapy alone, delivering approximately 5,500 cGy to point A, can control 100% of CIS and stage IA disease and is an acceptable alternative to surgery for patients who cannot undergo surgery due to their medical condition.

> RTOG 90-01 enrolled 390 patients with locally advanced cervical cancer. Extended-field radiotherapy (EFRT) was compared with pelvic radiotherapy and concomitant fluorouracil and cisplatin (CTRT). The median follow-up time for 228 surviving patients was 6.6 years. The overall survival rate for patients treated with CTRT was significantly greater than that for patients treated with EFRT (67% vs 41% at 8 years; *P* < .001). There was an overall reduction in the risk of disease recurrence of 51% for patients who received CTRT. The addition of fluorouracil and cisplatin to radiotherapy significantly improves the survival rate of women with locally advanced cervical cancer without increasing the rate of late treatment-related side effects (*Eifel PJ, Winter K, Morris M, et al: J Clin Oncol 22:872-880, 2004*).

Stage IB disease The most important prognostic factor associated with pelvic tumor control and survival following radiation therapy for stage IB cervical cancer is tumor size. The central pelvic control rate with radiotherapy alone is excellent for tumors < 8 cm (97%), with total pelvic control and survival rates of 93% and 82%, respectively. Therefore, many experts have argued that adjuvant hysterectomy following chemoradiation therapy is unnecessary for cervical cancer < 8 cm. For bulky cervical cancers ≥ 8 cm, pelvic control and survival rates decrease to 57% and 40%, respectively, with irradiation alone, and adjuvant hysterectomy may potentially improve local control and survival rates (Table 2).

An updated RTOG trial (RTOG 90-01) for advanced cervical cancer (stage IB or IIA with tumor ≥ 5 cm or with biopsy-proven pelvic lymph node involvement and stages IIB–IVA disease) compared external-beam pelvic irradiation plus concurrent fluorouracil (5-FU) and cisplatin with external-beam pelvic and para-aortic irradiation; in both arms, these therapies were followed by intracavitary irradiation. The addition of chemotherapy to irradiation improved 5-year survival from 55% to 79% and disease-free survival from 46% to 74% for stage IB/IIA disease by reducing the rates of both local recurrence and distant metastases. For stage III/IVA disease, chemoradiotherapy improved 5-year survival from 45% to 59% and disease-free survival from 37% to 54% (Figures 1 and 3).

GOG 123 randomized patients with stage IB bulky cervical cancer to receive either local treatment alone (external and intracavitary irradiation followed by hysterectomy) or local therapy plus weekly cisplatin. The combination of concurrent weekly cisplatin and irradiation significantly reduced the relapse rate and improved survival by 50%. The 3-year survival rate was significantly improved from 74% to 83% with the use of chemotherapy; this improvement was primarily due to a reduced risk of local recurrence (21% vs 9%).

On the other hand, an Australian gynecologic group randomized study with 76 patients and a Canadian randomized study with 127 patients with stages IB–IIB carcinoma of the cervix treated with chemotherapy and irradiation or irradiation alone showed no significant difference in tumor control or survival. A possible explanation for the discrepancy in the results between the five US trials and the National Cancer Institute (NCI) of Canada study has been analyzed by Lehman and Thomas. A review of 4,069 patients with invasive carcinoma of the cervix treated in Ontario, Canada, between 1992 and 2001 documented a significant increase in 3-year survival in patients treated with concurrent chemotherapy-radiotherapy (CT-RT) (75.9%) compared with those treated with irradiation alone (71.1%) (see Suggested Reading).

Current treatment recommendations Concurrent CT-RT (usually cisplatin-based) with or without adjuvant hysterectomy is standard treatment for bulky IB2 cervical cancer. An alternative approach is radical hysterectomy followed by tailored postoperative chemoradiation therapy.

The use of adjuvant hysterectomy is controversial for stage IB2 cervical cancer, since dose-intense external pelvic and intracavitary irradiation plus chemotherapy may obviate the need for adjuvant surgery. The GOG trial suggests that adjuvant hysterectomy reduces the recurrence rate but does not affect survival.

The use of weekly cisplatin for 6 cycles or 5-FU and cisplatin every 3 weeks × 2 cycles concurrently with radiotherapy is the standard treatment approach for bulky stage IB2 cervical cancer.

Stages IIA–IVA disease The most important prognostic factor associated with pelvic tumor control and survival is the bulk of pelvic disease within each stage. For stage IIB, bulky disease is variously defined as bilateral or lateral parametrial infiltration or central bulky disease > 4 cm. For stage IIIB, bulky disease is defined as bilateral sidewall involvement, lower-third vaginal involvement, or hydronephrosis.

In the previous GOG experience, in which para-aortic lymph node staging had been mandated, multivariate analysis testing revealed para-aortic lymph node involvement to be the most powerful negative prognostic factor, followed by pelvic lymph node involvement, larger tumor diameter, young age, advanced stage, and lower performance status for patients with negative para-aortic lymph nodes. Five-year survival rates for radiotherapy alone vary from 80% for stage I, 60% for stage II, and 45% for stage III disease, with corresponding pelvic control rates of 90%, 80%, and 50%, respectively.

Chemoradiation therapy A GOG phase III trial (GOG 120) compared standard pelvic external-beam irradiation/intracavitary brachytherapy plus hydroxyurea versus weekly cisplatin versus hydroxyurea, 5-FU, and cisplatin. Both the weekly cisplatin and the 5-FU–cisplatin–hydroxyurea arms produced significantly improved survival and relapse rates compared with hydroxyurea alone. Two-year disease progression-free survival rates were significantly improved from 47% to 67% and 64% with weekly cisplatin-irradiation and 5-FU–cisplatin–hydroxyurea–irradiation compared with hydroxyurea and radiotherapy (Figure 1). The improved outcome was due to the reduced rates of pelvic failure and lung metastases. Because of an improved therapeutic ratio, weekly cisplatin is the favored regimen. Updated results of this trial confirm the original observations.

A total of 294 patients with advanced cervical cancer were enrolled into a randomized phase III study to compare cisplatin and cisplatin + topotecan (Hycamtin). Patients receiving topotecan had statistically superior outcomes to those receiving cisplatin alone, with median overall survival of 9.4 and 6.5 months (P = .017), median PFS of 4.6 and 2.9 months (P = .014), and response rates of 27% and 13%, respectively (Long HJ 3rd, Bundy BN, Grendys EC Jr, et al: J Clin Oncol 23:4626-4633, 2005).

GOG 165 compared standard radiation therapy plus concurrent weekly cisplatin vs concurrent protracted venous infusion 5-FU (225 mg/m^2/d over 5 weeks) as radiation sensitizers. In this study, the dose of radiation to point A (in Figure 2) had been increased by 500 cGy, and the pelvic fields were redefined to improve the dose intensity and accuracy of radiotherapy. This recently reported study confirms the efficacy of pelvic radiotherapy with weekly cisplatin. The study was closed prematurely when a planned interim analysis indicated that the 5-FU arm had a 35% higher rate of treatment failure. An editorial published with the article highlighted the future difficulties with randomized trials for this population.

Current treatment recommendations In view of the multiple randomized trials documenting a survival benefit with concurrent CT-RT, the use of concurrent weekly cisplatin or cisplatin–5-FU every 3 weeks with irradiation is standard therapy for stages IB2–IVA cervical cancer (Figure 1).

Five of six large randomized clinical trials demonstrated a significant survival benefit for patients treated with concurrent CT-RT, using a cisplatin-based regimen, with a 28%–50% relative reduction in the risk of death. In addition, the results of a meta-analysis of 19 randomized clinical trials of concurrent CT-RT involving 4,580 patients showed that concurrent CT-RT significantly improved overall survival (hazard ratio [HR] = 0.71; $P < .001$), as well as disease progression-free survival (HR = 0.61; $P < .0001$). In line with these results, concurrent CT-RT is currently recommended as standard therapy (Table 3).

Based on the promising responses and acceptable toxicity reported in the phase I/II study, the current phase III GOG trial for advanced cervical cancer (stages IB2–IVA) is randomizing patients to undergo pelvic radiotherapy plus cisplatin weekly or pelvic radiotherapy, cisplatin, and tirapazamine (a hypoxic cell sensitizer).

For patients without para-aortic lymph node metastases, pelvic external irradiation (4,000–5,000 cGy) should be used, followed by intracavitary LDR brachytherapy (4,000–5,000 cGy) to point A, for a total dose of 8,000–9,000 cGy to point A.

Adjuvant radiotherapy following radical hysterectomy

Node-negative disease Local failure rates approach 20% following radical hysterectomy and pelvic lymphadenectomy when pelvic lymph nodes are not involved but the primary tumor has high-risk characteristics (primary tumor > 4 cm, outer-third cervical stromal invasion, and capillary-lymphatic space invasion). A GOG trial randomized these intermediate-risk patients with node-negative disease to receive pelvic external-beam radiation therapy (5,100 cGy/30 fractions) or no further therapy following radical hysterectomy-pelvic lymphadenectomy. Postoperative irradiation produced a significant 44% reduction in recurrence; the recurrence-free rate at 2 years was 88% with irradiation versus 79% without it. Survival analysis awaits further follow-up.

Node-positive disease For patients with positive pelvic lymph nodes following radical hysterectomy-pelvic lymphadenectomy, pelvic radiotherapy reduces the pelvic failure rate from approximately 50% to 25% but does not affect survival, since distant metastases are still seen in 30% of patients. A recently reported GOG/Southwest Oncology Group (SWOG 8797) trial randomized these high-risk patients with node-positive disease (or patients with positive surgical margins) to undergo pelvic external-beam irradiation (4,930 cGy/29 fractions) versus pelvic external-beam irradiation plus concurrent 5-FU and cisplatin for 4 cycles following radical hysterectomy-pelvic lymphadenectomy. A significant improvement in disease progression-free and overall survival was seen for concurrent 5-FU–cisplatin and radiation therapy compared with radiation therapy alone (4-year survival, 81% vs 71%).

Current treatment recommendations At present, the use of adjuvant pelvic radiotherapy should be considered for patients with negative nodes who are at risk for pelvic failure and remains the standard postoperative treatment for patients with positive lymph nodes. Treatment consists of external pelvic irradiation (45–50 Gy), with specific sites boosted with further external-beam or intracavitary irradiation as needed.

A prospective study comparing the accuracy of PET scan with that of CT and/or MRI scans has been presented. Eighteen patients underwent PET scans with CT or MRI scans prior to surgical exploration for pelvic exenteration. PET scan was reported to be the most accurate method of detecting extrapelvic metastasis, with a sensitivity of 100% and a specificity of 73% (*Husain A, Akhurst T, Larson S, et al: Gynecol Oncol* 106:177-180, 2007).

Since the combination of radical surgery and irradiation has greater morbidity than either modality alone, complete preoperative assessment is crucial to minimize the need for both.

Since concurrent CT-RT following radical hysterectomy provides a significant benefit in node-positive high-risk cervical cancer, it should be part of the postoperative treatment plan. Postoperative CT-RT following radical hysterectomy should be strongly considered for patients with negative nodes but positive margins or parametria, ≥ middle-third stro-

TABLE 3: Large randomized studies of concurrent chemoradiotherapy in cervical cancer

Author	Stage	Design	RT	CT (mg/m², except for HU)	No. of patients	Survival (%) CT/RT vs RT(follow-up)	P value
Whitney, GOG 85, 1999	IIB-IVA PAN(-), Washing cytology (-)	WP+PF × 3 vs WP+HU+PAN	IIB:40 Gy+Ra; III, IVA: WP, 51 Gy+Ra; III, IV: 61 Gy	P:50/day 1; F:1,000/days 2-5, every 4 weeks; HU:80 mg/kg/twice a week	388	55 vs 43 (8.7 years)	.018
Rose, GOG 120, 1999	IIIB-IVA, PAN(-)	WP+P weekly vs WP+PF+HU vs WP+HU	IIB: 40 Gy+Ra; III, IVA: WP, 51 Gy +Ra; III, IV: 61 Gy	P:40/week for 4 weeks vs P: 50/day 1+F:1,000/days 1-4 Hu:2,000/0/week, every 4 weeks vs HU:3,000/2/week of 6 weeks	176	66 vs 67 vs 50 (3 years); 8 vs 71 (4 years)	.0040 / .002
Keys GOG 123, 1999	IB ≥ 4 cm	WP+P weekly vs WP Adj TAH	WP:45 Gy + Ra	P:40/week for 6 weeks	369	83 vs 74 (3 years)	.008
Peters SWOG 8797, 2000	IA2-IIA Postsurgical pN1/pT2b/ stump(+)	WP+PF × 4 vs WP + PAN	WP:45 Gy WP+PAN	P:70/day 1 + F: 1,000/days 1-4, every 3 weeks	268	81 vs 71 (4 years)	.007
Pearcey NCI, Canada 2002	IB-IVA > 5 cm or pelvic LN (+)	WP+P weekly vs WP	WP 45 Gy + Ra	P:40 mg/m²	259	62 vs 58 (5 years)	.42
Eifel RTOG 90-01, 2004	IB-IVA > 5cm PAN(-)	WP+PF × 3 vs WP+PAN	WP: 45 Gy PAN:45 Gy	P:75/day 1F:1,000/days 2-5, every 3 weeks	403	67 vs 41 (8 years)	.0001

CT = chemotherapy; RT = radiotherapy; WP = whole pelvis; PAN = para-aortic lymph node; Adj = adjuvant; TAH = total abdominal hysterectomy; P = Platinol (cisplatin); F = 5-FU; Ra = radium therapy; HU = hydroxyurea; LN = lymph node
Adapted with permission from Kuzuya K: Chemotherapy for uterine cancer: Current status and perspective. Int J Clin Oncol 9:458–470, 2005.

mal invasion, and lymphovascular space invasion for tumors ≥ 5 cm.

SURGICAL MANAGEMENT OF RECURRENT OR METASTATIC DISEASE

Recurrent advanced disease

Pelvic exenteration For patients whose disease fails to respond to primary radiation therapy or for those with early invasive cervical carcinoma whose disease recurs after surgery or radiation therapy, pelvic exenteration offers the possibility of cure. Patients should be considered for pelvic exenteration only if they have locoregional disease that can be completely removed by this radical surgical procedure. In most cases, patients will require surgical removal of the bladder, uterus, cervix, vagina, and rectum.

Of all patients who are considered candidates for pelvic exenteration, only about half will be found to have resectable disease at the time of exploratory laparotomy. For patients who successfully undergo pelvic exenteration, 5-year survival rates range from 25% to 50%.

When the patient has central recurrence of squamous cell or adenocarcinoma of the cervix, the initial evaluation includes a complete physical examination, as well as a CT, MRI, or PET/CT scan.

Evidence of extrapelvic disease is a contraindication to pelvic exenteration. If no evidence of disease beyond the pelvis is found, the patient can be prepared for pelvic exenteration.

Preparation for exenteration includes complete bowel preparation, a visit with the stomal therapy nurse, and counseling regarding the radical nature of the surgery and the anticipated changes in body image after the operation. In most cases, we counsel the patient that vaginal reconstruction should be performed at the time of pelvic exenteration, both for maintenance of body image and improved healing.

Surgical procedure During surgery, a careful exploration is carried out to confirm that there is no evidence of unresectable disease beyond the pelvis. The pelvic sidewall spaces are opened and resectability is determined. An en bloc resection is usually performed; in some cases, especially when the recurrent tumor involves the lower vagina, a two-team approach can expedite the procedure. The actual exenterative portion of the procedure may take several hours and is usually accompanied by significant blood loss. In cases where surgical margin status may be questionable, the use of intraoperative radiation therapy is considered.

Reconstruction Following the exenterative procedure, the reconstructive portion of the procedure begins. We currently recommend to nearly all patients that they consider a continent urinary diversion. Although this step may add approximately 30–60 minutes to the surgical procedure, the improvement in quality of life is significant.

In patients who have undergone a supralevator pelvic exenteration, we frequently attempt a stapled reanastomosis of the colon. Unless there is excessive tension

TABLE 4: Active agents as defined by a response rate of at least 15%

Drug	No. of Patients	Responses	Response rate
Alkylating agents			
CCNU	5	1	20%
Chlorambucil	44	11	25%
Cyclophosphamide	251	38	15%
Dibromodulcitol	120	23	23%
Galactitol	36	7	19%
Ifosfamide	157	35	22%
Melphalan	20	4	20%
Heavy metal complexes			
Carboplatin	175	27	15%
Cisplatin	815	190	23%
Antibiotics			
Doxorubicin	266	45	17%
Mitomycin	18	4	22%
Porfiromycin	78	17	22%
Antimetabolites			
Baker's antifol	32	5	16%
5-Fluorouracil	142	29	20%
Methotrexate	96	17	18%
Plant alkaloids			
Vincristine	55	10	18%
Vindesine	21	5	24%
Vinorelbine	42	6	15%
Other agents			
Irinotecan	55	13	24%
Hexamethylmelamine	64	12	19%
ICRF-159	28	5	18%
Paclitaxel	52	9	17%
Teniposide	32	7	22%
Topotecan	43	8	19%

Adapted with permission from Thigpen T: The role of chemotherapy in the management of carcinoma of the cervix. Cancer J 9:425–432, 2003.

on the anastomosis or other problems, a diverting colostomy is not routinely indicated. About one-third of these patients suffer anastomotic breakdown in the postoperative period. At that time, a diverting colostomy can be performed. Unfortunately, Hatch et al found no benefit to the earlier use of colostomy.

Lung metastasis

For the rare patient who presents with a single isolated lung metastasis after treatment of invasive cervical carcinoma, pulmonary resection may offer the possibility of long-term disease-free survival or even cure in selected cases. For patients who have multiple lung metastases or unresectable pelvic disease, surgery offers little or no hope and produces significant morbidity and mortality.

THERAPY FOR RECURRENT OR METASTATIC DISEASE

Local recurrence after radical hysterectomy

Local recurrence confined to the pelvis following radical hysterectomy for cervical cancer can be treated with radiotherapy with curative intent. An experience with 5-FU–based chemotherapy and concurrent pelvic external-beam irradiation resulted in a 58% complete response rate and a 45% no-evidence-of-disease rate, at a median follow-up of 57 months. The total pelvic external-beam dose was 5,280 cGy plus a boost to sites of recurrence with twice-daily 160-cGy fractions during the 5-FU infusion. Therefore, radiotherapy, with or without chemotherapy, can provide durable local control, with better results attainable for small, central recurrences, for which brachytherapy is possible.

Local recurrence after definitive radiation therapy

Local recurrence confined to the pelvis following definitive radiation therapy rarely can be cured with exenteration. In a series of patients treated with definitive radiotherapy, 21% of recurrences (80 of 376) were isolated to the pelvis. Only 29% of these localized pelvic recurrences (23 of 80) were explored for curative exenteration, and for the 43% of patients (10 of 23) deemed operable, the 5-year survival rate was 16%.

Palliation of metastatic disease

Palliative radiation therapy to sites of metastatic cervical cancer is effective. The most common sites of metastasis are distant lymph nodes, bone, and lungs. Reirradiation of the pelvis is possible in selected patients to control local symptoms, such as bleeding, but carries an increased risk of bowel complications. For previously unirradiated sites of metastatic disease, 3,000 cGy in 10 fractions provides palliation of symptoms in the majority of patients.

CHEMOTHERAPY FOR ADVANCED/RECURRENT DISEASE

Chemotherapy has traditionally been used for the palliative management of advanced or recurrent disease that can no longer be managed by surgery or

TABLE 5: Combination chemotherapy for advanced or recurrent cervical carcinoma

Chemotherapy regimen	Number of patients	Overall response rate (%)
Doublets		
Cisplatin/5-FU	72	48
	32	47
	55	22
Cisplatin/gemcitabine	40	95
	40	75
Cisplatin/topotecan	32	28
Cisplatin/vinorelbine	67	30
	49	64
Cisplatin/paclitaxel	41	46
	34	47
Cisplatin/ifosfamide	30	50
	42	38
Cisplatin/irinotecan	29	59
	27	37
Cisplatin/bleomycin	24	54
Cisplatin/mitomycin	33	42
Cisplatin/tirapazamine	36	28
Carboplatin/paclitaxel	25	40
Carboplatin/ifosfamide	32	59
Triplets		
Bleomycin/cisplatin/ifosfamide	49	69
Bleomycin/carboplatin/ifosfamide	35	60
Paclitaxel/cisplatin/ifosfamide	45	67
	57	46
	45	47
Paclitaxel/cisplatin/5-FU	60	65
Ifosfamide/cisplatin/5-FU	30	53
Ifosfamide/cisplatin/mitomycin	44	34
Ifosfamide/leucovorin/5-FU	30	53
Vinblastine/bleomycin/cisplatin	33	66
Quartlets		
Bleomycin/vincristine/cisplatin/mitomycin	20	72
	90	76
Methotrexate/vinblastine/doxorubicin/cisplatin	29	66
	27	52

5-FU = fluorouracil

Modified from Cadron I, Leunen K, Amant F, et al: Gynecol Oncol 106:354–361, 2007; Long HJ 3rd: J Clin Oncol 25:2966–2974, 2007.

TABLE 6: Phase III clinical trials in advanced or recurrent cervical cancer

Protocol	Regimen	N	Response rate	PFS (months)	OS (months)
GOG	Cisplatin (50 mg/m²/d1)	150	21	3.7	7.1
	Cisplatin (20 mg/m²/d1-5)	128	25	3.9	6.1
	Cisplatin (100 mg/m²/d1)	166	31	4.6	7.0
GOG-110	Cisplatin	140	18	3.2	8.0
	Cisplatin/Mitolactol	147	21	3.3	7.3
	Cisplatin/Ifosfamide	151	31	4.6	8.3
GOG-149	Cisplatin/Ifosfamide	146	31	4.6	8.5
	Bleomycin/Ifosfamide/ Cisplatin	141	31	5.1	8.4
GOG-169	Cisplatin	134	19	2.8	8.8
	Cisplatin/Paclitaxel	130	36	4.8	9.7
GOG-179	Cisplatin	146	13	2.9	6.5
	Cisplatin/Topotecan	147	27	4.6	9.4

PFS = progression-free survival; OS = overall survival

Modified from Cadron I, Leunen K, Amant F, et al: Gynecol Oncol 106:354–361, 2007; Long HJ 3rd: J Clin Oncol 25:2966–2974, 2007.

radiation therapy (see Table 3). Various factors complicate the use of chemotherapy in such patients, however. Prior radiation treatment can affect the blood supply to the involved field, which may result in decreased drug delivery to the tumor site. Pelvic irradiation also reduces bone marrow reserve, thus limiting the tolerable doses of most chemotherapeutic agents. Moreover, irradiation may produce its cytotoxic effect, in part, through a mechanism similar to that of alkylating agents; thus, it is thought to be cross-resistant with some chemotherapeutic agents. A significant number of patients with advanced disease may also have impaired renal function, further limiting the use of certain chemotherapeutic regimens.

Single agents

Among the chemotherapeutic agents used for cervical cancer, cisplatin and ifosfamide (Ifex) have shown the most consistent activity as single agents (Table 4). The duration of response with any single agent is brief, ranging from 4 to 6 months, with survival ranging from 6 to 9 months.

Cisplatin has been the most extensively evaluated single agent for cervical carcinoma. A dose of 100 mg/m² was shown to have a higher response rate than a dose of 50 mg/m² (31% vs 21%), but the higher dose was associated with increased toxicity, and overall survival did not differ significantly between the two groups. A 24-hour infusion of cisplatin was tolerated better than a 2-hour infusion, with no difference in therapeutic efficacy.

Ifosfamide produces response rates ranging from 33% to 50% in various dose schedules. A dose of 1.5 g/m² over 30 minutes for 5 days (with mesna [Mesnex]) produced an overall response rate of 40% and a complete response rate of 20%.

Lower response rates are generally seen in patients who have had prior chemotherapy. Responses also are decreased in previously irradiated sites.

Taxanes Paclitaxel and docetaxel (Taxotere) have been reported to be active in cervical cancer. A study of paclitaxel (170 mg/m² over 24 hours) showed an objective response rate of 17%, and another study of paclitaxel (250 mg/m² over 3 hours) demonstrated an objective response rate of 27%. Docetaxel (100 mg/m² over 1 hour) has yielded a response rate of 19%.

Camptothecins Irinotecan (CPT-11 [Camptosar]) and topotecan (Hycamtin), semisynthetic camptothecins, have shown activity in patients with cervical cancer, even in patients who did not respond to prior chemotherapy and prior radiation therapy. The reported objective response rates were 21% and 19%, respectively.

Combination regimens

Various combination chemotherapy regimens have been evaluated in phase II trials, and high response rates (> 50%) were noted, even in patients who had received prior radiation therapy. The results of some of these trials are summarized in Tables 5 and 6. In one study, a subset analysis showed a response rate of 72% with the combination of bleomycin, ifosfamide, and cisplatin as treatment for tumors located in previously irradiated sites. Neoadjuvant regimens of cisplatin combined with gemcitabine (Gemzar) in patients with locally advanced cervical cancer demonstrated very high activity, with a clinical response rate of 95%. Neoadjuvant ifosfamide and cisplatin, with or without paclitaxel, produced 87% and 82% response rates, respectively, among 146 evaluable patients in a randomized study.

A randomized trial was reported by Long et al. A total of 146 patients with advanced persistent or recurrent cervical cancer were treated with cisplatin (50 mg/m² IV every 21 days), and 147 patients were treated with topotecan (.75 mg/m² IV during 30 minutes on days 1, 2, and 3 followed by cisplatin (50 mg/m² on day 1) repeated every 21 days. All regimens were administered for a maximum of 6 cycles for nonresponders or until disease progression or unacceptable toxicity prohibited additional chemotherapy. The complete response rate was 3% for cisplatin and 10% for the cisplatin-topotecan combination, and the complete and partial remission rates were 13% and 27%, respectively; the median progression-free survival was 2.9 and 4.6 months, respectively. Chemotherapy remains palliative, with no longevity prolongation of survival in recurrent or metastatic disease.

Palliative care

Palliation of the dying cervical cancer patient is difficult. Pain due to recurrent pelvic disease can be extreme and requires skillful use of combinations of narcotics, sedatives, and anxiolytics. Fistula from the bladder or rectum demands meticulous local skin care and occasionally surgical diversion procedures in patients with reasonable expected longevity. This patient population often has limited resources, with dependent children requiring careful social service planning. A small percentage has concurrent HIV infection, making the infectious disease specialist part of the palliative care team. The tripod of care in advanced cervical cancer is the judicious use of chemotherapy and radiation therapy, palliation of the symptoms of advancing disease, as well as emotional and social support for the patient and family members.

SUGGESTED READING

Cadron I, Van Gorp T, Amant F, et al: Chemotherapy for recurrent cervical cancer. Gynecol Oncol 107:S113–S118, 2007.

Choi CH, Kim TJ, Lee SJ, et al: Salvage chemotherapy with a combination of paclitaxel, ifosfamide, and cisplatin for the patients with recurrent carcinoma of the uterine cervix. Int J Gynecol Cancer 16:1157–1164, 2006.

Chou HH, Chang TC, Yen TC, et al: Low value of [18F]-fluoro-2-deoxy-D-glucose positron emission tomography in primary staging of early-stage cervical cancer before radical hysterectomy. J Clin Oncol 24:123–128, 2006.

Eifel PJ, Gershenson DM, Kavanagh JJ, et al: M.D. Anderson Cancer Care Series: Gynecologic Cancer. New York: Springer; 2006.

Eifel PJ, Winter K, Morris M, et al: Pelvic irradiation with concurrent chemotherapy versus pelvic and para-aortic irradiation for high-risk cervical cancer: An update of Radiation Therapy Oncology Group trial (RTOG) 90-01. J Clin Oncol 22:872–880, 2004.

FUTURE II Study Group: Quadrivalent vaccine against human papillomavirus to prevent high-grade cervical lesions. N Engl J Med 356:1915–1927, 2007.

Garland SM, Hernandez-Avila M, Wheeler CM, et al: Quadrivalent vaccine against human papillomavirus to prevent anogenital diseases. N Engl J Med 356:1928–1943, 2007.

Grigsby PW, Siegel BA, Dehdashti F, et al: Posttherapy [18F] fluorodeoxyglucose positron emission tomography in carcinoma of the cervix: Response and outcome. J Clin Oncol 22:2167–2171, 2004.

Grigsby PW, Siegel BA, Dehdashti F, et al: Posttherapy surveillance monitoring of cervical cancer by FDG-PET. Int J Radiat Oncol Biol Phys 55:907–913, 2003.

Husain A, Akhurst T, Larson S, et al: A prospective study of the accuracy of 18Fluorodeoxyglucose positron emission tomography (18FDG PET) in identifying sites of metastasis prior to pelvic exenteration. Gynecol Oncol 106:177–180, 2007.

Keys HM, Bundy BN, Stehman FB, et al: Radiation therapy with and without extrafascial hysterectomy for bulky stage IB cervical carcinoma: A randomized trial of the Gynecologic Oncology Group. Gynecol Oncol 89:343–353, 2003.

Kochanski JD, Roeske JC, Mell LK, et al: Outcome of FIGO stage I-II cervical cancer patients treated with intensity modulated pelvic radiation therapy [abstract]. Proc Am Soc Clin Oncol 23:454, 2004.

Kuzuya K: Chemoradiotherapy for uterine cancer: Current status and perspectives. Int J Clin Oncol 9:458–470, 2004.

Lai CH, Chang CJ, Huang HJ, et al: Role of human papillomavirus genotype in prognosis of early-stage cervical cancer undergoing primary surgery. J Clin Oncol 25:3628–3634, 2007.

Lanciano R, Calkins A, Bundy BN, et al: Randomized comparison of weekly cisplatin or protracted venous infusion of fluorouracil in combination with pelvic radiation in advanced cervix cancer: A Gynecologic Oncology Group Study. J Clin Oncol 23:8289–8294, 2005.

Long HJ 3rd: Management of metastatic cervical cancer: Review of the literature. J Clin Oncol 25:2966–2974, 2007.

Long HJ 3rd, Bundy BN, Grendys EC Jr, et al: Randomized phase III trial of cisplatin with or without topotecan in carcinoma of the uterine cervix: A Gynecologic Oncology Group Study. J Clin Oncol 23:4626–4633, 2005.

Maluf FC, Leiser AL, Aghajanian C, et al: Phase II study of tirapazamine plus cisplatin in patients with advanced or recurrent cervical cancer. Int J Gynecol Cancer 16:1165–1171, 2006.

Mitchell DG, Snyder B, Coakley F, et al: Early invasive cervical cancer: Tumor delineation by magnetic resonance imaging, computed tomography, and clinical examination, verified by pathological results, in the ACRIN 6651/GOG 183 Intergroup Study. J Clin Oncol 24:5687–5694, 2006.

Monk BJ, Huang HQ, Cella D, et al: Quality of life outcomes from a randomized phase III trial of cisplatin with or without topotecan in advanced carcinoma of the cervix: A Gynecologic Oncology Group Study. J Clin Oncol 23:4617–4625, 2005.

Moore D, Blessing J, McQuellon R, et al: Phase III study of cisplatin with or without paclitaxel in stage IVB, recurrent, or persistent squamous cell carcinoma of the cervix: A Gynecologic Oncology Group study. J Clin Oncol 222:3113–3119, 2004.

Nagao S, Fujiwara K, Oda T, et al: Combination chemotherapy of docetaxel and carboplatin in advanced or recurrent cervix cancer: A pilot study. Gynecol Oncol 96:805–809, 2005.

Odicino F, Pecorelli S, Zigliani L, et al: History of the FIGO cancer staging system. Int J Gynaecol Obstet 101:205–210, 2008.

Pearcey R, Miao Q, Kong W, et al: Impact of adoption of chemoradiotherapy on the outcome of cervical cancer in Ontario: Results of a population-based cohort study. J Clin Oncol 25:2383–2388, 2007.

Potter R, Haie-Meder C, Van Limbergen E, et al: Recommendations from gynaecological (GYN) GEC ESTRO working group (II): Concepts and terms in 3D image-based treatment planning in cervix brachytherapy-3D dose volume parameters and aspects of 3D image-based anatomy, radiation physics, radiobiology. Radiother Oncol 78:67–77, 2006.

Rose PG, Ali S, Watkins E, et al: Long-term follow-up of a randomized trial comparing concurrent single agent cisplatin, cisplatin-based combination chemotherapy, or hydroxyurea during pelvic irradiation for locally advanced cervical cancer: A Gynecologic Oncology Group Study. J Clin Oncol 25:2804–2810, 2007.

Rotman M, Sedlis A, Piedmonte MR, et al: A phase III randomized trial of postoperative pelvic irradiation in stage IB cervical carcinoma with poor prognostic features: Follow-up of a Gynecologic Oncology Group Study. Int J Radiat Oncol Biol Phys 65:169–176, 2006.

Sherris J, Castro W, Levin C, et al for The Alliance for Cervical Cancer Prevention: *The Case for Investing in Cervical Cancer Prevention,* Cervical Cancer Prevention Issues in Depth, No. 3. Seattle, ACCP, 2004.

Thigpen T: The role of chemotherapy in the management of carcinoma of the cervix. Cancer J 9:425–432, 2003.

Tierney J: Neoadjuvant chemotherapy for locally advanced cervical cancer: A systematic review and meta-analysis of individual patient data from 21 randomized trials. Eur J Cancer 39:2470–2486, 2003.

The authors would like to thank Dr. Xipeng Wang, Dr. Hye-Sook Chon, Dr. Xi Cheng, and Lora Lothringer for their assistance.

CHAPTER 21

Uterine corpus tumors

Kathryn M. Greven, MD, Maurie Markman, MD, and David Scott Miller, MD

ENDOMETRIAL CANCER

Carcinoma of the epithelial lining (endometrium) of the uterine corpus is the most common female pelvic malignancy. Factors influencing its prominence are the declining incidence of cervical cancer, longer life expectancy, and earlier diagnosis. Adenocarcinoma of the endometrium, the most prevalent histologic subtype, is currently the fourth most common cancer in women, with 39,080 new cases, ranking behind breast, lung, and bowel cancers. Endometrial adenocarcinoma is the eighth leading cause of death from malignancy in women, accounting for 7,400 deaths this year.

Epidemiology

Age Endometrial cancer is primarily a disease of postmenopausal women, although 25% of cases occur in premenopausal patients, with 5% of cases developing in patients < 40 years old.

Geography The incidence of endometrial cancer is higher in Western nations and very low in Eastern countries.

Immigrant populations tend to assume the risks of native populations, highlighting the importance of environmental factors in the genesis of this disease. Endometrial cancers tend to be more common in urban than in rural residents. In the United States, white women have a twofold higher incidence of endometrial cancer than black women.

Etiology and risk factors

Adenocarcinoma of the endometrium may arise in normal, atrophic, or hyperplastic endometrium. Two mechanisms are generally believed to be involved in the development of endometrial cancer. In approximately 75% of women, there is a history of exposure to unopposed estrogen, either endogenous or exogenous (type I). The tumors in these women begin as endometrial hyperplasia and progress to carcinomas, which usually are better differentiated and have a favorable prognosis.

In the other 25% of women, carcinomas appear spontaneously, are not clearly related to a transition from atypical hyperplasia, and rather arise in a background of atrophic or inert endometrium. These neoplasms tend to be associated with a more undifferentiated cell type and a poorer prognosis (type II).

Unopposed estrogen It has been hypothesized that long-term estrogenic stimulation of the endometrium unmodified by progesterone has a role in the development of endometrial carcinoma. This hypothesis derives from observations that women who are infertile or obese or who have dysfunctional bleeding due to anovulation are at high risk for this disease, as are women with estrogen-secreting granulosa theca cell ovarian tumors. Also, the recognition that atypical adenomatous (complex) hyperplasia is a precursor of cancer, and that it is associated with unopposed estrogen use in women, underscores the importance of the association among risk factors, estrogens, and cancer. In the late 1970s and early 1980s, several case-control studies demonstrated that the risk of endometrial cancer is increased 4- to 15-fold in long-term estrogen users, as compared with age-matched controls.

It is well established that past use of oral contraceptives (OCs) protects against endometrial cancer. Maxwell et al found that the use of OCs with either high-potency progestin (odds ratio [OR] for endometrial cancer = 0.21; 95% confidence interval [CI] = 0.10–0.43) or with low-potency progestin (OR = 0.39; 95% CI = 0.25–0.60) was associated with a decreased risk of endometrial cancer. Overall high-progestin potency OCs did not confer significantly more protection than low-progestin potency OCs (OR = 0.52; 95% CI = 0.24–1.14). However, among women with a body mass index (BMI) of at least 22.1 kg/m^2, those who used high-progestin potency OCs had a lower risk of endometrial cancer than those who used low-progestin potency OCs (OR = 0.31; 95% CI = 0.11–0.92), whereas those with a BMI below 22.1 kg/m^2 did not (OR = 1.36; 95% CI = 0.39–4.70). The potency of the progestin in most OCs appears adequate to provide a protective effect against endometrial cancer. Higher progestin-potency OCs may be more protective than lower progestin-potency OCs among women with a larger body habitus.

Diet The high rate of occurrence of endometrial cancer in Western societies and the very low rate in Eastern countries suggest a possible etiologic role for nutrition, especially the high content of animal fat in Western diets. There may be a relationship between high-fat diets and the higher incidence of endometrial carcinoma in women with conditions of unopposed estrogen. Endogenous estrogens rise in postmenopausal women because of increased production of androstenedione or a greater peripheral conversion of this hormone to estrone. In obese women, the extraglandular aromatization of androstenedione to estrone is increased in fatty tissue.

Obesity Phenotypically, the majority of women who develop endometrial cancer tend to be obese. Women who are 30 pounds over ideal weight have a 3-fold increased risk of developing endometrial cancer, whereas those 50 pounds or more over ideal weight have a 10-fold increased risk.

Parity Nulliparous women are at 2 times greater risk of developing endometrial cancer, females who undergo menopause after age 52 are at 2.5 times greater risk, and those who experience increased bleeding at the time of menopause are at 4 times greater risk.

Endometrial hyperplasia It is believed that the majority of endometrioid neoplastic lesions of the endometrium follow a continuum of histologically distinguishable hyperplastic lesions that covers a spectrum ranging from endometrial hyperplasia without atypia (EH) to endometrial hyperplasia with atypia (AEH) to well-differentiated endometrial cancer. Whereas patients found to have simple endometrial hyperplasia have a low risk of disease progression to cancer, 29% of those with complex atypical hyperplasia, if left untreated, will develop adenocarcinoma. However, the reproducibility of these diagnoses has been questioned by many.

As recently reported by Zaino et al and Trimble et al, a study by The Gynecologic Oncology Group (GOG), 0167, estimated the reproducibility of a referring institution's pathologists diagnosis of AEH and determined the frequency of concomitant adenocarcinoma in the hysterectomy obtained within 12 weeks of the initial diagnosis. The referring institution's pathologist's diagnosis of AEH was supported by the majority of the expert panel in only 38% of cases. The majority diagnosis was adenocarcinoma in 29%, cycling endometrium in 7%, and nonatypical hyperplasia in 18% of cases. Unanimous agreement for any diagnosis was reached among the entire expert panel in only 40% of cases. This study panel found that there was a high incidence (43%) of endometrial cancer in patients who had a community hospital biopsy demonstrating AEH.

Other risk factors Other known risk factors for endometrial cancer include diabetes mellitus; hypertension; endometrial hyperplasia; and a family history of endometrial, breast, and/or colon cancer. Diabetic females have a 3-fold increased risk, and hypertensive patients have a 1.5-fold greater risk of endometrial cancer.

Tamoxifen exerts its primary effect by blocking the binding of estrogen to estrogen receptors. It also exerts mild estrogenic effects on the female genital tract. This weak estrogenic effect presumably accounts for an increased frequency of endometrial carcinoma observed in women receiving prolonged adjuvant tamoxifen therapy for breast carcinoma.

Initially reported in 1985, the increased frequency of endometrial carcinoma in patients treated with tamoxifen was characterized more fully in a study of 1,846 women recorded in the Swedish Cancer Registry. This study reported a 6.4-fold increase in the relative risk of endometrial carcinoma with a daily dose of 40 mg of tamoxifen. The greatest cumulative risk was observed after 5 years of tamoxifen use.

The National Surgical Adjuvant Breast and Bowel Project (NSABP) subsequently reported on the incidence of other cancers in 2,843 women with node-negative, estrogen receptor-positive breast cancer treated with either tamoxifen or placebo in its B-14 randomized trial and an additional 1,220 patients treated with tamoxifen in another NSABP trial. The relative risk of endometrial carcinoma in the tamoxifen-treated patients was 7.5. The hazard rate was 0.2 per 1,000 cases with placebo and 1.6 per 1,000 cases with tamoxifen therapy. The mean duration of tamoxifen therapy for all patients was 35 months, and 36% of the cancers had developed by 2 years after the initiation of treatment. A more recent review of NSABP treatment and prevention trials revealed that the risk of uterine sarcomas was also increased with tamoxifen. The incidence of sarcomas was very low, however, with a rate of 0.17/1,000 women/year.

These data raise the question of whether tamoxifen should be used as adjuvant therapy for women at relatively low risk for breast cancer recurrence. First, it should be recognized that the endometrial cancers that develop in patients receiving tamoxifen exhibit the same stage, grade, and prognosis distribution as other endometrial cancers. There is some evidence that tamoxifen use is associated with an increased risk of uterine sarcoma; fortunately, this risk is low, and the cure rate should be high. Second, adjuvant tamoxifen reduces the cumulative rate of recurrence of breast cancer from 228 to 124 cases/1,000 women and the cumulative rate of second primary breast cancers from 40.5 to 23.5 cases/1,000 women.

When all of these facts are taken into account, there is an overall 38% reduction in the cumulative hazard rate for recurrence of breast cancer in tamoxifen-treated patients. Thus, the benefits of tamoxifen may outweigh the risks of endometrial cancer.

The current recommendations for screening women on tamoxifen are to educate patients about the significance of abnormal spotting, bleeding, or discharge and to investigate promptly any of these abnormalities.

Some experts have proposed that tamoxifen-treated women be screened with transvaginal ultrasonography. However, recent data suggest a high false-positive rate and a low frequency of significant findings, leading to the conclusion that endometrial screening is not warranted.

Signs and symptoms

Postmenopausal women Symptoms of early endometrial carcinoma are few. However, 90% of patients complain of abnormal vaginal discharge, and 80% of these women experience abnormal bleeding, usually after menopause. In the general population, 15% of postmenopausal women presenting with abnormal bleeding will be found to have endometrial carcinoma. Signs and symptoms of more advanced disease include pelvic pressure and other symptoms indicative of uterine enlargement or extrauterine tumor spread.

Premenopausal women The diagnosis of endometrial cancer may be difficult to make in premenopausal patients. The physician must maintain a high index of suspicion in this group of patients and perform endometrial sampling in any women who complain of prolonged, heavy menstrual periods or intermenstrual spotting.

Screening and diagnosis

Screening There is no role for screening of asymptomatic patients for endometrial cancer.

Outpatient endometrial sampling procedures, such as endometrial biopsy or aspiration curettage coupled with endocervical sampling, are definitive if results are positive for cancer. The results of endometrial biopsies correlate well with endometrial curettings, and these biopsy procedures have the advantage of avoiding general anesthesia. However, if sampling techniques fail to provide sufficient diagnostic information or if abnormal bleeding persists, formal dilation and curettage is required.

Dilation and curettage is the gold standard for assessing uterine bleeding and diagnosing endometrial carcinoma. Before dilating the cervix, the endocervix should be curetted. Next, careful sounding of the uterus is accomplished. Dilation of the cervix is then performed, followed by systematic curetting of the entire endometrial cavity. Cervical and endometrial specimens should be kept separate and forwarded for pathologic interpretation.

The American Cancer Society (ACS) recently concluded that there was insufficient evidence to recommend routine screening for endometrial cancer for average-risk women. However, the ACS recommends that at the time of menopause, all women should be informed about the risks and symptoms of endometrial cancer and strongly encouraged to report any unexpected bleeding or spotting to their physicians. Women at elevated risk for endometrial cancer from tamoxifen therapy should be informed about the risk and symptoms of endometrial cancer and strongly encouraged to report any unexpected bleeding or spotting to their physicians. In addition, results from three HNPCC (hereditary nonpolyposis colorectal cancer) registries have shown a 10-fold increased risk of endometrial cancer for women who carry the HNPCC genetic abnormality, with a cumulative risk for endometrial cancer of 43% by age 70. Women with or at risk for HNPCC can be offered endometrial screening annually beginning at age 35, but informed decision-making after a discussion of options, including benefits, risks, and limitations of testing, is appropriate. Additional investigation is needed to determine the appropriate monitoring for endometrial cancer in HNPCC carriers.

Pathology

Adenocarcinoma Endometrioid adenocarcinoma is the most common form of endometrial carcinoma, comprising 75% to 80% of cases. It varies from well differentiated to undifferentiated. The former demonstrates well-preserved glands in at least 95% of the tumor, whereas in the latter, less than half of the neoplasm shows glandular differentiation. Squamous differentiation can be seen in 30% to 50% of cases.

Adenoacanthoma Adenocarcinoma with benign squamous differentiation has been termed adenoacanthoma and generally has a good prognosis.

Adenosquamous carcinoma If the squamous component resembles squamous carcinoma, the tumor is designated an adenosquamous carcinoma. These lesions tend to have a worse prognosis due to their association with a poorly differentiated glandular component.

Serous carcinoma is an aggressive form of endometrial cancer that accounts for < 10% of these tumors. Serous cancer of the endometrium closely resembles serous carcinoma of the ovaries and fallopian tubes and is usually found in an advanced stage in older women.

Clear-cell carcinomas of the endometrium closely resemble their counterparts in the cervix, vagina, and ovaries. As with serous cancers, these tumors generally occur in older women and have a poor prognosis due to their propensity for early intraperitoneal spread.

Secretory adenocarcinoma is an uncommon endometrial cancer that resembles secretory endometrium with its associated progestational changes. These cancers tend to be of low grade and have a good prognosis.

Staging and prognosis

Two large prospective GOG surgical staging trials reported in 1984 and 1987 helped define the prognostic factors for endometrial carcinoma and the current treatment approach. In addition to evaluating the predictive value of such factors as age, race, and endocrine status, the studies confirmed that prognosis is directly related to the presence or absence of easily determined uterine and extrauterine risk factors.

Uterine prognostic factors include histologic cell type, tumor grade, depth of myometrial invasion, occult extension of disease to the cervix, and vascular space invasion.

Extrauterine prognostic factors include adnexal metastases, intraperitoneal spread of disease to other extrauterine structures, positive peritoneal cytology, pelvic lymph node metastases, and aortic node involvement.

Peritoneal cytology The current International Federation of Gynecology and Obstetrics (FIGO) staging system would classify the presence of malignant cells in the peritoneal fluid as stage IIIA disease, implying a worse prognosis, similar to that observed with cancer spread to the adnexa or serosa.

A study compared the outcome of patients with stages I versus IIIA endometrial cancer. The outcomes of the patients with stage IIIA disease were then reanalyzed by dividing the population into those based solely on the finding of a positive peritoneal cytology, "cytologic stage IIIA," and a group with histologic documentation of either serosal or adnexal involvement with cancer, "histologic stage IIIA."

The 5-year disease-specific survival for the patients with cytologic stage IIIA disease was 91%, remarkably similar to that of women in the series who presented with stage I endometrial cancer (92%). However, the 5-year disease-specific survival for the patients with histologic stage IIIA disease was only 50% ($P < .001$). This analysis was confirmed after controlling for other potential prognostic factors. These data raise the important question of whether the current endometrial cancer staging system, where the finding of a positive peritoneal cytologic result alone is considered a poor prognostic factor, should be reconsidered.

Uterine size was previously believed to be a risk factor and was part of the older clinical staging system. However, recent information indicates that uterine size is *not* an independent risk factor but rather relates to cell type, grade, and myometrial invasion.

TABLE 1: FIGO surgical staging for endometrial cancer

Stage	Grade	Characteristics
IA	G1,2,3	Tumor limited to the endometrium
IB	G1,2,3	Tumor invasion to less than half of the myometrium
IC	G1,2,3	Tumor invasion to more than half of the myometrium
IIA	G1,2,3	Endocervical glandular involvement only
IIB	G1,2,3	Cervical stromal invasion
IIIA	G1,2,3	Tumor invades serosa or adnexa or positive peritoneal cytology
IIIB	G1,2,3	Vaginal metastases
IIIC	G1,2,3	Metastases to pelvic or para-aortic lymph nodes
IVA	G1,2,3	Tumor invades the bladder and/or bowel mucosa
IVB		Distant metastases, including intra-abdominal and/or inguinal lymph nodes

Histopathology—Degree of differentiation[a]

G1		≤ 5% of a nonsquamous or nonmorular solid growth pattern
G2		6%-50% of a nonsquamous or nonmorular solid growth pattern
G3		> 50% of a nonsquamous or nonmorular solid growth pattern

FIGO = International Federation of Gynecology and Obstetrics

[a] Cases should be grouped by the degree of differentiation of the adenocarcinoma.

Surgical staging Cell type and grade can be determined before hysterectomy, although in some series, grade, as determined by dilation and curettage, has an overall inaccuracy rate of 31% compared with grade in the hysterectomy specimen, and grade 3 tumors have an inaccuracy rate of 50%. Recognition of all of the other factors requires an exploratory laparotomy, peritoneal fluid sampling, and hysterectomy with careful pathologic interpretation of all removed tissue. This primary surgical approach led the FIGO to define endometrial cancer as a surgically staged disease in 1988, incorporating many of the prognostic factors into the staging process (Table 1).

Treatment

Surgery

Approximately 90% of patients with a diagnosis of endometrial cancer are medically able to undergo surgery. Preparation for this surgery should include evaluation of such concurrent medical problems as hypertension and diabetes, which are frequently found in patients with endometrial cancer.

Open surgical procedure The operative procedure is performed through an adequate abdominal incision that allows for thorough intra-abdominal exploration and retroperitoneal lymph node removal if necessary. On entry into the peritoneal cavity, fluid samples are obtained for subsequent cytologic determination (intraperitoneal cell washings). Next, thorough intra-abdominal and pelvic exploration is undertaken, with biopsy or excision of any suspicious lesions. In particular, the uterus should be observed for tumor breakthrough of the serosal surface. The distal ends of the fallopian tubes are clipped or ligated to prevent possible tumor spillage during uterine manipulation.

These procedures should be followed by total extrafascial hysterectomy and bilateral salpingo-oophorectomy. The excised uterus is opened away from the operating table, and the depth of myometrial penetration is determined by clinical observation or microscopic frozen section. The depth of myometrial invasion can be accurately assessed in over 90% of cases.

Laparoscopic surgery An alternative method of surgically staging patients with clinical stage I endometrial cancer is gaining in popularity. This approach combines laparoscopically assisted vaginal hysterectomy with laparoscopic lymphadenectomy.

Laparoscopy-assisted surgical staging (LASS) is feasible in a select group of patients. However, it is not yet known whether this approach is applicable to all patients with clinical stage I disease. In particular, patients who are overweight or have intra-abdominal adhesions may not be ideal candidates. Para-aortic lymphadenectomy is technically more difficult through the laparoscope. To obtain adequate exposure, it is necessary to elevate the small bowel mesentery into the upper abdomen, which becomes increasingly difficult as the patient's weight increases, especially when weight exceeds 180 pounds.

Spirtos et al recently reported a feasibility trial by GOG on laparoscopic lymphadenectomy after incomplete surgical staging. A total of 69% of the women underwent complete endoscopic staging with photographic documentation, whereas 10% were incompletely staged. In addition, 20% needed laparotomy, of whom 6% had bowel complications and 11% were found to have more advanced disease. The safety, efficacy, and cost savings of LASS were reevaluated by GOG in a prospective randomized trial comparing LASS versus staging laparotomy. Data have recently matured and confirmed that laparoscopy is feasible, with longer operative times, comparable complications, shorter hospital stay, and better quality of life at 6 weeks than laparotomy. Patients who underwent laparoscopy had similar rates of intraoperative injuries as patients who underwent laparotomy (9.5% vs 7.6%; $P=.11$), fewer adverse events (27.5% vs 36.9%; $P<.001$), fewer moderate-to-severe (> CTC [Common Toxicity Criteria] grade 2) complications (14.3% vs 21.1%; $P<.001$), and shorter length of hospital stay (median 3 days vs 4 days; $P<.001$). Eight (0.5%) deaths within 6 weeks occurred in the laparoscopy arm and six (0.7%), in the laparotomy arm ($P=.579$).

Lymph node evaluation Any suspicious pelvic or para-aortic lymph nodes should be removed for pathologic evaluation. If there is no gross residual intraperitoneal tumor, pelvic and para-aortic lymph nodes should be removed for the following indications:

- invasion of more than one-half of the outer myometrium
- presence of tumor in the isthmus-cervix
- adnexal or other extrauterine metastases
- presence of serous, clear-cell, undifferentiated, or squamous types
- palpably enlarged lymph nodes.

Lymph nodes need not be removed in patients whose tumor is limited to the endometrium, regardless of grade, because < 1% of these patients have disease spread to pelvic or para-aortic lymph nodes. The decision of whether to perform lymph node sampling is less clear-cut for patients whose only risk factor is invasion of the inner half of the myometrium, particularly if the tumor grade is 1 or 2. This group has a ≤ 5% chance of node positivity.

Lymphadenectomy The extent of lymph node removal has been the subject of debate. Recently, GOG defined the extent of lymphadenectomy required for entry into its studies:

Pelvic lymphadenectomy

- The skin incision may be of the surgeon's choosing, including midline vertical, transverse, and lateral vertical. The procedure may be performed via laparoscopy or by a retroperitoneal approach.

- Identify the bifurcation of the common iliac, external iliac, and hypogastric arteries; veins; and the ureters bilaterally.

- Any enlarged or suspicious nodes will be excised or biopsied if unresectable.

- Remove bilaterally all nodal tissue and skeletonization of all vessels from the mid portion of the common iliac artery superiorly, to the circumflex iliac vein inferiorly.

- Remove bilaterally all nodal tissue from the mid portion of the psoas muscle laterally to the ureters medially, including the hypogastric arteries and veins and from the obturator fossas anterior to the obturator nerves.

- An adequate dissection requires that a minimum of four lymph nodes be demonstrated pathologically from each side (right and left) of the pelvis, preferably from multiple sites.

Para-aortic lymphadenectomy

- The bifurcation of the aorta, the inferior vena cava, the ovarian vessels, the inferior mesenteric artery, the ureters, and duodenum should be identified.

- The nodal tissue over the distal vena cava from the level of the inferior mesenteric artery to the mid right common iliac artery is removed.

- The nodal tissue between the aorta and the left ureter from the inferior mesenteric artery to the left mid common iliac artery is removed.

- An adequate dissection requires that lymphatic tissue be demonstrated pathologically from each side (right and left).

Surgical staging After these procedures, the patient is surgically staged according to the 1988 FIGO criteria. The overall surgical complication rate after this type of staging is approximately 20%. The rate of serious complications is 6%, and they include vascular, ureteral, and bowel injuries.

What defines an adequate lymphadenectomy has been controversial. Data from other disease sites suggest that a certain number of negative lymph nodes identify patients with a better prognosis who are less likely to benefit from adjuvant therapy. Phelps et al from the University of Texas Southwestern Medical Center at Dallas analyzed their experience in over 400 surgical stages I and II patients as it relates to the number of lymph nodes identified in the surgical specimen. Utilizing statistical analysis with receiver operator curves, they identified 13 negative lymph nodes as the best cutoff for assuring freedom from recurrence in patients at risk.

Grossly involved lymph nodes can often be completely resected. Havrilesky et al reported data for 96 patients with stage IIIC endometrial cancer and pelvic and/or aortic lymph node metastasis who underwent surgery between 1973 and 2002. Of these women, 45 had microscopic lymph node involvement and 51 had grossly enlarged nodes. Forty-four of the women with grossly involved lymph nodes underwent complete resection. Analysis revealed 5-year disease-specific survival rates of 50% in the patients with grossly positive lymph nodes who underwent complete resection, compared with 63% in those with microscopic metastatic disease, and 43% in the women with residual macroscopic lymph node metastasis.

Adjuvant radiation therapy

Following surgical staging, adjuvant radiation therapy is offered to patients based on prognostic factors found at the time of surgery. A pelvic recurrence rate of 7% to 14% is predictable for all stage I patients after surgery alone, although certain subgroups with more risk factors may have a higher incidence of recurrence of endometrial carcinoma. Well-described prognostic factors include disease extent (cervical involvement, extrauterine involvement of the serosa, adnexa, lymph nodes, peritoneal fluid, or intra-abdominal spread), as well as histologic grade of the tumor, depth of myometrial penetration, pathologic subtype, and presence of lymphovascular space invasion.

Teletherapy Adjuvant irradiation has been delivered primarily using external-beam irradiation directed to the pelvis, which allows for treatment of the pelvic nodes. There have now been three large randomized trials examining the role of external-beam radiation therapy for uterine-confined disease.

Review of more than 21,000 patients from SEER data demonstrated improved overall and relative survival rates for those with stage IC endometrial cancer who were treated with adjuvant radiation therapy compared with surgery alone (*Lee CM, Szabo A, Shrieve DC, et al: JAMA 295:389-397, 2006*).

A trial conducted by GOG compared the results of pelvic irradiation with those of observation following hysterectomy and lymphadenectomy. The estimated 2-year cumulative incidence of recurrence was 12% in the observation arm and 3% in those irradiated ($P = .007$). The treatment difference was particularly evident among a "high-intermediate risk" subgroup defined as those (1) with moderate to poorly differentiated tumor, presence of lymphovascular invasion, and outer-third myometrial invasion; (2) age 50 or older with any two risk factors previously listed; or (3) age of at least 70 with any risk factor previously listed, where the cumulative incidence of recurrence in the observed patients was 26% versus 6% in the treated patients. Overall survival rates at 3 years did not differ significantly between the two groups.

However, one-third of patients were found to be in a high-risk group that included patients who were older, had lymph-vascular space invasion, deep myometrial penetration, and high-grade disease. When outcomes were stratified by these factors, the addition of pelvic irradiation was found to reduce the recurrence and death rate from 36% to 17%, the cancer death rate from 17% to 10%, and the distant metastatic rate from 19% to 10%. This finding suggests that pelvic irradiation may not only influence pelvic recurrence in these patients, but that there is a subgroup of patients who may benefit in terms of distant metastasis and death. A larger trial with high-risk patients is needed to validate this assumption.

Of the 18 pelvic recurrences in the no adjuvant treatment arm, 13 were in the vagina. Thirteen other sites of recurrence were outside the pelvis. It has been speculated that vaginal irradiation alone could have controlled these vaginal recurrences, leading to interest in treatment with vaginal irradiation instead of pelvic irradiation.

The findings of a multicenter trial with 754 patients from the Netherlands called the Post Operative Radiation Therapy in Endometrial Carcinoma (PORTEC) study have been reported. Eligible patients had IC grade 1 (21%), IB or IC grade 2 tumors (69%), or IB grade 3 tumors (10%). After total abdominal hysterectomy without lymphadenectomy, patients were randomized to receive pelvic radiotherapy (46 Gy) or no further treatment.

Pelvic irradiation decreased the incidence of locoregional tumor recurrence but did not affect survival. Patients with grade 3 histology demonstrated the highest risk of distant metastases and death caused by endometrial cancer. Most of the locoregional relapses were located in the vagina (30 of 40 cases). It is possible that vaginal brachytherapy could have prevented the majority of these cases. When patients were subdivided into a high-risk subgroup with two or three risk factors, including age ≥ 60, grade 3 histology, and myometrial depth $\geq 50\%$, the 10-year locoregional relapse rate was 4.6% in the radiotherapy group versus 23.1% in the control group.

PORTEC also registered patients on a prospective trial who had deep myometrial invasion and grade 3 histology. All patients were treated with pelvic irradiation following hysterectomy. Notably, these patients had a distant recurrence rate at 5 years of 31%, and a pelvic recurrence rate at 5 years of 14%. The information from this report as well as from the subgroup of patients in the GOG 99 trial suggests that there may be a role for systemic therapy as well as pelvic irradiation in this high-risk subgroup.

A third randomized trial was presented at the 2007 Annual Meeting of the American Society of Clinical Oncology (ASCO). Over 900 patients with stage I or IIa endometrial cancer from the National Cancer Institute of Canada (NCIC) and the Medical Research Council (MRC) were randomized to receive pelvic radiation therapy or no pelvic radiation therapy. Notably, vaginal radiation therapy was optional, and 52% of patients in each arm received it. There was no difference in survival and only a minimal difference in local or regional tumor recurrence rates.

Brachytherapy A few reports have demonstrated excellent local tumor control with vaginal irradiation alone. A review of the world literature included 1,800 patients with low- to intermediate-risk disease. Overall, the vaginal control rate was 99.3% following adjuvant high-dose-rate (HDR) vaginal brachytherapy.

In a randomized study from the Norwegian Radium Hospital, pelvic irradiation significantly decreased the incidence of locoregional tumor recurrences compared with vaginal irradiation alone. Patients with deeply invasive, grade 3 tumors had lower death and recurrence rates when treated with pelvic plus vaginal irradiation than patients treated with vaginal irradiation alone.

Many women with endometrial cancer are being treated with lymphadenectomy at the time of hysterectomy. There has been some interest in using vaginal irradiation alone to treat women who have negative nodes but deep myometrial penetration or high-grade histology. Several small retrospective reports have demonstrated excellent outcomes for such patients. However, more experience is needed to determine whether vaginal irradiation alone is adequate.

> **A** randomized phase III trial compared pelvic radiation therapy with observation for 905 stage I/IIa endometrial cancer patients. There was no difference in survival. Pelvic recurrence was 7% versus 4% for external beam radiation therapy compared with observation *(Orton J, Blake P, on behalf of ASTEC/EN.5 collaborators: J Clin Oncol 25[18S]: 5504, 2007).*

The results of a phase III randomized trial from PORTEC were presented at ASCO 2008. This trial included patients that had a high-intermediate risk EC: age > 60 and stage IC grade 1/2 or stage IB grade 3; any age and stage IIA grade 1/2 or grade 3 with < 50% invasion. They were randomized to receive pelvic radiation or vaginal brachytherapy. 427 patients were randomized between 2002–2006. At a median follow-up of 34 months, 3-year actuarial rates of vaginal relapse were 0.9% in the VBT arm and 2.0% after EBRT ($P = .97$), with SE of the difference 1.4%. Three-year rates of PR were 3.6% and 0.7% ($P = .03$). There were no significant differences in 3-year OS (90.4% vs 90.8%, $P = .55$) and RFS (89.5% vs 89.1%, $P = .38$). As patient reported quality of life after VBT was shown to be better than after EBRT, VBT should be the treatment of choice for patients with high-intermediate risk endometrial carcinoma.

Vaginal irradiation alone is appropriate for patients at low risk for pelvic node metastasis. Because of increased rectal and vaginal sequelae, treatment of the entire length of the vagina is usually not recommended.

TABLE 2: Recommendations for adjuvant pelvic irradiation

Histologic grade	Stage		
	IA	IB	IC
G1	−	−	−
G2	−	−	+[b]
G3	+[b]	+[b]	+[b]
Vascular space invasion[a]	+	+	+

[a] Any grade; + = irradiation recommended; − = irradiation not recommended

[b] After full lymphadenectomy, consider brachytherapy alone because of excess complications

Irradiation of the pelvis and vagina has been combined for the adjuvant treatment of some patients. Patients with cervical involvement or extrauterine disease, who may have an increased incidence of local failure, may benefit from the two treatments combined, although there are no data to suggest that the addition of brachytherapy improves outcome over external-beam irradiation alone. Patients with uterine-confined disease have excellent local tumor control following treatment with either type of irradiation. Combining the two treatments has not been shown to benefit these patients.

Vaginal irradiation Vaginal irradiation can be delivered with HDR or low-dose-rate (LDR) equipment. Both techniques have resulted in excellent local tumor control rates and low morbidity when administered by experienced practitioners. Each technique has its advantages. HDR treatments require multiple insertions, generally with one insertion performed every week for 3 to 6 weeks. However, hospitalization is not required, and each insertion takes only a brief amount of time. LDR treatments are delivered once but require hospitalization for 2 to 3 days.

Stage I disease Current recommendations for the treatment of patients with pathologic stage I disease include adjuvant pelvic irradiation for women with deep myometrial penetration, grade 2 or 3 histology, or evidence of vascular space invasion (Table 2). Data support the use of vaginal irradiation alone for women with more superficial tumors and low-grade histology.

Radiation doses are generally 45 to 50 Gy with standard fractionation. The technique should include multiple fields treated daily, with attempts to protect the small bowel. Complications from adjuvant pelvic irradiation are related to technique and the extent of lymphadenectomy.

If full lymphadenectomy has been performed, the incidence of complications increases significantly with pelvic irradiation. For these patients, consideration should be given to adjuvant brachytherapy rather than pelvic irradiation.

Papillary serous histology The high rate of upper abdominal, pelvic, and vaginal recurrences in patients with uterine papillary serous cancers has led some clinicians to recommend that these patients receive whole abdominal irradiation (WAI, with doses up to 30 Gy) and additional treatments to bring the pelvic dose to 50 Gy. A vaginal cylinder or colpostats may be used to boost the surface dose with 40 Gy. This treatment has resulted in a 5-year survival rate of 50%.

Stage II disease Patients whose endometrial cancer extends to the cervix usually represent a heterogeneous group, with differing histologic grades and varying degrees of cervical involvement, myometrial penetration, and nodal involvement. Similar outcomes with preoperative and postoperative irradiation suggest that initial surgical treatment with tailored postoperative irradiation is a reasonable approach.

Current treatment recommendations frequently include adjuvant pelvic irradiation to a dose of 45 to 50 Gy, in addition to insertion of a vaginal cylinder or colpostats to raise the total dose to the vaginal surface to 80 to 90 Gy. This treatment should result in a 5-year disease-free survival rate of 80%, with a locoregional tumor control rate of 90%. Of course, outcome varies with the extent of myometrial penetration, degree of cervical involvement, and histologic grade of tumor.

Extensive cervical involvement Patients who have a large amount of cervical involvement that precludes initial hysterectomy are candidates for preoperative irradiation. A multiple-field technique is used to deliver a dose of 40 to 45 Gy with standard fractionation. A midline block may be inserted for the last 20 Gy to protect the rectum.

Intracavitary insertion with a standard Fletcher applicator, consisting of a uterine tandem and vaginal colpostats, delivers 20 to 25 Gy to point A (defined as 2 cm caudally and 2 cm laterally to the cervical os). Hysterectomy should follow in approximately 4 to 6 weeks. The expected 5-year disease-free survival rate for patients with extensive disease is 70% to 80%.

More favorable patients have an isolated extrauterine site (eg, adnexa or peritoneal cytology alone), low-grade histology, and/or disease confined to the pelvis. Greven et al reported that 17 patients with an isolated extrauterine site who had low-grade histology and received postoperative pelvic radiation therapy had a 100% disease-free survival rate. However, patients with grade 2 or 3 disease or more than one extrauterine site had progressively worse outcomes.

Isolated ovarian metastasis One subgroup found to have a relatively favorable prognosis includes women with isolated ovarian metastasis. Five-year disease-free survival rates ranging from 60% to 82% have been reported in these women after hysterectomy and pelvic irradiation, depending on the histologic grade of the tumor and the depth of myometrial penetration. Pelvic irradiation usually includes a dose of 45 to 50 Gy using standard fractionation. A vaginal boost with a cylinder or colpostats may add 30 to 35 Gy to the vaginal surface.

Extension to pelvic and periaortic nodes Patients with pelvic node involvement alone have much better outcomes than patients with extension to periaortic nodes, despite the fact that they are both considered stage IIIC patients. Morrow et al demonstrated 5-year recurrence-free survival rates of 70% and 35% for patients with pelvic nodes compared with patients with para-aortic nodes, respectively. Patients with pelvic nodes and negative para-aortic nodes are generally treated with adjuvant pelvic radiation therapy. Those with para-aortic nodes are treated with extended-field irradiation, which includes 45 to 50 Gy to a volume encompassing the pelvic and periaortic regions.

WAI Because upper abdominal failures have been reported previously in patients with stage III disease, attention has focused on the role of WAI. Although subsets of patients have done well with WAI, it is unclear whether this more aggressive therapy has any benefit over pelvic irradiation. A GOG phase II trial of WAI demonstrated a 3-year progression-free survival rate of 35%. GOG has completed a trial of WAI compared with chemotherapy. (The outcomes from this trial are discussed in the chemotherapy section.) Unfortunately, because most studies have combined patients who have favorable stage III disease with patients who have unfavorable stage IV disease, it is impossible to determine whether there are some subgroups of patients who might best be managed with a particular therapy.

Combining radiation therapy with chemotherapy Because many of these patients are at increased risk of pelvic recurrence as well as distant recurrence, there is interest in combining pelvic radiation therapy with systemic therapy. RTOG (Radiation Therapy and Oncology Group) 9708 combined pelvic radiation therapy with cisplatin and followed it with cisplatin and paclitaxel. Toxicity was predominantly hematologic. 4-year survival and disease-free survival rates for stage III patients were 77% and 72%, respectively. There were no recurrences for patients with IC, IIA or IIB disease.

GOG 0184 was instituted following the completion of GOG 0122 based on the assumption that combined-modality therapy with radiation therapy and chemotherapy in advanced but optimally cytoreduced endometrial carcinoma may lead to a better result than either modality used alone. Patients with stages III and IV adenocarcinoma of the endometrium with less than 2 cm of residual disease were treated with radiation therapy tailored to include the volume at risk followed by randomization to cisplatin plus doxorubicin or cisplatin, doxorubicin and paclitaxel. The addition of paclitaxel to cisplatin and doxorubicin did not improve progression-free survival.

Definitive radiation treatment

For patients who are poor operative risks, definitive treatment with irradiation has produced excellent local tumor control and survival rates. Such treatment is considered to be justified when the operative risk exceeds the 10% to 15% uterine recurrence rate expected with irradiation alone.

A more favorable outcome with definitive irradiation is related to low clinical tumor stage, less aggressive histologic variant, and use of brachytherapy for at least part of the treatment. Five-year disease-specific survival rates as high as 87%, 88%, and 49% have been reported in patients with stages I, II, and III or IV disease, respectively. Ten-year local tumor control rates in patients with stages I/II, III, and IV disease were 84%, 87%, and 68%, respectively.

Treatment techniques with irradiation alone for patients with early-stage disease and low-grade histology consist of uterine intracavitary insertions with Heyman or Simon capsules or an afterloading intrauterine tandem. Doses for intracavitary treatment range from 40 to 45 Gy prescribed to point A. Patients with more advanced disease, a large uterus, or aggressive histology generally receive both an intrauterine intracavitary insertion and external pelvic irradiation. External irradiation typically delivers 40 to 45 Gy to the pelvis, followed by intracavitary treatment that delivers 30 to 35 Gy to point A.

Complication rates Rates of serious complications attributable to irradiation range from 4% to 5% with intracavitary treatment alone to 10% to 15% with combined external and intracavitary irradiation.

Adjuvant systemic therapy

Only a few trials of adjuvant systemic therapy have been conducted in patients with early-stage endometrial cancer. At present, we believe that such therapy should not be recommended outside the clinical trial setting.

Endocrine therapy Early uncontrolled trials suggested that progestin therapy might prolong the disease progression-free interval and time to recurrence in patients with stages I and II lesions treated with initial surgery and irradiation. However, at least three subsequent randomized trials failed to show any survival benefit for progestins, and a meta-analysis has demonstrated no advantage of adjuvant progestin therapy.

Chemotherapy To date, there are emerging data suggesting a possible role for adjuvant chemotherapy. A recently reported European phase III randomized trial revealed that in patients with early-stage high-risk endometrial cancer, the addition of chemotherapy (most patients received either cisplatin plus an anthracycline or carboplatin plus paclitaxel) to external radiation therapy improved progression-free survival compared with the use of radiation therapy alone.

A Japanese Gynecologic Oncology Group study published by Susuma et al has suggested that chemotherapy may also be employed as an alternative to radiotherapy for more localized, intermediate-risk disease (> 50% myometrial invasion). Patients (n = 425) were randomized to receive either cisplatin/doxorubicin/cyclophosphamide (CAP) or whole pelvic radiotherapy. The study revealed no difference between the two regimens with respect to risk of local recurrence (15% to 16%) or survival (progression-free or overall). However, among patients in a high- to intermediate-risk group defined as (1) stage IC in patients older than age 70 years or with G3 endometrioid adenocarcinoma or (2) stage II or IIIA (positive cytology), the CAP group had a significantly higher progression-free

> A phase III trial of 382 patients randomized between radiation therapy and radiation therapy with chemotherapy demonstrated an improvement in 5-year progression-free survival and cause-specific survival for high-risk stage I-III patients *(Hogberg T, Rosenberg P, Kristensen G, et al: J Clin Oncol 25[18S]:5503, 2007).*

survival rate (84% vs 66%, log-rank test $P = .024$; hazard ratio, 0.44) and a higher overall survival rate (90% vs 74%, log-rank test $P = .006$; hazard ratio, 0.24). Adverse effects were not significantly increased in the CAP group versus the pelvic radiotherapy group. Thus, adjuvant chemotherapy may be a useful alternative to radiotherapy for intermediate-risk endometrial cancer.

Results from a GOG trial comparing adjuvant chemotherapy (doxorubicin plus cisplatin) with WAI were reported by Randall et al. The patient population included patients with stages III and IV disease (75% and 25%, respectively) with 50% endometrioid histologies. Patients treated with WAI had significantly improved progression-free (38% vs 50%) and overall (42 % vs 55%) survival at 5 years. However, serious adverse effects were also more common in the chemotherapy group than in the radiotherapy group, with treatment-related deaths twice as high in the former group, at 4% versus 2%. Pelvic and abdominal recurrences were the predominant pattern of recurrence for both treatment arms. Distant recurrences were slightly less frequent for patients treated with chemotherapy. This finding may support the concept of combining chemotherapy with involved-field irradiation. A GOG trial exploring this treatment strategy has recently closed to accrual. However, the results are not yet available.

Hormone replacement therapy (HRT) Whether HRT increases the likelihood of recurrence has been studied, with several retrospective reports showing no adverse outcomes. Thus, GOG undertook a large randomized placebo-controlled trial of HRT after treatment for earlier stage endometrial cancer. However, there were too few events, and it was closed after the findings of the Women's Health Initiative were released. In results published by Barakat et al, HRT was not associated with a significant incidence of recurrent disease, mortality, or new malignancy.

TREATMENT OF RECURRENT OR METASTATIC DISEASE

Patterns of recurrence

Recurrent endometrial cancer is initially confined to the pelvis in 50% of patients. The major sites of distant metastasis are the abdominal cavity, liver, and lungs.

Following diagnosis and initial treatment, periodic evaluation, including history, physical examination, and pelvic examination, is recommended at 3 to 6-month intervals for the first 5 years and yearly thereafter. More extensive and more costly procedures, such as chest x-ray, CT imaging, and marker studies, used in asymptomatic patients is of questionable value and is unlikely to have a major impact on survival. Symptomatic patients should be evaluated as is appropriately.

Radiation therapy

After hysterectomy alone for endometrial cancer, approximately 50% of recurrences are pelvic and 50% are extrapelvic. It is clear that locoregional recurrences can develop in isolation, without distant metastasis, and salvage can be accomplished with high-dose irradiation.

Pelvic recurrences Five-year disease-specific survival rates as high as 51% have been reported in patients with isolated locoregional recurrences treated with radiation therapy. Factors that have an adverse impact on outcome are increased size of tumor at recurrence, young age, pelvic versus vaginal involvement, and treatment of recurrence with external-beam irradiation only versus the addition of vaginal brachytherapy.

The PORTEC group has published its experience with salvage of vaginal recurrence in patients who did not receive adjuvant irradiation. At 5 years, the survival rate after vaginal relapse was 65% in the control group, compared with 43% in the irradiated group.

Radiation treatment for pelvic recurrence usually consists of external-beam irradiation with the addition of a brachytherapy boost that may include colpostats, a cylinder, interstitial needles, or seeds. Treatment must be individualized based on the location and size of the recurrence and the boost method selected. The tolerance of normal tissues must be respected, but combined doses > 60 Gy have been associated with improved local tumor control.

Extrapelvic recurrences For patients with recurrences outside the pelvis, irradiation is effective in producing responses in localized symptomatic lesions. Therefore, irradiation may be effective for palliation of such lesions in the lymph nodes, brain, or bones. Doses and protocols vary, depending on the site of recurrence.

Pelvic exenteration for pelvic recurrences after irradiation

Isolated pelvic central recurrence after irradiation is rare. Selected patients in whom it does occur may benefit from pelvic exenterative surgery. No large series have been published, but some long-term survivors have been reported.

Although the long-term survival rate after this procedure is only 20%, it remains the only potentially curative option for the few patients with central recurrence of endometrial cancer who have not responded to standard surgery and radiation therapy.

Endocrine therapy

Progestins produce complete and partial response rates of 15% to 25% in patients with locoregional recurrence or distant metastases. The route, type, and dose of progestins do not appear to be related to response; hence, oral therapy is preferred.

In clinical practice, oral administration of 200 mg of medroxyprogesterone or 160 mg of megestrol produces blood levels similar to those achieved with parenteral therapy (400 to 1,000 mg of medroxyprogesterone IM weekly). A phase III trial conducted by GOG comparing 200 mg and 1,000 mg of medroxyprogesterone given orally daily found no differences between the two regimens, although it is noteworthy that the trends all favored the low-dose regimen (Table 3). Doses higher than 200 mg/d of medroxyprogesterone, therefore, are clearly not warranted.

TABLE 3: Results of a phase III, dose-response trial of progestins in advanced or recurrent endometrial carcinoma

| Parameter | Oral medroxyprogesterone | |
	200 mg/d (n = 145)	1,000 mg/d (n = 154)
Response rate (%)	25	15
Complete response rate (%)	17	9
Median disease progression-free survival (mo)	3.2	2.5
Median survival (mo)	11.1	7.0

Several factors are predictive of a favorable response to progestin therapy. Patients with well-differentiated lesions are more likely to respond than those with poorly differentiated tumors. A related observation is that a much higher percentage of grade 1 tumors have significant levels of estrogen and progesterone receptors; data show that lesions with higher receptor levels respond much more frequently to progestins than those with lower receptor levels. Response is almost always associated with better progression-free and overall survival.

The median time to disease progression for all patients treated with progestins is 3 to 4 months, and the median survival is 10 months.

Tamoxifen has a 0% to 13% response rate, is not as active as progestins, and is of little value as second-line therapy in patients who do not respond to progestins.

GOG has evaluated combined therapy with tamoxifen plus a progestin given sequentially in the hope that tamoxifen may increase progesterone receptor expression and, thus, increase the likelihood of response to progestins. Continuous tamoxifen and medroxyprogesterone given every other week was an active treatment, with a 33% response rate. A subsequent study found a 27% response rate for alternating megestrol, with several prolonged responses. As with prior hormonal studies, patients with well-differentiated cancers were more likely to respond. Nevertheless, this trial was relatively unique in that 22% of patients with poorly differentiated tumors responded.

Other hormonal agents, such as gonadotropin-releasing hormone analogs and aminoglutethimide (Cytadren), have been studied to some extent in endometrial carcinoma. These agents do not appear to have sufficient activity to warrant further study.

Chemotherapy

Single agents Chemotherapy for advanced endometrial cancer focuses on three groups of agents with demonstrated activity: anthracyclines, platinum compounds, and taxanes.

Active agents The anthracyclines studied include doxorubicin and epirubicin. In a total of 298 patients, doxorubicin produced a 27% response rate. Epirubicin, primarily in European studies including 27 patients, yielded a 26% response rate. Two platinum compounds have activity. Cisplatin, in 86 patients, elicited responses in 29%. Carboplatin produced a 31% response rate in 52 patients. Paclitaxel, in two GOG studies, yielded responses in 36% of chemotherapy-naive and 27% of previously treated patients.

For all of these studies, the progression-free interval ranged from 4 to 7 months, with an overall survival range of 8 to 12 months. Approximately one-third of the responses were clinical complete responses, with a substantially longer duration and better survival than partial responders.

Agents with limited activity Other agents studied have included alkylating agents (cyclophosphamide, ifosfamide), altretamine (Hexalen), fluorouracil (5-FU), methotrexate, mercaptopurine (Purinethol), vinblastine, etoposide, teniposide (Vumon), and mitoxantrone. All these agents exhibited insufficient activity to warrant further study.

Combination regimens A number of phase II trials of combination regimens have been conducted. The combination of carboplatin and paclitaxel has been demonstrated to be active in advanced endometrial cancer (50% to 60% response rate). Further support for this approach was provided by a report from Sovak et al, who conducted a retrospective analysis of their experience with this combination chemotherapy regimen in endometrial cancer. The objective response rate in chemotherapy-naive patients was 47% (2% complete response rate), with a median progression-free survival of 4.2 months and a median overall survival of 11 months. Ultimately, the relative merits of combination chemotherapy with carboplatin and paclitaxel must be judged in the context of the randomized trial that is being performed by GOG.

Following encouraging phase II results, a phase III trial of circadian timed administration of cisplatin and doxorubicin found no significant benefit. GOG then compared this two-drug (cisplatin [50 mg/m^2]/doxorubicin [60 mg/m^2]) regimen with a three-drug combination of cisplatin (50 mg/m^2), doxorubicin (45 mg/m^2), and paclitaxel (160 mg/m^2 as a 3-hour infusion), with G-CSF (granulocyte colony-stimulating factor, filgrastim [Neupogen]) support (GOG protocol 177). The three-drug combination of the paclitaxel-containing program produced a higher response rate (57% vs 35%) and an improved progression-free survival (8.3 months vs 5.3 months). Overall survival was also modestly improved (15.3 months vs 12.3 months; $P = .037$) with the three-drug program but with considerably greater toxicity, particularly peripheral neuropathy (grade 3, 12% vs 1%).

There has been concern about the potential effect of "high-risk" endometrial histologies on response to chemotherapy. It has been suggested that papillary serous and clear cell tumor adenocarcinomas should be treated differently. McMeekin et al correlated histology with chemotherapy outcomes in several of the above-mentioned trials and found no significant difference in response or survival based on the histologic type of endometrial cancer.

Chemotherapy plus progestins Combinations of chemotherapy plus progestins have been studied in a number of phase II trials. The only large, randomized trial evaluating this approach (GOG protocol 29) allocated patients with advanced or recurrent disease to receive either cyclophosphamide, doxorubicin, cisplatin, and megestrol or melphalan (Alkeran), 5-FU, and megestrol. In pilot studies, these two regimens had been reported to yield response rates of 75% and 94%, respectively. The randomized trial produced response rates of 36% and 38%, respectively, with no evident advantage of either combination over prior studies of single-agent doxorubicin with regard to response rate, progression-free interval, or overall survival. These results do not suggest any advantage for the combined use of chemotherapy and progestins.

Treatment recommendations

Patients who have advanced or recurrent endometrial carcinoma should be considered for systemic therapy. Patients should first be offered the opportunity to participate in a clinical trial. Those who are ineligible or who choose not to participate should be treated according to current evidence.

Patients who have a grade 1 tumor and/or known progesterone receptor-positive disease clearly benefit from treatment with progestins (response rate, 40%; median progression-free interval, 9 months; overall median survival, 14 months) and should be so treated. Those with a grade 2 to 3 tumor and/or known progesterone receptor-negative disease do not do well with progestin therapy (response rate, 12%; median progression-free interval, 3 months; overall median survival, 10 months) and should be considered for initial treatment with single-agent chemotherapy (eg, paclitaxel, doxorubicin, carboplatin) or a combination regimen. Options include cisplatin/doxorubicin, cisplatin/paclitaxel, and carboplatin/paclitaxel. (It is difficult to justify the routine use of the three-drug paclitaxel-containing regimen noted previously despite the modest improvement in efficacy due to substantial toxicity.) Chemotherapy should also be considered for patients who do not respond to initial hormonal therapy.

Regimens that include both chemotherapy and hormonal therapy should not be considered outside a clinical trial because of the lack of data supporting any advantage of these combinations. Likewise, sequential use of tamoxifen and progestins is not indicated because of the absence of enhanced efficacy.

UTERINE SARCOMAS

Carcinosarcomas and other uterine sarcomas are uncommon tumors, accounting for less than 4% of all cancers of the uterine corpus. Carcinosarcomas, the most common histologic subtype, demonstrate both epithelial and stromal differentiation. Endometrial stromal sarcomas and leiomyosarcomas (LMSs) are characterized by differentiation toward one or more stromal tissues. LMSs occur at an earlier age than do carcinosarcomas, with a plateau observed in middle age. There is strong epidemiologic evidence that prior exposure to pelvic irradiation may increase the risk for the development of uterine sarcomas. Generally, these tumors are characterized by aggressive growth, with early lymphatic or hematogeneous spread. The overall survival rate is poor, with the majority of deaths occurring within 2 years of diagnosis.

Patterns of spread

Lymphatic metastases are a significant route of spread for carcinosarcoma, with a reported incidence of 40% to 60% occurring with stage I disease. LMS has a propensity for extra-abdominal spread, often involving the lungs. For carcinosarcoma, the initial site for recurrence after surgical resection is likely to be the pelvis or abdomen, whereas LMSs tend to fail to recur distantly. In a prospective surgical staging trial by GOG, the recurrence rate for early-stage carcinosarcoma was 53% and for LMS was 71%.

Treatment

Surgery

Surgery is the mainstay of treatment for uterine sarcomas. For carcinosarcoma, this usually consists of total abdominal hysterectomy and bilateral salpingo-oophorectomy, with washings to be obtained for peritoneal cytology. The GOG prospective staging study reported a 17% incidence of nodal metastasis for this histologic subtype, so retroperitoneal nodes should be sampled as for poorly differentiated endometrial cancers. For patients with advanced/recurrent disease, aggressive surgical debulking does not appear to improve outcome.

Hysterectomy with oophorectomy is also standard therapy for uterine LMS. Retroperitoneal nodal sampling is not usually performed, because lymph node involvement is unusual. For late recurrences of LMS, surgery must be individualized. Five-year survival rates of 30% to 50% have been reported following pulmonary resection for lung metastases. Patients with unilateral metastases have a significantly better prognosis than those with bilateral disease. Local and regional recurrences may also be amenable to surgical resection of disease.

Hysterectomy with oophorectomy is the standard of care for patients with low-grade endometrial stromal sarcomas. Removal of the ovaries was thought to be critical, as these tumors tend to have very high concentrations of estrogen and progesterone receptors and often respond to hormonal therapy. However, Li et al reviewed a multi-institutional experience and reported that bilateral salpingo-oophorectomy did not appear to affect time to recurrence or overall survival. Retention of ovarian function may be an option for premenopausal women with low-grade endometrial stromal sarcomas. Because these tumors have a tendency to spread via the lymphatics, resection of all disease, especially extension into the parametrium, should be attempted. This approach may require radical hysterectomy.

Adjuvant irradiation

Pelvic recurrence is a pattern of failure for most uterine sarcomas; isolated pelvic recurrences are uncommon. Adjuvant irradiation can decrease local recurrence, but there is no clear evidence that it improves survival. Patients will often experience recurrence distantly and treatment failure. Pelvic irradiation may be indicated for improvement of quality of life, however, because pelvic recurrence can be associated with pain, bleeding, and intestinal obstruction.

Radiotherapy

Uterine sarcomas represent only 2% to 5% of all uterine malignancies. These patients have a high incidence of distant, as well as pelvic, recurrences. In a nonrandomized prospective GOG study, patients with stages I and II mixed mesodermal sarcomas and LMSs had fewer pelvic recurrences following irradiation than did those patients who did not undergo pelvic irradiation. No difference in overall or disease-free survival was noted.

Several retrospective reports have suggested improved pelvic control rates following pelvic irradiation for stages I and II uterine sarcomas. Decreasing pelvic recurrences may improve symptom-free survival for these patients. As reported by Wolfson et al, GOG 0150 was a randomized study of patients with stages I–IV carcinosarcoma of the uterus with less than 1 cm of residual disease and no extra-abdominal spread. Patients were treated with either cisplatin (20 mg/m^2/d for 4 days) plus ifosfamide (1.5 g/m^2/d for 4 days every 3 weeks for 3 cycles) or whole abdominal irradiation (WAI) to a total dose of 3,000 cGy and the pelvis treated to a total dose of 4,980 cGy. The abdomen received 150 cGy per fraction with 5 fractions per week. The pelvis was boosted an additional 11 fractions at 180 cGy per fraction. The study tested whether patients treated with systemic treatment or locoregional treatment differ in progression-free interval, survival, and failure patterns. There were 105 patients in the WAI and 101 in the chemotherapy cohorts, respectively.

Of 206 study patients, there were 112 total recurrences (54%), with 60 (57%) in the radiotherapy and 52 (51%) in the chemotherapy treatment arms. Although patients may have had several different sites of failure, there were more vaginal failures in the chemotherapy group (10%) than in the WAI group (4%). However, there were more abdominal relapses in the WAI arm (28%) than in the chemotherapy cohort (19%). Pelvic and distant failures were essentially the same. Although acute toxicities of anemia and neuropathy were more frequent in the chemotherapy arm, there were more severe grade 3/4 gastrointestinal late effects in the WAI group, and two patients died as a direct result of radiation hepatitis. The estimated probability of surviving 5 years was 35% versus 45% for WAI versus chemotherapy. After adjusting for stage and age, there was no definite survival advantage but rather a trend favoring chemotherapy (the estimated death rate was 29% lower for chemotherapy patients than for WAI patients [RH = 0.712; 95% CI: 0.484–1.048; P = .085, two-tail test]).

GOG 0150 has shown that adjunctive chemotherapy has less toxic long-term side effects and is more likely than radiotherapy to improve the survival for these patients. Because chemotherapy did not reduce the risk of vaginal relapses, less toxic vaginal brachytherapy with chemotherapy would be an appropriate experimental arm for future adjuvant therapeutic trials in this group of patients.

GOG reported a randomized study for patients with stages I to IV mixed mesodermal sarcomas. Following resection of gross disease, patients were randomized to receive WAI (30 Gy) with a pelvic boost (19.8 Gy) or chemotherapy alone with cisplatin, ifosfamide, and mesna (Mesnex). There was no statistically significant difference in recurrence or survival rates between these two arms.

Chemotherapy

There is no proven role for adjuvant chemotherapy in stage I disease following complete surgical resection. A GOG study looking at adjuvant doxorubicin versus no further therapy showed no differences in recurrence rate, progression-free survival, or overall survival. As reported by Sutton et al, GOG 0117 showed that adjuvant ifosfamide and cisplatin after primary surgery for stage I or II carcinosarcoma of the uterus was tolerable. That combination was then compared with WAI in GOG 0150 (described in detail above), which showed a trend in survival favoring those treated with that chemotherapy combination.

For patients with advanced/recurrent disease, single-agent chemotherapy or combination chemotherapy can be used with a palliative intent. For carcinosarcomas, ifosfamide or paclitaxel appears to be the agent of choice. Because GOG 0108 showed that ifosfamide plus cisplatin had no greater progression-free interval or survival than ifosfamide alone, GOG 0161 randomized patients to receive ifosfamide (2.0 $g/m^2/d$ for 3 days every 3 weeks for 8 cycles) versus ifosfamide (1.6 $g/m^2/d$ for 3 days) plus paclitaxel (135 mg/m^2 by 3-hour infusion on day 1 repeated every 3 weeks for 8 cycles). Homesley et al reported that there was a survival advantage for combination chemotherapy (13.5 months vs 5.8 months). Doxorubicin has traditionally been used for LMSs. The GOG experience with gemcitabine (Gemzar) in patients previously treated for LMS, showed 20% of patients responded. A recently reported phase III trial conducted by GOG revealed a modest improvement in survival associated with the combination of ifosfamide plus paclitaxel compared with ifosfamide alone. Hormonal agents, specifically progestins, are the treatment of choice for advanced/recurrent endometrial stromal sarcomas.

GESTATIONAL TROPHOBLASTIC DISEASES

Gestational trophoblastic diseases (GTDs) encompass a spectrum of neoplastic disorders that arise from placental trophoblastic tissue after abnormal fertilization. In the United States, GTDs account for less than 1% of gynecologic malignancies. Forty years ago, women with choriocarcinoma had a 95% mortality rate. Today, with the advent of effective chemotherapy and the development of a reliable tumor marker (β-subunit human chorionic gonadotropin [β-hCG]), the cure rate for choriocarcinoma is 90% to 95%.

Clinical presentation

Complete mole

The classic signs of a molar pregnancy include the absence of fetal heart sounds, physical evidence of a uterus that is larger than expected for gestational age, and vaginal bleeding. Although an intact fetus may coexist with a partial mole, this occurs in fewer than 1 in 100,000 pregnancies.

The most common presenting symptom of molar pregnancy is vaginal bleeding, reported in up to 97% of patients. Intrauterine clots may undergo oxidation and liquefaction, producing pathognomonic prune juice-like fluid. Prolonged or recurrent bleeding may result in iron-deficiency anemia. Symptoms of anemia occur in approximately 50% of patients at the time of diagnosis. Early toxemia (hypertension, proteinuria, and edema) presenting during the first or second trimester is common (20% to 30%) in molar pregnancy.

Hyperthyroidism is seen clinically in approximately 7% of molar pregnancies. An elevation of triiodothyronine (T_3) and thyroxine (T_4) levels is observed more commonly than are the clinical manifestations of tachycardia, sweating, weight loss, and tremor. These hormonal elevations are presumed to be secondary to the structural similarity of hCG to thyroid-stimulating hormone (TSH).

Partial mole

Patients with partial mole have different clinical features than those with complete mole. Fewer than 10% of patients with partial mole have uterine enlargement. Patients with partial mole do not have prominent theca-luteal cysts, hyperthyroidism, or respiratory insufficiency. They experience toxemia only rarely. The diagnosis of partial mole is usually made after histologic review of curettage specimens.

Gestational trophoblastic neoplasia

GTD develops in 6% to 19% of patients after molar evacuation. Metastases sometimes have an identical histology to that of molar disease, but the vast majority are choriocarcinomas. Metastatic spread is hematogeneous. Because of its extensive vascular network, metastatic GTD often produces local, spontaneous bleeding. The New England Trophoblastic Disease Center (NETDC) reported that the common metastatic sites of GTD are the lungs (80%); vagina (30%); pelvis (20%); liver (10%); brain (10%); and bowel, kidneys, and spleen (5% each).

Pulmonary metastases are common (80% of patients with metastatic disease) and occur when trophoblastic tissue enters the circulation via uterine venous sinuses. The radiologic features may be protean or subtle and include alveolar, nodular, and miliary patterns. Pleural effusions may also be present. Pulmonary metastases can be extensive and can cause respiratory failure and death.

Right upper-quadrant pain has been observed when hepatic metastases stretch Glisson's capsule. GI lesions may result in severe hemorrhage or in perforation with peritonitis, both of which require emergency intervention. Vaginal examination may reveal bluish metastatic deposits; these and other metastatic sites should not undergo biopsy because severe uncontrolled bleeding may occur.

CNS involvement from metastatic GTD suggests widespread disease and has a poor prognosis. CNS metastases are clinically evident in 7% to 28% of patients with metastatic choriocarcinoma. Cerebral metastases tend to respond favorably to both radiotherapy and chemotherapy.

Diagnostic studies

Although the clinical presentation may suggest a diagnosis of GTD, certain laboratory studies, particularly a determination of the patient's β-hCG level, and radiographic studies are needed to confirm this diagnosis.

Laboratory studies Thyroid function studies should be performed in all patients with a clinical history or physical examination suggestive of hyperthyroidism. Abnormal thyroid function, manifested as an elevated T_4 level, is common in GTD. Metastatic deposits in the kidneys or GI tract may reveal themselves by hematuria or hematochezia.

Tumor markers A well-characterized glycoprotein hormone secreted by the syncytiotrophoblast, hCG is essential to maintaining normal function of the corpus luteum during pregnancy. Because all trophoblastic tumors secrete β-hCG, this hormone serves as an excellent marker for tumor activity in the nonpregnant patient. Serial β-hCG levels should be monitored during therapy to ensure adequate treatment. The level of β-hCG is roughly proportional to the tumor burden and inversely proportional to the therapeutic outcome.

Radiologic studies A chest x-ray should always be performed because 70% to 80% of patients with metastatic GTD have lung involvement. Although this x-ray usually demonstrates nodular metastases, the patterns of metastatic disease can range from atelectatic areas to subtle pleural abnormalities. A CT scan is often helpful in evaluating these nonspecific findings.

Since it has been demonstrated that 97% to 100% of patients with CNS disease from choriocarcinoma have concomitant pulmonary metastases, a CNS workup in asymptomatic patients with normal chest x-rays is not routinely warranted. If the chest x-ray is abnormal, or if β-hCG levels plateau or rise during treatment, a more thorough evaluation for metastatic disease is indicated. MRI of the brain, brain stem, and cerebellum as well as CT scans of the abdomen and pelvis should be performed to evaluate other likely sites of metastatic spread. The presence of intrauterine or ovarian disease also may be detected by MRI of the pelvis. Ultrasonography is a reliable, safe, economical, and relatively simple method for confirming the diagnosis of intrauterine GTD. It is also useful in identifying embryonic remnants.

The proposed FIGO 2000 anatomic staging system is a straightforward system based on anatomic criteria. In GTD, stage I disease is confined to the uterus; stage II disease is outside the uterus but limited to the genital structures; stage III disease extends to the lungs with or without known genital tract involvement; and stage IV disease includes all other metastatic sites. The FIGO 2000 scoring system is based on a method (adapted from the World Health Organization [WHO]) to identify patients at high risk for treatment failure. With the FIGO 2000 scoring system, patients are classified as being in a low-, middle-, or high-risk category. A total score of up to 4 is considered low risk; 5 to 7, middle risk; and 8 or greater, high risk. (Some centers recommend a low-risk score of 6 or less, a high-risk score of 7 or greater, and no middle-risk score.)

Treatment

The treatment strategy for GTD must be individualized for each patient. The stratification of risk groups enables physicians to direct an appropriate treatment strategy. Low-risk disease responds readily to single-agent chemotherapy and is virtually 100% curable. High-risk disease is not likely to be cured with single-agent therapy and therefore requires multidrug regimens.

Molar pregnancy

For patients with complete or partial hydatidiform mole, evacuation of the mole by suction and sharp curettage should be performed. Oxytocics also are given to produce uterine involution and to control bleeding. However, these agents should be used judiciously, as they may cause hyponatremia and fluid overload. A baseline chest x-ray and β-hCG measurement should be obtained prior to surgery. After molar evacuation, 80% of patients will need no further intervention.

Follow-up As mentioned previously, all patients with molar disease should obtain a baseline chest x-ray. Serial β-hCG levels should be obtained every 1 to 2 weeks until the level is normal for three consecutive assays. Complete remission is defined by three consecutive normal β-hCG levels. Once this has occurred, β-hCG levels should be checked monthly for 12 months, every 4 months for the following year, and then yearly for 2 years. However, Lavie et al showed that a single undetectable human chorionic gonadotropin level after evacuation is sufficient follow-up to ensure remission in patients with partial hydatidiform moles.

Although the use of OCs during the surveillance period remains controversial, strict contraception is required, because pregnancy would obviate the usefulness of β-hCG as a tumor marker. In general, once 12-month surveillance establishes a disease-free status, conception is acceptable. These women are always at high risk for future molar disease and will require close observation during future pregnancies. A pelvic ultrasonographic examination should be performed during the first trimester of all subsequent pregnancies to confirm that gestation is normal.

Chemotherapy is indicated when there is a plateau or increase in β-hCG levels on consecutive measurements, failure to reach normal levels by 16 weeks, or metastatic disease. Such patients are usually at low risk and will respond to single-agent chemotherapy. Methotrexate is the most commonly initiated single agent. Therapy is continued for one to two courses after a normal β-hCG level is achieved.

Low-risk metastatic disease

In more than 30 years of experience, single-agent chemotherapy with methotrexate has produced a high cure rate in patients with low-risk GTD. Likewise, methotrexate plus leucovorin induces remission in 90% of patients with low-risk metastatic disease with low toxicity. The use of dactinomycin (Cosmegen) in methotrexate-resistant patients increased the cure rate to more than 95%. Covens et al reported on the first prospective multicenter phase II trial of salvage therapy for failed low-risk gestational trophoblastic neoplasia, GOG 0176. Pulse actinomycin D (1.24 mg/m^2 IV every 2 weeks) is an active regimen.

GOG conducted two phase II trials; both showed that a single dose of dactinomycin every other week (GOG 0069) or weekly IM methotrexate (GOG 0079) had good compliance, comparable activity, and tolerable toxicity. GOG 0174 randomized patients to receive either 30 mg/m^2 weekly of IM methotrexate or "pulsed" intravenous actinomycin D (1.25 mg/m^2 every 2 weeks). "Pulsed" intravenous actinomycin D was the more active regimen.

High-risk metastatic disease

The discovery that etoposide is an effective agent against trophoblastic disease led to the development of the EMA-CO regimen (etoposide, methotrexate, actinomycin D [dactinomycin], cyclophosphamide, Oncovin [vincristine]) by Bagshawe, who reported a survival rate of 83% in patients with high-risk choriocarcinoma.

EMA-CO is the preferred regimen for high-risk GTD. This regimen is also used for patients with middle-risk GTD, as defined by the FIGO 2000 criteria. EMA-CO is generally well tolerated, with no life-threatening toxic effects. Alopecia occurs universally, and anemia, neutropenia, and stomatitis are mild. Reproductive function is preserved in approximately 75% of patients.

Within hours of receiving chemotherapy, patients with a significant tumor burden are at risk of hemorrhage into tumors and surrounding tissues. Thus, any acute organ toxicity that begins shortly after the induction of chemotherapy should be considered as possibly related to this phenomenon. Some researchers have advocated a reduction in dosage at the beginning of therapy in patients with large-volume disease to minimize these sequelae.

Salvage therapy

Unfortunately, about 25% of women with high-risk metastatic disease become refractory to EMA-CO and fail to achieve a complete remission. Currently, there is no standard salvage chemotherapy regimen for patients not responding to EMA-CO. However, salvage regimens that combine cisplatin, etoposide, vinca alkaloids, and bleomycin have been administered.

Early studies show cisplatin-based regimens to be an effective salvage therapy in GTD. A recent dose-intensive regimen, EMA-CE, utilizes cisplatin (100 mg/m^2) and etoposide (200 mg/m^2) combined with EMA, with favorable results.

Another alternative is to give cisplatin in the EMA-POMB regimen (Platinol [cisplatin], Oncovin [vincristine], methotrexate, bleomycin). POMB is administered as vincristine, 1 mg/m² IV, and methotrexate, 300 mg/m² IV (day 1); bleomycin, 15 mg IV over 24 h by continuous infusion (CI), and folinic acid, 15 mg twice daily for four doses (day 2); bleomycin, 15 mg IV over 24 h CI (day 3); and cisplatin, 120 mg/m² IV (day 4).

A new PEBA regimen (Platinol [cisplatin], etoposide, bleomycin, Adriamycin [doxorubicin]) was reported from China and was found to be effective in EMA-CO–resistant disease. A complete remission was achieved in 96% of the women, and 73% had a sustained complete remission that lasted at least 1 year. In a small study, ifosfamide alone and combined in the VIP regimen (VePesid [etoposide], ifosfamide, and Platinol [cisplatin]) showed promise as being an effective salvage drug in GTD. Lurain and Nejad reviewed the experience of the Brewer Trophoblastic Disease Center in patients with persistent or recurrent high-risk gestational trophoblastic neoplasia. They showed that those who develop resistance to methotrexate-containing treatment protocols should be treated with drug combinations employing a platinum agent and etoposide with or without bleomycin or ifosfamide.

Another consideration in the treatment of refractory GTD is the use of high-dose chemotherapy with autologous bone marrow transplantation.

SUGGESTED READING

ON ENDOMETRIAL CANCER

Barakat RR, Bundy BN, Spirtos NM, et al: Randomized double-blind trial of estrogen replacement therapy versus placebo in stage I or II endometrial cancer: A Gynecologic Oncology Group Study. J Clin Oncol 24:587–592, 2006.

Cragun JM, Havrilesky LJ, Calingaert B, et al: Retrospective analysis of selective lympadenectomy in apparent early-stage endometrial cancer. J Clin Oncol 23:3668–3675, 2005.

Fayed A, Mutch DG, Rader JS, et al: Comparison of high-dose-rate and low-dose-rate brachytherapy in the treatment of endometrial carcinoma. Int J Radiat Oncol Biol Phys 67:480–484, 2007.

Greven K, Winter K, Underhill K, et al: Final analysis of RTOG 9708: Adjuvant postoperative irradiation combined with cisplatin/paclitaxel chemotherapy following surgery for patients with high-risk endometrial cancer. Gynecol Oncol 103:155–159, 2006.

Hogberg T, Rosenberg P, Kristensen G, et al: A randomized phase-III study on adjuvant treatment with radiation (RT) ± chemotherapy (CT) in early-stage high-risk endometrial cancer (NSGO-EC-9501/EORTC 55991). J Clin Oncol 25[18S]:5503, 2007.

Johnson N, Cornes P: Survival and recurrent disease after postoperative radiotherapy for early endometrial cancer: Systematic review and meta-analysis. BJOG 114:1313–1320, 2007.

Lin LL, Mutch DG, Rader JS, et al: External radiotherapy versus vaginal brachytherapy for patients with intermediate risk endometrial cancer. Gynecol Oncol 106:215–220, 2007.

Maxwell GL, Schildkraut JM, Calingaert B, et al: Progestin and estrogen potency of combination oral contraceptives and endometrial cancer risk. Gynecol Oncol 103:535–540, 2006.

McMeekin DS, Filiaci VL, Thigpen JT, et al: The relationship between histology and outcome in advanced and recurrent endometrial cancer patients participating in first-line chemotherapy trials: A Gynecologic Oncology Group study. Gynecol Oncol 106:16–22, 2007.

Nout RA, Putter H, Jurgenliemk-Schulz IM, et al: Vaginal brachytherapy versus external beam pelvic radiotherapy for high-intermediate risk endometrial cancer: Results of the randomized PORTEC-2 trial. J Clin Oncol 26:[abstract LBA5503], 2008.

Patel S, Portelance L, Gilbert L, et al: Analysis of prognostic factors and patterns of recurrence in patients with pathologic stage III endometrial cancer. Int J Radiat Oncol Biol Phys 68:1438–1445, 2007.

Polyzos NP, Pavlidis N, Paraskevaidis E, et al: Randomized evidence on chemotherapy and hormonal therapy regimens for advanced endometrial cancer: An overview of survival data. Eur J Cancer 42:319–326, 2006.

Randall ME, Filiaci VL, Muss H, et al: Randomized phase III trial of whole-abdominal irradiation versus doxorubicin and cisplatin chemotherapy in advanced endometrial carcinoma: A Gynecologic Oncology Group Study. J Clin Oncol 234:36–44, 2006.

Scholten AN, van Putten WL, Beerman H, et al; PORTEC Study Group: Postoperative radiotherapy for stage 1 endometrial carcinoma: Long-term outcome of the randomized PORTEC trial with central pathology review. Int J Radiat Oncol Biol Phys 63:834–838, 2005.

Sovak MA, Chuai S, Anderson S, et al: Paclitaxel and carboplatin (TP) for treatment of advanced or recurrent endometrial cancer: A retrospective study (abstract). J Clin Oncol 23(suppl):460s, 2005.

Spirtos NM, Eisekop SM, Boike G, et al: Laparoscopic staging in patients with incompletely staged cancers of the uterus, ovary, fallopian tube, and primary peritoneum: A Gynecologic Oncology Group (GOG) study. Am J Obstet Gynecol 193:1645–1649, 2005.

Straughn JM Jr, Numnum TM, Kilgore LC, et al: The use of adjuvant radiation therapy in patients with intermediate-risk stages IC and II uterine corpus cancer: A patient care evaluation study from the Amerian College of Surgeons National Cancer Data Base. Gynecol Oncol 99:530–535, 2005.

Susumu N, Sagae S, Udagawa Y, et al: Randomized phase III trial of pelvic radiotherapy versus cisplatin-based combined chemotherapy in patients with intermediate- and high-risk endometrial cancer: A Japanese Gynecologic Oncology Group study. Gynecol Oncol 108:226–233, 2008.

Sutton G, Axelrod JH, Bundy BN, et al: Adjuvant whole abdominal irradiation in clinical stages I and II papillary serous or clear cell carcinoma of the endometrium: A phase II study of the Gynecologic Oncology Group. Gynecol Oncol 100:349–354, 2006.

Trimble CL, Kauderer J, Zaino R, et al: Concurrent endometrial carcinoma in women with a biopsy diagnosis of atypical endometrial hyperplasia: A Gynclogic Oncology Group study. Cancer 106:812–819, 2006.

Zaino RJ, Kauderer J, Trimble CL, et al: Reproducibility of the diagnosis of atypical endometrial hyperplasia: A Gynecologic Oncology Group study. Cancer 106:804–811, 2006.

ON GESTATIONAL TROPHOBLASTIC DISEASES

Covens A, Filiaci VL, Burger RA, et al: Phase II trial of pulse dactinomycin as salvage therapy for failed low-risk gestational trophoblastic neoplasia: A Gynecologic Oncology Group study. Cancer 107:1280–1286, 2006.

Lavie I, Rao GG, Castrillon DH, et al: Duration of human chorionic gonadotropin surveillance for partial hydatidiform moles. Am J Obstet Gynecol 192:1362–1364, 2005.

Lurain JR, Nejad B: Secondary chemotherapy for high-risk gestational trophoblastic neoplasia. Gynecol Oncol 97:618–623, 2005.

ON UTERINE SARCOMAS

Homesley HD, Filiaci V, Markman M, et al: Phase III trial of ifosfamide with or without paclitaxel in advanced uterine carcinosarcoma: A Gyncologic Oncology Group Study. J Clin Oncol 25:526–531, 2007.

Li AJ, Giuntoli RI 2nd, Drake R, et al: Ovarian preservation in stage I low-grade endometrial stromal sarcomas. Obstet Gynecol 106:1304–1308, 2005.

Sutton G, Kauderer J, Carson LF, et al: Adjuvant ifosfamide and cisplatin in patients with completely resected stage I or II carcinosarcomas (mixed mesodermal tumors) of the uterus: A Gynecologic Oncology Group study. Gynecol Oncol 96:630–634, 2005.

Wolfson AH, Brady MF, Rocereto T, et al: A gynecologic oncology group randomized phase III trial of whole abdominal irradiation (WAI) vs cisplatin-ifosfamide and mesna (CIM) as post-surgical therapy in stage I-IV carcinosarcoma (CS) of the uterus. Gynecol Oncol 107:177–185, 2007.

CHAPTER 22

Ovarian cancer

Stephen C. Rubin, MD, Paul Sabbatini, MD,
and Akila N. Viswanathan, MD, MPH

Despite the fact that it is highly curable if diagnosed early, cancer of the ovaries causes more mortality in American women each year than all other gynecologic malignancies combined. An estimated 21,650 new cases of this cancer will be diagnosed in the United States in 2008, and about 15,520 women will succumb to the disease.

Notable advances in chemotherapy and surgery over the past several decades have begun to translate into improved survival. According to American Cancer Society data, the overall 5-year survival rate from ovarian cancer has increased significantly, from 36% in the mid-1970s to 53% in the mid-1990s. Recent data from the National Cancer Institute show a similar increase in stage-specific survival. It is expected that data from the current decade, reflecting continued improvements in chemotherapy and surgery, will continue this trend.

This chapter will focus on epithelial cancers of the ovaries, which account for about 90% of ovarian malignancies.

Epidemiology

Age Ovarian cancer is primarily a disease of postmenopausal women, with the large majority of cases occurring in women between 50 and 75 years old. The incidence of ovarian cancer increases with age and peaks at a rate of 61.5 per 100,000 women in the 75–79-year-old age group.

Race The incidence of ovarian cancer appears to vary by race, although the effects of race are difficult to separate from those of environment related to culture, geography, and socioeconomic status. In the United States, the age-adjusted rate of ovarian cancer for Caucasians is estimated to be 17.9 per 100,000 population, which is significantly higher than 11.9 per 100,000 for the African-American population.

Geography There are distinct geographic variations in the incidence of ovarian cancer, with the highest rates found in industrialized countries and the lowest rates seen in underdeveloped nations. Japan, with an incidence of only about 3.0 per 100,000 population, is a notable exception to this observation. It has been postulated that geographic variations in the incidence of ovarian cancer are related, in part, to differences in family size.

Some of the highest rates are seen in women of Eastern European Jewish ancestry, who have an estimated incidence of 17.2 per 100,000 population, a probable result of the relatively high frequency of *BRCA1* and *BRCA2* mutations in this population.

Etiology and risk factors

The cause of epithelial ovarian cancer remains unknown. Although it now appears certain that, at the cellular level, ovarian cancer results from the accumulation of multiple discrete genetic defects, the mechanism(s) by which these defects develop have yet to be determined. Epidemiologic studies have identified a number of factors that may increase or decrease the risk of the disease. In addition, a small proportion of ovarian cancers in the United States, approximately 5%–10%, result from inherited defects in the *BRCA1* gene or other genes, including *BRCA2* and the hereditary nonpolyposis colorectal cancer *(HNPCC)* genes.

Diet It has been suggested that numerous dietary factors increase the risk of ovarian cancer, although the magnitude of the reported increase is relatively modest.

Fat A low-fat diet may reduce the incidence of ovarian cancer among postmenopausal women.

Lactose Populations with a high dietary intake of lactose who lack the enzyme galactose-1-phosphate uridyltransferase have been reported to be at increased risk.

Coffee Conflicting reports have been published regarding the role of coffee consumption and the risk of ovarian cancer.

Environmental factors Various environmental risk factors also have been suggested.

Talc Exposure to talc (hydrous magnesium trisilicate) used as dusting powder on diaphragms and sanitary napkins has been reported in some studies to increase the risk of ovarian cancer, although other studies have failed to find an association.

Radiation No association between exposure to ionizing radiation and the risk of ovarian cancer has been documented.

Viruses Several studies have examined the effect of viral agents, including mumps, rubella, and influenza viruses, on the risk of ovarian cancer. No clear relationship has been demonstrated.

Exercise Physical activity may decrease the risk of ovarian cancer.

Hormonal and reproductive factors In contrast to the conflicting data on dietary and environmental factors, some clear associations have been drawn between certain hormonal and reproductive factors and the risk of developing ovarian cancer.

Low parity and infertility Several analyses have documented that women with a history of low parity or involuntary infertility are at increased risk of ovarian cancer.

Tubal ligation significantly decreases the risk of ovarian cancer, as demonstrated by several epidemiologic studies.

Ovulation-inducing drugs Evidence suggests that treatment with ovulation-inducing drugs, particularly for prolonged periods, may be a risk factor, although it is difficult to separate the increased risk related to the infertility itself from the risk carried by use of ovulation-inducing agents.

Breastfeeding for long durations may decrease ovarian cancer risk.

Hormone replacement therapy Although the data are not consistent, some studies have shown an association between the use of postmenopausal hormone replacement and the development of ovarian cancer. Data from the Women's Health Initiative randomized trial of estrogen plus progestin showed a slight increase in the risk of ovarian cancer in users of hormone replacement therapy, although it was not statistically significant.

Oral contraceptives Several large case-controlled studies have documented a marked protective effect of oral contraceptives against ovarian cancer. Women who have used oral contraceptives for at least several years have approximately half the risk of ovarian cancer as do nonusers, and the protective effect of oral contraceptives appears to persist for years after their discontinuation. It is estimated that the routine use of oral contraceptives may prevent nearly 2,000 cases of ovarian cancer yearly in the United States. Evidence suggests that the protective effect of oral contraceptives also applies to women carrying *BRCA* mutations.

Hereditary cancer syndromes There has been a fascinating evolution in our understanding of the role of hereditary factors in the development of ovarian cancer. It has been recognized for many years that women with a family history of cancer, particularly cancer of the ovaries or breasts, are themselves at increased risk of ovarian cancer. In the 1980s, Lynch and colleagues refined these observations by delineating several apparently distinct syndromes of hereditary cancer involving the ovaries, including breast-ovarian cancer syndrome, site-specific ovarian cancer syndrome, and Lynch II syndrome (HNPCC).

Epidemiologically, these syndromes appear to be inherited as an autosomal-dominant trait with variable penetrance. During the past decade, the specific genes responsible for HNPCC (*MSH1* and *MLH2*) and for most cases of hereditary ovarian cancer have been identified, allowing fundamental observations to be made regarding their molecular pathophysiology.

BRCA1 mutations The *BRCA1* gene is classified as a tumor suppressor, since mutations in this gene increase the risk of breast and ovarian cancers. Definitive identification of the function of the protein translated from this gene remains to be elucidated, although evidence suggests that it plays a role in the repair of oxidative damage to DNA. Part of the protein appears to contain a DNA-binding domain, suggesting that it also functions as a transcriptional regulator.

The frequency of *BRCA1* mutations in the general population is estimated at approximately 1 in 800, and in Jewish women of eastern European descent, 1 in 100.

Women carrying a germline mutation of *BRCA1* have a significantly elevated risk of both breast and ovarian cancers compared with the general population. The average population risk of developing breast cancer is about 12.5% (one in eight) and of developing ovarian cancer, 1.5%. However, in the presence of a germline *BRCA1* mutation and a strong family history of cancer, these risks rise to about 90% and 40% for breast and ovarian cancers, respectively.

It is important to recognize that these risk estimates are derived from families identified with multiple cases of breast and/or ovarian cancer. The risk for women with *BRCA1* mutations from families with less impressive family histories is probably lower for ovarian cancer, perhaps in the range of 15%–20%.

Although the presence of germline mutations in *BRCA1* is not limited to women with a strong family history of breast cancer, data from several laboratories suggest that *BRCA1* mutations usually are not a feature of sporadic ovarian cancer. Mutations in this gene appear to play a role in the development of approximately 50% of familial breast cancer cases and may account for the majority of hereditary ovarian cancers. Evidence from multiple studies suggests that *BRCA1*-related ovarian cancers may have a less aggressive clinical course than do sporadic ovarian cancers.

BRCA2 mutations Hereditary ovarian cancers not related to *BRCA1* are most often related to mutations in the *BRCA2* gene.

For patients having a *BRCA1* or *BRCA2* mutation, laparoscopic prophylactic risk-reducing salpingo-oophorectomy after childbearing can reduce the risk of both breast and ovarian carcinomas.

Signs and symptoms

Early-stage disease In the early stages, ovarian cancer may be an insidious disease, but nonspecific symptoms that may be clues to the diagnosis are present more often than previously thought. A prospective case-controlled study by Goff et al evaluated 1,709 women with the diagnosis of ovarian cancer and compared their self-reported symptoms with those of women without ovarian cancer who attended a primary care clinic. The combination of bloating, increased abdominal size, and urinary symptoms was found in 43% of those with cancer but in only 8% of those without cancer. These symptoms are nonspecific, however, and will not likely yield the reliable discovery of early-stage disease in the majority of patients.

The impact of screening patients with serum CA-125 levels and transvaginal ultrasonography on mortality is being addressed in the Prostate, Lung, Colorectal, and Ovarian Trial (PLCO). In this study, 39,115 women were randomized to undergo screening. To date, screening has identified both early- and late-stage cancers, and the predictive value is low (3.7% for abnormal CA-125, 1.0% for abnormal transvaginal ultrasonography, and 23.5% for both). Follow-up is ongoing to determine whether there is an effect on mortality.

Early ovarian cancer also may be detected as a pelvic mass noted fortuitously at the time of a routine pelvic examination. Imaging with sonography, CT, or MRI will confirm the presence of a mass. The size, internal architecture, and blood flow of the mass can be used to make an educated guess as to whether it is benign or malignant, but imaging findings are not diagnostic in this regard. Approximately 50% of patients with early ovarian cancers have an elevated serum CA-125 level.

Advanced-stage disease Patients may complain of abdominal bloating or swelling if ascites is present, and large pelvic masses may produce bladder or rectal symptoms. Occasional patients may have respiratory distress as a result of a large pleural effusion, which is more common on the right side. Infrequently, there may be a history of abnormal vaginal bleeding.

Most patients with advanced disease have ascites detectable by physical examination or imaging. Complex pelvic masses and an omental tumor cake may be present, and nodules can frequently be palpated in the pelvic cul-de-sac on rectovaginal examination. It should be noted that some patients with advanced ovarian cancer have essentially normal-sized ovaries. Approximately 80% of patients with advanced ovarian cancer will have an elevated serum CA-125 level.

Screening and diagnosis

Screening Unfortunately, no effective strategy exists for screening of the general population for ovarian cancer. Imaging techniques, including abdominal and transvaginal sonography, have been studied extensively, as has the serum marker CA-125. None of these techniques, alone or in combination, is specific enough to serve as an appropriate screening test, even in populations targeted by age.

Both the National Institutes of Health Consensus Conference (see full page of NIH guidelines) and the American College of Obstetricians and Gynecologists have issued statements advising against routine screening for ovarian cancer, which, due to its high false-positive rate, leads to an unacceptable amount of invasive interventions in women without significant disease.

The NIH PLCO Screening Trial has accrued its full complement of 152,000 patients. For the ovarian cancer segment of the trial, half of the women will be screened via physical examination, CA-125 level, and vaginal ultrasonography and the other half, via standard medical care. Since patients will be followed for 13 years or more final results are not yet available. It is not expected that these screening modalities will have a significant impact in the general population.

Recent studies using serum proteomics to screen for early ovarian cancer have yielded promising results. Work in this area is ongoing and may result in a clinically useful assay in the near future.

High-risk patients Management of women from families with hereditary ovarian cancer is controversial. Evidence suggests that surveillance of such women with serum markers and sonography is of limited benefit in early detection of ovarian cancer. Most experts recommend prophylactic laparoscopic excision of the ovaries and fallopian tubes after age 35 if the woman has completed childbearing, as several studies have shown that it will dramatically reduce the risk of ovarian cancer. Evidence also suggests that prophylactic oophorectomy substantially lowers the risk of breast cancer in women from high-risk families.

Preoperative evaluation Patients with suspected ovarian cancer should undergo a thorough evaluation prior to surgery. This assessment should include a complete history and physical examination and serum CA-125 level determination. In women younger than age 30, determinations of β-human chorionic gonadotropin (β-hCG) and α-fetoprotein (AFP) levels are useful, as germ-cell tumors are more common in this age group.

Abdominal CT and MRI In apparent early-stage cases, abdominal scanning by CT or MRI adds little to the diagnostic evaluation, and, thus, these studies are not routinely necessary. CT and MRI may be useful in providing a preoperative assessment of disease extent in probable advanced-stage cases.

Exploratory laparotomy The diagnosis of ovarian cancer is generally made by histopathologic study following exploratory laparotomy. The stage of the disease can only be determined by surgery, as discussed later.

Preoperative endometrial sampling Women with abnormal vaginal bleeding should undergo preoperative endometrial sampling.

Preoperative cytologic or histologic evaluation of effusions or tumor masses is neither necessary nor desirable. Often, patients with ascites and large pelvic masses, for whom exploration is necessary, are subjected to paracentesis or needle biopsy. These procedures only delay definitive management and may lead to seeding of tumor cells along needle tracks.

Pathology

The ovaries are notable for their ability to give rise to a large variety of neoplasms with distinct embryologic origins and differing histologic appearances.

Epithelial adenocarcinoma Approximately 90% of all ovarian malignancies are of epithelial origin, arising from the cells on the surface of the ovaries. These cells give rise to a variety of adenocarcinomas, including serous, mucinous, endometrioid, and clear-cell types. These tumors have benign counterparts of similar histologic appearance and can also exist as "borderline" cancers, also known as "tumors of low malignant potential." There is some prognostic significance to the cell type of the tumor, with clear-cell and mucinous varieties tending to be especially virulent.

Histologic differentiation Pathologists also classify adenocarcinomas according to the degree of histologic differentiation. Those tumors retaining clear-cut glandular features are considered grade 1, or well differentiated, whereas those that are

NIH GUIDELINES ON SCREENING FOR OVARIAN CANCER

Until clinical trials gather enough information, no evidence supports routine screening for ovarian cancer in women without first-degree relatives affected by the disease, according to a consensus development panel convened by the NIH.

The panel did recommend that physicians take a comprehensive family history of their female patients. The panel also advised women to undergo routine annual rectovaginal pelvic examinations.

There are no conclusive data that screening is beneficial, even for women with two or more first-degree relatives with ovarian cancer, the panel stated. However, these women have a significant chance of having a hereditary ovarian cancer syndrome and should be counseled by a gynecologic oncologist or other qualified specialist regarding their individual risk.

Patients with hereditary ovarian cancer syndrome

Patients with hereditary ovarian cancer syndrome (assuming autosomal-dominant inheritance with 80% penetrance) have a 40% lifetime risk of developing ovarian cancer. Recent data suggest that screening these women reduces their mortality from ovarian cancer.

High-risk women

The three known hereditary syndromes that place a woman at exceedingly high risk are familial site-specific ovarian cancer syndrome, breast-ovarian cancer syndrome, and breast-ovarian-endometrial-colorectal cancer syndrome. Annual rectovaginal pelvic examinations, CA-125 level determinations, and transvaginal ultrasonography are recommended for these women until their childbearing is completed or until age 35, at which time prophylactic bilateral oophorectomy is recommended.

Prophylactic oophorectomy performed in women undergoing abdominal surgery for other indications, such as benign uterine disease, is also associated with a significant reduction in the risk of ovarian cancer. The appropriateness of hormonal replacement therapy is not straightforward given that many of these women are at higher risk for breast cancer. In addition, the report from the study by the Women's Health Initiative in postmenopausal women raised questions regarding the role of long-term hormonal replacement, particularly showing no benefit in terms of cardiovascular risk reduction. Women should discuss the potential for estrogen replacement vs other agents for the prevention of osteoporosis, for example, with their health care provider.

Other panel recommendations

Women with ovarian masses who have been identified preoperatively as having a significant risk of ovarian cancer should be advised to have their surgery performed by a gynecologic oncologist.

Aggressive attempts at cytoreductive surgery as the primary management of ovarian cancer will improve the chances for long-term survival.

Women with stage IA and IB, grade 1 ovarian cancer do not require postoperative adjuvant therapy, although many remaining patients with stage I disease do require chemotherapy. Subsets of stage I must be fully defined and ideal treatment determined.

Second-look laparotomy should not be employed as routine care for all patients but should be performed for patients enrolled in clinical trials or for patients in whom the surgery will affect clinical decision-making and the clinical course.

From Ovarian cancer: Screening, treatment and follow-up. NIH Consensus Statement. 12:1–30, 1994.

TABLE I: FIGO staging system for ovarian cancer

Stage	Characteristics
I	Growth limited to the ovaries
IA	Growth limited to one ovary; no ascites; no tumor on the external surfaces, capsule intact
IB	Growth limited to both ovaries; no ascites; no tumor on the external surfaces, capsule intact
IC	Tumor either stage IA or IB but on the surface of one or both ovaries; capsule ruptured; ascites containing malignant cells present; or positive peritoneal washings
II	Growth involving one or both ovaries with pelvic extension of disease
IIA	Extension of disease and/or metastases to the uterus and/or fallopian tubes
IIB	Extension of disease to other pelvic tissues
IIC	Tumor either stage IIA or IIB but on the surface of one or both ovaries; capsule(s) ruptured; ascites containing malignant cells present; or positive peritoneal washings
III	Tumor involving one or both ovaries with peritoneal implants outside the pelvis and/or positive retroperitoneal or inguinal nodes; superficial liver metastasis equals stage III; tumor is limited to the true pelvis but with histologically verified malignant extension to the small bowel or omentum
IIIA	Tumor grossly limited to the true pelvis with negative nodes but with histologically confirmed microscopic seeding of abdominal peritoneal surfaces
IIIB	Tumor of one or both ovaries; histologically confirmed implants on abdominal peritoneal surfaces, none > 2 cm in diameter; nodes negative
IIIC	Abdominal implants > 2 cm in diameter and/or positive retroperitoneal or inguinal nodes
IV	Growth involving one or both ovaries with distant metastases; if pleural effusion is present, there must be positive cytologic test results to allot a case to stage IV; parenchymal liver metastasis equals stage IV

FIGO = International Federation of Gynecology and Obstetrics

largely composed of solid sheets of tumor are considered grade 3, or poorly differentiated. Tumors showing both glandular and solid areas are assigned to grade 2. The histologic grade seems to correlate roughly with biologic aggressiveness.

Stromal and germ-cell tumors Malignancies can also arise from the ovarian stroma or the primordial germ cells contained within the ovaries. Stromal tumors are often hormone-producing and include such types as the granulosa tumor, Sertoli-Leydig tumor, and several variants. Germ-cell tumors, which tend to be highly aggressive, include the dysgerminoma, endodermal sinus tumor, malignant teratoma, embryonal carcinoma, and rare primary choriocarcinoma of the ovaries. Malignant germ-cell tumors occur primarily in younger patients, with an average age at diagnosis of about 19 years.

TABLE 2: Procedures for surgical staging for apparent early ovarian cancer

Vertical incision

Multiple cytologic washings

Intact tumor removal

Complete abdominal exploration

Removal of remaining ovaries, uterus, fallopian tubes[a]

Omentectomy

Lymph node sampling

Random peritoneal biopsies, including the diaphragm

[a] May be preserved in selected patients who wish to preserve fertility

Staging and prognosis

Staging system

The staging system for ovarian cancer shown in Table 1, developed by the International Federation of Gynecology and Obstetrics (FIGO), is used uniformly in all developed countries. It is based on the results of a properly performed exploratory laparotomy, a fact that bears emphasis, since inadequate surgical staging has been and continues to be a significant problem.

Surgical staging The surgical staging of ovarian cancer is based on an understanding of the patterns of disease spread and must be conducted in a systematic and thorough manner. It should include a complete evaluation of all visceral and parietal surfaces within the peritoneal cavity, omentectomy, and biopsy of aortic and pelvic lymph nodes. It generally includes removal of the internal reproductive organs as well, although exceptions to this rule can be made for younger women with limited disease who may wish to retain fertility.

The issue of adequate surgical staging becomes particularly acute in just the patient population likely to be operated upon by individuals with no specialized training in gynecologic oncology: patients with adnexal masses that are not obvious cancers on preoperative evaluation. At the time of exploration, if the mass is shown to be malignant on frozen section and there is no obvious metastatic disease, a complete staging operation is essential to search for occult metastatic spread, which may be present in 20%–30% of such cases. Also, if the tumor is documented to be stage IA by thorough staging and the patient wishes to preserve the potential for future fertility, it may be appropriate to conserve the uterus and uninvolved ovaries and fallopian tubes.

The elements of surgical staging for apparent early ovarian cancer are listed in Table 2.

Prognostic factors

The prognosis of epithelial ovarian cancer depends on a number of factors.

Disease stage Of primary importance is the disease stage, which, when properly determined, is of strong prognostic significance. The distribution of ovarian cancer cases by stage follows: stage I, 26%; stage II, 15%; stage III, 42%; stage IV, 17%. For patients with advanced ovarian cancer, the amount of residual tumor at the conclusion of the initial operation is of major importance. Patients with stage III disease who have minimal or no residual tumor may have a 30%–50% chance of 5-year survival, whereas those patients with stage III disease left with bulky tumor masses have a 5-year survival rate of only about 10%.

Histologic grade and type Most studies have found the histologic grade of the tumor to have prognostic significance; the histologic cell type of the tumor is of less importance, although patients with clear-cell and possibly mucinous tumors may have a worse prognosis.

Molecular markers In recent years, a great deal of effort has been devoted to the identification of molecular markers of prognosis in ovarian cancer. Studies of HER2, *p53*, *ras*, and other oncogenes and tumor-suppressor genes have had varying results relative to prognostic significance. Currently, the assessment of molecular markers of prognosis has no clinical utility, although much work continues in this area, particularly with the development of high-throughput techniques for determining gene and protein expression.

Predictors of chemosensitivity Despite a continued effort to assess in vitro methods to predict the sensitivity or resistance of ovarian cancers to various chemotherapeutic drugs, the clinical usefulness of such an approach remains under investigation. The American Society of Clinical Oncology (ASCO) recently reviewed the relevant literature on the subject and reached the same conclusion for cancers in general.

Treatment

Surgery plays a crucial role in all phases of the management of ovarian cancer and, when applied as part of a multidisciplinary approach, affords patients the highest likelihood of a favorable outcome. For most patients with ovarian carcinoma, surgery is not curative due to dissemination of tumor cells throughout the abdominal cavity. Therefore, successful management generally requires additional treatment.

The use of postoperative chemotherapy is standard for all patients with advanced-stage disease and for many patients with early-stage disease. Adjunctive chemotherapy significantly prolongs survival, with most current data supporting the use of platinum- and taxane-based regimens.

Despite a long history of the use of radiation therapy in ovarian carcinoma, due to the relatively high sensitivity of ovarian cancer to radiation in general, opinions on indications for use differ widely. Presumably, this controversy is due to the limited amount and adequacy of data comparing radiotherapy with modern chemotherapy regimens, as well as concerns regarding potential toxicities. Studies using radiation in both radical and palliative settings have been published, but standardization of the use of radiation varies significantly worldwide.

MANAGEMENT OF EARLY-STAGE DISEASE

Clearly, comprehensive surgical staging is necessary to properly identify patients with stages I and II ovarian carcinoma. Beyond surgery, the need for adjuvant treatment with chemotherapy has been recently supported, with the exception of patients with stage I disease and well-differentiated histology.

Surgery

Suspicious adnexal masses should be excised intact and submitted for frozen section. If a malignancy is confirmed and there is no obvious metastatic spread, complete surgical staging should be undertaken. As discussed previously (see section on "Staging and prognosis"), it is of critical importance that surgical staging be performed in a systematic and complete manner. Inadequate staging may result in inappropriate postoperative treatment, which can severely compromise the chances for cure.

Data from the American College of Surgeons community hospital-based tumor registry show that almost 75% of the primary surgeries for ovarian cancer performed in this country are done so without the involvement of a gynecologic oncologist. This finding is unfortunate given the fact that, with physical examination, measurement of CA-125 levels, and appropriate imaging tests, the majority of cases of ovarian cancer can be identified preoperatively. Results from other studies suggest that when a gynecologic oncologist is not present at the initial operation, staging is more often inadequate, cytoreduction is more often suboptimal, and long-term survival is poorer.

Conservation of reproductive organs In a woman of reproductive age with cancer limited to one ovary, it may be possible to conserve the uterus and opposite fallopian tube and ovary if she wishes to maintain the option of future fertility. To facilitate such intraoperative decision-making, it is essential that the surgeon's preoperative discussion with the patient and her family address the possibility of malignancy and review the surgical options for both benign and malignant diseases.

Operative laparoscopy Recent advances in the instrumentation for operative laparoscopy have led to an increase in the proportion of adnexal masses being managed with this technique. Physicians should exercise caution in selecting patients with adnexal masses for operative laparoscopic approaches. Unless the surgeon's laparoscopic skills are extraordinary, suspicious masses are best managed by laparotomy. For masses that are approached laparoscopically, the same surgical principles of removal without spill and complete surgical staging apply.

Systemic chemotherapy for early-stage disease

The current management of patients with early-stage disease focuses on comprehensive surgical staging and the identification of high-risk features. Patients with stage IA or IB tumors with well-differentiated histology have excellent 5-year survival rates, and adjuvant chemotherapy is generally not used in such patients. High-risk features include moderately to poorly differentiated tumors, stage IC or II disease, and clear-cell histology.

The reported survival rates of 60%–80% in patients who have early-stage tumors with high-risk features suggested a potential role for adjuvant therapy. The Italian Inter-Regional Cooperative Group conducted two randomized trials to evaluate the role of adjuvant therapy in patients with stage I disease. The first trial compared cisplatin, 50 mg/m^2 q28d $\times$ 6, with observation in 85 patients with stage IA or IB, grade 2–3 disease. The 5-year disease-free survival rate was higher in patients treated with cisplatin than in those who were observed (83% vs 63%), but the 5-year overall survival rate was similar in the two groups (88% vs 82%).

The second trial compared cisplatin (same dose) to phosphorus-32 (P-32) administration in 161 patients with stage IA–IB, grade 2, or stage IC disease. The 5-year disease-free survival rate again favored the platinum arm (85% vs 65%), but the 5-year overall survival rate was unchanged and similar to that reported in the previous trial. P-32 administration was associated with more long-term toxicity.

More recent data have provided support for a survival benefit to the immediate use of adjuvant chemotherapy in patients with early-stage disease. The results of the ACTION (European Organization for Research on the Treatment of Cancer [EORTC] Adjuvant Treatment in Ovarian Neoplasm) and International Collaborative on Ovarian Neoplasm (ICON) trials were combined and reported. A 5-year survival rate improvement of 8% was reported for those receiving immediate chemotherapy compared with reserving chemotherapy for those who relapsed (74% vs 82%; 95% confidence interval [CI], 2%–12%).

Improvements in systemic chemotherapy for advanced ovarian cancer with associated improvements in survival are relevant to the design of regimens for early-stage disease. A Gynecologic Oncology Group trial (GOG 157) evaluated 3 vs 6 cycles of paclitaxel and carboplatin (Paraplatin) in patients with stage IA or IB, grade 2–3; stage IC; or stage II disease. The trial completed accrual in 1995, and final results showed no significant benefit to the longer regimen. The GOG replacement trial is evaluating 3 cycles of paclitaxel plus carboplatin with or without additional weekly paclitaxel (40 mg/m^2) in patients with early-stage disease.

In the absence of additional data, taxane- and platinum-based systemic chemotherapy should be considered the standard approach for patients who have early-stage disease with the exception of well-staged IA or IB, grade 1 disease. The optimal number of cycles is currently unclear, but 3 cycles were considered the standard arm in the GOG 157 trial, although many clinicians offer 6 cycles of therapy in the absence of prohibitive toxicity.

Radiation therapy

Past GOG trials have established that patients with stage IA–IB, well-differentiated or moderately differentiated tumors have a 5-year survival rate of 90%–98%, which does not seem to improve with adjuvant chemotherapy. However, patients with less favorable neoplasms by virtue of higher grade or stage have poorer outcomes (80% 5-year survival rate among treated patients).

Whole-abdominal irradiation A study by Hepp et al found whole -abdominal irradiation (WAI) to be an effective adjuvant therapy in patients with optimally debulked tumors. In a series of 60 patients, the 5-year survival rate was 55%, with a median follow-up of 96.5 months. Patients who received chemotherapy (n = 41) fared slightly worse than those who received radiation therapy only. The abdominal control rate was 83%, and the grade 3 and 4 late toxicity rates were 7% and 3%, respectively.

The findings indicate that 5- and 10-year survival rates obtained with WAI are at least equivalent to results obtained using modern systemic agents. However, in view of the recognized limitations of these trials, more rigorously gathered data will be required to establish the role of WAI in these patients.

Collectively, existing data suggest that WAI should be studied further as a primary adjuvant treatment modality in patients thought to require treatment. The entire abdomen should be treated with an open-field technique using 100–150 cGy/d, to a total dose of 2,200–3,000 cGy, with careful attention paid to protecting the kidneys. Recent uses of intensity-modulated radiation therapy (IMRT) to the whole abdomen allow significant sparing of the kidneys, liver, heart, and other normal tissues. The utility of routine pelvic boosts is questionable in patients with completely debulked tumors.

MANAGEMENT OF ADVANCED DISEASE

Surgery

In the majority of cases, surgeons operating on patients with ovarian cancer find obvious evidence of widespread metastatic disease. Ascites is often present, with diffuse peritoneal tumor studding and extensive omental involvement. In such cases, it is still important to document the surgical stage (usually a substage of stage III) and carefully evaluate and describe the extent and location of tumor identified at both the beginning and conclusion of surgery.

Optimal cytoreduction The primary function of surgery in patients with advanced ovarian cancer is cytoreduction or debulking. When surgery is performed by experienced gynecologic cancer surgeons, at least 50% of patients with stage III ovarian cancer can be left with "optimal" residual tumor (ie, ≤ 1 cm). The morbidity associated with such surgery is low, and operative mortality is rare.

Patients with optimally debulked disease have an increased likelihood of achieving a complete clinical response to chemotherapy. Disease progression-free interval, median survival, and long-term survival are all improved in patients who have optimal cytoreduction.

Two GOG studies recently reported both indicated that the major survival benefit of cytoreductive surgery was in those patients who were optimally cytoreduced to no macroscopic residual disease.

In the first series, 1,895 patients with stage III disease received cisplatin and paclitaxel in standard intravenous regimens. Optimal cytoreduction to no macroscopic disease was achieved in 23%. This resulted in significantly better ($P < .001$) progression-free and overall survival rates (PFS = 33.0 months; OS = 71.9 months) vs patients with residual disease of 0.1 to 1 cm residual disease (PFS = 16.8 months; OS = 42.4 months) or residual disease greater than 1 cm (PFS = 14.1 months; OS = 35.0 months).

In a subsequent GOG report on 360 patients with stage IV disease who received cisplatin and paclitaxel in standard intravenous regimens, 8% were optimally cytoreduced to no macroscopic residual tumor, yielding a PFS of 20.1 months and OS of 64.1 months. For those patients with residual disease less than or equal to 1 cm, or between 1.1 and 5 cm, PFS and OS rates were similar (PFS = 13.0 months in both groups; OS = 28.7 and 31 months, respectively) *(Winter WE III, Maxell GL, Tian C, et al: J Clin Oncol 25:3621-3627, 2007; Winter WE III, Maxell GL, Tian C, et al: J Clin Oncol 26:83-89, 2008).*

Even among patients with suboptimal residual disease (> 1 cm) after primary surgery, those left with smaller tumor volumes (1–2 cm) have a survival advantage over those with a larger residuum. It is thus clear that aggressive surgical cytoreduction, if successful in reducing tumor to small volumes, improves several measures of outcome.

Interval cytoreduction In an EORTC trial, 299 patients with suboptimal advanced ovarian cancer were randomized to receive 6 cycles of cisplatin plus cyclophosphamide with or without interval surgical cytoreduction after the third cycle. Median survival for patients who underwent interval debulking surgery was 27 months, versus 19 months for patients who did not have interval debulking ($P = .01$). The GOG has recently completed a randomized trial of interval cytoreduction using a cisplatin-paclitaxel chemotherapy regimen. These results show no benefit for interval cytoreduction (median overall survival, 32 vs 33 months). The use of taxane-based chemotherapy and more standardized aggressive initial debulking by experienced gynecologic oncologists in the GOG trial have been offered as possible explanations for the discordant outcomes. If an aggressive initial surgical attempt is provided by a gynecologic oncologist, interval surgical cytoreduction cannot be routinely recommended.

Chemotherapy

Primary treatment The results of two randomized trials support a survival advantage for patients treated with combinations of IV platinum and paclitaxel, as compared with those given a platinum plus cyclophosphamide. McGuire et al found a 37- vs 24-month median survival advantage for the platinum-paclitaxel arm. Similarly, an analysis of the intergroup trial by Piccart et al showed an improvement in median survival from 25 to 35 months ($P = .001$) in favor of the paclitaxel arm. In contrast, the initial analysis of the ICON 3 trial evaluating a control arm (carboplatin or CAP [cyclophosphamide, Adriamycin (doxorubicin), Platinol (carboplatin)] chemotherapy) versus paclitaxel and carboplatin has failed to show a survival advantage for the taxane-containing arm. Many factors in the study have been proposed to

TABLE 3: Chemotherapy regimens for ovarian carcinoma

Drug/combination	Dose and schedule

Paclitaxel/carboplatin

Paclitaxel	175 mg/m^2 IV infused over 3 hours on day 1
Carboplatin	Dose calculated by the Calvert formula to an AUC between 5.0 and 7.5 mg/mL/min IV infused over 30 minutes
	Carboplatin is given after paclitaxel

Repeat cycle every 21 days for six courses.

PREMEDICATIONS: Dexamethasone, 20 mg PO, 12 and 6 hours prior to paclitaxel; as well as diphenhydramine, 50 mg IV, and ranitidine, 50 mg IV, both 30–60 minutes prior to paclitaxel.

Coleman RL, Bagnell KG, Townley PM: Cancer J Sci Am 3:246–253, 1997.

Paclitaxel/cisplatin

Paclitaxel	135 mg/m^2 IV over 24 hours on day 1
	60 mg/m^2 IP on day 8 for 6 total cycles
Cisplatin	100 mg/m^2 IP on day 2

Armstrong DK, Bundy B, Wenzel L, et al: N Engl J Med 354:34–43, 2006.

Single-agent topotecan[a] (refractory or recurrent disease)

Topotecan	1.5 mg/m^2 IV over 30 minutes daily for 5 days

Repeat cycle every 21 days.

Iva B, Ondrej B, Milan B, et al: Proc Am Soc Clin Oncol 19:1570a, 2000.

Single-agent liposomal doxorubicin[a] (refractory or recurrent disease)

Liposomal doxorubicin	50 mg/m^2 IV on day 1 at an initial rate of 1 mg/min; if tolerated, complete administration over 1 hour

Repeat cycle every 4 weeks.

Muggia FM, Hainsworth JD, Jeffers S, et al: J Clin Oncol 15:987–993, 1997.

[a]**NOTE:** Clinical experience is accumulating to suggest that liposomal doxorubicin (at doses of 40 mg/m^2 every 4 weeks) and topotecan (at 1.0 mg/m^2/d × 5 days or 4 mg/m^2/wk) are equally efficacious and better tolerated than these agents at initial phase II doses. Definitive trials are ongoing.

AUC = area under the curve

Table prepared by Ishmael Jaiyesimi, DO

---

explain this difference, and for the present, taxane- and platinum-based therapy remains the standard.

A randomized trial (GOG 158) comparing paclitaxel (175 mg/m^2 via a 3-hour infusion) plus carboplatin (dosed to achieve an area under the curve [AUC] of 7.5) versus the standard regimen of paclitaxel (135 mg/m^2 via a 24-hour infusion) plus cisplatin (75 mg/m^2) in patients with optimally debulked disease showed the shorter schedule with carboplatin to be as effective as the older regimen. Due to its decreased toxicity and ease of administration, the shorter schedule with carboplatin is the preferred treatment.

In addition, preliminary results from the SCOTROC (Scottish Randomized Trial in Ovarian Cancer) suggested that, as primary treatment, docetaxel (Taxotere) and paclitaxel have similar efficacy when combined with carboplatin and that docetaxel produces less neuropathy.

A five-arm international randomized study of primary therapy for patients with stage III or IV disease has recently been reported. This trial evaluated carboplatin and paclitaxel as the control arm and studied two triplets (carboplatin + paclitaxel with either gemcitabine [Gemzar] or liposomal doxorubicin [Doxil]) and two sequential doublets (topotecan [Hycamtin]/carboplatin + carboplatin/paclitaxel or carboplatin/gemcitabine + carboplatin/paclitaxel). No difference in progression-free or overall survival rates was seen among the arms, and therefore paclitaxel and carboplatin remain the standard. Based on the variety of phase III trials employing intravenous paclitaxel and carboplatin therapy following maximal surgical cytoreduction, the expected progression-free and overall survival rates of stage III patients follow: stage III optimal (progression-free survival, 21–28 months; overall survival, 52–57 months) and stage III suboptimal (progression-free survival, 18 months; overall survival, 38 months).

Intraperitoneal chemotherapy

The most recent randomized study by Armstrong et al employed intraperitoneal (IP) therapy as part of primary treatment. They showed a median overall survival of 65.6 months for the IP arm versus 49 months in the IV group. This finding represents the largest difference to date between two treatment arms in any study evaluating primary therapy. The study is the third in a series of studies supporting the IP administration of primary chemotherapy to optimally debulked stage III patients.

The first study by Alberts et al predated paclitaxel and carboplatin use and simply asked the question of whether the IV or IP administration of cisplatin was better, showing an advantage for the latter (median overall survival, 49 vs 41 mos; $P = .02$) This first IP study has been criticized because it does not contain paclitaxel and thus does not reflect contemporary treatment.

The second study by Markman et al included paclitaxel, but the experimental arm not only included IP delivery of cisplatin but also added high-dose IV carboplatin in an attempt to "chemically debulk" the tumor prior to IP administration. The Markman study, while also showing an advantage for the IP-containing experimental arm (overall survival, 52 vs 63 months; $P = .05$), was criticized because more than one variable was changed and the benefit could not be directly attributed to IP therapy.

As previously discussed, the third and well-designed trial by Armstrong et al showed a median overall survival of 65.6 months for the IP arm versus 49 months in the IV treated group. This study used IV paclitaxel (135 mg/m^2) IV over 24 hours on day 1, IP cisplatin (100 mg/m^2) on day 2, and IP paclitaxel (60 mg/m^2) on day 8 for 6 total cycles. Due to increased toxicity in the IP arm (metabolic, neuropathy), only 42% of patients completed all 6 cycles. However, a quality-of-life analysis at 12 months showed no difference between the IP and IV groups, suggesting the toxicity was reversible.

The general consensus opinion is that patients with stage III optimally debulked disease should be offered IP primary therapy. Studies are under way to modulate the regimen in an attempt to preserve the benefit and lessen toxicity. Initial modifications have included changing the IV paclitaxel to 135 mg/m^2 over 3 hours on day 1 and lowering the IP cisplatin dose to 75 mg/m^2 on day 2. If toxicity becomes prohibitive for a given patient, therapy is completed using IV paclitaxel and carboplatin. For patients not suited for IP treatment or for suboptimally debulked stage III patients or those with stage IV disease, IV paclitaxel with carboplatin also remains the standard.

Radiation therapy as a single modality

Patients not considered candidates for chemotherapy, or those in whom chemotherapy is indicated but refuse treatment, may consider whole abdominal irradiation (WAI). In ovarian cancer, no prospective randomized trial has compared WAI, performed with modern techniques and equipment, with a taxol-containing chemotherapy regimen. However, the ability of WAI to sterilize macroscopic deposits of ovarian carcinoma is limited. Patients with any site of residual disease > 1 cm have compromised outcomes; the limited radiation tolerance of the abdominal organs limits the radiation dose.

Chemotherapy plus radiation therapy

Sequential combined-modality therapy (CMT) employing chemotherapy and irradiation has been shown in one randomized trial to significantly increase survival over patients treated with chemotherapy alone. A phase III prospective randomized trial in patients with stage III ovarian cancer from the Swedish-Norwegian Group showed a significant 20% improvement in 5-year progression-free survival for patients treated with chemotherapy and whole abdominal radiation therapy versus chemotherapy alone.

In another European study, 64 of 94 patients with stages IC–IV disease who had undergone "radical" surgery and had no evidence of gross residual disease after 6 courses of chemotherapy (carboplatin, epirubicin [Ellence], and prednimustine [Sterecyt]) were randomized to receive either consolidation WAI (30 Gy), followed by a boost to the para-aortic region and pelvis (12.0 and 21.6 Gy, respectively), or no further therapy. Relapse-free survival rates were significantly higher in patients who received adjuvant chemoradiation therapy than in those who received adjuvant chemotherapy only (2- and 5-year relapse-free survival rates, 68% vs 56% and 49% vs 26%, respectively); the same was true of overall survival rates (2- and 5-year overall survival rates, 87% vs 61% and 59% vs 33%, respectively). The differences between the two treatment groups were more pronounced in patients with stage III disease (2- and 5-year relapse-free survival rates, 77% vs 54% and 45% vs 19%, respectively; 2- and 5-year overall survival rates, 88% vs 58% and 59% vs 26%, respectively).

Einhorn et al, from the Karolinska Hospital in Stockholm, treated 75 patients with stages IIB–IV ovarian carcinoma with combined surgery, chemotherapy, and WAI to 40 Gy, utilizing a "six-field" approach. Outcomes were compared with those of 98 patients treated in subsequent years with only surgery and chemotherapy. After different prognostic factors were controlled statistically, it was found that patients who received WAI had a significantly better survival rate than those who did not. The authors suggest that, given the results of this and other studies combined with the limited success of modern combination chemotherapy regimens, the role of abdominal radiation therapy should be further investigated in a prospective fashion.

Despite these successful European trials, the regimen of chemotherapy and radiation in the upfront management of stage III ovarian cancer has not been implemented in the U.S. due to many factors. Taxol-based chemotherapy provides a significant benefit for patients, as does intraperitoneal chemotherapy. The use of radiation may increase potential bowel toxicity, particularly with intraperitoneal chemotherapy, and in some patients may cause bone marrow suppression, which theoretically may hinder future administration of chemotherapy.

Recurrent disease

Patients who respond to primary chemotherapy with paclitaxel and platinum agents and who relapse ≥ 6 months after the completion of treatment often have additional responses when retreated with the same agents. Response rates to repeat treatment with carboplatin are ~30% in those patients who relapse 12 months after primary therapy and 57% if the relapses occur > 24 months after primary therapy. In addition, a plethora of new agents have demonstrated modest phase II activity in patients with refractory disease.

Topotecan has received FDA (US Food and Drug Administration) approval for the treatment of patients with refractory disease (Table 3). An oral preparation is in phase III trials.

An open, randomized study compared topotecan (1.5 mg/m^2/d for 5 days) with paclitaxel (175 mg/m^2 q21d) in 226 women whose ovarian cancer had recurred after first-line platinum therapy. There were no statistically significant differences between the treatment groups with respect to response rate (20.5% vs 14.0%), response duration (25.9 vs 21.6 weeks), or median survival (63 vs 53 weeks).

Topotecan has efficacy comparable to that of paclitaxel in this setting and is being evaluated in combination with platinum and other agents.

Liposomal doxorubicin also has received FDA approval for the treatment of patients with metastatic platinum- and paclitaxel-refractory disease (Table 3). A randomized trial by Gordon et al compared liposomal doxorubicin with topotecan in this setting; similar response rates, time to disease progression, and overall survival (60.0 vs 56.7 weeks) were seen with these two agents.

Other agents Phase II trials have demonstrated the activity of other agents in patients with recurrent ovarian cancer. They include gemcitabine, vinorelbine (Navelbine), oral altretamine (Hexalen), and oral etoposide. In general, these agents have similar response rates, ranging from 10%–15% in patients with platinum-resistant disease and 30% in patients with platinum-sensitive disease, with a median duration of response ranging from 4 to 8+ months. With the judicious selection and dosing of available agents to keep symptoms from disease and treatment to a minimum, a good quality of life can be maintained throughout much of the disease course.

A randomized ICON 4/AGO-OVAR 2.2 study addressed the issue of using single-agent carboplatin versus paclitaxel with carboplatin for patients with platinum-sensitive recurrent disease (defined generally as patients relapsing more than 6 months from prior platinum therapy). Both disease progression-free (hazard ratio, 0.76; CI, 0.66–0.80; $P = .0004$) and 1-year overall survival rates (50% vs 40%) favored combination therapy. An AGO study evaluating carboplatin versus carboplatin with gemcitabine in a similar population was reported. This study likewise showed an improved response rate (47.2% vs 30.9%; $P = .0016$) and disease progression-free survival (8.6 vs 5.8 months; $P = .0031$) favoring the combination. Taken together, these data suggest a benefit for platinum-based combination therapy over single-agent carboplatin in patients with platinum-sensitive recurrence. Other combinations such as topotecan or liposomal doxorubicin with carboplatin are being investigated.

Salvage and palliative radiotherapy after chemotherapy

In the setting of small-volume residual disease detected after chemotherapy, external-beam irradiation has been used with some success. Favorable experiences with salvage radiation therapy in chemotherapy-refractory ovarian carcinomas continue to be reported. Table 4 lists possible prognostic variables in these patients.

In a report of 20 patients who received multiple chemotherapy regimens for recurrent disease located in the pelvis, surgical debulking of the recurrent mass was followed by postoperative radiation therapy to 50.4Gy. Patients that were able to have a complete debulking and radiation had a 3-year overall survival of 50%, disease-free survival of 72% and local relapse free survival rate of 89%. Those with residual disease had corresponding values of 19% OS, 22% DFS, and 42% LRFS. Radiation should be considered for patients with a localized recurrence of ovarian cancer who have failed multiple chemotherapy regimens, given the general sensitivity of ovarian cancer to radiation.

Sedlacek et al described 27 patients who had not responded to aggressive cytoreductive surgery followed by multiple-drug platinum-based chemotherapy and who received WAI (30–35 Gy at 100–150 cGy/fraction, with a pelvic boost to a total dose of 45 Gy). The 5-year survival rate was 15%. The extent of residual disease at the initiation of radiation therapy strongly correlated with the length of survival.

Baker et al analyzed the efficacy of salvage WAI in 47 patients with ovarian cancer who had not responded to one or more chemotherapy regimens. Actuarial 4-year survival and disease-free survival rates were 48% and 37%, respectively, in patients with microscopic residual disease, vs 11% and 5%, respectively, in patients with macroscopic residual disease. In addition, patients with disease limited to the pelvis after laparotomy (including gross disease) had a

TABLE 4: Possible prognostic factors for salvage radiation therapy following chemotherapy

Residual tumor before WAI	Lymph node status
Location of residual disease	Chemotherapy duration
Initial FIGO stage	Type of prior chemotherapy
Histologic grade	Completion of WAI
Disease bulk at diagnosis	Response to chemotherapy
Patient age	Histologic type
Disease-free interval from	CA-125 level
initial treatment to relapse	CA-125 level trend
Performance status	Parameters of WAI
Number of sites of residual disease	Interval debulking/second-look surgery

FIGO = International Federation of Gynecology and Obstetrics; WAI = whole-abdominal irradiation

4-year actuarial survival rate of 60% and disease-free survival rate of 54%, as compared with 16% and 4%, respectively, in patients with upper abdominal involvement.

This finding was confirmed by Firat and Erickson, who described their experience with selective radiotherapy in 28 patients with recurrent or persistent disease involving the vagina and/or rectum. Pelvic radiotherapy was uniformly successful in palliating vaginal bleeding. Furthermore, there were eight long-term survivors (five with no evidence of disease), implying that pelvic radiotherapy alone can be effective salvage therapy, particularly when there is no extrapelvic disease.

Fujiwara and colleagues reported high rates of objective and symptomatic responses using local radiotherapy in 20 patients (42 evaluable lesions) with recurrent ovarian cancer following chemotherapy. Lymph node metastases appeared to be particularly responsive.

Tinger et al reported an overall response rate of 73% in 80 patients with advanced and recurrent disease treated with palliative intent. Responses were maintained until death in all but 10 patients. Toxicity was limited, and there was no grade 4 toxicity. It was suggested that response rate, survival, and toxicity with palliative radiotherapy compared favorably with those of second- and third-line chemotherapy.

Based on these and other studies, certain treatment guidelines can be suggested:

- Palliation of vaginal bleeding, pelvic pain, or bowel or bladder blockage due to tumor compression may be feasible.
- Salvage radiation may also be considered in selected patients after a localized pelvic recurrence following maximal debulking.

Novel approaches

Recent data have supported the efficacy of antivascular strategies for patients with ovarian cancer. Two studies reported in abstract form evaluated the activity of bevacizumab (Avastin). A phase II trial evaluating bevacizumab (15 mg/kg every 3 weeks) as second- or third-line therapy showed a single-agent response rate of 17%, with a median progression-free interval of approximately 10 months. A second phase II study evaluated bevacizumab in conjunction with oral cyclophosphamide; it showed partial responses in 28% of patients and stable disease in an additional 59% with a median progression-free interval of 5.8 months (95% CI, 3.8–8.1 months). The progression-free interval at 6 months was 57%. An advanced ovarian cancer trial evaluating bevacizumab in refractory ovarian cancer patients with measurable disease was halted due to an excess in bowel perforation, which is a known side effect. GOG currently has an ongoing randomized study evaluating bevacizumab in addition to paclitaxel and carboplatin for patients who are suboptimally debulked.

Other studies with anti-VEGF strategies, such as PTK (an oral VEGF inhibitor), VEGF-TRAP, sorafenib (Nexavar), and sunitinib (Sutent) are currently under way to define both toxicity and efficacy. For many patients, ovarian cancer becomes a chronic disease characterized by a series of relapses followed by partial or complete remission.

High-dose chemotherapy In a trial conducted largely in patients with platinum-resistant (66%) and bulky disease (61%), the median disease progression-free and overall survival intervals were short (7 and 13 months, respectively) in patients treated with high-dose chemotherapy and stem-cell support, suggesting no benefit. There is no role for high-dose chemotherapy in the standard management of patients with epithelial ovarian cancer.

Treatment recommendations and unresolved issues

For advanced ovarian cancer, current frontline management should incorporate a taxane with platinum-based therapy. Results also support the use of a taxane and platinum-based therapy in patients with high-risk early-stage disease.

Issues that are evolving include (1) considering a variety of IP doses and schedules to reduce the toxicity of this approach, which has been shown to prolong overall survival; (2) the role of maintenance or consolidation treatment with standard chemotherapy or with novel agents following primary therapy; (3) the optimal use of platinum versus nonplatinum agents, and whether used as single agents or in combination, for patients with recurrent disease; and (4) the role of novel drugs, notably bevacizumab and other antivascular agents, in both the adjuvant and recurrent disease settings.

SUGGESTED READING

Albuquerque KV, Singla R, Potkul RK, et al: Impact of tumor volume-directed involved field radiation therapy integrated in the management of recurrent ovarian cancer. Gynecol Oncol 96:701–704, 2005.

Anderson GL, Judd HL, Kaunitz AM, et al: Effects of estrogen plus progestin on gynecologic cancers and associated diagnostic procedures: The Women's Health Initiative randomized trial. JAMA 290:1739–1748, 2003.

Armstrong DK, Bundy B, Wenzel L, et al: Intraperitoneal cisplatin and paclitaxel in ovarian cancer. N Engl J Med 354:34-43, 2006.

Burger RA, Sill MW, Monk BJ, et al: Phase II trial of bevacizumab in persistent or recurrent epithelial ovarian cancer or primary peritoneal cancer: A Gynecologic Oncology Group Study. J Clin Oncol 25:5165–5171, 2007.

Buys SS, Partridge E, Greene MH, et al: Ovarian cancer screening in the Prostate, Lung, Colorectal and Ovarian (PLCO) cancer screening trial: Findings from the initial screen of a randomized trial. Am J Obstet Gynecol 193:1630–1639, 2005.

Cannistra SA, Matulonis UA, Penson RT, et al: Phase II study of bevacizumab in patients with platinum resistant ovarian cancer or peritoneal serous cancer. J Clin Oncol 25:5180–5186, 2007.

Goff BA, Mandel LS, Melancon CH, et al: Frequency of symptoms of ovarian cancer in women presenting to primary care clinics. JAMA 291:2705–2712, 2004.

ICON and AGO collaborators: Paclitaxel plus platinum based chemotherapy versus conventional platinum based chemotherapy in women with relapsed ovarian cancer: The ICON 4/AGO-OVAR 2.2 trial. Lancet 361:2099–2106, 2003.

ICON and EORTC-ACTION investigators: International Collaborative on Ovarian Neoplasm Trial 1 and Adjuvant Treatment in Ovarian Neoplasm Trial: Two parallel randomized phase III trials of adjuvant chemotherapy in patients with early stage ovarian cancer. J Natl Cancer Inst 95:105–112, 2003.

Kauff ND, Domchek SM, Friebel TM, et al: Risk-reducing salpingo-oophorectomy for the prevention of BRCA1- and BRCA2-associated breast and gynecologic cancer: A multicenter, prospective study. J Clin Oncol 26:1331–1337, 2008.

Kauff ND, Satagopan JM, Robson ME, et al: Risk-reducing salpingo-oophorectomy in women with a BRCA1 or BRCA2 mutation. N Engl J Med 346:1609–1615, 2002.

Markman M, Liu PY, Wilczynski S, et al: Phase III randomized trial of 12 versus 3 months of maintenance paclitaxel in patients with advanced ovarian cancer after complete response to platinum and paclitaxel based chemotherapy: A Southwest Oncology Group and Gynecologic Oncology Group Trial. J Clin Oncol 21:2460–2465, 2003.

Martin L and Schilder R: Novel approaches in advancing the treatment of epithelial ovarian cancer: The role of angiogenesis inhibition. J Clin Oncol 25:2894–2901, 2007.

Ozols RF, Bundy BN, Greer E, et al: Phase III trials of carboplatin and paclitaxel compared with cisplatin and paclitaxel in patients with optimally resected stage III ovarian cancer: A Gynecologic Oncology Group Study. J Clin Oncol 21:3194–3200, 2003.

Pfisterer J, Plante M, Vergote I, et al: Gemcitabine/carboplatin (GC) vs carboplatin (C) in platinum-sensitive recurrent ovarian cancer (OVCA): Results of a Gynecologic Cancer Intergroup randomized phase III trial of the AGO OVAR, the NCIC CTG, and the EORTC GCG (abstract). J Clin Oncol 24:4699–1707, 2006.

Rose PG, Nerenstone S, Brady MF, et al: Secondary surgical cytoreduction for advanced ovarian carcinoma. N Engl J Med 351:2489–2497, 2004.

Sorbe B, for the Swedish-Norwegian Ovarian Cancer Study Group: Consolidation treatment of advanced (FIGO stage III) ovarian carcinoma in complete surgical remission after induction chemotherapy: A randomized, controlled clinical trial comparing whole abdominal radiotherapy, chemotherapy, and no further treatment. Int J Gynecol Cancer 13:278–286, 2003.

Vasey PA, Jayson GC, Gordon A, et al; Scottish Gynaecological Cancer Trials Group: Phase III randomized trial of docetaxel-carboplatin versus paclitaxel-carboplatin as first-line chemotherapy for ovarian cancer. J Natl Cancer Inst 96:1682–1691, 2004.

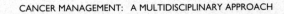

CHAPTER 23

Melanoma and other skin cancers

Richard Essner, MD, Aradhana Kaushal, MD, and Keith Flaherty, MD

Skin cancer is the single most common form of cancer, accounting for more than 75% of all cancer diagnoses. More than 1 million cases of squamous cell and basal cell carcinoma are diagnosed annually, with a lifetime risk of more than one in five. The vast majority of skin cancers can be cured with surgery alone; resection is the mainstay of therapy, even for skin cancer involving regional lymph nodes or, in some cases, more distant metastatic sites.

Sun exposure is the predominant risk factor for squamous cell and basal cell skin cancers, and is the only known predisposing exposure for melanoma. It accounts for 90% of all skin cancer-related mortality. Melanoma accounts for 4% of all skin cancer diagnoses (60,000 new cases of invasive melanoma per year) but contributes to 75% of deaths from skin cancer. The natural history of melanoma that has spread to regional lymph nodes or beyond is minimally impacted by available systemic therapies.

Unlike many other cancers, the incidence of melanoma and death rates from melanoma continue to rise. The superficial nature of melanoma and other skin cancers supports campaigns to raise public awareness and healthcare provider expertise in detecting skin cancers at the earliest possible stage. Screening initiatives would be less likely to benefit the 10% of melanomas that are nonpigmented or arise from the choroid of the eyes or mucosal surfaces.

Epidemiology

Age The relationship between the incidence of melanoma and age is somewhat unique in comparison to other common cancers. There is not an exponential increase in risk with age but rather a more even distribution across age groups. The highest incidence is among people between the ages of 45 and 54. Forty-two percent of cases present in people younger than age 55, contributing to the third highest number of years of life lost across all cancers. The incidence of squamous cell and basal cell carcinomas increases exponentially with age.

Acknowledgment: Portions of this chapter are reprinted from the 10th Edition of *Cancer Management: A Multidisciplinary Approach*, chapter 23, written by Eric H. Jensen, Kim A. Margolin, and Vernon Sondak.

Gender Men are more likely than women to develop melanoma (60% higher incidence), and their prognosis is worse (130% higher risk of death from melanoma). The risk of recurrence in the setting of resected primary melanoma is higher, and their expected survival in the setting of regionally advanced disease is significantly shorter.

Location Basal cell cancers arise exclusively from cutaneous sites and are closely related to sites of skin that receive the most sun exposure, such as the scalp, face, neck, and arms. Squamous cell cancers can arise from numerous sites in the body, but the term squamous cell skin cancer is reserved for cutaneous sites. The vast majority of melanomas arise from cutaneous sites, but most cases of melanoma and most fatal cases arise from intermittently sun-exposed skin. A small percentage of melanomas arise on acral surfaces of the hands and feet, which tend to be diagnosed at a later stage. Melanoma can arise from melanocytes adjacent to the retina or within mucosal surfaces in the oropharynx, sinuses, rectum, or vulva. These lesions typically present with greater local invasion and risk of distant spread than cutaneous melanoma.

Geography The rates of melanoma and other skin cancers are highest where fair-skinned Caucasians migrated to lower latitudes, with annual sun exposure that is substantially higher than their historically native climates. Australia, New Zealand, South Africa, and Israel bear a disproportionate burden of skin cancer. In Australia, melanoma is the third most common cancer. In the United States, Hawaii and the desert Southwest have the highest rates of skin cancer of all kinds and melanoma.

Race Caucasians are by far the most susceptible race for melanomas, as well as squamous cell and basal cell cancers. Hispanics have a lower incidence but represent the group at next highest risk. Asians and African-Americans have the lowest rates of skin cancer. For those populations, cutaneous melanomas arising from sun-exposed sites are uncommon but not unseen. All racial groups are equally likely to develop melanoma on the acral surfaces of the hands and feet or mucosal surfaces. Therefore, melanomas arising from these sites represent nearly all cases of melanoma in these more darkly pigmented racial groups.

Survival Skin cancers that are confined to the skin at presentation and with adequate staging evaluation have a high rate of cure. The 10-year survival rate for melanomas that are less than 1 mm in thickness and that lack ulceration is 97%. Melanoma that is microscopically or macroscopically evident in regional nodes is associated with only a 30% likelihood of survival after 10 years. The presence of more distant metastatic disease is associated with only a 10% possibility of survival 10 years from initial recognition.

Etiology and risk factors

Genetic predisposition Although there are families in which melanoma can occur with high likelihood, an underlying genetic predisposition can only be found in 3% all cases. The pedigrees have been identified because of their high likelihood of a mutation carrier developing melanoma. Lower penetrance genotypes remain to be elucidated. Nonetheless, the identification of the genes responsible for familial melanoma has contributed greatly to the understanding of the molecular pathophysiology of melanoma.

The clinical observations that patients with multiple dysplastic nevi were at greater risk of developing melanoma and that many such patients came from families with multiple affected individuals provided the first insight into a melanoma progression model that might be accelerated based on inborn genetic abnormalities. Two highly related genes were discovered to harbor germline mutations in roughly 50% of melanoma pedigrees: *CDKN2A* and *CDK4*. *CDKN2A* enocodes two products via alternate splicing of messenger RNA: $p16^{INK4A}$ and $p14^{ARF}$. Each of these tumor suppressor genes exerts an inhibitory effect on cell cycle progression.

Xeroderma pigmentosum is a rare inherited disorder in which DNA repair mechanisms are compromised, particularly in response to ultraviolet (UV) light. Mutations in *XP* genes A though G have been identified as the underlying molecular event. Squamous cell and basal cell carcinomas and melanoma are prevalent in this population and at a young age. The near-complete penetrance of melanoma in these patients emphasizes the critical balance between UV-induced DNA damage and repair in risk for skin cancer. As DNA damage repair is mediated by a complex network of sensor and effector proteins, variability in the function of this system almost certainly underlies the variability in risk among the fair-skinned population.

Genetic variability in melanocortin-1 receptor (MC1R) has been clearly implicated in pigmentation of skin and hair and, more recently, to melanoma predisposition. It has been known for decades that melanoma is more prevalent among fair-skinned individuals with red or blond hair. Furthermore, blond-haired individuals with an inability to tan are at substantially greater risk of developing melanoma than blond-haired individuals who tan readily. Polymorphisms, distinct from mutations, in MC1R appear to account for skin and hair color differences among Caucasians. It appears that individuals with melanocortin receptors that have a muted response to increased melanocortin expression following sun exposure suffer the greatest UV-induced genetic damage, leading to a greater risk of melanoma.

Exposure Even the inheritance of CDKN2A and CDK4 mutations is insufficient to lead to melanoma in all carriers. It is clear that multiple genetic changes are required to give rise to invasive disease. UV damage is the best-described modifiable risk factor for melanoma, as well as squamous cell and basal cell skin cancers. It is believed that the acquired or somatic genetic changes that give rise to melanoma occur as a consequence of UV-induced genetic damage.

Epidemiologic data relate the risk of melanoma most closely to a connection between cumulative sun exposure, severe sun burns, or sun exposure during childhood, depending on the study. The disagreement between studies likely stems from methodologic differences in obtaining a sun exposure history, a heterogeneous effect of sun exposure and risk depending on the underlying genetic composition of the study population, or both. It has been recently clarified that melanoma arising on intermittently sun-exposed skin (such as the trunk) has its peak incidence among younger individuals and declines severely with increasing age. On the other hand, melanoma arising from chronically sun-damaged skin (such as the face, neck, and upper extremities) has the highest incidence in older individuals. With the rise in popularity of indoor tanning salons, data indicate that those who use them are at higher risk of melanoma than those who are sun exposed. There is little dispute regarding the causal link between sun exposure or tanning salon use and risk of melanoma; however, there is disagreement regarding the constituents of light (UV-A or UV-B) that contribute most to genetic damage. Laboratory studies support a connection for both, and suggest that prevention strategies must take the entire UV light spectrum into account.

Prevention With the incidence of melanoma still rising, it is clear that primary prevention efforts have not yet taken hold. The only approach firmly rooted in evidence is to minimize sun exposure. The use of sun-protective clothing appears to be the next best strategy. There are conflicting data regarding the protective effect of suncreens for melanoma, although there is no controversy regarding their ability to prevent squamous cell and basal cell carcinomas. Protection against UV-A has been a long-standing feature of widely available suncreens, whereas UV-B protection has more recently been engineered into all mainstream products. It is possible that the more widespread of these wide-spectrum sunscreens will provide more meaningful protective effects over the coming decades.

Immunosuppression There is incontrovertible evidence linking immunosuppression and squamous cell skin cancer. This increased risk applies to patients with acquired immunodeficiency syndrome as well as transplant recipients on chronic immunosuppressive medications. The risk of developing primary melanoma in the setting of immunosuppression is less well established, but there is some evidence that patients who have a history of melanoma are more likely to develop disease recurrence in the setting of immunosuppression.

Nevi Patients with numerous benign nevi (small, regularly shaped, and uniformly pigmented moles) are at increased risk of melanoma, as are patients with relatively few dysplastic nevi (large, irregularly shaped, and heterogeneously pigmented moles). Patients in either group may have a five-fold increased risk of developing melanoma compared with those with few benign nevi or without dysplastic nevi. However, it is critical to recognize that these preexisting moles represent a risk factor for melanoma, rather than precursor lesions, in most cases. The majority of melanomas do not arise from preexisting melanocytic lesions. There seems to be little value in resecting every nevus that appears dysplastic on clinical grounds. Surveying the skin regularly for new or changing moles has been most widely adapted for educating patients and healthcare providers. Beyond the age of 25 to 30, new mole formation warrants examination by a provider who is comfortable making the diagnosis of melanoma.

Congenital nevi are relatively rare compared with acquired nevi. In general, they do not suggest a predisposition to melanoma. A small number of children are born with so-called giant congenital nevi, also referred to as bathing trunk nevi.

History of melanoma Perhaps the single greatest clinical risk factor for melanoma is a personal history of melanoma. In addition to having surveillance for local and distant recurrence related to their prior melanoma, these individuals require lifelong observation for the emergence of a new primary melanoma; their risk is 10 times greater than the general population.

Actinic keratoses represent the precursor lesion for the vast majority of squamous cell skin cancers. They manifest as raised, nonpigmented lesions with a plaque-like surface. Typically, they have an erythematous base and arise on heavily sun-exposed skin. These lesions are typically treated with either excision, cryotherapy, topical chemotherapy (5-fluorouracil [5-FU]), or immunotherapy (imiquimod). It is unclear what effect nonsurgical therapy has on the long-term risk of progression to squamous cell carcinoma, but the relatively indolent nature of most actinic keratoses suggests that nonsurgical therapy followed by close observation is reasonable, particularly for lesions arising on cosmetically sensitive areas such as the face.

Burns (unrelated to sun exposure) predispose to the formation of squamous cell carcinoma on permanently scarred areas. Although not particularly prevalent among those with a burn history, a high clinical suspicion for malignancy must be taken for the patient with a new nonpigmented lesion or an area of ulceration on a preexisting healed burn.

Signs and symptoms The diagnosis of melanoma is based on complete pathologic evaluation of the skin. A growing skin lesion is the easiest description that a patient can provide a physician to assist in determining which skin lesions should be biopsied. ABCDs is a simple learning method (see below for more information) also to assist patients. This system, which is based on asymmetry of the skin lesion, irregular edges, color appearance, and diameter, can be helpful to patients but may lead to some melanomas being missed.

Diagnosis

Early diagnosis of melanoma Beyond prevention, early detection is the next priority in limiting the life-threatening potential of melanoma. Although tumor invasion into the dermis (the definition of invasive melanoma) cannot be assessed clinically, there are hallmarks of melanoma that can be appreciated by visual inspection. The "ABCD" algorithm, promoted by the American Cancer Society, has not proven to be a particularly effective method of educating the general population, but healthcare providers are better suited to implementing this system in clinical practice. (See the color atlas following this chapter.) 'A' indicates gross asymmetry of a pigmented lesion. 'B' refers to irregular or indistinct borders. 'C' regards color, which, in the case of melanoma, refers to black, dark brown, or blue color for newly formed lesions. In the case of preexisting moles, the loss of pigmentation in a portion of the lesion can indicate regression, which is worrisome for melanoma. Additionally, a focus of darker pigmentation within a preexisting mole is grounds for concern. 'D', or diameter of 6 mm or greater, raises concern for melanoma, whereas smaller lesions are rarely indicative of invasive lesions. None of these single criteria can be considered as grounds for performing a biopsy, rather lesions that satisfy multiple criteria warrant either close observation or biopsy of the most abnormal portion. Not included in the ABCD system is the papular or nodular characteristic of most melanomas. If melanoma arises within a preexisting mole, the raised element of an otherwise flat or macular lesion should be considered suspicious for melanoma. Some primary melanomas do not produce melanin and therefore lack the classic appearance.

Atypical nevi represent a risk factor for melanoma in that individual lesions can occasionally progress to invasive melanoma. More commonly, the presence of dysplastic nevi suggests an individual at risk for melanoma formation at other sites. The clinical definition of atypical nevi has never been formally established but generally refers to the presence of one or two of the ABCD features. Cutaneous photography has been routinely incorporated in the follow-up of patients with multiple clinically dysplastic nevi in specialized pigmented lesion clinics. Full-body cutaneous photography (dermoscopy) is increasingly available to patients and provides an objective baseline from which to judge change of preexisting lesions or the appearance of new lesions. In general, excision of all atypical nevi is impractical and does not adequately address the risk that patients face of developing melanoma in sites where no precursor lesion is found.

Nodular melanoma represents the most difficult subset of melanomas to diagnose at an early stage. These lesions are more rapidly proliferative than typical melanomas and are generally not pigmented. Furthermore, they are generally raised early in their development and have symmetric and well-demarcated boundaries. Thus, they do not meet the ABCD criteria. Nodular melanomas account for approximately 10% of melanoma cases but account for a disproportionate percentage of fatalities. The most useful clinical rule to apply in the assessment of lesions that have these features is that the de novo appearance of such lesions over a short time (months) warrants consideration of biopsy. As the features of nodular melanoma are common to some benign skin lesions, as well as basal cell carcinoma, the yield of biopsies for such lesions may be relatively low. Nonetheless, heightened awareness of this small but lethal subset of melanoma is needed.

Nonmelanoma skin cancers Classically, basal cell skin cancers are nodular and have a pearly, nonpigmented surface. Squamous cell carcinomas typically have a scaly, nonpigmented surface and can occasionally be ulcerated. Both types are generally slow to evolve. In most cases, squamous cell carcinomas are believed to arise from actinic keratoses in most cases. The differentiation between the two is based largely on size, with actinic keratoses being less than 1 cm in diameter. The appearance of nodularity or induration in preexisting keratinized lesions raises concern for tumor invasion into the dermis and warrants biopsy.

Skin examination of the entire body should be performed for any patient who presents with numerous benign-appearing nevi, any dysplastic nevi, or a history of even a single melanoma. The entire skin is at risk in these individuals and must be investigated for the appearance of new or changing lesions. Patients who fit into any of these risk groups should be instructed to perform monthly skin self-examination. Two mirrors are required to adequately examine the back if a partner is not available to assist in examining the back longitudinally.

Skin examination should be performed in a well-lit room with the patient completely disrobed. For patients with numerous moles, full-body cutaneous photography is extremely helpful to provide an objective baseline from which to judge change. For patients with only a few atypical moles, close-up photographs of those lesions may facilitate careful evaluation of those lesions while the remainder of the skin is surveyed for new lesions. A focused method for examining individual lesions, dermoscopy employs low-level magnification of the epidermis with tangential light applied to a liquid-skin interface. Examination of pigmented lesions with dermoscopy allows more precise visualization of patterns of pigmentation than is possible with the unaided eye. This method requires some degree of training and the availability of appropriate equipment. When regression of part or all of a preexisting mole is suspected, a Wood's lamp can be helpful in bringing out the contrast in pigmentation between normally pigmented surrounding skin and an area where immunologic destruction of melanocytes has occurred.

Lymph node examination should be performed in all patients who are suspected of having invasive melanoma or large squamous cell, basal cell, or Merkel cell carcinomas. The closest lymph node basin is the most essential area to examine. The presence of a palpable lymph node mandates biopsy of the suspicious node, generally with fine needle aspiration. Whereas sentinel lymph node biopsy is performed routinely for patients with primary melanomas greater than 1 mm in thickness, palpable lymphadenopathy with histologic evidence of melanoma, or nonmelanoma skin cancer, warrants proceeding directly to a regional lymph node dissection.

Biopsy techniques

Excisional biopsy is recommended for any lesion that is suspected of being melanoma, squamous cell cancer, or basal cell carcinoma. This is especially true for lesions that can be entirely excised without concern for causing an unacceptable cosmetic result. Local anesthesia is generally all that is required. Narrow margins of 1 to 2 mm are sufficient when making an initial diagnosis of skin cancer. The biopsy should extend to the subcutaneous tissue to provide an adequate estimate of the depth of invasion, particularly for melanoma. Biopsy specimens should be placed in formalin and submitted for expert pathologic preparation including embedding in paraffin.

Incisional biopsy is an acceptable alterative for large lesions (greater than 1 cm in diameter). In the case of possible melanoma lesions, the most abnormal appearing area should be biopsied. As with excisional biopsies, the biopsy should include subcutaneous tissue to allow an estimation of thickness. A punch biopsy, of sufficient diameter to encompass the most abnormal appearing area, is the preferred method.

Techniques to avoid For lesions that are suspected to represent melanoma, every attempt should be made to preserve the ability to assess involvement of margins and to perform immunohistochemistry of the primary tumor. The latter is critically important in borderline cases, where the diagnosis of melanoma is uncertain. Thus, shave biopsies and serial thin section techniques (such as Mohs surgery) are strictly contraindicated. Frozen biopsy assessment is inadequate for the diagnosis of melanoma and does not allow adequate material for review in difficult pathologic cases.

Pathology

Nonmelanoma skin cancers The two most common skin cancers are basal and squamous cell carcinomas. Both of these skin cancers arise predominately on sunexposed areas and may be considered in the differential diagnosis with melanoma. The diagnosis of these skin cancers should be made after pathologic analysis of the skin specimen. There are a variety of other skin cancers that may be mistaken for melanoma. Merkel cell carcinoma, a rare neuroendocrine tumor of the skin, appears to have a similar propensity as melanoma to spread locally and to regional lymph nodes.

Staging and prognosis of melanoma

A great deal of information is available regarding factors that correlate with clinical outcome in patients with melanoma. In the absence of known distant metastatic disease, the most important prognostic factor is regional lymph node involvement. Overall, however, 85% of melanoma patients present with clinically normal lymph nodes. In clinically node-negative patients, most investigators have found the microscopic degree of invasion of the melanoma, or microstaging, to be of critical importance in predicting outcome (Tables 1–3).

Microstaging

Two methods have been described for microscopic staging of primary cutaneous melanomas.

Clark's level Wallace Clark and associates devised a system to classify melanomas according to the level of invasion relative to histologically defined landmarks in the skin. Although Clark's levels correlate with prognosis (lesions with deeper levels of invasion have a greater propensity for recurrence), the inherent problem with Clark's system is that the thickness of the skin and hence the distance between the various landmark dermal layers varies greatly in different parts of the body. Furthermore, except for Clark's level I (melanoma in situ), there is no scientific rationale for considering these landmarks to be biologic barriers to tumor growth. For example, there is no a priori reason to suspect that a lesion that reaches but does not invade the reticular dermis is inherently less aggressive than a similar melanoma that penetrates the reticular dermis in an area where the skin is thinner.

Breslow's thickness An alternative microstaging method, described by Alexander Breslow, obviates some of the problems associated with Clark's levels. In this method, the thickness of the primary tumor is measured from the top of the granular layer of the epidermis to the deepest contiguous tumor cell at the base of the lesion using a micrometer in the microscope eyepiece.

Ulceration The presence of ulceration in a primary melanoma has been recognized as one of the strongest negative predictive factors for long-term survival. Ulceration is defined as the lack of a complete epidermal layer overlying the melanocytic lesion. The presence of ulceration essentially upstages affected patients to the next highest T level. In other words, a patient with a 1.1–2-mm melanoma that is ulcerated will carry the same long-term prognosis as a patient with a 2.1–4-mm melanoma that does not have ulceration. The likelihood of finding ulceration is directly related to tumor depth: Patients with thin melanomas (≤ 1 mm) have a 6% rate of ulceration, whereas those with > 4-mm melanomas have a 63% incidence of ulceration. Along with tumor depth, ulceration is integral in determining a patient's long-term prognosis and is an independent predictor of patient outcome.

TABLE 1: TNM classification of melanoma

Primary tumor (T)

Tx	Primary tumor cannot be assessed (eg, shave biopsy or regressed melanoma)
T0	No evidence of primary tumor
Tis	Melanoma in situ
T1	Melanoma ≤ 1.0 mm in thickness, with or without ulceration
T1a	Melanoma ≤ 1.0 mm in thickness and Clark's level II or III, no ulceration
T1b	Melanoma ≤ 1.0 mm in thickness and Clark's level IV or V or with ulceration
T2	Melanoma 1.01-2.0 mm in thickness, with or without ulceration
T2a	Melanoma 1.01-2.0 mm in thickness, no ulceration
T2b	Melanoma 1.01-2.0 mm in thickness, with ulceration
T3	Melanoma 2.01-4.0 mm in thickness, with or without ulceration
T3a	Melanoma 2.01-4.0 mm in thickness, no ulceration
T3b	Melanoma 2.01-4.0 mm in thickness, with ulceration
T4	Melanoma > 4.0 mm in thickness, with or without ulceration
T4a	Melanoma > 4.0 mm in thickness, no ulceration
T4b	Melanoma > 4.0 mm in thickness, with ulceration

Regional lymph nodes (N)

Nx	Regional lymph nodes cannot be assessed
N0	No regional lymph node metastasis
N1	Metastasis in one lymph node
N1a	Clinically occult (microscopic) metastasis
N1b	Clinically apparent (macroscopic) metastasis
N2	Metastasis in two to three regional nodes or intralymphatic regional metastasis without nodal metastases
N2a	Clinically occult (microscopic) metastasis
N2b	Clinically apparent (macroscopic) metastasis
N2c	Satellite or in-transit metastasis without nodal metastasis
N3	Metastasis in four or more regional nodes, or matted metastatic nodes, or in-transit metastasis or satellite(s) with metastasis in regional node(s)

Distant metastasis (M)

Mx	Distant metastasis cannot be assessed
M0	No distant metastasis
M1	Distant metastasis
M1a	Metastasis to skin, subcutaneous tissues, or distant lymph nodes
M1b	Metastasis to lungs
M1c	Metastasis to all other visceral sites or distant metastasis at any site associated with an elevated serum lactic dehydrogenase (LDH) level

From Greene FL, Page DL, Fleming ID, et al (eds): AJCC Cancer Staging Manual, 6th ed. New York, Springer-Verlag, 2002.

TABLE 2: Stage groupings for cutaneous melanoma

Clinical staging[a]				Pathologic staging[b]			
0	Tis	N0	M0	0	Tis	N0	M0
IA	T1a	N0	M0	IA	T1a	N0	M0
IB	T1b	N0	M0	IB	T1b	N0	M0
	T2a	N0	M0		T2a	N0	M0
IIA	T2b	N0	M0	IIA	T2b	N0	M0
	T3a	N0	M0		T3a	N0	M0
IIB	T3b	N0	M0	IIB	T3b	N0	M0
	T4a	N0	M0		T4a	N0	M0
IIC	T4b	N0	M0	IIC	T4b	N0	M0
III	Any T	N1	M0				
		N2					
		N3					
				IIIA	T1-4a	N1a	M0
					T1-4a	N2a	M0
				IIIB	T1-4b	N1a	M0
					T1-4b	N2a	M0
					T1-4a	N1b	M0
					T1-4a	N2b	M0
					T1-4a/b	N2c	M0
				IIIC	T1-4b	N1b	M0
					T1-4b	N2b	M0
					Any T	N3	M0
IV	Any T	Any N	Any M1	IV	Any T	Any N	Any M1

[a]Clinical staging includes microstaging of the primary melanoma and clinical/radiologic evaluation for metastases; by convention, it should be used after complete excision of the primary melanoma with *clinical* assessment for regional and distant metastases.

[b]Pathologic staging includes microstaging of the primary melanoma and pathologic information about the regional lymph nodes after partial or complete lymphadenectomy, except for pathologic stage 0 or stage IA patients, who may not need pathologic evaluation of their lymph nodes.

Adapted from Balch CM, Buzaid AC, Soong SJ, et al: J Clin Oncol 19:3635–3648, 2001.

TABLE 3: Five-year survival rates of pathologically staged patients[a, b]

	IA	IB	IIA	IIB	IIC	IIIA	IIIB	IIIC
Ta: Nonulcerated melanoma	T1a	T2a	T3a	T4a	–	N1a	N1b	N3
	95%	89%	79%	67%	–	N2a	N2b	–
	–	–	–	–	–	67%	54%	28%
Tb: Ulcerated melanoma	–	T1b	T2b	T3b	T4b	–	N1a	N1b
	–	91%	77%	63%	45%	–	N2a	N2b
	–	–	–	–	–	–	–	N3
	–	–	–	–	–	–	52%	24%

a Adapted from Balch CM, et al: Melanoma of the skin, in Greene FL, Page DL, Fleming ID, et al (eds): AJCC Cancer Staging Manual, 6th ed. New York, Springer-Verlag, 2002.

b See Table 2 for staging details. N1 = 1 node; N2 = ≥ 2 nodes; Na = microscopic; Nb = macroscopic.

Many investigators have documented an inverse correlation between Breslow's tumor thickness and survival. More important, several studies have demonstrated that tumor thickness conveys more prognostic information than does Clark's level of invasion. In addition, the measurement of tumor thickness is generally more reproducible and less subjective than is the determination of Clark's level.

Occasionally, Breslow's thickness is impossible to determine and only the Clark's level is available for microstaging, usually because of technical factors related to the performance of the biopsy or the preparation of the histologic specimen. These situations, which inevitably result in the loss of important prognostic information, can be largely avoided by the performance of full-thickness (not shave) biopsies and by careful attention to detail when preparing specimens.

Regional lymph node involvement

In clinically localized disease, lymph node involvement is the strongest prognostic indicator in the staging of melanoma. Patients with nodal involvement at the time of their diagnosis have significantly decreased survival when compared with those who do not, independent of the primary lesion. There is a direct relationship between the depth of invasion of the primary lesion and the potential for lymph node involvement. The number of involved lymph nodes is inversely related to long-term survival. Patients with a single lymph node with metastatic disease have a better 5-year survival rate of approximately 60% than those who have multiple nodes (20%–25%). Also, patients with clinically enlarged or matted nodes at the time of diagnosis have a worse prognosis than those with microscopic disease.

An unknown primary

Melanoma of an unknown primary (MUP) is identified in up to 5% of patients who present with a newly diagnosed lesion. Lymphadenopathy is the most common presenting feature, followed by identification of visceral metastases and cutaneous nodules. In cases of MUP, consultations (such as ophthalmology, gastroenterology, otolaryngology, and gynecology) should be considered for appropriate evaluation of retinal and mucosal surfaces that may harbor a primary lesion. CT scan of the chest, abdomen, and pelvis should also be performed. PET scan may be considered, although its utility in the evaluation of melanoma is not yet clear. Surgical management of MUP should include lymphadenectomy for nodal disease and consideration of visceral resection if no other foci of disease are identified. Single dermal nodules with no identifiable primary lesion are typically treated in similar fashion to primary melanomas, with wide local excision and regional nodal evaluation (sentinel lymph node biopsy [SLNB]) if appropriate. If a primary lesion is identified, it should be excised widely. The prognosis for patients who present with MUP is similar to that for patients with metastatic disease from a known primary.

Clinical and pathologic staging

TNM staging system The melanoma staging committee of the American Joint Committee on Cancer (AJCC) has revised the TNM staging system to reflect more accurately the impact of statistically significant prognostic factors that were validated on a multi-institution sample of over 17,000 melanoma patients. The new system is shown in Tables 1 and 2.

For patients with stage IV disease (distant metastases), there are few but significant differences in prognosis for disease limited to the skin, for subcutaneous and nodal sites versus visceral sites, and for levels of lactic dehydrogenase (LDH) in the serum.

Some of the most significant changes include new cutoff points for T classification (T1 = ≤ 1.0 mm, T2 = 1.01–2.0 mm, T3 = 2.01–4.0 mm, T4 = > 4 mm), inclusion of ulceration as a factor in T stage (a: no ulceration, b: ulceration), placement of node size with node number for N stage, inclusion of node size (microscopic vs macroscopic) as a factor in N stage, and inclusion of LDH level as a factor in M stage. When incorporated into new clinical protocols, the new system will undoubtedly improve the value of data from clinical trials in this disease (Table 2).

Other prognostic factors

Age Overall, patients who are ≥ 65 years old have a survival rate that is decreased by 10%–15% compared with their younger counterparts. Although this trend has been demonstrated in numerous studies, whether age is truly an independent predictor of survival remains unclear. A different relationship between age and risk of lymph node involvement, however, is emerging. Data from the prospective Sunbelt Melanoma Trial and retrospective studies reveal that younger patients are significantly more likely to harbor nodal disease than older patients with similar lesions. Age, therefore, deserves consideration in management decisions regarding surgical evaluation of nodal basins.

Gender Many studies have identified a trend toward improved survival in women compared with men with melanoma. As an independent predictor of survival, however, this has frequently not reached statistical significance.

Anatomic location There is a correlation between anatomic location and prognosis of primary melanoma. Those with lesions on the back, upper arms, neck, and scalp (BANS area) have a worse prognosis than those with lesions on the extremities. This may be due to the simple fact that these lesions cannot be evaluated easily by the patient because of their inopportune location rather than a manifestation of true differences in tumor biology. In fact, location of the primary melanoma has not stood out as an independent predictor of prognosis in multivariate analysis. Men are more likely to develop truncal melanomas, whereas women are most likely to develop melanoma on their extremities. Acral lesions carry a worse prognosis than other extremity lesions.

Desmoplastic melanoma Desmoplastic melanomas represent a less common but clinically distinct spindle cell variant of melanoma with dense fibrosis and frequent neurotropism. Clinically, they are raised, firm nodules that are amelanotic in up to 40% of patients, leading to a common delay in diagnosis. Likely because of their neurotropism, these tumors have local recurrence rates as high as 40%, which has led many clinicians to advocate local radiation therapy following excision of these lesions. However, whether desmoplastic melanomas that lack neurotropism are truly at high risk for local recurrence, and whether radiation therapy helps control local recurrence if they are, remains an area of debate.

Additionally, although many of these lesions are deeply invasive at the time of diagnosis, desmoplastic melanomas are less likely to involve regional lymph node basins and more commonly develop distant metastases without lymphatic involvement. This observation should not deter sentinel lymph node biopsy in appropriate patients, as approximately 12% will harbor nodal disease. Despite these seemingly adverse prognostic factors, patients with desmoplastic and neurotropic melanomas tend to have overall survival rates that are slightly favorable compared with other melanomas.

Angiolymphatic invasion Defined as invasion of tumor cells into the wall and/or lumen of vessels or lymphatics of the dermis or deeper structures, angiolymphatic invasion is uncommon in malignant melanoma. However, this finding is clearly associated with more aggressive tumors and signifies likely poor outcomes for these patients. Multiple large studies have shown worsened long-term survival and more frequent lymph node involvement in patients with angioinvasive melanomas. In fact, risk of lymphatic involvement increases as much as threefold, whereas 5-year survival is reduced by as much as 50%, in patients with vascular invasion compared to matched patients without vascular invasion.

Regression The finding of regression represents host immune response to invasive melanoma. Areas where invasive cells may have once existed are replaced by inflammatory reaction and fibrosis, which may make it impossible to determine the precise depth of the initial lesion histologically. There is continuing debate regarding the prognostic importance of regression; however, many clinicians believe that thin lesions that show signs of regression should be given higher consideration for surgical nodal staging, given the fact that the initial lesion may have originally been more deeply invasive. Although some studies have shown that regressed lesions have a higher propensity for lymph node metastases than nonregressed primary tumors of the same thickness, this finding has not been universally observed.

Variable numbers of tumor infiltrating lymphocytes (TILs) are observed in melanoma. Tumors with a high number of TILs should carry an improved prognosis because of the active host response to tumor. In fact, many studies have shown this tendency.

Angiogenesis Studies have found angiogenesis to be an independent factor in long-term survival as well as local recurrence. More commonly identified as tumor depth increases, angiogenesis is a marker of invasive potential. Deep lesions with ulceration and high mitotic rates are typically associated with angiogenesis, and the combination of all of these factors is associated with poor outcome.

Treatment of melanomas

SURGICAL TREATMENT OF CUTANEOUS MELANOMA

Excision of primary lesion It was recognized over a century ago that tumor cells could extend within the skin for several centimeters beyond the visible borders of a melanoma, so that the risk of local recurrence relates to the width of normal skin excised around the primary tumor. Only much more recently was it realized that the thickness of the primary tumor influenced the likelihood of contiguous spread and that not all melanomas require the same excision margin. This realization prompted a number of randomized trials to determine the optimal excision margins for melanomas of different Breslow's thicknesses.

Initially, a "one-size-fits-all" approach of taking a 5-cm margin around all cutaneous melanomas was adopted. With such wide margins, skin grafts were required after removal of melanomas on most parts of the body. Melanomas < 1 mm thick had low recurrence rates, however, even when less than the full 5-cm margin was excised.

A randomized trial found that when a 1-cm margin of normal skin was taken around a melanoma < 1 mm thick, the local recurrence rate was exceedingly low (< 1%), and patient survival was just as good as if 3-cm margins were taken. For melanomas 1–2 mm in thickness, patient survival was the same for both margins of excision, but the local recurrence rate was higher with the 1-cm margin (3.3% after 10-year follow-up).

Another randomized trial compared 2- vs 4-cm margins for all cutaneous melanomas between 1 and 4 mm in thickness. In this trial, both local recurrence and survival were the same regardless of whether 2- or 4-cm margins were taken. Skin grafts were less frequent and hospital stays shorter with the narrower margin.

In one phase III trial, 2-cm margins were compared with 5-cm margins for primary tumors ≤ 2 mm deep. Again, there was no difference in the local or distant relapse rate or overall survival.

Current recommendations Based on these three important studies, it is possible to make rational recommendations for excision margins for melanoma patients.

- For lesions > 1 mm in thickness, the recommended excision margin is 1 cm.
- For lesions 1–4 mm in thickness, a 2-cm margin is recommended.
- At least a 2-cm margin should be taken for lesions > 4 mm in thickness.

Several facts should be considered regarding these recommendations:

- Regardless of the recommended margin, a histologically negative margin is necessary. Thus, if a 2-cm margin is taken and the pathology report reveals melanoma cells or atypical melanocytic hyperplasia at the margins, further excision is indicated.
- When the anatomic location of the primary tumor precludes excision of the desired margin (eg, on the hands and feet or the face), at least 1 cm should be taken as long as the margins are histologically negative.
- If a minor compromise in excision margin can allow primary closure without a skin graft, it is worthwhile.

Management of regional lymph nodes

Physical examination is the primary screening tool for lymphatic involvement with melanoma. All potentially involved basins should be examined as part of a thorough history and physical examination. Patients who present with clinically negative nodes will have their further evaluation defined by the depth and characteristics of their primary melanoma. Currently, those patients with melanoma having Breslow depth ≥ 1 mm are candidates for surgical evaluation of nodal involvement using SLNB techniques. Patients with thinner melanomas may also be candidates for SLNB if adverse prognostic factors are identified in their primary tumor.

The first step in evaluating palpable nodes is generally FNA. Positive cytology is sufficient to mandate complete nodal dissection. A negative or inadequate sample FNA may be repeated, with image guidance if necessary, or may lead directly to an open node biopsy, followed by complete lymphadenectomy in the event of a positive frozen section or touch-prep cytologic determination of metastasis.

Clinically enlarged nodes Melanoma patients with clinically enlarged nodes and no evidence of distant disease (AJCC stage III) should undergo complete regional lymphadenectomy. Physical examination may be inaccurate in its prediction of nodal involvement, however, and so other techniques may be utilized to identify positive nodes. FNA of palpable nodes may assist in further decision-making. If positive cytology is identified, lymphadenectomy should be performed. A negative FNA should not preclude further surgical evaluation. Touch-prep cytology may also be a useful adjunct for intraoperative evaluation of suspicious nodes during SLNB or open biopsy.

Clinically normal nodes The surgical management of clinically normal nodes is determined by the characteristics of the primary lesion. A direct relationship between thickness of the primary lesion and nodal involvement has long been recognized. In addition, the Sunbelt Melanoma Trial has identified additional prognostic factors that increase the risk of nodal disease.

Thin melanomas Patients with thin melanomas (< 1 mm Breslow depth) have a low risk of occult nodal involvement (< 5%) and therefore generally undergo wide excision with 1-cm margins and no nodal staging procedure. Some patients with melanomas 0.76–1 mm have a high enough risk of lymph node involvement to justify consideration of SLNB in addition to wide excision.

Multiple risk factors that confer an increased risk for lymph node metastases in patients with thin melanomas have been identified. If they are present, consideration may be given to SLNB in patients with thin melanomas (between 0.76 and 1 mm). Historically, Clark's level of IV or V was considered to be a significant prognostic indicator and continues to be included in the AJCC staging system. Emerging data, however, suggest that this criterion is probably the least satisfactory in discriminating those patients with thin melanomas who should undergo lymph node biopsy.

Intermediate-thickness melanomas Melanomas 1–4 mm in thickness are associated with an overall risk of occult lymph node involvement of 20%–25%. However, relative risk rises significantly with increasing depth of invasion. Patients with a 1-mm-thick melanoma have approximately a 15% chance of involvement, whereas those with a 4-mm melanoma have up to a 55% risk of nodal metastases. For these reasons, wide excision of the primary tumor is generally accompanied by SLNB for evaluation of the nodal basin involved. An alternative approach of wide excision alone with observation and serial physical examination of nodal basins has been advocated by some clinicians and has not been shown to reduce long-term survival if complete lymph node dissection is performed at the identification of clinically positive nodes. The use of SLNB vs observation continues to be an area of intense debate.

Selective lymphadenectomy The identification and management of nodal disease have evolved significantly over the past 20 years. The evolution of SLNB has led to an improved ability to accurately stage patients earlier in their disease process. Historically, complete lymph node dissections were performed electively on patients with intermediate and thick melanomas with the belief that they would lead to a survival benefit. With elective node dissection, however, a significant percentage (80%–85%) of patients underwent complete lymphadenectomy only to find that their nodal basin was free of disease.

Currently, node dissection is used selectively, only on those melanoma patients who have been shown to have nodal involvement by SLNB. SLNB was described by Morton et al, who found that dermal injection of vital blue dye (Lymphazurin) surrounding the primary melanoma site allowed for visualization of the draining lymphatics and the "sentinel" node, which was defined to be the first draining lymph node receiving lymph from the primary tumor bed. The original dye-based technique allowed for identification of the "sentinel" node in approximately 85% of cases.

To increase the success rate for sentinel node identification, technetium^{99m}–labeled sulfur colloid is injected into the primary site preoperatively, and the potentially involved lymph basins are identified with a gamma camera. The patient is then taken to the operating room, where a hand-held gamma probe is used to identify the sentinel node(s). This technique, in combination with the use of vital blue dye, has led to a success rate exceeding 99% in most large current trials.

The ability to accurately detect or rule out disease in the sentinel lymph node has allowed many patients to forego the higher morbidity of complete node dissection. In addition, patients can be more accurately staged and treated earlier in the course of their disease. The intuitive hope that this ability could lend itself to improved survival in patients who undergo SLNB remains to be determined in prospective, randomized trials. Even in the absence of a proven survival benefit, however, the staging advantages of SLNB are sufficiently compelling to justify its routine use in healthy patients with melanomas and a significant risk of nodal involvement. Current data also support the watch-and-wait approach to nodal evaluation, with lymph node dissection (LND) reserved for those who develop clinically positive nodes, which still has a place in the treatment of melanoma and likely does not negatively impact survival. The prospective clinical trials are currently investigating the role of complete lymphadenectomy following positive SLNB.

The evolution of reverse transcriptase-PCR (RT-PCR) has allowed for identification of submicroscopic metastatic nodal disease. It is unknown whether submicroscopic metastatic disease has clinical relevance in the long-term survival of patients with melanoma. These issues are currently being prospectively investigated in the Sunbelt Melanoma trial. Although a number of retrospective studies have suggested that RT-PCR analysis has a role to play in predicting outcome for patients with histologically negative sentinel nodes, a recent study with longer follow-up suggested that this prognostic value was lost over time. This observation stresses the importance of prospective evaluation of candidate prognostic tests such as RT-PCR.

Thick melanomas Primary melanomas > 4 mm in thickness are treated with a 2-cm excision margin. In addition, because deep melanomas harbor nodal metastases in up to 60% of patients, surgical evaluation of the nodal basin is generally pursued. Although elective LND has not proven beneficial in these patients, SLNB has been used extensively to guide diagnostic, prognostic, and therapeutic decision-making.

SURGICAL TREATMENT OF NONCUTANEOUS MELANOMA

Noncutaneous melanomas generally present at a more advanced stage than cutaneous lesions. The site of the lesion greatly affects the approach to the primary tumor and regional lymph nodes.

Ocular melanomas generally do not have access to lymphatic channels, so the surgical principles outlined previously do not apply here. However, the unique propensity to metastasize hematogenously, often to the liver after a long relapse-free interval, warrants further study of this primary site's unique biology. Advances in understanding the biology of ocular melanomas may lead to adjuvant approaches different from therapies now under investigation for cutaneous primaries.

A diagnosis of ocular melanoma with no evidence of distant disease signifies that a decision must be made as to whether or not the eye can be spared. Some small melanomas situated peripherally in the retina can be excised with minimal loss of vision, but most cannot. For larger lesions, treatment options are enucleation (total removal of the eye) or implanted radiotherapy with a radioactive gold plaque fitted to the back of the eyeball immediately behind the tumor. A multi-institution, randomized trial comparing implanted radiotherapy with enucleation for local disease control and overall survival was completed by the Collaborative Ocular Melanoma Study Group; it appears that both techniques provide similar outcomes for all sizes of tumors.

Melanomas of the anus and vulva pose challenges in the treatment of both the primary lesion and regional nodes. Excision of primary tumors in these areas should not be overly radical: Abdominoperineal resection or radical vulvectomy is unnecessarily deforming and is not associated with improved survival compared with wide local excision. Abdominoperineal resection, with its attendant permanent colostomy, is indicated only for locally recurrent melanomas after prior sphincter-conserving excision or for melanomas with radiographic evidence of mesorectal node involvement.

Anal and vulvar melanomas often present with inguinal lymph node metastases; if there is no evidence of distant disease, both the primary site and regional nodes should be removed.

Nasal sinuses or nasopharyngeal melanomas Melanomas arising in the nasal or nasopharyngeal mucosa should be widely excised to include adjacent bony structures, if needed. Node dissection is reserved for patients who have proven nodal involvement. Radiation therapy should be considered for those patients whose primary tumor cannot be fully removed from this site with adequate margins.

ADJUVANT THERAPY FOR MELANOMA

Interferon-alpha-2b (IFN-α; Intron A) was established as a standard therapy on the basis of an adjuvant therapy trial conducted in patients with high-risk stages II and III disease (Eastern Cooperative Oncology Group [E1684]). Interferon-alpha-2b was administered by intravenous infusion, 20 mU/m^2 for 5 consecutive days every 7 days for 4 weeks during the "induction" phase. For a subsequent 48 weeks, 10 mU/m^2 were administered by subcutaneous injection on alternate days for a total of three doses every 7 days in the "maintenance" phase.

This "high-dose" regimen was compared with observation. A statistically significant 25% improvement in overall survival was demonstrated with interferon, compared with the observation arm; relapse-free survival was improved by 50%. Three-quarters of the interferon-treated patients experienced severe toxicities, most commonly fatigue, asthenia, fever, depression, and elevated liver transaminase levels. A quality-of-life analysis found that the toxicity associated with this regimen was largely compensated for by the prevention of disease relapse.

Due to uncertainty regarding the optimal dose and schedule of interferon, a second trial was initiated comparing the high-dose regimen and a low-dose regimen (3 mU by subcutaneous injection 3 times weekly for 24 months) as well as observation. No significant improvement in overall survival for either the high-dose or low-dose arms was observed compared with observation; relapse-free survival was improved by 22% in the high-dose arm compared with observation. A pooled analysis of E1684 and E1690, with longer follow-up for both trials, revealed a continued, statistically significant impact on relapse-free survival but not on overall survival.

Two additional randomized trials were conducted comparing high-dose interferon with vaccination with ganglioside GM2/keyhole limpet hemocyanin (E1694 and E2696). Although these trials did not include an observation control arm, the relative superiority of high-dose interferon to the experimental arm has been marshaled as further evidence of the benefit of interferon therapy. A 34% improvement in overall survival and a 32% improvement in relapse-free survival were observed in the larger of the two trials, E1694. However, the recent study from EORTC (European Organization for Research on the Treatment of Cancer) that a GM2 vaccine resulted in a significantly worse survival compared with observation among patients with resected stage II melanoma diminishes the value of these trials in supporting the efficacy of interferon. High-dose interferon has been consistently shown to improve relapse-free survival compared with either observation or ganglioside GM2/keyhole limpet hemocyanin vaccination but does not confer a clear survival advantage.

Intermediate-dose regimens with interferon have been evaluated in several trials; they have less consistently demonstrated a relapse-free survival advantage compared with observation and have never resulted in a survival advantage. The largest such trial employed conventional interferon-alpha-2b whereas the other administered pegylated interferon. In E18952, interferon 10 mU daily for 5 days out of 7 repeated for 4 weeks followed by 10 mU three times weekly for 1 year was compared with interferon 10 mU daily for 5 days out of 7 repeated for 4 weeks followed by 5 mU three times weekly for 2 years or observation. In E18991, patients were treated with pegylated interferon (6 μg/kg once weekly for 8 weeks by subcutaneous injection) followed by maintenance, at 3 μg/kg weekly for 5 years. These regimens are not considered standard adjuvant treatment in the United States, but are offered in Europe.

Chemotherapy Single-agent chemotherapy or combination chemotherapy regimens have not been systematically evaluated for the adjuvant treatment of melanoma. The largest randomized trial compared an intravenously administered regimen of carmustine (BiCNU; 80 mg/m^2) every 4 weeks, actinomycin D (10 μg/kg), and vincristine (1.0 mg/m^2) every 2 weeks for 6 months with observation among patients with resected stage III or IV melanoma. A significant improvement in relapse-free survival, but not overall survival, was observed in this small study. A randomized trial comparing dacarbazine and observation failed to demonstrate an improvement in either relapse-free or overall survival. A biochemotherapy regimen, consisting of cisplatin, vincristine, dacarbazine, interferon and interleukin-2, is being compared with high-dose interferon among patients with stage III melanoma in a cooperative group phase III trial (S0008).

There is currently no standard adjuvant therapy following resection of metastatic melanoma. Interferon has not been thoroughly evaluated in this setting. Therefore, observation remains the standard of care for patients in this setting, and investigational vaccines are currently being evaluated among these patients.

Neoadjuvant therapy for resectable stage IIIC or IV melanoma remains an investigational approach. Unlike systemic therapies breast and rectal cancers, for which chemotherapy regimens are associated with high response rates, systemic therapies for melanoma are not sufficiently active to support their incorporation into neoadjuvant treatment.

Radiation therapy in the adjuvant setting is controversial. Given the high risk of recurrence in the regional node basin among patients with numerous (greater than 10) positive lymph nodes or a single node with extracapsular extension, some experts advocate the use of radiation therapy following complete lymph node dissection to prevent regional recurrences. In the neck, this approach is associated with relatively little long-term morbidity, but the increased risk of debilitating lymphedema in the axilla or groin limits the routine application of this approach.

Reports have demonstrated that the pessimistic impression that melanoma is a "nonradioresponsive" tumor is not justified. A study at M. D. Anderson Cancer Center suggested that postoperative radiation therapy to the neck after radical or modified radical neck dissection decreased regional recurrence rates over those of historic controls in node-positive patients or in those with a primary tumor that is greater than 1.5 mm thick.

Formal investigation of the role of adjuvant irradiation in patients thought to be at uniquely high risk for locoregional disease has been hampered by technical challenges to protocol design and changes in the practical approach to these patients. Nevertheless, it seems reasonable to consider the use of postoperative radiation therapy in patients with high-risk nodal disease defined as follows: more than four lymph nodes, gross extracapsular extension, a lymph node greater than 3 cm, cervical lymph node location, recurrent nodal disease, sentinel lymph node involved, and an unplanned complete dissection. Those patients with a high-risk primary disease such as: a desmoplastic variant, positive surgical margins, locally recurrent disease, and a Breslow depth of greater then 4 mm accompanied by either ulceration or satellitosis are also reasonable candidates to discuss the role of adjuvant radiation therapy for the benefit of decreasing local recurrence.

Because these patients are also candidates for IFN-a or investigational studies of adjuvant therapy, the optimal schedule for integrating radiation therapy with IFN-a will need to be determined. In the absence of definitive data, we defer the start of radiation therapy until after the completion of the initial month of intravenous IFN-a. One goal of the new agents is to provide radiosensitization, so radiation therapy can be a more useful adjunct either in the adjuvant setting, as addressed here, or in the advanced setting, as addressed later in the chapter.

Radiation therapy can provide some benefit and should be considered in the palliative treatment of melanoma metastatic to bone or other symptomatic sites.

Vaccines remain an investigational approach, which are currently being tested among patients with resected stages II, III, and IV melanoma. The goal of this approach is to reverse immune tolerance of microscopic residual melanoma following surgery through the amplification of melanoma-specific cytolytic T cells. This approach is distinct from conventional immunization against pathogens to which the host is naïve, where long-lasting, antibody-mediated immunity is sought by induction of memory B cells.

A single randomized trial administering a melanoma cell lysate to patients following resection of stage III melanoma demonstrated a modest, statistically insignificant improvement in overall survival. However, two recently reported trials using a mixture of three irradiated allogeneic melanoma cell lines demonstrated a detrimental effect on overall survival for either resected stage III or stage IV patients. Another randomized trial compared a ganglioside vaccine with observation in patients with resected stage II melanoma and demonstrated inferior survival among the vaccinated patients. Although each of these approaches was associated with little toxicity, the possibility exists that some attempts to immunize against melanoma can be distracting to productive immune surveillance and can compromise long-term outcome.

Melanoma peptide vaccines are currently being intensely evaluated in clinical trials. Peptides have been selected from two classes for clinical development: melanocyte-specific proteins and so-called cancer-testis antigens. The latter are proteins that have a restricted spatiotemporal expression and are not detectable in adult tissues outside the immunologic sanctuary site of the testes. The most widely studied peptides are derived from gp-100, tyrosinase, melan-A (all melanocyte-specific), and NY-ESO-1 and MAGE proteins (cancer-testis antigens). Preliminary evidence suggests that this approach may successfully engender specific and potent immunologic responses to the protein fragments being administered. Protection against disease recurrence in patients at high risk following surgery has not yet been demonstrated. Notably, no randomized data suggesting a detrimental effect from peptide vaccination in melanoma have been presented.

TREATMENT OF ADVANCED MELANOMA

Surgery The treatment of advanced-stage melanoma is controversial, as there are only a few systemic agents with demonstrated tumor responses, and only a few patients may be eligible for surgery. The concept of resection of metastatic disease is based primarily on clinical data demonstrating up to 40% 5-year survival rates in patients with a variety of malignancies that spread to the lungs and had complete resection of the metastases. Resection should be confined to patients with a good performance status who can physiologically tolerate the procedure and who have favorable tumor biology with slow-growing tumors (tumor doubling times greater than 60 days). A number of retrospective studies have shown the validity of resecting pulmonary metastases in melanoma, and more recent studies have shown similar survival rates for patients undergoing resection of limited number and sites of disease (usually up to four) for metastases to distant lymph nodes, skin and subcutaneous tissue, and lungs. Patients with metastases in the liver, adrenal, brain, and gastrointestinal tract can undergo resection, but generally the survival of these patients is poor, based on the presence of subclinical disease and rapid tumor progression in the postoperative period.

Surgery can also be performed for palliation of systems. Large skin and subcutaneous or lymph node disease can cause significant pain or bleeding and may be effectively palliated with surgery. Bleeding or obstruction from small intestine metastases are best managed by resection. Although palliative resection can provide short-term effective relief of patient symptoms, numerous studies have shown that incomplete resection does nothing to enhance survival time.

Single-agent chemotherapy Melanoma is regarded as a relatively chemotherapy-refractory tumor. Durable objective responses have been observed in a small minority of patients with metastatic melanoma treated with single-agent chemotherapy, providing perhaps the most compelling reason to offer these agents routinely.

In a phase III trial comparing temozolomide (Temodar) and dacarbazine as first-line therapy, 3% of patients on either arm experienced complete responses. The highest response rates have been observed with alkylating agents, platinum analogues, and mictrotubule interactive drugs (Table 4). The reference standard to which novel agents and regimens are compared is dacarbazine. In the majority of trials, dacarbazine was administered intravenously at daily doses of 200 mg/m^2 for 5 days every 3 or 4 weeks; however, 1,000 mg/m^2 once every 3 or 4 weeks has been given in recent trials. The most common toxicities are myelosuppression and nausea. The severity of myelosuppression rarely requires the use of growth factor support, and the advent of potent antiemetics in recent years has significantly improved the tolerability of this agent. In the largest phase III trial that included a single-agent dacarbazine arm, the objective response rate was 3.5%, and the median progression-free survival was 1.5 months. Overall survival for dacarbazine-treated patients is 6 to 9 months and does not clearly differ from the natural history of metastatic melanoma. Fotemustine, a nitrosourea with modestly superior activity compared with dacarbazine, is available for clinical use in Europe but not in the United States.

Combination chemotherapy regimens As with other types of cancer, combinations of agents with some measurable single-agent activity in melanoma have been empirically developed. Clinical trials combining chemotherapy have produced promising response rates in single-arm, single-institution studies but have never demonstrated an improvement in overall survival compared with single-agent chemotherapy in multicenter, randomized trials. Given the increased toxicity associated with such regimens, the absence of a survival advantage limits their consideration as standard therapies. These treatments include cisplatin, vinblastine, and dacarbazine (CVD) and the Dartmouth regimen (cisplatin, carmustine, dacarbazine, and tamoxifen). Inpatient treatment is standard for these regimens, and the severity of myelosuppression often requires growth factor support not needed for single-agent chemotherapies. Given that longevity is not impacted for these patients who have such a short life

TABLE 4: Selected chemotherapy agents – Results from phase II and phase III trials in melanoma

Chemotherapy	Patients (N)	Objective response rate
Alkylating agents		
Dacarbazine	2470	18%
Temozolomide	350	15%
Nitrosoureas		
Lomustine	270	13%
Fotemustine	153	24%
Platinum analogues		
Cisplatin	188	23%
Carboplatin	43	16%
Microtubule stabilizing/destabilizing		
Paclitaxel	85	13%
Docetaxel	105	11%
Vincristine	52	12%
Vinblastine	62	13%
Vindesine	273	14%

expectancy, the quality-of-life detriment associated with combination therapy cannot be justified.

Tamoxifen Based on anecdotes of tumor regression associated with single-agent tamoxifen and laboratory evidence suggesting synergy with chemotherapy, clinical trials were undertaken combining tamoxifen with individual chemotherapy agents or combination regimens. As with other combination chemotherapy trials, single-arm trials of regimens containing tamoxifen appeared promising. However, in randomized trials where the same chemotherapy regimen was administered to all patients, and tamoxifen given only to the experimental arm, no evidence of clinical benefit was observed with the addition of tamoxifen.

Biologic therapies Interleukin-2 (IL-2) was approved by the US Food and Drug Administration (FDA) as a treatment for metastatic melanoma on the basis of durable complete and partial remissions associated with the "high-dose" regimen. This regimen requires patients to be in excellent overall health to tolerate the physiologic stress of 5 days of inpatient therapy. The standard dose is 200,000 U/m^2 repeated every 8 hours, for a maximum of 14 doses. This treatment is followed by a 10 to 14 day treatment break and readmission for another course of therapy. Patients who demonstrate some degree of tumor regression are offered additional courses of therapy. Typical toxicities include fever, malaise, hypotension complicated by renal dysfunction, elevated liver transaminases levels, and mood alterations. Clinical expertise among physicians and nurses is required to safely and effectively administer this therapy. As a consequence, the use of high-dose IL-2 has largely been restricted to high-volume referral centers.

Interferon-alpha-2b has demonstrated single-agent activity in metastatic melanoma that is comparable to chemotherapy, including occasional durable responses. A randomized trial comparing interferon-alpha-2b with dacarbazine in metastatic disease has never been conducted. Given the significant toxicity associated with chronic administration of interferon, its use in the metastatic setting is limited.

Biochemotherapy regimens The distinct mechanism of action of biologic agents and evidence of single-agent activity have led investigators to combine these agents with chemotherapy for the treatment of metastatic melanoma. Given the toxicity associated with high-dose IL-2, it is not possible to safely administer chemotherapy concurrently. However, lower-dose IL-2 regimens can be safely coadministered with combination chemotherapy. Likewise, the high-dose interferon regimen that is the current standard therapy for adjuvant treatment of stages II and III melanoma cannot be easily combined with chemotherapy, whereas modified schedules of interferon can.

The first biochemotherapy regimens tested in phase II trials and then subsequently in large, randomized phase III trials combined interferon alpha with dacarbazine. Despite early evidence suggesting a substantially higher response rate associated with the combination, definitive phase III trials failed to identify a survival advantage to this regimen compared with dacarbazine alone.

More intensive regimens combining chemotherapy with biologic agents, requiring inpatient administration, have more recently been evaluated. A regimen containing cisplatin, vinblastine, dacarbazine, with concurrent interferon and IL-2 was evaluated in several phase II trials, a small, single-institution phase III trial, and a multicenter phase III trial in comparison to multiagent chemotherapy without the biologic agents. Although progression-free survival appeared modestly superior to that of the chemotherapy backbone alone, no improvement in overall survival could be demonstrated. Likewise, a trial in which the contribution of IL-2 to a regimen of cisplatin, dacarbazine, and interferon-alpha was isolated failed to demonstrate a significant improvement in outcome.

Targeted therapy The discovery of somatic genetic mutations in melanoma, underlying aberrant signal transduction in melanoma cells, has provided leads for the development of molecularly targeted therapy. The MAP kinase pathway, which is activated in the vast majority of melanoma due to mutations in BRAF, NRAS, and c-kit, has been the focus of most clinical investigations of signal transduction (kinase) inhibitors. Angiogenesis, necessary for the progression of all solid tumors, has proven to be a valuable therapeutic target in the treatment of other metastatic cancers and is currently being investigated in randomized trials in melanoma.

Combinations of targeted therapy with chemotherapy are currently being extensively studied. Sorafenib (Nexavar) has been approved by the FDA for treatment of renal cell carcinoma and hepatocellular carcinoma as a single agent, and is currently being evaluated in combination with chemotherapy in phase III trials in melanoma. This agent offers the potential to inhibit both the MAP kinase pathway and tumor angiogenesis. Bevacizumab (Avastin), proven to enhance the efficacy of chemotherapy in colon, non-small cell lung, and breast cancers is currently being evaluated in combination with chemotherapy in melanoma in a randomized trial.

Treatment of CNS metastasis

Unfortunately, many patients with melanoma develop brain metastases, second behind only breast and lung primary malignancies. The treatment of brain metastases from melanoma is an area under active investigation and research. For this group of patients, whole-brain radiation therapy is one of the few treatments available for palliation of unresectable CNS metastases. Additionally, techniques of stereotactic irradiation, either alone or in combination with whole-brain radiation therapy, have shown encouraging results in patients with melanoma metastatic to the CNS.

Patients with metastatic melanoma to the brain were included among the patients enrolled in the Radiation Therapy Oncology Group (RTOG) 95-08 trial, which examined whole-brain radiotherapy versus whole-brain radiotherapy plus a stereotactic boost. In this trial, patients with a single lesion had a statistically significant survival advantage with the boost. Those with more than one lesion had an improved performance status and decreased steroid use. Alternative fractionation schedules of whole-brain radiotherapy have been investigated but have not proved to be superior to standard regimens of whole-brain irradiation, and more research needs to be done to improve the efficacy, role, and administration of radiation therapy as a whole.

The benefit of adding whole-brain irradiation therapy to focal radiation therapy or surgery for patients with brain metastases is an area that awaits new modulations of the available therapies, such as safe and effective radiosensitizers, in an effort to potentiate efficacy. Some preliminary studies have shown patient tolerability and response for concurrent temozolomide and whole-brain radiation therapy, but this is an area that needs additional research and should not be used widely as standard care practice. Various phase II and III trials sponsored by the North Central Cancer Treatment Group, the European Organization for Research and Treatment of Cancer, and the Japan Clinical Oncology Group are investigating the role of stereotactic radiosurgery and whole brain radiotherapy and surgery in various combinations.

In addition to radiotherapy, corticosteroids are often given concomitantly with brain irradiation to minimize intracranial swelling and are tapered off rapidly after the completion of therapy. Because melanoma is often associated with intracranial hemorrhage, excision should be considered for brain metastases that can be removed safely.

The somewhat limited success in treating brain metastases with chemotherapy reflects the lack of activity of available cytotoxic agents, including those that efficiently penetrate the CNS, such as nitrosoureas and temozolomide. Therapies with higher reported response rates have failed to reduce the rate of CNS metastatic disease, presumably due to their lack of CNS penetration and the emergence of metastases in a "sanctuary" site from a disease with a high propensity to seed the CNS. Thus, therapeutic success in this setting will require highly active combinations that can be used in the adjuvant setting before CNS metastases develop from recurrent disease, therapies with sufficient antitumor activity and CNS penetration, and agents with high antitumor activity and CNS penetration to treat those with established CNS metastatic disease.

Initial treatment of nonmelanoma skin cancer

Surgery
Surgical excision Most nonmelanoma skin cancers can be conservatively excised with much narrower margins than are required for cutaneous melanomas. Excision margins of 0.5–1.0 cm are adequate for most nonrecurrent basal cell and squamous cell cancers and yield local recurrence rates under 5%, provided that histologically negative margins are achieved. For most tumors in most anatomic sites, these excision margins can be achieved using standard surgical techniques with local anesthesia and primary closure.

Radiation therapy
Radiation therapy is effective for the treatment of squamous cell and basal cell skin cancers, and is associated with a similar likelihood of cure as surgery. However, this practice is only considered standard in areas of the body where surgery would be disfiguring or debilitating. In instances where negative margins cannot be obtained without an unacceptable cosmetic result, adjuvant radiation therapy to treat microscopic residual disease appears effective. This practice is also typically extended to Merkel cell skin cancers and sarcomas of the skin. The use of radiation therapy to the surgical bed when negative margins have been obtained is more controversial and is not well supported by data.

Topical and intralesional therapy
Topical therapy is a consideration for patients with large areas of skin affected by numerous or recurrent squamous cell or basal skin cancers. Immunocompromised patients and occasional patients with extremes of cumulative lifetime sun exposure are candidates for topical 5-fluorouracil (5-FU) or imiquimod. These therapies are generally not offered to patients who are

otherwise good candidate for surgical resection. 5-FU is an antimetabolite chemotherapy that is effective in eradicating both actinic keratoses and squamous cell skin cancers. Following treatment, patients typically develop significant erythema in treated skin lasting for several weeks until the treated skin has adequately regenerated its epithelium. Imiquimod stimulates the activity of antigen-presenting cells in the skin when applied topically, which engenders an immune response in treated tumors. Complete regression of treated tumors is typically achieved. However, patients who are offered this therapy are typically at high risk for local recurrence and appearance of new lesions elsewhere and thus require lifelong surveillance and, potentially, repeated treatment.

Intralesional therapy for unresectable or recurrent basal cell skin cancers has been investigated. The only readily available agent that has been employed for this purpose is interferon-alpha. Comparative trials have not been conducted with intralesional versus topical therapies.

Management of recurrent nonmelanoma skin cancer

Local recurrence complicates approximately 5% of cases of nonmelanoma skin cancer; if possible, surgical resection should be performed. In areas of skin where surgery would result in an unacceptable cosmetic result, radiation therapy can be offered. The vast majority of recurrent nonmelanoma skin cancers can be cured with re-excision or radiation therapy.

Regional lymph node involvement Among nonmelanoma skin cancers, Merkel cell carcinoma is the most likely to be associated with regional lymph node involvement. The prognosis of patients with lymph node involvement appears to be significantly worse than that of patients with localized disease. Thus, sentinel lymph node biopsy is justified as a staging procedure in patients with primary tumors greater than 2 cm. Squamous cell skin cancer is less likely to involve regional lymph nodes (5% of all cases), and sentinel lymph node biopsy is generally reserved for patients with large primary tumors (greater than 5 cm). Palpable lymph nodes should be evaluated with fine needle biopsy to determine the need for lymph node dissection. Basal cell carcinoma infrequently spreads to regional lymph nodes, leaving assessment of palpable nodes with fine needle aspiration as the only evaluation indicated.

Distant metastases occur infrequently in squamous cell carcinoma (2% of all cases) and generally are limited to patients who are immunocompromised. Fewer than 1 in 1,000 cases of basal cell carcinoma develop metastatic disease. Therefore, clinical trials in these patients have not been conducted. Combination chemotherapy regimens employed for squamous cell carcinoma from other sites are typically employed for patients with metastatic squamous cell carcinoma of the skin, although responses appear to be infrequently and usually short-lived.

SUGGESTED READING

ON SKIN CANCERS

Swetter SM, Geller AC, Kirkwood JM: Melanoma in the older person. Oncology 18:1187–1196, 2004.

Tsao H, Atkins MB, Sober AJ: Management of cutaneous melanoma. N Engl J Med 351:998–1012, 2004.

ON BIOLOGY AND EPIDEMIOLOGY OF MELANOMA

Chao C, McMasters KM: Relationship between age and other prognostic factors in melanoma. Am J Oncol Rev 3:446–454, 2004.

Curtin JA, Fridlyand J, Kgeshita T, et al: Distinct sets of genetic alterations in melanoma. N Engl J Med 353:2135–2147, 2005.

Demierre MF, Merlino G: Chemoprevention of melanoma. Curr Oncol Rep 6:406–413, 2004.

Kashani-Sabet M: Melanoma genomics. Curr Oncol Rep 6:401–405, 2004.

Tucker MA, Fraser MC, Goldstein AM, et al: A natural history of melanomas and dysplastic nevi: An atlas of lesions in melanoma-prone families. Cancer 94:3192–3209, 2002.

ON SURGICAL TREATMENT AND IMAGING

Ballo MT, Ang KK: Radiotherapy for cutaneous malignant melanoma: Rationale and indications. Oncology 18:99–108, 2004.

Bonnen MD, Ballo MT, Myers JN, et al: Elective radiotherapy provides regional control for patients with cutaneous melanoma of the head and neck. Cancer 100:383–389, 2004.

DuBay D, Cimmino V, Lowe L, et al: Low recurrence rate after surgery for dermatofibrosarcoma protuberans: A multidisciplinary approach from a single institution. Cancer 100:1008–1016, 2004.

Kammula US, Ghossein R, Bhattacharya S, et al: Serial follow-up and the prognostic significance of reverse transcriptase-polymerase chain reaction–Staged sentinel lymph nodes from melanoma patients. J Clin Oncol 22:3989–3996, 2004.

McMasters KM, Reintgen DS, Ross MI, et al: Sentinel lymph node biopsy for melanoma: Controversy despite widespread agreement. J Clin Oncol 19:2851–2855, 2001.

Mijnhout GS, Hoekstra OS, van Lingen A, et al: How morphometric analysis of metastatic load predicts the (un)usefulness of PET scanning: The case of lymph node staging in melanoma. J Clin Pathol 56:283–286, 2003.

Pawlik TM, Sondak VK: Malignant melanoma: Current state of primary and adjuvant treatment. Crit Rev Oncol Hematol 45:245–264, 2003.

Statius Muller MG, van Leeuwen PA, de Lange-de Klerk ES, et al: The sentinel lymph node status is an important factor for predicting clinical outcome in patients with stage I or II cutaneous melanoma. Cancer 91:2401–2408, 2001.

Thomas JM, Newton-Bishop J, A'Hern R, et al: Excision margins in high-risk malignant melanoma. N Engl J Med 350:757–766, 2004.

ON ADJUVANT THERAPY

Andrews DW, Scott CB, Sperduto PW, et al: Whole brain radiation therapy with or without stereotactic radiosurgery boost for patients with one to three brain metastases: Phase III results of the RTOG 9508 randomised trial. Lancet 363:1665–1672, 2004.

Ang KK, Byers RM, Peters LJ, et al: Regional radiotherapy as adjuvant treatment for head and neck malignant melanoma: Preliminary results. Arch Otolaryngol Head Neck Surg 116:169–172, 1990.

Ang KK, Peters LJ, Weber RS, et al: Postoperative radiotherapy for cutaneous melanoma of the head and neck region. Int J Radiat Oncol Biol Phys 30:795–798, 1994.

Buchsbaum JC, Suh JH, Lee SY, et al: Survival by radiation therapy oncology group recursive partitioning analysis class and treatment modality in patients with brain metastases from malignant melanoma: A retrospective study. Cancer 94:2265–2272, 2002.

Kirkwood JM, Manola J, Ibrahim J, et al: A pooled analysis of Eastern Cooperative Oncology Group and Intergroup trials of adjuvant high-dose interferon for melanoma. Clin Cancer Res 10:1670–1677, 2004.

ON SYSTEMIC THERAPY

Eichler AF, Loeffler JS: Multidisciplinary management of brain metastases. Oncologist 12:884–898, 2007.

Panelli MC, Wang E, Monsurro V, et al: Overview of melanoma vaccines and promising approaches. Curr Oncol Rep 6:414–420, 2004.

Ribas A, Butterfield LH, Glaspy JA, et al: Current developments in cancer vaccines and cellular immunotherapy. J Clin Oncol 21:2415–2432, 2003.

Rosenberg SA: Shedding light on immunotherapy for cancer. N Engl J Med 350:1461–1463, 2004.

Rosenberg SA, Dudley ME: Cancer regression in patients with metastatic melanoma after the transfer of autologous antitumor lymphocytes. Proc Natl Acad Sci 101(suppl 2):14639–14645, 2004.

The ABCDEs of moles and melanomas

Concept and photographs:
The Skin Cancer Foundation, www.skincancer.org

People at high risk of developing melanoma are those who have:

- A family history of melanoma, or who have had a melanoma in the past
- Unusual moles on the skin, or changing moles
- Fair skin, light hair and eye color, and who sunburn easily or tan with difficulty
- A record of painful or blistering sunburns as children or in their teenage years
- Indoor occupations and outdoor recreational habits

When you inspect moles, pay special attention to their sizes, shapes, edges, and color. A handy way to remember these features is to think of the A, B, C, D, and E of skin cancer–asymmetry, border, color, diameter, and evolving.

Asymmetry: If you draw a line through an asymmetrical mole, the two halves will not match.

Border: The borders of an early melanoma tend to be uneven. The edges may be scalloped or notched.

Color: Having a variety of colors is another warning signal. A number of different shades of brown, tan or black could appear. A melanoma may also become red, blue, or some other color.

Diameter: Melanomas usually are larger in diameter than the size of the eraser on your pencil (1/4 inch or 6 mm), but they may sometimes be smaller when first detected.

Evolving: Any change in a mole – in size, shape, color, elevation, or another trait, or any new symptom such as bleeding, itching, or crusting – points to suspicion and possible danger.

A
Asymmetry

Benign   Symmetrical

Malignant   Asymmetrical

B
Border

Benign   Even edges

Malignant   Uneven edges

C
Color

Benign   One shade

Malignant   Two or more shades

D
Diameter

Benign   Smaller than 6 mm

Malignant   Larger than 6 mm

MOLES/MELANOMAS

E
Evolving

Benign

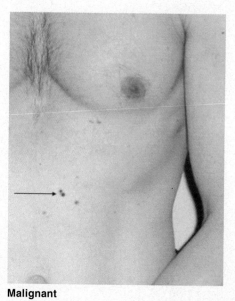

Malignant

A color atlas of skin lesions

Prepared by The Skin Cancer Foundation, www.skincancer.org, and the American Academy of Dermatology

SKIN LESIONS

FIGURE 1: Malignant melanoma
The heterogeneous color and asymmetry of the lesion point to
the diagnosis of melanoma. Particularly note the black color of
the right side of the lesion. (Figures 1 and 2 courtesy of the
American Academy of Dermatology)

FIGURE 2: Malignant melanoma
There are several colors clearly visible in this lesion, consistent
with melanoma. There are mottled black areas of the lesion,
with central tumor growth that is eroded and less pigmented.

FIGURE 3: Thick melanoma
Thick melanomas (> 4 mm in thickness) tend to have a nodular shape. While this lesion is dark, some thick melanomas may be pale. (Figures 3 through 11 courtesy of The Skin Cancer Foundation)

FIGURE 4: Thin melanoma
Thin melanomas (1 mm or less in thickness) are frequently diagnosed and are considered highly curable.

FIGURE 5: Squamous cell carcinoma
This infiltrated red plaque has central erosion and crust.

FIGURE 6: Squamous cell carcinoma
Erythematous and infiltrated lesion in a maximally
sun-exposed area, with an erosive center.

FIGURE 7: Actinic keratosis
Actinic keratosis is considered the earliest stage in skin cancer development.

FIGURE 8: Actinic keratosis
Actinic keratosis may present as a dry, rough-textured patch on the skin.

FIGURE 9: Basal cell carcinoma

Basal cell carcinoma is a type of non-melanoma. It begins as a papule and enlarges into a crater.

FIGURE 10: Basal cell carcinoma

Basal cell carcinoma is the most common type of skin cancer and often presents on the face and head.

FIGURE 11: Basal cell carcinoma
Basal cell carcinoma may crust and bleed. Metastasis is rare.

CHAPTER 24

Bone sarcomas

Alan W. Yasko, MD, Warren Chow, MD, and Deborah Frassica, MD

Bone sarcomas are extremely rare neoplasms, which precludes determination of their true incidence. Approximately 2,400 new cases are identified annually in the United States. Population-based tumor registries seldom separate bone sarcomas into various histologic types.

Osteosarcoma is the most common malignant primary bone tumor (excluding multiple myeloma), comprising 30% of all such malignancies. The annual incidence of osteosarcoma is approximately 800 cases per year in the United States. Chondrosarcoma is the second most common malignant primary tumor of bone; its annual incidence is approximately half that of osteosarcoma. Ewing's sarcoma represents approximately 6% of all primary malignant bone tumors, with an annual incidence of 200 cases. Malignant fibrous histiocytoma (MFH) comprises < 1% of primary bone sarcomas.

Epidemiology

Gender The incidence of primary bone sarcomas is higher in males than in females regardless of histologic type. A low-grade variant of osteosarcoma (parosteal osteosarcoma) is observed more frequently in females.

Age Osteosarcoma and Ewing's sarcoma develop primarily in children and adolescents. A biphasic pattern of incidence of osteosarcoma has been observed; peaks in adolescents (rapid growth of long bones) and in the elderly (secondary tumors arising in association with Paget's disease or within previously irradiated tissue). Chondrosarcomas are rarely seen in skeletally immature patients. They usually develop in middle-aged and older adults. MFH is observed in adults.

Race No predilection has been noted in any particular race. However, Ewing's sarcoma is extremely rare in American and African blacks.

Disease site Any bone and any site within a given bone may be affected. Most osteosarcomas occur in the metaphyseal region of skeletally immature long bones (ie, distal femur, proximal tibia, and proximal humerus), which have the greatest growth potential. Ewing's sarcoma is classically described as a diaphyseal lesion but may arise in any region within an involved long bone. It commonly arises in the flat bones of the pelvis and scapula. Primary bone tumors of any histologic type are extremely rare in the spine and sacrum.

Survival Low-grade sarcomas are associated with the most favorable survival, which approaches 90% in patients with adequately treated tumors. With regard to high-grade sarcomas, survival has improved dramatically in patients with osteosarcoma or Ewing's sarcoma due to the advent of effective multiagent chemotherapy regimens. Survival has improved with multimodality therapy from historic rates of < 20% to current rates of 50% to 75%.

Etiology and risk factors

For the majority of bone sarcomas, no specific etiology has been established. A few predisposing factors have been identified.

Genetic factors Children with familial retinoblastoma have a 13q chromosome deletion and an increased incidence of osteosarcoma. Li-Fraumeni syndrome is also associated with an increased risk of bone sarcomas, as well as other cancers such as breast, leukemia, soft-tissue sarcoma, brain, and adrenal cortical tumors. Li-Fraumeni syndrome results from a genetic loss of p53.

Radiation therapy Bone sarcomas constitute a rare but devastating consequence of therapeutic irradiation. Radiation-associated sarcomas develop within the radiation field, usually after a latent period of at least 3 years. The majority of these tumors are osteosarcomas. MFH and other histologies also can arise within a radiation field.

Chemotherapy Alkylating agents and anthracyclines administered for unrelated cancers have been implicated as etiologic factors in the development of second malignant neoplasms, particularly osteosarcoma.

Preexisting benign tumors/conditions Osteosarcomas can arise in association with Paget's disease and rarely in association with benign bone tumors (ie, fibrous dysplasia). Chondrosarcomas can develop in the cartilaginous component of osteochondromas (solitary and multiple hereditary exostosis) and in patients with enchondromatosis (Ollier's disease and Maffucci's syndrome). MFH can arise in association with bone infarcts.

Trauma A traumatic event often prompts medical intervention, at which time the bone sarcoma is detected. The short temporal relationship between the traumatic event and the diagnosis of the tumor usually rules out a causal relationship.

Orthopedic implants Case reports of bone sarcomas arising in the region in which a metallic prosthetic device has been implanted have been published. The rarity of these clinical situations relative to the vast number of devices implanted makes a causal relationship unlikely.

Signs and symptoms

Local symptoms Localized pain and swelling are the hallmark clinical features of bone sarcomas. The pain, which initially is insidious and transient, becomes progressively more severe and unremitting. Localized soft-tissue swelling, with or without associated warmth and erythema, may be present. A joint effusion may be observed, and range of motion of the adjacent joint may be limited and painful. Movement or weight-bearing of the involved extremity may exacerbate local symptoms.

Patients with tumors arising in the lower extremities can present with a painful limp. The neurovascular examination of the affected extremity is usually normal. Regional lymph nodes are rarely involved.

Pathologic fracture may also be a presenting sign, although a history of pain prior to fracture usually can be elicited.

Constitutional symptoms are rare in patients with bone sarcoma, but such symptoms as fever, malaise, and weight loss can be observed in those with Ewing's sarcoma.

Screening and diagnosis

Currently, there is no screening test for primary bone sarcomas. The diagnosis must be made by clinical and radiographic evaluations and confirmed by histopathologic analysis of biopsy-obtained tissue.

Physical examination should include an assessment of the local extent of the soft-tissue mass, if present, and its relationship to the adjacent joint.

Laboratory studies A CBC may demonstrate anemia and/or leukocytosis associated with Ewing's sarcoma, but, in general, results of these studies fall within the normal range. Alkaline phosphatase and lactic dehydrogenase (LDH) levels may be elevated in patients with osteosarcoma or Ewing's sarcoma. An abnormal glucose tolerance test may be observed in patients with chondrosarcomas.

X-rays Biplanar (AP and lateral) plain radiographs of the affected extremity provide critical information on the nature of the bone lesion. The specific site of involvement within the bone, pattern and extent of bone destruction, type of periosteal changes, presence of matrix mineralization within the tumor, and presence of soft-tissue extension may be gleaned from plain films.

CT Standard CT scans provide further delineation of many of these changes.

MRI is the imaging study of choice for the evaluation of the extent of an associated soft-tissue mass and the relationship of the tumor to the neurovascular structures, surrounding soft tissues, and the adjacent joint. The intramedullary extent of the tumor and presence of skip metastases within the bone are best demonstrated by MRI.

Bone scan A bone scan is performed to screen for distant osseous metastases.

Chest radiographic studies A plain film of the chest is required in any patient suspected of having a bone sarcoma. Once the diagnosis of malignancy has been established, a CT scan of the chest is a critical part of initial staging.

Biopsy With few exceptions, a biopsy must be obtained to confirm the diagnosis. Tissue may be obtained by percutaneous (closed) or surgical (open) techniques. The biopsy should be performed by personnel expert in percutaneous biopsy techniques who are familiar with bone tumors and their treatment.

Stage	Grade	Site
IA	Low	Intracompartmental
IB	Low	Extracompartmental
IIA	High	Intracompartmental
IIB	High	Extracompartmental
III	Any regional or distant metastasis	Any

Enneking WF, Spanier SS, Goodman MA: A system for the surgical staging of musculoskeletal sarcoma. Clin Orthop 153:106–120, 1980.

Biopsies performed at referring institutions have been reported to be associated with a higher incidence of misdiagnosis and complications, which may affect patient outcome. Optimally, the biopsy should be performed at the institution where definitive treatment will be given.

Pathology

Histologic subtypes Current histopathologic classification of bone neoplasms is based on the putative cell of origin. Malignant tumors may arise from any cellular constituent present in bone, including osteogenic (osteosarcoma), chondrogenic (chondrosarcoma), hematopoietic (multiple myeloma, lymphoma), vascular (angiosarcoma, hemangioendothelioma, leiomyosarcoma), lipogenic (liposarcoma), neurogenic (neurofibrosarcoma, chordoma), and histiocytic and fibrohistiocytic (MFH, Ewing's sarcoma) elements. Histologic subtyping is based on the predominant cellular pattern present within the tumor, degree of anaplasia, and relationship of the tumor to the bone (intramedullary vs surface).

A monoclonal antibody (CD99) that recognizes a cell-surface glycoprotein (p30/32MIC2) in human Ewing's sarcoma and primitive neuroectodermal tumor (PNET) has been developed. There is strong immunoreactivity of CD99 in Ewing's sarcoma and PNET that aids in distinguishing these tumors from other small round-cell tumors of childhood and adolescence. Additional experience with CD99, however, demonstrates that it is not exclusively specific for Ewing's sarcoma and PNET.

Dedifferentiation Primary bone sarcomas can exhibit the phenomenon of "dedifferentiation." These neoplasms demonstrate a dimorphic histologic pattern, which is characterized by the presence of a borderline malignant or low-grade malignant tumor juxtaposed against a high-grade, histologically different sarcoma. Enchondromas, low-grade chondrosarcomas, low-grade variants of osteosarcoma (surface and intramedullary), and chordomas may all develop an area of high-grade spindle-cell tumor, usually MFH.

Metastatic spread Approximately 10% to 20% of patients with osteosarcoma and 15% to 35% of patients with Ewing's sarcoma have evidence of metastatic disease at initial presentation. In approximately 90% of patients with bone sarcomas, the initial site of distant metastasis is the lungs. Distant osseous sites, bone marrow, and viscera may also be involved as a manifestation of advanced disease, but involvement of these sites is less common and usually occurs after the development of pulmonary metastases. Regional lymph node involvement is rare.

Staging and prognosis

Staging system The staging system of the Musculoskeletal Tumor Society (MTS) is currently used (Table 1). This system is based on tumor grade (I = low or II = high), tumor extent (A = intraosseous involvement only or B = extraosseous extension), and presence of distant metastases, regardless of the extent of local disease (III). Patients with a localized tumor may have stage IA, IB, IIA, or IIB disease.

Prognostic factors Many studies have demonstrated that tumor response to preoperative chemotherapy, as determined by histologic analysis of the resected specimen, is the most powerful predictor of survival for patients with osteosarcoma. Adverse prognostic indicators, such as an axial primary tumor or elevated LDH and alkaline phosphatase levels, signal an even worse outcome.

Tumor size (low volume) and anatomic site (peripheral), absence of metastases at initial presentation, and good histologic response to chemotherapy are prognostic variables associated with better outcome in patients with osteosarcomas and Ewing's sarcoma. The translocation t(11;22), which results in the type 1 EWS-FLI1 fusion, is also a significant positive predictor of overall survival in Ewing's sarcoma.

For low-grade malignant tumors, adequacy of surgery is the most significant predictor of outcome.

Treatment

PRIMARY TREATMENT OF BONE SARCOMAS

Surgical excision is the mainstay of treatment for patients with low-grade sarcomas. For high-grade tumors, multimodality therapy is indicated. For most high-grade bone sarcomas, excluding chondrosarcoma, preoperative multiagent chemotherapy (3 to 4 cycles) is followed by surgical extirpation of the primary tumor. Chemotherapy is reinitiated postoperatively after wound healing has occurred (usually 2–3 weeks after surgery).

For patients with Ewing's sarcoma, the optimal therapy for local tumor control is less well defined. Historically, radiotherapy has been a mainstay of local treatment. However, there has been a recent trend toward surgery, with or without radiotherapy, to achieve local tumor control. No prospective, randomized studies have been performed to define the relative role of each of these treatment modalities, but several retrospective studies suggest improvements in local tumor control and patient survival when surgery is satisfactorily performed. Patients with unresectable tumors or microscopic or macroscopic residual disease following tumor excision clearly require adjuvant radiotherapy to consolidate their local treatment.

Surgical treatment strategy

The MTS recognizes wide excision, either by amputation or a limb-salvage procedure, as the recommended surgical approach for high-grade sarcomas. A wide excision removes the primary tumor en bloc along with its reactive zone and a cuff of normal tissue in all planes. Conceptually, this strategy is applicable to all high-grade sarcomas. Wide excision successfully controls local disease in ≥ 90% of patients.

The timing of surgery must be coordinated with the patient's chemotherapy schedule and with bone marrow recovery to minimize the period of systemic therapy. Generally, surgical intervention is postponed until the patient's absolute neutrophil count (ANC) has recovered to a level of ≥ 1,500/μL and platelet count, to a level of ≥ 70,000/μL.

Limb-salvage procedures

Wide tumor excision with limb preservation has supplanted amputation as the principal surgical method for eradicating local disease in patients with primary sarcomas of bone, regardless of histology or grade. Local tumor control and patient survival have not been compromised by this more conservative operative strategy. Refinements in surgical techniques and advances in bioengineering have increased the number of patients eligible for limb-salvage surgery. Currently, 75% to 80% of patients may be treated with conservative surgery.

Successful limb-salvage surgery for the patient with a high-grade bone sarcoma is predicated on complete extirpation of the tumor, effective skeletal reconstruction, and adequate soft-tissue coverage. Planning for the operative procedure must begin far in advance to permit adequate time to procure the implant for reconstruction.

Types of resection Limb-sparing tumor resection falls into one of three types based on the anatomic site and extent of involved bone to be excised. Resection can involve (1) tumor-bearing bone and the adjacent joint (osteoarticular), (2) tumor-bearing bone only (intercalary), or (3) whole bone and adjacent joints (whole bone).

Since most bone sarcomas arise in the metaphysis of the long bone near the joint, the majority of procedures performed for these tumors involve resection of both the segment of tumor-bearing bone and the adjacent joint (osteoarticular resection). Most of these resections are performed through the adjacent joint (intra-articular). When the tumor extends along the joint capsule or ligamentous structures and/or invades the joint, the entire joint should be resected (extra-articular) to avoid violating areas that have tumor involvement.

Reconstruction Prosthetic arthroplasty is the most common method by which the skeletal defect and adjacent joint are reconstructed. Osteoarticular allografts, intercalary allografts, and vascularized and nonvascularized autografts are also used, depending on the extent of resection and requirements for successful reconstruction.

Tumors in the immature skeleton

Tumors arising in the immature skeleton pose a unique problem for the orthopedic oncologist, particularly in patients with substantial projected growth of the involved extremity. The surgical management of bone sarcomas in young patients, with few exceptions, has entailed amputation or rotationplasty.

Custom-manufactured expandable metallic joint prostheses can be implanted to allow for skeletal growth in those children deemed candidates for limb-salvage surgery. The long-term outcome of this technique has been promising. However, multiple operative procedures should be anticipated to maintain a functional extremity.

Soft-tissue coverage

Adequate soft-tissue coverage is critical to the success of any limb-salvage procedure. Local transposition muscle flaps and free tissue transfers are extremely useful for providing a healthy, well-vascularized soft-tissue envelope to cover the reconstruction and reduce the risk of deep infection.

SURGICAL TREATMENT OF METASTATIC DISEASE

The most common site of metastatic involvement for bone sarcoma is the lungs. Patients who present with pulmonary metastases (10%–20% of patients with osteosarcoma) have a poor prognosis (5-year survival rate < 15%). Approximately 30% to 40% of patients who present with localized disease and who subsequently develop resectable pulmonary metastases can undergo salvage treatment with reinduction chemotherapy and metastasectomy (see section on "Treatment of advanced osteosarcoma"). Patients with extrapulmonary metastases or unresectable pulmonary metastases have a uniformly poor prognosis. The objective of any surgical intervention in these patients, therefore, would be palliative.

Long-term follow-up is necessary for patients treated for osteosarcoma. Late side effects of neoadjuvant chemotherapy for osteosarcoma were assessed in a retrospective review performed by investigators at the Rizzoli Institute in Italy. Of the 755 patients with localized osteosarcoma treated with 6 subsequent protocols, the following side effects were noted: symptomatic cardiomyopathy (1.7%), second malignant neoplasms (2.1% after a median of 7 years), permanent azoospermia (100% in men who received 60–75 g/m^2 of ifosfamide), subclinical renal impairment (48% in those who received > 60 g/m^2 of ifosfamide), and hearing impairment (40% of those who received cisplatin; *Bacci G, Ferrari C, Longhi A, et al: J Clin Oncol 28:774-780, 2006*).

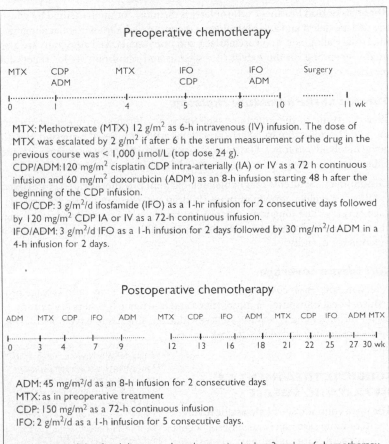

Preoperative chemotherapy

MTX	CDP ADM	MTX	IFO CDP	IFO ADM	Surgery
0	1	4	5	8 10	11 wk

MTX: Methotrexate (MTX) 12 g/m² as 6-h intravenous (IV) infusion. The dose of MTX was escalated by 2 g/m² if after 6 h the serum measurement of the drug in the previous course was < 1,000 μmol/L (top dose 24 g).
CDP/ADM: 120 mg/m² cisplatin CDP intra-arterially (IA) or IV as a 72 h continuous infusion and 60 mg/m² doxorubicin (ADM) as an 8-h infusion starting 48 h after the beginning of the CDP infusion.
IFO/CDP: 3 g/m²/d ifosfamide (IFO) as a 1-hr infusion for 2 consecutive days followed by 120 mg/m² CDP IA or IV as a 72-h continuous infusion.
IFO/ADM: 3 g/m²/d IFO as a 1-h infusion for 2 days followed by 30 mg/m²/d ADM in a 4-h infusion for 2 days.

Postoperative chemotherapy

ADM	MTX	CDP	IFO	ADM	MTX	CDP	IFO	ADM	MTX	CDP	IFO	ADM MTX
0	3	4	7	9	12	13	16	18	21	22	25	27 30 wk

ADM: 45 mg/m²/d as an 8-h infusion for 2 consecutive days
MTX: as in preoperative treatment
CDP: 150 mg/m² as a 72-h continuous infusion
IFO: 2 g/m²/d as a 1-h infusion for 5 consecutive days.

In patients with localized disease and total necrosis, the last 3 cycles of chemotherapy were omitted.

FIGURE 1: The IOR/OS-4 protocol for neoadjuvant/adjuvant chemotherapy for osteosarcoma of the extremities, from the Rizzoli Institute, Bologna, Italy.

Bacci G, Briccoli A, Ferrari S, et al: Eur J Cancer 37:2030-2039, 2001.

CHEMOTHERAPY FOR OSTEOSARCOMA

The probability of 5-year disease-free survival for patients with osteosarcoma of the extremities treated with either amputation or limb-salvage surgery alone is < 20%. Although the incidence of local recurrence is low, microscopic dissemination is likely to be present in 80% of patients at the time of diagnosis, leading to distant metastases, mostly in the lungs and bones, within the first 6 to 12 months. The incorporation of chemotherapy as part of the standard therapeutic plan for osteosarcoma (Figure 1) has improved both relapse-free and overall survival.

Neoadjuvant/adjuvant chemotherapy

To achieve better systemic control and decrease the degree of functional defect following surgery, neoadjuvant (presurgical) treatment programs have been developed by several centers. Early trials incorporated high doses of methotrexate, given weekly for 4 weeks with leucovorin rescue, prior to surgery. Subsequent modifications included the incorporation of bleomycin, dactinomycin (Cosmegen), and cyclophosphamide into the regimen, with the further addition of doxorubicin.

The next generation of trials adjusted the adjuvant (postoperative) chemotherapeutic regimen, depending on the degree of tumor necrosis found at the time of surgery. Patients who had a good tumor response (> 90% necrosis) were treated with additional cycles of the neoadjuvant regimen; those who had a poor response received cisplatin and doxorubicin. It remains controversial whether altering the adjuvant chemotherapeutic regimen for patients with poor histologic response truly changes their event-free survival.

The addition of ifosfamide did not improve survival in pediatric patients with osteosarcoma in one study. A Children's Oncology Group (COG) study reported no difference in outcome between a three-drug combination of cisplatin, doxorubicin, and high-dose methotrexate and a four-drug regimen of the same drugs plus ifosfamide. The European Osteosarcoma Intergroup (EOI) reported no difference in histopathologic response to preoperative chemotherapy and overall survival in patients randomized to receive a two-drug regimen with doxorubicin and cisplatin or a complex multidrug protocol containing doxorubicin, cisplatin, and high-dose methotrexate among other agents.

The EOI also investigated standard-dose versus increased-dose intensity (dose-dense) cisplatin and doxorubicin for patients with operable osteosarcoma of the extremity. The overall dose intensity was increased by 24% for cisplatin and 25% for doxorubicin. Good histologic response (≤ 10% viable tumor) was significantly higher in the intensified arm (51% vs 36%). Unfortunately, overall survival at 4 years was not significantly different (61% for standard and 64% for intensified).

The actuarial 5-year event-free survival rate in patients presenting with localized, primarily extremity osteosarcoma is > 70%. Regardless of the multidrug therapy used, event-free survival correlates with histologic response. Patients with > 90% tumor necrosis have a > 80% probability of 5-year event-free survival. Complete responses are more likely to occur in patients with the nonchondroblastic subtype and in those whose peak serum methotrexate levels are > 700 μmol/L. Chemosensitivity also seems to be diminished in patients with metastatic disease at presentation.

A joint protocol of four of the world's leading multi-institutional osteosarcoma groups (COG, EOI, Cooperative Osteosarcoma Study Group [COSG], and Scandinavian Sarcoma Group) is currently accruing patients with localized osteosarcoma (European and American Osteosarcoma Study Group [EURAMOS]. All patients will receive induction chemotherapy with two cycles of cisplatin and doxorubicin along with four cycles of high-dose methotrexate (MAP). Patients will then proceed to surgical resection. Postoperative therapy will be determined by histologic response. Good responders will be randomized to continue with MAP or receive MAP with pegylated interferon alfa-2b as maintenance therapy after MAP. Poor responders will be randomized to continue with MAP or receive the same regimen with the addition of ifosfamide and etoposide.

TREATMENT OF ADVANCED OSTEOSARCOMA

Axial primary tumor For the 10% to 15% of patients who present with axial primary osteosarcoma, neoadjuvant chemotherapy should be considered to reduce the tumor burden prior to surgery or radiation therapy. The COSG reported that 11.4% of its patients treated before 1999 had proven metastases at diagnosis. Actuarial survival at 5 and 10 years was 29% and 24%, respectively, when treated with preoperative and postoperative multiagent chemotherapy as well as aggressive surgery for all resectable lesions. Multivariate Cox regression analysis demonstrated that multiple metastases at diagnosis and macroscopically incomplete surgical resection are significantly associated with inferior outcomes in patients with primary metastatic osteosarcoma.

Pulmonary metastasis Patients with metastatic disease to the lungs should be evaluated for resection. Following aggressive pulmonary metastasectomy, < 25% of patients will achieve prolonged relapse-free survival. Hence, these patients may also benefit from aggressive "secondary" adjuvant chemotherapy.

Chemotherapy should also be considered for patients whose pulmonary metastases are unresectable, with the intention of performing surgery in those who have a sufficient response; approximately 10% of such patients may become long-term survivors.

Poor-risk patients or patients with recurrent disease are candidates for clinical trials that evaluate newer therapeutic agents. The POG demonstrated stabilization of disease in patients with recurrent or refractory osteosarcoma employing the combination of cyclophosphamide and topotecan (Hycamtin), although objective responses were rare. The University of Michigan reported that the combination of gemcitabine (Gemzar) and docetaxel (Taxotere) is moderately active in recurrent osteosarcoma, Ewing's sarcoma, and other soft-tissue sarcomas.

The prognosis for patients who develop metachronous skeletal osteosarcoma has been considered grave compared with that for patients with relapse limited to the lungs. Investigators at Memorial Sloan-Kettering Cancer Center reported that in a small subset of patients who developed metachronous osteosarcoma at 24 months or more from the initial diagnosis (11 of 23 patients with osteosarcoma), combined-modality therapy with surgery and aggressive chemotherapy resulted in a 5-year postmetachronous survival rate of 83%, versus 40% for patients receiving monotherapy (usually surgery) only. These results refute an earlier pessimistic sentiment.

RADIOTHERAPY FOR OSTEOSARCOMA

Although the routine use of adjuvant radiotherapy for osteosarcoma is unnecessary, certain patients may benefit from treatment. Patients with positive margins and poor response to chemotherapy are particularly at risk for local recurrence. Primary lesions in the axial skeleton are more likely to be difficult to resect with wide margins. DeLaney et al have reported a local control rate of 78% in patients with subtotal resections followed by radiotherapy. Doses in the range of 60 Gy or more are recommended. Patients who have unresectable disease should be considered for high-dose radiotherapy following chemotherapy. Local tumor control may be achieved in 40% to 55% of patients. Sophisticated planning with intensity-modulated radiotherapy and/or proton therapy may be required for lesions located adjacent to radiosensitive structures such as the spinal cord.

Investigators at the Mayo Clinic reported significant palliation of pain in patients with osteosarcoma and symptomatic bone metastases who were treated with high doses of Samarium SM 153 ethylene diamine tetramethylene phosphonate ([153]SM EDTMP), a bone-seeking radiopharmaceutical, in conjunction with stem-cell rescue. Escalating doses up to 30mCi/kg were studied. Nonhematologic side effects were minimal. [153]SM at a dose of 1 mCi/kg has been used for palliation of bone pain from skeletal metastases without the need for stem-cell support. Investigators at the Johns Hopkins Hospital have also been studying the utility of samarium in combination with external-beam radiotherapy in the management of those with high-risk osteosarcoma, including patients with lung metastases and multifocal bone lesions.

CHEMOTHERAPY FOR EWING'S SARCOMA

Prior to the availability of effective chemotherapeutic agents, < 10% of patients with Ewing's sarcoma survived beyond 5 years. The first intergroup Ewing's sarcoma study demonstrated an improved survival rate for patients receiving systemic therapy with the VACA regimen (vincristine, Actinomycin D [dactinomycin], cyclophosphamide, Adriamycin [doxorubicin]), for those receiving the first three drugs only, and for patients receiving VAC plus bilateral pulmonary irradiation. In the future, selection of a specific therapeutic regimen may be influenced by the presence of molecular markers in addition to standard clinical criteria.

In the second intergroup study, the addition of doxorubicin to VAC, when given on an intermittent schedule and at a higher dose, improved the 5-year relapse-free survival rate to 73%; this rate was almost double that of the cohort of patients not receiving doxorubicin as part of their treatment. The worst results were observed in patients with pelvic, proximal extremity, and lumbar vertebral lesions.

In a phase III study, the addition of ifosfamide and etoposide to standard chemotherapy (doxorubicin, vincristine, cyclophosphamide, and dactinomycin) for patients with Ewing's sarcoma and PNET of the bone significantly improved overall survival for patients with localized disease (72% vs 61%), but it did not affect the outcome for patients with metastatic disease (overall survival 34% vs

35%). In addition to biologic adverse features at presentation (male sex, age, high LDH levels, anemia, fever, axial locations, non-type 1 fusion transcripts, and lack of feasibility of surgical resection), independent prognostic factors also include the type of chemotherapy and degree of tumor necrosis.

CHEMOTHERAPY FOR ADVANCED EWING'S SARCOMA

Aggressive combination chemotherapy and irradiation can lead to prolonged progression-free survival, even in patients with metastatic disease. The combination of ifosfamide (1.6 g/m^2) and etoposide (100 mg/m^2 given on days 1–5) results in high response rates of > 80%. Unfortunately, late recurrences are not uncommon.

Dose intensification of active chemotherapeutic compounds, including those employing autologous stem-cell rescue, has not been definitively shown to significantly improve survival of patients with poor-risk and metastatic Ewing's sarcoma and PNET. However, dose-dense chemotherapy is postulated to improve outcome in localized Ewing's sarcoma and is the focus of a randomized phase III trial by COG. The arms studied were standard chemotherapy with growth factor support given every 3 weeks versus every 2 weeks. Newer therapeutic agents should be tested.

In patients with recurrent or refractory Ewing's sarcoma, the combination of cyclophosphamide and topotecan was shown to possess significant antitumor activity by POG.

RADIOTHERAPY FOR EWING'S SARCOMA

Local control Definitive radiotherapy is recommended for patients with unresectable primary tumors or when the morbidity from resection is judged to be excessive. Patients treated with radiotherapy alone tend to have larger, less favorable tumors. In modern series of patients treated without surgery, local failure rates are on the order of 20%, compared with 4% to 10% with surgery or surgery plus radiotherapy. Patients treated definitively with chemotherapy and radiation therapy alone generally receive 45 Gy to the initial prechemotherapy volume plus a 2 cm margin, followed by a 10.8-Gy boost to a smaller volume, including the site of the original lesion plus any residual soft-tissue disease after chemotherapy.

When microscopic or gross positive margins remain following resection, postoperative radiotherapy is indicated. A dose of 45 Gy is recommended for microscopic positive margins. Lower doses appeared to be associated with higher recurrence rates, based on data from two Cooperative Ewing's Sarcoma Study trials. If gross disease is left, total doses similar to those used for definitive radiotherapy are utilized.

Metastatic disease Patients with lung metastases at presentation should be considered for "consolidative" low-dose whole-lung irradiation following chemotherapy. Doses in the range of 15 to 18 Gy are typically utilized in 1.5-Gy fractions. Radiotherapy may also be used to treat isolated bone metastases following chemotherapy. Patients with painful bone metastases can benefit from palliative radiotherapy for pain control, with up to 55% achieving complete pain relief and an additional 30% achieving partial relief.

SUGGESTED READING

Bölling T, Schuck A, Paulussen M, et al: Whole lung irradiation in patients with exclusively pulmonary metastases of Ewing tumors. Toxicity analysis and treatment results of the EICESS-92 trial. Strahlenther Onkol 184:193–197, 2008.

Chow WA: Update on chondrosarcomas. Curr Opin Oncol 19:371–376, 2007.

DeLaney TF, Spiro IJ, Suit HD, et al: Neoadjuvant chemotherapy and radiotherapy for large extremity soft-tissue sarcomas. Int J Radiat Oncol Biol Phys 56:1117–1127, 2003.

Ferrari S, Smeland S, Mercuri M, et al: Neoadjuvant chemotherapy with high-dose ifosfamide, high-dose methotrexate, cisplatin, and doxorubicin for patients with localized osteosarcoma of the extremity: A joint study by the Italian and Scandinavian Sarcoma Groups. J Clin Oncol 23:8845–8852, 2005.

Frink SJ, Rutledge J, Lewis VO, et al: Favorable long-term results of prosthetic arthroplasty of the knee for distal femur neoplasms. Clin Orthop Relat Res 438:65–70, 2005.

Grier HE, Krailo MD, Tarbell NJ, et al: Addition of ifosfamide and etoposide to standard chemotherapy in Ewing's sarcoma/primitive neuroectodermal tumor of bone. N Engl J Med 384:694–701, 2003.

Grimer RJ, Carter SR, Tillman RM, et al: Chondrosarcoma of bone: An assessment of outcome. J Bone Joint Surg Am 82:1203–1204, 2000.

Indelicato DJ, Keole SR, Shahlaee AH, et al: Long-term clinical and functional outcomes after treatment for localized Ewing's tumor of the lower extremity. Int J Radiat Oncol Biol Phys 70:501–509, 2008.

Jeys LM, Kulkarni A, Grimer RJ, et al: Endoprosthetic reconstruction for the treatment of musculoskeletal tumors of the appendicular skeleton and pelvis. J Bone Joint Surg Am 90:1265–1271, 2008.

Kager L, Zoubek A, Pötschger U, et al: Primary metastatic osteosarcoma: Presentation and outcome of patients treated on neoadjuvant Cooperative Osteosarcoma Study Group protocols. J Clin Oncol 21:2011–2018, 2003.

Koontz BF, Clough RW, Halperin EC: Palliative radiation therapy for metastatic Ewing sarcoma. Cancer 106:1790–1793, 2006.

La TH, Meyers PA, Wexler LH, et al: Radiation therapy for Ewing's sarcoma: Results from Memorial Sloan-Kettering in the modern era. Int J Radiat Oncol Biol Phys 64:544–550, 2006.

Ladanyi M: EWS-FLI1 and Ewing's sarcoma: Recent molecular data and new insights. Cancer Biol Ther 1:330–336, 2002.

Lewis IJ, Nooij MA, Whelan J, et al: Improvement in histologic response but not survival in osteosarcoma patients treated with intensified chemotherapy: A randomized phase III trial of the European Osteosarcoma Intergroup. J Natl Cancer Inst 99:112–128, 2007.

Longhi A, Ferrari S, Bacci G, et al: Long-term follow-up of patients with doxorubicin-induced cardiac toxicity after chemotherapy for osteosarcoma. Anticancer Drugs 18:737–744, 2007.

Machak GN, Tkachev SI, Solovyev YN, et al: Neoadjuvant chemotherapy and local radiotherapy for high-grade osteosarcoma of the extremities. Mayo Clin Proc 78:147–155, 2003.

Meyers PA, Schwartz CL, Krailo M, et al: Osteosarcoma: A randomized, prospective trial of the addition of ifosfamide and/or muramyl tripeptide to cisplatin, doxorubicin, and high-dose methotrexate. J Clin Oncol 23:2004–2011, 2005.

Miser JS, Goldsby RE, Chen Z, et al: Treatment of metastatic Ewing sarcoma/primitive neuroectodermal tumor of bone: Evaluation of increasing the dose intensity of chemotherapy--a report from the Children's Oncology Group. Pediatr Blood Cancer 49:894–900, 2007.

Rodriguez-Galindo C, Navid F, Liu T, et al: Prognostic factors for local and distant control in Ewing sarcoma family of tumors. Ann Oncol 19:814–820, 2008.

Schuck A, Ahrens S, Paulussen M, et al: Local therapy in localized Ewing tumors: Results of 1058 patients treated in the CESS 81, CESS 86, and EICESS 92 trials. Int J Radiat Oncol Biol Phys 55:168–177, 2003.

Yock TI, Krailo M, Fryer CJ, et al: Local control in pelvic Ewing sarcoma: Analysis from INT-0091--a report from the Children's Oncology Group. J Clin Oncol 24:3838–3843, 2006.

CHAPTER 25

Soft-tissue sarcomas

Peter W. T. Pisters, MD, Mitchell Weiss, MD, Robert Maki, MD, PhD, and Gary N. Mann, MD

The soft-tissue sarcomas are a group of rare but anatomically and histologically diverse neoplasms. This is due to the ubiquitous location of the soft tissues and the nearly three dozen recognized histologic subtypes of soft-tissue sarcomas. In the United States, approximately 9,500 new cases of soft-tissue sarcoma are identified annually, and about 3,500 patients die of the disease each year. The age-adjusted incidence is 2 cases per 100,000 persons.

Epidemiology

Unlike the more common malignancies, such as colon cancer, little is known about the epidemiology of soft-tissue sarcomas. This, again, reflects the uncommon nature of these lesions.

Gender There is a slight male predominance, with a male-to-female ratio of 1.1:1.0.

Age The age distribution in adult soft-tissue sarcoma studies is < 40 years, 20.7% of patients; 40 to 60 years, 27.6% of patients; and > 60 years, 51.7% of patients.

Race Studies in large cohorts of patients demonstrate that the race distribution of soft-tissue sarcomas mirrors that of the American population (86% Caucasian, 10% African-American, 1% Asian-American, and 3% other).

Geography Studies have suggested that the incidence and mortality of soft-tissue sarcomas may be increasing in New Zealand. There are no currently available data addressing this possibility in the United States.

Etiology and risk factors

In the majority of cases of patients with soft-tissue sarcoma, no specific etiologic agent is identifiable. However, a number of predisposing factors have been recognized.

Radiation therapy Soft-tissue sarcomas have been reported to originate in radiation fields following therapeutic irradiation for a variety of solid tumors. Frequently, they are seen in the lower-dose regions at the edge of the radiation target volume. By definition, radiation-induced sarcomas arise no sooner than 3 years after radiation therapy and often develop decades later. The majority of these sarcomas are high-grade lesions (90%), and osteosarcoma is a predominant histology. High-grade undifferentiated pleomorphic sarcoma (HGUPS), formerly called malignant fibrous histiocytoma (MFH), angiosarcoma, and other histologic subtypes have also been reported.

Chemical exposure Exposure to various chemicals in specific occupations or situations has been linked with the development of soft-tissue sarcoma. These chemicals include the phenoxy acetic acids (forestry and agriculture workers), chlorophenols (sawmill workers), Thorotrast (diagnostic x-ray technicians), vinyl chloride (individuals working with this gas, used in making plastics and as a refrigerant), and arsenic (vineyard workers).

Chemotherapy Soft-tissue sarcomas have been reported after previous exposure to alkylating chemotherapeutic agents, most commonly after treatment of pediatric acute lymphocytic leukemia. The drugs implicated include cyclophosphamide, melphalan (Alkeran), procarbazine (Matulane), nitrosoureas, and chlorambucil (Leukeran). The relative risk of sarcoma appears to increase with cumulative drug exposure.

Chronic lymphedema Soft-tissue sarcomas have been noted to arise in the chronically lymphedematous arms of women treated with radical mastectomy for breast cancer (Stewart-Treves syndrome). Lower-extremity lymphangiosarcomas have also been observed in patients with congenital lymphedema or filariasis complicated by chronic lymphedema.

Trauma and foreign bodies Although a recent history of trauma is often elicited from patients presenting with soft-tissue sarcoma, the interval between the traumatic event and diagnosis is often short; thus, a causal relationship is unlikely. Chronic inflammatory processes, however, may be a risk factor for sarcoma. Foreign bodies, such as shrapnel, bullets, and implants, have also been implicated.

Signs and symptoms

Signs and symptoms of soft-tissue sarcoma depend, in large part, on the anatomic site of origin. Due to the ubiquitous location of the soft tissues, these malignancies may arise at any site in the body where soft tissues are located. Since 50% of soft-tissue sarcomas arise in an extremity, the majority of patients present with a palpable soft-tissue mass. Pain at presentation is noted in only one-third of cases.

Extremity and superficial trunk Extremity and superficial trunk sarcomas account for 60% of all soft-tissue sarcomas. The majority of patients present with a painless primary soft-tissue mass.

Retroperitoneum Retroperitoneal sarcomas account for 15% of all soft-tissue sarcomas. Most patients (80%) present with an abdominal mass, with 50% of patients reporting pain at presentation. Due to the considerable size of the retroperitoneum and the relative mobility of the anterior intra-abdominal organs, these tumors often grow to substantial size before the patient's nonspecific complaints are evaluated or even before an abdominal mass is noted on physical examination.

Viscera Visceral soft-tissue sarcomas, which comprise 15% of all soft-tissue sarcomas, present with signs and symptoms unique to their viscus of origin. For example, GI leiomyosarcomas or gastrointestinal stromal tumors (GISTs) present with GI symptoms that are usually indistinguishable from those of the more common adenocarcinomas. Similarly, uterine leiomyosarcomas frequently present with painless vaginal bleeding, such as that often noted in patients with more common uterine malignancies.

Head and neck Head and neck sarcomas comprise 10% of all soft-tissue sarcomas. Although generally smaller than sarcomas in other sites, they may present with important mechanical problems related to compression or invasion of adjacent anatomy (eg, orbital contents, airway, or pharynx). In addition, their proximity to critical anatomy can pose management difficulties due to compromise in the delivery of both surgery and radiotherapy.

Pathology

Histopathologic classification As a consequence of the wide spectrum of soft tissues, a variety of histologically distinct neoplasms have been characterized. The current histopathologic classification is based on the putative cell of origin of each lesion. Such classification based on histogenesis is reproducible for the more differentiated tumors. However, as the degree of histologic differentiation declines, it becomes increasingly difficult to determine cellular origin.

In addition, many of these tumors dedifferentiate. This process results in a variety of overlapping patterns, making uniform classification difficult. Experienced soft-tissue pathologists frequently disagree as to the cell of origin of an individual tumor. Comparative studies have demonstrated concordance in histopathologic diagnosis in only two-thirds of cases. MFH used to be the most common histologic subtype of soft-tissue sarcoma. However, in one study, reanalysis histologically, immunohistochemically, and ultrastructurally allowed reclassification in 84% of tumors to a specific line of differentiation. GIST is now recognized as the most common form of sarcoma.

Assignment of a specific histologic subtype is of secondary importance. This is because, with the possible exceptions of certain small-cell sarcomas, rhabdomyosarcoma, fibrosarcoma, and some forms of angiosarcoma, histogenesis is not directly related to biologic behavior. The propensity for distant metastases and disease-related mortality are best predicted on the basis of histologic grade and tumor size.

Staging and prognosis

AJCC/UICC staging system

The relative rarity of soft-tissue sarcomas, the anatomic heterogeneity of these lesions, and the presence of more than 30 recognized histologic subtypes of variable grade have made it difficult to establish a functional system that can accurately stage all forms of this disease. The revised staging system (6th edi-

TABLE 1: AJCC/UICC staging system for soft-tissue sarcomas

Primary tumor (T)

Tx		Primary tumor cannot be assessed
T0		No evidence of primary tumor
T1		Tumor ≤ 5 cm in greatest dimension
	T1a	Superficial tumor[a]
	T1b	Deep tumor[a]
T2		Tumor > 5 cm in greatest dimension
	T2a	Superficial tumor[a]
	T2b	Deep tumor[a]

Regional lymph nodes (N)

Nx	Regional lymph nodes cannot be assessed
N0	No regional lymph node metastasis
N1	Regional lymph node metastasis

Grade (G)

Gx	Grade cannot be assessed
G1	Well differentiated
G2	Moderately differentiated
G3	Poorly differentiated
G4	Poorly differentiated or undifferentiated (four-tiered systems only)

Stage grouping

Stage I	T1a-T2b	N0	M0	G1,2	G1	Low
Stage II	T1a-T2a	N0	M0	G3,4	G2,3	High
Stage III	T2b	N0	M0	G3,4	G2,3	High
Stage IV	Any T	N1	M0	Any G	Any G	High or low
	Any T	N0	M1	Any G	Any G	High or low

[a] Superficial tumor is located exclusively above the superficial fascia without invasion of the fascia; deep tumor is located either exclusively beneath the superficial fascia or superficial to the fascia with invasion of or through the fascia. Retroperitoneal, mediastinal, and pelvic sarcomas are classified as deep tumors.

AJCC = American Joint Committee on Cancer; UICC = International Union Against Cancer

From Greene FL, Page DL, Fleming ID, et al (eds): AJCC Cancer Staging Manual, 6th ed. New York, Springer-Verlag, 2002.

tion) of the American Joint Committee on Cancer (AJCC) and the International Union Against Cancer (UICC) is the most widely employed staging classification for soft-tissue sarcomas (Table 1). All soft-tissue sarcoma subtypes are included, except dermatofibrosarcoma protuberans. Four distinct histologic grades are recognized, ranging from well differentiated to undifferentiated.

Histologic grade and tumor size are the primary determinants of clinical stage. Tumor size is further substaged as "a" (a superficial tumor that arises outside the investing fascia) or "b" (a deep tumor that arises beneath the fascia or invades the fascia).

The AJCC/UICC system is designed to optimally stage extremity tumors but is also applicable to torso, head and neck, and retroperitoneal lesions. It should not be used for sarcomas of the GI tract.

A major limitation of the current staging system is that it does not take into account the anatomic site of soft-tissue sarcomas. Anatomic site, however, is an important determinant of outcome. Patients with retroperitoneal, head and neck, and visceral sarcomas have a worse overall prognosis than do patients with extremity tumors. Although the anatomic site is not incorporated as a specific component of any current staging system, outcome data should be reported on a site-specific basis.

At Memorial Sloan-Kettering Cancer Center, a retrospective review of 369 patients with high-grade soft-tissue sarcoma of the extremity treated with postoperative radiation therapy was conducted to evaluate the influence of tumor site on local control and complications. The tumor site was upper extremity in 103 of patients (28%) and lower extremity in 266 patients (72%). With a median follow-up of 50 months, the 5-year actuarial rate of local control, distant relapse-free, and overall survival for the entire population was 82%, 61%, and 71%, respectively. The 5-year local control rates in patients with upper extremity lesions vs lower extremity lesions was 70% and 86%, respectively ($P = .0004$). On multivariate analysis, upper extremity site ($P = .001$) and positive resection margin ($P = .02$) were significant predictors of poor local control.

Prognostic factors

Understanding relevant clinicopathologic prognostic factors is important in treatment planning for patients with soft-tissue sarcoma. Several reports document the adverse prognostic significance of tumor grade, anatomic site, tumor size, and depth relative to the investing fascia (for extremity and body wall tumors). Patients with high-grade lesions, large (T2) sarcomas, a nonextremity subsite, or deep tumor location are at increased risk for disease relapse and sarcoma-specific death.

Sarcoma-specific nomogram Kattan and colleagues from Memorial Sloan-Kettering Cancer Center have developed a sarcoma-specific nomogram for estimation of sarcoma-specific 12-year survival. The nomogram takes into account pretreatment clinicopathologic factors, including anatomic site, histologic subtype, tumor size, histologic grade, tumor depth, and patient age. The nomogram is based on prospectively collected data and has been validated in a population of 2,136 patients with sarcoma. The nomogram can be found on www.nomograms.org and is available in a handheld personal digital assistant version. The sarcoma nomogram may be useful for patient stratification for clinical trials and for risk assessment and treatment planning for individual patients.

Prognostic factors for local vs distant recurrence Unlike other solid tumors, the adverse prognostic factors for local recurrence of a soft-tissue sarcoma differ from those that predict distant metastasis and tumor-related mortality. In other words, patients with a constellation of adverse prognostic factors for local recurrence are not necessarily at increased risk for distant metastasis or tumor-related death.

This concept has been validated by an analysis of the Scandinavian Sarcoma Group prospective database. In 559 patients with soft-tissue sarcomas of the extremities and trunk treated with surgery alone, inadequate surgical margin was found to be a risk factor for local recurrence but not for distant metastasis. Therefore, staging systems that are designed to stratify patients for risk of distant metastasis and tumor-related mortality using these prognostic factors (such as the AJCC/UICC system) do not stratify patients for risk of local recurrence.

Screening and diagnosis

Currently, there are no screening tests for soft-tissue sarcomas. Since the majority of patients with soft-tissue sarcoma have lesions arising in the extremities or superficial trunk, most of the comments here apply to soft-tissue lesions in those sites. A separate algorithm is usually employed for the evaluation of a primary retroperitoneal mass or visceral sarcoma.

Physical examination should include an assessment of the size of the mass and its mobility relative to the underlying soft tissues. The relationship of the mass to the investing fascia of the extremity (superficial vs deep) and nearby neurovascular and bony structures should be noted. Site-specific neurovascular examination and assessment of regional lymph nodes should also be performed.

Biopsy Any soft-tissue mass in an adult extremity should be biopsied if it is symptomatic or enlarging, is > 5 cm, or has persisted beyond 4 to 6 weeks.

Percutaneous approaches Percutaneous tissue diagnosis can usually be obtained with fine-needle aspiration (FNA) for cytology or by percutaneous core biopsy for histology. The needle track should be placed in an area to be excised or that can be encompassed in adjuvant radiotherapy fields if they are to be used. In most instances, when an experienced cytopathologist and/or histopathologist examines the specimen, a diagnosis of malignant soft-tissue sarcoma can be made. FNA is often viewed as a suboptimal method of establishing an initial diagnosis of soft-tissue sarcoma. Histology is usually preferred to cytology because more tissue is obtained, which allows for a more accurate delineation of tumor type and grade. Percutaneous tissue diagnosis is preferred to facilitate subsequent treatment planning and to permit surgical resection to be performed as a one-stage procedure.

Open biopsy In some cases, an adequate histologic diagnosis cannot be secured by percutaneous means. Open biopsy is indicated in these instances, with the exception of relatively small superficial masses, which can be easily removed by excisional biopsy with clear margins.

Biopsies should be incisional and performed with a longitudinal incision parallel to the long axis of the extremity. This approach facilitates subsequent wide local excision of the tumor and the incisional scar and results in minimal difficulties in wound closure. It also facilitates inclusion of any scars within the area of the tumor in adjuvant radiation fields without the excessive morbidity of large-field radiotherapy planning. The incision should be centered over the mass at its most superficial location. It is important to note that care should be taken not to raise tissue flaps. Meticulous hemostasis should be ensured after the biopsy to prevent dissemination of tumor cells into adjacent tissue planes by hematoma.

Retroperitoneal or intra-abdominal mass Biopsy of primary retroperitoneal soft-tissue masses is generally not required for radiographically resectable masses, nor is biopsy recommended for suspected GISTs. The circumstances under which percutaneous or preoperative biopsy of retroperitoneal masses should be strongly considered include:

- tissue diagnosis for radiographically unresectable disease
- clinical suspicion of lymphoma or germ-cell tumor
- tissue diagnosis for neoadjuvant treatment, including radiotherapy and/or chemotherapy
- suspected metastases from another primary tumor.

Primary tumor imaging Optimal imaging of the primary tumor depends on the anatomic site. For soft-tissue masses of the extremities, MRI has been regarded as the imaging modality of choice because it enhances the contrast between tumor and muscle and between tumor and adjacent blood vessels and also provides multiplanar definition of the lesion. However, a study by the Radiation Diagnostic Oncology Group that compared MRI and CT in 183 patients with malignant bone and 133 patients with soft-tissue tumors showed no specific advantage of MRI over CT from a diagnostic standpoint.

For pelvic lesions, the multiplanar capability of MRI may provide superior single-modality imaging. In the retroperitoneum and abdomen, CT usually provides satisfactory anatomic definition of the lesion. Occasionally, MRI with gradient sequence imaging can better delineate the relationship of the tumor to midline vascular structures, particularly the inferior vena cava and aorta. In the future, MRI-CT fusion techniques may facilitate treatment planning using conformal radiotherapy techniques.

More invasive studies, such as angiography and cavography, are almost never required for the evaluation of soft-tissue sarcomas. The role of PET scan in sarcoma management is not well defined, although it correlates well with contrast enhanced CT scans in patients with GIST.

Imaging for metastatic disease Cost-effective imaging to exclude the possibility of distant metastatic disease depends on the size, grade, and anatomic location of the primary tumor. In general, patients with low-grade soft-tissue sarcomas < 10 cm in size or intermediate-/high-grade tumors < 5 cm in diameter require only a chest x-ray for satisfactory staging of the chest. This reflects the fact that these patients are at comparatively low risk of presenting with pulmonary metastases. In contrast, patients with very large (≥ 10 cm) low-grade tumors or high-grade tumors ≥ 5 cm should undergo more thorough staging of the chest by CT.

Patients with retroperitoneal and intra-abdominal visceral sarcomas should undergo single-modality imaging of the liver to exclude the possibility of synchronous hepatic metastases. The liver is a common site for a first metastasis from these lesions.

Treatment

TREATMENT OF LOCALIZED DISEASE

Surgical resection is the cornerstone of therapy for patients with localized disease. Over the past 20 years, there has been a gradual shift in the surgical management of soft-tissue sarcoma of the extremities away from radical ablative surgery, such as amputation or compartment resection, and toward limb-sparing approaches combining wide local resection with preoperative or postoperative radiotherapy. The development of advanced surgical techniques (eg, microvascular tissue transfer, bone and joint replacement, and vascular reconstruction) and the application of multimodality approaches have allowed most patients to retain a functional extremity without any compromise in survival.

Surgery

The surgical approach to soft-tissue sarcomas depends on careful preoperative staging with MRI or CT for lesions of the extremities and a percutaneous histologic diagnosis and assessment of grade. In most instances, preoperative imaging studies allow for accurate prediction of resectability.

The surgical approach to soft-tissue sarcomas is based on an awareness that these lesions tend to expand and compress tissue planes, producing a pseudocapsule comprising normal host tissue interlaced with tumor fimbriae. Conservative surgical approaches in which the plane of dissection is immediately adjacent to this pseudocapsule, such as intracapsular or marginal excision, are associated with prohibitive local recurrence rates of 33% to 63%.

Wide local resection encompassing a rim of normal tissue around the lesion has led to improvements in local control, with local recurrence rates of approximately 30% in the absence of adjuvant therapies. However, studies indicate that carefully selected patients with localized, small (T1), low-grade soft-tissue sarcomas of the extremity can be treated by wide resection alone, with local recurrence rates of < 10%. For example, in a cohort of 56 patients with primarily subcutaneous or intramuscular lesions treated with wide local excision without adjuvant irradiation, 4 local recurrences were noted.

The need for adjuvant irradiation in small (< 5 cm), high-grade lesions has been studied. A retrospective review of 204 patients with stage IIB soft-tissue sarcoma of the extremity

A prospective trial examining local recurrence rates for T1 primary soft-tissue sarcomas of the trunk and extremities was recently completed. Patients underwent function-preserving surgery. Postoperative radiation was delivered for microscopically positive margins (R1 resection). No radiation was delivered if margins were negative (R0 resection). Eighty-eight patients were evaluated in this trial. A total of 16% had R1 resection and received adjuvant radiation therapy, while 84% had R0 resection and did not receive radiation therapy. With a median follow-up 75 months, isolated local recurrence was observed in six patients in the R1 arm (43%) and six patients in the R0 arm (8%). The 5- and 10-year local recurrence rates in the R0 arm were 7.9% and 10.6%, respectively, and the sarcoma-specific death rates were 3.2% at both 5 and 10 years in the R0 arm *(Pisters PW, Pollock RE, Lewis VO, et al: Ann Surg 246:675-682, 2007).*

treated at Memorial Sloan-Kettering Cancer Center has been completed. A total of 57% of patients did not receive adjuvant radiation therapy, whereas 43% received either brachytherapy or external-beam radiation therapy. With a median follow-up of 67 months, there was no significant difference in 5-year local control, distant relapse-free survival, or disease-specific survival when adjuvant irradiation was delivered.

Further studies will be required to define which subsets of patients with primary extremity sarcoma can be treated by wide excision surgery alone. Preoperative or postoperative radiotherapy should be employed for patients with primary T1 sarcomas in whom a satisfactory gross surgical margin cannot be attained without compromise of functionally important neurovascular structures.

Limb-sparing surgery plus irradiation Limb-sparing surgery employing adjuvant irradiation to facilitate maximal local control has become the standard approach for large (T2) soft-tissue sarcomas of the extremities. In most centers, upward of 90% of patients are treated with limb-sparing approaches. Amputation is reserved as a last-resort option for local control and is used with the knowledge that it does not affect survival. This approach was validated in a prospective National Cancer Institute (NCI) study, in which patients with a limb-sparing surgical option were randomized to receive limb-sparing surgery with postoperative radiation therapy or amputation. Both arms of the study included postoperative therapy with doxorubicin, cyclophosphamide, and methotrexate.

Surgical procedure The planned resection should encompass the skin, subcutaneous tissues, and soft tissues adjacent to the tumor, including the previous biopsy site and any associated drain sites. The tumor should be excised with a 2- to 3-cm margin of normal surrounding tissue whenever possible. Since good adjuvant approaches are available to facilitate local control, this ideal margin is sometimes compromised rather than attempting resection of adjacent, possibly involved bone or neurovascular structures that would result in significant functional loss. In the rare circumstance of gross involvement of neurovascular structures or bone, they can be resected en bloc and reconstructed.

Metal clips should be placed at the margins of resection to facilitate radiation field planning, when and if external irradiation is indicated. Drain sites should be positioned close to the wound to allow inclusion in radiation therapy fields. As noted earlier, avoidance of transverse incisions greatly facilitates the ability to include the tissues at risk in radiation target volume without unduly large fields.

Regional lymphadenectomy Given the low, 2% to 3%, prevalence of lymph node metastasis in adult sarcomas, there is no role for routine regional lymphadenectomy. Patients with angiosarcoma, embryonal rhabdomyosarcoma, synovial sarcoma, and epithelioid histologies have an increased incidence of lymph node metastasis and should be carefully examined and radiographically imaged for lymphadenopathy. Clinically apparent lymphadenopathy should be treated with therapeutic lymphadenectomy. A recent analysis suggested that select patients undergoing lymphadenectomy, particularly in the absence of systemic metastases, may have a 5-year survival rate of 57%.

Radiotherapy

Scheduling Radiation therapy is usually combined with surgical resection in the management of patients with soft-tissue sarcomas of the extremities. The decision of whether to use preoperative (neoadjuvant) or postoperative (adjuvant) irradiation remains controversial and has been addressed in a phase III randomized trial.

Preoperative irradiation has a number of theoretic and practical advantages: (1) Smaller radiation portals can be utilized, as the scar, hematomas, and ecchymoses do not need to be covered. (2) Preoperative irradiation may produce tumor encapsulation, facilitating surgical resection from vital structures. (3) It is easier to spare a strip of skin and thereby reduce the risk of lymphedema. (4) The size of the tumor may be reduced, thus decreasing the extent of surgical resection. (5) Lower radiation doses can be utilized, as there are fewer relatively radioresistant hypoxic cells.

Preoperative irradiation also has several drawbacks, however. They include (1) the inability to precisely stage patients based on pathology due to downstaging and (2) increased problems with wound healing.

Studies of preoperative irradiation from the University of Florida, M. D. Anderson Cancer Center, and Massachusetts General Hospital demonstrated local control rates of 90% using doses of approximately 50 Gy. Survival depended on the size and grade of the primary tumor. Distant metastases were the primary pattern of failure.

Postoperative irradiation A number of retrospective reports, as well as a randomized trial from the NCI, have demonstrated that limb-sparing surgery plus postoperative irradiation produces local control rates comparable to those achieved with amputation. Five-year local control rates of 70% to 90%, survival rates of 70%, and limb-preservation rates of 85% can be expected.

Equivocal or positive histologic margins are associated with higher local recurrence rates, and, therefore, adjuvant external-beam irradiation should be considered in all patients with sarcoma of the extremities with positive or close microscopic margins in whom reexcision is impractical. Postoperative doses of 60–65 Gy should be used.

Interstitial therapy with iridium-192 is used at some institutions as a radiation boost to the tumor bed following adjuvant external-beam irradiation. At Memorial Sloan-Kettering Cancer Center, adjuvant brachytherapy is often used in place of external irradiation. In a randomized trial, the 5-year local control rate was 82% in patients who received adjuvant brachytherapy, versus 69% in those treated with surgery alone. On subset analysis, the local control rate was found to be 89%, versus 66% for those patients with high-grade lesions. This study and further studies have indicated that brachytherapy has no impact on local control for low-grade lesions.

If an implant alone is used, the dose is 40–45 Gy to a volume that includes all margins; when a boost is combined with additional external-beam irradiation, a dose of 20–25 Gy is utilized. Some data suggest a higher rate of wound complications and a delay in healing when implants are afterloaded prior to the third postoperative day. Although some centers load implants sooner, this step must be performed with caution and strict attention to the incision site.

Over a 15-year period, 202 patients with high-grade sarcoma of the extremities underwent complete gross resection and adjuvant brachytherapy to a median dose of 45 Gy, delivered over 5 days. With a median follow-up of 61 months, the 5-year local control, distant relapse-free survival, and overall survival rates were 84%, 63%, and 70%, respectively. These rates compared favorably with data on external-beam irradiation. Morbidity of brachytherapy was considered acceptable, with reoperation rates of 12%, bone fractures in 3%, and nerve damage in 5%.

Comparison of irradiation techniques Comparable local control results (90%) are obtained with preoperative, postoperative, and interstitial techniques, although rates of wound complications are higher with preoperative techniques. Brachytherapy can offer a number of advantages. When brachytherapy is employed as the sole adjuvant, the entire treatment (surgery and irradiation) is completed in a 10- to 12-day period, compared with the 10 to 12 weeks required for typical external-beam irradiation (6 to 7 weeks) and surgery (4- to 6-week break before or after irradiation). Generally, smaller volumes can be irradiated with brachytherapy, which could improve functional results. However, smaller volumes may not be appropriate, depending on the tumor size, grade, and margin status.

The NCI of Canada Clinical Trials Group published 3-year median follow-up results of a randomized phase III trial comparing preoperative and postoperative radiotherapy for limb soft-tissue sarcoma (Figures 1A–1D). Wound complications were observed in 31 of 88 patients (35%) in the preoperative group and 16 of 94 patients (17%) in the postoperative group (difference, 18% [95% confidence interval: 5–30]; $P = .01$). Tumor size and anatomic site were also significant risk factors in multivariate analysis. Local control was identical in both arms of the trial. Five-year outcomes have been reported, and no difference in metastases, cause-specific survival, or overall survival was noted. Because preoperative radiotherapy is associated with a greater risk of wound complications than postoperative radiotherapy, but less late fibrosis and edema, the choice of regimen for patients with soft-tissue sarcoma should take into account the timing of surgery and radiotherapy and the size and anatomic site of the tumor.

Regardless of the technique employed, local control is a highly achievable and worthwhile endpoint, as demonstrated in a study of 911 patients treated by various techniques at Memorial Sloan-Kettering Cancer Center. Of the 116 patients who developed local recurrence, 38 patients subsequently developed metastases and 34 patients died. Metastases after local recurrence were predicted in patients with high-grade or large (> 5 cm) tumors.

Treatment recommendations Adjuvant radiotherapy should be employed for virtually all high-grade sarcomas of the extremities and larger (≥ 5 cm) low-grade lesions. If small (T1) lesions can be resected with clear margins, radio-

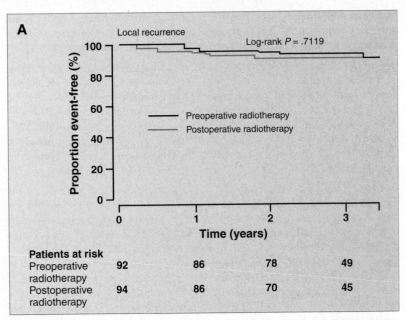

FIGURE 1A: Kaplan-Meier plots for probability of local recurrence in the National Cancer Institute of Canada Clinical Trials Group phase III trial.

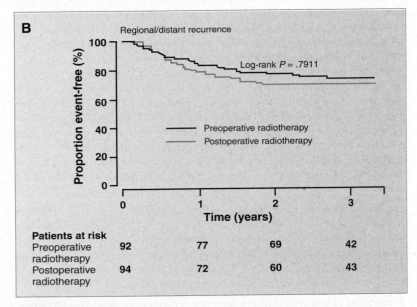

FIGURE 1B: Kaplan-Meier plots for probability of metastatic (regional and distant) recurrence in the National Cancer Institute of Canada Clinical Trials Group phase III trial.

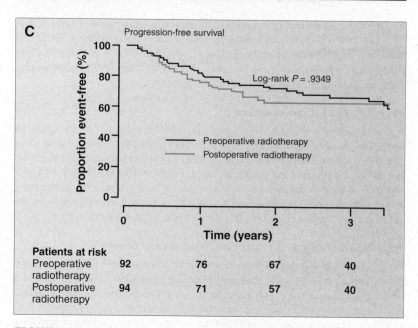

FIGURE 1C: Kaplan-Meier plots for probability of progression-free survival in the National Cancer Institute of Canada Clinical Trials Group phase III trial.

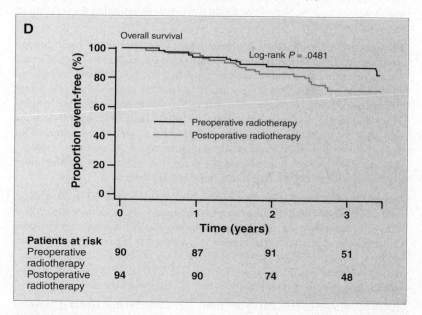

FIGURE 1D: Kaplan-Meier plots for probability of overall survival in the National Cancer Institute of Canada Clinical Trials Group phase III trial.

From O'Sullivan R, Davis AM, Turcotte R, et al: Lancet 359:2235–2241, 2002.

therapy can be omitted. Postoperative therapy with either external-beam irradiation (with or without an interstitial implant boost) or an implant alone will achieve a high likelihood of local control and, therefore, limb preservation. Preoperative irradiation, although equally efficacious, does carry a higher wound complication rate than the postoperative approach.

Primary radiation therapy

Several studies on radiation therapy alone in the treatment of unresectable or medically inoperable soft-tissue sarcomas have reported 5-year survival rates of 25% to 40% and local control rates of 30%. Local control depends largely on the size of the primary tumor. Radiation doses should be at least 65–70 Gy, if delivery of such doses is feasible. The tumor's location may be particularly important in determining this dose because of the potential for damage to critical structures (eg, the spinal cord) with the higher doses normally used.

Radiation therapy in retroperitoneal sarcomas

Only 50% of patients with retroperitoneal sarcomas are able to undergo complete surgical resection. Of patients undergoing complete resection, one-half develop local recurrence. This significant local failure rate suggests a potentially important role for adjuvant treatment in all patients with retroperitoneal sarcomas. However, the role of radiation therapy for retroperitoneal sarcomas remains controversial due to the rarity of the tumor, the paucity of data, the retrospective nature of available studies, the low doses of radiation used in many studies, and the lack of consistent policies in determining the indications for radiation therapy.

Preoperative irradiation The advantages of preoperative radiotherapy have already been discussed for soft-tissue sarcomas of the extremities. In the retroperitoneum, an additional advantage is that bowel is frequently displaced significantly by the tumor. In contrast to the postoperative setting, the bowel being treated is also unlikely to be tethered by adhesions from prior surgery. These features significantly offset acute toxicity of large-field intra-abdominal radiotherapy (eg, nausea, vomiting, and diarrhea) as well as the potential for late-onset bowel toxicity. Conformal techniques capable of sparing normal tissues are also more easily applied in the preoperative setting, when the tumor can be visualized and the target area more readily defined.

Intraoperative irradiation In a prospective trial from the NCI, 35 patients with completely resected retroperitoneal sarcomas were randomized to receive either intraoperative electron-beam irradiation (IORT) followed by low-dose (30–40 Gy) postoperative external-beam irradiation or high-dose postoperative external-beam irradiation (35–40 Gy plus a 20-Gy boost). Absolute local recurrence rates were significantly lower in the IORT group ($P < .05$), but disease-specific and overall survival rates did not differ between the two groups.

Similarly, a nonrandomized series from the Massachusetts General Hospital has suggested improved local control with IORT for patients with retroperitoneal sarcoma. In 16 patients who underwent irradiation, complete gross resection, and IORT, overall survival and local control rates were 74% and 83%, respectively. These numbers diminished to 30% and 61%, respectively, in the 13 patients treated with irradiation and complete gross resection without IORT. Although these local control results are encouraging, IORT remains investigational and cannot be advocated on a routine basis at this time.

Postoperative irradiation Two-year local control rates of 70% have been reported with the addition of postoperative irradiation. However, irradiation of the retroperitoneum/abdomen in doses that have effected local control in soft-tissue sarcoma of the extremities (50–65 Gy) is usually associated with significant GI toxicity. Obviously, the incidence of GI toxicity depends on the exact fields and technique used. However, as most retroperitoneal sarcomas are > 10–15 cm, the radiation fields employed are generally also quite large, and bowel is often located and/or tethered in the high-risk area. Three-dimensional treatment planning and conformal techniques can now be utilized to maximize the radiation dose to the tumor bed while minimizing the dose to the surrounding normal tissues.

Isolated limb perfusion

Recent studies have evaluated the role of isolated limb perfusion (ILP) in the management of sarcomas of the extremities. These studies have generally been extrapolations from protocols initially designed to treat locally advanced melanoma.

The agents most commonly employed for ILP have been melphalan and tumor necrosis factor-alpha (TNF-α), with or without interferon-gamma (IFN-γ-1b [Actimmune]). The results of the largest series of ILP in patients with locally advanced soft-tissue sarcoma of the extremities were reported by Eggermont and colleagues. TNF-α has now been approved in Europe for ILP in patients with locally advanced, grade 2/3 soft-tissue sarcomas of the extremities.

The Netherlands Cancer Institute published its results in patients with unresectable soft-tissue sarcoma of the extremities who were perfused with melphalan and TNF-α. A total of 49 patients were treated and followed for a median of 26 months. One patient died shortly after perfusion, but 31 patients (63%) were able to undergo resection of the tumor. Based on clinical and pathologic grounds, an overall response was seen in 31 patients (63%), and a complete response was seen in 4 patients (8%). A total of 28 patients (57%) had local control with limb preservation. Toxicity was frequent but usually mild.

ROLE OF ADJUVANT CHEMOTHERAPY

The striking success of combined-modality therapy in children with osteogenic sarcoma, rhabdomyosarcoma, and the Ewing's sarcoma family of tumors has provided the stimulus for the use of aggressive combined-modality approaches in adults. The literature is replete with reports of the apparent benefit of combined-modality therapy in patients with resectable soft-tissue sarcoma. Yet most series are either retrospective or small nonrandomized trials.

Preoperative chemotherapy

Preoperative chemotherapy has been adopted at many centers for patients with large high-grade sarcoma. The specific regimens employed have evolved over the years but generally contain both an anthracycline and ifosfamide.

Aside from theoretic considerations, there are several pragmatic reasons to favor preoperative over postoperative treatment. First, a reduction in the size of a large lesion may permit surgical resection with less morbidity. Second, compliance may be better with preoperative therapy. One observation that supports the neoadjuvant approach is that response to preoperative chemotherapy, whether pathologic or radiographic, predicts improved tumor control and survival.

Neoadjuvant chemotherapy has been explored in a prospective randomized trial initiated by the EORTC (European Organization for Research on the Treatment of Cancer). The trial was open to patients who had a sarcoma measuring at least 8 cm (of any grade), a primary or recurrent intermediate- to high-grade (grade 2/3) sarcoma of any size, or a locally recurrent or inadequately excised grade 2/3 sarcoma. In spite of these broad eligibility criteria, accrual was slow, and the trial was closed after only 150 patients entered.

Patients were randomized to receive either immediate surgery, followed by radiation therapy for close or positive margins, or 3 cycles of chemotherapy with doxorubicin (50 mg/m^2 by IV bolus) plus ifosfamide (5 g/m^2 by 24-hour continuous infusion) with mesna (Mesnex). Among the 134 eligible patients, over 80% had primary tumors of the extremities, but only 4% had grade 2/3 lesions > 8 cm. Among 49 patients evaluable for response, 29% had major objective responses, including four complete responses. Only 18% had progression of disease before surgery. Chemotherapy was generally well tolerated and never prevented surgery. With a median follow-up of 7.3 years, the estimated 5-year survival rate was similar for both groups.

Trials have explored the role of neoadjuvant chemotherapy and radiation therapy to decrease the rate of distant failure and possibly impact survival. A study reported from Massachusetts General Hospital enrolled patients with high-grade soft-tissue sarcomas (8 cm or larger). Patients were treated with 3 cycles of preoperative chemotherapy consisting of MAID (mesna, doxorubicin [Adriamycin], ifosfamide, dacarbazine) interdigitated with 44 Gy of radiation therapy. This reigmen was followed by surgical resection and 3 cycles of postoperative MAID chemotherapy. In cases with positive surgical margins, an additional 16 Gy of radiation therapy was delivered.

This regimen resulted in a significant improvement in 5-year freedom from distant metastasis (75% vs 44%; $P = .0016$) when compared with historic control patients. Additionally, 5-year disease-free and overall survival rates were 70% versus 42% ($P = .0002$) and 87% versus 58% ($P = .0003$) for the MAID and control groups, respectively. There was a 29% rate of wound healing complications in the MAID group.

These data have been extended in a follow-up study of similar interdigitated chemotherapy/radiation therapy in a phase II study from the Radiation Therapy

Oncology Group (RTOG). In this study, 66 patients with primary high-grade soft-tissue sarcoma ≥ 8 cm in diameter received a modified MAID regimen plus granulocyte colony-stimulating factor (G-CSF [Neupogen]) and radiation therapy, followed by resection and postoperative chemotherapy. Preoperative radiotherapy and chemotherapy were successfully completed by 89% and 79% of patients, respectively. Grade 4 hematologic and nonhematologic toxicities affected 80% and 23% of patients, respectively. Two patients developed late myelodysplasia. Delayed wound healing was noted in 31%. The estimated 3-year survival, disease-free survival, and local control rates were 75%, 55%, and 79%, respectively.

The M. D. Anderson Cancer Center conducted a phase I trial to define the maximum tolerated dose of continuous infusion doxorubicin administered with preoperative radiation therapy to a dose of 50 Gy. In total, 27 patients with intermediate- or high-grade sarcomas were enrolled in the trial. The maximum tolerated dose of doxorubicin was $17.5 \text{ mg/m}^2/\text{wk}$. Twenty-six patients underwent surgery, and all had a macroscopic complete resection (R0 or R1). Two patients had a pathologic complete response. These studies suggest that further investigation of a preoperative approach combining chemotherapy and radiation therapy is warranted.

Postoperative chemotherapy

A number of published trials have compared postoperative chemotherapy with observation alone in adults who had undergone resection of a primary or recurrent soft-tissue sarcoma. Most of these trials included fewer than 100 patients, and even the largest trial had inadequate statistical power to detect a 15% difference in survival. Other flaws confound the interpretation of many of the studies. Some trials included low-risk patients with small and/or low-grade sarcomas. In some trials, patient ineligibility rates were as high as 20%, and in none of the trials published before 2000 was ifosfamide part of the combination evaluated.

In five of the six trials in which doxorubicin monotherapy was studied, including one study limited to patients with uterine sarcoma, a significant improvement in survival could not be demonstrated. Among the trials of combination chemotherapy, most used the combination known as CyVADIC (cyclophosphamide, vincristine, doxorubicin [Adriamycin], dacarbazine). A significant survival advantage was seen in only one combination chemotherapy trial.

Nonetheless, some of the trials showed a trend or a statistically significant improvement in disease-free survival among patients who were administered adjuvant chemotherapy, especially among those with high-grade sarcomas of the extremities. Analyses of the pooled results of the published literature are consistent with this observation.

SMAC meta-analysis A formal meta-analysis of individual data from 1,568 patients who participated in randomized trials of postoperative adjuvant chemotherapy versus no chemotherapy control patients was performed by the Sarcoma Meta-Analysis Collaboration (SMAC). Although not all data were available for all patients, the analysis demonstrated a significant reduction in the risk of local or distant recurrence in patients who received adjuvant chemotherapy.

The overall hazard ratio for distant relapse-free survival was 0.70; ie, the risk of distant relapse (metastasis) was reduced by 30% in treated patients. The absolute benefit at 10 years was 10%, so the recurrence-free survival rate at 10 years was improved from 60% to 70%. Also, the hazard ratio for local recurrence-free survival was 0.73 (27% reduction in the risk of local recurrence), and the absolute benefit was 6%.

The hazard ratio for overall survival, however, was 0.89, which did not meet the criteria for statistical significance. The observed survival at 10 years was 54% for patients who received chemotherapy and 50% for those who did not. Subset analysis failed to show that the effects of chemotherapy differed by primary site, although the best evidence for an effect of adjuvant chemotherapy was seen in patients with sarcoma of the extremities.

Ifosfamide-containing trials Only one trial included in the meta-analysis used an ifosfamide-containing regimen; that trial involved only 29 patients. An attempt to conduct a large prospective trial of postoperative chemotherapy with the MAID regimen in the United States failed because of insufficient patient accrual.

An Italian cooperative group conducted a trial in which patients 18 to 65 years old with high-grade (> 5 cm) or any recurrent sarcoma of the extremities were randomized to receive postoperative chemotherapy or observation alone. The treatment consisted of 5 cycles of epirubicin, 60 mg/m^2 on days 1 and 2, plus ifosfamide, 1.8 g/m^2 on days 1–5. G-CSF was used to support the granulocyte counts during therapy.

The trial had been planned for 200 patients but was interrupted after accrual of 104 patients, when an interim analysis showed a significant survival advantage for the chemotherapy-treated group. At 36 months after the last randomization, with a median follow-up of 59 months, median overall survival among the patients who received adjuvant chemotherapy was 75 months, versus 46 months for control patients ($P = .03$). In a longer-term follow-up analysis, survival was not improved on an intention-to-treat analysis, although 5-year overall survival rates still favored the patients receiving chemotherapy.

A recently completed analysis of adjuvant chemotherapy using doxorubicin and ifosfamide was conducted by the EORTC and reported at ASCO 2007. This study examined surgery and adjuvant radiation therapy versus the same local therapy and adjuvant chemotherapy with 5 cycles of doxorubicin (75 mg/m^2) and ifosfamide (5 g/m^2) every 21 days. The data indicated no benefit in overall survival for the chemotherapy arm and tempered some of the enthusiasm regarding adjuvant chemotherapy as demonstrated in a positive Italian study of epirubicin and ifosfamide.

Two other randomized studies since the time of the original Italian study have been performed. They do not indicate a benefit for chemotherapy but are underpowered to detect small differences in outcome.

Analyses of other collected prospective data regarding adjuvant chemotherapy from large referral centers have yielded somewhat conflicting data. In two analyses of patients with synovial sarcoma and one involving myxoid/round cell liposarcoma, chemotherapy appeared to improve overall survival. In a large analysis of two prospective databases, patients receiving chemotherapy initially had superior survival but then suffered inferior survival compared with those who received no adjuvant chemotherapy. Notably, patients were not randomized as part of their treatment. In fact, given this was a registry instead of a randomized study, there was by definition a bias to treat patients who had higher-risk tumors with chemotherapy, although this did not appear to correlate with a specific single variable in the analysis. Thus, if there is a benefit to adjuvant chemotherapy, it is a small one, and patients should be managed on a case-by-case basis.

Treatment recommendations

- Multidisciplinary treatment planning should precede the initiation of any therapy. An experienced multidisciplinary team should evaluate pathologic material and imaging studies and coordinate the integration of surgical resection, irradiation, and systemic therapy.

- Ideally, patients should be offered participation in clinical trials. Unfortunately, there are no active trials in the United States that will definitively answer the most important questions. Thus, a decision to treat must be made on an individual basis.

- Preoperative chemotherapy should be considered for fit, high-risk patients after a discussion of the risks and potential benefits. Older patients, especially those with cardiac or renal disease, are not optimal candidates for such treatment.

- Patients who do not receive preoperative chemotherapy may still be offered postoperative treatment. Adjuvant doxorubicin/ifosfamide combinations may improve relapse-free survival in carefully selected patients and can be considered for the treatment of those with tumor size > 5 cm, deep tumor location, and high histologic grade.

- For patients who opt for preoperative or postoperative chemotherapy, a regimen that includes doxorubicin (60–75 mg/m²) or epirubicin (120 mg/m²) plus ifosfamide (9–10 g/m²), given for a total of 5 cycles, is a reasonable choice for subjects younger than age 60.

- Outside the context of a clinical trial, concurrent doxorubicin-based chemotherapy and irradiation should be avoided.

TREATMENT OF LOCAL RECURRENCE

Despite optimal multimodality therapy, local recurrence develops in 10% to 50% of patients, with a median local recurrence-free interval of ~24 months. Local recurrence rates are a function of the primary site and are highest for retroperitoneal and head and neck sarcomas, for which adequate surgical margins are difficult to attain. In addition, high-dose adjuvant irradiation of these sites is often limited by the relative radiosensitivity of surrounding structures. These factors result in local recurrence rates of 40% for retroperitoneal sarcomas and up to 50% for head and neck sarcomas, which are substantially higher than the 10% proximity typically seen for extremity sarcomas.

A large retrospective analysis of patients with high-grade sarcoma of the extremities was reported from UCLA. Local recurrence required amputation in 38% of cases and was associated with a threefold decrement in survival. This finding accentuates the necessity for adequate local therapy for sarcomas presenting primarily as well as for multidisciplinary management of local recurrence.

Reoperation Following staging evaluation, patients with isolated local recurrence should undergo reoperation. The results of reoperation in this setting are good, with two-thirds of patients experiencing long-term survival.

Adjuvant radiation therapy If no prior radiation therapy was employed, adjuvant irradiation (50–65 Gy) should be used before or after surgery for locally recurrent disease. Radiation therapy (external-beam irradiation or brachytherapy) should be considered in patients for whom previous radiation doses were subtherapeutic or the previous radiation field design permitted additional treatment.

Reports from Memorial Sloan-Kettering Cancer Center, M. D. Anderson Cancer Center, and Princess Margaret Hospital suggest that patients who develop local recurrence following previous full-dose irradiation represent a difficult local control challenge. A report from Memorial Sloan-Kettering Cancer Center suggests that limb-sparing surgery combined with adjuvant brachytherapy may produce excellent local control and function in this group.

ILP Ongoing clinical investigations are defining the role of ILP in the management of patients with locally recurrent sarcoma.

TREATMENT OF LIMITED PULMONARY METASTASIS

Thoracotomy and metastasectomy The most common site of metastatic disease involvement of soft-tissue sarcoma is the lungs. Rates of 3-year survival following thoracotomy for pulmonary metastasectomy range from 23% to 42%. This fact, combined with the limited efficacy of systemic therapy, is the basis for the recommendation that patients with limited pulmonary metastases and no extrapulmonary disease should undergo thoracotomy and metastasectomy.

Appropriate patient selection for this aggressive therapeutic approach to metastatic disease is essential. The following are generally agreed upon criteria: (1) the primary tumor is controlled or controllable; (2) there is no extrathoracic metastatic disease; (3) the patient is a medical candidate for thoracotomy; and (4) complete resection of all disease appears to be possible.

Preresection chemotherapy Chemotherapy is often recommended before resection of pulmonary metastases. However, there are no convincing data to support this approach.

CHEMOTHERAPY FOR UNRESECTABLE LOCALLY ADVANCED OR METASTATIC DISEASE

Single agents

Doxorubicin Early trials of doxorubicin reported major responses in approximately 30% of patients with advanced soft-tissue sarcoma. In more recent randomized series, however, the rate of response has been closer to 17%.

Subset analysis of patients with soft-tissue sarcoma from a broad phase II trial in which patients were randomized to receive various doses of doxorubicin demonstrated a steep dose-response relationship; patients treated with doses below 60 mg/m^2 rarely responded. Whether dose intensification of doxorubicin is associated with improved survival remains an open question (see section on "Intensifying chemotherapy").

Pegylated liposomal doxorubicin (Doxil in the United States, Caelyx in Europe) has demonstrated limited activity in phase II trials, especially in patients whose disease is refractory to standard doxorubicin. In a randomized comparison among 95 previously untreated patients, however, the response rates to pegylated liposomal doxorubicin (50 mg/m^2 every 4 weeks; 10%) and to standard doxorubicin (75 mg/m^2 every 3 weeks; 9%) were similar, with no significant difference in time to disease progression or survival. Response rates improved to 14% and 12%, respectively, when GIST cases were excluded.

Ifosfamide In a randomized phase II trial conducted by EORTC, 18% of patients treated with ifosfamide (5 g/m^2) experienced major responses, in contrast to 12% of patients treated with cyclophosphamide (1.5 g/m^2), despite the greater myelosuppression with the latter agent. In a large American phase II trial, 17 of 99 patients with soft-tissue sarcoma responded to ifosfamide (8 g/m^2). All of the patients had been treated previously with doxorubicin-based therapy, suggesting a degree of non–cross-resistance.

Increasing ifosfamide dose Responses to ifosfamide ($\geq$ 12 g/m^2) have been observed in patients whose disease progressed while receiving lower doses, supporting the concept of a dose-response relationship.

In a randomized trial, the response to 9 g/m^2 of ifosfamide (17.5%) was superior to the 3% response observed among patients treated with 5 g/m^2. The reason for the low response to the lower dose was unclear. In a subsequent trial by the same investigators, the response to 12 g/m^2 was only 14%, however.

Among 45 evaluable patients enrolled in a Spanish phase II trial of ifosfamide (14 g/m^2 given by continuous infusion over 6 days), the response rate was 38%, but 47% of patients developed febrile neutropenia and 32%, grade 3 neurotoxicity.

At M. D. Anderson Cancer Center, ifosfamide (14 g/m^2 given by continuous infusion over 3 days) yielded responses in 29% of 37 patients with soft-tissue sarcoma and 40% of patients with bone sarcoma. Also within that report was a small cohort of patients in whom the response to the same total dose of ifosfamide was higher when the drug was given by an intermittent bolus rather than a continuous infusion; this finding led the authors to suggest that bolus therapy is more efficacious than continuous infusion. Pharmacokinetic studies, however, have shown no difference between a 1-hour infusion and bolus injection of ifosfamide with respect to the area under the curve for serum ifosfamide or its metabolites or the levels of ifosfamide metabolites in urine.

In an EORTC phase II trial, ifosfamide (12 g/m^2 given as a 3-day continuous infusion every 4 weeks) yielded a response rate of 17% among 89 chemotherapy-naive patients and 16% among 25 previously treated patients.

Ifosfamide doses as high as $14-20 \text{ g/m}^2$ have been given with hematopoietic growth factor support; reported response rates are high, but neurologic and renal toxicities often are dose-limiting. The available data suggest that synovial sarcoma is particularly sensitive to ifosfamide.

Dacarbazine The activity of dacarbazine in soft-tissue sarcoma has been recognized since the 1970s and was confirmed in a formal phase II trial. This marginally active agent has been used mostly in doxorubicin-based combinations. In particular, patients with leiomyosarcoma respond better to dacarbazine than do patients with other sarcoma subtypes.

Ecteinascidin (ET-743, trabectedin [Yondelis]), a novel compound derived from a marine organism, has demonstrated promising activity as well. In phase I trials, trabectedin demonstrated activity in heavily pretreated patients with advanced sarcoma. Three phase II trials of trabectedin ($1,500 \text{ mg/m}^2$ over 24 hours every 3 weeks) in refractory non-GIST soft-tissue sarcoma have been reported.

In one trial, 2 partial responses and 4 minor responses were seen among 52 patients; 9 additional patients had stable disease for at least 6 months. Twenty-four percent of patients were free of disease progression at 6 months. The median survival was 12.8 months, with 30% of patients alive at 2 years.

In a second trial, responses were observed in 3 of 36 patients, with 1 complete response and 2 partial responses, for an overall response rate of 8% (95% confidence interval: 2–23). Responses, however, were durable, lasting up to 20 months.

Finally, a phase II study of patients treated in first line with the 24-hour infusion schedule of trabectedin demonstrated a 17% response rate. These data confirm that trabectedin is an active compound in the treatment of soft-tissue sarcomas, with a response rate similar to the 10% to 30% range seen for either doxorubicin or ifosfamide. The predominant toxicities were neutropenia and elevation of transaminase levels. Two phase II trials of trabectedin in patients with GIST showed no therapeutic activity. Trabectedin was approved for use in chemotherapy-refractory sarcomas in Europe in 2007.

Other agents Gemcitabine (Gemzar) has demonstrated modest activity in several phase II trials, although results of a recent Southwest Oncology Group (SWOG) trial were disappointing. Taxanes, vinca alkaloids, and platinum compounds have demonstrated only marginal activity, however. It should be noted that the taxanes, gemcitabine, and vinorelbine have been observed to be active in angiosarcoma, especially involving the scalp and face.

Combination chemotherapy

Combination chemotherapy regimens have been used widely in the management of patients with soft-tissue sarcoma (Table 2). High response rates have been reported in a number of single-arm phase II trials. Most combination regimens include an anthracycline (either doxorubicin or epirubicin) plus an alkylating agent, dacarbazine, or both agents. Overall response rates are higher in these single-arm trials than when the same regimens are tested in larger, randomized studies.

CyVADIC and doxorubicin/dacarbazine regimens Combinations of doxorubicin with other agents have not proved to be superior to doxorubicin alone in terms of overall survival. Also, for over a decade, the CyVADIC regimen was widely accepted as the standard of care. In a prospective, randomized trial, however, CyVADIC did not prove to be superior to doxorubicin alone.

Doxorubicin (or epirubicin) plus ifosfamide Combinations of doxorubicin (or epirubicin) plus ifosfamide have consistently yielded responses in over 25% of patients in single-arm trials. In sequential trials conducted by the EORTC, doxorubicin at 75 mg/m^2 plus ifosfamide (5 g/m^2) was superior to doxorubicin at 50 mg/m^2 plus ifosfamide (5 g/m^2). A prospective randomized EORTC trial with 314 patients compared the two regimens. There was no difference in response rate or overall survival, but disease progression-free survival favored the more intensive regimen.

The strategy of intensifying the dosing of ifosfamide within the context of combination chemotherapy was explored in a randomized phase II trial. This study included both patients with localized disease treated with 4 cycles of preoperative chemotherapy as well as patients with metastatic disease. Overall, there was no survival benefit for patients treated with doxorubicin (60 mg/m^2) plus 12 g/m^2 of ifosfamide over those treated with doxorubicin (60 mg/m^2) plus 6 g/m^2 of ifosfamide. Also, there was no advantage to the patients with localized disease in terms of disease-free survival.

MAID regimen The MAID regimen yielded an overall response rate in 47% of patients in a large phase II trial. In a randomized comparison of AD (doxorubicin/dacarbazine) versus MAID regimens, the response to MAID was 32%, versus 17% with the two-drug regimen ($P < .002$). However, the price paid for the higher response was toxicity; of 8 toxic deaths reported in this trial, 7 occurred among the 170 patients treated with MAID. All treatment-related deaths occurred in patients > 50 years old. During the study, the doses of MAID were reduced to lessen toxicity. The median survival did not differ significantly between the two regimens, although a trend favoring the AD regimen was noted.

Combination chemotherapy vs single-agent doxorubicin Combination chemotherapy has been compared with single-agent doxorubicin in eight randomized phase III trials. Two trials were limited to patients with uterine sarcoma. Some of these studies showed superior response rates with combination chemotherapy, but none of the trials found a significant survival advantage. Kaplan-Meier plots of survival are virtually superimposable within each trial and from trial to trial.

TABLE 2: Chemotherapy regimens for soft-tissue sarcoma

Drug/combination	Dose and schedule
AIM	
Adriamycin (doxorubicin)	30 mg/m^2 IV on days 1 and 2 by rapid IV infusion
Ifosfamide	3,750 mg/m^2 on days 1 and 2 by IV infusion over 4 hours
Mesna	750 mg/m^2 IV infused immediately preceding and 4 and 8 hours after ifosfamide administration on days 1 and 2

Repeat cycle every 21 days.

NOTE: IV hydration at 300 mL/h beginning 3 hours before each treatment cycle and for 3 days at 100 mL/h after each day-1 ifosfamide infusion. Granulocyte colony-stimulating factor, 5 μg/kg subcutaneously, may be given starting 24 to 48 hours daily for 10 days or until a granulocyte count of 1,500/μL is reached. Appropriate supportive measures should be given.

Edmonson JH, Ryan LM, Blum RH, et al: J Clin Oncol 11:1269–1275, 1993.

EIM	
Epirubicin	60 mg/m^2 IV infused on days 1 and 2, total dose of 120 mg/m^2 per cycle
Ifosfamide	1.8 g/m^2/d on days 1-5, total dose of 9 g/m^2 per cycle
Mesna	360 mg/m^2 IV infused immediately before and 4 and 8 hours after ifosfamide infusion

Repeat cycle every 3 weeks for a total of 5 cycles.

Granulocyte colony-stimulating factor, 300 μg subcutaneously given on days 8 through 15.

Hydration (1,500-2,000 mL) of fluids IV given after ifosfamide.

Frustaci S, Gherlinzoni F, De Paoli A, et al: J Clin Oncol 19:1238–1247, 2001.

Gemcitabine and docetaxel	
Gemcitabine	900 mg/m^2 IV on days 1 and 8
Docetaxel	100 mg/m^2 on day 8

Repeat cycle every 21 days.

NOTE: Granulocyte colony-stimulating factor is given subcutaneously on days 9 and 15. Patients who have undergone prior pelvic radiation therapy receive 25% dose reduction of both agents. Gemcitabine is delivered over 30 to 90 minutes in cycles 1 and 2 and by 90-minute infusion in all subsequent cycles. Lower docetaxel doses are typically used off-study.

Hensley ML, Maki R, Venkatraman E, et al: J Clin Oncol 20:2824–2831, 2002.

Table prepared by Ishmael Jaiyesimi, DO

It should be emphasized that approximately 20% to 25% of patients entered into such trials are alive 2 years after therapy was initiated. Complete responses are uncommon and do not appear to translate into prolonged survival.

Gemcitabine plus docetaxel In a phase II study of 34 patients with unresectable leiomyosarcoma, mostly uterine in origin, 53% responded to a combination of gemcitabine (given by 90-minute infusion) plus docetaxel (Taxotere), with G-CSF support. An additional 20% had stable disease. Almost half of the patients had disease progression after anthracycline-based therapy. The median time to disease progression was 5.6 months, and grade 3/4 toxicity was uncommon. The activity of the gemcitabine-docetaxel combination was confirmed in a variety of other sarcoma subtypes in another study, which also confirmed the rationale for the sequence used in the study in vitro.

Intensifying chemotherapy Hematopoietic growth factors have facilitated the evaluation of dose-intensive chemotherapy in patients with sarcoma. The nonhematologic toxicities (cardiac, neurologic, and renal) of the agents most active in soft-tissue sarcoma prevent dramatic dose escalation.

> A prospective, randomized trial comparing gemcitabine (Gemzar)-docetaxel (Taxotere) with gemcitabine alone in a spectrum of histologic types of sarcoma has been completed. The response rates were 8% for gemcitabine alone and 16% for gemcitabine-docetaxel. Time to disease progression and overall survival were superior with gemcitabine-docetaxel (17.9 months vs 11 months). Although this is one of the few studies in metastatic sarcoma to show a survival advantage, enthusiasm is tempered by toxicity, causing treatment discontinuation in up to 50% of patients after 6 months of gemcitabine-docetaxel chemotherapy. These data suggest that a dose reduction is needed in the off-study use of the therapy (*Maki RG, Wathen JK, Patel SR, et al: J Clin Oncol 25:2755-2763, 2007*).

Phase I/II trials of dose-intense anthracycline/ifosfamide regimens with hematopoietic growth factor support have shown that doxorubicin (70–90 mg/m^2) can be used in combination with ifosfamide (10–12 g/m^2) in selected patients. Response rates as high as 69% have been reported. Although toxicity increases, often dramatically, with these relatively modest dose escalations, the clinical benefit in terms of survival or palliation in patients with metastatic disease remains uncertain.

No randomized trial has demonstrated a survival advantage for patients treated with these more aggressive regimens. In one randomized trial, however, the French Federation of Cancer Centers Sarcoma Group demonstrated that, in comparison with standard doses, a 25% escalation in doses of MAID with G-CSF support did not improve outcome.

High-dose therapy with autologous stem-cell transplantation Most trials are small and presumably involve highly selected patients. In one trial involving 30 patients with metastatic or locally advanced sarcoma accrued over 6 years, more than 20% were free of disease progression at 5 years after high-dose therapy with stem-cell rescue. Complete response to standard induction chemotherapy predicted superior 5-year survival. Based on these favorable results, the investigators suggested a prospective randomized trial examining this approach. Although some groups are still exploring this approach, the appropriateness of generalizing these results to most patients with soft-tissue sarcoma remains speculative.

Prognostic factors for response to therapy Over the past 20 years, the EORTC has collected data on more than 2,000 patients with metastatic disease who participated in first-line anthracycline-based chemotherapy trials. Multivariate analysis of these data indicated that the patients most likely to respond to chemotherapy are those without liver metastases ($P < .0001$), younger patients, individuals with high histologic grade, and those with liposarcoma. In this Cox model, the factors associated with superior survival were good performance status, absence of liver metastases, low histologic grade, a long time to metastasis after treatment of the primary tumor, and young age.

More recently, these same investigators have reported that the observed response rate is superior in patients who have pulmonary metastases only, as compared with those who have metastases to the lungs and other sites or to other sites only. These findings highlight the danger of reaching broad conclusions based on extrapolations from small trials that include highly selected patients. The EORTC data are also consistent with the observation that patients with metastatic GI sarcoma rarely respond to standard chemotherapy regimens. This increasingly recognized observation has been used to explain the low response rates seen in some trials.

Targeted therapy for GISTs

Advances in our understanding of the biology of GIST, and the availability of an effective therapy for patients with advanced disease, have resulted in intense interest in this entity and rapid expansion of this disease. Because this entity had not been recognized, the incidence of GIST was underappreciated. GIST is the most common nonepithelial tumor of the GI tract, with an estimated annual incidence of 3,000 to 3,500 cases in the United States. Approximately 50% to 60% of GISTs arise in the stomach and 25%, in the small bowel. Other sites include the rest of the GI tract, the omentum, mesentery, and retroperitoneum. These tumors may range in size from millimeters to huge masses. It is not clear how many of these GISTs become clinically relevant and how many are noted anecdotally at the time of endoscopic ultrasonography or other abdominal procedures.

The demonstration of the efficacy of imatinib (Gleevec) in GIST has been among the most dramatic and exciting observations in solid-tumor oncology. A randomized multicenter trial evaluated two doses of oral imatinib (400 vs 600 mg) in 147 patients with advanced GISTs. With a median follow-up of 288 days, 54% had a partial response, and 28% had stable disease, but there were no complete responses. Response was sustained, with a median duration over 6 months. Most patients had mild grade 1 or 2 toxicity, but only 21% had severe grade 3 or 4 toxicity. GI or intra-abdominal hemorrhage occurred in 5% of patients. There was no difference in response or toxicity between the two doses.

These observations were expanded in two parallel, multi-institution trials in which patients with GISTs were randomized to receive imatinib (400 or 800 mg daily). The results were remarkably similar. In the American trial, among 746 registered patients, the overall response rate was 43% for patients treated with 400 mg and 41% for those treated with 800 mg. There were no differences in survival between the two arms. At 2 years, disease progression-free and overall survival rates in the 400-mg arm were 50% and 78%, respectively. In the 800-mg arm, the rate of disease progression-free survival at 2 years was 53%, and the rate of overall survival was 73%.

In a large European trial, 946 patients were randomized to receive imatinib (400 mg daily or twice a day). Among the 615 patients whose response could be evaluated, there was no difference in response frequency (43%) or survival between the two arms. Complete responses were seen in 3% and 2% of the lower-dose and higher-dose patients, respectively. Sixty-nine percent of patients whose disease was progressing on 400 mg of imatinib were allowed to cross over to the higher dose (800 mg). Further therapeutic activity was seen, with 26% of these patients free of disease progression at 1 year.

Based on these results, the EORTC, in conjunction with the Italian Sarcoma Group and the Australasian Gastrointestinal Group, has recently reported its results to further identify factors predicting early and late resistance to imatinib in patients with GIST. Initial resistance was defined as disease progression within 3 months of randomization, and late resistance was disease progression beyond 3 months. Initial resistance was noted in 116 of 934 patients (12%). Low hemoglobin level, high granulocyte count, and presence of lung and absence of liver metastases were independent predictors of initial resistance. Late resistance occurred in 347 of 818 patients. Independent predictors were high baseline granulocyte count, primary tumor outside the stomach, large tumor size, and low initial imatinib dose. The impact of the dose on late resistance was significant in patients with high baseline granulocyte counts and in patients with GI tumors originating outside the stomach and small intestine.

Among a group of 127 patients with advanced GISTs, activating mutations of KIT or PDGFRA (platelet-derived growth factor receptor-alpha) were identified in 87.4% and 3.9% of patients, respectively. In patients harboring an exon 11 mutation of KIT, the partial remission rate was 83.5%, whereas in patients without a discernible mutation in KIT or PDGFRA, the partial remission rate was 9.1%. The presence of an exon 11 mutation in KIT correlated with clinical response, decreased risk of treatment failure, and improved overall survival.

The National Comprehensive Cancer Network (NCCN) recently established a GIST Task Force to develop guidelines for the evaluation and treatment of patients with GIST. This group recommended 400 mg daily as the initial starting dose of imatinib. Dose escalation should be considered in patients who do not respond initially or who demonstrate unequivocal disease progression. Surgery remains the primary modality for treatment of primary GIST, but adjuvant and neoadjuvant trials are ongoing. The efficacy, dose, and duration of imatinib therapy in these settings have not been established, so participation of patients in such trials should be encouraged.

Recent data indicate that sunitinib malate (Sutent) is an active agent in imatinib-refractory GIST. In both phase I/II and III studies, the response rate is on the order of 10%, with a greater than 60% chance of these patients remaining on treatment for 6 months or longer. Notably, the patients with the most benefit

The results of the American College of Surgeons Oncology Group (ACOSOG) phase III study of adjuvant imatinib (Gleevec) for 48 weeks versus placebo were recently reported at ASCO 2007. The study examined patients with any gastrointestinal stromal tumor (GIST) of at least 3 cm maximum dimension. DeMatteo et al indicated that there was only a 3% chance of disease progression after the 48 weeks of therapy, in comparison to 17% in those who underwent surgery alone. However, there was a decay in the progression-free survival curve after approximately 2 to 2.5 years of therapy back toward that of the untreated patients. Furthermore, overall survival was no different between the two study arms, although median survival was only 15 months at the time of the report. These data indicate that imatinib is a good salvage strategy for patients with recurrent GIST but cannot be considered a new standard of care, given the lack of overall survival benefit noted with evidence of disease progression after therapy is complete. Thus, longer exposure to imatinib may be necessary, and is the subject of two studies in Europe (0 vs 2 years imatinib, 1 vs 3 years imatinib) and future studies by ACOSOG. Greater follow up is needed to make definitive conclusions about this important topic (DeMatteo R, Owzar K, Maki R, et al: J Clin Oncol 25[18S]:10079, 2007).

were those with the converse c-Kit genetic phenotype (exon 9 mutation or wild type c-Kit) to that seen as sensitive to imatinib (exon 11 mutation). Nonetheless, imatinib remains the first line of therapy regardless of mutation type, because there is still a response rate seen for imatinib in patients with wild-type or exon 9 c-Kit mutations and since because imatinib is less toxic than sunitinib in its present schedule (4 weeks on at 50 mg by mouth daily, 2 weeks off). Some studies are examining new schedules of sunitinib (eg, 37.5 mg oral daily continuously), whereas other studies are evaluating the benefit of other small-molecule inhibitors of c-Kit. Newer tyrosine kinase inhibitors such as sorafenib (Nexavar) and nilotinib (Tasigna) and novel agents such as heat shock protein inhibitor IPI-504 are in phase I and II studies as agents that may have some activity in the imatinib- and sunitinib- refractory settings.

The French Sarcoma Group has initiated a phase III randomized trial looking at intermittent versus continuous imatinib therapy after completion of 1 year of continuous imatinib therapy. A total of 159 patients have enrolled in the trial. A partial or complete response was achieved in 52% of patients. Twenty-three patients were randomized to join the intermittent arm and 23, the continuous arm. After 3 months, five patients (21%) in the intermittent arm had evidence of disease progression, versus no patients in the continuous arm. Reintroduction of imatinib resulted in tumor control in all patients.

Assessment of response and treatment after disease progression on imatinib The use of standard (RECIST) response criteria in patients with GIST may be misleading. On CT or MR imaging, large tumor masses may become completely necrotic without a reduction in size for months in spite of dramatic clinical improvement. Indeed, such masses may actually increase in size. ^{18}F-FDG (^{18}F-fluorodeoxyglucose)-PET imaging may be extremely useful in selected patients, because response may be seen as early as 24 hours after a dose of imatinib. It should be noted that the survival of patients with stable disease parallels that of patients with major objective responses using RECIST criteria.

Surgery does not cure GIST that recurs after resection of primary disease and should be managed as metastatic disease. However, multimodality therapy should be considered in patients with limited sites of disease. It has also been recognized that patients with disease progression in limited sites of disease, occasionally with a growing nodule within a previously necrotic metastasis, may experience rapid disease progression of previously controlled areas. Thus, imatinib should be continued indefinitely in such patients, who should be referred for investigational therapy.

It is promising that other rare forms of sarcoma, such as dermatofibrosarcoma protuberans and desmoid tumors, have been reported to respond to imatinib, indicating the potential utility of these and many other kinase-targeted therapies now in phase I and II studies (eg, sorafenib], temsirolimus [Torisel], and everolimus [RAD001]). The finding of mTOR inhibitor deforolimus as effective for at least some sarcomas will spur further analysis of combinations of targeted agents as well as targeted agents with cytotoxic chemotherapy.

Recommendations for the treatment of metastatic sarcoma

- For patients with rapidly progressive disease or with symptoms, combination chemotherapy with an anthracycline/ifosfamide combination is indicated. For most patients, however, sequential single-agent therapy is less toxic and not inferior in terms of survival.

- The management of metastatic GIST involves imatinib as first-line therapy, and increasing doses of imatinib, when feasible, before changing to sunitinib. Some patients can be maintained with good responses to imatinib for 6 years or longer.

- Schedules other than the 50 mg oral daily dose of sunitinib (4 weeks on, 2 off) can be considered in an attempt to minimize the drug's toxicity.

- Surgery is increasingly being performed at the time of best response (typically 6 to 9 months) and at the time of limited disease progression. There are no data that indicate that early surgery (at the time of best response) leads to superior survival than later surgery (at the time of limited disease progression). Surgery should generally be avoided in patients with multifocal progressive disease; a change in medical therapy is appropriate in this setting.

- The importance of histology relevant to selection of therapy is increasingly being appreciated. It is especially significant to distinguish GISTs from GI leiomyosarcomas. Patients with GIST progressive on standard therapy should be referred to subspecialty centers experienced in the multimodality management of this disease.

- Periods of watchful waiting may be appropriate for many patients with metastatic sarcoma who have no or only minimal symptoms.

SUGGESTED READING

Blay JY, Le Cesne A, Ray-Coquard I, et al: Prospective multicentric randomized phase III study of imatinib in patients with advanced gastrointestinal stromal tumors comparing interruption versus continuation of treatment beyond 1 year: The French Sarcoma Group. J Clin Oncol 25:1107–1113, 2007.

Chawla SP, Sankhala KK, Chua V, et al: A phase II study of AP23573 (an mTOR inhibitor) in patients with advanced sarcomas (abstract). J Clin Oncol 23(16S):833s, 2005.

Corless CL, Fletcher JA, Heinrich MC, et al: Biology of gastrointestinal stromal tumors. J Clin Oncol 22:3813–3825, 2004.

Cormier JN, Huang X, Xing Y, et al: Cohort analysis of patients with localized, high-risk, extremity soft tissue sarcoma treated at two cancer centers: Chemotherapy-associated outcomes. J Clin Oncol 22:4567–4574, 2004.

DeLaney TF, Spiro IJ, Suit HD, et al: Neoadjuvant chemotherapy and radiotherapy for large extremity soft-tissue sarcomas. Int J Radiat Oncol Biol Phys 56:1117–1127, 2003.

Demetri GD, van Oosterom AT, Garrett CR, et al: Efficacy and safety of sunitinib in patients with advanced gastrointestinal stromal tumour after failure of imatinib: A randomised controlled trial. Lancet 368:1329–1338, 2006.

Eilber FC, Eilber FR, Eckardt J, et al: The impact of chemotherapy on the survival of patients with high-grade primary extremity liposarcoma. Ann Surg 240:686–695, 2004.

Eilber FC, Rosen G, Nelson SD, et al: High-grade extremity soft-tissue sarcomas: Factors predictive of local recurrence and its effect on morbidity and mortality. Ann Surg 237:218–226, 2003.

Ferrari A, Gronchi A, Casanova M, et al: Synovial sarcoma: A retrospective analysis of 271 patients of all ages treated at a single institution. Cancer 101:627–634, 2004.

Fletcher JA, Corless CL, Dimitrijevic S, et al: Mechanisms of resistance to imatinib mesylate (IM) in advanced gastrointestinal stromal tumor (GIST) (abstract). Proc Am Soc Clin Oncol 22:815, 2003.

Frustaci S, De Paoli A, Bidoli E, et al: Ifosfamide in the adjuvant therapy of soft tissue sarcomas. Oncology 65(suppl 2):80–84, 2003.

Garcia-Carbonero R, Supko JG, Maki RG, et al: Ecteinascidin-743 (ET-743) for chemotherapy-naive patients with advanced soft tissue sarcomas: Multicenter phase II and pharmacokinetic study. J Clin Oncol 23:5484–5492, 2005.

Grobmyer SR, Maki RG, Demetri GD, et al: Neo-adjuvant chemotherapy for primary high-grade extremity soft tissue sarcoma. Ann Oncol 15:1667–1672, 2004.

Heinrich MC, Maki RG, Corless CL, et al: Sunitinib response in imatinib-resistant GIST correlates with *KIT* and *PDGFRA* mutation status (abstract). J Clin Oncol 24(18S):520s, 2006.

Kraybill WG, Harris JH, Spiro I, et al: Radiation Therapy Oncology Group 95-14: A phase II study of neoadjuvant chemotherapy and radiation therapy in the management of high-risk, high grade, soft tissue sarcomas of the extremities and body wall (abstract). Proc Am Soc Clin Oncol 22:815, 2003.

Le Cesne A, Blay J, Judson I, et al: Phase II study of ET-743 in advanced soft tissue sarcomas: A European Organisation for the Research and Treatment of Cancer (EORTC) soft tissue and bone sarcoma group trial. J Clin Oncol 23:5276, 2005.

Leu KM, Ostruszka LJ, Shewach D, et al: Laboratory and clinical evidence of synergistic cytotoxicity of sequential treatment with gemcitabine followed by docetaxel in the treatment of sarcoma. J Clin Oncol 22:1706–1712, 2004.

Maki RG, Fletcher JA, Heinrich MC, et al: Results from a continuation trial of SU11248 in patients with imatinib-resistant gastrointestinal stromal tumor (GIST) (abstract). J Clin Oncol 23(16S):818s, 2005.

Noorda EM, Vrouenraets BC, Nieweg OE, et al: Isolated limb perfusion with tumor necrosis factor-alpha and melphalan for patients with unresectable soft tissue sarcoma of the extremities. Cancer 98:1483–1490, 2003.

O'Sullivan B, Bell RS, Bramwell VHC: Sarcomas of the soft tissues, in Souhami RL, Tannock I, Hohenberger P, et al (eds): Oxford Textbook of Oncology, 2nd ed, pp 2495–2523. Oxford, Oxford University Press, 2002.

O'Sullivan B, Davis A, Turcotte R, et al: Five-year results of a randomized phase III trial of preoperative vs post-operative radiotherapy in extremity soft tissue sarcoma (abstract). J Clin Oncol 22:(14S):9007, 2004.

O'Sullivan B, Davis AM, Turcotte R, et al: Preoperative versus postoperative radiotherapy in soft-tissue sarcoma of the limbs: A randomized trial. Lancet 359:2235–2241, 2002.

Pisters PW, Patel SR, Prieto VG, et al: Phase I trial of preoperative doxorubicin-based concurrent chemoradiation and surgical resection for localized extremity and body wall soft tissue sarcomas. J Clin Oncol 22:3375–3380, 2004.

Pisters PW, Pollock RE, Lewis VO, et al: Long-term results of prospective trial of selective use of radiation for patients with T1 extremity and trunk soft tissue sarcomas. Ann Surg 246:675–682, 2007.

Riad S, Griffin AM, Liberman B, et al: Lymph node metastasis in soft tissue sarcoma in an extremity. Clin Orthop Sep:129–134, 2004.

Van den Abbeele AD, Badawi RD Cliche J-P, et al: 18F-FDG-PET predicts response to imatinib mesylate (Gleevec) in patients with advanced gastrointestinal stromal tumors (GIST) (abstract). Proc Am Soc Clin Oncol 21:403a, 2002.

Wendtner C-M, Abdel-Rahman S, Krych M, et al: Response to neoadjuvant chemotherapy combined with regional hyperthermia predicts long-term survival for adult patients with retroperitoneal and visceral high-risk soft-tissue sarcomas. J Clin Oncol 20:3156–3164, 2002.

Zalcberg JR, Verweij J, Casali PG, et al: Outcome of patients with advanced gastrointestinal stromal tumours crossing over to a daily imatinib dose of 800 mg after progression on 400 mg. Eur J Cancer 41:1751–1757, 2005.

CANCER MANAGEMENT: A MULTIDISCIPLINARY APPROACH

Important Safety Information

SPINAL/EPIDURAL HEMATOMAS

When neuraxial anesthesia (epidural/spinal anesthesia) or spinal puncture is employed, patients anticoagulated or scheduled to be anticoagulated with low molecular weight heparins or heparinoids for prevention of thromboembolic complications are at risk of developing an epidural or spinal hematoma which can result in long-term or permanent paralysis.

The risk of these events is increased by the use of indwelling epidural catheters for administration of analgesia or by the concomitant use of drugs affecting hemostasis such as non steroidal anti-inflammatory drugs (NSAIDs), platelet inhibitors, or other anticoagulants. The risk also appears to be increased by traumatic or repeated epidural or spinal puncture.

Patients should be frequently monitored for signs and symptoms of neurological impairment. If neurological compromise is noted, urgent treatment is necessary.

The physician should consider the potential benefit versus risk before neuraxial intervention in patients anticoagulated or to be anticoagulated for thromboprophylaxis (also see **WARNINGS, Hemorrhage** and **PRECAUTIONS, Drug Interactions**).

- FRAGMIN® is contraindicated in patients with active major bleeding or with known hypersensitivity to the drug, heparin, or pork products, or with thrombocytopenia associated with a positive antiplatelet antibody test

- Patients undergoing regional anesthesia should not receive FRAGMIN® for unstable angina or non–Q-wave myocardial infarction, and patients with cancer undergoing regional anesthesia should not receive FRAGMIN® for extended treatment of symptomatic VTE, due to an increased risk of bleeding associated with the dosage of FRAGMIN® recommended for these indications

- FRAGMIN® Injection is not intended for intramuscular administration

- FRAGMIN® cannot be used interchangeably (unit for unit) with unfractionated heparin or other low–molecular-weight heparins

- FRAGMIN®, like other anticoagulants, should be used with extreme caution in patients who have an increased risk of hemorrhage; bleeding can occur at any site during therapy. An unexpected drop in hematocrit or blood pressure should lead to a search for a bleeding site

- **FRAGMIN® should be used with extreme caution in patients with history of heparin-induced thrombocytopenia**

- In a clinical trial of patients with cancer and acute symptomatic VTE treated for up to 6 months in the FRAGMIN® treatment arm, platelet counts of <100,000/mm^3 occurred in 13.6% of patients, including 6.5% who also had platelet counts less than 50,000/mm^3. In the same clinical trial, thrombocytopenia was reported as an adverse event in 10.9% of patients in the FRAGMIN® arm and 8.1% of patients in the oral anticoagulant arm. FRAGMIN® dose was decreased or interrupted in patients whose platelet counts fell below 100,000/mm^3

- Thrombocytopenia of any degree should be monitored closely. Heparin-induced thrombocytopenia can occur with administration of FRAGMIN®. The incidence of this complication is unknown at present. In clinical practice, rare cases of thrombocytopenia with thrombosis have also been observed

- FRAGMIN® should be used with caution in patients with bleeding diathesis, thrombocytopenia or platelet defects; severe liver or kidney insufficiency, hypertensive or diabetic retinopathy, and recent gastrointestinal bleeding

- Each multiple-dose vial of FRAGMIN® contains benzyl alcohol as a preservative [which] has been reported to be associated with a fatal "Gasping Syndrome" in premature infants. Because benzyl alcohol may cross the placenta, FRAGMIN® preserved with benzyl alcohol should be used with caution in pregnant women and only if clearly needed. If anticoagulation with FRAGMIN® is needed during pregnancy, preservative-free formulations should be used, where possible

- FRAGMIN® should be used with care in patients receiving oral anticoagulants, platelet inhibitors, and thrombolytic agents because of increased risk of bleeding (see **PRECAUTIONS, Laboratory Tests**). Aspirin, unless contraindicated, is recommended in patients treated for unstable angina or non–Q-wave myocardial infarction (see **DOSAGE AND ADMINISTRATION**)

- Allergic reactions (i.e., pruritus, rash, fever, injection site reaction, bulleous eruption) have occurred rarely. A few cases of anaphylactoid reactions have been reported

- The most commonly reported side effect is hematoma at the injection site

Fragmin®
(dalteparin sodium injection)

FRAGMIN

(dalteparin sodium injection)

For *Subcutaneous* Use Only

BRIEF SUMMARY: For full prescribing information, see package insert.

SPINAL/EPIDURAL HEMATOMAS

When neuraxial anesthesia (epidural/spinal anesthesia) or spinal puncture is employed, patients anticoagulated or scheduled to be anticoagulated with low molecular weight heparins or heparinoids for prevention of thromboembolic complications are at risk of developing an epidural or spinal hematoma which can result in long-term or permanent paralysis. The risk of these events is increased by the use of indwelling epidural catheters for administration of analgesia or by the concomitant use of drugs affecting hemostasis such as non steroidal anti-inflammatory drugs (NSAIDs), platelet inhibitors, or other anticoagulants. The risk also appears to be increased by traumatic or repeated epidural or spinal puncture. Patients should be frequently monitored for signs and symptoms of neurological impairment. If neurological compromise is noted, urgent treatment is necessary. The physician should consider the potential benefit versus risk before neuraxial intervention in patients anticoagulated or to be anticoagulated for thromboprophylaxis (also see **WARNINGS, Hemorrhage** and **PRECAUTIONS, Drug Interactions**).

INDICATIONS AND USAGE
FRAGMIN Injection is indicated for the prophylaxis of ischemic complications in unstable angina and non-Q-wave myocardial infarction, when concurrently administered with aspirin therapy (as described in **CLINICAL TRIALS, Prophylaxis of Ischemic Complications in Unstable Angina and Non-Q-Wave Myocardial Infarction**).
FRAGMIN is also indicated for the prophylaxis of deep vein thrombosis (DVT), which may lead to pulmonary embolism (PE):
• In patients undergoing hip replacement surgery;
• In patients undergoing abdominal surgery who are at risk for thromboembolic complications;
• In medical patients who are at risk for thromboembolic complications due to severely restricted mobility during acute illness.
FRAGMIN is also indicated for the extended treatment of symptomatic venous thromboembolism (VTE) (proximal DVT and/or PE), to reduce the recurrence of VTE in patients with cancer.

CONTRAINDICATIONS
FRAGMIN Injection is contraindicated in patients with known hypersensitivity to the drug, active major bleeding, or thrombocytopenia associated with positive *in vitro* tests for antiplatelet antibody in the presence of FRAGMIN. Patients undergoing regional anesthesia should not receive FRAGMIN for unstable angina or non-Q-wave myocardial infarction, and patients with cancer undergoing regional anesthesia should not receive FRAGMIN for extended treatment of symptomatic VTE, due to an increased risk of bleeding associated with the dosage of FRAGMIN recommended for these indications. Patients with known hypersensitivity to heparin or pork products should not be treated with FRAGMIN.

WARNINGS
FRAGMIN Injection is not intended for intramuscular administration. FRAGMIN cannot be used interchangeably (unit for unit) with unfractionated heparin or other low molecular weight heparins. **FRAGMIN should be used with extreme caution in patients with history of heparin-induced thrombocytopenia.**
Hemorrhage: FRAGMIN, like other anticoagulants, should be used with extreme caution in patients who have an increased risk of hemorrhage, such as those with severe uncontrolled hypertension, bacterial endocarditis, congenital or acquired bleeding disorders, active ulceration and angiodysplastic gastrointestinal disease, hemorrhagic stroke, or shortly after brain, spinal or ophthalmological surgery. **Spinal or epidural hematomas can occur with the associated use of low molecular weight heparins or heparinoids and neuraxial (spinal/epidural) anesthesia or spinal puncture, which can result in long-term or permanent paralysis. The risk of these events is higher with the use of indwelling epidural catheters or concomitant use of additional drugs affecting hemostasis such as NSAIDs (see boxed WARNING and ADVERSE REACTIONS, Ongoing Safety Surveillance).** As with other anticoagulants, bleeding can occur at any site during therapy with FRAGMIN. An unexpected drop in hematocrit or blood pressure should lead to a search for a bleeding site.
Thrombocytopenia: In FRAGMIN clinical trials supporting non-cancer indications, platelet counts of <100,000/mm^3 and <50,000/mm^3 occurred in <1% and <1% of patients, respectively. In the clinical trial of patients with cancer and acute symptomatic venous thromboembolism treated for up to 6 months in the FRAGMIN treatment arm, platelet counts of <100,000/mm^3 occurred in 13.6% of patients, including 6.5% who also had platelet counts less than 50,000/mm^3. In the same clinical trial, thrombocytopenia was reported as an adverse event in 10.9% of patients in the FRAGMIN arm and 8.1% of patients in the OAC arm. FRAGMIN dose was decreased or interrupted in patients whose platelet counts fell below 100,000/mm^3. Thrombocytopenia of any degree should be monitored closely. Heparin-induced thrombocytopenia can occur with the administration of FRAGMIN. The incidence of this complication is unknown at present. In clinical practice, rare cases of thrombocytopenia with thrombosis have also been observed.
Miscellaneous: Each multiple-dose vial of FRAGMIN contains benzyl alcohol as a preservative. Benzyl alcohol has been reported to be associated with a fatal "Gasping Syndrome" in premature infants. Because benzyl alcohol may cross the placenta, FRAGMIN preserved with benzyl alcohol should be used with caution in pregnant women and only if clearly needed. If anticoagulation with FRAGMIN is needed during pregnancy, preservative-free formulations should be used, where possible (see **PRECAUTIONS, Pregnancy Category B, Nonteratogenic Effects**).

PRECAUTIONS
General: FRAGMIN Injection should not be mixed with other injections or infusions unless specific compatibility data are available that support such mixing. FRAGMIN should be used with caution in patients with bleeding diathesis, thrombocytopenia or platelet defects; severe liver or kidney insufficiency, hypertensive or diabetic retinopathy, and recent gastrointestinal bleeding. If a thromboembolic event should occur despite dalteparin prophylaxis, FRAGMIN should be discontinued and appropriate therapy initiated.
Drug Interactions: FRAGMIN should be used with care in patients receiving oral anticoagulants, platelet inhibitors, and thrombolytic agents because of increased risk of bleeding (see **PRECAUTIONS, Laboratory Tests**). Aspirin, unless contraindicated, is recommended in patients treated for unstable angina or non-Q-wave myocardial infarction (see **DOSAGE AND ADMINISTRATION**).
Laboratory Tests: Periodic routine complete blood counts, including platelet count, blood chemistry, and stool occult blood tests are recommended during the course of treatment with FRAGMIN. No special monitoring of blood clotting times (i.e., APTT) is needed. When administered at recommended prophylaxis doses, routine coagulation tests such as Prothrombin Time (PT) and Activated Partial Thromboplastin Time (APTT) are relatively insensitive measures of FRAGMIN activity and, therefore, unsuitable for monitoring the anticoagulant effect of FRAGMIN. Anti-Factor Xa may be used to monitor the anticoagulant effect of FRAGMIN, such as in patients with severe renal impairment or if abnormal coagulation parameters or bleeding should occur during FRAGMIN therapy.
Drug/Laboratory Test Interactions: Elevations of Serum Transaminases: In FRAGMIN clinical trials supporting non-cancer indications where hepatic transaminases were measured, asymptomatic increases in transaminase levels (SGOT/AST and SGPT/ALT) greater than three times the upper limit of normal of the laboratory reference range were seen in 4.7% and 4.2%, respectively, of patients during treatment with FRAGMIN. In the FRAGMIN clinical trial of patients with cancer and acute symptomatic venous thromboembolism treated with FRAGMIN for up to 6 months, asymptomatic increases in transaminase levels, AST and ALT, greater than three times the upper limit of normal of the laboratory reference range were reported in 8.9% and 9.5% of patients, respectively. The frequencies of Grades 3 and 4 increases in AST and ALT, as classified by the National Cancer Institute, Common Toxicity Criteria (NCI-CTC) Scoring System, were 3% and 3.8%, respectively. Grades 2, 3 & 4 combined have been reported in 12% and 14% of patients, respectively.
Carcinogenicity, Mutagenesis, Impairment of Fertility: Dalteparin sodium has not been tested for its carcinogenic potential in long-term animal studies. It was not mutagenic in the *in vitro* Ames Test, mouse lymphoma cell forward mutation test and human lymphocyte chromosomal aberration test and in the *in vivo* mouse micronucleus test. Dalteparin sodium at subcutaneous doses up to 1200 IU/kg (7080 IU/m^2) did not affect the fertility or reproductive performance of male and female rats.
Pregnancy: Pregnancy Category B. Teratogenic Effects: Reproduction studies with dalteparin sodium at intravenous doses up to 2400 IU/kg (14,160 IU/m^2) in pregnant rats and 4800 IU/kg (40,800 IU/m^2) in pregnant rabbits did not produce any evidence of impaired fertility or harm to the fetuses. There are, however, no adequate and well-controlled studies in pregnant women. Because animal reproduction studies are not always predictive of human response, this drug should be used during pregnancy only if clearly needed.
Nonteratogenic Effects: Cases of "Gasping Syndrome" have occurred when large amounts of benzyl alcohol have been administered (99–404 mg/kg/day). The 9.5 mL and the 3.8 mL multiple-dose vials of FRAGMIN contain 14 mg/mL of benzyl alcohol.
Nursing Mothers: Limited data are available for excretion of dalteparin in human milk. One study in 15 lactating women receiving prophylactic doses of dalteparin detected small amounts of anti-Xa activity in breast milk, equivalent to a milk/plasma ratio of <0.025-0.224. As oral absorption of LMWH is extremely low, the clinical implications, if any, of this small amount of anticoagulant activity on the nursing infant are unknown. Caution should be exercised when FRAGMIN is administered to nursing women.
Pediatric Use: Safety and effectiveness in pediatric patients have not been established.
Geriatric Use: Of the total number of patients in clinical studies of FRAGMIN, 5516 patients were 65 years of age or older and 2237 were 75 or older. No overall differences in effectiveness were observed between these subjects and younger subjects. Some studies suggest that the risk of bleeding increases with age. Postmarketing surveillance and literature reports have not revealed additional differences in the safety of FRAGMIN between elderly and younger patients. Careful attention to dosing intervals and concomitant medications (especially antiplatelet medications) is advised, particularly in geriatric patients with low body weight (<45 kg) and those predisposed to decreased renal function (see also **CLINICAL PHARMACOLOGY** and **General** and **Drug Interactions** subsections of **PRECAUTIONS**).

ADVERSE REACTIONS

Hemorrhage: The incidence of hemorrhagic complications during treatment with FRAGMIN Injection has been low. The most commonly reported side effect is hematoma at the injection site. The incidence of bleeding may increase with higher doses; however, in abdominal surgery patients with malignancy, no significant increase in bleeding was observed when comparing FRAGMIN 5000 IU to either FRAGMIN 2500 IU or low dose heparin. In a trial comparing FRAGMIN 5000 IU once daily to FRAGMIN 2500 IU once daily in patients undergoing surgery for malignancy, the incidence of bleeding events was 4.6% and 3.6%, respectively (n.s.). In a trial comparing FRAGMIN 5000 IU once daily to heparin 5000 U twice daily, the incidence of bleeding events was 3.2% and 2.7%, respectively (n.s.) in the malignancy subgroup.

Unstable Angina and Non-Q-Wave Myocardial Infarction: Table 8 summarizes major bleeding events that occurred with FRAGMIN, heparin, and placebo in clinical trials of unstable angina and non-Q-wave myocardial infarction.

Table 8: Major Bleeding Events in Unstable Angina and Non-Q-Wave Myocardial Infarction

Indication	Dosing Regimen		
Unstable Angina and Non-Q-Wave MI	FRAGMIN 120 IU/kg/12 hr. s.c.[1] n(%)	Heparin i.v. and s.c.[2] n(%)	Placebo every 12 hr s.c. n(%)
Major Bleeding Events[3,4]	15/1497 (1.0)	7/731 (1.0)	4/760 (0.5)

[1]Treatment was administered for 5 to 8 days.
[2]Heparin i.v. infusion for at least 48 hours, APTT 1.5 to 2 times control, then 12,500 U s.c. every 12 hours for 5 to 8 days.
[3]Aspirin (75 to 165 mg per day) and beta blocker therapies were administered concurrently.
[4]Bleeding events were considered major if: 1) accompanied by a decrease in hemoglobin of ≥2 g/dL in connection with clinical symptoms; 2) a transfusion was required; 3) bleeding led to interruption of treatment or death; or 4) intracranial bleeding.

Hip Replacement Surgery: Table 9 summarizes: 1) all major bleeding events and, 2) other bleeding events possibly or probably related to treatment with FRAGMIN (preoperative dosing regimen), warfarin sodium, or heparin in two hip replacement surgery clinical trials.

Table 9: Bleeding Events Following Hip Replacement Surgery

Indication	FRAGMIN vs Warfarin Sodium		FRAGMIN vs Heparin	
	Dosing Regimen		Dosing Regimen	
Hip Replacement Surgery	FRAGMIN[2] 5000 IU once daily s.c. n(%)	Warfarin Sodium[1] oral n(%)	FRAGMIN[4] 5000 IU once daily s.c. n(%)	Heparin 5000 U three times a day s.c. n(%)
Major Bleeding Events[3]	7/274 (2.6)	1/279 (0.4)	0	3/69 (4.3)
Other Bleeding Events[5]				
Hematuria	8/274 (2.9)	5/279 (1.8)	0	0
Wound Hematoma	6/274 (2.2)	0	0	0
Injection Site Hematoma	3/274 (1.1)	NA	2/69 (2.9)	7/69 (10.1)

[1]Warfarin sodium dosage was adjusted to maintain a prothrombin time index of 1.4 to 1.5, corresponding to an International Normalized Ratio (INR) of approximately 2.5.
[2]Includes three treated patients who did not undergo a surgical procedure.
[3]A bleeding event was considered major if: 1) hemorrhage caused a significant clinical event, 2) it was associated with a hemoglobin decrease of ≥2 g/dL or transfusion of 2 or more units of blood products, 3) it resulted in reoperation due to bleeding, or 4) it involved retroperitoneal or intracranial hemorrhage.
[4]Includes two treated patients who did not undergo a surgical procedure.
[5]Occurred at a rate of at least 2% in the group treated with FRAGMIN 5000 IU once daily.

Six of the patients treated with FRAGMIN experienced seven major bleeding events. Two of the events were wound hematoma (one requiring reoperation), three were bleeding from the operative site, one was intraoperative bleeding due to vessel damage, and one was gastrointestinal bleeding. None of the patients experienced retroperitoneal or intracranial hemorrhage nor died of bleeding complications. In the third hip replacement surgery clinical trial, the incidence of major bleeding events was similar in all three treatment groups: 3.6% (18/496) for patients who started FRAGMIN before surgery; 2.5% (12/487) for patients who started FRAGMIN after surgery; and 3.1% (15/489) for patients treated with warfarin sodium.

Abdominal Surgery: Table 10 summarizes bleeding events that occurred in clinical trials which studied FRAGMIN 2500 and 5000 IU administered once daily to abdominal surgery patients.

Table 10: Bleeding Events Following Abdominal Surgery

Indication	FRAGMIN vs Heparin				FRAGMIN vs Placebo		FRAGMIN vs FRAGMIN	
	Dosing Regimen				Dosing Regimen		Dosing Regimen	
Abdominal Surgery	FRAGMIN 2500 IU once daily s.c. n(%)	Heparin 5000 U twice daily s.c. n(%)	FRAGMIN 5000 IU once daily s.c. n(%)	Heparin 5000 U twice daily s.c. n(%)	FRAGMIN 2500 IU once daily s.c. n(%)	Placebo once daily s.c. n(%)	FRAGMIN 2500 IU once daily s.c. n(%)	FRAGMIN 5000 IU once daily s.c. n(%)
Postoperative Transfusions	26/459 (5.7)	36/454 (7.9)	81/508 (15.9)	63/498 (12.7)	14/182 (7.7)	13/182 (7.1)	89/1025 (8.7)	125/1033 (12.1)
Wound Hematoma	16/467 (3.4)	18/467 (3.9)	12/508 (2.4)	6/498 (1.2)	2/79 (2.5)	2/77 (2.6)	1/1030 (0.1)	4/1039 (0.4)
Reoperation Due to Bleeding	2/392 (0.5)	3/392 (0.8)	4/508 (0.8)	2/498 (0.4)	1/79 (1.3)	1/78 (1.3)	2/1030 (0.2)	13/1038 (1.3)
Injection Site Hematoma	1/466 (0.2)	5/464 (1.1)	36/506 (7.1)	47/493 (9.5)	8/172 (4.7)	2/174 (1.1)	36/1026 (3.5)	57/1035 (5.5)

Medical Patients with Severely Restricted Mobility During Acute Illness: Table 11 summarizes major bleeding events that occurred in a clinical trial of medical patients with severely restricted mobility during acute illness.

Table 11: Bleeding Events in Medical Patients with Severely Restricted Mobility During Acute Illness

Indication	Dosing Regimen	
Medical Patients with Severely Restricted Mobility	FRAGMIN 5000 IU once daily s.c. n(%)	Placebo once daily s.c. n(%)
Major Bleeding Events[1] at Day 14	8/1848 (0.4)	0/1833 (0)
Major Bleeding Events[1] at Day 21	9/1848 (0.5)	3/1833 (0.2)

[1]A bleeding event was considered major if: 1) it was accompanied by a decrease in hemoglobin of ≥2 g/dL in connection with clinical symptoms; 2) intraocular, spinal/epidural, intracranial, or retroperitoneal bleeding; 3) required transfusion of ≥2 units of blood products; 4) required significant medical or surgical intervention; or 5) led to death.

Three of the major bleeding events that occurred by Day 21 were fatal, all due to gastrointestinal hemorrhage (two patients in the group treated with FRAGMIN and one in the group receiving placebo). Two deaths occurred after Day 21: one patient in the placebo group died from a subarachnoid hemorrhage that started on Day 55, and one patient died on day 71 (two months after receiving the last dose of FRAGMIN) from a subdural hematoma.

Patients with Cancer and Acute Symptomatic Venous Thromboembolism

Table 12 summarizes the number of patients with bleeding events that occurred in the clinical trial of patients with cancer and acute symptomatic venous thromboembolism. A bleeding event was considered major if it: 1) was accompanied by a decrease in hemoglobin of ≥2 g/dL in connection with clinical symptoms; 2) occurred at a critical site (intraocular, spinal/epidural, intracranial, retroperitoneal, or pericardial bleeding); 3) required transfusion of ≥2 units of blood products; or 4) led to death. Minor bleeding was classified as clinically overt bleeding that did not meet criteria for major bleeding. At the end of the six-month study, a total of 46 (13.6%) patients in the FRAGMIN arm and 62 (18.5%) patients in the OAC arm experienced any bleeding event. One bleeding event (hemoptysis in a patient in the FRAGMIN arm at Day 71) was fatal.

Table 12: Bleeding Events (Major and Any) (As treated population)[1]

Study period	FRAGMIN 200 IU/kg (max. 18,000 IU) s.c. once daily x 1 month, then 150 IU/kg (max 18,000 IU) s.c. once daily x 5 months			OAC FRAGMIN 200 IU/kg (max 18,000 IU) s.c. once daily x 5-7 days and OAC for 6 months (target INR 2-3)		
	Number at risk	Patients with Major Bleeding n(%)	Patients with Any Bleeding n(%)	Number at Risk	Patients with Major Bleeding n(%)	Patients with Any Bleeding n(%)
Total during study	338	19 (5.6)	46 (13.6)	335	12 (3.6)	62 (18.5)
Week 1	338	4 (1.2)	15 (4.4)	335	4 (1.2)	12 (3.6)
Weeks 2-4	332	9 (2.7)	17 (5.1)	321	1 (0.3)	12 (3.7)
Weeks 5-28	297	9 (3.0)	26 (8.8)	267	8 (3.0)	40 (15.0)

[1]Patients with multiple bleeding episodes within any time interval were counted only once in that interval. However, patients with multiple bleeding episodes that occurred at different time intervals were counted once in each interval in which the event occurred.

Thrombocytopenia: See WARNINGS: Thrombocytopenia.

Other: Allergic Reactions: Allergic reactions (i.e., pruritus, rash, fever, injection site reaction, bulleous eruption) have occurred rarely. A few cases of anaphylactoid reactions have been reported. Local Reactions: Pain at the injection site, the only non-bleeding event determined to be possibly or probably related to treatment with FRAGMIN and reported at a rate of at least 2% in the group treated with FRAGMIN, was reported in 4.5% of patients treated with FRAGMIN 5000 IU once daily vs 11.8% of patients treated with heparin 5000 U twice daily in the abdominal surgery trials. In the hip replacement trials, pain at injection site was reported in 12% of patients treated with FRAGMIN 5000 IU once daily vs 13% of patients treated with heparin 5000 U three times a day.

Ongoing Safety Surveillance: Since first international market introduction in 1985, there have been more than 15 reports of epidural or spinal hematoma formation with concurrent use of dalteparin sodium and spinal/epidural anesthesia or spinal puncture. The majority of patients had postoperative indwelling epidural catheters placed for analgesia or received additional drugs affecting hemostasis. In some cases the hematoma resulted in long-term or permanent paralysis (partial or complete). Because these events were reported voluntarily from a population of unknown size, estimates of frequency cannot be made.

Post-Marketing Experience: Skin necrosis has occurred rarely. There have been isolated cases of alopecia reported that improved on drug discontinuation.

OVERDOSAGE

Symptoms/Treatment: An excessive dosage of FRAGMIN Injection may lead to hemorrhagic complications. These may generally be stopped by the slow intravenous injection of protamine sulfate (1% solution), at a dose of 1 mg protamine for every 100 anti-Xa IU of FRAGMIN given. A second infusion of 0.5 mg protamine sulfate per 100 anti-Xa IU of FRAGMIN may be administered if the APTT measured 2 to 4 hours after the first infusion remains prolonged. Even with these additional doses of protamine, the APTT may remain more prolonged than would usually be found following administration of conventional heparin. In all cases, the anti-Factor Xa activity is never completely neutralized (maximum about 60 to 75%). Particular care should be taken to avoid overdosage with protamine sulfate. Administration of protamine sulfate can cause severe hypotensive and anaphylactoid reactions. Because fatal reactions, often resembling anaphylaxis, have been reported with protamine sulfate, it should be given only when resuscitation techniques and treatment of anaphylactic shock are readily available. For additional information, consult the labeling of Protamine Sulfate Injection, USP, products. A single subcutaneous dose of 100,000 IU/kg of FRAGMIN to mice caused a mortality of 8% (1/12) whereas 50,000 IU/kg was a non-lethal dose. The observed sign was hematoma at the site of injection.

Manufactured for and Marketed by Eisai Inc., Woodcliff Lake, NJ 07677

FR080231

Printed February 2008

©2008 Eisai Inc.

CHAPTER 26

Primary and metastatic brain tumors

Lisa M. DeAngelis, MD, Jay S. Loeffler, MD, and Adam N. Mamelak, MD

Intracranial neoplasms can arise from any of the structures or cell types present in the cranial vault, including the brain, meninges, pituitary gland, skull, and even residual embryonic tissue. The overall annual incidence of primary brain tumors in the United States is 14 cases per 100,000 population.

The most common primary brain tumors are meningiomas, representing 27% of all primary brain tumors, and glioblastomas, representing 23% of all primary brain tumors; many of these tumors are clinically aggressive and high grade. Primary brain tumors are the most common of the solid tumors in children and the second most frequent cause of cancer death after leukemia in children.

Brain metastases occur in approximately 15% of cancer patients as a result of hematogenous dissemination of systemic cancer, and the incidence may be rising due to better control of systemic disease. Lung and breast cancers are the most common solid tumors that metastasize to the central nervous system (CNS). Melanoma and testicular and renal carcinomas have the greatest propensity to metastasize to the brain, but their relative rarity explains the low incidence of these neoplasms in large series of patients with brain metastases. Patients with brain metastases from nonpulmonary primaries have a 70% incidence of lung metastases. Although many physicians presume that all brain metastases are multiple, in fact, half are single and many are potentially amenable to focal therapies.

Epidemiology

Gender There is a slight predominance of primary brain tumors in men.

Age Primary brain tumors have a bimodal distribution, with a small peak in the pediatric population and a steady increase in incidence with age, beginning at age 20 years and reaching a maximum of 20 cases per 100,000 population between the ages of 75 and 84 years.

Etiology and risk factors

The cause of primary brain tumors is unknown, although genetic and environmental factors may contribute to their development.

Genetic factors Clear heritable factors play a minor role in the genesis of primary brain tumors; less than 5% of patients with glioma have a family history of brain tumor. Several inherited diseases, such as tuberous sclerosis, neurofibromatosis type I, Turcot syndrome, and Li-Fraumeni cancer syndrome, predispose patients to the development of gliomas. However, these tumors tend to occur in children or young adults and do not account for the majority of gliomas that appear in later life.

Loss of heterozygosity (LOH) on chromosomes 9p and 10q and p16 deletions are frequently observed in high-grade gliomas, with low-grade gliomas having the fewest molecular abnormalities. In oligodendrogliomas, 1p and 19q LOH is associated with significantly improved survival.

Molecular markers One of the most useful markers, the epigenetic silencing of the MGMT (06-methylguanine-DNA methyltransferase) DNA-repair gene by promoter methylation is an independent prognostic factor in patients with glioblastoma and has been associated with longer survival in patients who received the alkylating agent temozolomide. Molecular markers of brain tumors can predict survival and will become increasingly important in the diagnosis and treatment of glioma.

Environmental factors Prior cranial irradiation is the only well-established risk factor for intracranial neoplasms.

Lifestyle characteristics Brain tumors are not associated with lifestyle characteristics such as cigarette smoking, alcohol intake, or cellular phone use.

Signs and symptoms

Brain tumors produce both nonspecific and specific signs and symptoms.

Nonspecific symptoms include headaches, which occur in about half of patients but are rarely an isolated finding of intracranial tumors, and nausea and vomiting, which are caused by an increase in intracranial pressure. Because of the widespread availability of CT and MRI, papilledema is now seen in < 10% of patients, even when symptoms of raised intracranial pressure are present.

Specific signs and symptoms are usually referable to the particular intracranial location of the tumor and are similar to the signs and symptoms of other intracranial space-occupying masses.

Lateralizing signs, including hemiparesis, aphasia, and visual-field deficits, are present in ~50% of patients with primary and metastatic brain tumors.

Seizures are a common presenting symptom, occurring in ~25% of patients with high-grade gliomas, at least 50% of patients with low-grade tumors, and 50% of patients with metastases from melanoma, perhaps due to their hemorrhagic nature. Otherwise, seizures are the presenting symptom in 15% to 20%

of patients with brain metastases. Seizures may be generalized, partial, or focal.

Stroke-like presentation Hemorrhage into a tumor may present like a stroke, although the accompanying headache and alteration of consciousness usually suggest an intracranial hemorrhage rather than an infarct. Hemorrhage is usually associated with high-grade gliomas, occurring in 5% to 8% of patients with glioblastoma multiforme. However, oligodendrogliomas have a propensity to bleed, and hemorrhage occurs in 7% to 14% of these low-grade neoplasms. Sudden visual loss and fatigue may be seen with bleeding into or infarction of pituitary tumors, termed *pituitary apoplexy*.

Altered mental status Approximately 75% of patients with brain metastases, and as many as half of patients with malignant gliomas, have impairment of consciousness or cognitive function. Some patients with multiple bilateral brain metastases may present with an altered sensorium as the only manifestation of metastatic disease; this finding can be easily confused with metabolic encephalopathy.

Screening for metastatic brain tumors

Screening for brain metastases is performed in only a few clinical situations.

Lung cancer Approximately 10% of patients with small-cell lung cancer (SCLC) have brain metastases at diagnosis, and an additional 20% to 25% develop such metastases during their illness. Therefore, cranial CT or MRI is performed as part of the initial evaluation for extent of disease.

Occasionally, patients with non–small-cell lung cancer (NSCLC) undergo routine cranial CT or MRI prior to definitive thoracotomy, since the presence of brain metastases may influence the choice of thoracic surgical procedure. This approach is particularly valuable in patients with suspected stage IIB or III disease for whom thoracotomy is considered following neoadjuvant therapy.

Diagnosis

Radiographic appearance of primary lesions

MRI The diagnosis of a brain tumor is best made by cranial MRI. This should be the first test obtained in a patient with signs or symptoms suggestive of an intracranial mass. MRI is superior to CT and should always be obtained with and without contrast material such as gadolinium (Figure 1).

High-grade or malignant primary brain tumors appear as contrast-enhancing mass lesions that arise in white matter and are surrounded by edema (Figure 2). Multifocal malignant gliomas are seen in ~5% of patients.

Low-grade gliomas typically are nonenhancing lesions that diffusely infiltrate and tend to involve a large region of the brain. Low-grade gliomas are usually best appreciated on T2-weighted or fluid-attenuated inversion recovery (FLAIR) MRI scans (Figure 3).

CT A contrast-enhanced CT scan may be used if MRI is unavailable or the patient cannot undergo MRI (eg, because of a pacemaker). CT is adequate to exclude brain metastases in most patients, but it can miss low-grade tumors or small lesions located in the posterior fossa. Tumor calcification is often better appreciated on CT than on MRI.

PET Body positron emission tomography (PET) scans performed for staging of systemic malignancies have a sensitivity of only 75% and a specificity of 83% for identification of cerebral metastases. Therefore, they are less accurate than MRI, which remains the gold standard.

Radiographic appearance of metastatic lesions On CT or MRI, most brain metastases are enhancing lesions surrounded by edema, which extends into the white matter (Figure 1). Unlike primary brain tumors, metastatic lesions rarely involve the corpus callosum or cross the midline.

The radiographic appearance of brain metastases is nonspecific and may mimic other processes, such as infection. Therefore, the CT or MRI scan must always be interpreted within the context of the clinical picture of the individual patient, particularly since cancer patients are vulnerable to opportunistic CNS infections or may develop second primaries, which can include primary brain tumors.

Other imaging tools Magnetic resonance spectroscopy and perfusion imaging can help differentiate low-grade from high-grade brain tumors but cannot distinguish different tumor types of the same grade.

FIGURE 1: Gadolinium-enhanced MRI scan demonstrating multiple brain metastases. Note the edema surrounding each lesion.

FIGURE 2: T1-weighted MRI with gadolinium contrast showing a typical appearance of a glioblastoma multiforme. Non–contrast-enhanced images of this lesion (not shown) revealed the presence of some hemorrhage.

Pathology

Glial tumors arise from astrocytes, oligodendrocytes, or their precursors and exist along a spectrum of malignancy. The astrocytic tumors are graded, using the four-tier World Health Organization (WHO) system. Grade I tumors are localized tumors called pilocytic astrocytomas, which are usually found in children and may be associated with neurofibromatosis type I. Grade II tumors are low-grade diffuse fibrillary astrocytomas. Grade III (anaplastic astrocytoma) and IV (gliobastoma) tumors are high-grade malignant neoplasms. Grading is based on pathologic features, such as endothelial proliferation, cellular pleomorphism, mitoses, and necrosis. The oligodendroglial neoplasms are classified as either the low-grade oligodendroglioma (grade II) or the anaplastic oligodendroglioma (grade III).

Low-grade glial tumors (such as astrocytoma and oligodendroglioma) and mixed neuronal-glial tumors (such as ganglioglioma) grow slowly but have a propensity to transform into malignant neoplasms over time. Transformation is usually associated with progressive neurologic symptoms and the appearance of enhancement on MRI.

The high-grade gliomas include glioblastoma, gliosarcoma, anaplastic astrocytoma, and anaplastic oligodendroglioma. These tumors are extremely invasive, with tumor cells often found up to 4 cm away from the primary tumor.

FIGURE 3: T2-weighted MRI demonstrating a diffusely infiltrating, low-grade oligodendroglioma involving the left frontal and temporal lobes. This lesion did not enhance with gadolinium.

Ependymomas Intracranial ependymomas are relatively rare, accounting for < 2% of all brain tumors. They are most frequently seen in the posterior fossa or spinal cord, although they may also arise in the supratentorial compartment. Ependymomas are typically low grade histologically, but their high rate of recurrence indicates malignant behavior.

Medulloblastomas are uncommon in adults but are one of the two most common primary brain tumors in children (the other being cerebellar astrocytomas). Medulloblastomas arise in the cerebellum and are always high-grade neoplasms.

Primitive neuroectodermal tumors (PNETs) are high-grade, aggressive tumors that usually occur in children. They include pineoblastoma and neuroblastoma. Histologically, they are identical to medulloblastomas, but their prognosis is usually worse than that for medulloblastomas. Thus, their biology is different, even though they may be similar pathologically.

Extra-axial tumors The most common extra-axial tumor is the meningioma. Meningiomas are usually benign tumors that arise from residual mesenchymal cells in the meninges. They produce neurologic symptoms by compressing the underlying brain. Meningiomas rarely are malignant or invade brain tissue.

Other common extra-axial tumors include pituitary adenoma, epidermoid or dermoid tumors, and acoustic neuroma (vestibular schwannoma). Most extra-axial tumors have a benign histology but can be locally invasive. Many extra-axial benign tumors are incidentally identified on MRI imaging performed for non-specific symptoms such as headache. Most of these tumors do not require therapy and do not enlarge. Many benign extra-axial tumors identified in this way can be observed with serial imaging studies alone.

Metastatic brain tumors The pathology of metastatic brain lesions recapitulates the pathology of the underlying primary neoplasm. This feature often enables the pathologist to suggest the primary source in patients whose systemic cancer presents as brain metastasis. However, even after a complete systemic evaluation, the site of the primary tumor remains unknown in 5% to 13% of patients with brain metastases.

Staging and prognosis

Staging is not applicable to most primary brain tumors because they are locally invasive and do not spread to regional lymph nodes or distant organs. Staging with an enhanced complete spinal MRI and cerebrospinal fluid (CSF) evaluation is important for a few primary tumor types, such as medulloblastoma, ependymoma, and PNET, because they can disseminate via the CSF. All systemic cancers are stage IV when they present with brain metastasis.

Prognostic factors For patients with primary brain tumors, prognosis is inversely related to several important factors, including pathologic grade and patient age, and is directly related to the overall clinical condition at diagnosis. Several molecular markers that correlate well with prognosis have been identified recently, such as LOH on chromosomes 1p and 19q in anaplastic oligodendroglioma.

With conventional treatment, including surgical resection, radiotherapy, and chemotherapy, median survival is 3 years for patients with an anaplastic astrocytoma and 1 year for those with glioblastoma multiforme. In a population of patients with low-grade tumors, including astrocytoma and oligodendroglioma, median survival is 5 to 10 years; most of these individuals die of malignant transformation of their original tumor. Patients with low-grade oligodendroglioma can survive a median of 16 years in some series. Patients ≥ 40 years old with low-grade glioma generally have a more aggressive disease; their median survival is usually < 5 years. Prognosis for patients with low-grade tumors is significantly better than for those with malignant tumors, with > 80% of patients experiencing long-term survival.

For a large proportion of patients with brain metastases, median survival is only 4 to 6 months after whole-brain radiotherapy. However, some patients (ie, those who are < 60 years old, have a single lesion, or have controlled or controllable systemic disease) can achieve prolonged survival, and these individuals warrant a more aggressive therapeutic approach. Furthermore, most of these patients qualify for vigorous local therapy for their brain metastases, such as surgical resection or, possibly, stereotactic radiosurgery. These approaches can achieve a median survival of 40 weeks or longer.

Treatment

Treatment of primary brain tumors and brain metastases consists of both supportive and definitive therapies.

SUPPORTIVE THERAPY

Supportive treatment focuses on relieving symptoms and improving the patient's neurologic function. The primary supportive agents are anticonvulsants and corticosteroids.

Anticonvulsants

Anticonvulsants are administered to ~25% of patients who have a seizure at presentation. Phenytoin (300–400 mg/d) is the most commonly used medication, but carbamazepine (Tegretol [600–1,000 mg/d]), phenobarbital (90–150 mg/d), and valproic acid (750–1,500 mg/d) are equally efficacious. Doses of all these anticonvulsants can be titrated to the appropriate serum levels to provide maximal protection.

Newer anticonvulsants, such as levetiracetam (Keppra), gabapentin, lamotrigine (Lamictal), and topiramate (Topamax), are also effective. Most of these agents have the advantages of causing few cognitive side effects, and because they do not induce the hepatic microsomal system, they do not alter the metabolism of chemotherapeutic agents. These agents are replacing the older drugs as first-line antiepileptic therapy.

Prophylaxis Prospective studies have failed to show the efficacy of prophylactic anticonvulsants for patients with brain tumors who have not had a seizure. Consequently, prophylactic anticonvulsants should not be administered, except during the perioperative period, when their use may reduce the incidence of postoperative seizures; the drugs can be tapered off within 2 weeks of surgery. Increasingly, the new agents are being used for prophylaxis.

Corticosteroids

Corticosteroids reduce peritumoral edema, diminishing mass effect and lowering intracranial pressure. This effect produces prompt relief of headache and improvement of lateralizing signs. Dexamethasone is the corticosteroid of choice because of its minimal mineralocorticoid activity. The starting dose is ~16 mg/d, but this dose is adjusted upward or downward to reach the minimum dose necessary to control neurologic symptoms.

Long-term corticosteroid use is associated with hypertension, diabetes mellitus, a nonketotic hyperosmolar state, myopathy, weight gain, insomnia, and osteoporosis. Thus, the steroid dose in patients with a brain tumor should be tapered as rapidly as possible once definitive treatment has begun. Most patients can stop taking steroids by the time they have completed cranial irradiation. All patients taking corticosteroids for more than 6 weeks should be on antibiotic prophylaxis for *Pneumocystis carinii* pneumonia. Prophylaxis should continue for 1 month after the steroids have been discontinued.

DEFINITIVE THERAPY: PRIMARY BRAIN TUMORS

Definitive treatment of brain tumors includes surgery, radiation therapy, and chemotherapy. The first step is to devise an overall therapeutic plan that should outline the sequence and elements of multidisciplinary therapy.

Surgery

Various surgical options are available, and the surgical approach should be carefully chosen to maximize tumor resection while preserving vital brain structures and minimizing the risk of postoperative neurologic deficits. The goals of surgery include (1) obtaining an accurate histologic diagnosis; (2) reducing tumor burden and associated mass effect caused by the tumor and/or peritumoral edema; (3) maintaining or re-establishing pathways for CSF flow; (4) achieving a potential "cure" by gross total removal; and (5) reducing tumor burden prior to adjuvant irradiation or chemotherapy. Surgery for a primary brain tumor rarely achieves cure but can reduce tumor burden so that the tumor becomes more amenable to adjuvant irradiation or chemotherapy.

Surgical tools A variety of tools are available to help the neurosurgeon achieve these goals, including stereotactic and image-based guidance systems and electrophysiologic brain mapping.

Stereotactic frames provide a rigid, three-dimensional (3D) coordinate system for accurate targeting of brain lesions identified on CT or MRI scans and are particularly well suited for obtaining tissue for biopsy from tumors located in deep structures or in other sites where aggressive tissue removal would produce unacceptable neurologic deficits. A limitation of stereotactic biopsy is that small volumes of tissue are obtained, and tissue sampling errors may result in failure to reach a correct diagnosis. Stereotactic biopsy may be nondiagnostic in 3% to 8% of cases and has a surgical morbidity of approximately 5%.

Image-based guidance system "Frameless" or "image-guided" stereotactic systems use computer technology to coregister preoperative imaging studies with intraoperative head position, thereby establishing stereotactic accuracy without the need for a frame. These systems are useful for stereotactic biopsy or achieving maximal resections of predefined tumor volumes and minimizing surgical morbidity. Intraoperative MRI accomplishes similar goals but is limited by a requirement for specialized operating suites.

Intraoperative brain mapping, also termed cortical mapping, uses electrical stimulation of the cortical surface to define the primary motor, sensory, or speech cortex. By identifying the exact location of these areas prior to tumor resection, the surgeon can avoid these structures, thereby preserving neurologic function. These tools enable the neurosurgeon to perform more complete removal of tumors with less morbidity.

Pathology-based surgical approach for primary brain tumors The surgical approach to an intracranial lesion is strongly influenced by the suspected or previously confirmed pathology. Guidelines for the management of the most common tumors are discussed.

Meningiomas and other extra-axial tumors Benign extra-axial tumors, such as meningiomas, usually have a well-defined plane separating them from the surrounding brain parenchyma. In general, total extirpation can be achieved by open craniotomy, particularly when the tumor is located over the convexity. Firm attachment of the tumor to the dura, cranial nerves, vascular structures, or skull base may make this impossible. Subtotal resections that preserve neural or vascular structures while reducing mass effect are often favored for extensive skull base tumors.

The surgical management of other benign extra-axial tumors, such as acoustic neuroma, pineocytoma, choroid plexus papilloma, and pituitary adenoma, closely parallels that of meningiomas. Gross total resection is generally curative and should be attempted whenever safe.

Low-grade gliomas Gross total resection, whenever possible, is the goal of surgery for low-grade gliomas and mixed neuronal-glial tumors (eg, astrocytoma, oligodendroglioma, pilocytic astrocytoma, and ganglioglioma). Long-term survival is generally considered better in patients who have undergone a gross total resection than in those who have had a subtotal resection (5-year survival rates > 80% for gross total resection vs ~50% for subtotal resection).

If a radiographically proven gross total resection is attained, postoperative irradiation or chemotherapy can often be withheld until there is evidence of tumor progression (see section on "Radiation therapy"). If a postoperative scan reveals a small but surgically accessible residual lesion, immediate reoperation should be considered, particularly in children or in those with pilocytic astrocytomas (WHO grade I).

When low-grade tumors are found in patients with medically refractory chronic epilepsy, surgical management should be oriented toward curing the epilepsy, as well as achieving total tumor removal.

Ependymomas Gross total resection is the goal of surgery whenever possible for ependymomas. Because ependymomas arise in the ventricular system, they can disseminate in the CSF. Therefore, all patients should be assessed for subarachnoid metastases with complete cranial and spinal MRI performed with gadolinium.

High-grade gliomas More extensive resections improve the quality of life and neurologic function of patients with high-grade gliomas (glioblastoma, anaplastic astrocytoma, and anaplastic oligodendroglioma) by reducing mass effect, edema, and steroid dependence. Resection of > 98% of the tumor volume prolongs survival relative to subtotal or partial resections, but extensive subtotal resections do not appear to confer any survival advantage over biopsy alone or limited resection. For this reason, most neurosurgeons attempt to achieve maximal resection while minimizing the risk to critical areas of the brain.

Recurrent or progressive tumors When a brain tumor recurs or enlarges, reoperation is often necessary to reduce mass effect. Although rarely curative, these procedures can improve quality of life and modestly extend survival. In general, reoperation is not considered in patients with a Karnofsky performance status (KPS) score ≤ 60 or in those patients who are not candidates for adjuvant therapy following initial surgery. A recurrent tumor cannot be distinguished from radiation necrosis on routine MRI. Both disorders may cause severe mass effect and edema, and resection is the optimal treatment for both. However, PET or magnetic resonance spectroscopy (MRS) can often distinguish tumor from treatment effect.

Initial resection or reoperation followed by intracavitary or intraparenchymal administration of chemotherapy, immunotherapy, or liquid I-125 radiotherapy (GliaSite) is being explored but is still investigational. Carmustine (BiCNU)-impregnated wafers (Gliadel) are the only form of intracavitary chemotherapy currently approved by the US Food and Drug Administration (FDA) for glioblastoma.

Radiation therapy

Radiation therapy plays a central role in the treatment of brain tumors in adults. It is the most effective nonsurgical therapy for patients with malignant gliomas and also has an important role in the treatment of patients with low-grade gliomas and metastatic brain tumors.

Whole-brain vs partial-brain irradiation Whole-brain irradiation is reserved for multifocal lesions, lesions with significant subependymal or leptomeningeal involvement, and metastatic brain tumors. For the majority of patients with unifocal disease, limited-field treatment results in less morbidity and appears to produce equal, albeit poor, overall survival.

Intensity-modulated radiotherapy (IMRT) is an advanced technique to deliver high-precision radiotherapy to a tumor. Treatment is planned using 3D CT images to design a dose that will conform to the 3D shape of the tumor. Using multiple beams, a uniform dose of RT is delivered to the whole tumor while sparing normal tissues.

Radiation therapy for low-grade gliomas Retrospective studies suggest a limited radiation dose response in low-grade gliomas. However, selection bias may play a role in these studies.

Several recently completed randomized studies addressed the question of optimal timing and dose of radiotherapy in patients with low-grade gliomas. An American intergroup randomized trial compared 50.4 versus 64.8 Gy of radiation in patients with low-grade glioma. A European Organization for Research on the Treatment of Cancer (EORTC) trial compared 45.0 versus 59.4 Gy of radiation in patients with low-grade astrocytoma. Both studies confirmed the superiority or equivalent efficacy of the lower radiation dose.

A second EORTC trial tested immediate versus delayed radiotherapy in individuals with low-grade glioma. Although immediate radiotherapy significantly improved 5-year disease progression-free survival, overall survival was identical in the two treatment arms. Furthermore, quality of life was better in patients whose radiotherapy was deferred until clinical or radiographic disease progression was evident.

Recommended treatment approach for low-grade astrocytomas The role of postoperative radiotherapy in the management of incompletely resected low-grade astrocytomas has not been firmly established. However, based on the available data, the following principles appear reasonable:

- A complete surgical resection of hemispheric astrocytomas should be attempted.

- If a complete surgical resection has been attained, radiation therapy can be withheld until MRI or CT studies clearly indicate a recurrence that cannot be approached surgically.

- When a complete surgical resection is not performed, postoperative irradiation may be recommended, depending upon the patients' clinical condition. Patients with controlled seizures and no neurologic deficit can be followed and radiation therapy deferred until clinical or radiographic disease progression occurs. Patients with progressive neurologic dysfunction, such as language or cognitive difficulties, require immediate therapy. Astrocytomas must be treated with radiotherapy, but oligodendrogliomas or mixed gliomas may benefit from chemotherapy as initial treatment (see later in this chapter).

- Radiation therapy should be delivered, using a megavoltage machine, in 1.7- to 2.0-Gy daily fractions, to a total dose of about 50 Gy. The treatment fields should include the primary tumor volume only, as defined by MRI, and should not encompass the whole brain.

- In low-grade astrocytomas, radiation therapy can be expected to produce a 5-year survival rate of 50% and a 10-year survival rate of 20%. Patients with low-grade oligodendrogliomas survive even longer.

- Cognitive impairment may develop in long-term survivors of low-grade gliomas treated with radiotherapy.

Radiation therapy for high-grade gliomas An analysis of three studies of high-grade gliomas performed by the Brain Tumor Study Group (BTSG) showed that postoperative radiotherapy doses > 50 Gy were significantly better in improving survival than no postoperative treatment and that 60 Gy resulted in significantly prolonged survival compared with 50 Gy. Doses used in the American Intergroup protocol greater than 60 Gy resulted in competing morbidity.

Based on these data, involved-field radiotherapy to 60 Gy in 30 to 33 fractions is standard treatment for high-grade histologies; this amount corresponds to a dose just above the threshold for radionecrosis. About half of patients with anaplastic astrocytomas exhibit radiographic evidence of response following 60 Gy of radiation, compared with 25% of patients with glioblastoma. Complete radiographic response is rare in either case.

Alternatives to conventional radiotherapy

The results of standard radiation treatment in patients with malignant gliomas are poor. Patients with glioblastoma multiforme have a median survival of 9 to 12 months, whereas patients with anaplastic astrocytomas survive a median of 3 years. In an attempt to improve these poor results, a number of new approaches have been tried, including hyperfractionated radiotherapy (HFRT), focal dose escalation with interstitial brachytherapy, and radiosurgery, but none improves survival. Brachytherapy and HFRT have been abandoned.

Radionecrosis Both brachytherapy and stereotactic radiosurgery can induce focal radionecrosis. This complication produces symptoms of mass effect in about 50% of patients with malignant glioma, requiring resection to remove the necrotic debris. (Fewer than 5% of patients with other lesions [eg, brain metastases] require reoperation for radionecrosis.) Occasionally, treatment with corticosteroids can control the edema around the radionecrotic area, but often the patient becomes steroid-dependent, with all of the attendant complications of chronic steroid use. Radionecrosis can be a significant limitation of the focal radiotherapy techniques.

Additional radiotherapeutic approaches

A new technology has been developed to fill a surgical cavity with an inflatable balloon that contains radioactive iodine (GliaSite). The temporary source of radiation appears to increase local control without leading to radionecrosis.

Recommended approach for extra-axial tumors Surgery alone is curative in the vast majority of patients with benign tumors. However, in certain subsets of patients, postoperative radiotherapy may control further growth of these lesions.

Pituitary adenomas For hormonally inactive pituitary adenomas that persist or recur after surgery, 45 to 50 Gy is delivered in 25 to 28 fractions to the radiographic boundaries of the tumor. For Cushing disease and acromegaly, higher doses are required for biochemical remission. Coronal-enhanced MRI is critical for treatment planning, because CT often does not visualize the skull base and the entire extent of disease.

The most common indications for radiotherapy are invasion of the cavernous sinus or the suprasellar space and incomplete resection of macroadenomas (> 1.5 cm). Most pituitary lesions do not grow following radiotherapy, and hormonally active tumors usually demonstrate a hormonal response, with a reduction in hormone hypersecretion in 1 to 3 years. Following radiation therapy, 20% to 50% of patients develop panhypopituitarism, requiring hormone replacement therapy. Other significant complications (ie, damage to the visual apparatus) are rare today.

Older patients with newly diagnosed glioblastoma are often treated with an abbreviated radiotherapy regimen or none at all due to their poor prognosis. However, there are now definitive data that focal RT to 50 Gy gives a significantly longer survival (median, 29.1 weeks) than supportive care alone (median, 16.9 weeks) without deterioration in quality of life in patients 70 years of age or older *(Keime-Guibert F, Chinot O, Taillandier L, et al: N Engl J Med 356:1527-1535, 2007).*

Meningiomas are readily curable with complete surgical resection. However, base of skull lesions and lesions involving a patent venous sinus often cannot be resected completely. For some patients with these lesions, a course of post-operative radiotherapy is indicated. In general, 54 Gy is delivered in 30 fractions to the radiographic tumor region utilizing 3D treatment planning. Malignant meningiomas always require postoperative radiotherapy, even after gross total resection. Radiosurgery may also be useful in treating meningiomas, and doses of 13 to 18 Gy are associated with a high rate of control 10 years following therapy.

Acoustic neuroma has classically been considered a surgical disease. Following total resection, recurrence rates are < 5%. When only subtotal resection is possible, disease recurs in at least 60% of patients.

Radiosurgery has been used as an alternative to surgery for acoustic neuroma. Control rates of > 80% at 20 years have been reported. For patients with useful hearing prior to radiosurgery, that function is preserved in < 50%. After radiosurgery, 10% of patients experience facial weakness and 25%, trigeminal neuropathy. The risk of cranial neuropathies is related to the size of the lesion treated.

Chemotherapy

Malignant gliomas Chemotherapy has a limited but measurable benefit in the treatment of patients with malignant gliomas and temozolomide is the most active agent.

In a large phase III trial, patients with newly diagnosed glioblastoma were randomized to receive radiotherapy alone or radiotherapy with concurrently administered temozolomide (Temodar) followed by adjuvant temozolomide. A total of 573 patients were studied, and median survival was significantly prolonged from 12.1 months to 14.6 months with the addition of temozolomide to radiotherapy. The 2-year survival rate was only 10.4% in those treated with radiotherapy alone compared with 26.5% in those who received radiotherapy plus temozolomide. The combined-modality regimen was well tolerated and associated with minimal additional toxicity. This regimen has now become the standard for all newly diagnosed patients with glioblastoma and combines the potential radiosensitizing effect of concurrent temozolomide with the benefit of adjuvant chemotherapy.

This study demonstrates clear benefit in patients with glioblastoma, and many investigators have extrapolated this regimen for use in patients with gliomas of all grades. This regimen is currently under study in patients with grade III glioma. The current practice is to adopt combined-modality therapy for patients with malignant gliomas.

Despite initial treatment, virtually all malignant gliomas recur. At relapse, patients may benefit from re-resection or different chemotherapeutic agents. Most patients will have received temozolomide as part of initial therapy, so procarbazine (Matulane) or a nitrosourea would be a reasonable conventional choice at recurrence. Hydroxyurea and imatinib (Gleevec) may also provide durable antitumor activity in some patients. Clinical trials employing signal transduction inhibitors, or epidermal growth factor receptor inhibitors, may also be available at tumor relapse, but initial results have been disappointing. Current studies are using multitargeted approaches to enhance efficacy.

There has been considerable interest in the potential use of antiangiogenic agents in malignant gliomas. Thalidomide (Thalomid) is a weak antiangiogenic drug and as a single agent, it has produced few responses, but stable disease was seen in one-third of patients. Data on bevacizumab (Avastin) and chemotherapy in patients with recurrent malignant glioma demonstrate a 60% response rate with prolonged survival. This has become standard second-line treatment for many patients if the agents are available. There has been no increase in intratumoral hemorrhage with the antiangiogenic agents, which makes them safe for use in patients with malignant gliomas.

Astrocytomas Chemotherapy has no role in the initial treatment of low-grade astrocytomas, and often they have progressed to malignant tumors at the time of recurrence.

Oligodendroglioma In contrast, the oligodendroglioma is now recognized as a particularly chemosensitive primary brain tumor. This finding was first observed with the anaplastic oligodendroglioma but has recently been seen with the more common low-grade oligodendroglioma. Chemosensitivity of anaplastic and low-grade tumors is associated with loss of chromosomes 1p and 19q.

Several alkylating agents are active, but the best studied regimen is procarbazine, lomustine (CeeNu), and vincristine (PCV), which produces response rates of 75% and 90% in malignant and low-grade oligodendrogliomas, respectively. PCV is an active regimen but has largely been supplanted by temozolomide because of the significant myelosuppression, neuropathy, and asthenia associated with PCV. Consequently, chemotherapy is an important therapeutic modality and may be used as initial treatment in patients with low-grade tumors who require therapeutic intervention. This approach defers or eliminates the late cognitive toxicity associated with cranial irradiation in patients with low-grade tumors who can have relatively prolonged survival. Patients with malignant oligodendrogliomas require radiotherapy with or without chemotherapy for initial treatment.

Temozolomide has activity against recurrent brain metastases, particularly from NSCLC and melanoma.

DEFINITIVE THERAPY: BRAIN METASTASES

Surgery

Surgical approach for metastatic tumors Most patients with brain metastases have a life expectancy of < 6 months, but the majority who undergo resection of a metastatic lesion followed by irradiation will die of systemic rather than intracranial disease.

Excision of metastatic brain tumors is rarely curative, however, as microscopic cells may be left behind. Nevertheless, the reduced tumor burden becomes more amenable to adjuvant irradiation and/or chemotherapy.

Criteria The decision whether to recommend surgery for metastatic brain tumors should be based on the following factors:

Extracranial oncologic status A comprehensive work-up of the patient's extracranial oncologic status is necessary. Extensive critical organ metastases preclude surgery in favor of palliative irradiation as the sole therapy. Brain surgery should not be performed in patients with limited expected survival (3 to 6 weeks) based on extracranial disease.

Number of metastases In general, only patients harboring a single metastasis are considered for resection. Occasionally, a large tumor will be removed in the presence of multiple smaller nodules if the edema and mass effect of this lesion are causing a substantial neurologic deficit that could be improved by tumor removal.

If brain metastasis is the presenting sign of systemic cancer and no clear primary source can be identified with routine staging, surgery may also be required to establish a tissue diagnosis and plan further therapy.

In addition, surgical removal of a brain metastasis often reverses the neurologic deficits caused by compression of local structures by tumor and reduces intracranial hypertension.

Three studies have concluded that when multiple (up to three distinct locations) metastases are resected, either with or without radiotherapy, survival times are identical to those in patients with a surgically resected single metastasis and almost twice as long as those in patients treated by radiation therapy or radiosurgery alone. These studies suggest that a more aggressive surgical approach may be justified in patients with multiple brain metastases who have stable systemic disease.

Recurrence of solitary metastases Up to 20% of single metastases may recur in long-term survivors. In these cases, a second operation may be warranted to remove the recurrent lesion and confirm the histologic diagnosis (ie, exclude radionecrosis).

Radiotherapy

Radiation therapy for metastatic brain tumors For symptomatic patients with brain metastases, median survival is about 1 month if untreated and 3 to 6 months if whole-brain radiation therapy is delivered, with no significant differences among various conventional radiotherapy fractionation schemes (20 Gy in 5 fractions, 30 Gy in 10 fractions, 40 Gy in 20 fractions). A more protracted schedule is used for patients who have limited or no evidence of systemic disease or for those who have undergone resection of a single brain metastasis, since these patients have the potential for long-term survival or even cure. The use of hypofractionated regimens is associated with an increased risk of neurologic toxicity.

The addition of the radiosensitizer motexafin gadolinium to whole-brain radiotherapy (130 Gy) did not improve survival or time to neurologic disease progression in a randomized phase III trial. Subgroup analysis suggested prolonged time to neurocognitive disease progression in patients with brain metastases from lung cancer.

Relief of neurologic symptoms The major result of whole-brain radiation therapy is an improvement in neurologic symptoms, such as headache, motor loss, and impaired mentation. The overall response rate ranges from 70% to 90%. Unfortunately, symptomatic relief is not permanent, and symptoms recur with intracranial tumor progression.

Multiple lesions Patients with multiple lesions are generally treated with whole-brain radiation therapy alone. Retreatment with a second course of whole-brain radiation therapy can provide further palliation for patients with progressive brain metastases (who have at least a 6-month or longer remission of symptoms after the initial course of cranial irradiation).

Concomitant steroid therapy Since the radiographic and clinical responses to whole-brain irradiation take several weeks, patients with significant mass effect should be treated with steroids during whole-brain radiation therapy. Dexamethasone (16 mg/d) is started prior to therapy, and the dose may be tapered as tolerated during treatment. Occasionally, higher doses are necessary to ameliorate neurologic symptoms. However, most patients can be safely tapered off corticosteroids at the completion of whole-brain radiotherapy.

Radiosurgery for metastatic brain tumors

In patients with one to three brain metastases, aggressive local therapy (surgical resection or radiosurgery) produces superior survival and quality of life compared with whole-brain radiation therapy alone. Radiosurgery may be the optimal choice for elderly patients at greater risk for surgical morbidity. Radiosurgery has been used as sole therapy, as a boost to whole-brain radiation therapy, or for recurrent lesions in patients with brain metastases. Radiosurgery has the advantage of delivering effective focal treatment, usually in a single dose, without irradiating the normal brain. Radiosurgery of brain metastases $\leq$ 1 cm achieves 1- and 2-year local control rates of 86% and 78%, respectively, significantly better than 56% and 24% for lesions $>$ 1 cm. It is particularly useful for patients who have one to three lesions, each $<$ 4 cm in diameter. Patients with numerous lesions are not good candidates for radiosurgery because some of the ports may overlap, and, more importantly, these patients likely harbor other microscopic lesions in the brain that are not being treated effectively with such focal therapy.

Brain metastases are particularly amenable to treatment with radiosurgery. Metastatic tumors do not infiltrate the brain and tend to have well-circumscribed borders; therefore, they can be targeted effectively with highly focused irradiation techniques that maintain a sharp delineation between the enhancing tumor seen on neuroimaging and normal brain. Furthermore, radiosurgery

Bevacizumab combined with irinotecan was well tolerated in 32 patients with recurrent malignant glioma. Response rate was 63% and median progression-free survival was 24 weeks (Vredenburgh JJ, Desjardins A, Herndon JE 2nd, et al: *Clin Cancer Res* 13:1253-1259, 2007).

does not have the operative morbidity that may be associated with resection of a brain metastasis. Consequently, it can be used safely in many patients who are not surgical candidates, and it can even treat lesions in surgically unapproachable locations such as the brainstem.

Radiosurgery can achieve crude local control rates of 73% to 98% over a median follow-up of 5 to 26 months. Radiosurgery was initially used as a boost after treatment with whole-brain radiotherapy. Three randomized trials have reported on the value of radiosurgery in addition to whole-brain radiotherapy for patients with multiple brain metastases. Although all three studies show a local control advantage and an improvement in quality-of-life endpoints with the addition of a radiosurgery boost, none shows a statistical advantage in survival. For patients with multiple brain metastases, adding radiosurgery to whole-brain radiotherapy only offers an improved neurologic quality of life with no impact on survival.

A prospective, randomized RTOG trial compared whole-brain radiotherapy alone versus whole-brain radiotherapy plus radiosurgery in patients with one to three metastases. Local control, neurologic function, and steroid doses were improved in patients with a single lesion treated with radiosurgery. Although there was no statistical improvement in overall survival in the two arms of the trial, a subset analysis showed improved survival for those patients with a single lesion.

Radiosurgery is often considered an alternative to standard surgical resection, but it is unclear whether they are equivalent. Most retrospective studies suggest that the two techniques produce similar results; however, some reports indicate that surgery offers improved local control, whereas others suggest that radiosurgery is superior.

Increasingly, radiosurgery is being used as sole therapy for one to three brain metastases. A prospective randomized trial compared radiosurgery with or without whole-brain radiotherapy in patients with one to four brain metastases. Results were similar to those of the phase III trial of surgical resection of a single brain metastasis with or without radiotherapy: improved local control but no survival benefit. Therefore, whole-brain radiotherapy reduced CNS relapse but had no impact on survival.

Median survival from the time of radiosurgery is 6 to 15 months, and some patients can live for years without recurrence. Most patients exhibit clinical improvement and decreased steroid requirement after radiosurgery, and only 11% to 25% of patients eventually die of neurologic causes.

Chemotherapy

Metastatic brain tumors Chemotherapy usually has a limited role in the treatment of brain metastases and has not proven to be effective as an adjuvant therapy after irradiation or surgery. However, it may have some efficacy in patients with recurrent brain metastases who are not eligible for further whole-brain radiation therapy or stereotactic radiosurgery. In addition, chemotherapy has proven active in patients with asymptomatic brain metastases, discovered on screening neuroimaging who are scheduled to receive chemotherapy for their systemic disease. We have seen patients with brain metastases from a variety of primary tumors respond in this situation. A recent phase III trial of chemotherapy with early versus delayed whole-brain radiotherapy in NSCLC patients with brain metastases showed an identical intracranial response rate and survival. Thus, systemic chemotherapy had some efficacy against brain metastases.

A recently completed phase II trial of temozolomide (75mg/m2/d) and concurrent whole-brain radiotherapy (40 Gy in 20 fractions) versus whole-brain radiotherapy alone demonstrated improved response rates and neurologic improvement in the combined-modality arm. In addition, there is growing recognition that systemic chemotherapy can be effective against brain metastases when the drugs are selected based on the primary tumor. Capecitabine (Xeloda) is effective against brain metastases from breast cancer. High-dose methotrexate has activity against a number of primaries.

> Newly diagnosed patients with anaplastic oligodendroglioma were randomized to receive radiotherapy alone vs preradiotherapy PCV (procarbazine, lomustine [CeeNu], and vincristine) followed by radiotherapy. Preradiotherapy PCV prolonged progression-free survival (1.7 yrs vs 2.6 yrs; P = .004) but did not affect survival. PCV was associated with grade 3/4 toxicity in 65% of patients (*Cairncross G, Berkey B, Shaw E, et al: J Clin Oncol 24:2707-2714, 2006*).

Temozolomide has activity against recurrent brain metastases, particularly from NSCLC and melanoma.

SUGGESTED READING

ON PRIMARY INTRACRANIAL TUMORS

Abrey LE, Louis DN, Paleologos N, et al: Survey of treatment recommendations for anaplastic oligodendroglioma. Neuro Oncol 9:314–318, 2007.

Chang SM, Parney IF, Huang W, et al: Patterns of care for adults with newly diagnosed malignant glioma. JAMA 293:557–564, 2005.

Correa DD: Cognitive functions in brain tumor patients. Hematol Oncol Clin North Am 20:1363–1376, 2006.

Kaloshi G, Benouaich-Amiel A, Diakite F, et al: Temozolomide for low-grade gliomas: Predictive impact of 1p/19q loss on response and outcome. Neurology 68:1831–1836, 2007.

Keime-Guibert F, Chinot O, Taillandier L, et al: Radiotherapy for glioblastoma in the elderly. N Engl J Med 356:1527–1535, 2007.

Liau LM, Prins RM, Kiertscher SM, et al: Dendritic cell vaccination in glioblastoma patients induces systemic and intracranial T-cell responses modulated by the local central nervous system tumor microenvironment. Clin Cancer Res 11:5515–5525, 2005.

Park I, Tamai G, Lee MC, et al: Pattern of recurrence analysis in newly diagnosed glioblastoma multiforme after three-dimensional conformal radiation therapy with respect to pre-radiation therapy magnetic resonance spectroscopic findings. Int J Radiat Oncol Biol Phys 69:381–389, 2007.

Pope WB, Lai A, Nghiemphu P, et al: MRI in patients with high-grade gliomas treated with bevacizumab and chemotherapy. Neurology 66:1258–1260, 2006.

Reardon DA, Egorin MJ, Quinn JA, et al: Phase II study of imatinib mesylate plus hydroxyurea in adults with recurrent glioblastoma multiforme. J Clin Oncol 23:9359–9368, 2005.

Reijneveld JC, van der Grond J, Ramos LM, et al: Proton MRS imaging in the follow-up of patients with suspected low-grade gliomas. Neuroradiology 47:887–891, 2005.

Stupp R, Mason WP, van den Bent MJ, et al: Radiotherapy plus concomitant and adjuvant temozolomide for glioblastoma. N Engl J Med 352:987–996, 2005.

Tsao MN, Mehta MP, Whelan TJ, et al: The American Society for Therapeutic Radiology and Oncology (ASTRO) evidence-based review of the role of radiosurgery for malignant glioma. Int J Radiat Oncol Biol Phys 63:47–55, 2005.

ON PRIMARY EXTRA-AXIAL TUMORS

Yang SY, Park CK, Park SH, et al: Atypical and anaplastic meningiomas: Prognostic implication of clinicopathological features. J Neurol Neurosurg Psychiatry Aug 31; [Epub ahead of print] 2007.

ON METASTATIC BRAIN TUMORS

Aoyama H, Shirato H, Tago M, et al: Stereotactic radiosurgery plus whole-brain radiation therapy vs stereotactic radiosurgery alone for treatment of brain metastases: A randomized controlled trial. JAMA 295:2483–2491, 2006.

Aoyama H, Tago M, Kato N, et al: Neurocognitive function of patients with brain metastasis who received either whole brain radiotherapy plus stereotactic radiosurgery or radiosurgery alone. Int J Radiat Oncol Biol Phys 68:1388–1395, 2007.

Eichler AF, Loeffler JS: Multidisciplinary management of brain metastases. Oncologist 12:884–898, 2007.

Ekenel M, Hormigo AM, Peak S, et al: Capecitabine therapy of central nervous system metastases from breast cancer. J Neurooncol 85:223–227, 2007.

Mehta MP, Tsao MN, Whelan TJ, et al: The American Society for Therapeutic Radiology and Oncology (ASTRO) evidence-based review of the role of radiosurgery for brain metastases. Int J Radiat Oncol Biol Phys 63:37–46, 2005.

Ohashi K, Kiura K, Takigawa N, et al: Radiation necrosis mimicking progressive brain metastasis in a patient with non-small cell lung cancer. J Thorac Oncol 2:762–763, 2007.

Pan M, Santamaria M, Wollman DB: CNS response after erlotinib therapy in a patient with metastatic NSCLC with an EGFR mutation. Nat Clin Pract Oncol 4:603–607, 2007.

Varlotto JM, Flickinger JC, Niranjan A, et al: The impact of whole-brain radiation therapy on the long-term control and morbidity of patients surviving more than one year after gamma knife radiosurgery for brain metastases. Int J Radiat Oncol Biol Phys 62:1125–1132, 2005.

Vredenburgh JJ, Desjardins A, Herndon JE 2nd, et al: Phase II trial of bevacizumab and irinotecan in recurrent malignant glioma. Clin Cancer Res 13:1253–1259, 2007.

CHAPTER 27

AIDS-related malignancies

Ronald T. Mitsuyasu, MD, and Jay S. Cooper, MD

Malignancies have been detected in approximately 40% of all patients with acquired immunodeficiency syndrome (AIDS) sometime during the course of their illness. These cancers have been both a primary cause of death in some patients and also a source of considerable morbidity. In the current era of protease inhibitors and highly active antiretroviral therapy (HAART), patients infected with the human immunodeficiency virus (HIV) are surviving longer than ever. HAART appears to have substantially reduced the incidence of Kaposi's sarcoma (KS) and non-Hodgkin lymphoma (NHL) and may enhance the efficacy of treatment for those patients who do develop these tumors. Unfortunately, HAART has not shown a similar effect on the development of other types of neoplasms, and caring for patients who develop malignancies in the setting of HIV remains a challenge. Furthermore, HAART is not available universally, with many patients in resource-poor developing countries not having access to antiretroviral drugs.

In a multicenter national study of causes of death among HIV-infected adults in France in 2005, the proportion of underlying causes of death due to AIDS decreased (36% in 2005 vs 47% in 2000) and the proportion of cancer not related to AIDS or hepatitis increased (17% vs 11%), such that cancer was the second leading cause of death among HIV patients in 2005 (ANRS EN19 and Mortavic). Similar findings of cancer being the most frequent non-AIDS-defining cause of death has been reported from Australia and the United States (Lewden C, May T, Rosenthal E, et al: J Acquir Immune Defic Syndr 48:590-598, 2008; Petoumenos K, Law MG: Sex Health 3:103-12, 2006; Palella FJ Jr, Baker RK, Moorman AC, et al: J Acquir Immune Defic Syndr 43:27-34, 2006).

KAPOSI'S SARCOMA

KS has been the most common tumor associated with HIV infection, but it currently develops in < 10% of homosexual men with AIDS in the United States and in 1% to 2% of other HIV-infected persons. The incidence of KS has declined substantially, from 4.8 per 100 person-years in 1990 to 1.5 per 100 person-years in 1997. In 2003, a European study found that the incidence of KS among HIV-infected individuals was less than 10% of the incidence seen a decade earlier in 1994.

Epidemiology

Gender Among AIDS patients in the United States, the incidence of KS is higher in males than in females. There is also a higher incidence of KS in men than in women in Africa (male-female ratio, 2:1), despite the equal prevalence of HIV infection among men and women.

Age The age distribution of AIDS-related KS follows the distribution of HIV infection. As such, AIDS-related KS can occur in all age groups. In American adult males, the most common age of onset of AIDS-related KS is 30 to 40 years old. No peak age has been reported.

Race No racial or ethnic differences in the incidence of AIDS-related KS have been observed.

Geography In the United States, KS is seen in < 10% of homosexual men with AIDS. The proportion of KS among AIDS-defining diagnoses is lower in parts of Europe, where there are proportionately fewer male homosexual AIDS cases (eg, 6.8% of Italian AIDS patients), and higher in parts of Africa, where KS is endemic in the non–HIV-infected population. Among AIDS cases in the United States, the proportion of patients with KS has declined from the beginning of the AIDS epidemic, possibly as a result of changes in high-risk sexual behavior among homosexual men and the wider use of more effective antiretroviral combination regimens.

Etiology and risk factors

Viruses In 1994, unique viral DNA sequences were identified in tumor tissues from patients with AIDS-related KS, which led to the identification of a new virus called KS-associated herpesvirus (KSHV) or human herpesvirus type 8 (HHV-8). HHV-8 has been found in > 90% of AIDS-KS tumors, as well as in classic KS, endemic African KS, and post–organ transplant-related KS. It has also been identified in body cavity–based lymphoma/primary effusion lymphoma, multicentric Castleman's disease, and angio-immunoblastic lymphadenopathy with dysproteinemia (AILD) in HIV-infected patients.

HHV-8 may be transmitted through sexual contact, blood products, or organ transplantation. The seroprevalence of HHV-8 in AIDS-related KS is nearly 100%. HHV-8 has been found in high concentration in saliva in patients with KS.

HHV-8 is critical in the pathogenesis of AIDS-related KS. The mechanism by which HHV-8 induces KS in susceptible individuals is the subject of intense current investigations.

Environmental and host factors Various environmental and host factors, including HIV- and HHV-8–induced cytokines, AIDS-associated infections, the host's hormonal milieu, immunosuppression, and antiretroviral therapy, may induce or suppress the development of KS and alter its growth.

Signs and symptoms

The manifestations of KS in patients with AIDS are variable and range from small innocuous-looking cutaneous lesions to symptom-producing visceral or oral lesions, which may be troublesome and even life-threatening. Although just about every internal organ can occasionally be involved with KS, it is rarely seen in the bone marrow or CNS.

Skin lesions KS tumors typically begin as flat or raised lesions that may progress to plaque-like or nodular tumors. Lesions vary in size and shape but are generally nonpruritic and painless. They range in color from light pink to red to deep purple. KS lesions may be cosmetically disfiguring and may result in social stigmatization that far exceeds any actual physical impairment.

Dermal and lymphatic infiltration with tumor can result in edema of the extremities, periorbital areas, and genitals and may be complicated by skin breakdown and bacterial cellulitis. Edema can be marked and may prevent patients from wearing shoes and/or walking.

Lesions on the feet can cause pain and hamper walking.

Oral lesions are often asymptomatic but can produce pain and swallowing difficulties.

GI tract involvement with KS is seen in up to 50% of patients. Most lesions are asymptomatic; however, obstruction, bleeding, or enteropathy can occur occasionally.

Pulmonary KS usually presents as dyspnea without fever and may become severely debilitating and rapidly fatal if untreated.

Screening and diagnosis

Currently, there are no screening tests for KS. Although most KS lesions are readily recognized, early lesions may be difficult to diagnose, and the lesions of other diseases (eg, bacillary angiomatosis) may mimic those of KS. Once clinically suspected, the diagnosis of KS is made by biopsy and histologic examination of skin lesions, an excised lymph node, or other tissue or by presumptive diagnosis based on the bronchoscopic or endoscopic appearance of a visceral lesion. Staining for HHV8 antigen in biopsy specimen can confirm diagnosis of KS.

GI KS has a typical red, raised appearance and is difficult to diagnose by biopsy because of the submucosal location of many lesions.

Pulmonary KS In patients with pulmonary KS, chest radiographs typically demonstrate diffuse, reticular-nodular infiltrates, mediastinal enlargement, and, sometimes, pleural effusion. Bronchoscopy may reveal extensive endobronchial involvement with tumor. Definitive diagnosis requires transbronchial or open-lung biopsy. Transbronchial biopsies, however, often yield negative results. A presumptive diagnosis of pulmonary KS may be made, in the absence of fever, based on typical radiographic and endobronchial findings of KS-appearing lesions and after the exclusion of infections.

Thallium and technetium-99m scanning may help differentiate KS from other pulmonary diseases. Patients with KS have been found to have thallium– and technetium–avid scans, whereas pulmonary lymphomas and infections are more typically gallium–avid.

Pathology

Cutaneous KS is a lesion of the dermis composed of a proliferation of aberrant vascular structures lined by abnormal-appearing, spindle-shaped endothelial cells and with extravasated erythrocytes and leukocytes within the structures. These spindle cells are generally sparse in early stages but become more numerous and "stack up" between the vascular structures as the tumor advances. Infiltration of mononuclear leukocytes, including plasma cells, T cells, and monocytes, is more prominent in earlier lesions. The histologic appearance of KS in AIDS patients is similar to that seen in non–HIV-infected patients.

Cell of origin The KS tumor cell is believed to be of mesenchymal, endothelial origin. Several endothelial cell markers are positive in KS, including stains for CD31, CD34, and EN-4. In addition, the tumor stains with factor VIIIa, CD68, and α-actin but not with PAL-E.

Staging and prognosis

Prognostic factors Although it is difficult to predict from the initial presentation which patients are most likely to have rapidly progressive tumors, several retrospective studies have shown a correlation of survival with the degree of T-cell immunodeficiency, as reflected in the absolute number of T-helper cells. Prior opportunistic infections or the presence of such symptoms as fevers, night sweats, and weight loss (B symptoms) also portend a poor prognosis. Patients who develop KS or whose tumor growth accelerates after an opportunistic infection often have a more aggressive clinical course. Patients with pulmonary involvement generally have a poor prognosis.

Staging system A tumor classification system has been proposed for AIDS-related KS by the oncology committee of the AIDS Clinical Trials Group (ACTG). This system segregates patients into good or poor prognostic groups based on tumor characteristics, immune system function, and systemic illness (the TIS system; see Table 1). A retrospective analysis of 294 patients with AIDS-related KS has shown that the TIS system is a valid predictor for survival.

Gauging response to therapy Given the heterogeneity and unpredictable growth of this tumor, it is often difficult to gauge objective responses. The peculiarities of this multicentric tumor make some subjectivity almost inevitable in gauging treatment responses.

Treatment

The treatment of AIDS-related KS requires an individualized approach, based on the extent and location of the lesions, the wishes and treatment needs of the patient, the presence of tumor-associated symptoms (eg, pain, bleeding, edema), the presence of other AIDS-associated illnesses, and the patient's tolerance of medications. Nevertheless, the following general statements can be made:

- Patients with widespread symptomatic disease or life-threatening visceral involvement require prompt, cytoreductive treatment with one or more chemotherapeutic drugs.

- Even in the absence of symptomatic visceral disease, the disfigurement and emotional distress of having these visible reminders of AIDS may mandate treatment for psychological reasons.

- For patients with asymptomatic indolent lesions, aggressive treatment is not mandatory, but these patients may derive substantial benefits from local treatment or investigational therapies that are directed against HIV or HHV-8 or that may interrupt the pathogenesis of KS and/or restore immune competence.

Treatment options

With the introduction of protease inhibitors and non-nucleoside reverse transcriptase inhibitors for HIV, cases of KS regression with combination antiretroviral therapy have been reported. Because KS seems to be influenced by the state of HIV infection, we believe that all patients with AIDS-related KS should have their HIV infection under optimal control. There is no one best anti-HIV regimen, and oncologists should consult with infectious disease specialists familiar with the treatment of HIV infection. Occasionally, a flare in KS tumor progression may be seen when antiretroviral therapy is initiated. Eventually, even with good anti-HIV therapy, many patients with AIDS-related KS

TABLE 1: Staging classification for AIDS-related KS[a]

Characteristic	Risk status	
	Good risk (0)	Poor risk (1)
	All of the following:	Any of the following:
Tumor (T)	Tumor confined to skin and/or lymph nodes and/or minimal oral disease[b]	Tumor-associated edema or ulceration; extensive oral KS; GI KS; KS in other non-nodal viscera
Immune system (I)	CD4 cells $\geq 150/\mu L$	CD4 cells $< 150/\mu L$
Systemic illness (S)	No history of opportunistic infection or thrush; no B symptoms[c]; performance status ≥ 70 (Karnofsky scale)	History of opportunistic infection and/or thrush; B symptoms; performance status < 70 (Karnofsky scale); other HIV-related illness (eg, neurologic disease, lymphoma)

Adapted from Krown SE, Metroka C, Wernz JC: J Clin Oncol 7:1201, 1989, as modified by Krown SE, et al: J Clin Oncol 15:3085, 1997.

[a] Patients are assigned a disease state TXIXSX, where X corresponds to the risk designation (0 or 1) for each risk category.

[b] Minimal oral disease is non-nodular KS confined to the palate.

[c] B symptoms: unexplained fever, night sweats, > 10% involuntary weight loss, or diarrhea persisting for more than 2 weeks.

will require some form of treatment for their tumor.

Local treatments, including cryotherapy, topical retinoic acid, intralesional chemotherapy and other sclerosing agents, and local irradiation, can produce good local control of tumors. Interferon-alfa (IFN-α [Intron A, Roferon-A]) and cytotoxic chemotherapy are effective systemic treatments for patients with more extensive or symptomatic disease. Single-agent or combination chemotherapy is effective in controlling tumors, even in patients with extensive disease and severe immune deficiencies (Table 2). The use of hematopoietic growth factors has facilitated the administration of myelosuppressive treatments, such as IFN-α and chemotherapy.

IFN-α

The first treatment licensed for AIDS-related KS was recombinant IFN-α. Tumor responses have been seen in approximately 30% of patients treated with SC interferon given either daily or 3 times weekly. Current practice is to administer IFN-α 3 times weekly by SC injection. Unmaintained response durations in trials of IFN-α monotherapy have ranged from 12 to 24 months in complete responders and from 8 to 12 months in partial responders.

Duration of therapy The optimal duration of IFN-α treatment is unknown; however, many patients relapse within a few months after discontinuation of therapy. Reinduction of second responses with IFN-α after relapse may be unreliable and often is of short duration. It is therefore generally recommended that treatment with IFN-α be continued for as long as drug tolerance and tumor responses continue.

Dose The optimal dose of IFN-α also has not been clearly established. IFN-α is generally administered at either 3 or 5 million units SC 3 times weekly together with antiretroviral therapy.

Major dose-limiting toxicities of IFN-α include fever, chills, rigor, and other flu-like symptoms. They are dose-related and often observed at the initiation of treatment but lessen somewhat with continued use. Neutropenia, elevation of transaminase levels, depression, peripheral neuropathy, and other neuropsychiatric abnormalities may also occur.

Other side effects include headaches, cognitive impairments, paresthesias, and mild thrombocytopenia. As the subjective side effects of IFN-α are also common in HIV-related or other conditions, care must be taken to avoid ascribing all of these symptoms to drug toxicity and overlooking treatable infections and other conditions.

Retinoids

Alitretinoin gel 0.1% (9-*cis*-retinoic acid [Panretin]) has received approval of the US Food and Drug Administration (FDA) for the topical treatment of localized cutaneous KS. This compound inhibits the growth of KS and induces apoptosis of KS cells by binding to retinoic acid receptors on the cell surface.

Phase II clinical trials comparing 3 to 4 times daily application of alitretinoin versus placebo gel demonstrated a 35% rate of complete and partial responses in the alitretinoin-treated patients, as compared with a rate of 18% in controls.

The median time to response to alitretinoin was 29 to 34 days, with a median duration of response of 12 to 16 weeks. Responses were seen in both previously untreated and previously treated KS patients and were not dependent on patients' CD4 cell count.

Local cutaneous adverse reactions to alitretinoin include erythema, skin irritation, skin cracking, flaking, peeling, and desquamation. The severity of these reactions can be mitigated by less frequent dosing, thinner application, or use of topical vitamin E.

Alitretinoin should be reserved for patients who do not require systemic treatment for visceral disease. However, it may be used in conjunction with other treatments for cutaneous disease.

Oral alitretinoin has been investigated in patients with AIDS-related KS and found to have a 37% response rate.

Bexarotene (Targretin), an oral retinoid X receptor (RXR)-selective agonist, has been studied in patients with AIDS-related KS, with an overall response rate of 33% in one study.

TABLE 2: Chemotherapy for AIDS-related KS

Regimen	Dose	Response rate[a] (%)
Vincristine	2 mg/wk IV	20-60
Vinblastine	0.05-0.1 mg/kg/wk IV	25-30
Doxorubicin	20 mg/m^2 IV every other wk	50-60
Etoposide	150 mg/m^2 IV every d × 3 q3-4wk	75
Vinorelbine	30 mg/m^2 IV q2wk	47
Liposomal daunorubicin	40 mg/m^2 IV q2-4wk	25-70
Liposomal doxorubicin	20 mg/m^2 IV q2-4wk	58-63
Paclitaxel	100-135 mg/m^2 IV over 3 h q2-4 wk	60-72
Irinotecan	150 mg/m^2 IV days 1-10	75
Vincristine + vinblastine	2 mg IV vincristine alternating with 0.1 mg/kg IV vinblastine every other wk	45
Vincristine + bleomycin	2 mg IV vincristine + 10 mg/m^2 IV bleomycin q2wk	23-70
Doxorubicin + bleomycin + vincristine	10 mg/m^2 IV doxorubicin + 10 mg/m^2 IV bleomycin + 1-2 mg IV vincristine q2wk	87

[a] Complete responses plus partial responses

Chemotherapy

For patients with more widely disseminated, rapidly progressive, or symptomatic disease, systemic chemotherapy is generally warranted. Chemotherapy drugs are included in Table 2.

Antiretroviral drugs A total of 21 anti-HIV drugs have received FDA approval, and more are in various stages of clinical development. When evaluated by an oncologist, the majority of HIV-infected individuals will be taking some anti-HIV drugs. The interactions between cytotoxic chemotherapy and the various anti-HIV drugs have not been fully studied. Thus, oncologists treating patients with AIDS-related KS should continue to monitor them frequently for side effects. Withholding antiretroviral therapy during chemotherapy and then immediately restarting it after giving the chemotherapy drugs may avoid some toxic effects of drug interactions, especially with high-dose therapy.

Combination regimens The two most frequently utilized combination chemotherapy regimens are Adriamycin (doxorubicin), bleomycin, and vincristine (ABV) and bleomycin and vincristine (BV). These regimens were initially reported to yield tumor response rates in excess of 70% to 90%, with good palliation of symptoms, including decreased edema, decreased pain, and, in patients with pulmonary KS, respiratory improvement and alleviation of obstructive symptoms. A beneficial effect of these combinations on survival has not been clearly demonstrated, however.

Early reports of a high response rate with these combination regimens have not been reproduced by later multicenter trials. A conservative response rate of 50% to 60% has been reported in more contemporary phase III trials. The discrepancy in response rates most likely stems from differences in the response criteria used.

Liposomal anthracyclines (eg, liposomal doxorubicin [Doxil] and liposomal daunorubicin [DaunoXome]) are also effective in inducing tumor regression in KS. Clinical trials have shown that liposomal anthracyclines as single agents can achieve a response rate equal to or better than that obtained with the ABV (Adriamycin [doxorubicin], bleomycin, vinblastin) combination regimen. As such, the liposomal anthracyclines have become first-line chemotherapy for AIDS-related KS.

The dose-limiting toxicity is neutropenia, and many patients will require the use of granulocyte colony-stimulating factor (G-CSF, filgrastim [Neupogen]) after several cycles of treatment. Other common side effects include nausea, fatigue, anemia, and thrombocytopenia. A palmar-plantar syndrome, characterized by acute painful erythematous swelling of the hands and feet, has been reported with the use of liposomal doxorubicin. Once the symptoms resolved, readministration of liposomal doxorubicin did not necessarily reproduce the syndrome. Neither of the liposomal anthracyclines has been reported to depress left ventricular function.

Paclitaxel has been shown to produce responses in both chemotherapy-naive KS patients and patients with refractory tumors, including those refractory to liposomal anthracyclines. The dosage is typically 100 to 135 mg/m^2 IV given over 3 hours every 2 to 4 weeks. This agent is widely considered the primary second-line chemotherapy for KS.

The dose-limiting toxicity is neutropenia. Other reported toxicities include anemia, stomatitis, alopecia, and fatigue. Neuropathy has not been a major problem with this low-dose approach.

Investigational agents Other drugs under investigation for the treatment of KS include Col-3 and other antiangiogenesis compounds. Compounds that may affect HHV-8 gene expression (eg, valproic acid) or signal transduction pathways in KS-infected cells (eg, imatinib [Gleevec] and sunitinib) and m-Tor inhibitor (eg rapamycin) are also in development or in early clinical testing in KS patients. Cidofovir (Vistide) does not appear to be clinically active.

Radiation therapy

Although radiation therapy can easily produce sufficient regression of KS to be useful for palliation of symptomatic disease or cosmetic improvement of disfiguring lesions, this practice has become less common as HAART has changed the natural history of AIDS. More than 90% of lesions will respond (complete responses [CRs] and partial responses [PRs]). Local radiation therapy commonly alleviates pain and bleeding, lessens edema, and shrinks obstructing lesions.

Treatment technique For most superficial lesions, a single, shaped, en face beam of relatively limited penetration (approximately 100 kV) works well. A relatively low-energy electron beam (eg, 6 MeV) often can be used with shielding as an alternative to superficial x-rays.

Large lesions For large lesions, electron beams are used more often, due to the limited penetration of kilovoltage x-ray beams and the limited width of the treatment cones attached to most superficial x-ray units. For patients with more widespread tumors of the legs with edema, parallel opposed megavoltage x-ray beams and overlying bolus material are often used to provide homogeneous irradiation to the entire area.

Dose fractionation regimens Several dose fractionation regimens have proven effective in AIDS-related KS. As this tumor is radiosensitive, almost any dose of radiation therapy can produce some response. Interestingly, in vitro irradiation of KS cell cultures induces the cells to produce interleukin-6 (IL-6) and oncostatin M (OSM), which, in turn, make the cells more sensitive to radiation therapy.

For most cutaneous lesions, a single treatment of 800 cGy will produce a short-term response. For lesions on sensitive structures (eg, penis, hands, conjunctivae), some radiation oncologists attenuate treatment to a total dose of 2,000 cGy administered in 300 cGy increments (accepting a 50% decrease in CR rate), whereas 3,000 cGy delivered over 2 weeks is more typically used for lesions in general.

Prospectively acquired data clearly demonstrate a dose-response relationship for radiation therapy in AIDS-related KS. A dose of 4,000 cGy delivered in 20 fractions over 4 weeks was significantly more effective than 2,000 cGy in 10 fractions or 800 cGy in 1 fraction, as measured by a higher response rate, longer duration of tumor control, and the absence of residual hyperpigmentation. However, the short- and medium-term effects of moderately intense but briefer regimens, such as 3,000 cGy in 10 fractions over 2 weeks, probably are equivalent to those of higher total dose, more protracted regimens, and the moderately intense regimens require only half the time to deliver.

For patients with an anticipated survival of < 3 months, in whom the response duration may be of less overall importance, a single fraction of 800 cGy is likely to provide the same benefit as the more intensive regimens. In contrast, small lesions in patients who are expected to survive for at least 1 year should be treated with fractionated radiation therapy, such as 3,000 cGy in 10 fractions over 2 weeks.

NON-HODGKIN LYMPHOMA

The incidence of NHL is 60 times higher in individuals with HIV infection than in the general population. The overall occurrence of lymphoma as a manifestation of AIDS has declined somewhat as treatment of HIV has improved.

Although NHL currently comprises < 5% of all initial AIDS-defining conditions, it accounts for as many as 28% of all AIDS-related deaths. The majority of patients present with advanced-stage, high- or intermediate-grade, B-cell lymphoma and have a high frequency of extranodal involvement. Primary CNS lymphoma occurs in approximately 0.5% of patients with AIDS.

The majority of patients with AIDS-related lymphoma have advanced HIV disease. Median CD4 cell counts in patients with systemic lymphoma range from 100 to 200 cells/mm^3, although NHL can occur at any CD4 count.

Epidemiology

At-risk groups NHL occurs with approximately equal frequency in all population groups infected by HIV, including IV drug users, homosexual-bisexual men, transfusion recipients, and patients with hemophilia.

Gender and race AIDS-related NHL is seen more frequently in men than in women and occurs more often in whites than in blacks.

Age The age distribution of AIDS-related NHL follows the distribution of HIV infection. Primary CNS lymphoma occurs with the same frequency in all age groups.

Geography Current data do not indicate any geographic differences in the incidence of AIDS-related NHL.

Etiology and risk factors

AIDS-related NHL is believed to arise as a consequence of continued stimulation of B-cell proliferation as a result of HIV, Epstein-Barr virus (EBV), and other infections, all of which occur in the setting of profound T-cell immunodeficiency. An association between the polyomavirus, simian virus 40 (SV40), and diffuse large B-cell and follicle-type lymphoma has been detected. HIV also induces the expression of a number of cytokines (eg, IL-6 and IL-10) that can further increase B-cell activation.

Small noncleaved lymphomas Genetic errors are increased in the setting of chronic B-cell proliferation, and a variety of chromosomal translocations resulting in oncogene activation can lead to polyclonal and monoclonal B-cell expression. Other molecular biological abnormalities associated with small noncleaved lymphomas include expression of an abnormal *TP53* (alias *p53*) tumor-suppressor gene and the c-*myc* or *ras* oncogene.

Immunoblastic lymphoma The pathogenesis of AIDS-related immunoblastic lymphoma appears to be distinct from that of small noncleaved lymphoma and is more likely related to EBV infection without c-*myc* dysregulation. Clonal integration of EBV within tumor cells, with expression of various latent EBV proteins, has been demonstrated in essentially all cases of AIDS-related primary CNS lymphoma and in as many as two-thirds of systemic lymphomas.

Diffuse large cell lymphoma The specific molecular aberrations described in patients with AIDS-related diffuse large cell lymphoma appear distinct as well, with recent descriptions of abnormal *bcl*-6 expression in approximately 40% of cases.

Body cavity–based lymphoma/primary effusion lymphoma appears to be highly associated with HHV-8 and EBV. The tumor cells stain positive for CD45. The disease appears to occur predominantly in males and may coexist with KS in patients with AIDS.

Signs and symptoms

B symptoms (ie, fever, weight loss, and night sweats) are seen in approximately 80% of patients with systemic AIDS-related NHL. In these patients, it is mandatory to exclude the presence of occult opportunistic infections before ascribing B symptoms to the lymphoma itself.

Extranodal involvement Advanced-stage disease is expected in the majority of patients, with extranodal involvement reported in 60% to 90% of patients in most series. Common sites of extranodal involvement include the CNS (occurring in approximately 30% of patients), GI tract (25%), and bone marrow (25%). Essentially any other site in the body can also be involved, including the rectum, soft tissue, oral cavity, lungs, and heart.

CNS lymphoma Patients with primary CNS lymphoma often present with focal neurologic deficits, seizures, and/or altered mental status. Any site in the brain may be involved, and one to four space-occupying lesions are usually seen on MRI or CT scan.

Other sites Changes in bowel habits, GI bleeding, weight loss, pain, and hepatomegaly are common presenting symptoms in patients with GI involvement. Pancytopenia may indicate bone marrow involvement.

Primary effusion lymphoma Patients usually present with pleural or pericardial effusion without an identifiable mass. Pain, shortness of breath, and B symptoms are the main initial complaints.

Screening and diagnosis

Diagnosis of NHL in patients with AIDS requires histologic confirmation by biopsy with immunophenotypic and/or molecular gene-rearrangement studies.

A complete staging evaluation should be done. This should include:

- CT or MRI of the head
- PET/CT scan of whole body
- bone marrow aspiration and biopsy
- liver function studies
- spinal fluid analysis.

Assessing spinal fluid for EBV The presence of EBV DNA in cerebrospinal fluid, as determined by polymerase chain reaction (PCR), appears to have a high specificity and sensitivity for the diagnosis of primary CNS lymphoma.

Pathology

Common tumor types Over 95% of AIDS-related NHL cases are of B-lymphocyte origin. Most AIDS-related NHL tumors are high-grade types, including the immunoblastic and small noncleaved lymphomas. Diffuse large cell lymphoma constitutes up to 30% of AIDS lymphomas.

Less common tumor types Although not considered part of the AIDS epidemic, several cases of T-cell lymphoma occurring in HIV-infected patients have been described. In addition, cases of Ki-1–positive, large cell anaplastic lymphoma and plasmablastic lymphoma have been reported in HIV-infected patients. The clinical and pathologic characteristics of these forms of lymphoma are similar to those seen in non–HIV-infected individuals.

CNS lymphomas are typically of the immunoblastic or large cell type.

GI and oral cavity lymphomas Large cell or immunoblastic lymphomas are also more likely to involve the GI tract and oral cavity than are small noncleaved lymphomas.

Primary effusion lymphomas The cells are large and pleomorphic with prominent nucleoli and immunoblastic morphology. Clonal immunoglobulin DNA rearrangement demonstrates clonality of the tumor cells but not surface immunoglobulin expression.

Staging and prognosis

Staging system Staging of AIDS-related NHL is the same as that for non–AIDS-related NHL. The Ann Arbor classification system for staging of NHL is utilized (see chapter 30), and the staging work-up includes imaging studies, as well as bone marrow and CNS evaluation for lymphomas.

Prognostic factors Five factors have been shown to correlate most closely with a shorter survival in patients with systemic AIDS-related NHL:

- a history of opportunistic infection prior to the lymphoma
- CD4 cell count < 100 cells/μL
- International Prognostic Index (IPI) score
- Karnofsky performance score < 70
- stage IV disease, especially if due to bone marrow or meningeal involvement.

In patients without these findings, the median survival is typically 11 to 12 months, as compared with a median survival of approximately 4 to 5 months in those with one or more of these adverse prognostic features.

Three factors correlate with *better* survival in patients with primary CNS lymphoma:

- Karnofsky performance score > 70
- age < 35 years
- adequate dose of radiation therapy.

Type of lymphoma To date, no major differences have been seen in response or survival among the various pathologic types of systemic AIDS-related NHL. Patients with polyclonal lymphomas appear to have better tumor responses to chemotherapy and better survival. Patients with primary CNS lymphoma have an extremely poor prognosis, with a median survival of only 2 to 3 months despite therapy; treatment with potent antiretroviral therapy does seem to improve survival. The prognosis for patients with primary effusion lymphoma is also poor, with a median survival of only 5 months.

Treatment

TREATMENT OF SYSTEMIC NHL

Chemotherapy

The mainstay of treatment for patients with systemic AIDS-related NHL is chemotherapy. As the likelihood of tumor dissemination is great, AIDS patients who develop NHL must be assumed to have widespread disease at presentation and should be treated with systemic chemotherapy, even if tumor dissemination is not confirmed on routine staging evaluation.

Some of the commonly used regimens designed for AIDS-related NHL are listed in Table 3. No regimen appears to be superior to any other, although early findings show that the EPOCH regimen (etoposide, prednisone, Oncovin [vincristine], cyclophosphamide, doxorubicin) gives the best results to date.

TABLE 3: Chemotherapy for AIDS-related NHL

Regimen	Drugs and dosage	Cycle length	CR rate (%)	Median survival
m-BACOD	Methotrexate, 500 mg/m^2 IV on day 15, with leucovorin, 25 mg PO q6h × 4, after completion of methotrexate	q28d	41	35 wk
	Bleomycin, 4 U/m^2 IV on day 1			
	Adriamycin (doxorubicin), 25 mg/m^2 IV on day 1			
	Cyclophosphamide, 300 mg/m^2 IV on day 1			
	Oncovin (vincristine), 1.4 mg/m^2 IV on day 1 (maximum, 2 mg)			
	Dexamethasone, 3 mg/m^2 PO on days 1-5			
CDE	Cyclophosphamide, 800 mg/m^2/96 h IV	q28d	46	8.2 mo
	Doxorubicin, 50 mg/m^2/96 h IV			
	Etoposide, 240 mg/m^2/96 h IV			
R-EPOCH	Rituximab, 375 mg/m^2 IV day 1	q3-4wk	79	53 mo+
	Etoposide, 200 mg/m^2/96 h IV			
	Prednisone, 60 mg/m^2 PO on days 1-6			
	Oncovin (vincristine), 1.6 mg/m^2/96 h IV			
	Cyclophosphamide, 187 mg/m^2 IV on day 5 (if CD4 cell count < 100 cells/μL) or 375 mg/m^2 IV on day 5 (if CD4 cell count ≥ 100 cells/μL)*			
	Doxorubicin, 40 mg/m^2/96 h IV			
CEOP	Cyclophosphamide, 750 mg/m^2 IV on day 1	q3-4wk	47	10 mo
	Epirubicin, 50 mg/m^2 IV on day 1			
	Oncovin (vincristine), 2 mg IV on day 1			
	Prednisone, 100 mg PO on days 1-5			
R-CHOP	Rituximab, 375 mg/m^2 IV day 1	q21d	63	9 mo
	Cyclophosphamide, 750 mg/m^2 IV on day 1			
	Doxorubicin, 50 mg/m^2 IV on day 1			
	Oncovin (vincristine), 1.4 mg/m^2 IV on day 1 (maximum, 2 mg)			
	Prednisone, 60 mg PO on days 1-5			

CR = complete response
* With dose escalation as tolerated with each subsequent cycle, to a maximum of 750 mg/m^2

CNS prophylaxis with either intrathecal cytarabine (Ara-C; 50 mg) or intrathecal methotrexate (10–12 mg) every week for four treatments has been shown to be effective in reducing the incidence of CNS relapse.

In an Italian study, rituximab (Rituxan), an anti-CD 20 monoclonal antibody, also has been studied in combination with CDE (cyclophosphamide, doxorubicin, etoposide) at lower doses and has been shown to have an overall response rate of 86% and an actuarial 2-year survival rate of 80%.

Dose intensity Standard-dose chemotherapy (eg, CHOP [cyclophosphamide, doxorubicin, Oncovin, prednisone]) is generally recommended for most patients with AIDS-related NHL. Results from trials using continuous infusion therapy (eg, EPOCH or CDE) have shown better CR rates and long disease progression-free and overall survival.

Certain subsets of patients with high CD4 cell counts (> 100 cells/μL), no B symptoms, lower disease stage at presentation (stage I or II), and good performance status (0 or 1) may enjoy prolonged survival (> 2 years) when treated with either a standard-dose or intensive, high-dose regimen.

Growth factor and other support The major dose-limiting toxic effect of multiagent chemotherapy regimens is myelosuppression. Studies of m-BACOD (methotrexate with leucovorin, bleomycin, Adriamycin [doxorubicin], cyclophosphamide, Oncovin [vincristine], dexamethasone) or CHOP chemotherapy demonstrated that coadministration of myeloid hematopoietic growth factors enhanced patient tolerance of these regimens. In addition, prophylactic antibiotics with TMP/SMZ, azithromycin, fluconazole, valganciclovir and ciprofloxacin can also reduce the risk of infection during intensive chemotherapy and rituximab.

Salvage chemotherapy Patients in whom initial treatment fails or relapse occurs after initial remission rarely achieve a prolonged second remission. Studies of various salvage regimens with or without autologous stem-cell support have demonstrated some early promising results.

Second-line chemotherapy (eg, ESHAP [etoposide, methylprednisolone, high-dose Ara-C, Platinol (cisplatin)]) has been shown to produce a CR of up to 31% and a PR of 23%, with a median survival of 7.1 months, in patients with refractory or relapsed AIDS-related NHL.

Radiation therapy

The role of radiotherapy in systemic lymphoma is limited to consolidation of the effects of chemotherapy. Treatment principles are similar to those used for aggressive NHL in the non-HIV setting and typically involve the use of involved or extended fields only.

While previous studies initially suggested that rituximab may cause more infectious complications and greater mortality in the treatment of AIDS-NHL with chemotherapy, a recent study by the AIDS Malignancy Consortium (AMC 034) demonstrated that when rituximab is added either concomitantly or sequentially to EPOCH chemotherapy with HAART and prophylactic antibiotics, that CR rates of 53% to 69% can be achieved with few infectious complications and no increase in treatment related death (Levine AM, Lee J, Kaplan L et al: J Clin Oncol 26:[abstract 8527], 2008).

Lymphomatous meningitis For patients with lymphomatous meningitis and/or radiographically detectable cerebral deposits, "step-brain" irradiation (including the covering meninges) is administered along with intrathecal chemotherapy to control microscopic spinal disease. Focal radiation therapy may be required for known tumor deposits in the spine. Unfortunately, many such patients develop multiple deposits anywhere along the spinal axis, either synchronously or metachronously.

Fractionated doses of 3,000 to 4,500 cGy may be used to control local lymphoma deposits in nodal areas. Patients who have lymphomatous meningitis typically have a poor prognosis and are best treated with regimens that do not unduly occupy their time (eg, 3,000 cGy in 10 fractions over 2 weeks).

TREATMENT OF PRIMARY CNS LYMPHOMA

An effective therapy for patients with AIDS-related CNS lymphoma has not yet been found, although many AIDS oncologists find high dose methotrexate with leucovorin rescue more effective than radiation therapy.

Radiation therapy

The conventional standard of treatment is step-brain irradiation, which can result in response rates of 50% and improve survival, as compared with untreated patients, even when adjusted for antiretroviral therapy, CD4 cell count, and time to diagnosis. Treatment is directed to the entire cranial contents, including the meninges down to C2.

Doses equivalent to 3,900 cGy (or more) delivered at 200 cGy/fraction appear to be associated with increased survival. Better Karnofsky performance scores and younger age at the time of treatment are also associated with longer survival. Mean survival ranges from 2 to 6 months, with death often due to complicating opportunistic infections.

CERVICAL CARCINOMA

Cervical carcinoma in the setting of HIV infection has been recognized as an AIDS-defining malignancy since 1993. Unfortunately, in some women, cervical carcinoma may be the first indication that they have HIV infection.

Cervical intraepithelial neoplasia (CIN) is also seen in association with HIV infection. These premalignant lesions, also known as squamous intraepithelial lesions (SILs), may foretell a higher incidence of cervical carcinoma among HIV-infected women. SILs have been associated with human papillomavirus (HPV), particularly those subtypes with greater oncogenic potential, such as serotypes 16, 18, 31, 33, and 35.

Epidemiology

Prevalence of HIV infection and cervical abnormalities The risk of HIV infection in women with an abnormal Pap smear varies with the prevalence of HIV infection in the given population. Screening in clinics in high-prevalence areas has yielded HIV-positivity rates of between 6% and 7% (and up to 10% in parts of Africa). In such high-prevalence areas, among women younger than age 50 with cervical carcinoma, up to 19% of women were found to be HIV positive. HIV-positive women have up to a 10-fold increased risk of abnormal cervical cytology. Several centers have reported abnormal cytology rates of 30% to 60% in HIV-positive women and Pap smears consistent with cervical dysplasia in 15% to 40%. The prevalence of cervical dysplasia increases with declining CD4 cell counts in HIV-infected women.

Nationwide, invasive cervical carcinoma was found in 1.3% of women with AIDS. In New York, invasive cervical carcinoma constitutes 4% of AIDS-defining illnesses in women. Recent findings from linkage studies in the US and Italy clearly have shown increased rates of cervical cancer in women with HIV.

Race and geography The prevalence of invasive cervical carcinoma among American Hispanic and black women is lower than that in white women. However, this difference may stem from a difference in access to health care. The southern and northeastern sections of the United States have a higher reported number of cases of HIV-associated invasive cervical carcinoma.

Etiology and risk factors

The severe cellular immunodeficiency associated with advanced HIV infection may allow oncogenic viruses to flourish and may also compromise the body's immunologic defenses that control the development of these tumors.

HPV There is abundant evidence that HPV infection is related to malignant and premalignant neoplasia in the lower genital tract. HPV serotypes 16, 18, 31, 33, and 35 are the most oncogenic strains and have been associated with invasive cervical carcinoma and progressive dysplasia. The prevalence of cervical SILs among HIV-infected women may be as high as 20% to 30%, with many having higher cytologic and histologic grade lesions.

Signs and symptoms

The majority of cervical SILs are detected on routine cytologic evaluation of Pap smears in women with HIV infection.

Advanced invasive disease Postcoital bleeding with serosanguineous and/or foul-smelling vaginal discharge is usually the first symptom of more advanced invasive disease. Lumbosacral pain or urinary obstructive symptoms may indicate advanced disease.

Screening and diagnosis

Because the majority of patients with cervical dysplasia or early invasive cancer are asymptomatic, frequent cytologic screening of women at risk for HIV infection must be undertaken. The role of newly developed HPV vaccines in preventing HPV infection or disease progression in HIV-infected women has yet to be determined.

Screening of HIV-positive women Current screening recommendations call for women with HIV infection to have pelvic examinations and cytologic screening every 6 months. Pap smears indicating cervical SILs must be taken seriously, and abnormalities justify immediate colposcopy. Although abnormalities are sometimes missed by relying solely on cytologic screening, recommendations for routine colposcopy have not yet been established.

Screening of women with a history of cervical SILs For women who have a history of cervical SILs, more frequent reevaluation and cytologic screening should be undertaken. Since these women are at high risk for recurrence or development of lesions in other areas of the lower genital tract, post-therapy surveillance with repeat colposcopy also is warranted.

Work-up of women with invasive carcinoma For women with invasive carcinoma, complete staging should be undertaken; this should include pelvic examination, CT of the pelvis and abdomen, chest x-ray, and screening laboratory tests for hepatic and bone disease. In addition, full evaluation and treatment for HIV and related complications should be initiated.

Pathology

Squamous cell carcinoma Most cases of cervical carcinoma are of the squamous cell type.

Staging and prognosis

The staging classification for cervical carcinoma (see chapter 20), as adopted by the International Federation of Gynecology and Obstetrics (FIGO), also applies to AIDS patients.

Cervical dysplasia in HIV-infected women is often of higher cytologic and histologic grade. These women are more likely to have CIN II-III lesions with extensive cervical involvement, multisite (vagina, vulva, and anus) involvement, and endocervical lesions.

HIV-infected women with cervical carcinoma typically present with more advanced disease and appear to have a more aggressive clinical course. Tumors are typically high grade with a higher proportion of lymph node and visceral involvement at presentation. Mean time to recurrence after primary treatment is short, and many patients have persistent disease after primary therapy. The median time to death in one series was 10 months in HIV-infected women, as compared with 23 months in HIV-negative patients.

Treatment

TREATMENT OF PREINVASIVE DISEASE

Cryotherapy, laser therapy, cone biopsy, and loop electrosurgical excision procedure (LEEP) have all been used to treat preinvasive disease in HIV-infected patients. Short-term recurrence rates of 40% to 60% have been reported.

Determinants of recurrence Immune status of the patient seems to be the most important determining factor for recurrence. Close surveillance after initial therapy is critical, and repetitive treatment may be necessary to prevent progression to more invasive disease.

TREATMENT OF CERVICAL CARCINOMA

The same principles that guide oncologic management of the immunocompetent patient with cervical carcinoma (see chapter 20) are utilized in AIDS patients with this cancer.

Surgery can be undertaken for the usual indications, and surgical decisions should be based on oncologic appropriateness and not on HIV status.

Radiation therapy As most AIDS patients with cervical cancer present with advanced disease, radiation therapy is indicated more often than surgery. If the patient's overall physical condition permits, treatment regimens are identical to those used for the same stage disease in uninfected individuals (see chapter 20). It is important to note that the standard of care for advanced carcinoma of the cervix (stages III–IV, without hematogeneous dissemination) now includes a combination of irradiation and concurrent cisplatin-based chemotherapy. At present, there is insufficient evidence to suggest that irradiation or other treatments for cervical carcinoma in AIDS patients is any less effective than in similar non–HIV-infected individuals.

Chemotherapy regimens, such as cisplatin (50 mg/m^2) or carboplatin (200 mg/m^2), bleomycin (20 U/m^2; maximum, 30 U), and vincristine (1 mg/m^2), have been used in patients with metastatic or recurrent disease. Vigorous management of side effects and complications of these treatments and of AIDS itself must be provided.

ANAL CARCINOMA

Although anal carcinoma is not currently an AIDS-defining illness, the incidence of this tumor is increasing in the population at risk for HIV infection. The incidence of anal carcinoma in homosexual men in a San Francisco study was estimated at between 25 and 87 cases per 100,000, compared with 0.7 case per 100,000 in the entire male population.

Etiology and risk factors

HPV Precursor lesions of anal intraepithelial neoplasia (AIN), also known as anal SILs, have been found to be associated with HPV infection, typically with oncogenic serotypes, eg, types 16 and 18. Cytologic abnormalities occur in nearly 40% of patients, especially those with CD4 cell counts < 200 cells/μL. Abnormal cytology may predict the later development of invasive carcinoma.

Other STDs and sexual practices Individuals with a history of perianal herpes simplex, anal condylomas, or practice of anal-receptive behavior with multiple sexual partners are at higher risk of developing this tumor than those without such a history.

Signs and symptoms

Rectal pain, bleeding, discharge, and symptoms of obstruction or a mass lesion are the most frequent presenting symptoms.

Screening and diagnosis

Studies to evaluate the usefulness of anoscopy with frequent anal cytology have been undertaken to determine whether early detection of AIN may result in interventions that would prevent the development of invasive tumors.

Work-up of patients with anal carcinoma For patients with anal carcinoma, determination of the extent of local disease, as well as full staging for dissemination, should be undertaken (see chapter 16).

Pathology

Squamous cell carcinoma The majority of anal carcinomas are of the squamous cell type.

Histologic grading The grading for AIN is similar to that for CIN, with AIN-1 denoting low-grade dysplasia and AIN-2 and AIN-3, higher grade dysplastic lesions. The gross appearance of lesions on anoscopy does not predict histologic grade. Higher grade dysplastic lesions are seen in patients with lower CD4 cell counts.

Staging and prognosis

The staging of squamous cell carcinoma of the anus in HIV-infected individuals is the same as that in non–HIV-infected patients (see chapter 16). Patients with severe immunosuppression, ie, CD4 cell counts < 50 cells/μL, may present with more advanced, more aggressive disease. The true natural history of this tumor in the AIDS population has yet to be defined, however.

Treatment

TREATMENT OF AIN AND CARCINOMA IN SITU

Treatment of patients with local AIN is similar to that of women with CIN. Ablative therapy may be used.

TREATMENT OF INVASIVE ANAL SQUAMOUS CELL CARCINOMA

Anal cancer can be controlled with chemotherapy and radiation therapy despite HIV infection. However, patients who have low CD4 cell counts appear to be more likely to experience severe toxicity and to require colostomy for salvage therapy than those with higher CD4 cell counts. For patients with squamous cell carcinoma of the anus, chemotherapy with mitomycin (10 mg/m^2 on day 1) and fluorouracil (5-FU; 1,000 mg/m^2 by continuous infusion on days 1–4) combined with radiation therapy can produce high rates of complete remission.

Concomitant radiation therapy, 5-FU, and mitomycin have been reported to produce a CR in 9 of 11 patients with AIDS-associated invasive anal carcinoma (median CD4 cell count at diagnosis of 209 cells/μL) and a 60% 2-year actuarial survival rate. Two patients remain alive more than 8 years following treatment, but severe toxicity (three grade 3 hematologic, one grade 3 dermatologic, one grade 4, and one grade 5 gastrointestinal toxicity) and one death resulted from treatment.

Evidence appears to suggest that 5-FU plus cisplatin may be better tolerated than 5-FU plus mitomycin in HIV patients. Tolerance to treatment seen in patients who have relatively intact immune systems is similar to that seen in HIV-infected patients. The role of cetuximab (Erbitux) and other target therapies in this disease population also has not yet been determined. However, the appropriate dose of radiation therapy for patients with anal carcinoma in the context of HIV infection remains unsettled. Patients who are unable to tolerate chemoradiation therapy and those in whom treatment fails (defined as a positive biopsy after a CR) should be considered for abdominoperineal resection.

OTHER NON–AIDS-DEFINING MALIGNANCIES

A growing number of reports from around the world now indicate that other malignant tumors are occurring in HIV-infected individuals, including Hodgkin lymphoma (HL), nonmelanomatous skin cancers, lung cancer, germ-cell tumors, myeloid or lymphoid leukemias, multiple myeloma, renal cell carcinoma, head and neck cancer, brain tumors, squamous tumor of the conjunctiva, and leiomyosarcoma in pediatric patients.

Rates of other non–AIDS-defining cancers appear to be increasing among HIV-infected individuals. In an Australian cancer data base, 196 cases of non–AIDS-defining cancers were noted in 13,067 individuals (1.5%) among 8,351 HIV-infected-only patients and 8,118 patients with AIDS.

As HIV-infected individuals are surviving longer with currently available combination anti-HIV drugs, clinicians should anticipate seeing the development of more tumors in these patients. Greater vigilance for these tumors is warranted.

HL Studies showing a possible increased incidence of HL in HIV-infected individuals have been reported from Europe, Australia, and the United States. The most common histology is mixed cellularity and lymphocyte-depleted. Male predominance, a higher prevalence of B symptoms, and more extranodal disease on presentation are the main characteristics of HL in HIV patients.

Chemotherapy is recommended for this group of patients, due to the high proportion of stage III or IV disease. Standard treatments include ABVD (Adriamycin, bleomycin, vinblastine, and dacarbazine) or ABVD alternating with MOPP (mechlorethamine [Mustargen], Oncovin [vincristine], procarbazine [Matulane], and prednisone). More recently, early results with BEACOPP [bleomycin, etoposide, doxorubicin (Adriamycin), cyclophosphamide, Oncovin (vincristine), procarbazine, prednisone] and the Stanford V regimen look promising.

Nonmelanomatous skin cancers As in the general population, basal cell carcinoma is more common than squamous cell carcinoma in the setting of HIV infection. The risk factors for the development of these tumors are the same as in the general population: namely, fair skin, history of sun exposure, and family history.

Lung cancer Patients with HIV appear to have a higher relative risk of developing lung cancer than do age-matched controls (relative risk = 4.5; 95% confidence interval = 4.2–4.8). These tumors tend to present at later stages than do tumors with a similar histologic distribution in the general population.

Pediatric leiomyosarcoma Cases of aggressive leiomyosarcoma developing in HIV-positive children have been reported. Leiomyosarcoma is a rare tumor, occurring in < 2 cases per 10 million non–HIV-infected children. However, a much higher than expected frequency of leiomyosarcoma has been reported in HIV-infected children. Visceral sites are commonly involved, eg, the lungs, spleen, and GI tract.

SUGGESTED READING

ON KAPOSI'S SARCOMA

El Amari EB, Toutous-Trellu L, Gayet-Ageron A, et al: Predicting the evolution of Kaposi sarcoma, in the highly active antiretroviral therapy era. AIDS 22:1019–1028, 2008.

Franceschi S, Maso LD, Rickenbach M, et al: Kaposi sarcoma incidence in the Swiss HIV Cohort Study before and after highly active antiretroviral therapy. Br J Cancer 99:800–804, 2008.

Dittmer DP, Krown SE: Targeted therapy for Kaposi's sarcoma and Kaposi's sarcoma-associated herpesvirus. Curr Opin Oncol 19:452–457, 2007.

Spano JP, Costagliola D, Katlama C, et al: AIDS-related malignancies: State of the art and therapeutic challenges. J Clin Oncol 26:4834–4842, 2008.

Sullivan RJ, Pantanowitz L, Casper C, et al: HIV/AIDS: Epidemiology, pathophysiology and treatment of Kaposi sarcoma-associated herpes virus disease: Kaposi sarcoma, primary effusion lymphoma and multicentric Castleman disease. Clin Infect Dis 47:1209–1215, 2008.

ON NON-HODGKIN LYMPHOMA

Lewden C, May T, Rosenthal E, et al: Changes in causes of death among adults infected by HIV between 2000 and 2005: The "Mortalite 2000 and 2005" surveys (ANRS EN19 and Mortavic). J Acquir Immune Defic Synd 48:590–598, 2008.

Levine A, Lee J, Kaplan L, et al: Efficacy and toxicity of concurrent rituximab plus infusional EPOCH in HIV-associated lymphoma: AIDS Malignancy Consortium Trial 034. J Clin Oncol 26:8527, 2008.

Levine AM: Management of AIDS-related lymphoma. Curr Opin Oncol 20:522–528, 2008.

Spitzer TR, Ambinder RF, Lee JY, et al: Dose-reduced busulfan, cyclophosphamide and autologous stem cell transplantation for HIV associated lymphoma: AIDS Malignancy Consortium Study 020. Biol Blood Marrow Transplant 14:59–66, 2008.

Berenguer J, Miralles P, Ribera JM, et al: Characteristics and outcome of AIDS-related Hodgkin lymphoma before and after the introduction of highly active antiretroviral therapy. J Acquir Immune Defic Syndr 47:422–428, 2008.

ON CERVICAL AND ANAL CARCINOMAS

Kitchener H, Nelson L, Adams J, et al: Colposcopy is not necessary to assess the risk to the cervix in HIV-positive women: An international cohort study of cervical pathology in HIV-1 positive women. Int J Cancer 121:2484–2491, 2007.

Cranston RD, Hart SD, Gornbein JA, et al: The prevalence and predictive value of abnormal anal cytology to diagnose anal dysplasia in a population of HIV-positive men who have sex with men. Int J STD AIDS, 18:77–80, 2007.

Stier EA, Goldstone SE, Berry JM, et al: Infrared coagulator treatment of high-grade anal dysplasia in HIV-infected individuals: An AIDS malignancy consortium pilot study. J Acquir Immune Defic Syndr 47:56–61, 2008.

Salama JK, Mell LK, Schomas DA, et al: Concurrent chemotherapy and intensity-modulated radiation therapy for anal canal cancer patients: a multicenter experience. J Clin Oncol 25:4581-86, 2007.

ON NON-AIDS-DEFINING MALIGNANCIES

Grulich AE, van Leeuwen MT, Falster MO, et al: Incidence of cancers in people with HIV/AIDS compared with immunosuppressed transplant recipients: A meta-analysis. Lancet 370:59–67, 2007.

Hakimian R, Fang H, Thomas L, et al: Lung cancer in HIV-infected patients in the era of highly active antiretroviral therapy. J Thorac Oncol 2:268–272, 2007.

Patel P, Hanson DL, Sullivan PS, et al: Incidence of types of cancer among HIV-infected persons compared with the general population in the United States, 1992-2003. Ann Intern Med 148:728–736, 2008.

Bräu N, Fox RK, Xiao P, et al: Presentation and outcome of hepatocellular carcinoma in HIV-infected patients: A US-Canadian multicenter study. J Hepatol 47:527–537, 2007.

Acknowledgment: Supported, in part, by grants from the State of California, University-wide Task Force on AIDS to the UCLA California Collaborative HIV/AIDS Research Center (CHO5-LA-608) and USPHS, NIH grants AI-69424, CA-121947, and RR00865.

CHAPTER 28

Carcinoma of an unknown primary site

John D. Hainsworth, MD, and Lawrence M. Weiss, MD

Carcinoma of an unknown primary site is a common clinical syndrome, accounting for approximately 3% of all oncologic diagnoses. Patients in this group are heterogeneous, having a wide variety of clinical presentations and pathologic findings. A patient should be considered to have carcinoma of an unknown primary site when a tumor is detected at one or more metastatic sites, and routine evaluation (see below) fails to define a primary tumor site.

Although all patients with cancer of an unknown primary site have advanced, metastatic disease, universal pessimism and nihilism regarding treatment are inappropriate. Subsets of patients with specific treatment implications can be defined using clinical and pathologic features. In addition, trials of empiric chemotherapeutic regimens incorporating new antineoplastic agents have suggested improved response rates and survival in unselected groups of patients with carcinoma of an unknown primary site.

Epidemiology

Gender Unknown primary cancer occurs with approximately equal frequency in men and women and has the same prognosis in the two genders.

Age As with most epithelial cancers, the incidence of unknown primary cancer increases with advancing age, although a wide age range exists. Some evidence suggests that younger patients are more likely to have poorly differentiated histologies.

Disease sites Autopsy series performed prior to the availability of CT resulted in the identification of a primary site in 70%-80% of patients. Above the diaphragm, the lungs were the most common primary site, whereas various GI sites (pancreas, colon, stomach, liver) were most common below the diaphragm. Several frequently occurring cancers, particularly breast and prostate cancers, were rarely identified in autopsy series.

With improved radiologic diagnosis, the spectrum of unknown primary cancer has probably changed. Limited recent autopsy data suggest a lower percentage of primary sites identified, particularly in patients with poorly differentiated histology.

TABLE 1: Immunohistochemical studies useful in the differential diagnosis of carcinoma vs another neoplasm

Tumor type	Immunoperoxidase stains			
	Pan-keratin	CD45 and other markers	S-100 protein	Vimentin
Carcinoma	+	–	–	–/+
Malignant lymphoma	–	+	–	–/+
Malignant melanoma	–	–	+	+
Sarcoma	–	–	–	+

Signs and symptoms

Patients with unknown primary cancer usually present with symptoms related to the areas of metastatic tumor involvement.

Sites of metastatic involvement include the lungs, liver, and skeletal system; therefore, symptoms referable to these areas are common.

Constitutional symptoms such as anorexia, weight loss, weakness, and fatigue are common.

Physical findings include peripheral adenopathy, pleural effusions, ascites, and hepatomegaly.

Pathologic evaluation

Optimal pathologic evaluation is critical in the evaluation of patients with carcinoma of an unknown primary site and can aid with the following:

- distinguishing carcinoma from other cancer types
- determining histologic type
- identifying the primary site
- identifying specific characteristics that may direct specific treatments.

Initial approach Although cytologic evaluation, including fine-needle aspiration biopsy, can often determine whether a lesion is malignant, a tissue biopsy will probably be needed to further evaluate the neoplasm. Tissue is required for paraffin-section immunohistochemistry, which is currently the usual methodology of choice in the work-up. Electron microscopy, which optimally requires glutaraldehyde fixation, is usually no longer required. Nucleic acid microarray analysis represents a technology of the future.

TABLE 2: Most useful organ-specific markers

Organ or type of cancer	Antibody
Breast	GCDFP-15, estrogen receptor
Lung	TTF-1
Gastrointestinal carcinoma	CDX-2
Stomach	CDX-2 + Hep-Par
Colon	CDX-2 + CK20
Liver	Hep-Par
Pancreas	CK17
Kidney	CD10
Prostate	Prostate-specific antigen
Serous/endometrioid gynecologic	ER
Urinary bladder	CK7, CK20, CK5/6
Seminoma/embryonal carcinoma	OCT-4
Mesothelioma	Calretinin
Thyroid	TTF-1 + thyroglobulin
Neuroendocrine	Chromogranin + synaptophysin

Carcinoma vs other neoplasms It is important to rule out the possibility of malignant lymphoma, malignant melanoma, and sarcoma. A battery of antibodies is utilized in an attempt to distinguish carcinoma from other types of neoplasms, as summarized in Table 1. The staining result obtained with any single marker is unreliable, as exceptions may occur for each individual antibody. For example, although keratin is a relatively reliable marker of carcinoma, some carcinomas (eg, adrenal cortical carcinoma or undifferentiated carcinoma of the thyroid) may be keratin-negative, whereas some types of sarcoma are characteristically keratin-positive (eg, epithelioid sarcoma).

Determination of histologic type There may be clues on initial histologic examination. For example, the presence of gland formation or mucin production would indicate an adenocarcinoma, whereas the presence of keratinization would indicate a squamous cell carcinoma. Evidence of neuroendocrine differentiation may be suggested by the presence of a characteristic relatively fine chromatin pattern. Immunohistochemistry can also be of use, as expression of keratin subtypes 7 and 20 would favor adenocarcinoma, and expression of keratin subtypes 5/6 and 14 would favor squamous cell carcinoma. Reliable neuroendocrine markers include chromogranin A and synaptophysin.

Identification of specific treatment target characteristics Even if the primary site is not determined, characteristics of the carcinoma may suggest specific treatment options or impart prognostic information. Examples of the former may include determination of estrogen or progesterone receptors or expression of members of the epidermal growth factor receptor family (eg, HER2/neu). Examples of the latter may include Ki-67, which is a surrogate marker of the proliferation rate of a neoplasm.

Clinical evaluation

After a biopsy has established metastatic carcinoma, a relatively limited clinical evaluation is indicated to search for a primary site. Recommended evaluation includes a complete history, physical examination, chemistry profile, CBC, chest radiograph, and CT scan of the abdomen.

Symptomatic areas Specific radiologic and/or endoscopic evaluation of symptomatic areas should be pursued. In addition, mammography, ultrasonography, and breast MRI should be performed in women with clinical features suggestive of metastatic breast cancer (eg, estrogen receptor-positive tumor and/or specific metastatic involvement including axillary nodes, bones, or pleura), and serum prostate-specific antigen (PSA) level should be measured in men with features suggestive of prostate cancer (eg, blastic bone metastasis; Table 2). In young men with poorly differentiated carcinoma, serum human chorionic gonadotropin (hCG) and alpha-fetoprotein (AFP) levels should always be measured.

Asymptomatic areas In general, radiologic or endoscopic evaluation of asymptomatic areas is not productive and should be avoided. An exception is positron emission tomography (PET) scanning, which detects a primary site in almost 40% of cases and frequently changes the approach to treatment. The PET scan is now considered a standard part of the initial evaluation of patients with carcinoma of an unknown primary site.

Cervical lymphadenopathy Metastatic squamous carcinoma in cervical lymph nodes usually involves upper or mid-cervical locations. All patients should undergo a thorough search for a primary site in the head and neck region, including direct endoscopic examination of the oropharynx, hypopharynx, nasopharynx, larynx, and upper esophagus. Any suspicious areas should be biopsied. Fiberoptic bronchoscopy should be considered in patients with involvement of low cervical or supraclavicular nodes. This type of evaluation will identify a primary site, usually in the head and neck, in 85%-90% of these patients. Further evaluation with PET scanning can identify a primary site in 15%-30% of the remaining patients and should be considered. Low cervical adenopathy (level IV, supraclavicular) may also represent an upper gastrointestinal primary.

Inguinal lymphadenopathy Patients with metastatic squamous cell cancer presenting in inguinal lymph nodes almost always have an identifiable primary site in the perineal area. Women should undergo careful examination of the vulva, vagina, and cervix; men should have careful inspection of the penis. Anoscopy should be performed to exclude lesions in the anorectal area.

TABLE 3: Recommended treatment for recognized clinicopathologic subsets

Histopathology	Clinical subset	Treatment
Adenocarcinoma	Women with isolated axillary adenopathy	Treat as stage II breast cancer
	Women with peritoneal carcinomatosis	Treat as stage III ovarian cancer
	Men with blastic bone metastases or elevated serum PSA level	Treat as metastatic prostate cancer
	Colon cancer "profile"	Treat as metastatic colon cancer
	Single metastatic site	Local excision and/or radiation therapy
Squamous cell carcinoma	Cervical adenopathy	Treat as head/neck primary (combined-modality therapy)
	Inguinal adenopathy	Node dissection ± radiation therapy
Poorly differentiated carcinoma	Young men with a mediastinal/retroperitoneal mass	Treat as extragonadal germ-cell tumor
	Neuroendocrine features by immunoperoxidase staining or electron microscopy	Treat with platinum/etoposide-based regimen
	All others with good performance status	Treat with taxane/platinum or platinum/etoposide-based regimen
Neuroendocrine carcinoma	Well differentiated (low grade)	Treat as advanced carcinoid tumor
	Poorly differentiated or small cell	Treat with platinum/etoposide-based regimen

PSA = prostate-specific antigen

Treatment

Table 3 summarizes the recommended treatment for various recognized clinicopathologic subsets.

Adenocarcinoma

When evaluating patients with adenocarcinoma of an unknown primary site, several clinical subsets should be identified and treated specifically. Empiric therapy for patients not included in any of these subsets is outlined in the final section of this chapter.

Women with isolated axillary adenopathy Treatment appropriate for stage II breast cancer should be administered. Mastectomy reveals an occult primary cancer in 50%-60% of these patients, even when physical examination and mammography are normal. Axillary dissection with breast irradiation is also a reasonable treatment, although there are no definitive comparisons of this approach versus mastectomy. Adjuvant systemic therapy, following standard guidelines for stage II breast cancer, is also indicated.

Women with peritoneal carcinomatosis Often, the histopathology in these patients suggests ovarian cancer (ie, serous cystadenocarcinoma or papillary adenocarcinoma). However, all women with this syndrome should be treated as if they had stage III ovarian cancer. Initial cytoreductive surgery should be followed by chemotherapy with a taxane/platinum combination, as recommended for advanced ovarian cancer. In these patients, serum CA-125 can often be used as a tumor marker.

Men with bone metastasis Metastatic prostate cancer should be suspected and usually can be diagnosed with either an elevated serum PSA level or positive tumor staining for PSA. In such patients, androgen deprivation therapy, as recommended for advanced prostate cancer, is often of palliative benefit.

Patients with a colon cancer "profile" Treatment with modern regimens for advanced colon cancer (eg, FOLFOX/bevacizumab [Avastin]) should be considered for patients with a metastatic pattern (liver +/– peritoneal involvement) and pathologic findings (adenocarcinoma, CK20+/CK7–) strongly suggestive of metastatic colorectal cancer. Although clinical data to support this recommendation are still developing, the improved efficacy of advanced colon cancer regimens (versus the taxane/platinum regimens used empirically for carcinoma of an unknown primary site) provides a strong rationale.

Patients with a single metastatic site Surgical resection or radiation therapy should be administered to patients who present with clinical evidence of a single metastasis. Prior to proceeding with local therapy in these patients, PET scanning should be considered to rule out additional metastatic sites. Some of these patients have prolonged survival after local therapy, particularly those who present with a sole metastasis in an isolated peripheral lymph node group. The role of "adjuvant" systemic therapy is undetermined in these patients.

Squamous cell carcinoma

Squamous cell cancer accounts for only 10% of light microscopic diagnoses in patients with unknown primary cancer. Isolated cervical adenopathy is the most common presentation for squamous cell carcinoma of an unknown primary site; other patients have isolated inguinal adenopathy at presentation. Specific management is essential for both of these subgroups, since both have the potential for long-term survival following treatment.

Patients with cervical lymphadenopathy in whom no primary site is identified should be treated as if they had a primary site in the head and neck. Concurrent treatment with chemotherapy and radiation therapy has recently proved superior to local treatment alone and to these treatment modalities used sequentially. Radiation therapy doses and techniques should be identical to those used in treating patients with known head and neck primaries. In addition to the involved neck, the nasopharynx, oropharynx, and hypopharynx should be included in the radiation field. Radical neck dissection should be considered in patients who have any evidence of residual cancer following combined-modality therapy.

Five-year survival rates with combined-modality therapy are 60%-70% and appear superior to results with local modalities alone (30%-50%). The extent of cervical lymph node involvement is the most important prognostic factor. (For additional discussion, see "Unknown head and neck primary site" in chapter 4 on "Head and Neck Tumors.")

Patients with inguinal lymphadenopathy Identification of a primary site in the perineal area is important in patients with inguinal lymphadenopathy, as curative therapy is available for some patients, even after metastasis to inguinal lymph nodes. In the uncommon patient for whom no primary site is identified, inguinal node dissection, with or without radiation therapy, can result in long-term survival. Although limited data exist on this uncommon subgroup, the demonstrated superiority of combined-modality therapy versus local treatment alone for primary squamous cell cancers in the perineal area (eg, cervix, anus) has led to a suggestion that the addition of platinum-based chemotherapy may improve treatment results.

Poorly differentiated carcinoma

This heterogeneous group includes a minority of patients with highly responsive neoplasms and therefore requires special attention in initial clinical and pathologic evaluations. Specialized pathologic techniques can identify some patients with tumor types known to be treatable; these patients should be treated using standard guidelines for the appropriate tumor type.

In the remaining patients, several investigators have documented an increased responsiveness to platinum-based chemotherapy when compared with patients with adenocarcinoma of an unknown primary site. In addition, several series have described a small cohort of long-term survivors following platinum-based treatment. Patients with poorly differentiated adenocarcinoma have usually been included in this group when making treatment decisions. Although most patients in this group should receive an empiric trial of treatment, several specific subsets can be recognized.

Men with extragonadal germ-cell cancer syndrome Young men with a predominant tumor location in the mediastinum and retroperitoneum and/or high levels of serum hCG or AFP should be treated as if they had a poor prognosis germ-cell tumor (ie, four courses of chemotherapy with cisplatin/etoposide/bleomycin, followed by surgical resection of residual radiographic abnormalities).

Molecular genetic analysis can identify an i(12p) chromosomal abnormality diagnostic of a germ-cell tumor in some of these patients, even when the diagnosis cannot be made by any other pathologic evaluation. Patients with

TABLE 4: Results of empiric chemotherapy for carcinoma of an unknown primary site[a]

Regimen	Number of patients	Response rate (%)	Median survival (mo)
Old regimens			
FAM	120	20	8
AM	197	29	5
CAF/CMeF	72	17	5
Cisplatin/5-FU–based	186	24	6
Other cisplatin-based	90	30	5
New regimens			
Paclitaxel/carboplatin/etoposide	71	46	11
Paclitaxel/carboplatin	72	41	12
Docetaxel/platinum	76	24	8
Paclitaxel/carboplatin/gemcitabine	120	25	9
Gemcitabine/cisplatin	40	42	8
Gemcitabine/docetaxel	35	40	10

F = 5-FU (fluorouracil); A = Adriamycin (doxorubicin); M = mitomycin; C = cyclophosphamide; Me = methotrexate

[a]Reported series using similar regimens have been compiled; response rates and median survivals are averages.

germ-cell tumors diagnosed in this manner have been shown to be as responsive to treatment as patients with extragonadal germ-cell tumors of typical histology.

Patients with poorly differentiated neuroendocrine carcinoma With the improved immunoperoxidase stains now available, neuroendocrine features are recognized more frequently in patients with poorly differentiated carcinoma. These tumors are distinct in biology and therapeutic implications from well-differentiated neuroendocrine tumors (eg, carcinoid tumors, islet-cell tumors) of an unknown primary site, which almost always present with multiple liver metastases. In contrast to typical carcinoid tumors, poorly differentiated neuroendocrine tumors are difficult to recognize by light microscopic examination alone, although some of the latter tumors have neuroendocrine or "small-cell" features.

Patients with poorly differentiated neuroendocrine carcinoma of an unknown primary site should receive a trial of chemotherapy with a regimen containing a platinum and etoposide. In a group of 51 such patients, the complete response rate was 28% following treatment with cisplatin and etoposide, with or without bleomycin; the overall response rate was 71%. Eight patients (16%) had durable complete remissions.

The combination of paclitaxel, carboplatin (Paraplatin), and etoposide is also highly active in the treatment of poorly differentiated neuroendocrine tumors (response rate, 53%; 2-year survival, 33%). However, the addition of paclitaxel increases myelosuppression and is not clearly superior to platinum/etoposide therapy.

Although the identity of most poorly differentiated neuroendocrine tumors remains unknown, this group of chemotherapy-responsive patients can be reliably identified using specialized, but widely available, pathologic evaluation.

Other patients with poorly differentiated carcinoma Most patients with poorly differentiated carcinoma do not have neuroendocrine features or clinical features of germ-cell tumor. Patients in this group should receive an empiric trial of chemotherapy, unless an extremely poor performance status precludes this possibility. In a group of 220 such patients treated with cisplatin-based regimens effective for germ-cell tumor at a single institution, the overall response rate was 64%, with 27% complete responses. Median survival of this group was 20 months, and 13% of patients have been disease free for more than 8 years and are considered cured. Although the young median age of 39 years indicates that this was a select patient group, the extreme chemosensitivity of some patients in this large, heterogeneous group is clearly demonstrated.

Empiric chemotherapy - adenocarcinoma - non-specific subgroup

Systemic therapy for patients not included in any specific treatable subgroup has been difficult. Unfortunately, this group includes the majority of patients with adenocarcinoma of an unknown primary site; some patients with poorly differentiated carcinoma and no "favorable" clinical features also respond poorly to current therapy.

'Old' regimens Table 4 summarizes results compiled from phase II trials of empiric chemotherapy. Most patients in these trials had adenocarcinoma, but 5%-10% had poorly differentiated carcinoma. Regimens initially evaluated included historic regimens for GI malignancy and breast cancer, as well as various cisplatin-based regimens. Most of these regimens have produced response rates of 20%-35% and median survival durations of 5-8 months. There is little evidence of prolongation of median survival or long-term complete remission with any of these regimens, and none is considered "standard treatment" in this group of patients.

Regimens incorporating new agents The recent availability of several new antineoplastic agents with broad-spectrum activity has renewed interest in the empiric therapy of carcinoma of an unknown primary site. The taxanes, gemcitabine (Gemzar), and the topoisomerase I inhibitors are all agents with potential efficacy in the treatment of an unknown primary cancer.

Most experience to date has been with taxane/platinum-based regimens. Results of phase II trials suggest higher response rates and longer median survivals along with a moderate decrease in toxicity with these regimens versus previous cisplatin-based regimens (Table 4). Long-term follow-up of patients treated with paclitaxel/carboplatin/etoposide shows actual 2-year and 3-year survival rates of 20% and 14%, respectively. Recently, other combinations of new agents (eg, gemcitabine/cisplatin and gemcitabine/docetaxel) have also shown substantial activity, but further experience is required before comparisons are possible. Targeted agents have undergone limited evaluation in patients with carcinoma of an unknown primary site. In a recent phase II trial, the combination of bevacizumab/erlotinib (Tarceva) showed activity in a group of previously treated patients (objective response or stable, 71%; 1-year survival, 33%). Additional evaluation of various targeted agents is ongoing.

At present, paclitaxel/carboplatin, with or without etoposide, should be considered for empiric therapy for patients with adenocarcinoma of an unknown primary site and a good performance status.

SUGGESTED READING

Culine S, Lortholary A, Voigt J, et al: Cisplatin in combination with either gemcitabine or irinotecan in carcinomas of unknown primary site: Results of a randomized phase II study. Trial for the French Study Group in Carcinomas of Unknown Primary (GEFCAPI 01). J Clin Oncol 21:3479–3482, 2003.

Hainsworth JD, Spigel DR, Farley C, et al: Phase II trial of bevacizumab and erlotinib in carcinomas of unknown primary site: The Minnie Pearl Cancer Research Network. J Clin Oncol 25:1747–1752, 2007.

Hainsworth JD, Spigel DR, Litchy S, et al: Phase II trial of paclitaxel, carboplatin, and etoposide in advanced poorly differentiated neuroendocrine carcinoma: A Minnie Pearl Cancer Research Network study. J Clin Oncol 24:3548–3554, 2006.

Park SY, Yim BH, Kim JH, et al: Panels of immunohistochemical markers help determine primary sites of metastatic adenocarcinoma. Arch Pathol Lab Med 131:1561–1567, 2007.

Pouessel D, Culine S, Becht C, et al: Gemcitabine and docetaxel as front-line chemotherapy in patients with carcinoma of an unknown primary site. Cancer 100:1257–1261, 2004.

Seve P, Billotey C, Brousolle C, et al: The role of 2-deoxy-2-[F-18]fluoro-D-glucose positron emission tomography in disseminated carcinoma of unknown primary site. Cancer 109:292–299, 2007.

CHAPTER 29

Hodgkin lymphoma

Joachim Yahalom, MD, and David Straus, MD

In the year 2008, approximately 8,200 new cases of Hodgkin lymphoma (HL) will be diagnosed in the United States. Over the past 4 decades, advances in radiation therapy and the advent of combination chemotherapy have tripled the cure rate of patients with HL. In 2008, more than 80% of all newly diagnosed patients can expect a normal, disease-free life span.

Epidemiology

Gender The male-to-female ratio of HL is 1.3:1.0.

Age The age-specific incidence of the disease is bimodal, with the greatest peak in the third decade of life and a second, smaller peak after the age of 50 years.

Race HL occurs less commonly in African-Americans (2.3 cases per 100,000 persons) than in Caucasians (3.0 per 100,000 persons).

Geography The age-specific incidence of HL differs markedly in various countries. In Japan, the overall incidence is low and the early peak is absent. In some developing countries, there is a downward shift of the first peak into childhood.

Etiology and risk factors

The cause of HL remains unknown, and there are no well-defined risk factors for its development. However, certain associations have been noted that provide clues to possible etiologic factors.

Familial factors For example, same-sex siblings of patients with HL have a 10 times higher risk for the disease. Patient-child combinations are more common than spouse pairings. Higher risk for HL is associated with few siblings, single-family houses, early birth order, and fewer playmates—all of which decrease exposure to infectious agents at an early age. The monozygotic twin sibling of a patient with HL has a 99 times higher risk of developing HL than a dizygotic twin sibling of a patient with HL. These associations suggest a genetic predisposition and/or a role for an infectious or environmental agent during childhood or early adolescence in the etiology of the disease.

Viruses Familial aggregation may imply genetic factors, but other epidemiologic findings mentioned previously suggest an abnormal response to an infective agent. Both factors may play a role in the pathogenesis of the disease. The

HODGKIN

Epstein-Barr virus (EBV) has been implicated in the etiology of HL by both epidemiologic and serologic studies, as well as by the detection of the EBV genome in 20% to 80% of tumor specimens.

There have been no conclusive studies regarding the possible increased frequency of HL in patients with human immunodeficiency virus (HIV) infection. However, HL in HIV-positive patients is associated with an advanced stage and poor therapeutic outcome. (For further discussion of HL in patients with HIV infection, see chapter 27.)

Signs and symptoms

HL is a lymph node-based malignancy and commonly presents as an asymptomatic lymphadenopathy that may progress to predictable clinical sites.

Location of lymphadenopathy More than 80% of patients with HL present with lymphadenopathy above the diaphragm, often involving the anterior mediastinum; the spleen may be involved in about 30% of patients. Less than 10% to 20% of patients present with lymphadenopathy limited to regions below the diaphragm. The commonly involved peripheral lymph nodes are located in the cervical, supraclavicular, and axillary areas; para-aortic pelvic and inguinal areas are involved less frequently. Disseminated lymphadenopathy is rare in patients with HL, as is involvement of Waldeyer's ring and occipital, epitrochlear, posterior mediastinal, and mesenteric sites.

Systemic symptoms About 30% of patients experience systemic symptoms. They include fever, night sweats, or weight loss (so-called B symptoms) and chronic pruritus. These symptoms occur more frequently in older patients and have a negative impact on prognosis (see section on "Staging and prognosis").

Extranodal involvement HL may affect extranodal tissues by direct invasion (contiguity; the so-called E lesion) or by hematogeneous dissemination (stage IV disease). The most commonly involved extranodal site is the lungs. Liver, bone marrow, and bone may also be involved.

Diagnosis

The initial diagnosis of HL can only be made by biopsy. Because reactive hyperplastic nodes may be present, multiple biopsies of a suspicious site may be necessary. Needle aspiration is inadequate because the architecture of the lymph node is important for diagnosis and histologic subclassification.

Pathology

Reed-Sternberg cell

In a biopsied lymph node, the Reed-Sternberg (R-S) cell is the diagnostic tumor cell that must be identified within the appropriate cellular milieu of lymphocytes, eosinophils, and histiocytes. HL is a unique malignancy pathologically in that the tumor cells constitute a minority of the cell population, whereas normal inflammatory cells are the major cell component. As a result, it may be difficult to identify R-S cells in some specimens. Also, other lymphoproliferations may have cells resembling R-S cells.

The R-S cell is characterized by its large size and classic binucleated structure with large eosinophilic nucleoli. Two antigenic markers are thought to provide diagnostic information: CD30 (Ber-H2) and CD15 (Leu-M1). These markers are present on R-S cells and their variants but not on background inflammatory cells. It is also important to obtain a stain for CD20, since it may be positive in the minority of patients with classic HL (nodular sclerosis or mixed cellularity). The prognostic significance of CD20-positive R-S cells in classic HL is controversial.

Studies have confirmed the B-cell origin of the R-S cell. Single-cell polymerase chain reaction (PCR) analysis of classic R-S cells shows a follicular center B-cell origin for these cells with clonally rearranged but crippled V heavy-chain genes, presumably leading to inhibition of apoptosis. Also, high levels of the nuclear transcription factor-kappa-B (NF-kB) have been found in R-S cells; these high NF-kB levels may play a role in pathogenesis by interfering with apoptosis. A molecular link between R-S cells and tumor cells of mediastinal diffuse large B-cell lymphoma has been recently found in gene-profiling studies.

Histologic subtypes

According to the Rye classification (based on the number and appearance of R-S cells, as well as the background cellular milieu), there are four histologic subtypes of HL.

Nodular sclerosis, the most common subtype, is typically seen in young adults (more commonly in females) who have early-stage supradiaphragmatic presentations. Its distinct features are the presence of (1) broad birefringent bands of collagen that divide the lymphoid tissue into macroscopic nodules and (2) an R-S cell variant, the lacunar cell.

Mixed cellularity is the second most common histology. It is more often diagnosed in males, who usually present with generalized lymphadenopathy or extranodal disease and with associated systemic symptoms. R-S cells are frequently identified; bands of collagen are absent, although fine reticular fibrosis may be present; and the cellular background includes lymphocytes, eosinophils, neutrophils, and histiocytes.

Lymphocyte-predominant HL is an infrequent form of HL in which few R-S cells or their variants may be identified. The cellular background consists primarily of lymphocytes in a nodular or sometimes diffuse pattern. The R-S variants express a B-cell phenotype (CD20-positive, CD15-negative). B-cell clonality has also been demonstrated by PCR of the immunoglobulin heavy-chain genes in single R-S variant cells in biopsy material from patients with lymphocyte-predominant HL.

This finding has led investigators to propose that lymphocyte-predominant HL is a B-cell malignancy with a mature B-cell phenotype, distinct from the other three histologic types of HL. Lymphocyte-predominant HL is often clinically localized, is usually treated effectively with irradiation alone, and may relapse late (a clinical feature reminiscent of low-grade lymphoma). The 15-year disease-specific survival is excellent (> 90%).

The World Health Organization (WHO) classification recognizes a new subtype of lymphocyte-rich classic HL that has morphologic similarity to nodular lymphocyte-predominant HL. However, the R-S cells have a classic morphology and phenotype (CD30-positive, CD15-positive, CD20-negative), and the surrounding lymphocytes are reactive T cells. This disease subtype does not show a tendency toward late relapse and should be managed like other classic HL histologies.

Lymphocyte depletion is a rare diagnosis, particularly since the advent of antigen marker studies, which led to the recognition that many such cases represented T-cell non-HLs (NHLs). R-S cells are numerous, the cellular background is sparse, and there may be diffuse fibrosis and necrosis. Patients usually have advanced-stage disease, extranodal involvement, an aggressive clinical course, and a poor prognosis.

The International Working Group (IWG) updated the recommendation for staging and response criteria of lymphomas, including Hodgkin lymphoma. PET or (preferably) PET/CT is strongly recommended prior to treatment and is essential for post-treatment evaluation, yet altering treatment based on interim PET is experimental and recommended only for clinical trials. Response criteria have also been changed. A change from a positive PET to a negative PET, even in the presence of residual CT mass, is considered a complete response. Yet, if pre-treatment PET was not obtained, a negative post-treatment PET indicates a CR only in the presence of a normal CT. The category of CR(u) has been omitted by the use of PET (Cheson BD, Pfistner B, Juweid ME et al: J Clin Oncol 25:579-586, 2007).

Staging and prognosis

Precise definition of the extent of nodal and extranodal involvement with HL according to a standard staging classification system is critical for selection of the proper treatment strategy.

Staging system

The staging system is detailed in Table 1, and the anatomic regions that provide the basis for the staging classification are illustrated in Figure 1. The assignment of stage is based on:

■ the number of involved sites

■ whether lymph nodes are involved on both sides of the diaphragm and whether this involvement is bulky (particularly in the mediastinum)

■ whether there is contiguous extranodal involvement (E sites) or disseminated extranodal disease

- whether typical systemic symptoms (B symptoms) are present.

In defining the disease stage, it is important to note how the information was obtained, since this fact reflects on remaining uncertainties in the evaluation for extent of disease. Clinical staging refers to information that has been obtained by initial biopsy, history, physical examination, and laboratory and radiographic studies only. A pathologic stage is determined by more extensive surgical assessment of potentially involved sites, eg, by surgical staging laparotomy and splenectomy.

Also, various designations relating to the presence or absence of B symptoms or bulky disease (see Table 1) can be applied to any disease stage. For example, a patient with no B symptoms

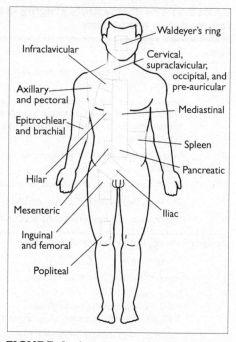

FIGURE 1: Anatomic regions for staging of Hodgkin lymphoma

but with a bulky mediastinal mass and involvement of the cervical lymph nodes would be defined as having CS IIAX disease. A patient with axillary disease and fever who underwent a staging laparotomy that revealed involvement of the para-aortic lymph nodes and spleen would be staged as PS III$_2$B.

Most recent studies in stage I/II disease distinguish between favorable and unfavorable early-stage disease, according to the European Organization for Research and Treatment of Cancer (EORTC) definitions outlined in Table 2.

Clinical staging evaluation

Disease-associated symptoms As mentioned previously, disease-associated symptoms may occur in up to one-third of patients. They may include B symptoms, pruritus, and, less commonly, pain in involved regions after ingestion of alcohol. In each anatomic stage, the presence of B symptoms is an adverse prognostic indicator and may strongly affect treatment choices. B symptoms are carefully defined in the staging system. Unexplained fever should be > 38°C and recurrent during the previous month, night sweats should be drenching and recurrent, and unexplained weight loss should be significant only if > 10% of body weight has been lost within the preceding 6 months. Although pruritus is no longer considered to be a B symptom, the presence of generalized itching may be considered to be an adverse prognostic symptom.

TABLE 1: The Cotswald's staging classification for Hodgkin lymphoma

Stage	Description
I	Involvement of a single lymph node region or lymphoid structure (eg, spleen, thymus, Waldeyer's ring)
II	Involvement of two or more lymph node regions on the same side of the diaphragm (ie, the mediastinum is a single site, hilar lymph nodes are lateralized). The number of anatomic sites should be indicated by a subscript (eg, II$_2$).
III	Involvement of lymph node regions or structures on both sides of the diaphragm:
	III$_1$: With or without involvement of splenic, hilar, celiac, or portal nodes
	III$_2$: With involvement of para-aortic, iliac, or mesenteric nodes
IV	Involvement of extranodal site(s) beyond that designated E

Designations applicable to any disease stage[a]

A	No symptoms
B	Fever, drenching sweats, weight loss
X	Bulky disease: > 1/3 the width of the mediastinum > 10 cm maximal dimension of nodal mass
E	Involvement of a single extranodal site, contiguous or proximal to a known nodal site
CS	Clinical stage
PS	Pathologic stage

[a] For examples of how these designations are applied to disease stage, see text discussion.

Certain combinations of B symptoms are more prognostically significant than others. For example, the combination of fever and weight loss has a worse prognosis than do night sweats alone.

Physical examination should carefully determine the location and size of all palpable lymph nodes. Inspection of Waldeyer's ring, detection of splenomegaly or hepatomegaly, and evaluation of cardiac and respiratory status are important.

Laboratory studies should include a complete blood count (CBC) with white blood cell (WBC) differential and platelet count, the erythrocyte sedimentation rate (ESR), tests for liver and renal function, and assays for serum alkaline phosphatase and lactate dehydrogenase (LDH). A moderate to marked leukemoid reaction and thrombocytosis are common, particularly in symptomatic patients, and usually disappear with treatment.

C*ESR* The ESR may provide helpful prognostic information. At some centers, treatment programs for patients with early-stage disease are influenced by the

TABLE 2: EORTC prognostic definition of early-stage disease

Favorable	CS I and II (maximum 3 involved areas) and < 50 years *and* ESR < 50 mm/h (no B symptoms) *or* ESR < 30 mm/h (B symptoms present) *and* MT ratio < 0.33
Unfavorable	CS II ≥ 4 nodal areas involved *or* age ≥ 50 years *or* ESR ≥ 50 mm/h (no B symptoms) *or* ESR ≥ 30 mm/h (B symptoms present) *or* MT ratio ≥ 0.33

CS = Cotswald's staging; EORTC = European Organization for Research and Treatment of Cancer; ESR = erythrocyte sedimentation rate; MT = mediastinal/thoracic

degree of ESR elevation. In addition, changes in the ESR following therapy may correlate with response and relapse.

Abnormalities of liver function studies should prompt further evaluation of that organ, with imaging and possible biopsy.

Alkaline phosphatase An elevated alkaline phosphatase level may be a nonspecific marker, but it may also indicate bone involvement that should be appropriately evaluated by a radionuclide bone scan and directed skeletal radiographs.

Imaging studies Radiologic studies should include a chest x-ray and computed tomography (CT) scan of the chest, abdomen, and pelvis with IV contrast. Positron emission tomography (PET) scan will provide important information on the extent of disease and a baseline for evaluation of response to treatment. Radionuclide bone scan, magnetic resonance imaging (MRI) of the chest or abdomen, and CT scan of the neck are contributory only under special circumstances.

Evaluation for supradiaphragmatic disease The thoracic CT scan details the status of intrathoracic lymph node groups, the lung parenchyma, pericardium, pleura, and chest wall. Since the chest CT scan may remain abnormal for a long time after the completion of therapy, the evaluation of pretreatment involvement and response to therapy is the use of a PET scan.

Evaluation of the abdomen and pelvis A CT scan and PET are the basic imaging studies for evaluation of the abdomen and pelvis.

Bone marrow biopsy Bone marrow involvement is relatively uncommon with HL, but because of the impact of a positive biopsy on further staging and treatment, unilateral bone marrow biopsy should be part of the staging process of patients with stage IIB disease or higher.

Lymphangiography and staging laparotomy

These two old methods of staging have been replaced by modern imaging techniques using high-resolution CT scanning and ^{18}F-fluorodeoxyglucose (FDG)-PET.

TABLE 3: Results of prospective randomized studies with short chemotherapy followed by IFRT for early-stage HL

Study (# of patients)	Prognostic group	Treatment	RFS or FFTF	OS (median follow-up)
Milan (133)	Favorable and unfavorable	ABVD (4) + IFRT (36 Gy)	94%	94% (12 years)
GHSG HD8 (1,064)	Unfavorable	COPP/ABVD (4) + IFRT (30 Gy + 10 Gy to bulk)	84%	92% (5 years)
EORTC H8U (995)	Unfavorable	MOPP/ABV (4) + IFRT (36 Gy)	96%	93% (4 years)
GHSG HD10 (1,131)	Favorable	ABVD (2 or 4) + IFRT (20 or 30 Gy)	97%	99% (2 years)
GHSG HD11 (1,363)	Unfavorable	ABVD (4) or BEACOPP (4) + IFRT (20 or 30 Gy)	90%	97% (2 years)

Abbreviations: For chemotherapy, see Table 4
EORTC = European Organization for Research and Treatment of Cancer; FFTF = freedom from treatment failure; GHSG = German Hodgkin's Study Group; HL = Hodgkin lymphoma; IFRT = involved-field radiation therapy; OS = overall survival; RFS = relapse-free survival

The possibility of eliminating consolidation radiotherapy after CR chemotherapy and a negative PET scan was tested in a prospective randomized study. A total of 160 patients who were converted to PET negative (that was positive prior to treatment) after chemotherapy but with a small residual CT abnormality were randomized to receive either involved-field radiotherapy (32 Gy) or no further treatment. At a median follow-up of 40 months, significantly more patients failed in the no radiotherapy arm (P = .03). Patients who were PET-negative and CT-negative post chemotherapy were not randomized and only observed. They also had a relatively high rate of failures compared to the irradiated group (Picardi M, De Renzo A, Pane F, et al: Leuk Lymphoma 48:1721-1727, 2007).

Treatment

HL is sensitive to radiation and many chemotherapeutic drugs, and, in most stages, there is more than one effective treatment option. Disease stage is the most important determinant of treatment options and outcome. All patients, regardless of stage, can and should be treated with curative intent.

TREATMENT OF STAGE I/II DISEASE

The treatment of choice for favorable and unfavorable early-stage classic HL is brief chemotherapy followed by involved-field radiotherapy (IFRT). Most of the experience that yielded excellent treatment results with low toxicity was with ABVD (Adriamycin [doxorubicin], bleomycin, vinblastine, and dacarbazine) for 4 cycles and IFRT of 30 to 36 Gy. Table 3 summarizes data from randomized studies that reported on the combination of short chemotherapy (4 or even only 2 cycles) followed by IFRT. The three top randomized studies have also indicated that adding extended-field radiotherapy to chemotherapy is not necessary and the small involved field is adequate.

The most recent (and as yet not fully mature) excellent results are with shortening the duration of chemotherapy to only 2 cycles of ABVD in favorable patients and reducing the IFRT dose to 20 Gy (Table 3). If the excellent results obtained by the German Hodgkin's Study Group prevail with additional follow-up, brief ABVD and low-dose IFRT will become the standard of care for favorable early-stage HL.

The Stanford group reported on an effective brief combined-modality regimen for the treatment of bulky or non-bulky but unfavorable (see Table 2) early-stage patients. They used the full Stanford V regimen (see Table 4) for patients with bulky early-stage and an abbreviated Stanford V (8 weeks chemotherapy and involved-field radiation therapy of only 20-30 Gy) for non-bulky unfavorable early-stage patients. At a median follow-up of 7 years, the 10-year estimated freedom-from progression was 91%, and overall survival was 89% for bulky disease and 97% for nonbulky unfavorable patients. Acute and long-term toxicity was minimal *(Advani RH, Hoppe RT, Rosenberg SA, et al: 7th International Symposium on Hodgkin Lymphoma, Cologne, Germany 2007. Haematologica 2007, S5, p. 27).*

Subtotal lymphoid irradiation (ie, treatment of the mantle and para-aortic fields only) remains an adequate alternative treatment of clinically or pathologically staged favorable (nonbulky and without B symptoms) early-stage HL (stage I/II). Yet this option is no longer the treatment of choice due to the risk of second tumors and (to a lesser degree) coronary artery disease in long-term survivors of extensive radiotherapy alone as practiced in the past. In classic (non–lymphocyte- predominant) HL, subtotal lymphoid irradiation is adequate for patients who are not candidates for a chemotherapy-containing strategy.

In patients who underwent pathologic staging (laparotomy) and were treated with primary irradiation alone, several large series reported a 15- to 20-year survival rate of nearly 90% and a relapse-free survival rate of 75% to 80%. Most relapses (75%) occurred within 3 years after the completion of therapy; late relapses were uncommon. More than half of the patients who relapsed after radiotherapy alone were still curable with standard chemotherapy.

Canadian and European studies have reported excellent overall survival results in patients selected for radiotherapy on the basis of clinical prognostic factors alone. Thus, irradiation alone can be safely offered to clinically staged patients with favorable prognostic factors who are not candidates for combined-modality treatment.

Chemotherapy alone In two prospective, randomized studies, radiotherapy alone was as effective as or superior to MOPP (mechlorethamine [Mustargen], Oncovin [vincristine], procarbazine [Matulane], and prednisone) chemotherapy in improving the survival of patients with early-stage disease. Although the re-

In the recent EORTC/GELA study H9, 1,591 patients with stage I/II HL were enrolled into two trials based on four prognostic factors: age, symptoms, number of involved areas, and mediastinal mass to thoracic ratio. The H9-F trial compared 36 Gy IFRT vs 20 Gy IFRT vs no RT in patients in complete remission after 6 cycles of EBVP. In the H9-F trial for favorable patients, of the 783 patients enrolled, 619 (79%) achieved a CR and were randomized to receive treatment. After a median follow-up of 33 months, the 4-year event-free survival rates were 87% in the 36 Gy and 84% in the 20 Gy arms; it was 70% in the 0 Gy arm ($P <$ .001). The 4-year overall survival rate was 98% in all three arms. The group concluded that in patients with favorable HL who achieved CR after 6 cycles of EBVP, omission of IFRT leads to an unacceptable failure rate; in contrast, an IFRT dose reduced to 20 Gy provides equivalent early results to an IFRT dose of 36 Gy (*Thomas J, Ferme C, Noordijk EM, et al: 7th International Symposium on Hodgkin Lymphoma, Cologne, Germany 2007. Haematologica 2007, S5, p. 27*).

lapse rate after chemotherapy is similar to that after radiotherapy, conventional-dose salvage chemotherapy used after failure of chemotherapy produces poor results, which translates into an inferior overall survival.

More recently, five prospective randomized studies compared chemotherapy alone with chemotherapy followed by IFRT or regional radiotherapy in patients with early-stage HL. The Children's Cancer Group (CCG) tested the role of radiation therapy in young patients (< 21 years old) who attained a complete response with risk-adapted chemotherapy (mostly COPP [cyclophosphamide, Oncovin (vincristine), procarbazine, and prednisone)/ABV [Adriamycin (doxorubicin), bleomycin, and vinblastine], 4 to 6 cycles). They enrolled 829 patients into the study (68% had early-stage disease); 501 patients who achieved a complete response were then randomized to receive either low-dose (21 Gy) IFRT or no further treatment. The accrual was stopped earlier than planned because of a significantly higher number of relapses on the no-radiotherapy arm. The 3-year event-free survival rate with an intent-to-treat analysis was 92% for patients randomized to receive radiotherapy and 87% for those randomized to receive no further treatment ($P = $.057).

The EORTC/Groupe d'Etude des Lymphomes de l'Adulte (GELA) conducted a large randomized trial in patients with favorable early-stage classic HL. All patients received 6 cycles of EBVP (epirubicin, bleomycin, vinblastine, and prednisone). Only patients who achieved a complete response were randomized to receive either IFRT of 36 Gy, IFRT of 20 Gy, or no irradiation. After an interim analysis, the EORTC/GELA groups closed the entry to the no-radiotherapy arm because of the excessive number of relapses. It should be noted that in previous EORTC studies, EBVP with IFRT was found to be inferior to MOPP/ABV with IFRT hybrid in patients with unfavorable disease but provided excellent results when combined with radiotherapy and was compared with radiotherapy alone in patients with favorable disease.

The National Cancer Institute of Canada and the Eastern Cooperative Oncology Group (ECOG) included 405 patients with nonbulky stage I/II disease. They were randomized to receive either "standard therapy," namely, subtotal nodal irradiation (STNI) for favorable patients, and ABVD (2 cycles) followed by STNI for unfavorable (B, elevated ESR, ≥ 3 sites, age ≥ 40, mixed cellularity histology) patients or experimental therapy consisting of 6 cycles or 4 cycles (if complete response was attained after 2 cycles) of ABVD and no radiotherapy. At a median follow-up of 4.2 years, progression-free survival with ABVD alone was significantly inferior ($P =$ .006; hazard ratio = 2.6; 5-year estimates of disease progression-free survival, 87% vs 93%). At 5 years, no event-free or overall survival difference has been detected. The study was planned for 12 years' analysis of survival.

The Memorial Sloan-Kettering Cancer Center trial included 152 patients with nonbulky early-stage HL. Patients were randomized up front to receive either ABVD × 6 alone or ABVD × 6 followed by radiotherapy. At 60 months, the duration of complete response and freedom from disease progression for ABVD and radiotherapy versus ABVD alone were 91% versus 87% ($P =$ .61) and 86% versus 81% ($P =$ .61), respectively. Overall survival was 97% with ABVD and radiotherapy vs 90% with ABVD alone ($P =$ .08). Although the differences between the outcome of the two treatment groups were not statistically significant, the study was not powered to detect differences between the treatment strategies that were smaller than 20%, due to the small number of patients and events.

> Long-term follow-up has been reported from two large randomized controlled trials comparing extended-field radiation therapy (EFRT) with combined-modality treatment (CMT) for early stage favorable HL. Both demonstrated significantly fewer relapses in the CMT arm as compared with EFRT, but neither demonstrated a difference in survival. In the EORTC H7-F trial, patients were randomized to EFRT or CMT with 6 cycles of epirubicin, bleomycin, vinblastine, and prednisone (EBVP) and involved field radiation therapy (IFRT). The 10-year event-free survivals were 88% for EBVP + IFRT as compared with 78% for EFRT (P = .0113); (Noordjik EM, Carde P, Dupouy N, et al: J Clin Oncol 24:3128-3135, 2006).

In a prospectively randomized study reported from India, patients with HL who achieved a complete response after ABVD were randomized to receive either IFRT or no further therapy. The 8-year event-free and overall survival rates were significantly better for the patients who received consolidation with IFRT than for those who received ABVD alone. Subset analysis indicated that the benefit from added IFRT was more prominent in advanced-stage than in early-stage disease.

The National Comprehensive Cancer Network (NCCN) guidelines recommend combined-modality therapy as the treatment of choice for favorable or unfavorable classic HL. Opinions differ as to the use of chemotherapy alone, and it remains highly controversial.

TECHNICAL ASPECTS OF RADIATION THERAPY

IFRT and involved-node radiotherapy (INRT)

In a combined-modality setting, irradiation of the involved lymph node chain, with or without adjacent sites, and tailoring of the field borders to the postchemotherapy tumor volume (in critical areas such as the mediastinum) are recommended. IFRT is the most appropriate irradiation approach after chemotherapy. IFRT or regional radiotherapy alone is used for lymphocyte-predominant HL. Recommendations for IFRT for HL are detailed in an article by Yahalom and Mauch. Recently, further reduction in IFRT has been introduced and implemented in EORTC/GELA studies. The INRT field is limited to the prechemotherapy lymph node(s) volume, and in the mediastinum, it also accounts for the reduction of mass after chemotherapy. Although it decreases the radiation exposure to normal organs, data comparing its efficacy with those of the traditional IFRT are not yet available.

FIGURE 2: Extended radiation fields used for treatment of classic Hodgkin lymphoma with irradiation alone

Extended radiation fields

Successful therapy with irradiation alone in classic HL requires treatment of all clinically involved lymph nodes and all nodal and extranodal regions at risk for subclinical involvement (Figure 2). The HL radiation fields were designed to conform to the philosophy of treating regions beyond the immediately involved area while accounting for normal tissue tolerance and the technical constraints of field size. The extended radiation fields are inappropriate when radiation is administered as consolidation following chemotherapy and thus are rarely used today.

Researchers from the University of Toronto employed a radiobiological model to individually estimate breast cancer and lung cancer from radiotherapy. When they used a mantle-field design and a dose of 30 Gy, the risk found was similar to that obtained in epidemiological studies of second cancer risk. When the field was reduced to the currently used involved field, the excess relative risk was reduced by 63% for breast cancer and by 21% for lung cancer. When the dose was also lowered from 30 Gy to 20 Gy, the excess risk was reduced by 77% and 57%, respectively. The study supports other research that indicates a decrease in second cancer risk with modern smaller radiation fields and lower dose (Hodgson DC, Koh ES, Tran TH, et al: Cancer 110:2576-2586, 2007).

Dose considerations

When irradiation alone is used to treat HL, the standard total dose to each field is 3,600 cGy, delivered in daily fractions of 180 cGy over 4 weeks. In addition, clinically involved areas are given a boost of 360 to 540 cGy in 2 to 3 fractions to bring the total dose to these areas up to 3,960 to 4,140 cGy. Patients who receive irradiation as consolidation after chemotherapy receive a total dose of 2,000 to 3,600 cGy in 150 to 180-cGy fractions. We normally use opposed anterior and posterior fields that are evenly weighted and treat both fields daily. Three-dimensional conformal radiotherapy and intensity-modulated radiation therapy (IMRT) are employed for selected cases.

SIDE EFFECTS AND COMPLICATIONS OF RADIOTHERAPY

Side effects of radiotherapy depend on the irradiated volume, dose administered, and technique employed. They are also influenced by the extent and type of prior chemotherapy, if any, and by the patient's age.

Acute effects The potential acute side effects of involved fields in the upper body include mouth dryness, change in taste, pharyngitis, nausea, dry cough, dermatitis, and fatigue. These side effects are usually mild and transient.

The main potential side effects of subdiaphragmatic irradiation are loss of appetite, nausea, and increased bowel movements. These reactions are usually mild and can be minimized with standard antiemetic medications.

A recent meta-analysis was performed on all randomized studies comparing chemotherapy alone with combined-modality treatment in adult early-stage patients with Hodgkin Lymphoma. A total of 1,005 patients from 5 studies were analyzed. The analysis showed a statistically significant difference in overall survival in favour of using combined-modality therapy compared to chemotherapy alone (hazard ratio, 0.60; $P = .009$) *(Rehan FA, Billant C, Knaul I, et al: 7th International Symposium on Hodgkin Lymphoma, Cologne, Germany 2007. Haematologica 2007, S5, p. 30).*

Irradiation of more than one field, particularly after chemotherapy, can cause myelosuppression, which may necessitate treatment delays.

Delayed effects Delayed side effects may develop anywhere from several weeks to several years after the completion of radiotherapy.

Lhermitte's sign Approximately 15% of patients who receive the full dose of radiation to the neck may note an electric shock sensation radiating down the backs of both legs when the head is flexed (Lhermitte's sign) 6 weeks to 3 months after mantle-field radiotherapy. Possibly secondary to transient demyelinization of the spinal cord, Lhermitte's sign resolves spontaneously after a few months and is not associated with late or permanent spinal cord damage.

Pneumonitis and pericarditis During the same period, radiation pneumonitis and/or acute pericarditis may occur in < 5% of patients who receive large fields of radiation to the mediastinum; these side effects occur more often in those who have extensive mediastinal disease. Both inflammatory processes have become rare with modern radiation techniques.

Herpes zoster infection Patients with HL, regardless of treatment type, have a propensity to develop herpes zoster infection within 2 years after therapy. Usually, the infection is confined to a single dermatome and is self-limited. If the cutaneous eruption is identified promptly, treatment with systemic acyclovir will limit its duration and intensity.

Subclinical hypothyroidism Radiotherapy of the neck can induce subclinical hypothyroidism in about one-third of patients. This condition is detected by elevation of thyroid-stimulating hormone (TSH). Thyroid replacement with levothyroxine (T_4) is recommended, even in asymptomatic patients, to prevent overt hypothyroidism and decrease the risk of benign thyroid nodules.

Infertility Irradiation of the pelvis may have deleterious effects on fertility. In most patients, this problem can be avoided by appropriate gonadal shielding. In females, the ovaries can be moved into a shielded area laterally or inferomedially near the uterine cervix. Irradiation fields that spare the pelvis do not increase the risk of sterility.

Secondary malignancies Patients with HL who were cured with radiotherapy and/or chemotherapy have an increased risk of secondary solid tumors (most commonly, lung, breast, and stomach cancers, as well as melanoma) and NHL 10 or more years after treatment. Chemotherapy combinations that do not include alkylating agents or a new brief program (such as Stanford V) as well as the smaller involved fields and lower doses are less likely to have the increased risk observed with extended fields and/or MOPP or MOPP-like chemotherapy.

Lung cancer Patients who are smokers should be strongly encouraged to quit the habit because the increase in lung cancer that occurs after irradiation or chemotherapy with alkylating agents has been detected mostly in smokers. Alkylating agents (such as in the MOPP regimen) and radiation therapy were associated with an increased risk of lung cancer in an additive and dose-dependent fashion. These effects were multiplied by tobacco use (see Suggested Reading).

Breast cancer The increase in breast cancer risk is inversely related to the patient's age at HL treatment; no increased risk has been found in women irradiated after 30 years of age. The risk of breast cancer is increased with higher radiation breast dose and is reduced in patients who received chemotherapy or ovarian irradiation that induced early menopause.

In most situations, modern IFRT should spare the breast. Breast cancer is curable in its early stages, and early detection has a significant impact on survival. Breast examination should be part of the routine follow-up for women cured of HL, and routine mammography should begin about 8 years after treatment.

Cardiovascular disease An increased risk of cardiovascular morbidity has been reported among patients who have received mediastinal irradiation. In a retrospective study evaluating the cardiac risks of 450 patients cured of HL with radiotherapy alone or in combination, 42 patients (10%) developed coronary artery disease (CAD) at a median of 9 years after treatment, 30 patients (7%) developed carotid and/or subclavian artery disease at a median of 17 years after treatment, and 25 patients (6%) developed clinically significant valvular dysfunction at a median of 22 years after treatment. The most common valve lesion was aortic stenosis, which occurred in 14 valves. The only treatment-related factor associated with the development of CAD was use of a radiation technique that resulted in a higher total dose to a portion of the heart (RR = 7.8; 95% confidence interval [CI] = 1.1–53.2; P=.04). No specific treatment-related factor was associated with carotid or subclavian artery disease or valvular dysfunction. Freedom from cardiovascular morbidity was 88% at 15 years and 84% at 20 years.

To reduce this hazard, radiation fields should conform to the involved postchemotherapy volume, and the dose should be reduced to 20 to 30 Gy if possible. Patients who have received radiation to the mediastinum should be monitored and advised about other established CAD risk factors, such as smoking, hyperlipidemia, hypertension, and poor dietary and exercise habits. Cholesterol levels should be monitored and treated if elevated.

Effects on bone and muscle growth In children, high-dose irradiation will affect bone and muscle growth and may result in deformities. Current treatment programs for pediatric HL are chemotherapy-based; radiotherapy is limited to low doses.

TREATMENT OF STAGE III/IV DISEASE

Chemotherapy has become curative for many patients with advanced stages of HL. MOPP has been the primary effective combination chemotherapy regimen for advanced-stage disease since the 1960s. Over the past several years, ABVD has been shown to be more effective and less toxic than MOPP, particularly with respect to sterility and secondary leukemia.

Combination chemotherapy regimens

Doxorubicin-containing regimens A doxorubicin-containing regimen, such as ABVD (Table 4), is the treatment of choice for patients presenting with stage III or IV disease, as demonstrated by a randomized phase III trial undertaken by the Cancer and Leukemia Group B (CALGB). This trial showed higher complete response rates with ABVD and ABVD/MOPP (82% and 83%, respectively) than with MOPP alone (65%).

One reason for the improved response rate in the groups treated with doxorubicin-containing regimens was the higher percentage of patients who were able to receive ≥ 85% of the expected chemotherapy dose, particularly in the ABVD group. In addition, rates of significant and life-threatening neutropenia were higher in patients treated with the MOPP-containing regimens than in those treated with other regimens.

Subsequent trials compared ABVD, alternating MOPP/ABVD, and a MOPP/ABV hybrid. Alternating MOPP/ABVD and the MOPP/ABV hybrid was found to be equally effective in treating advanced-stage HL. However, a recent intergroup study that compared ABVD with MOPP/ABV hybrid (without irradiation) was closed early because of concerns of excess treatment-related deaths and second malignancies (mostly acute myelogenous leukemia and lung can-

A large cohort collaborative of 7,033 British patients was used to determine the mortality risk from myocardial infarction (MI) after treatment for Hodgkin lymphoma. A total of 166 deaths from MI occurred in the cohort, statistically significantly more than expected. Standardized mortality ratios decreased sharply with older age at first treatment, but absolute excess risks of death from MI increased with older age, up to age 65 years at first treatment. The statistically significantly increased risk of MI mortality persisted through to 25 years after first treatment. Risks were increased statistically significantly and independently for patients who had been treated with supradiaphragmatic radiotherapy, anthracyclines, or vincristine. Interestingly, risk was significantly increased in patients treated with ABVD, even when they had not received radiotherapy (*P* = .01) and when radiotherapy was included (*P* = .004); *(Swerdlow AJ, Higgins CD, Smith P, et al: J Natl Cancer Inst 99:206-214, 2007).*

TABLE 4: Chemotherapeutic regimens used for the treatment of Hodgkin lymphoma

Regimen	Dosage and schedule	Frequency
MOPP		
Mechlorethamine	6 mg/m^2 IV on day 1	
Oncovin	1.4 mg/m^2 IV on day 1 (maximum dose, 2.0 mg)	
Procarbazine	100 mg/m^2 PO on days 1-7	*Repeat cycle*
Prednisone[a]	40 mg/m^2 PO on days 1-14	*every 28 days.*
ABVD		
Adriamycin	25 mg/m^2 IV on days 1 and 15	
Bleomycin	10 mg/m^2 IV on days 1 and 15	
Vinblastine	6 mg/m^2 IV on days 1 and 15	*Repeat cycle*
Dacarbazine	375 mg/m^2 IV on days 1 and 15	*every 28 days.*
BEACOPP		
Bleomycin	10 mg/m^2 IV on day 8	
Etoposide	100 mg/m^2 (200 mg/m^2)[b] IV on days 1-3	
Adriamycin	25 mg/m^2 (35 mg/m^2)[b] IV on day 1	
Cyclophosphamide	650 mg/m^2 (1,200 mg/m^2)[b] IV on day 1	
Oncovin	1.4 mg/m^2 IV on day 8[c]	
Procarbazine	100 mg/m^2 PO on days 1-7	
Prednisone	40 mg/m^2 PO on days 1-14	*Repeat cycle*
G-CSF from day 8		*every 21 days.*
Stanford V		
Doxorubicin	25 mg/m^2 IV on days 1 and 15	*Repeat cycle*
Vinblastine[d]	6 mg/m^2 IV on days 1 and 15	*every 28 days for*
Mechlorethamine	6 mg/m^2 IV on day 1	*a total of 3 cycles.*
Vincristine[d]	1.4 mg/m^2 IV on days 8 and 22	*Radiotherapy to*
Bleomycin	5 U/m^2 IV on days 8 and 22	*initial sites ≥ 5 cm*
Etoposide	60 mg/m^2 IV on days 15 and 16	*(dose: 36 cGy).*
Prednisone[e]	40 mg/m^2 PO every other day	

[a] In the original report, prednisone was given only in cycles 1 and 4.
[b] Increased dose for BEACOPP
[c] Maximal dose of 2 mg
[d] Vinblastine dose was decreased to 4 mg/m^2 and vincristine dose to 1 mg/m^2 during cycle 3 for patients ≥ 50 years of age.
[e] Tapered by 10 mg every other day starting at week 10

G-CSF = granulocyte colony-stimulating factor

cer) in the MOPP/ABV hybrid arm. ABVD and MOPP/ABV hybrid yielded similar 5-year failure and overall survival rates.

Shortened dose-intense regimens Shortened dose-intense regimens have shown promise. For example, the 12-week Stanford V regimen (see Table 4) combined with IFRT produced a 5-year overall survival rate of 96% and a freedom-from-disease-progression rate of 89%. The freedom-from-disease-progression rate was significantly superior among patients with a prognostic score of 0–2, compared with those with a score of 3 and higher (94% vs 75%; P = .0001). Of interest, in 142 patients from Stanford, no secondary leukemia was observed, and 42 pregnancies were reported.

An escalated dose version of BEACOPP (bleomycin, etoposide, Adriamycin [doxorubicin], cyclophosphamide, Oncovin [vincristine], procarbazine, and prednisone) was found to have a statistically significant superior freedom from treatment failure at 5 years compared with standard-dose BEACOPP and alternating monthly COPP and ABVD for patients with advanced stages of HL. Short-term hematologic toxicity was greatest for escalated BEACOPP, and a significant increased risk for secondary acute leukemias was also seen as compared with standard-dose BEACOPP and COPP/ABVD.

Combined-modality therapy

Although the role of consolidation radiotherapy after induction chemotherapy remains controversial, irradiation is routinely added in patients with advanced-stage disease who present with bulky disease or who remain in uncertain complete remission after chemotherapy. Retrospective studies have demonstrated that adding low-dose radiotherapy to all initial disease sites after chemotherapy-induced complete response decreases the relapse rate by ~25% and significantly improves overall survival.

Interpretation of the impact of irradiation in prospective studies has been controversial. However, a Southwest Oncology Group (SWOG) randomized study of 278 patients with stage III or IV HL suggested that the addition of low-dose irradiation to all sites of initial disease after a complete response to MOP-BAP (mechlorethamine, Oncovin [vincristine], prednisone-, bleomycin, Adriamycin [doxorubicin], and procarbazine) chemotherapy improves the duration of remission in patients with advanced-stage disease. An intention-to-treat analysis showed that the advantage of combined-modality therapy was limited to patients with nodular sclerosis. No survival differences were observed.

In a recent study, 260 previously untreated patients with Hodgkin lymphoma with stages IIB-IV or IIA with adverse prognostic features were treated with 6 cycles of chemotherapy, mostly ABVD, and radiation therapy to patients with initial bulky or residual masses after chemotherapy. PET scans were performed prior to treatment and after 2 cycles of chemotherapy. The 2-year progression-free survival (PFS) for patients with a positive PET scan after 2 cycles was 12.8% and for patients with a negative PET scan, 95% (P < .0001). In a multivariate analysis post-cycle 2 PET was significant (P < .0001), but pretreatment features in the International Prognostic Score were not significant for PFS (*Gallamini A, Hutchings M, Rigacci L, et al: J Clin Oncol 25:3746-3752, 2007*).

A meta-analysis demonstrated that the addition of radiotherapy to chemotherapy reduces the rate of relapse but did not show a survival benefit for the combined-modality approach.

The EORTC conducted a randomized trial in patients with stages III and IV HL in which those achieving a complete remission with MOPP/ABV hybrid were randomized to receive either low-dose IFRT or no radiotherapy. Of the 739 patients enrolled, 421 achieved a complete remission. The median follow-up was 79 months. There was no statistically significant difference in 5-year event-free or overall survival. Partial responders received low-dose IFRT, and their event-free and overall survival rates were similar to those patients who achieved a complete remission.

LONG-TERM TOXICITIES OF COMBINATION CHEMOTHERAPY

The CALGB trial and the intergroup trials mentioned previously (see section on "Combination chemotherapy regimens") noted differences in the long-term toxicities of various combination chemotherapeutic regimens (Table 5).

Myelodysplasia and acute leukemia MOPP therapy is known to be related to the development of myelodysplastic syndromes (MDS) and acute leukemia. These secondary hematologic malignancies begin 2 years following therapy and decline by 10 years, with the maximum risk between 5 and 9 years. Patients with these malignancies have a poor prognosis.

The incidence of secondary leukemia appears to increase with cumulative doses of chemotherapy, age > 40 years when receiving chemotherapy for HL, and splenectomy. It is controversial whether combined-modality therapy increases the risk of leukemia compared with chemotherapy alone.

Cytogenetic studies of secondary leukemias reveal a loss of the long arm of chromosome 5 and/or 7. Less frequently, there is a loss of chromosome 18 or rearrangement of the short arm of chromosome 17. A balanced rearrangement of 11q23 and 2lq22 also has been described with etoposide therapy.

Other malignancies also are being observed with increasing frequency after chemotherapy (most regimens included alkylating agents), particularly for lung cancer and NHL. These malignancies have a longer latency period and usually are not observed until 15 years after therapy.

Infertility is another long-term complication seen with combination chemotherapy. At least 80% of males are found to have permanent azoospermia or oligospermia following more than 3 cycles of MOPP chemotherapy; < 10% of men will have recovery of spermatogenesis within 1–7 years following the end of chemotherapy. The risk of infertility with ABVD chemotherapy is significantly lower than that with MOPP chemotherapy, approximately 15% to 25%. All men who desire childbearing potential following therapy should be counseled regarding sperm banking.

In females, there is a 50% rate of primary ovarian failure overall. The risk is 25% to 30% in patients treated at age 25 or younger but increases to 80% to

100% in women older than age 25. Many women who do maintain ovarian function during chemotherapy will have premature menopause following therapy.

Pulmonary complications have been reported with ABVD chemotherapy and are related to bleomycin-induced lung toxicity. In a Memorial Sloan-Kettering Cancer Center study of 60 patients with early-stage HL receiving ABVD chemotherapy with or without mediastinal irradiation, bleomycin was discontinued in 23% of patients. Following ABVD therapy, there was a significant decline in median forced vital capacity (FVC) and diffusing capacity of the lungs for carbon monoxide (DLCO). Radiotherapy following ABVD chemotherapy resulted in a further decrease in FVC but did not significantly affect functional status. In a study from the Mayo Clinic, bleomycin pulmonary toxicity (BPT) was observed in 18% of patients. Increasing age, and use of ABVD and granulocyte colony-stimulating factor were associated with development of BPT. Patients

> Recent reports have confirmed the adverse effects of alkylating agent-containing chemotherapy but the relative sparing of non-alkylating agent chemotherapy on both male and female fertility. Female fertility is well preserved following treatment with ABVD *(Hodgson DC, Pintilie M, Gitterman L, et al: Hematol Oncol 25:11-15, 2007; Brusamolino E, Baio A, Orlandi E, et al: Clin Cancer Res 12:6487-6493, 2006).* Male fertility is poorly preserved following alkyating agent-containing chemotherapy (MOPP/ABV hybrid, BEACOPP), as measured both by semen analysis and FSH determinations, but well preserved with nonalkylating agent containing chemotherapy (ABVD, EBVP) by FSH determination *(van der Kaaij MA, Heutte N, Le Stang N, et al: J Clin Oncol 25:2825-2832, 2007; Sieniawski M, Reineke T, Nogova L, et al: Blood 111:71-76, 2008).*

with BPT had a 5-year overall survival of only 63% compared with 90% ($P=$ .001) in patients without BPT. Mortality from BPT was 4.2% in all patients and 24% in those who developed BPT. The omission of bleomycin had no effect on obtaining complete remission or on progression-free or overall survival.

In the CALGB trial, there were 3 fatal pulmonary complications in 238 patients; all 3 patients were older than age 40.

Pulmonary fibrosis has also been described after combined-modality therapy. Pulmonary function testing usually reveals a decreased diffusion capacity and restrictive changes prior to the onset of symptoms.

Cardiomyopathy is a recognized complication of doxorubicin therapy but is not commonly seen in patients receiving ABVD chemotherapy. Patients who are treated with 6 cycles of ABVD chemotherapy receive a total doxorubicin dose of 300 mg/m^2; cardiac toxicity is rarely seen in patients who receive a total dose $\leq$ 400 mg/m^2.

MANAGEMENT OF RELAPSED DISEASE

Relapse after radiation therapy

Patients with early-stage HL who relapse after initial therapy with irradiation alone have excellent complete remission rates and 50% to 80% long-term survival rates when treated with MOPP or ABVD. The dose regimens used for salvage therapy are the same as those outlined in Table 4.

Relapse after combination chemotherapy

Among patients with advanced-stage HL, 70% to 90% will have complete response to treatment; however, up to one-third of patients with stage III or IV disease will relapse, usually within the first 3 years after therapy.

Various studies have identified the following poor prognostic factors for response to first-line chemotherapy: B symptoms, age > 45 years, bulky mediastinal disease, extranodal involvement, low hematocrit, high ESR, high levels of CD30, and high levels of serum interleukin-10 (IL-10) and soluble IL-2 receptor.

An International Prognostic Index (IPI) has been devised for advanced HL based on a retrospective analysis of 1,618 patients from 25 centers. In the final model, seven factors were used: albumin < 4 g/dL, hemoglobin < 10.5 g/dL, male gender, stage IV disease, age ≥ 45 years, WBC ≥ 15,000/μL, and lymphocytes < 600/μL (or 8% of the WBC count). The worst prognostic group (7%) had a 5-year overall survival rate of 56% and a failure-free survival rate of 42%.

In a comparison of seven well-known prognostic models for HL applied retrospectively to a population of patients with advanced-stage disease, three were found to be the most predictive of outcome. One was the IPI, mentioned previously. The other two were the Memorial Sloan-Kettering Cancer Center model (employing age, LDH, hematocrit, inguinal nodal involvement, and mediastinal mass bulk) and the Database on Hodgkin Lymphoma model (employing stage, age, B symptoms, albumin level, and gender). Integration of the three models in a linear model improved their predictive power.

High-dose therapy with autologous stem-cell transplantation The preferred salvage method for patients who relapsed after combined-modality therapy or chemotherapy alone or remained refractory to those programs is high-dose chemoradiotherapy with autologous stem-cell transplantation (ASCT).

Two randomized studies (from Great Britain and Germany) demonstrated an event-free survival advantage with the high-dose therapy approach. Although a significant survival advantage was not observed due to the crossover design of the studies, most patients with refractory disease or postchemotherapy relapse are currently managed with high-dose chemoradiation therapy and ASCT.

No standard conditioning regimen has been used in this setting, as patients have had prior treatment with a variety of combinations of chemotherapy and radiation therapy. Although most patients who have received bone marrow have been treated with several regimens or have had poorly responsive disease from initial diagnosis, the complete response rate has ranged from 50% to 80%, with approximately 40% to 80% of responding patients achieving durable remission.

Analysis of prognostic factors in patients receiving high-dose salvage therapy indicated that B symptoms at relapse, extranodal disease, and short (< 1 year) remission or no remission are factors associated with a poor outcome.

A study from Memorial Sloan-Kettering Cancer Center reported the results of high-dose chemotherapy with ASCT in 65 patients with relapsed or refractory HL. At a median follow-up of 43 months, overall survival was estimated to be 73% and event-free survival was estimated to be 58% by intent-to-treat analysis. In a multivariate logistic regression model, there were three adverse prognostic factors: extranodal sites of relapse or refractory disease, complete remission duration of less than 1 year or refractory disease, and B symptoms. Patients with no or one adverse factor had an overall survival of 90% and an event-free survival of 83%; those with two adverse factors had an overall survival of 57% and an event-free survival of 27%; and those with three adverse factors had an overall survival of 25% and an event-free survival of 10%. A follow-up study of a risk-adapted approach based on the study previously described suggested that patients with adverse prognostic factors may benefit from further augmentation of high-dose programs, including a "double-transplant" for selected patients.

SUGGESTED READING

Aleman BM, Raemaekers JM, Tomisic R, et al: Involved-field radiotherapy for patients in partial remission after chemotherapy for advanced Hodgkin's lymphoma. Int J Radiat Oncol Biol Phys 67:19–30, 2007.

Aleman BM, van den Belt-Dusebout AW, De Bruin ML, et al: Late cardiotoxicity after treatment for Hodgkin lymphoma. Blood 109:1878–1886, 2007.

Cheson BD, Pfistner B, Juweid ME, et al: Revised response criteria for malignant lymphoma. J Clin Oncol 25:579–586, 2007.

Franklin J, Pluetschow A, Paus M, et al: Second malignancy risk associated with treatment of Hodgkin's lymphoma: Meta-analysis of the randomised trials. Ann Oncol 17:1749–1760, 2006.

Goodman KA, Toner S, Hunt M, et al: Intensity-modulated radiotherapy for lymphoma involving the mediastinum. Int J Radiat Oncol Biol Phys 62:198–206, 2005.

Hoppe RT, Advani RH, Bierman PJ, et al: Hodgkin disease/lymphoma: Clinical practice guidelines in oncology. J Natl Compr Canc Netw 4:210–230, 2006.

Lorigan P, Radford J, Howell A, et al: Lung cancer after treatment for Hodgkin's lymphoma: A systematic review. Lancet Oncol 6:773–779, 2005.

Meyer RM, Gospodarowicz MK, Connors JM, et al: Randomized comparison of ABVD chemotherapy with a strategy that includes radiation therapy in patients with limited-stage Hodgkin's lymphoma: National Cancer Institute of Canada Clinical Trials Group and the Eastern Cooperative Oncology Group. J Clin Oncol 23:4634–4642, 2005.

Tsai HK, Mauch PM: Nodular lymphocyte-predominant hodgkin lymphoma. Semin Radiat Oncol 17:184–189, 2007.

Yahalom J: Favorable early-stage Hodgkin lymphoma. J Natl Compr Canc Netw 4:233–240, 2006.

CHAPTER 30

Non-Hodgkin lymphoma

Steven T. Rosen, MD, Jane N. Winter, MD, Leo I. Gordon, MD,
Andrew M. Evens, DO, MS, Brian C. -H Chiu, PhD, and Richard Tsang, MD

The incidence rates of non-Hodgkin lymphoma (NHL) in the United States have almost doubled since the early 1970s, representing one of the largest increases of any cancer. Some of this increase may be artifactual, resulting from improved diagnostic techniques and access to medical care, or directly related to the development of NHL in 25- to 54-year-old men with human immunodeficiency virus (HIV) infection. However, additional factors must be responsible for this unexpected increase in frequency of NHL that has been observed throughout the United States.

The incidence of NHL per 100,000 persons has risen from 8.8 in 1972–1974 to 19.3 in 1995–1999 (all histologic subtypes) in the United States. The increases have been more pronounced in whites, males, the elderly, and those with NHL diagnosed at extranodal sites. Similar findings have been reported in other developed countries. NHL rates have decreased among American males aged 25 to 54 years in the middle to late 1990s (6% to 16% per year), although this may be in part due to improved HIV treatment.

Currently, NHL represents approximately 4% of all cancer diagnoses (4% in males and 4% in females), being the fifth most common cancer in women and the sixth in men. Estimates from the American Cancer Society indicate that in 2008, some 66,120 new cases of NHL will be diagnosed in the United States and approximately 19,160 people will die of this disease.

Epidemiology

Gender The overall incidence of lymphoma is higher in men than in women. The incidence rate (per 100,000 population) between 2000 and 2004 was 40% higher in males (23.2) than in females (16.3). Only thyroid NHL is more common in women than in men.

Age Overall, the incidence of NHL rises exponentially with increasing age. In persons older than age 65, the incidence is 87.2 per 100,000 population. Except for high-grade lymphoblastic and Burkitt lymphomas (the most common types of NHL seen in children and young adults), the median age at presentation for all subtypes of NHL exceeds 50+ years. Low-grade lymphomas account for 37% of NHLs in patients between the ages of 35 and 64 years at diagnosis but for only 16% of cases in those younger than age 35.

Race The incidence varies by race, with whites at higher risk than blacks and Asian-Americans (incidence rates increased 40% to 70% in whites compared with blacks). Most histologies, particularly low-grade small lymphocytic and follicular lymphomas, are more common in whites than in blacks. Only peripheral T-cell lymphoma, mycosis fungoides, and Sézary syndrome are more common in blacks than in whites.

Geography NHL is most common in developed countries, with the United States having the highest rate worldwide. The lowest NHL rates are found in Eastern and south central Asia (2–3 per 100,000 population). Certain endemic geographic factors appear to influence the development of NHL in specific areas.

HTLV-1–associated NHL Human T-cell lymphotrophic virus-1 (HTLV-1)–associated adult T-cell lymphoma/leukemia (ATLL) occurs more frequently where HTLV-1 is endemic, in southern Japan and the Caribbean, and occurs sporadically in Brazil, sub-Saharan Africa, the Middle East, and the southeastern United States. The seroprevalence in southwest Japan is 16%, although the lifetime risk of ATLL for these persons is 2% to 6%.

Burkitt lymphoma in Africa The incidence (per 100,000 population) of Burkitt NHL in Africa (Nigeria and Tanzania) is 6 to 8, as compared with 0.1 in the United States. The clinical features of Burkitt lymphoma in Africa differ from those of cases reported to the American Burkitt Lymphoma Registry. Etiologic endemic factors include malaria as a source of chronic B-cell antigenic stimulation and Epstein-Barr virus (EBV)-induced immortalization of B lymphocytes.

Immunoproliferative small intestinal disease (α-chain disease) Heavy-chain disease is a disorder of B-lymphoid cells characterized by diffuse thickening of the small intestine due to a lymphoplasmacytic infiltrate with secretion of incomplete IgA heavy chains. Pathologically, it is a mucosa-associated lymphoid tissue (MALT) lymphoma of the small bowel. This clinicopathologic entity is rarely encountered in individuals other than those of Mediterranean ethnic origin.

Follicular lymphomas are more common in North America and Europe but are rare in the Caribbean, Africa, China, Japan, the Middle East, and Latin America.

Peripheral T-cell lymphomas are more common in Europe and China than in North America. They represent 7% to 12% of lymphomas in Western countries.

A recent study reported that NHL confers a stronger familial association among men than among women. Siblings are also a more powerful marker of personal risk of NHL than is history of NHL in a parent. Overall, the pattern of NHL heritability is similar across histologic subtypes (Wang SS, Slager SL, Brennan P, et al: Blood 109:3479-3488, 2007).

Disease site Malignant lymphomas are a heterogeneous group of neoplasms that usually arise or present in lymphoid tissues, such as lymph nodes, spleen, and bone marrow, but they may arise in almost any tissue. The most frequent sites for extranodal lymphomas, which constitute about 20% to 30% of all lymphomas (peripheral T-cell NHL 80%; extranodal, follicular 9%), are the stomach, skin, oral cavity and pharynx, small intestine, and central nervous system (CNS). Although primary CNS lymphomas are rare, there has been a threefold increase in incidence, even if patients with HIV infection and other types of immunosuppression are excluded.

Survival The 5-year relative survival rate of patients with NHL increased from 28% between 1950 and 1954 to 63% between 1990 and 2003. These improvements in survival occurred mainly in patients with intermediate-high-grade histologies. The potential for cure varies among the different histologic subtypes and is directly related to stage at presentation and response to initial therapy. The natural history (survival rates) for indolent lymphomas has been unchanged from the 1950s to the early 1990s, although a recent analysis from Iowa of Surveillance, Epidemiology, and End Results (SEER) data (1979–1999) shows improving survival rates of patients with follicular lymphoma.

Etiology and risk factors

Chromosomal translocations and molecular rearrangements Nonrandom chromosomal and molecular rearrangements play an important role in the pathogenesis of many lymphomas and correlate with histology and immunophenotype (Table 1). The most commonly associated chromosomal abnormality in NHL is the t(14;18)(q32;q21) translocation, which is found in 85% of follicular lymphomas and 28% of higher grade NHLs. This translocation results in the juxtaposition of the *bcl-2* apoptotic inhibitor "oncogene" at chromosome band 18q21 to the heavy-chain region of the immunoglobulin locus within chromosome band 14q32.

The t(11;14)(q13;q32) translocation results in overexpression of *bcl-1* (cyclin D1/PRAD 1), a cell-cycle–control gene on chromosome 11q13, and is characteristically associated with mantle cell lymphoma. The t(3;16)(q27;p11) translocation makes the gene for the IL-2 (interleukin-2) receptor a partner of *bcl-6*, which is expressed in diffuse large cell lymphoma.

Chromosomal translocations involving 8q24 lead to c-*myc* deregulation and are frequently seen in Burkitt and Burkitt-like lymphomas, including those associated with HIV infection.

Environmental factors also may play a role in the development of NHL.

Occupations Certain workers have a slightly increased risk of developing NHL, including farmers; pesticide applicators; grain (flour) millers; meat workers; wood and forestry workers; chemists; painters; mechanics; machinists; and workers in the petroleum, rubber, plastics, and synthetics industries.

Chemicals that have been linked to the development of NHL include a variety of pesticides and herbicides (2,4-D-organophosphates, chlorophenols), solvents and organic chemicals (benzene, carbon tetra-chloride), wood preservatives, and some components in hair dye. There is evidence that the association between pesticides and NHL risk was limited to t(14;18)-positive NHL cases.

TABLE 1: Correlation of chromosomal abnormalities in NHL with histology, antigen rearrangement, and oncogene expression

Cytogenetic abnormality	Histology	Antigen rearrangement	Oncogene expression
B-cell lymphoma			
t(14;18)(q32;q21)	Follicular lymphoma, diffuse large B-cell lymphoma	IgH	bcl-2
	MALT lymphoma	IgH	MALT-1
t(11;14)(q13;q32)	Mantle cell	IgH	bcl-1
t(1;14)(p22;q32)	MALT lymphoma	IgH	bcl-10
t(11;18)(q21;q21)	MALT lymphoma		API-2 on chromosome 11 MALT-1on chromosome 18
t(9;14)(p13;q32)	Lymphoplasmacytic lymphoma	IgH	PAX-5
8q24 translocations	Burkitt lymphoma		c-myc
t(8;14)(q24;q32)	and variants	IgH	
t(2;8)(p11-12;q24)		Ig-λ	
t(8;22)(q24;q11)		Ig-κ	
(3;22)(q27;q11)	Diffuse (large cell, small cleaved cell)	Ig-κ	bcl-6 (LAZ-3)
T-cell lymphoma			
14q11 abnormalities			
inv 14(q11;q32)	Variable	TCR-α	tcl-1
t(10;14)(q24;q11)	Variable	TCR-α	hox-11 (tcl-3)
i(7q)(q10)	Hepatosplenic	TCR-δ	
2p23 translocations			alk
t(2;5)(p23;q35)	ALCL	TCR-α	NPM
t(1;2)(p21;p23)	ALCL	TCR-α	TPM3
t(2;3)(p23;p20)	ALCL	TCR-α	TFG
t(2;22)(p23;q11)	ALCL	TCR-α	CLTCL
inv(2)(p23;q35)	ALCL	TCR-α	ATIC

ALK = anaplastic lymphoma kinase; ALCL = anaplastic large cell lymphoma; ATIC = 5-aminoimidazole-4-carboxamide-1-beta-D-ribonucleotide transformylase/inosine monophosphate cyclohydrolase; INPM = nucleophosmin gene; TPM3 = nonmuscle tropomyosin; TFG = tropomyosin receptor kinase-fused gene; CLTCL = clathrin heavy polypeptide-like gene; ATIC = 5-aminoimidazole-4-carboxamide-1-beta-D-ribonucleotide transformylase/inosine monophosphate cyclohydrolase; inv = inversion; MALT = mucosa-associated lymphoid tissue

Chemotherapy and radiotherapy Patients who receive chemotherapy and/or radiation therapy are also at increased risk of developing NHL.

Viruses Several viruses have been implicated in the pathogenesis of NHL, including EBV; HTLV-1; Kaposi's sarcoma-associated herpesvirus (KSHV, also known as human herpesvirus 8, or HHV-8); and hepatitis C virus (HCV). Meta-analyses have shown 13% to 15% HCV seroprevalence in certain geographic regions among persons with B-cell NHL.

EBV is a DNA virus that has been associated with Burkitt lymphoma, particularly in endemic areas of Africa; Hodgkin lymphoma; lymphomas in immunocompromised patients (ie, organ transplantation and HIV infection); sinonasal lymphoma (Asia and South America); and sporadically in other B- and T-cell lymphomas. In contrast to studies performed in European patients, Mexican patients with intestinal lymphomas show a high frequency of EBV positivity; this finding is not limited to T-cell NHLs but rather includes a significant portion of B-cell NHLs. EBV can transform lymphocytes in culture. B lymphocytes from normal EBV-positive subjects have been shown to grow as tumors in mice with severe combined immunodeficiency.

HTLV-1 is a human retrovirus that establishes a latent infection via reverse transcription in activated T-helper cells. A minority (5%) of carriers develop ATLL. An HTLV-1–like provirus has been detected in some patients with mycosis fungoides, although conflicting findings have been reported.

KSHV or HHV-8: KSHV-like DNA sequences are frequently detected in primary effusion lymphomas in patients with HIV infection and in those with multicentric (plasma cell variant) Castleman's disease.

HCV infection is associated with the development of clonal B-cell expansions and certain subtypes of NHL, particularly in the setting of essential (type II) mixed cryoglobulinemia. HCV may predispose B cells to malignant transformation by enhancing signal transduction upon binding to the CD81 (TAPA-1) molecule.

Bacterial infections Infection with *Borrelia burgdorferi*, the etiologic agent in Lyme disease, has been detected in about 35% of patients with primary cutaneous B-cell lymphoma in Scotland. A near-complete clinical and histologic remission of a primary marginal zone B-cell lymphoma was observed after eradication of *B burgdorferi* with antibiotic treatment. Gastric MALT lymphoma is seen most frequently, but not exclusively, in association with *Helicobacter pylori* infection. Recent studies indicate that *Campylobacter jejuni* and immunoproliferative small intestinal disease (α-chain disease) are related.

Chlamydial infections Some reports noted an association between infection with *Chlamydia psittaci* and ocular adnexal lymphoma. The infection was found to be highly specific and does not reflect a subclinical infection widespread among the general population. Responses to antibiotics have been reported. Attempts to confirm this association in the Western hemisphere have been unsuccessful.

Immune modulation *Congenital immunodeficiencies* Congenital and acquired states of immunosuppression that are at increased risk include ataxia-telangiectasia, Wiskott-Aldrich syndrome, common variable hypogamma-globulinemia, X-linked lymphoproliferative syndrome, and severe combined immunodeficiency.

Acquired immunodeficiency states, such as HIV infection (relative risk of NHL is 150–250 increased among patients with AIDS, usually high grade and extranodal), iatrogenic immunosuppression (ie, organ or blood stem-cell transplantation recipients, long-term survivors of Hodgkin lymphoma), and a variety of collagen vascular and autoimmune diseases (eg, Sjögren's syndrome, rheumatoid vasculitis and Felty's syndrome, systemic lupus erythematosus, chronic lymphocytic thyroiditis), also pose an increased risk of NHL.

Autoimmune disorders An increased incidence of GI lymphomas is seen in patients with celiac (nontropical) sprue and inflammatory bowel disease, particularly Crohn's disease. An aberrant clonal intraepithelial T-cell population can be found in up to 75% of patients with refractory celiac sprue prior to the development of overt T-cell lymphoma using immunophenotyping and T-cell receptor gamma gene rearrangement PCR (polymerase chain reaction) techniques. Systemic lupus erythematosus and rheumatoid arthritis have been associated with B-cell lymphoma. Sjögren's syndrome has been associated with NHL overall and diffuse large B-cell lymphoma (DLBCL).

Lifestyle factors Several studies have reported an excess risk of NHL in association with diets high in fat and meat products. Some studies have suggested that ultraviolet radiation exposure and alcohol intake may be linked inversely with NHL risk

Signs and symptoms

Fever, weight loss, and night sweats, referred to as systemic B symptoms, as well as fatigue and weakness, are more common in advanced or aggressive NHL but may be present in all stages and histologic subtypes.

Low-grade lymphomas Painless, slowly progressive peripheral adenopathy is the most common clinical presentation in patients with low-grade lymphomas. Patients sometimes report a history of waxing and waning adenopathy before seeking medical attention. Spontaneous regression of enlarged lymph nodes can occur and can cause a low-grade lymphoma to be confused with an infectious condition.

Primary extranodal involvement and B symptoms are uncommon at presentation; however, both are common in advanced or end-stage disease. Bone marrow is frequently involved, sometimes in association with cytopenias. Splenomegaly is seen in about 40% of patients, but the spleen is rarely the only involved site at presentation.

Intermediate- and high-grade lymphomas The clinical presentation of intermediate- and high-grade lymphomas is more varied. Although the majority of patients present with adenopathy, more than one-third present with extranodal involvement, the most common sites being the GI tract (including Waldeyer's ring), skin, bone marrow, sinuses, genitourinary (GU) tract, thyroid, and CNS.

B symptoms are more common, occurring in about 30% to 40% of patients.

Lymphoblastic lymphoma often presents with an anterior superior mediastinal mass, superior vena cava syndrome, and leptomeningeal disease with cranial nerve palsies.

American patients with Burkitt lymphoma often present with a large abdominal mass and symptoms of bowel obstruction.

Screening and diagnosis

No effective methods are available for screening or identifying populations at high risk of developing NHL. A definitive diagnosis can be made only by biopsy of pathologic lymph nodes or tumor tissue. It is critical to perform an excisional node biopsy (fine-needle aspiration [FNA] is insufficient for diagnostic purposes) to avoid false-negative results and inaccurate histologic classification. One study showed that when FNAs and biopsy results for the diagnosis of NHL and Hodgkin lymphoma were directly compared, only 12% of FNAs correlated with subsequent excisional biopsy results. When clinical circumstances make surgical biopsy of involved lymph nodes or extranodal sites prohibitive, a core biopsy obtained under CT or ultrasonographic guidance may suffice but often requires the integration of histologic examination and immunophenotypic and molecular studies for diagnosis. A formal review by an expert hematopathologist is mandatory. Additional studies, such as immunophenotyping and genotyping, are often necessary.

Initial diagnostic evaluation of patients with lymphoproliferative malignancy should include the following:

- Careful history (night sweats, weight loss, fever; neurologic, musculoskeletal, or GI symptoms)
- Physical examination (lymph nodes, including submental, infraclavicular, epitrochlear, iliac, femoral, and popliteal nodes; pericardial rub, pleural effusion, distended neck and/or upper extremity veins in superior vena cava syndrome; breast masses; hepatosplenomegaly, bowel obstruction, renal mass, and testicular or ovarian mass; focal neurologic signs, such as plexopathy, spinal cord compression, nerve root infiltration, and meningeal involvement; skin lesions)
- Biopsy of peripheral lymphadenopathy (excisional biopsy)
- Chest x-ray (mediastinal or hilar adenopathy, pleural effusions, parenchymal lesions)
- CT scan of the neck (cervical lymph nodes, Waldeyer's ring) and chest (mediastinal, hilar, or parenchymal pulmonary disease)
- CT scan of the abdomen and pelvis (enlarged lymph nodes, splenomegaly, filling defects in liver and spleen)
- Bilateral bone marrow biopsy and aspirate

TABLE 2: Immunophenotypic and histochemical diagnosis of B-cell lymphomas/leukemias

Marker	Follicular	CLL	Mantle	MZL/ MALT	PLL*	DLBCL	HCL	BL/BLL	LPL
SIg	+	dim+	+	+/+	+	+(–)	+	+	+
CIg	–	–(+)	–	–(+)	–	–(+)	–	–	+
CD5	–	+	+	–/–	–(+)	–	–	–	–
CD10	+	–	–	–/–	–	–(+)	–	+	–
CD20	+	dim+	+	+/+	+	+	+	+	+
CD23	–(+)	+	–	–/–	+(–)	–	–	–	–
CD43	–	+	+	–(+)/–(+)	–	–(+)	+	–	+(–)
CD103	–	–	–	+/–	–	NA	+	NA	–
Cyclin D1	–	–	+	–/–	–	–	–(+)	–	–

+, > 90% positive; +(–), > 50% positive; –(+), < 50% positive; –, < 10% positive; MZL/MALT = splenic marginal zone/mucosa-associated lymphoid tissue; CLL = chronic lymphocytic leukemia; PLL = prolymphocytic leukemia; HCL = hairy cell leukemia; BL/BLL = Burkitt lymphoma/Burkitt-like lymphoma, DLBCL = diffuse large B-cell lymphoma; LPL = lymphoplasmacytic lymphoma; SIg = surface immunoglobulin; CIg = cytoplasmic immunoglobulin

* A T-cell variant is present in approximately 20% to 30% of PLL cases.

- PET scans (selected cases: B-cell follicular and aggressive histologies) for staging at diagnosis, response, assessment, and relapse

- CBC with differential and platelet count (peripheral blood lymphocytosis with circulating malignant cells is common in low-grade and mantle cell lymphomas). Bone marrow and peripheral blood involvement may be present, and the distinction between leukemia and lymphoma is difficult to make in some cases.

- General chemistry panel (including lactic dehydrogenase [LDH] level determination) is mandatory.

- HIV serology in at-risk patients with diffuse large cell and other aggressive and Burkitt histologies; HTLV-1 serology in select patients with cutaneous T-cell lymphoma, especially if they have hypercalcemia

- Cytogenetic and molecular analyses of lymph node, bone marrow, and peripheral blood (selected cases)

- Immunophenotyping can be of particular benefit in distinguishing B-cell chronic leukemia/small lymphocytic lymphoma from other lymphomas (Table 2).

- Examination of CSF and consideration of intrathecal chemotherapy prophylaxis in patients with (1) diffuse aggressive NHL with bone marrow, epidural, testicular, paranasal sinus, breast, or multiple extranodal sites; (2) high-grade lymphoblastic lymphoma and Burkitt lymphoma and its variants; (3) primary CNS lymphoma if no evidence of increased intracranial pressure

- Upper GI endoscopy and/or GI series with small bowel follow-through in patients with head and neck involvement (tonsil, base of tongue, nasopharynx) and those with a GI primary; mantle cell lymphoma is associated with a high incidence of occult GI involvement.

- Ultrasonography of opposite testis in patients with a testicular primary

- Spinal MRI scan for epidural disease when clinically indicated (useful in the evaluation of suspected spinal cord involvement).

Pathology

The Working Formulation was proposed in 1982 as a modification of the Rappaport classification of NHL based on morphology and biologic aggressiveness. Although many subtypes were not recognized, including T-cell lineage lymphomas, a revised European-American classification of lymphoid neoplasms (REAL classification) was introduced in 1994 incorporating T-cell malignancies, subtypes of Hodgkin lymphoma and newer defined lymphoma-proliferative disorders. The WHO (World Health Organization) classification for lymphomas (introduced in 1999) uses the principles of the REAL classification and defines each entity according to morphologic features, immunophenotype, genetic features, postulated normal counterpart, and clinical features. The WHO classification is similar to the REAL classification, with some modifications based on current data (Table 3).

WHO CLASSIFICATION

The most frequently occurring clinical entities recognized by the REAL/WHO classification are DLBCL (31%), follicular lymphoma (22%), lymphoma of MALT type (8%), small lymphocytic lymphoma (7%), mantle cell lymphoma (6%), peripheral T-cell lymphoma (7%), primary mediastinal large B-cell lymphoma (2%), anaplastic large T-/null-cell lymphoma (2%), lymphoblastic lymphoma of T- or B-cell lineage, marginal zone (monocytoid) B-cell lymphoma (2%), lymphoplasmacytic lymphoma (2%), Burkitt lymphoma (2%), and other (9%).

The WHO classification includes three types of follicular lymphoma (grades 1–3). Grades 1 and 2 correspond to follicular small-cleaved cell and follicular mixed small-cleaved and large cell lymphoma, which are considered to be low-grade lymphomas by the Working Formulation. Grade 3 corresponds to follicular large cell lymphoma, which is considered an intermediate-grade NHL in the Working Formulation, and is generally treated as a large cell lymphoma. The WHO classification considers B-cell small lymphocytic lymphoma to be synonymous with chronic lymphocytic leukemia (CLL).

TABLE 3: WHO classification of lymphoid neoplasms

B-cell neoplasms
    Precursor B-cell neoplasm
        Precursor B-lymphoblastic leukemia/lymphoma (precursor B-cell acute lymphoblastic leukemia)
    Mature (peripheral) B-cell neoplasms
        B-cell chronic lymphocytic leukemia/small lymphocytic lymphoma
        B-cell prolymphocytic leukemia
        Lymphoplasmacytic lymphoma
        Splenic marginal zone B-cell lymphoma (± villous lymphocytes)
        Hairy cell leukemia
        Plasma cell myeloma/plasmacytoma
        Extranodal marginal zone B-cell lymphoma of MALT type
        Nodal marginal zone B-cell lymphoma (± monocytoid B cells)
        Follicular lymphoma
        Mantle cell lymphoma
        Diffuse large B-cell lymphoma
            Mediastinal large B-cell lymphoma
            Primary effusion lymphoma
        Burkitt lymphoma/Burkitt-like lymphoma

T-cell and NK-cell neoplasms
    Precursor T-cell neoplasm
        Precursor T-lymphoblastic lymphoma/leukemia (precursor T-cell acute lymphoblastic leukemia)
    Mature (peripheral) T-cell neoplasms
        T-cell prolymphocytic leukemia
        T-cell granular lymphocytic leukemia
        Aggressive NK-cell leukemia
        Adult T-cell lymphoma/leukemia (HTLV-1+)
        Extranodal NK/T-cell lymphoma, nasal type
        Enteropathy-type T-cell lymphoma
        Hepatosplenic γ/δ T-cell lymphoma
        Subcutaneous panniculitis-like T-cell lymphoma
        Mycosis fungoides/Sézary syndrome
        Anaplastic large cell lymphoma, T-/null-cell, primary cutaneous type
        Peripheral T-cell lymphoma, unspecified
        Angioimmunoblastic T-cell lymphoma
        Anaplastic large cell lymphoma, T-/null-cell, primary systemic type

Hodgkin lymphoma (Hodgkin disease)
    Nodular lymphocyte-predominant Hodgkin lymphoma
    Classic Hodgkin lymphoma
        Nodular sclerosis Hodgkin lymphoma (grades 1 and 2)
        Lymphocyte-rich classic Hodgkin lymphoma
        Mixed cellularity Hodgkin lymphoma
        Lymphocyte-depletion Hodgkin lymphoma

Italic type denotes more common clinical entities. WHO = World Health Organization; MALT = mucosa-associated lymphoid tissue; NK = natural killer; HTLV-1 = human T-cell lymphotrophic virus-1

Other indolent lymphomas recognized by the WHO classification, but not by the Working Formulation, include lymphoplasmacytic lymphoma, splenic marginal zone B-cell lymphoma, extranodal marginal zone lymphoma of MALT type, and nodal marginal zone B-cell lymphoma.

The WHO classification has recognized marginal zone lymphomas (MZLs) as unique clinical and pathologic entities, ie, extranodal (MALT), nodal, and splenic NHL subtypes. MALT NHL is extremely indolent and presents as localized stages I to II disease, infrequently disseminating. The stomach is the most frequent site, but low-grade NHLs (and former pseudo-lymphomas) of the lungs, thyroid, salivary gland, and orbit are of this type.

Staging and prognosis

Determining the extent of disease in patients with NHL provides prognostic information and is useful in treatment planning. However, histologic subclassification (WHO classification) is the primary determinant of survival and potential for cure. Compared with patients with limited disease, those with extensive disease usually require different therapy, and certain extranodal sites of involvement, such as the CNS and testes, require specific treatment modalities.

Ann Arbor system Although initially devised for Hodgkin lymphoma, the Ann Arbor system has been routinely applied to NHL (Table 4). Because Hodgkin lymphoma commonly spreads via contiguous lymph node groups, this system is based primarily on the distribution of lymphatic involvement with respect to the diaphragm and the presence of extralymphatic organ involvement. The Ann Arbor system does not reflect the noncontiguous nature of disease spread in NHL, does not discriminate well between stages III and IV disease, and fails to account for tumor bulk or number of extranodal sites.

Some trials in Burkitt and Burkitt-like lymphoma use the St. Jude/Murphy staging system (Table 5), in part to more completely describe the extent of extranodal disease. Unlike the current WHO classification, this staging system recognizes Burkitt leukemia as a separate entity. Moreover, this system was developed

The anti-CD20 monoclonal antibody rituximab (Rituxan) has markedly changed the approach and prognosis of patients with follicular lymphoma (FL) and diffuse large B-cell lymphoma (DLBCL). The original International Prognostic Index (IPI) and Follicular Lymphoma International Prognostic Index (FLIPI) scoring systems were reported among patients who had not received rituximab. Given the improved results with rituximab, revisions using the same factors as the original IPI and FLIPI have been reported. Sehn et al showed that using the revised IPI for rituximab-treated DLBCL patients produced groups of very good (IPI score of 0), good (score of 1 or 2), and poor (score of 3 or more) risk groups with associated 4-year overall survival rates of 94%, 79%, and 55%, respectively. In addition, Buske et al showed that among advanced FL patients treated with R-CHOP in a phase III randomized trial, a modified separation of distinct FL IPI risk groups was achieved. Patients with 1 or 2 risk factors (55% of the patients), 3 risk factors (27% of patients), and 4 or 5 risk factors (18% of patients) had associated 2-year time to treatment failure rates of 90%, 74%, and 57%, respectively (P < .001); (Sehn LH, Berry B, Chhanabhai M, et al: Blood 109:1857-1861, 2007; Buske C, Hoster E, Dreyling M, et al: Blood 108:1504-1508, 2006).

TABLE 4: Ann Arbor staging classification for NHL[a]

Stage	Area of involvement
I	One lymph node region
I$_E$	One extralymphatic organ or site
II	Two or more lymph node regions on the same side of the diaphragm
II$_E$	One extralymphatic organ or site (localized) in addition to criteria for stage II
III	Lymph node regions on both sides of the diaphragm
III$_E$	One extralymphatic organ or site (localized) in addition to criteria for stage III
III$_S$	Spleen in addition to criteria for stage III
III$_{SE}$	Spleen and one extralymphatic organ or site (localized) in addition to criteria for stage III
IV	One or more extralymphatic organs with or without associated lymph node involvement (diffuse or disseminated); involved organs should be designated by subscript letters
	(P, lung; H, liver; M, bone marrow)

[a]Class A patients experience no symptoms; class B patients experience unexplained fever of $\geq$ 101.5°F; unexplained, drenching night sweats; or loss of >10% body weight within the previous 6 months.

TABLE 5: St. Jude/Murphy staging system for Burkitt lymphoma

Stage	Description
I	A single tumor (extranodal) or a single anatomic area (nodal) with the exclusion of the mediastinum or abdomen
II	A single extranodal tumor with regional node involvement
	Two single extranodal tumors on the same side of the diaphragm with or without regional node involvement
	Primary gastrointestinal tumor with or without involvement of associated mesenteric nodes only
	Two or more nodal areas on the same side of the diaphragm
IIR	Completely resected intra-abdominal disease
III	Two single extranodal tumors on opposite sides of the diaphragm
	All primary intrathoracic tumors (mediastinal, pleural, thymic)
	All paraspinal or epidural tumors, regardless of other tumor sites
	All extensive primary intra-abdominal diseases
	Two or more nodal areas on opposite sides of the diaphragm
IIIA	Localized but nonresectable intra-abdominal disease
IIIB	Widespread multiorgan abdominal disease
IV	Any of the above with initial CNS and/or bone marrow involvement (less than 25% involvement; greater than 25% involvement is defined as L3 A/LL)

TABLE 6: International Prognostic Index

Parameter	Adverse factor
Age	≥ 60 years
Ann Arbor stage	III or IV
Serum LDH level	Above normal
Number of extranodal sites of involvement	≥ 2
Performance status	≥ ECOG 2 or equivalent

LDH = lactic dehydrogenase; ECOG = Eastern Cooperative Oncology Group

From International non-Hodgkin's Lymphoma Prognostic Factors Project: N Engl J Med 329:987–994, 1993.

when surgery was used for diagnostic and therapeutic purposes. Patients are also typically stratified into two risk groups, with low-risk patients defined as having a normal LDH level and a single focus of disease measuring less than 10 cm and all others considered to be high risk.

Prognostic factors Histology and morphology remain the major determinants of treatment outcome and prognosis, but gene expression signatures are likely to be the principal determinants in the future. Some patients with slow-growing low-grade lymphoma may remain well for many years with minimal or no initial therapy, whereas survival of patients with some types of high-grade lymphoma is measured only in weeks unless aggressive treatment is initiated promptly. The biologic and clinical behaviors of these disorders vary among the different histologic subtypes.

The International Prognostic Index (IPI) was developed by 16 institutions and cooperative groups in the United States, Europe, and Canada as a prognostic factor model for aggressive NHL treated with doxorubicin-containing regimens. Clinical features that have been independently predictive of survival are included in Table 6.

TABLE 7: Follicular Lymphoma International Prognostic Index

Parameter	Adverse factor
Age	> 60 years
Ann Arbor stage	III or IV
Hemoglobin level	< 120 g/L
Serum LDH level	> ULN
Number of nodal sites	> 4

Low risk: 0–1 factors; intermediate risk: 2–3 factors; high risk: 4–5 factors

LDH = lactic dehydrogenase; ULN = upper limit of normal

From Solal-Celigny P, Roy P, Colombat P, et al: Follicular Lymphoma International Prognostic Index. Blood 104:1258–1265, 2004.

This index appears to be a useful guide for selecting treatment for patients with aggressive, diffuse large cell NHL, by identifying subsets of patients in whom intensified primary therapy may be warranted. Because younger and older patients have markedly different prognoses and younger patients are more likely to be considered for more intensive investigational regimens, an age-adjusted model for patients ≤ 60 years old has been proposed. In younger patients, stage (III or IV), high LDH level, and nonambulatory performance status are independently associated with decreased survival. In the post-rituximab (Rituxan) era, persons with no risk factors have a predicted 5-year overall survival of 94%, compared with 55% for high-risk patients with three to five risk factors.

The IPI also appears to be useful in predicting outcome in patients with low-grade lymphoma, mantle cell lymphoma, and relapsed or refractory large B-cell lymphoma in patients undergoing autologous stem-cell transplantation (SCT).

A prognostic factor model has been devised based on a study of 919 cases of follicular lymphoma, known as the Follicular Lymphoma IPI (FLIPI; Table 7). Multivariate analysis showed that age (> 60 vs ≤ 60 years), Ann Arbor stage (III–IV vs I–II), number of extranodal sites (> 4 vs ≤ 4), LDH level (above normal vs normal/below normal), and hemoglobin level (< 120 g/L vs ≥ 120 g/L) were predictors of overall survival.

Treatment-related factors Time to complete remission has been identified as an important treatment-related prognostic factor in aggressive NHL. Patients who require more than 5 cycles of standard chemotherapy to achieve remission have a high risk of relapse. Similarly, patients with PET-avid tumors who have persistent PET uptake at the midpoint of treatment are less likely to have durable remissions.

Immunobiologic factors Various immunobiologic factors have been suggested as predictors of outcome in NHL.

Immunophenotype Several studies have suggested that patients with aggressive T-cell NHL not of the anaplastic subtype have a higher relapse rate and decreased overall survival than do patients with B-cell disease. These observations have been confirmed in updated REAL/WHO studies involving large numbers of patients.

Tumor cell proliferation Studies using the Ki-67 antibody, a marker of nuclear proliferation, have shown that increased tumor cell proliferation is a poor prognostic factor in diffuse large cell lymphoma and mantle cell lymphoma.

Cytogenetic abnormalities and oncogene expression Patients with lymphomas with abnormalities involving chromosomes 1, 7, and 17 have a worse prognosis than do patients with other lymphomas of similar stage and bulk that do not exhibit these changes. Mutations of *p53* are associated with histologic transformation in follicular NHL, which is a phenomenon frequently associated with a poor prognosis. Expression of *bcl-2* in diffuse large cell lymphoma has also been associated with inferior survival, whereas *bcl-6* expression is a marker of germinal center derivation, a predictor of a favorable outcome with CHOP-like therapy. Dual expression of *bcl-2* and c-myc in B-cell lymphomas is also a poor prognostic sign.

Molecular profiling DNA microarray technology for gene expression profiling has identified distinct prognostic subgroups in DLBCL and follicular NHL. Studies in DLBCL have characterized patients into the following subgroups: germinal center B-like DLBCL, activated B-like DLBCL, and a heterogeneous subgroup termed type-3 DLBCL. In the pre-rituximab era, patients with germinal center B-like DLBCL had a significantly improved overall survival compared with the other molecular profiles. Although in the post-rituximab era, this prognostic difference is much less apparent. Recent studies in follicular NHL have identified two gene expression signatures that also predicted survival: immune-response 1 and immune-response 2. Interestingly, the genes that defined the prognostic signatures were not expressed in the tumor cells but were expressed by the nonmalignant tumor-infiltrating cells (primarily T cells, macrophages, and dendritic cells). A variety of immunologically active cell types including specific T-cell subsets and tumor-associated macrophages, have been associated with prognosis in some studies.

Treatment

The therapeutic approach for NHL differs for each subtype. Chemotherapy remains the most important modality (Tables 8 and 9). However, in select instances, radiation therapy or surgical resection plays a critical role. Biologic approaches, including interferons, monoclonal antibodies (Table 10), and recombinant toxins have shown significant activity and are now incorporated into treatment paradigms. Autologous and allogeneic SCTs, traditionally reserved for recurrent or refractory disease, are being evaluated as part of initial therapy in high-risk settings. This section will be organized by NHL subtype to best illustrate the biologic characteristics and therapeutic considerations that determine the management strategy for individual patients. Common NHLs will be covered in depth, whereas less frequent entities will be described in limited detail.

FOLLICULAR LYMPHOMA

Follicular lymphoma comprises 22% of all NHLs; only DLBCL is more common. The clinical presentation may be nodal or extranodal, and bone marrow involvement occurs in the majority of cases. Extensive intra-abdominal adenopathy without peripheral node enlargement is not uncommon. Clinical behavior is variable, reflecting the heterogeneity of the underlying biology; some patients survive decades, whereas others progress rapidly to resistant disease or transform to a more aggressive histology. There are rare spontaneous remissions. Transformation is common, occurring in 3% to 6% of patients each year and ultimately 30% to 50% of all patients. Although generally responsive to treatment, the clinical course is characterized by repeated relapses. Median survival for advanced-stage disease is 6 years. Although there was no improvement in survival for patients with follicular lymphoma for many years, there is new evidence that outcomes have improved, independent of the introduction of rituximab. It is likely that there will be further improvement associated with the use of rituximab in combination with chemotherapy.

TABLE 8: Chemotherapeutic regimens for NHL

Regimen	Dose	Route and frequency
CVP ± rituximab		
Cyclophosphamide	750-1,000 mg/m^2	IV on day 1
Vincristine	1.4 mg/m^2	IV on day 1 (maximum, 2 mg)
Prednisone	100 mg or 100 mg/m^2	PO on days 1-5
Rituximab	375 mg/m^2	IV on day 1
Repeat treatment every 21 days.		
CHOP ± rituximab		
Cyclophosphamide	750 mg/m^2	IV on day 1
Doxorubicin	50 mg/m^2	IV on day 1
Oncovin (vincristine)	1.4 mg/m^2	IV on day 1 (maximum, 2 mg)
Prednisone	40 mg/m^2 or 100 mg/d or 100 mg/m^2/d	PO on days 1-5
Rituximab	375 mg/m^2	IV on day 1
Repeat treatment every 21 days or every 14 days (with granulocyte colony-stimulating factor).		
F ± rituximab		
Fludarabine	25 mg/m^2	IV on days 1-3
Rituximab	375 mg/m^2	(see *J Clin Oncol* 23:694, 2005)
Repeat treatment every 28 days.		
FCR		
Fludarabine	25 mg/m^2	IV on days 1-3
Cyclophosphamide	300 mg/m^2	IV on days 1-3
Rituximab	375 mg/m^2	IV on day 1
Repeat treatment every 28 days.		
FCM + R		
Fludarabine	25 mg/m^2	IV on days 1-3
Cyclophosphamide	200 mg/m^2	IV on days 1-3
Mitoxantrone	6 mg/m^2	IV on day 1
Rituximab	375 mg/m^2	IV on day 0
Repeat treatment every 28 days.		

It is crucial to distinguish between reactive follicular hyperplasia and follicular lymphoma, as the former is a benign condition. Morphologic features as well as the absence of Bcl-2 staining within the follicle and the absence of CD10 and/or Bcl-6 protein expression in the interfollicular areas help to distinguish reactive follicular hyperplasia from follicular lymphoma. Follicular lymphoma is graded according to the number of admixed centroblasts within the neoplastic follicles. Grade 3 follicular lymphoma, previously known as follicular large cell lymphoma, is now subdivided into two subtypes: Grade 3a is characterized by a mixture of centrocytes and centroblasts within the follicle, whereas grade

TABLE 9: Commonly used salvage regimens for NHL

Regimen	Dose	Route and frequency
EPOCH[a]		
Etoposide	50 mg/m^2/d	Continuous 96-h IV infusion on days 1-4
Oncovin (vincristine)*	0.4 mg/m^2/d	Continuous 96-h IV infusion on days 1-4
Doxorubicin	10 mg/m^2/d	Continuous 96-h IV infusion on days 1-4
Cyclophosphamide	750 mg/m^2	IV on day 5
Prednisone	60 mg	PO on days 1-5

Oncovin is NOT capped. Repeat treatment every 21 days. Doses of etoposide, doxorubicin, and cyclophosphamide are adjusted 20% each cycle to achieve an absolute neutrophil count below 0.5 x 10^9/L.

Regimen	Dose	Route and frequency
DHAP[a]		
Platinol (cisplatin)	100 mg/m^2	Continuous 24-h IV infusion on day 1
Cytarabine	2 g/m^2	3-h IV infusion q12h for 2 doses on day 2
Dexamethasone	40 mg	IV on days 1-4

Repeat treatment every 21-28 days depending on hematologic recovery.

Regimen	Dose	Route and frequency
ESHAP[a]		
Etoposide	40 mg/m^2	1-h IV infusion on days 1-4
Solu-Medrol (MPS)	250-500 mg	15-min IV infusion on days 1-5
Cytarabine	2 g/m^2	2-h IV infusion on day 5
Platinol (cisplatin)	25 mg/m^2	Continuous 96-h IV infusion on days 1-4 (total dose, 100 mg/m^2)

Regimen	Dose	Route and frequency
GEMOX[a]		
Gemcitabine	1,000 mg/m^2	IV on day 1
Oxaliplatin	100 mg/m^2	IV on day 1

Repeat treatment every 14-21 days depending on hematologic recovery.

Regimen	Dose	Route and frequency
ICE[a]		
Ifosfamide	5,000 mg/m^2	Continuous IV × 24 h on day 2
Mesna	5,000 mg/m^2	Continuous IV × 24 h on day 2
Carboplatin	AUC 5 mg/mL/min	IV on day 2
Etoposide	100 mg/m^2	IV on days 1-3

[a] ± Rituximab
AUC = area under the curve; MPS = methylprednisolone

3b has only sheets of centroblasts with no residual centrocytes. The neoplastic lymphocytes in follicular lymphoma express the pan-B markers CD19, CD20, CD22, and CD79a and antigens of the germinal center (including CD10 and Bcl-6). Most follicular lymphomas express Bcl-2 protein, which is highly correlated with the t(14;18)(q32;q21), the cytogenetic hallmark of the disease. This translocation results in the juxtaposition of the *bcl*-2 oncogene into the immunoglobulin H heavy-chain locus on chromosome 14, resulting in its constitutive expression. Follicular lymphoma grade 3b with *bcl-6* rearrangement but no t(14;18)(q32;21) may be more closely related to DLBCL than to other follicular lymphomas.

TABLE 10: Monoclonal antibodies for lymphoid malignancies

Antigen	Antibody	Type	Investigational status
CD20	Rituximab (Rituxan)	Chimeric	FDA approved
	Ibritumomab (Zevalin)	Y-90-murine	FDA approved
	Tositumomab (Bexxar)	I-131 murine	FDA approved
	Ofatumumab (HuMaxCD20)	Humanized	Phase III planned
	Ocrelizumab	Humanized	Phase I/II
CD52	Alemtuzumab (Campath)	Humanized	FDA approved
CD22	Epratuzumab	Humanized	Phase II/III
CD80	Galiximab (IDEC-114)	Primatized	Phase II
CD23	Lumiliximab (IDEC-152)	Primatized	Phase I
CD30	SGN-30	Chimeric	Phase II
CD40	SGN-40	Humanized	Phase III

FDA = Food and Drug Administration

As previously mentioned, the FLIPI is a prognostic index designed specifically for follicular lymphomas based on five adverse prognostic factors (Table 7). Age is the most important factor. Three risk categories have been defined, each consisting of approximately one-third of patients. More than two-thirds of low-risk patients but only one-third of high-risk patients survive 10 years. Whereas clinical parameters are surrogates for biologic characteristics, DNA expression profiling using microarray technology may soon supersede clinical prognostic indicators such as the FLIPI.

Investigators from the National Cancer Institute (NCI) have described two gene expression signatures associated with vastly different clinical outcomes in follicular lymphoma. These two signatures represent the expression of immunoregulatory genes in the nonmalignant cells infiltrating the malignant lymphoma at the time of diagnosis. Others have reported that the number of tumor-associated macrophages, tumor-infiltrating mast cells, or specific T-cell subsets was an independent predictor of overall survival in follicular lypmphoma, also underscoring the importance of host response in follicular lymphoma.

Treatment of early-stage disease

For the relatively small number of patients with stage I or II follicular lymphoma, radiotherapy continues to be the standard of care. A recent update from the Princess Margaret Hospital's series of involved-field radiotherapy (IFRT) for early-stage disease showed cumulative relapse rates of 54% and 56% at 15 and 25 years, with only a 2% risk of relapse beyond 15 years. Combined-modality therapy has also resulted in excellent disease control, and a randomized trial comparing IFRT with combined-modality therapy is ongoing. Use of functional imaging with PET may improve the results of IFRT by more accurately identifying patients with truly localized disease.

For clinical stages I and IIA low-grade follicular lymphoma, irradiation alone is directed to the entire involved lymphoid region, as defined by Kaplan and coworkers, or the involved region plus one additional uninvolved region on each side of the involved nodes. The recommended dose is approximately 30 Gy for nonbulky disease showing prompt regression and 36 Gy for bulky or slowly regressive disease, in 1.75 to 2.0 Gy daily fractions. As the majority of subsequent relapses occur outside previous radiation fields, often in adjacent or distal lymph nodes, extended-field or total lymphoid irradiation has been used to try to improve cure rates. Clinical series have shown improvement in freedom from relapse only, with no significant difference in long-term survival.

Treatment of advanced-stage disease

Watch and wait The standard management of asymptomatic patients with follicular lymphoma has been a "watch-and-wait" approach. Treatment is delayed until symptoms or cytopenias intervene or there is impending compromise of vital organs. In the pre-rituximab era, multiple phase III randomized trials comparing immediate chemotherapy with observation for asymptomatic patients with advanced-stage follicular lymphoma have shown no difference in outcome. In fact, for patients older than age 70, the chances of not requiring chemotherapy were 40% at 10 years in a recently published trial. The median time to first systemic therapy for patients randomized to the observation arm was 2.6 years. Complete remission rates, however, were higher in the patients treated immediately after diagnosis than in those who were observed and later treated (63% vs 27%). The achievement of a complete remission may prove to be important if the ultimate goal is to administer postremission therapy (eg, vaccine) that is likely to be most effective in the presence of minimal residual disease. A phase III trial comparing the watch-and-wait approach with rituximab therapy for asymptomatic advanced-stage disease is ongoing in Europe. At the same time, an American Intergroup trial comparing two different rituximab dosing regimens is enrolling patients with low tumor burden indolent lymphoma who are asymptomatic.

Irradiation Irradiation for clinical stages III and IV, low-grade, extensive-stage NHL is used locally for palliation of symptomatic sites of disease and is extremely effective. Abbreviated fractionated schedules (25 to 30 Gy in 2.5 to 3 Gy daily fractions, respectively) are often used. A low-dose regimen of 4 Gy in 2 fractions has been shown to be effective, with an overall response rate of approximately 80% in the palliation of symptoms, and is well tolerated. Total-body irradiation, usually consisting of 12 Gy in 2 Gy fractions twice a day, is used as part of preparative regimens for bone marrow transplantation.

Rituximab For patients with symptoms or other reasons for treatment, there are many treatment options, including single or multiagent chemotherapy, monoclonal antibodies or radioimmunoconjugates, combinations of chemotherapy and immunotherapy with anti-idiotype vaccines, and new agents such as bortezomib (Velcade). Treatment with rituximab results in overall response rates of nearly 50%, with a median response duration of approximately 1 year, in relapsed or refractory indolent lymphomas. In previously untreated patients, however, the overall response rate was 80%, and the median progression-free survival is 18 months in one trial from France. Of note, 28% of all treated patients and 34% of all complete and partial responders maintained their responses for 5 or more years. Similar results have been reported by the US North Central Cancer Treatment Group (NCCTG).

To improve on response rates and duration of response, additional doses of rituximab have been administered as "maintenance therapy." The median event-free survival is prolonged with this approach, especially for previously untreated patients. In previously treated patients, the total duration of benefit from rituximab appears to be the same whether patients receive maintenance rituximab on a scheduled basis or reinduction with rituximab only at the time of disease progression. A confirmatory trial (Eastern Cooperative Oncoogy Group [ECOG] 4402) in untreated patients is in progress in patients with a low tumor burden. Maintenance regimens have varied, and the impact of the frequency of administration on the duration of response is unknown. Questions also remain regarding the impact of maintenance rituximab on the quality of life and the cost of care.

Rituximab maintenance also impacts progression-free survival among patients treated with chemotherapy alone and those receiving rituximab plus chemotherapy. Compared with observation, maintenance rituximab improved progression-free survival in previously untreated patients with follicular lymphoma who responded to cyclophosphamide, vincristine, prednisone (progression-free survival, 56% vs 33%). Among relapsed/refractory patients treated with CHOP (cyclophosphamide, doxorubicin, vincristine [Oncovin], prednisone) or rituximab-CHOP (R-CHOP) maintenance, rituximab also improved progression-free survival. Whether these results will translate into an overall survival benefit remains to be seen.

Interferon-α The use of interferon (IFN)-α in follicular lymphoma has been extensively investigated both in combination with chemotherapy and as maintenance therapy, with varying results. In most studies, IFN-α was associated with a prolongation of remission but not overall survival. A notable exception was the GELF86 (Group d'Etude des Lymphomes Folliculaires) trial, in which overall survival was prolonged. The Southwest Oncology Group (SWOG) recently reported the results of a large phase III trial in which patients with indolent lymphomas were randomized to receive IFN-α or observation following induction with an intensive anthracycline-containing regimen and in some cases radiotherapy. Postremission therapy did not prolong progression-free or overall survival. Although these results, along with the toxicities associated with IFN-α, have led many physicians to abandon its use altogether, a large phase

III study is currently ongoing in Germany comparing standard versus intensive dose maintenance.

Chemotherapy with and without rituximab Studies comparing single-agent chemotherapy with multiagent therapy in patients with advanced-stage follicular lymphoma have not shown meaningful differences in outcomes. Fludarabine (Fludara), identified in the 1980s as an active agent in follicular lymphoma, has been incorporated into combination regimens with high response rates (including molecular remissions) but has not been shown to prolong the duration of remission when compared with other multiagent regimens. Secondary myelodysplastic syndromes and acute leukemias have now been associated with the fludarabine, mitoxantrone, dexamethasone (FND) regimen. High response rates and durable remissions have resulted when rituximab was combined with CHOP chemotherapy in a small number of patients with follicular lymphoma, some of whom were treatment-naive. Four phase III trials comparing combinations of chemotherapy and rituximab with chemotherapy alone in previously untreated patients have now been reported. Overall response rates and either median time to treatment failure or event-free survival were superior in the chemoimmunotherapy arm in every series. An overall survival benefit has been demonstrated in three of the four trials and in the high-risk subset of the fourth study.

Radioimmunotherapy The anti-CD20 radioimmunoconjugates Y-90 ibritumomab (Zevalin) and I-131 tositumomab (Bexxar) both deliver ionizing radiation to target cells and their neighbors and have proven to be relatively easy to administer, safe, and effective. Response rates are higher and remissions more durable when radioimmunoconjugates are used early in the clinical course. Both agents are likely to have their greatest impact when used in previously untreated patients.

In previously treated patients, Y-90 ibritumomab, a high-energy beta-emitter, yielded an overall response rate of 80% for relapsed or refractory follicular or transformed CD20+ B-cell NHL, with a median duration of response of 14 months. For patients refractory to rituximab, response rates with Y-90 ibritumomab are high (74% overall response rate), but the median duration of response is relatively short (6.4 months; range 0.5–25+ months). The dose-limiting feature of this approach is hematologic toxicity. Short-lived myelosuppression occurs 7 to 9 weeks post treatment. Dosing is based on weight (0.4 mCi/kg), with a reduction (0.3 mCi/kg) for those with mild thrombocytopenia (< 100,000/μL).

I-131 tositumomab is both a gamma- and beta-emitter and is individually dosed on the basis of dosimetry to deliver 75 cGy of total-body irradiation. Similar to Y-90 ibritumomab, it is effective in both heavily pretreated relapsed and refractory patients. Heavily pretreated patients with refractory low-grade or transformed NHL had an overall response rate of 65% (20% complete response rate), with a median duration of response of 6.5 months. These rates were notable in view of a response rate of only 28% in the preceding chemotherapy regimen. Like Y-90 ibritumomab, I-131 tositumomab is associated with predictable mye-losuppression. Secondary myelodysplasia and leukemia have oc-

Consolidation therapy with Y-90 ibritumomab (Zevalin) prolonged progression-free survival from 13.5 months to 37 months in patients with follicular lymphoma in first complete response (CR) or partial remission. Only 14% of the 414 patients enrolled on this randomized phase III trial received a rituximab-containing regimen for induction. Now that the addition of rituximab to chemotherapy has become standard of care based on demonstrated improvements in progression-free and overall survival, the benefit of consolidation with radioimmunotherapy will need to be evaluated in patients treated first with chemoimmunotherapy (Morschhauser F, Radford J, Van Hoof A, et al: J Clin Oncol Oct 14, 2008 [Epub ahead of print]).

curred in patients treated with radioimmunotherapy, but only in patients previously treated with chemotherapy and thereby already at risk. In previously untreated patients, the complete response rate was 75%, with a 5-year progression-free survival of 59%. These data must be interpreted carefully, as this study enrolled a relatively young patient population (median age, 49 years), with low-bulk disease, a group that some physicians would choose to observe rather than treat.

I-131 tositumomab has been used to consolidate responders following induction with CHOP chemotherapy. In a phase II trial of previously untreated patients with follicular lymphoma, the percentage of complete response/unconfirmed complete response increased from 39% following CHOP chemotherapy to 69% following consolidation with I-131 tositumomab. With a median follow-up of 5.1 years, 66% of patients are alive and disease-free. Based on these phase II results and the encouraging outcome of patients treated with R-CHOP, the American Intergroup is currently comparing CHOP followed by I-131 tositumomab with R-CHOP in treatment-naive patients.

Anti-idiotype vaccines Lymphoma-specific idiotypes serve as tumor-specific antigens in follicular lymphoma and constitute the basis for vaccine therapy. In early vaccine trials, immunized patients who generated an anti-idiotype response experienced longer remissions than those who failed to mount a response. Anti-idiotype vaccine has been shown to clear minimal residual disease detectable only by PCR after intensive chemotherapy. In phase I trials, vaccination resulted in tumor shrinkage in some patients. One phase III placebo-controlled trial investigating this strategy showed no difference in disease progression rates following induction chemotherapy (cyclophosphamide, vincristine, prednisone [CVP]) between patients receiving anti-idiotype vaccine and those receiving a control. The results of two other phase III trials are expected in late 2008. While we await the results of these important studies, alternative methodologies, including DNA vaccines and dendritic cell-based vaccination, are under investigation.

Novel agents New agents targeting specific molecular targets such as the ubiquitin-proteasome pathway have shown promise in the treatment of follicular lymphoma. In recently reported phase II trials, bortezomib has shown activity in follicular lymphoma as well as in mantle cell lymphoma. New combinations including bortezomib are now being investigated. Bendamustine (Treanda) is a novel alkylator with activity in both rituximab-refractory and rituximab-sensitive indolent NHL that has recently been approved by the US

Food and Drug Administration (FDA) for relapsed disease that is refractory to rituximab.

Other new agents are also showing activity, including the histone deacetylase inhibitors, lenalidomide (Revlimid), and mammalian target of rapamycin (mTOR) inhibitors. Novel antibodies such as anti-CD80 and combinations of antibodies have also shown promise in the treatment of follicular lymphoma.

Stem cell transplantation The natural history of follicular lymphoma is characterized by response to therapy but repeated relapses and progressively shorter and shorter remissions, ultimately resulting in death from progressive disease. Autologous and allogeneic stem cell transplantations (SCTs) are alternative strategies often associated with durable remissions that may impact overall survival. Unfortunately, immediate and long-term toxicities are significant and must be considered when assessing the appropriate role of transplantation in the overall treatment plan for individual patients. The only phase III trial to address the role of autologous SCT in patients with relapsed follicular lymphoma closed prematurely because of poor accrual. Nonetheless, progression-free and overall survival rates were significantly longer with high-dose chemotherapy (HDCT) and autologous SCT (with purged or unpurged autografts) than with conventional alkylator therapy. Whether any of the new therapeutic strategies will prove to be as effective as autologous SCT in the relapsed setting remains to be seen.

Several groups have investigated the role of autologous SCT as consolidation therapy for patients in first complete or partial remission. Although progression-free survival may be prolonged, an impact on survival has not been demonstrated consistently. Contemporary trials evaluating the role of autologous SCT for follicular lymphoma in first remission induced with rituximab-containing regimens are needed. The results of a German Lymphoma Study Group trial comparing interferon maintenance with myeloablative chemotherapy with autologous SCT after induction with CHOP or R-CHOP are awaited. An increased incidence of secondary myelodysplasia following autologous SCT in first remission has reduced enthusiasm for this approach. An alternative approach to consolidating complete and partial remissions achieved with conventional induction therapy is the use of a sequential HDCT program, which culminates in an autologous SCT. The Italian cooperative groups have recently reported results of a phase III randomized trial comparing R-CHOP for 6 cycles with a sequential HDCT with autologous SCT. There was a significant difference in event-free survival but no difference in overall survival.

> Bendamustine (Treanda) plus rituximab (Rituxan) proved equally effective as rituximab-CHOP in previously untreated patients with follicular, indolent, and mantle cell lymphoma, according to the first interim analysis. In a multicenter randomized phase III trial that enrolled 439 patients, there were no differences in response rates or rates of disease progression or deaths between the two arms, albeit the median observation time was only 17 months. Bendamustine-rituximab was less myelosuppressive than R-CHOP and overall more tolerable (Rummel MJ, von Gruenhagen U, Niederle N, et al: Blood 110:[abstract 385], 2007).

Single-institution studies as well as analysis of registry data suggest that a tumor-free graft is an important determinant of outcome in follicular lymphoma. Administration of rituximab during stem-cell mobilization provides an "in vivo" purge, reducing contamination of the autograft with malignant lymphocytes. The long-term benefit of such an approach has not yet been demonstrated.

Allogeneic SCT has been investigated primarily in young patients with HLA-identical sibling donors and extensive disease and/or marrow involvement. Low relapse rates suggest that this approach is potentially curative but is associated with high treatment-related morbidity and mortality. Reduced-intensity transplantation is based on the assumption that a graft-versus-lymphoma effect is operative and has the potential to cure follicular lymphoma. Whether this approach will reduce toxicity while maintaining the low relapse rates associated with standard myeloablative allotransplants remains to be established. A randomized trial comparing this strategy with autologous SCT in relapsed follicular lymphoma has been initiated in the United States.

Overall treatment strategy

Whereas treatment choices were once limited to single or combination alkylator-based treatment, we now are faced with choosing among a wide variety of strategies. There are many unanswered questions that can only be addressed through well-designed clinical trials. Hence, whenever possible, every patient with follicular lymphoma should be enrolled in prospective clinical studies. In the absence of symptoms or other indications for treatment, patients should be observed. A combination of rituximab and chemotherapy is recommended in the absence of a clinical trial. Selected patients with comorbidities may be best served with rituximab alone. Radioimmunotherapy is a good option at the time of relapse, with transplantation reserved for selected patients in first or subsequent relapse.

CHRONIC LYMPHOCYTIC LEUKEMIA/SMALL LYMPHOCYTIC LYMPHOMA

Chronic lymphocytic leukemia/small lymphocytic lymphoma (CLL/SLL) is a malignancy of small, round, B lymphocytes involving peripheral blood, bone marrow, and lymph nodes. The term "SLL" is reserved for cases in which there are no circulating malignant lymphocytes. SLL generally presents with lymph node and splenic involvement. Involvement of the bone marrow and peripheral blood may develop later in the course of disease. At the time of presentation, patients may be asymptomatic, complain of only fatigue, or have symptoms related to cytopenias (including autoimmune hemolytic anemia, lymphadenopathy, or splenomegaly). The immunophenotype helps to distinguish CLL/SLL from other B-cell leukemias/lymphomas, including mantle cell and leukemic forms of follicular lymphoma. Typically, the malignant lymphocytes stain weakly with surface immunoglobulin, CD20, CD22, and CD79b; they are CD5+, CD23+, and FMC7–. Cytogenetic abnormalities are detected in the majority of cases when fluorescence in situ hybridization (FISH) analysis is used. Trisomy 12, deletions at 13q14, and deletions at 11q22-23 are common. Many molecular markers of prognosis have been studied in CLL, including Zap-70, but their value in SLL is unknown.

Given the relatively small numbers of patients with SLL, they have generally been included in clinical trials of "indolent lymphoma." Conventional alkylator-based regimens with rituximab as well as purine analogues and combinations thereof have been used when patients become symptomatic. Anthracyclines have not been shown to benefit patients with CLL/SLL. When compared with follicular lymphoma, CLL/SLL is less likely to respond to rituximab as a single agent. Alemtuzumab (Campath), a potent therapy for CLL, is less effective in treating nodal disease than peripheral blood and bone marrow involvement. SCT, both autologous and allogeneic, has been studied in selected patient populations but should be reserved for relapsed young patients with a good performance status.

SPLENIC MARGINAL ZONE LYMPHOMA

Splenic marginal zone lymphoma (SMZL) is a rare disorder comprising less than 1% of NHLs. Clinically, this lymphoma most often presents as splenomegaly with splenic hilar node involvement but without peripheral adenopathy. The bone marrow is commonly involved, and malignant villous lymphocytes may be detected in the peripheral blood. Cytopenias are a common presenting feature, often related to hypersplenism and less frequently to an autoimmune process or marrow replacement. Sometimes confused with CLL or mantle cell lymphoma, SMZL may be distinguished by its immunophenotype. Typically, cells are CD20+, CD79a+, CD5–, CD10–, CD23–, and CD43–. Staining for cyclin D1 is negative, excluding mantle cell lymphoma. The absence of CD103 helps to exclude hairy cell leukemia. Complex karyotypes are common. The clinical course is indolent. Cytopenias respond to splenectomy with long-lasting remissions. Anecdotal remissions have been seen following rituximab therapy. Transformation to more aggressive histologies may occur. Fludarabine alone or with rituximab appears to be more effective than alkylators.

NODAL MARGINAL ZONE LYMPHOMA

Nodal marginal zone lymphoma (NMZL) is a primary nodal B-cell disorder that resembles lymph nodes involved by MZLs of extranodal or splenic origin without extranodal or splenic involvement. Lymphadenopathy (either localized or generalized) is the presenting complaint in most cases. Extranodal lymphoma may be uncovered in the evaluation of many cases of suspected NMZL. The clinical course is usually indolent, similar to that of other MZLs.

EXTRANODAL MARGINAL ZONE B-CELL LYMPHOMA OF MALT TYPE

MALT lymphomas comprise only 7% to 8% of B-cell lymphomas but nearly 50% of all gastric lymphomas. Although the GI tract is most often involved, other common sites include the lungs, head and neck, ocular adnexae, skin, thyroid, and breasts. There often is an associated history of autoimmune disorders, such as Sjögren's syndrome or Hashimoto's thyroiditis or chronic inflammatory processes secondary to infectious agents (*H pylori*, *B burgdorferi*, or *C psittaci*). A form of MALT involving the small bowel (immunoproliferative small intestinal disease, previously known as α-chain disease) has been associated with *C jejuni*. The majority of patients present with stage I or II disease. The frequency of bone marrow involvement appears to differ depending on the primary site of involvement. Multiple extranodal sites may be involved at the time of presentation. Transformation to a high-grade lymphoma may occur in approximately 8% of cases.

The malignant lymphocytes of MALT lymphoma are typically CD20+, CD79a+, CD5–, CD10–, and CD23–. The t(11;18)(q21;q21) is characteristic of MALT lymphomas, particularly those involving the stomach or lungs. The translocation creates a fusion between the MALT-1 gene, which is an essential regulator of *bcl-10*–mediated NF-kB signaling, and the API2 gene, which inhibits apoptosis. This genetic abnormality is a marker of MALT lymphomas that do not respond to antibiotic therapy for *H pylori* infection, are associated with a more advanced stage, and do not transform into more aggressive histologic subtypes. This translocation has not been associated with nodal or splenic MZLs or other types of lymphoma. Additional characteristic translocations have been discovered (Table 1), but their clinical significance is uncertain at this time.

Treatment of *H pylori* infection with triple therapy (eg, omeprazole [Prilosec], metronidazole, and clarithromycin [Biaxin]) results in regression in the majority of early lesions. However, tumors invading beyond the submucosa and lesions with t(11;18) are associated with a failure to respond to *H pylori* eradication, deep penetration, and distant spread.

Localized MALT gastric lymphoma that does not respond to antibiotics may be cured with local irradiation, with a field including the stomach and perigastric lymph nodes. This treatment is safe, extremely effective, and preserves the stomach. A single-institution experience reported a 96% complete response rate and a 90% freedom-from-treatment-failure rate, at a median follow-up of 4 years. If local irradiation fails, chemotherapy or rituximab, and in some instances surgery, can be used. Alkylator-based therapy or purine analogues have been used with success for persistent or disseminated disease. The typical dose of radiotherapy is 30 Gy in 20 fractions directed to the stomach and perigastric lymph nodes. Localized non-gastric MALT lymphomas also respond well to local radiotherapy.

LYMPHOPLASMACYTIC LYMPHOMA/WALDENSTRÖM'S MACROGLOBULINEMIA

Lymphoplasmacytic lymphoma/Waldenström's macroglobulinemia is a disorder of small B lymphocytes; plasmacytoid lymphocytes; and plasma cells, typically involving the bone marrow, lymph nodes, and spleen. It is usually associated with a serum monoclonal protein (usually IgM) with associated hyperviscosity or cryoglobulinemia. The clinical presentation is usually related to hyperviscosity with visual symptoms, stroke, or congestive heart failure. Peripheral neuropathies occur in approximately 10% of patients related to reactivity of IgM with myelin-associated glycoprotein or gangliosides. An association with HCV infection has been demonstrated. Characteristically, the immunophenotypic analysis reveals surface and cytoplasmic immunoglobulin, usually IgM type, and B-cell–associated antigens (such as CD19, 20, 22, and 79a). The malignant cells are CD5–, CD10–, and CD23–.

The clinical course is generally indolent. Asymptomatic patients may be observed. Plasmapheresis may be appropriate first therapy for those who present with hyperviscosity. The clinical status of the patient, not the level of the protein, determines when treatment is initiated. Choice of therapy depends on many individual factors, including age, comorbidities, and the particular indication for therapy. Rituximab and nucleoside analogues (cladribine and fludarabine) as well as the traditional oral alkylators have shown efficacy. Combinations of these agents are also under study. Bortezomib, thalidomide (Thalomid), and alemtuzumab have shown activity in Waldenström's macroglobulinemia. SCT, both autologous and allogeneic, is being investigated in younger patients with relapsed or refractory disease.

DIFFUSE LARGE B-CELL LYMPHOMA

Clinical presentation Diffuse large B-cell lymphoma (DLBCL) makes up about one-third of the cases of NHL and is classified as a mature peripheral B-cell neoplasm by WHO. The clinical presentation is variable, but generally patients present with either peripheral lymphadenopathy (neck, axillae) or enlarged nodes in the mediastinum, the mesenteric region, or the retroperitoneum. These sites predict symptoms, which may include chest pain; facial swelling and suffusion of the eyelids (superior vena cava [SVC] syndrome from mediastinal disease); abdominal discomfort, ascites (mesenteric), or back pain; or renal obstruction (retroperitoneal presentations). More than 30% of patients present with disease in extranodal sites, such as the GI tract (including Waldeyer's ring), skin, bone marrow, sinuses, GU tract, thyroid, and CNS. B symptoms, consisting of fever, sweats, and weight loss, are more common in DLBCL than in the indolent lymphomas and occur in about 30% of patients. The median age at presentation is 60 years.

Once the diagnosis is clearly established, staging studies are carried out to determine treatment and define parameters for follow-up. Generally, imaging studies of the chest, abdomen, and pelvis are obtained, and CT scans provide the most accurate anatomic information. Recently, functional imaging using PET scans (which have largely replaced gallium scans) has shown promise as a means

TABLE 11: International Prognostic Index (IPI) in diffuse large B-cell lymphoma in the pre-rituximab era

Risk group	No. of risk factors	% of patients	Overall survival (2 yr)	Overall survival (5 yr)
Low	0, 1	35%	84%	73%
Low-intermediate	2	27%	66%	51%
High-intermediate	3	22%	54%	43%
High	4, 5	16%	34%	26%

of distinguishing between residual scar and active disease after treatment. Further, some investigators have shown that early response by PET scan (after 2 to 3 cycles) is a good prognostic indicator. In addition to CT and PET scans, bone marrow aspirate and biopsy, serum LDH level, and serum beta-2 microglobulin level have been described as important predictors of outcome.

Pathology/immunology The diagnosis should be made by incisional or excisional biopsy of an available lymph node, with adequate tissue for immunologic studies, such as flow cytometry or immunohistochemistry (IHC), to identify the characteristic B-cell clonality (kappa or lambda restriction). In many cases of DLBCL, CD10 is present, indicating a germinal center origin. The CD20 antigen is present in almost all cases of B-cell lymphomas and on almost all normal B cells. In addition, markers for *bcl*-2 and *bcl*-6 offer prognostic information and are part of most diagnostic evaluations of DLBCL. The use of FNA or core biopsy should be discouraged and is acceptable only when tissue cannot be safely obtained by other means and only if flow cytometry is used to help classify the disease and distinguish it from epithelial malignancies that can masquerade as lymphoma.

Prognostic factors Clinical predictors of response have been identified and are now widely used to help design therapeutic plans and clinical trials. These predictors include patient age (< or > age 60), performance status (0, 1 vs 2–4), number of extranodal sites (more than two), Ann Arbor stage (I or II vs III or IV), and serum LDH level (> normal; Table 6). Older patients, higher stage, poorer performance status, higher number of extranodal sites, and higher LDH level all predict a worse outcome, and this model has been validated in more than 3,000 patients. These parameters have been called the IPI; this index is used to plan therapy and clinical trials in the United States and abroad and may be used to predict survival (Table 11).

More recently, genomics have been used to help predict outcome based on molecular signature (see subsection on Molecular profiling). This molecular system provides prognostic information independent of the IPI. Several investigators using similar statistical methodologies have yielded comparable results, and recently these analyses have been extended to other lymphomas.

Treatment Prior to the 1970s, most patients with stage I/II large cell lymphoma (intermediate grade in the Working Formulation) were treated with irradiation alone, with overall cure rates of 40% to 50%. Patients with pathologically favorable stage I/II disease had even better outcomes, but relapse rates, even in these patients, were still 20% to 30%. Pathologic staging, therefore, selected a group suitable for irradiation alone. This approach is no longer appropriate, in view of the success of combined chemotherapy and irradiation in clinically staged patients.

Coiffier et al found that the addition of rituximab improved results in elderly patients with DLBCL, and recent data confirm these observations for younger patients as well. For patients with clinical stage I or II disease (by the Ann Arbor criteria), most studies suggest that chemotherapy (CHOP and most would add rituximab) for 3 to 4 cycles followed by localized radiation therapy is preferred. Excellent local and systemic control is obtained with combined-modality therapy.

In an ECOG phase III trial, Horning et al showed that 8 cycles of CHOP and irradiation produced a 10-year disease-free survival rate of 57%, compared with 46% with CHOP alone ($P = .04$). Overall survival was 64% versus 60%, respectively ($P = .23$), and time to disease progression was 73% versus 63%, respectively ($P = .07$).

Miller et al showed that CHOP (3 cycles of CHOP and irradiation) produced a progression-free survival at 5 years of 77%, versus 64% for 8 cycles of CHOP alone ($P = .03$). Overall survival at 5 years was 82% versus 72%, respectively ($P = .02$). A recent update of this SWOG study was reported by Miller et al, with an 8.2-year median follow-up. The 5-year estimates for CHOP (3 cycles plus irradiation) versus CHOP (for 8 cycles) remained unchanged. Kaplan-Meier estimates now show overlapping curves at 7 years for failure-free survival and 9 years for overall survival. The treatment advantage for CHOP (for 3 cycles plus irradiation) for the first 7 to 9 years was diminished because of excess late relapses and NHL deaths occurring between 5 and 10 years. Patients with good IPI risk factors had a 5-year overall survival of 94%; patients with one adverse risk factor had an overall survival of 70%; those with three adverse risk factors had a 5-year survival of 50%.

These results were confirmed by a single-arm (doxorubicin-containing chemotherapy) approach followed by IFRT conducted by the British Columbia Cancer Agency. However, two reports from European investigators question the value of consolidation irradiation in early-stage disease. These studies did not use rituximab or ^{18}fluorodeoxyglucose (FDG)-PET staging, and details on the irradiation technique used were not available. The necessity of consolidation radiation therapy after complete response to R-CHOP chemotherapy is now being tested in a randomized study in Germany.

Until further studies define the optimal therapy for stages IA to IIA DLBCL (nonbulky), many investigators consider 3 to 4 cycles of R-CHOP and IFRT the initial treatment of choice. For patients with bulky disease, a minimum of 6 cycles of R-CHOP is typically administered. Irradiation doses of 30 to 36 Gy, delivered in 1.75 to 1.8 Gy over 3 to 4 weeks after completion of systemic therapy, appear to be adequate. Radiation fields usually include involved lymph node sites or an involved extranodal site and its immediate lymph node drainage areas. Furthermore, the disease should be easily encompassed in a radiation field with acceptable toxicity.

Disease site or potential toxicities may influence the treatment plan:

- Lymphomas of the head and neck may be managed with chemotherapy alone to avoid the acute mucositis and long-term xerostomia associated with radiation therapy fields that are large and include both parotid glands. Alternatively, precise radiation therapy techniques can be employed with intentional sparing of salivary glands, using intensity-modulated radiation therapy (IMRT).

- Fully resected gastric or small intestinal lymphoma may be treated with chemotherapy alone. Patients at high risk of perforation or life-threatening hemorrhage may require surgical resection. Alternatively, chemotherapy followed by local irradiation allows gastric preservation and is preferred in most patients.

For patients with more advanced stage (III or IV) disease, CHOP has been the standard (now with rituximab) for 6 to 8 cycles or 2 cycles beyond remission. Recent data suggest an advantage to "dose-dense" therapy, shortening the interval between cycles from 3 to 2 weeks with growth factor support. More data are needed to validate these results. Many studies now suggest an advantage to the addition of immunotherapy in the form of rituximab, and in almost every study, the combination of rituximab and chemotherapy has improved the response rate and disease-free survival. There appears to be no advantage to maintenance therapy with rituximab in this setting, however, as long as rituximab is included in the induction. Responses are seen in upward of 80% of patients, and approximately 50% to 60% achieve a complete remission. It appears that 50% of these patients (30% to 50% overall) are likely cured.

For patients who either do not have a complete remission or who relapse, alternative therapies are possible, but long-term responses have been seen mostly with autologous or allogeneic SCT. Patients who do not have responsive disease prior to SCT generally do poorly. The IPI has been used to predict outcome for transplantation in DLBCL. The role of autologous SCT for high-risk patients remains open to debate. A randomized clinical trial of early versus delayed high-dose therapy for patients with high- and high-intermediate risk diffuse aggressive lymphoma conducted by the US Intergroup is just completing accrual. If this trial confirms the benefit of early SCT in poor-risk patients with chemosensitive diffuse aggressive NHL, subsequent studies will focus on increasing the number of patients who become eligible for transplant consolidation. Investigational treatments include novel antibodies, radioimmunotherapy, and single-agent chemotherapy drugs. Nonmyeloablative SCT is being evaluated in patients with recurrent or refractory disease.

Some investigators believe that irradiation for stages III and IV (advanced or extensive) DLBCL may be added after the completion of definitive chemotherapy if there is localized residual disease to improve local tumor control. Irradiation may also be delivered after chemotherapy to areas of initially bulky disease, again to enhance local tumor control. These recommendations are based on the observation that when DLBCL relapses after definitive chemotherapy, it usually does so in initially involved or bulky areas of disease. The benefits and potential side effects of irradiation should be weighed against the use of alternative chemotherapy salvage regimens.

MANTLE CELL LYMPHOMA

Clinical presentation By comparison with low-grade NHL, patients with mantle cell lymphoma are older (median age is 64 years), mostly male (75%), and more likely to have peripheral blood involvement (about 30%) and extranodal involvement (mostly the GI tract and CNS, as discussed below). The clinical course in mantle cell lymphoma is characterized by the worst features of the aggressive lymphomas (an aggressive course) and the indolent lymphomas (frequent recurrences). The disease is often widespread at diagnosis, and marrow involvement and splenomegaly are common. GI tract involvement is also common, and many centers suggest evaluation of the GI tract at the time of diagnosis. CNS recurrences are frequent (up to 20%), but isolated CNS disease is a rare occurrence. Leukemic presentations have been described.

Pathology/immunology This disorder was originally classified as diffuse, small, cleaved lymphoma by the REAL classification and represents less than 10% of all NHLs. In this disease, a homogeneous population of small lymphoid cells with irregular nuclear borders arises from and expands the mantle zone surrounding the germinal centers of the lymph nodes, spreading diffusely through the node as the germinal centers are overrun. The lymphocytes express IgM or IgD, as in CLL, but in much greater density. It was recognized that the cells carry a translocation of the long arms of chromosomes 11 and 14 notated as t(11;14)(q13;q23). This molecular event juxtaposes the *bcl-1* gene on chromosome 11 to the immunoglobulin heavy-chain gene on chromosome 14, leading to overexpression of *bcl-1*. This gene encodes the cell-cycle regulatory protein cyclin D1, which is believed to play a role in checkpoint control in DNA synthesis. The immunophenotype is characteristic, and mantle cell lymphomas are usually CD5+, CD20+, CD10-, CD23-, and FMC7+. This immunophenotype is similar to that seen with CLL/SLL, except that CD23 is most often expressed in CLL/SLL but usually is not expressed in mantle cell lymphoma. The key to the diagnosis is the demonstration in tumor tissue or peripheral blood of the t(11;14) by FISH or the cyclin D1 protein by IHC. Inactivation of the *ATM* gene has been described in mantle cell lymphoma.

Treatment Responses to aggressive chemotherapy (CHOP or R-CHOP) are seen, but patients relapse frequently, and median survival is short. Recent data suggest an advantage to SCT while patients are in remission, but more data are required to validate these results. Patients who have relapsed after autologous SCT have been "rescued" by allogeneic SCT.

The National Comprehensive Cancer Network (NCCN) guidelines recommend clinical trials for patients with mantle cell lymphoma (there is no "standard" therapy), and ongoing trials are investigating a short course of R-CHOP followed by radioimmunotherapy with ibritumomab. The complete response/unconfirmed complete response rate is 55% after R-CHOP plus ibritumomab, compared with 13% after R-CHOP alone; however, further follow-up is needed. Investigators have found that aggressive hyperfractionated chemotherapy with rituximab (R-hyper-CVAD) may result in long-term responses in patients with mantle cell lymphoma (Table 12). Anti-idiotype vaccine studies are also under way in this disease, and novel chemotherapy regimens/agents designed to take advantage of the molecular biology of this disease (flavopiridol, bortezomib, cladribine) are being tested. In addition, recent data suggest that a combination of rituximab and the novel hybrid alkylating agent bendamustine produces high response rates in patients with recurrent mantle cell lymphoma.

Recently, the Nordic group presented data that suggest it is possible to achieve long-term disease-free survival in patients with mantle cell lymphoma. They compared their prior experience (1996–2000) using a high-dose CHOP regimen for 4 cycles followed by an autologous SCT with BEAM (carmustine [BiCNU], etoposide, cytarabine [Ara-C], methotrexate) or BEAC (carmustine [BiCNU], etoposide, cytarabine [Ara-C], cyclophosphamide) conditioning with a newer regimen (2000–2006). With the newer regimen, patients received Ara-C in between cycles of CHOP, and then rituximab was added starting at week 10. This regimen was followed by an autologous SCT with BEAM or BEAC. The results of the two trials were compared and showed that 5-year event-free survival improved from 15% to 41% and overall survival, from 63% to 75%. These data suggest that there may be a plateau in the curve in mantle cell lymphoma and that the addition of Ara-C and rituximab may have contributed to that improvement. Further studies are needed to verify these data

BURKITT AND BURKITT-LIKE LYMPHOMA

Clinical presentation These diseases present as three distinct clinical entities: endemic, sporadic, and immunodeficiency-related types. Endemic Burkitt lymphoma most often presents in young children or adolescents with large nodes in the neck, often involving the maxilla or mandible. These cases are most often seen in equatorial Africa and follow the distribution of endemic malaria, hence its designation as "endemic Burkitt lymphoma." In American, or sporadic, Burkitt or Burkitt-like lymphomas, the disease presents in the abdomen and extranodal sites, especially in the GI tract. Sporadic Burkitt lymphoma accounts for 1% to 2% of all adult lymphomas in Western Europe and the United States. The immunodeficiency type is seen in the setting of HIV infection but can be seen in patients with CD4 cell counts > 200 cells/μL. In both endemic and sporadic Burkitt and in Burkitt-like lymphomas, males are affected more often than females.

The LDH level is often elevated, owing to the high turnover rate of these cells and the bulk of disease. The bone marrow and CNS are often involved, and if not involved initially, they are at risk, so CNS prophylaxis is needed. A staging system for Burkitt and Burkitt-like lymphomas has been developed by Murphy and associates (Table 5).

TABLE 12: M. D. Anderson regimen (hyper-CVAD/Ara-C–MTX) for mantle cell lymphoma, lymphoblastic lymphoma, and acute lymphoblastic leukemia

Agent	Dose and frequency
Cyclophosphamide	300 mg/m^2 infused over 3 h q12h × 6 doses (days 1-3) with mesna
Doxorubicin	50 mg/m^2/d on day 4
Vincristine	1.4 mg/m^2 (max 2 mg) IV on days 4 and 11
Dexamethasone	40 mg/d days 1-4 and 11-14
	Alternate every 21 days with
Methotrexate (MTX)	1 g/m^2 continuous infusion over 24 h (day 1)
Ara-C	3 g/m^2 over 2 h q12h × 4 doses (days 2 and 3)
Leucovorin rescue	50 mg PO at the end of MTX infusion and then 25 mg PO q6h × 48 h

Aggressive supportive care, including administration of cytokines, fluconazole (Diflucan), acyclovir, and trimethoprim-sulfamethoxazole, is strongly recommended.

Pathology/immunology These lymphomas are the most rapidly proliferating NHLs. Under the microscope, it is difficult to distinguish Burkitt from Burkitt-like lymphomas and from the B-cell French-American-British (FAB) L3 variant of acute lymphoblastic leukemia. Indeed, the WHO classification recognizes the lymphoma and leukemic phases as a single entity, a mature B-cell neoplasm. The disease is characterized by medium-sized cells with an abundant basophilic cytoplasm with lipid vacuoles. There are round nuclei with clumped chromatin and multiple nucleoli; a diffuse pattern of infiltration is seen and is classic for Burkitt lymphoma. The numerous macrophages that are usually seen in the lymph node biopsy specimens give rise to the so-called starry-sky appearance.

The proliferative rate of this tumor is high, and there are frequent apoptotic cells. In the Burkitt-like variant, there is greater pleomorphism in nuclear size and shape, and the nuclei have fewer nucleoli. There is a low level of concordance among pathologists (about 53%) when they attempt to distinguish Burkitt from Burkitt-like lymphomas, and even by clinical criteria, that distinction is difficult. The cells express surface IgM, CD19, CD20, CD22, CD10, and CD79a and do not express CD5, CD23, and TdT. Bcl-6, a zinc finger protein, is usually expressed. The major consideration in the differential diagnosis is precursor B-cell lymphoma/leukemia, which in contrast expresses TdT; surface immunoglobulin is mostly negative. CD20 may also be negative in this disorder. In Burkitt lymphoma, the expression of CD10 and Bcl-6 protein suggests that these cells originate from the germinal center, and indeed, this is confirmed by sequence analysis of the immunoglobulin variable heavy-chain and light-chain genes. Somatic hypermutation of these genes has been described.

TABLE 13: Cyclophosphamide, vincristine, doxorubicin, high-dose methotrexate (CODOX-M) regimen

Day	Drug	Dose	Method	Time
1	Cyclophosphamide	800 mg/m^2	IV	–
	Vincristine	1.5 mg/m^2 (max 2 mg)	IV	–
	Doxorubicin	40 mg/m^2	IV	–
	Cytarabine	70 mg/m^2	IT	–
2-5	Cyclophosphamide	200 mg/m^2	IV	Daily
3	Cytarabine	70 mg	IT	–
8	Vincristine	1.5 mg/m^2 (max 2 mg)	IV	–
10	Methotrexate	1,200 mg/m^2	IV	Over 1 h
		240 mg/m^2	IV	Each hour over 23 h
11	Leucovorin	192 mg/m^2	IV	At hour 36
		12 mg/m^2	IV	Every 6 h until methotrexate level is < 5 x 10^{-8} M
13	G-CSF	5 µg/kg (or 1 x 263 µg ampule)	SC	Daily until AGC 1 x 10^9/L
15	Methotrexate	12 mg	IT	–
16	Leucovorin	15 mg	PO	24 h after IT methotrexate

Ifosfamide, etoposide, and high-dose cytarabine (IVAC) regimen[a]

Day	Drug	Dose	Method	Time
1-5	Etoposide	60 mg/m^2	IV	Daily over 1 h
	Ifosfamide	1,500 mg/m^2	IV	Daily over 1 h
	Mesna	360 mg/m^2 (mixed with ifosfamide)	IV	Over 1 h
		then 360 mg/m^2	IV	3 h (7 doses/ 24 h)
1 & 2	Cytarabine	2 g/m^2	IV	Over 3 h, 12 hourly (total of four doses)
5	Methotrexate	12 mg	IT	–
6	Leucovorin	15 mg	PO	24 h after IT methotrexate
7	G-CSF	5 µg/kg	SC	Daily until AGC > 1.0 x 10^9/L

[a] Commence next cycle (CODOX-M) on the day that the unsupported AGC is > 1.0 x 10^9/L, with an unsupported platelet count of > 75 x 10^9/L.

AGC = absolute granulocyte count; G-CSF = granulocyte colony-stimulating factor; IT = intrathecal; IV = intravenous; PO = oral; SC = subcutaneous

Genetics The almost constant genetic abnormality in Burkitt lymphoma is overexpression of the c-*myc* oncogene; in 80% of cases, this abnormality results from a balanced translocation between chromosomes 8 and 14, notated as t(8;14), where the c-*myc* oncogene on chromosome 8 is juxtaposed to immunoglobulin heavy-chain enhancer elements on chromosome 14. In the remaining 20% of cases, there are other translocations, including t(2;8)(p12;q24) and t(8;22)(q24;q11). There have been different breakpoints identified in Burkitt lymphoma, and they have been associated with the sporadic and immunodeficiency subtypes.

EBV One cannot discuss these highly aggressive NHLs without discussing the role of EBV. This virus, a member of the herpesvirus family, has the ability to infect resting B cells and transform them into proliferating blasts, most likely by bypassing antigens on lymphocytes and activating signaling molecules. By contrast, certain viruses (HCV) and bacteria (*H pylori*) may cause lymphoma by activating lymphocytes in an antigen-specific manner. EBV infection results in a polyclonal proliferation of lymphoblasts that are latently infected with the virus, as opposed to the infection seen in infectious mononucleosis, which is a lytic infection. This process is regulated by the expression of up to nine latent viral proteins, which are under the control of the transcription factor EBV nuclear antigen 2 (EBNA-2). It appears that the type and result of EBV infection in lymphoid tissue are controlled by various "growth programs," each causing expression of different viral proteins, which then determine the fate of the infected cell. These in vitro events are different from what occurs in healthy carriers of EBV (up to 90% of the population has been exposed), where the viral proteins are not expressed because all of the latently infected cells are resting memory B cells. It is in the germinal center of the lymph node, however, that virally infected cells can transform into memory B cells, as the viral proteins are expressed within the B cells of the germinal center.

Although EBV was found in patients with Burkitt lymphoma over 40 years ago, the role of EBV in the disease still remains uncertain. The exact role of c-*myc* overexpression in the pathogenesis of the disease is also not known, but c-*myc* is known to play a role in cell-cycle progression and cellular transformation. EBV is found in over 95% of cases of "endemic Burkitt lymphoma," which occurs in Africa, but its role in the pathogenesis of the disease is still not clear. The reason therapy with antiviral agents (ganciclovir or acyclovir) cannot be used to treat EBV-associated lymphomas is that the required thymidine kinase (TK) gene is not expressed in latent EBV infection. Recent studies using the small molecule arginine butyrate to upregulate the TK gene and protein expression with concomitant antiviral antibiotics have met with some success.

Treatment Patients must be treated quickly after diagnosis, which should be made on a full biopsy so that adequate tissue is obtained. Tumor lysis syndrome occurs most often with Burkitt lymphoma, and attempts to reduce uric acid production with allopurinol or to degrade it with the enzyme rasburicase (Elitek) should be part of the management, as should aggressive hydration. Patients should be managed in a facility with access to support such as urgent dialysis, because it may be necessary if tumor lysis syndrome occurs.

Treatment includes aggressive chemotherapy, with anthracyclines and cyclophosphamide as the cornerstone. Regimens incorporating hyperfractionated cyclophosphamide such as hyper-CVAD, developed by Murphy and adopted by the M. D. Anderson group, have been used. Other published regimens include CODOX-M/IVAC (cyclophosphamide, vincristine, doxorubicin, high-dose methotrexate/ifosfamide, etoposide, and high-dose Ara-C; Table 13) and the French regimen, which incorporate intensive therapy given weekly in various combinations and intrathecal chemotherapy, and systemic high-dose methotrexate or high-dose Ara-C to facilitate CNS penetration. In children, the results are excellent, and about 80% of patients can be cured. In adults, the outcome is not as favorable, but with newer more intensive regimens, 40% to 60% of patients survive 5 years without disease. New approaches using rituximab and early SCT are being investigated, as are new agents (flavopiridol and an analog of resveratrol) with unique mechanisms of action, which may have relevance to Burkitt and Burkitt-like lymphoma. Addition of rituximab to hyper-CVAD has resulted in marked improvement in outcome in adults with Burkitt lymphoma.

PRIMARY MEDIASTINAL LARGE B-CELL LYMPHOMA

Clinical presentation Primary mediastinal large B-cell lymphoma (PMLBCL) occurs most often in young women (female:male ratio is 2:1) who present with mediastinal masses only. These masses are usually bulky and often invade surrounding structures, such as the pleura, lungs, pericardium, and chest wall, but disease is infrequently found outside the chest cavity. At recurrence, however, extranodal sites such as the lungs, adrenal glands, liver, or kidneys may be involved. Because of the location and bulk of the disease, patients complain of chest pain, cough and shortness of breath and are often found to have superior vena cava (SVC) syndrome. This can be subtle, with unexplained breast enlargement the only symptom in some cases. The diagnosis can be delayed if the clinician does not recognize the signs and symptoms of SVC. This clinical presentation is similar to classic Hodgkin lymphoma, and indeed, that is the primary differential diagnostic consideration when these patients are evaluated.

Pathology/immunology The pathology is characterized by a diffuse proliferation of large cells with clear cytoplasm, often accompanied by extensive sclerosis. The cells are mostly of B-cell origin and express CD20 and other B-cell markers but do not express surface immunoglobulin (Ig). Indeed, the discordant expression of CD79a and Ig expression are distinguishing features of PMLBCL. There are data that describe gains of chromosomal material in tissue specimens, most often 2p, 9p, 12q, and Xq. The *rel*, *mal*, and *fig1* (interleukin-4 [IL-4] gene) oncogenes are overexpressed in tissue specimens. Ig genes have a high level of somatic hypermutation. All of these observations suggest that this entity is unique, especially compared with B-cell lymphomas that arise in peripheral nodes. IL-13 expression and downstream effectors of IL-13 signaling pathways are overexpressed, along with tumor necrosis factor (TNF) family members and TNF receptor-associated factor-1.

The overexpression of the *rel* oncogene, previously described, has been associated almost exclusively with the nucleus, consistent with NF-κB pathway activation, and the *mal* overexpression has been confirmed in gene array studies. These data help us to reorder our thinking about these clinically unique lymphomas and to begin to build a molecular story that is consistent with the clinical observation that PMLBCL is more like classic Hodgkin lymphoma than like DLBCL. Further, the observations that certain signaling pathways are involved provide a rationale to attack these pathways specifically in a targeted approach.

Treatment The clinical course is variable; some report a poor outcome with conventional, CHOP-based chemotherapy regimens and irradiation, and some report an excellent outcome. It seems clear that bulk of disease and LDH level are important prognostic factors and that prediction of the outcome by the IPI is useful. A variety of chemotherapy regimens have been evaluated, including CHOP and MACOP-B/VACOP-B (methotrexate or etoposide, Adriamycin, cyclophosphamide, Oncovin, prednisone, bleomycin), and more recently rituximab has been incorporated into the management. Usually, radiation therapy is a part of the initial treatment; however, recent data suggest that radiation therapy may not be necessary in all patients. In general, in 2008, patients receive anthracycline-containing chemotherapy with rituximab and after 4 to 6 courses, radiation therapy may be given to patients with bulky disease. There are no randomized trials comparing radiation therapy with no radiation therapy in this setting. PET scanning may influence the use of consolidation radiation therapy in the future.

PERIPHERAL T-CELL LYMPHOMA, UNSPECIFIED

Peripheral T-cell lymphoma, unspecified (PTCL) is predominantly a nodal lymphoma that represents the most common T-cell lymphoma subtype in Western countries, comprising approximately 50% to 60% of T-cell lymphomas and 5% to 7% of all NHLs. PTCL usually affects male adults (1.9:1 male-to-female ratio) with a median age of 61 years (range, 17–90), with 25% of patients presenting in stage I or IIE; 12%, in stage III; and 63%, in stage IV. Patients with PTCL from this study commonly presented with unfavorable characteristics, including B symptoms (40%), elevated LDH level (66%), bulky tumor ≥ 10 cm (11%), nonambulatory performance status (29%), and extranodal disease (56%), leading to the majority of patients (53%) falling into the unfavorable IPI category (score of 3 to 5).

Most T-cell NHL patients are treated in the same manner as aggressive B-cell patients, with anthracycline-based combination chemotherapy such as CHOP. Randomized trials comparing CHOP with other combination regimens confirmed CHOP as a standard regimen for aggressive B-cell NHL; unfortunately, these trials do not allow for subset analysis of T-cell patients. Rituximab should not be included in the treatment of PTCL (unless other conditions such as immune thrombocytopenic purpura exist), as CD20 is not expressed. Other therapeutic agents being tested in T-cell NHL include purine and pyrimidine analogs, denileukin diftitox (Ontak), and a retinoic acid/IFN-α (interferon-) combination.

Denileukin diftitox is a novel recombinant fusion protein consisting of peptide sequences for the enzymatically active and membrane translocation domains of diphtheria toxin with recombinant IL-2 (CD25 receptor); it has been studied mostly in cutaneous T-cell NHL, although clinical benefit has been reported in other T-cell NHL patients. Recently, the histone deacetylase inhibitors SAHA and depsipeptide have shown activity against PTCL.

ANGIOIMMUNOBLASTIC T-CELL LYMPHOMA

Angioimmunoblastic T-cell lymphoma (AITL), also known as angio-immunoblastic lymphadenopathy with dysproteinemia, is one of the more common T-cell lymphomas, accounting for 15% to 20% of cases and 3% to 4% of all lymphomas. The mean age at presentation is 57 to 65 years, with a slight male predominance, and the majority of patients present with stage III or IV disease. AITL is commonly a systemic disease with nodal involvement with various associated disease features, such as organomegaly, B symptoms (50%–70%), skin rash, pruritus, pleural effusions, arthritis, eosinophilia, and varied immunologic abnormalities (positive Coombs' test, cold agglutinins, hemolytic anemia, antinuclear antibodies, rheumatoid factors, cryoglobulins, and polyclonal hypergammaglobulinemia).

Spontaneous disease regression is seen on rare occasions, although AITL typically follows an aggressive clinical course. Treatment with anthracycline-based combination chemotherapy results in complete remission rates of 50% to 70% of AITL patients, although only 10% to 30% of patients are long-term survivors. One prospective, nonrandomized multicenter study treated newly diagnosed "stable" AITL patients with single-agent prednisone and combination chemotherapy for relapsing/refractory patients or initially if "life-threatening" disease was present at diagnosis. The complete remission rate was 29% with single-agent prednisone, whereas the complete remission rate for relapsed/refractory patients or patients treated initially with combination chemotherapy was 56% and 64%, respectively. With a median follow-up of 28 months (range, 7 to 53), the overall and disease-free survival rates were 40.5% (confidence interval [CI], 24% to 56%) and 32.3% (CI, 17% to 47%), respectively, although the median overall survival was 15 months. There are anecdotal reports of relapsed AITL patients who have responded to immunosuppressive therapy, such as low-dose methotrexate/prednisone, as well as reported responses to purine analog treatment. Furthermore, cyclosporine has demonstrated activity in relapsed AITL patients in case reports, and the ECOG is evaluating this agent in a prospective study. There are anecdotal reports of thalidomide plus steroid responses in AITL.

ANAPLASTIC LARGE-CELL LYMPHOMA, T-/NULL-CELL, PRIMARY SYSTEMIC TYPE

Anaplastic large cell lymphoma (ALCL), primary systemic type, accounts for approximately 2% to 3% of all NHLs. This disease mainly involves lymph nodes, although extranodal sites may be involved (not exclusively the skin; see sub-section on ALCL, CD30+ cutaneous type). This disease may be divided in part based on the expression of the TK anaplastic lymphoma kinase (ALK), created from a balanced chromosomal translocation t(2;5) and other less common translocations involving 2p23 (see Table 1). When heterogeneous patient populations are analyzed, the prevalence of ALK positivity in primary systemic ALCL cases is 50% to 60%. ALK-positive ALCL is typically diagnosed in men prior to age 35 (male-to-female ratio, 1.7:1), with frequent systemic symptoms and extranodal and advanced-stage disease. ALK-negative patients are usually older (median age, 61 years), with a male-to-female ratio of 1.5:1, with a similar high incidence of extranodal disease. In addition to the prognostic importance of ALK positivity, the IPI has been identified as an independent prognostic factor within the group of ALK-positive ALCL patients, with a reported 5-year overall survival of 94% versus 41% for IPI 0 or 1 and 2 to 4, respectively. This better prognosis is apparent despite ALK-positive patients more commonly presenting with poorer performance status and more advanced-stage disease compared with ALK-negative patients.

Therapy for pediatric ALCL is often based on prognostic risk factors, with treatment regimens modeled after high-grade B-cell NHL protocols. Following a brief cytoreductive prephase, short, intensified polyagent chemotherapy is administered, with the number of cycles dependent on the stage of disease. Therapy for adult ALCL, systemic type, has commonly included anthracycline-based regimens such as CHOP. Autologous hematopoietic SCT in first complete remission for ALK-negative ALCL has been advocated by some groups, although this approach warrants prospective validation.

HEPATOSPLENIC T-CELL LYMPHOMA

Hepatosplenic T-cell lymphoma (HSTCL) is an uncommon T-cell lymphoma that is seen mainly in young males (median age, 35) presenting with B symptoms, prominent hepatosplenomegaly, mild anemia, neutropenia, thrombocytopenia (commonly severe), significant peripheral blood lymphocytosis, and rare lymphadenopathy and is associated with an aggressive clinical course (median survival, 12 to 14 months).

The tumor cells are usually negative for CD4 and CD8 (85%); positive for CD2, CD3, and CD7 (negative for CD5); and express CD56 in 70% to 80% of cases. TIA-1 is present in almost all cases, but commonly granzyme B and perforin are not present, an indication of a nonactivated cytotoxic T-cell phenotype. Cells usually express the γ/δ T-cell receptor (Vd1+/Vd2–/Vd3–) but are negative for EBV.

Historically, patients with HSTCL have been treated with CHOP-like regimens. Early autologous SCT has been favored by some investigators based on anecdotal cases. A recent report described activity with the purine analog pentostatin in relapsed HSTCL patients. Approximately 10% to 20% of HSTCL cases arise in immunocompromised patients, predominantly in the solid-organ transplant setting.

EXTRANODAL NK/T-CELL LYMPHOMA AND NASAL-TYPE

Extranodal NK/T-cell lymphoma, and nasal-type, formerly known as angiocentric lymphoma, is rare in Western countries, being more prevalent in Asia and Peru. The disease commonly presents in men at the median age of 50 years. This entity is associated with EBV and is typically characterized by extranodal presentation and localized stage I/II disease but with angiodestructive proliferation and an aggressive clinical course. These tumors have a predilection for the nasal cavity and paranasal sinuses ("nasal"), although the "nasal-type" designation encompasses other extranodal sites of NK/T-cell lymphomatous disease (skin, GI, testis, kidneys, upper respiratory tract, and rarely orbit/eye).

Combined-modality therapy incorporating doxorubicin-based chemotherapy (minimum of 6 cycles for patients with stage III or IV disease), IFRT (minimum 50 Gy), and intrathecal prophylaxis are recommended for patients with extranodal NK/T-cell lymphoma, nasal, although the benefit of the addition of chemotherapy to radiation therapy has not been confirmed for limited-stage disease.

Patients with systemic disease have poor long-term survival (5-year overall survival, 20%–25%), with high locoregional (over 50%) and systemic failure rates (over 70%).

ENTEROPATHY-TYPE INTESTINAL T-CELL LYMPHOMA

Enteropathy-type intestinal T-cell lymphoma (EITCL; also known as intestinal T-cell lymphoma) is a rare T-cell lymphoma of intraepithelial lymphocytes that commonly presents with multiple circumferential jejunal ulcers in adults with a brief history of gluten-sensitive enteropathy. EITCL accounts for less than 1% of NHLs, according to the International Lymphoma Study Group, and has been recognized to have a poor prognosis, with reported 5-year overall and disease-free survival rates of 20% and 3%, respectively. This finding is in part related to many patients presenting with a poor performance status and varied complications of locally advanced disease by the time a diagnosis of EITCL has been confirmed.

EITCL may present without an antecedent celiac history, but most patients have abdominal pain and weight loss. Evidence of celiac serologic markers such as positive antigliadin antibodies and/or HLA types such as DQA1*0501/DQB1*0201/DRB1*0304 may be present at diagnosis of EITCL. Moreover, these genotypes may represent celiac patients at higher risk for development of EITCL. Small bowel perforation or obstruction, GI bleeding, and enterocolic fistulae are recognized complications of this disease. The immunophenotype consists of pan–T-cell antigens, usually CD8+, and the mucosal lymphoid antigen CD103 is often expressed.

Following diagnosis of EITCL, doxorubicin-based combination chemotherapy should be considered for each patient, and aggressive nutritional support with parenteral or enteral feeding is critical in the care of these patients. Patients with known celiac disease should adhere to a gluten-free diet.

ADULT T-CELL LEUKEMIA/LYMPHOMA

The retrovirus HTLV-1 has been documented to be critical to the development of adult T-cell leukemia/lymphoma (ATLL). HTLV-1 is known to cause diseases other than ATLL, including tropical spastic paraparesis/HTLV-1–associated myelopathy, infective dermatitis, and uveitis. In endemic areas in Japan, approximately 10% to 35% of the population is infected with HTLV-1. Among these carriers, the overall risk of ATLL is approximately 2.5% in patients who live to age 70. Of the Caribbean population, 2% to 6% are HTLV-1 carriers, whereas less than 1% of the population in lower-risk areas, such as the United States and Europe, are seropositive. HTLV-1 is transmitted through sexual intercourse, transfused blood products (products containing white blood cells, not fresh frozen plasma), shared needles, breast milk, and vertical transmission. Transfusion of HTLV-1–contaminated blood products results in seroconversion in approximately 30% to 50% of patients, at a median of 51 days.

The clinical features of 187 ATLL patients included a median age at onset of 55 years, lymphadenopathy (72%), skin lesions (53%), hepatomegaly (47%), splenomegaly (25%), and hypercalcemia (28%) present at diagnosis. The differential diagnosis between cutaneous ATLL and mycosis fungoides is often difficult. ATLL is separated into four subtypes divided by clinicopathologic features and prognosis: acute, lymphoma, chronic, and smoldering. Shimoyama and colleagues reported on the characteristics of 818 ATLL patients. Patients with acute-type ATLL present with hypercalcemia, leukemic manifestations, and tumor lesions and have the worst prognosis, with a median survival of approximately 6 months. Patients with lymphoma-type ATLL present with low circulating abnormal lymphocytes (< 1%) and nodal, liver, splenic, CNS, bone, and GI disease; the median survival is 10 months. Patients with the chronic type present with > 5% abnormal circulating lymphocytes and have a median survival of 24 months, whereas the median survival of patients with the smoldering type has not yet been reached.

ATLL is an aggressive neoplasm with resistance to conventional chemotherapy, in part due to the viral protein tax-mediated resistance to apoptosis and overexpression of p-glycoprotein (the product of the multidrug resistance-1 gene). Patients may initially respond to combination chemotherapy, but unfortunately, response durations are brief (5 to 7 months). El-Sabban and colleagues combined arsenic trioxide (Trisenox) with IFN-α, which induced cell-cycle arrest and apoptosis. Response rates of 70% to 90% to combination IFN-α and zidovudine (Retrovir) therapy have been demonstrated in ATLL, with associated increased median survival rates compared with those of historic controls (11 to 18 vs 4 to 8 months, respectively). A clinical trial that investigated initial cytoreductive therapy with CHOP followed by antinucleoside, IFN-α, and oral etoposide therapy demonstrated encouraging results. Other agents with anecdotal activity in ATLL include irinotecan and the purine analogues (pentostatin [Nipent] and 2-chlorodeoxyadenosine), although pentostatin did not appear to improve outcomes when added to combination chemotherapy. Future research should include the investigation of recombinant toxins and antibodies, such as denileukin diftitox (Ontak) and alemtuzumab (Campath).

A phase III clinical trial to evaluate the overall efficacy and safety of denileukin diftitox (Ontak) in CD25+ patients with refractory CTCL (stages IA–III) was recently completed. A total of 144 patients with CD25+ CTCL were randomized to receive either of two doses of denileukin diftitox (18 μg/kg/d [n = 55] or 9 μg/kg/d [n = 45]), or placebo (n = 44), for up to 8 cycles. Treatment was administered via IV infusion on d 1 to 5 of each 21-day cycle. The median number of cycles for all treated patients was six for the 18 μg/kg/d group (range 1–11) and seven for the 9 μg/kg/d group (range 1–10). The primary endpoint was overall response rate (ORR).

For patients receiving 18 μg/kg/d of denileukin diftitox, ORR was 46% vs 15% for placebo (P = .002) and for the 9 μg/kg/d group, ORR was 37% (P = .03 vs placebo).

Analysis of a secondary endpoint, progression-free survival (PFS), suggested a 73% reduction in risk of disease progression in the 18 μg/kg/d group (hazard ratio = 0.27; P = .0002; 95% CI = 0.14, 0.54) and a 58% reduction in risk of disease progression in the 9 μg/kg/d group (hazard ratio = 0.42; P = .02; 95% CI = 0.20, 0.86) compared to placebo.

This was the largest randomized, double-blind, placebo-controlled trial ever conducted in CTCL. Based on results of the trial, in October 2008, FDA granted Ontak full approval in CD25+ CTCL.

CUTANEOUS T-CELL LYMPHOMAS

Cutaneous T-cell lymphomas (CTCLs) constitute a group of cutaneous NHLs with clonal expansion of T lymphocytes into the skin. Several entities are recognized by the combined European Organization for Research and Treatment of Cancer (EORTC) and WHO classification, which is based on morphologic, histopathologic, and molecular features (Table 14). The frequency and disease-specific survival differ for each entity.

MYCOSIS FUNGOIDES/SÉZARY SYNDROME

Mycosis fungoides and its variants represent the most common type of CTCL, comprising 50% of CTCLs, with a male predominance of approximately 2:1 and a predominance of African-American patients of 1.6:1. It has a yearly incidence of 0.36 cases per 100,000 population that has remained constant over the past decade. Clinical and histologic diagnosis of mycosis fungoides has proved to be difficult, because in early stages, it may resemble other dermatoses such as eczematous dermatitis, psoriasis, and parapsoriasis.

Clinically, mycosis fungoides is characterized by erythematous patches, evolving into plaques or tumors; however, the progress is variable. It is classified as an indolent lymphoma by the EORTC. The neoplastic cells have a mature CD3+, CD4+, CD45RO+, CD8– memory T-cell phenotype. Sézary syndrome is the aggressive, leukemic, and erythrodermic form of CTCL, which is characterized by circulating, atypical, malignant T lymphocytes with cerebriform nuclei (Sézary cells), and lymphadenopathy. Circulating Sézary cells also have a mature memory T-cell phenotype with loss of CD7 and CD26. For staging purposes, the tumor node metastasis (TNM) system is most commonly used (Table 15).

Investigative and approved options that have shown activity against mycosis fungoides/Sézary syndrome include the histone deacetylase inhibitors vorinostat (FDA approved), depsipeptide, and panobinostat; the proteasome inhibitor bortezomib and monoclonal antibodies targeting CD4 (zanolimumab), CD2 (siplizumab), and CD30 (SGN-30).

TABLE 14: The new World Health Organization-European Organization for Research and Treatment of Cancer (WHO-EORTC) consensus classification for primary cutaneous lymphomas with relative frequency and 5-year survival

WHO-EORTC	Frequency	5-year survival
Cutaneous T-cell and NK-cell lymphomas		
Indolent		
Mycosis fungoides (MF)	44%	88%
• Follicullar MF	4%	80%
• Pagetoid reticulosis	< 1%	100%
• Granulomatous slack skin	< 1%	100%
CD30+ lymphoproliferative disorders		
• Anaplastic large cell lymphoma	8%	95%
• Lymphomatoid papulosis	12%	100%
Subcutaneous panniculitis-like T-cell lymphoma	1%	82%
CD4+ small/medium pleomorphic T-cell lymphoma	2%	72%
Aggressive		
Sézary syndrome	3%	24%
Cutaneous peripheral T-cell lymphoma, unspecified	2%	16%
• Cutaneous aggressive CD8+ T-cell lymphoma	< 1%	18%
• Cutaneous γ/δ T-cell lymphoma	< 1%	–
Cutaneous NK/T-cell lymphoma, nasal type	< 1%	–
Cutaneous B-cell lymphomas		
Indolent		
Follicle center cell lymphoma	11%	95%
Marginal zone lymphoma	7%	99%
Intermediate clinical behavior		
Large B-cell lymphoma of the leg	4%	55%
Cutaneous diffuse large B-cell lymphoma, other	< 1%	50%
Intravascular large B-cell lymphoma	< 1%	65%

EORTC = European Organization for Research and Treatment of Cancer; NK = natural killer; WHO = World Health Organization

TABLE 15: Stage classification for mycosis fungoides and Sézary syndrome

Stage	T	N	NP	M
IA	1	0	0	0
IB	2	0	0	0
IIA	1/2	1	0	0
IIB	3	0/1	0	0
III	4	0/1	0	0
IVA	1–4	0/1	1	0
IVB	1–4	0/1	0/1	1

T (Skin)

T1	Limited patch/plaque (< 10% of BSA)
T2	Generalized patch/plaque (> 10% of BSA)
T3	Tumors
T4	Generalized erythroderma

N (Nodes)

N0	No clinically abnormal peripheral lymph nodes
N1	Clinically abnormal peripheral lymph nodes
NP0	Biopsy performed, not CTCL
NP1	Biopsy performed, CTCL
LN0	Uninvolved
LN1	Reactive lymph node
LN2	Dermatopathic node, small clusters of convoluted cells (< 6 cells per cluster)
LN3[a]	Dermatopathic node, large clusters of convoluted cells (> 6 cells per cluster)
LN4[a]	Lymph node effacement

M (Viscera)

M0	No visceral metastasis
M1	Visceral metastasis

B (Blood)

B0	Atypical circulating cells not present (< 5%)
B1	Atypical circulating cells present (> 5%)

[a]Pathologically involved lymph nodes

BSA = body surface area; CTCL = cutaneous T-cell lymphoma; TNMB = tumor, node, metastasis, blood
M = viscera; N = node; NP1 = biopsy performed, not cutaneous T-cell lymphoma; NP2 = biopsy performed, cutaneous T-cell lymphoma; T = tumor

TABLE 16: Treatment options for cutaneous T-cell lymphoma by stage

Stage	Clinical features	Treatment options
IA	Limited patch, plaque (< 10% BSA)	Topical steroids, nitrogen mustard, or BiCNU, bexarotene gel[a], spot electron-beam irradiation, PUVA
IB-IIA	Extensive patch, plaque (> 10% BSA)	Topical nitrogen mustard or BiCNU, PUVA, bexarotene gel,[a] total skin electron-beam irradiation, methotrexate, IFN, PUVA + IFN, bexarotene capsules, PUVA + bexarotene capsules, vorinostat
IIB	Tumors	Spot electron-beam irradiation, PUVA ± IFN, methotrexate, bexarotene capsules, denileukin diftitox, vorinostat
III	Erythroderma without Sézary cells	PUVA, total skin electron-beam irradiation, topical Sézary cells, nitrogen mustard, or BiCNU, bexarotene capsules, IFN, PUVA + IFN or bexarotene capsules, alemtuzumab, methotrexate, purine analogues, photopheresis, vorinostat
III	Erythroderma with Sézary cells	Extracorporeal photopheresis, PUVA + IFN, bexarotene capsules ± PUVA, methotrexate, purine analogues, denileukin diftitox, alemtuzumab, vorinostat
IV	Lymph node or visceral organ	Bexarotene capsules, IFN, denileukin diftitox, purine analogues, visceral involvement cytotoxic chemotherapy ± skin-directed therapies, vorinostat

[a]Topical bexarotene may cause irritation if applied to a large body surface area.

BSA = body surface area; BiCNU = carmustine; PUVA = psoralen plus ultraviolet A; IFN = interferon

Treatment of early-stage disease

At present, CTCLs are regarded as incurable. In early CTCL, the cell-mediated immune response is usually normal. Therefore, the majority of these cases can be treated successfully with topical modalities. Early aggressive therapy does not improve the prognosis of patients with CTCL. The skin-targeted modalities include psoralen plus ultraviolet A (PUVA); narrow-band–ultraviolet B (NB-UVB); skin electron-beam radiation therapy; spot radiation therapy; as well as topical preparations of steroids, retinoids, carmustine, or nitrogen mustard (Table 16). Radiation therapy prescriptions may be similar to those for other lymphomas or may be delivered at high dose in limited fractions.

Both the EORTC (Trautinger F, Knobler R, Willemze R, et al: Eur J Cancer 42:1014-1030, 2006) and NCCN (www.nccn.org) have published consensus recommendations for the treatment of mycosis fungoides/Sézary syndrome.

Treatment of advanced-stage disease

A limited number of patients progress to more aggressive and advanced disease with either cutaneous or extracutaneous tumor manifestations. Treatment goals in advanced stages should be to reduce the tumor burden, relieve symptoms, and decrease the risk of transformation into aggressive lymphoma. Established treatment options include mono- or polychemotherapy including COP (cyclophosphamide, vincristine [Oncovin], prednisone) or CHOP regimens, extracorporeal photopheresis, interferons, retinoids and rexinoids (bexarotene [Targretin] capsules), histone deacetylase inhibitors (vorinostat [Zolinza]), monoclonal antibodies (alemtuzamab), and recombinant toxins (denileukin diftitox). Combinations are frequently used (Table 16). Select patients with progressive and recalcitrant disease have been cured with an allogeneic SCT.

PRIMARY CUTANEOUS CD30-POSITIVE LYMPHOPROLIFERATIVE DISORDERS

Primary cutaneous CD30-positive lymphoproliferative disorders are the second most common group of CTCL, representing approximately 30% of CTCLs. This spectrum of diseases includes lymphomatoid papulosis, ALCL CD30+ cutaneous type, and borderline cases. The distinction between these entities can be challenging and is often made on clinical behavior.

LYMPHOMATOID PAPULOSIS

Lymphomatoid papulosis is most commonly associated with mycosis fungoides, CD30+ large T-cell lymphoma, and Hodgkin lymphoma. Three histologic types have been identified, characterized as types A, B, and C. Types A and C consist of large lymphocytes resembling Reed-Sternberg cells. Type A cells are embedded in a dense inflammatory background, whereas type C cells form large sheets imitating CD30+ large T-cell lymphoma. Type B simulates classic features of mycosis fungoides, with epidermotropism and a dermal band-like infiltrate composed of small to medium cells. Lymphomatoid papulosis lesions occasionally exhibit clonal gene rearrangements.

Lymphomatoid papulosis represents a benign, chronic recurrent, self-healing, papulonodular, and papulonecrotic CD30+ skin eruption. However, 10% to 20% of patients may develop a lymphoid malignancy, but the prognosis for patients with lymphomatoid papulosis is otherwise excellent, with a 5-year survival of 100%. There is no curative treatment available. Lymphomatoid papulosis is managed by observation, intralesional steroid injection, topical bexarotene, ultraviolet light therapy, or low-dose methotrexate.

ANAPLASTIC LARGE CELL LYMPHOMA, CD30+ CUTANEOUS TYPE

Primary systemic CD30+ anaplastic large cell lymphoma (ALCL) and primary cutaneous CD30+ ALCL represent identical morphologic entities, but they are clinically distinct diseases.

The neoplastic cells of primary cutaneous CD30+ ALCL are of the CD4+ helper T-cell phenotype with CD30 expression. It represents 9% of CTCLs and typically presents with solitary or localized nodules. This tumor has an excellent prognosis, as confirmed in several studies, in contrast to the transformation of mycosis lymphoma to a CD30− large cell variant. It shows histologic and immunophenotypic overlap with lymphomatoid papulosis. In most cases, tumor cells show anaplastic features, less commonly a pleomorphic or immunoblastic appearance. However, there is no difference in the prognosis and survival rate. Primary CD30+ ALCL rarely carries the t(2;5) translocation and is usually ALK-negative. These lesions may undergo spontaneous regression, as do the lesions of lymphomatoid papulosis. The mechanism of tumor regression remains unknown.

Spot radiation therapy or surgical excision is the preferred treatment, with systemic chemotherapy reserved for cases with large tumor burden and extracutaneous involvement. More recently, there has been reported efficacy of recombinant IFN-γ-1b (Actimmune) and combined treatment with bexarotene and IFN-α-2a (Roferon-A).

SUBCUTANEOUS PANNICULITIS-LIKE T-CELL LYMPHOMA

Subcutaneous panniculitis-like T-cell lymphoma (SCPTCL) is a rare T-cell lymphoma that infiltrates the subcutaneous fat without dermal and epidermal involvement, causing erythematous to violaceous nodules and/or plaques. Systemic symptoms are frequent and include weight loss, fever, and fatigue. The disease may be complicated by the hemophagocytic syndrome. SCPTCL may be preceded by a benign-appearing panniculitis for years. The infiltrate is pleomorphic and associated with inflammation and necrosis. The T-cell phenotype is α/β+ with CD4(+/−), CD8+, and CD56(−/+). Standard treatment has historically included CHOP-like chemotherapy. However, recent data suggest patients can be controlled for long periods with local radiation treatment and/or steroids. Five-year survival rates exceed 80%.

CUTANEOUS γ/δ T-CELL LYMPHOMA

Cutaneous γ/δ T-cell lymphoma is a rare panniculitis presenting with disseminated (ulcerated) plaques, nodules, or tumors. Involvement of mucosal or extranodal sites is common. Systemic symptoms, including weight loss, fever, and fatigue, are almost always present. The hemophagocytic syndrome is often noted. The γ/δ+ T cells are characteristically CD2+, CD3+, CD4−, CD5−, CD7(−/+), CD8(−/+), and CD56+. Aggressive chemotherapy is indicated, with consideration of autologous or allogeneic SCT incorporated into the initial treatment schema. The median survival is less than 2 years.

PLEOMORPHIC T-CELL LYMPHOMAS WITH SMALL/MEDIUM CELLS

The small/medium pleomorphic CTCL type appears clinically with single erythematous to violaceous nodules or tumors and accounts for less than 3% of CTCL cases. Most cases have an unfavorable prognosis, with a median survival of ≤ 24 months; however, the CD3+, CD4+, CD8–, CD30– subtype with limited lesions might be associated with a better prognosis, with a reported 45% 5-year survival rate.

The optimal therapy for pleomorphic T-cell lymphomas with small/medium cells has not been defined. Localized lesions have been treated with radiation therapy or surgical excision. Only short-term outcome has been reported. Patients with generalized skin disease or progression have been treated effectively with systemic treatments, including multiagent chemotherapy, retinoids, interferons, and monoclonal antibodies.

CUTANEOUS B-CELL LYMPHOMAS

Primary cutaneous B-cell lymphomas (CBCLs) are rare entities. They constitute up to 25% of all cutaneous lymphomas. However, the incidence of CBCLs has been underestimated due to the absence of immunologic and molecular markers. In addition, their terminology and classification remain controversial, with until recently separate and distinct terminology promoted by WHO and EORTC. Primary CBCLs are distinct from nodal lymphomas, and the majority of them have an excellent prognosis. Several types are recognized, with the most common types being follicle center cell lymphoma and marginal zone lymphoma.

Follicle center cell lymphoma Follicle center cell lymphoma (FCCL) is defined as a proliferation of centrocytes (small to large cleaved cells) and centroblasts (large round cells with prominent nuclei), showing a nodular or diffuse infiltrate in the majority of cases and presenting only rarely a true follicular pattern. FCCL is the most common subtype, comprising 40% of CBCLs. FCCL shows a predilection for the head, neck, and trunk in elderly patients, with a median age of 60 years and a male predominance of approximately 1.5:1. The clinical course is usually indolent, with an excellent overall survival of up to 97%. However, relapses occur frequently. The large round cell morphology might be associated with a higher rate of disease progression and poorer prognosis.

Small centrocytes predominate in low-grade FCCL, whereas an increased number of large cells occurs in high-grade FCCL; however, lesions with pure high-grade disease may behave indolently and should not by themselves drive the treatment administered. In contrast to their nodal counterpart, bcl-2 is usually not expressed in neoplastic cells, and the t(14;18) translocation is rarely detected. More recently, low rates of bcl-2 expression have been reported. In addition to CD10+ and bcl-6+ expression, FCCL also has an aberrant expression of CD45 RA and CD43 and thus provides a helpful clue to distinguish it from pseudolymphomas. Radiation therapy is often the preferred therapy for solitary or localized group lesions. Surgical excision can be considered for small lesions. Chemotherapy, though effective, rarely results in cure. Rituximab has proven to be effective for palliation. Observation is a reasonable alternative in many instances.

Immunocytoma /marginal zone lymphoma Immunocytoma (IC)/marginal zone lymphoma (MZL) is a recently recognized low-grade lymphoma and represents the second most common subtype of CBCLs. It predominantly occurs on the upper and lower extremities. The median age at presentation is 55 years, and females are affected more often than males. The reported survival rates are 97% to 100%, although relapses commonly occur. Histologically, IC/MZL has features of MALT lymphomas and shows a nodular or diffuse dermal infiltrate with a heterogeneous cellular infiltrate of small lymphocytes, lymphoplasmacytoid cells, plasma cells, intranuclear inclusions (Dutcher bodies), and reactive germinal centers that may be infiltrated by neoplastic cells. Diagnosis can be difficult, because of the variable composition of the infiltrate that may be interpreted as a reactive process or as FCCL. In contrast to FCCL, MZL is negative for *bcl*-6 and CD10. In 50% of cases, CD43 is highly expressed. Large cell transformation and a head and neck presentation may be associated with a worse prognosis. Therapeutic alternatives are similar to those described for FCCL.

LARGE B-CELL LYMPHOMA OF THE LEG

Primary cutaneous large B-cell lymphoma of the leg (LBCLL) forms a separate category in the WHO–EORTC classification, as a more aggressive type seen in elderly patients, with a median age of 76 years at diagnosis and a female predominance of 7:2. Most cases have a follicle center cell origin, and histologic evaluation shows a diffuse dermal infiltrate with predominance in large B cells with multilobulated nuclei, comprised of centroblasts and immunoblasts, with presence of small, cleaved cells and a minor admixed infiltrate component. Eosinophilic intranuclear (Dutcher body) or intracytoplasmic (Russell body) inclusions of immunoglobulin are common. Unlike FCCL, LBCLLs consistently express *bcl*-2, although they are not associated with the t(14;18) translocation.

The prognosis is less favorable for LBCLL than for other CBCLs, with a 5-year survival rate of 50% to 60%. Prognostic factors identified with a poor outcome include the predominance of round cells (centroblasts/immunoblasts) over cleaved cells (centrocytes) in the tumor infiltrate, MUM-1 expression, and multiple lesions at presentation. The use of an IPI-based model is required to investigate whether LBCLL is associated with a poorer prognosis. These lymphomas should be treated as systemic DLBCL with anthracycline-based chemotherapy. In patients presenting with a single, small skin tumor, radiotherapy is a consideration. Rituximab has also been incorporated into combination regimens.

Intravascular large B-cell lymphoma WHO and EORTC have proposed intravascular large B-cell lymphoma (IVLBCL) or angiotropic B-cell lymphoma as a provisional entity. This subtype is rare and corresponds to the proliferation of malignant lymphocytes within lumina of small vessels, involving most frequently the skin and CNS. It was previously considered a vascular tumor and referred to as malignant angioendotheliomatosis. Although the majority of cases are of B-cell origin, few cases of T-cell lineage have been reported. The reason for intravascular localization is not clear, but association with an unknown surface receptor or dysfunction of lymphocyte-endothelial interaction affecting adhesion molecules has been suspected.

IVLBCL is clinically characterized by tender erythematous, purpuric, indurated patches and plaques located on the trunk and thighs, where it can resemble panniculitis. Cases of generalized telangiectasia over normal skin have been reported. Cytomorphology reveals intravascular occlusion of small vessels, filled with large atypical centroblast-like B lymphocytes. IHC shows CD19, CD20, CD45, and CD79a expression. Genotypic analysis has demonstrated clonality, although it may not be positive in every case. Generally, the prognosis of this aggressive type of lymphoma is poor despite the use of combination chemotherapy, because of the initial or secondary CNS involvement. Prognosis appeared better in some reports, if isolated cutaneous involvement was present. However, no large series permitting a precise prognosis to be determined are available.

CD4+/CD56+ HEMATODERMIC NEOPLASM (BLASTIC NK-CELL LYMPHOMA)

The CD4+/CD56+ hematodermic neoplasm commonly presents in the skin, with nodular and extracutaneous systemic involvement. This rare disorder appears to be derived from a plasmacytoid dendritic cell precursor. T-cell receptor genes are in germline configuration. This entity causes a dismal prognosis (median survival, 14 months) despite intensive chemotherapy.

PLASMACYTOMA

Primary cutaneous involvement of plasmacytoma is uncommon and generally develops as a consequence of direct spread from an underlying multiple myeloma. It represents 4% of extramedullary plasmacytomas and affects predominantly elderly men with a median age of 60 years at diagnosis. It is characterized by a monoclonal proliferation of mature plasma cells. Cutaneous plasmacytomas are potentially curable, with a 5-year survival rate of > 90%. However, the presentation of multiple lesions is an important adverse prognostic factor. Histopathology shows a dense monomorphous dermal infiltrate of plasma cells with a varying degree of maturation and atypia, admixed with few lymphocytes and histiocytes. Neoplastic plasma cells express clonal immunoglobulin, CD38, and CD79a but are negative for CD20. Rarely, amyloid deposition within the tumor is demonstrated, which is more common in secondary cutaneous involvement of plasmacytoma. A recent organized workshop on plasma cell dyscrasias questioned whether these cases are true cutaneous plasmacytomas, represent reactive B-cell infiltrates associated with an infectious etiology, or represent a variant of MZL with a predominant population of plasma cells. Diagnosis may rely on demonstration of monoclonality by restriction of Ig light-chain expression. Excision or radiation treatment is most commonly used.

HIV-RELATED LYMPHOMAS

Most lymphomas seen in patients who have HIV infection are of an aggressive histology and advanced stage at presentation. Extranodal disease is common, with unusual sites of presentation, including the GI tract, CNS, and multiple soft-tissue masses. Some patients present with primary CNS lymphoma. Poor-risk factors include a high LDH level, large tumor bulk, extranodal disease, and low CD4 cell counts (< 100 cells/μL). Because of their increased risk of opportunistic infections and impaired hematologic reserve, historically many patients with HIV-related lymphomas have been unable to tolerate aggressive chemotherapy regimens. Current antiviral medications have allowed for the use of more traditional regimens, including R-CHOP and R-EPOCH (rituximab -etoposide, prednisone, vincristine [Oncovin], cyclophosphamide, doxorubicin [hydroxydaunorubicin]), with results comparable to those of other NHL patients with similar histologies and presentations.

CNS prophylaxis with intrathecal chemotherapy is necessary to prevent meningeal dissemination. (For a more detailed discussion of HIV-related NHL, see chapter 27.)

POST-TRANSPLANTATION NHL

Post-transplantation lymphoproliferative disorders (PTLDs) comprise a histologic spectrum, ranging from hyperplastic-appearing lesions to frank NHL or multiple myeloma histology. The incidence varies from 1% in renal transplant recipients to 8% in lung transplant recipients, who require more potent immunosuppressive therapy.

PTLD is typically subdivided into several diesease categories, as described by Harris et al (Table 17). Furthermore, monomorphic PTLD, similar to classic DLBCL, should be further characterized by the WHO lymphoma classification.

The median onset of disease in solid organ recipients is 6 months, whereas in

TABLE 17: Disease categories of post-transplantation lymphoproliferative disorders

PTLD disease category	Category description
Plasmacytic or atypical lymphoid hyperplasia	Infectious mononucleosis-like syndrome; nodal disease with preservation of lymph node architecture; typically 3–6 months post transplantation; polyclonal
Polymorphic	Nodal disease with effacement of lymph node architecture or extranodal disease; full range of B-cell maturation; monoclonal; normal cytogenetics/no oncogenic mutations
Monomorphic (non-Hodgkin B- or T-cell lymphoma)	Nodal disease with effacement of lymph node architecture or invasive extranodal disease; monomorphic sheets of transformed B cells; monoclonal; some with abnormal cytogenetics or mutations in ras or p53
T-cell-rich, large B-cell lymphoma	Nodal disease; background of small T cells with superimposed Reed–Sternberg-like cells; monoclonal
Plasmacytoma-like lesions	Nodal disease with effacement of lymph node architecture by mature plasma cells with monoclonal immunoglobulin; monoclonal

PTLD = post-transplantation lymphoproliferative disorders

SCT patients it is 70 to 90 days. A total of 80% of cases occur within 1 year of transplant. The others occur a year or more after transplant and are often defined as "late-onset" PTLD. Cases have been seen as early as 1 week and as late as 9 years following transplant. Overall mortality, though unclear, has been estimated between 40% and 70%. Early PTLD cases are typically EBV-positive, whereas late-onset cases are more likely to be EBV-negative (median onset 50 months after transplantation) and have been reported to behave more aggressively clinically.

Treatment strategies for PTLD most importantly focus on reduction of immunosuppression (usually by at least 50%), especially for "early" EBV-positive cases. EBV-negative PTLD will respond to immunosuppression reduction but less frequently (15% to 25%) than EBV-positive cases (50% to 65%). In addition, the status of the transplanted organ will in part dictate the amount of immunosuppression safely allowable to avoid organ rejection. Rituximab is often given at initial diagnosis of EBV-positive PTLD along with reduction in immunosuppression, although there are no controlled studies that have proven this strategy.

Anecdotal reports have described the activity of TK inhibitor antiviral therapies such as ganciclovir (Cytovene) and acyclovir (Zovirax) to prevent and/or treat PTLD, although the data are not convincing. This finding is not surprising, as EBV survives as an episome outside the lymphocyte genome, and these drugs do not eradicate latently infected B cells. However, one group has shown that arginine butyrate was able to induce EBV TK activity in EBV-immortalized B cells and convert patient-derived latently infected B-cell lymphoma tumor cells that were resistant to ganciclovir to a sensitive phenotype. A phase I/II study with encouraging clinical results was recently reported .

For patients who fail to experience reduction in immunosuppression, for those with untreated EBV-negative PTLD, and/or for patients who need a rapid reduction/response of disease, anthracycline-based chemotherapy (eg, R-CHOP) is commonly used. Of note, during chemotherapy, immunosuppressant medication doses should be either significantly reduced or carefully stopped completely, to avoid infectious complications. Other therapeutic options include EBV-specific donor T cells and cytokines such as IFN-α. Carefully selected patients with relapsed/refractory monomorphic PTLD are able to receive high-dose chemotherapy followed by autologous SCT, with long-term survival reported in some series.

PRIMARY CNS LYMPHOMA

Primary CNS lymphoma is a rare form of NHL, arising within and confined to the CNS. Histologically, primary CNS lymphomas are indistinguishable from systemic NHLs. More than 40% of patients have evidence of leptomeningeal dissemination, and 15% have ocular disease at presentation. A stereotactic needle biopsy is the procedure of choice for diagnosis. Resection does not appear to improve survival.

The two most important prognostic factors in primary CNS lymphoma are age (> 50 years) and poor performance status (Karnofsky Performance Score < 70).

Retrospective studies have documented that treatment of primary CNS lymphoma with whole-brain radiotherapy (WBRT) alone (with or without corticosteroids) results in a median survival of 10 to 15 months, with a 5-year survival of 3% to 4%. Current standard therapy for newly diagnosed primary CNS lymphoma is systemic chemotherapy, including high-dose intravenous methotrexate-based therapy (at least 2,500 mg/m^2 per cycle) alone or more commonly combined with agents that penetrate the CNS (vincristine, procarbazine [Matulane], and high-dose Ara-C). This regimen results in median survival rates of 50 months to 60 months. WBRT has been considered a standard component following chemotherapy; however, long-term neurotoxicity remains a major concern, especially for patients older than 60 years.

A recent study reported encouraging results for primary CNS lymphoma patients who achieved complete remission following 5 to 7 cycles of high-dose methotrexate-based chemoimmunotherapy and subsequently received reduced-dose WBRT (23.4 Gy) compared with standard WBRT of 45 Gy. Long-term survival data are available using autologous or allogeneic SCT for relapsed/refractory primary CNS lymphoma, although an important factor is control of CNS disease immediately prior to transplant.

Treatment complications

Tumor lysis syndrome is a common complication after treatment of high-grade, bulky NHLs (due to their exquisite sensitivity to therapy and high proliferative capacity). The syndrome is characterized by renal failure, hyperkalemia, hyperphosphatemia, and hypocalcemia.

Measures to prevent this complication include aggressive hydration; allopurinol; alkalinization of the urine; and frequent monitoring of electrolytes, uric acid, and creatinine. Dialysis is sometimes required. Rasburicase, a recombinant urateoxidase enzyme, is now available for the prevention and treatment of hyperuricemia. (For a more comprehensive discussion of the tumor lysis syndrome, see chapter 44.)

Follow-up of long-term survivors

Relapse The most important risk to patients with NHL is relapse. Among patients with diffuse aggressive lymphomas, most recurrences are seen within the first 2 years after the completion of therapy, although later relapses may occur. Physical examination and laboratory testing at 2- to 3-month intervals and follow-up CT scans (with or without PET scan) at 6-month intervals for the first 2 years following diagnosis are recommended. However, it is recognized that upon relapse of disease, the patient usually presents with symptoms rather than the relapse being diagnosed purely on the basis of surveillance scans or routine clinic visits.

Early detection of recurrent disease is important because these patients may be candidates for potentially curative high-dose therapy and SCT. Patients with advanced low-grade NHL are at a constant risk of relapse, and late recurrence of disease may be seen, sometimes after more than a decade-old remission.

Secondary malignancies Long-term survivors are at increased risk of second cancers. In a survey of 6,171 patients with NHL who survived 2 or more years, nearly 1,000 patients lived 15 or more years after diagnosis. Second cancers were reported in 541 subjects, with significant excesses seen for all solid tumors; acute myeloid leukemia; melanoma; Hodgkin lymphoma; and cancers of the lungs, brain, kidneys, and bladder. The actuarial risk of developing a second malignancy at 3 to 20 years after diagnosis of NHL was 21%, compared with a population-expected cumulative risk of 15%.

Treatment complications There has been a more selective use of irradiation as part of the initial therapy for NHL; therefore, the risk of certain radiation-induced complications has been reduced or eliminated in more recently diagnosed patients. Nevertheless, total-body irradiation may be used as a component of myeloablative conditioning regimens. Also, transplant recipients are at increased risk of secondary myelodysplasia and acute myeloid leukemia, regardless of whether they received a radiation-containing conditioning regimen. All individual chemotherapy agents have their own potential long-term morbidity.

Long-term survivors need continued follow-up for possible treatment-related complications. Some of these toxicities may still be unknown. Careful documentation of late complications will be important in the design of future treatment strategies aimed at preserving or improving response rates and the duration of remission while reducing toxicity.

SUGGESTED READING

Alexander DD, Mink PJ, Adami HO, et al: The non-Hodgkin lymphoma: A review of the epidemiologic literature. Int J Cancer 120(suppl 12):1–39, 2007.

Arneshna KM, Smith P, Norton A, et al: Long-term effect of a watch and wait policy versus immediate systemic treatment for asymptomatic advanced-stage non-Hodgkin lymphoma: A randomized controlled trial. Lancet 362:516–522, 2003.

Bendandi M: The role of idiotype vaccines in the treatment of human B-cell malignancies. Expert Rev Vaccines 3:163–170, 2004.

Bonnet C, Fillet G, Mounier N, et al: CHOP alone compared with CHOP plus radiotherapy for localized aggressive lymphoma in elderly patients: A study by the Groupe d'Etude des Lymphomes de l'Adulte. J Clin Oncol 25:787–792, 2007.

Cheson BD, Pfistner B, Juweid ME, et al: Revised response criteria for malignant lymphoma. J Clin Oncol 25:579–586, 2007.

Coiffier B, Lepage E, Briere J, et al: CHOP chemotherapy plus rituximab compared with CHOP alone in elderly patients with diffuse large B-cell lymphoma. N Engl J Med 346:235–242, 2002.

Dal Col J, Zancai P, Terrin L, et al: Distinct functional significance of Akt and mTOR constitutive activation in mantle cell lymphoma. Blood 111:5142–5151, 2008.

Dave SS, Wright G, Tan B, et al: Prediction of survival in follicular lymphoma based on molecular features of tumor-infiltrating immune cells. N Engl J Med 351:2159–2169, 2004.

De Falco G, Leucci E, Lenze D, et al: Gene-expression analysis identifies novel RBL2/p130 target genes in endemic Burkitt lymphoma cell lines and primary tumors. Blood 110:1301–1307, 2007.

Evens AM, Winter JN, Hou N, et al: A phase II clinical trial of intensive chemotherapy followed by consolidative stem cell transplant: Long-term follow-up in newly diagnosed mantle cell lymphoma. Br J Haematol 140:385–393, 2008.

Fisher RI, Bernstein SH, Kahl BS, et al: Multicenter phase II study of bortezomib in patients with relapsed or refractory mantle cell lymphoma. J Clin Oncol 24:4867–4874, 2006.

Galicier L, Fieschi C, Borie R, et al: Intensive chemotherapy regimen (LMB86) for St Jude stage IV AIDS-related Burkitt lymphoma/leukemia: A prospective study. Blood 110:2846–2854, 2007.

Kis LL, Takahara M, Nagy N, et al: IL-10 can induce the expression of EBV-encoded latent membrane protein-1 (LMP-1) in the absence of EBNA-2 in B lymphocytes and in Burkitt lymphoma- and NK lymphoma-derived cell lines. Blood 107:2928–2935, 2006.

Lossos IS, Czerwinski DK, Alizadeh AA, et al: Prediction of survival in diffuse large-B-cell lymphoma based on the expression of six genes. N Engl J Med 350:1828–1837, 2004.

Milpied N, Deconinck E, Gailland T, et al: Initial treatment of aggressive lymphoma with high-dose chemotherapy and autologous stem cell support. N Engl J Med 350:1287–1295, 2004.

Nyman H, Adde M, Karjalainen-Lindsberg ML, et al: Prognostic impact of immunohistochemically defined germinal center phenotype in diffuse large B-cell lymphoma patients treated with immunochemotherapy. Blood 109:4930–4935, 2007.

Park IW, Reddy MV, Reddy EP, et al: Evaluation of novel cell cycle inhibitors in mantle cell lymphoma. Oncogene 26:5635–5642, 2007.

Pérez-Galán P, Roué G, Villamor N, et al: The BH3-mimetic GX15-070 synergizes with bortezomib in mantle cell lymphoma by enhancing Noxa-mediated activation of Bak. Blood 109:4441–4449, 2007.

Petersen PM, Gospodarowicz M, Tsang R, et al: Long-term outcome in stage I and II follicular lymphoma following treatment with involved field radiation therapy alone (abstract). Proc Am Soc Clin Oncol 23:561, 2004.

Pfreundschuh M, Schubert J, Ziepert M, et al: Six versus eight cycles of bi-weekly CHOP-14 with or without rituximab in elderly patients with aggressive CD20+ B-cell lymphomas: A randomised controlled trial (RICOVER-60). Lancet Oncol 9:105–116, 2008.

Pfreundschuh M, Trümper L, Osterborg A, et al: CHOP-like chemotherapy plus rituximab versus CHOP-like chemotherapy alone in young patients with good-prognosis diffuse-large-B-cell lymphoma: A randomised controlled trial by the MabThera International Trial (MinT) Group. Lancet Oncol 7:379–391, 2006.

Popov SW, Moldenhauer G, Wotschke B, et al: Target sequence accessibility limits activation-induced cytidine deaminase activity in primary mediastinal B-cell lymphoma. Cancer Res 67:6555–6564, 2007.

Querfeld C, Guitant T, Kuzel T, et al: A Guide for the Community Oncologist. Manhasset, NY; CMPMedica; 2006.

Querfeld C, Kuzel TM, Guitart J, et al: Primary cutaneous CD30+ lymphoproliferative disorders: New insights into biology and therapy. Oncology 21:689–700, 2007.

NON-HODGKIN LYMPHOMA **773**

Reyes F, Lepage E, Ganem G, et al: ACVBP versus CHOP plus radiotherapy for localized aggressive lymphoma. N Engl J Med 352:1197–1205, 2005.

Rizvi MA, Evens AM, Tallman MS, et al: T-cell non-Hodgkin lymphoma. Blood 107:1255–1264, 2006.

Rodig SJ, Savage KJ, LaCasce AS, et al: Expression of TRAF1 and nuclear c-Rel distinguishes primary mediastinal large cell lymphoma from other types of diffuse large B-cell lymphoma. Am J Surg Pathol 31:106–112, 2007.

Rodriguez J, Caballero MD, Gutierrez A, et al: Autologous stem-cell transplantation in diffuse large B-cell non-Hodgkin's lymphoma not achieving complete response after induction chemotherapy: The GEL/TAMO experience. Ann Oncol 15:1504–1509, 2004.

Rosado MF, Byrne GE Jr, Ding F, et al: Ocular adnexal lymphoma: A clinicopathologic study of a large cohort of patients with no evidence for an association with *Chlamydia psittaci.* Blood 107:467–472, 2006.

Rosenwald A, Wright G, Leroy K, et al: Molecular diagnosis of primary mediastinal B cell lymphoma identifies a clinically favorable subgroup of diffuse large B cell lymphoma related to Hodgkin lymphoma. J Exp Med 198:851–862, 2003.

Sampson VB, Rong NH, Han J, et al: MicroRNA let-7a down-regulates MYC and reverts MYC-induced growth in Burkitt lymphoma cells. Cancer Res 67:9762–9770, 2007.

Savage KJ, Harris NL, Vose JM, et al: ALK-anaplastic large-cell lymphoma is clinically and immunophenotypically different from both ALK+ and ALCL and peripheral T-cell lymphoma, not otherwise specified: Report from the International Peripheral T-Cell Lymphoma Project. Blood 111(12):5496–5504, 2008.

Schouten HC, Quan W, Kvaloy S, et al: High-dose therapy improves progression-free survival and survival in relapsed follicular non-Hodgkin's lymphoma: Results from the randomized European CUP trial. J Clin Oncol 21:3918–3927, 2003.

Sehn LH, Berry B, Chhanabhai M, et al: The revised International Prognostic Index (R-IPI) is a better predictor of outcome than the standard IPI for patients with diffuse large B-cell lymphoma treated with R-CHOP. Blood 109:1857–1861, 2007.

Shah GD, Yahalom J, Correa DD, et al: Combined immunochemotherapy with reduced whole-brain radiotherapy for newly diagnosed primary CNS lymphoma. J Clin Oncol 25:4730–4735, 2007.

Solal-Celigny P, Roy P, Colombat P, et al: Follicular Lymphoma International Prognostic Index. Blood 104:1258–1265, 2004.

Trautinger F, Knobler R, Willemze R, et al: EORTC consensus recommendations for the treatment of mycosis fungoides/Sézary syndrome. Eur J Cancer 42:1014–1030, 2006.

Weniger MA, Gesk S, Ehrlich S, et al: Gains of REL in primary mediastinal B-cell lymphoma coincide with nuclear accumulation of REL protein. Genes Chromosomes Cancer 46:406–415, 2007.

Willemze R, Jaffe ES, Burg G: WHO-EORTC classification for cutaneous lymphomas. Blood 105:3768–3785, 2005.

Winter JN, Gascoyne RD, Van Besien K: Low grade lymphoma. In: Broudy VC, Berliner N, Larson RA, et al (eds): Hematology 2004, pp 203–220. Washington, DC, American Society of Hematology, 2004.

Witzig TE, Molina A, Gordon LI, et al: Long-term responses in patients with recurring or refractory B-cell non-Hodgkin lymphoma treated with yttrium 90 ibritumomab tiuxetan. Cancer 109:1804–1810, 2007.

CHAPTER 31

Multiple myeloma and other plasma cell dyscrasias

Sundar Jagannath, MD, Paul Richardson, MD, and Nikhil C. Munshi, MD

MULTIPLE MYELOMA

Multiple myeloma is a disseminated malignancy of monoclonal plasma cells that accounts for 15% of all hematologic cancers. In 2008, an estimated 19,920 new cases will be diagnosed in the United States, and 10,690 Americans will die of this disease. Incidence rates for myeloma (5.3 in men and 3.5 in women) and mortality rates (3.7 in men and 2.5 in women) per 100,000 population have remained stable for the past decade.

Epidemiology

Gender Men are affected more frequently than women (1.4:1.0 ratio).

Age The median age at presentation is 71 years, according to most tumor registries, although the median age reported in studies is approximately 66 years.

Race The annual incidence per 100,000 population is 6.4 among white men and 4.1 among white women. Among black men and women, the frequency doubles to 12.7 and 10.0, respectively, per 100,000 population. This racial difference is not explained by socioeconomic or environmental factors and is presumably due to unknown genetic factors.

Geography There is no clear geographic distribution of multiple myeloma. In Europe, the highest rates are noted in the Nordic countries, the United Kingdom, Switzerland, and Israel. France, Germany, Austria, and Slovenia have a lower incidence, and developing countries have the lowest incidence. This higher relative incidence in more developed countries probably results from the combination of a longer life expectancy and more frequent medical surveillance.

Survival The 5-year survival rate for all patients treated with conventional therapy is approximately 33%. The 5-year survival rate is lower among patients ≥ age 65 (20% to 25%) than in those < age 65 (30% to 35%).

Etiology and risk factors

No predisposing factors for the development of multiple myeloma have been confirmed.

Environment Some causative factors that have been suggested include radiation exposure (radiologists and radium dial workers), occupational exposure (agricultural, chemical, metallurgical, rubber plant, pulp, wood and paper workers, and leather tanners), and chemical exposure to formaldehyde, epichlorohydrin, Agent Orange, hair dyes, paint sprays, and asbestos. None of these associations has proven to be statistically significant, and some have been contradicted by negative correlations. The initial report that survivors of the atomic bombings in Japan had an increased risk of developing myeloma has been refuted by longer follow-up.

Viruses A preliminary report in a limited number of patients noted the presence of herpesvirus 8 in the dendritic cells of patients with multiple myeloma. However, further evaluation by a number of investigators has failed to confirm this result. Patients with myeloma also do not appear to have a significant immune response against this virus.

Cytogenetics Karyotypic abnormalities in myeloma are complex, with both numeric and structural abnormalities. DNA aneuploidy is observed in more than 90% of cases, which are predominantly hyperdiploid, with less than 10% hypodiploid (which carries a poor prognosis). Recurrent nonrandom structural abnormalities have been identified and linked to the pathogenesis and prognosis of myeloma. The immunoglobulin (Ig) heavy-chain gene at 14q32 is frequently involved in translocations with partner chromosomes 4, 6, 8, 11, and 16. The location and oncogenes involved are shown in Table 1. Translocations involving chromosomes 4 and 16 as well as del17p13 (p53) have been associated with a poor prognosis. Del13q or monosomy 13 is observed in 15% to 20% of patients with conventional cytogenetics and also carries a poor prognosis across standard and high-dose therapies. Interphase fluorescence in situ hybridization (FISH) with a specific probe for chromosome 13q34 (retinoblastoma gene, *Rb 1*) identifies this abnormality in up to 50% of patients, with a less clear prognostic implication.

> Interactions between multiple myeloma (MM) cells and their microenvironment, the extracellular matrix and the bone marrow stromal cells (BMSCs), allow MM cells to survive, grow, migrate, and resist apoptosis induced by traditional chemotherapies. These effects are partially mediated through adhesion-mediated signalling and partly through various cytokines, including IL-6, VEGF, IGF-1, and IL-2. The molecular signals mediating the proliferative effects include the *ras/raf* MAPK pathway, whereas the PI3K/Akt pathway provides cell survival and drug resistance signals. Improved understanding of these interactions and the molecular mechanisms mediating them has now allowed us to evaluate novel therapies that directly target MM cells as well as act on the bone marrow microenvironment.

Genetic factors Although multiple myeloma is not an inherited disease, there have been numerous reports of multiple cases in the same family. However, a case-control study revealed no significant increase in the inci-

TABLE 1: The location and oncogenes involved in multiple myeloma

Locus	Oncogene	Incidence
11q13	Cyclin D1	15%-20%
6p21	Cyclin D3	5%
4p16.3	FGFR3 and MMSET	12%
16q23	c-maf	5%-10%
8q24	c-myc	< 10%
6p25	MUM1/IRF4	5%
20q11	MAFB	5%
1q21-34	bcl-9, IL-6R, mcl-1	Frequent

dence among relatives of patients who had multiple myeloma, other hematologic malignancies, or other cancers.

Monoclonal gammopathy of unknown significance (MGUS) Patients with MGUS develop myeloma, macroglobulinemic lymphoma, or amyloidosis at a rate of 1% per year.

Signs and symptoms

The clinical features of multiple myeloma are variable. Findings that suggest the diagnosis include lytic bone lesions, anemia, azotemia, hypercalcemia, and recurrent infections. Approximately 30% of patients are free of symptoms and are diagnosed on routine physicals with abnormal laboratory studies including elevation of serum protein.

Bone disease Bone pain, especially from compression fractures of the vertebrae or ribs, is the most common symptom. At diagnosis, 70% of patients have lytic lesions, which are due to accelerated bone resorption. These changes are induced by factors modulating osteoclastic activity and produced by the bone marrow microenvironment and, to a lesser extent, myeloma cells. These factors include interleukin (IL)-1B, tumor necrosis factor (TNF)-α, and IL-6 as well as newly identified factors such as osteoprotogerin, TNF-related activation-induced cytokine (TRANCE), MIP-1–alpha, and receptor activator of nuclear factor kappa B (RANK) ligand. DKK-1 has been described as a soluble factor produced by multiple myeloma cells inhibiting osteoblastic activity.

Anemia Normocytic, normochromic anemia is present in 60% of patients at diagnosis. It is due primarily to the decreased production of red blood cells by marrow, infiltration with plasma cells, and the suppressive effect of various cytokines. Patients with renal failure may also have decreased levels of erythropoietin, which can worsen the degree of anemia.

Hypercalcemia Among newly diagnosed patients, 20% have hypercalcemia (corrected serum calcium level > 11.5 mg/dL) secondary to progressive bone destruction, which may be exacerbated by prolonged immobility. Hypercalcemia should be suspected in patients with myeloma who have nausea, fatigue, confusion, polyuria, or constipation. It may suggest high tumor burden. It should be considered an oncologic emergency and requires prompt treatment.

Renal failure Approximately 20% of patients present with renal insufficiency and another 20% to 40% develop this complication in later phases of the disease. Light-chain cast nephropathy is the most common cause of renal failure. Additional causes include hypercalcemia, dehydration, and hyperuricemia. Less commonly, amyloidosis, light-chain deposition disease, nonsteroidal anti-inflammatory agents taken for pain control, intravenous radiographic contrast administration, and calcium stones may contribute to renal failure. More recently, bisphosphonate therapy has been associated with renal failure.

Infections Many patients with myeloma develop bacterial infections that may be serious, and infectious implications remain the most common cause of death in myeloma patients. In the past, gram-positive organisms (eg, *Streptococcus pneumoniae, Staphylococcus aureus*) and *Haemophilus influenzae* were the most common pathogens. More recently, however, gram-negative organisms, anaerobes, and fungi have become frequent. The increased susceptibility of patients with myeloma to bacterial infections, specifically with encapsulated organisms, has been attributed to impairments of host-defense mechanisms, such as hypogammaglobulinemia, granulocytopenia, decreased cell-mediated immunity, and the prolonged use of steroids.

Screening and diagnosis

No screening measures for multiple myeloma have demonstrated any benefit.

The diagnosis usually requires the presence of bone marrow plasmacytosis and a monoclonal protein in the urine and/or serum (Table 2). One immunoglobulin class is produced in excess, whereas the other classes are usually depressed.

Initial work-up The initial work-up for patients suspected of having a plasma cell dyscrasia should include:

- CBC with differential count and platelet count
- Routine serum chemistry panel (eg, calcium, BUN, creatinine)
- Bone marrow aspirate and biopsy to assess plasmacytosis
- Serum protein electrophoresis and immunofixation to define protein type
- Serum free light chain
- 24-hour urine protein, electrophoresis, and immunofixation
- Quantitative serum immunoglobulin levels
- Skeletal survey (bone scans contribute little since isotope uptake is often low in purely lytic bone disease)
- Cytogenetics, including FISH.

TABLE 2: Common laboratory features of plasma cell dyscrasias

Multiple myeloma
Marrow plasmacytosis ≥ 10%
Monoclonal immunoglobulin peak (usually > 3.0 g/dL)
Suppressed uninvolved immunoglobulins
Clonal plasma cells
Presence of Bence Jones protein
Lytic bone lesions or diffuse osteopenia
Related organ or tissue impairment

Smoldering myeloma
Monoclonal immunoglobulin level > 3.0 g/dL and/or bone marrow plasma cells > 10%
No symptoms due to plasma cell dyscrasia
No bone lesion
Normal calcium and renal function
No anemia

Solitary plasmacytoma of bone (SPB)
Solitary bone lesion due to plasma cell tumor
Normal skeletal survey and MRI of the skull, spine, and pelvis
Normal bone marrow plasmacytosis
No anemia, hypercalcemia, or renal disease
Preserved levels of uninvolved immunoglobulins

Monoclonal gammopathy of unknown significance (MGUS)
Monoclonal immunoglobulin level < 3.0 g/dL
Bone marrow plasma cells < 10%
No bone lesions
No symptoms due to plasma cell dyscrasia
Usually preserved levels of uninvolved immunoglobulins
No related organ or tissue impairment

Amyloidosis without myeloma
Same as MGUS plus evidence of amyloidosis on biopsy

The recently available serum free light-chain assay is useful especially in patients with light-chain–only disease, oligo- or nonsecretory myeloma, patients with renal failure, and amyloidosis.

MRI is an excellent tool for evaluation of spinal cord compression/impingement. In addition, MRI identifies generalized signal abnormalities and focal lesions that can be monitored after therapy. MRI is especially useful in staging nonsecretory disease presenting as macrofocal lesions. ^{18}F-fluorodeoxyglucose (FDG)-PET scan is becoming more widely used, as it provides details of axial and appendicular skeletal involvement but also identifies extramedullary soft-tissue plasmacytomas.

In addition, prognostic factors, such as β_2-microglobulin (β2M), serum albumin, C-reactive protein, lactate dehydrogenase (LDH) levels, plasma cell labeling index, and ploidy, may provide additional useful data.

Laboratory and pathologic features

Peripheral blood The peripheral blood smear may reveal a normocytic, normochromic anemia with rouleaux formation. Plasma cells may also be seen.

Bone marrow Bone marrow examination usually reveals an increased number of plasma cells. These cells are strongly positive for CD38, CD138, and cytoplasmic immunoglobulin (cIg). The majority of myeloma cells also express CD40 and CD56. Myeloma cells are negative for CD5, CD19, CD20, and surface immunoglobulin (sIg) expression. CD10 expression is generally negative but has sometimes been noted in advanced disease. Monoclonality may be demonstrated by immunoperoxidase staining with κ and λ antibodies.

The pattern of bone marrow involvement in plasma cell myeloma may be macrofocal. As a result, plasma cell count may be normal when an aspirate misses the focal aggregates of plasma cells that are better visualized radiographically or on direct needle biopsy.

Monoclonal proteins The types of monoclonal protein produced are IgG (60%), IgA (20%), IgD (2%), IgE (< 0.1%), or light-chain κ or λ only (18%). Biclonal elevations of myeloma proteins occur in < 1% of patients, and < 5% of patients are considered to have nonsecretory disease because their plasma cells do not secrete detectable levels of monoclonal Ig.

Staging and prognosis

The Durie-Salmon staging system is employed most frequently to stage multiple myeloma (Table 3). However, the variability in interpretation of staging criteria resulting, in part, from imprecise quantification of the extent of bone lesions and from factors other than myeloma that contribute to hypercalcemia (eg, immobility) or anemia (eg, renal failure) has decreased its utility. Moreover, the Durie-Salmon staging system was devised for assessment of tumor burden but is not as good for prognosis following high-dose therapy or novel agent therapy. An alternate staging system is proposed using simple laboratory measurements of serum β2M and albumin (International Staging System [ISS]). The ISS staging has been validated for prognosis in the context of conventional therapy and stem cell transplant.

Prognosis

Cytogenetic abnormalities Chromosomal abnormalities, especially loss of whole chromosome 13 (monosomy) or deletions of parts of chromosome 13 (13q), with hypodiploid have been associated with inferior survival after both standard chemotherapy and high-dose therapy. Primary translocations involving 14q32 and 6p21 (cyclin D3), 4p16 (FGFR3), and 16q23 (c-*maf*) in multivariate analysis have been shown to be important predictors of survival.

β2M Serum β2M level is an important and convenient prognostic indicator. When cytogenetic changes are not studied, β2M is consistently the most important prognostic indicator on multivariate analysis. As β2M is excreted by

TABLE 3: Durie-Salmon staging system for multiple myeloma

Stage	Criteria	Myeloma cell mass ($\times 10^{12}$ cells/m^2)
I	Hemoglobin > 10 g/dL	< 0.6 (low)
	Serum calcium level ≤ 12 mg/dL (normal)	
	Normal bone or solitary plasmacytoma on x-ray	
	Low M-component production rate:	
	IgG < 5 g/dL	
	IgA < 3 g/dL	
	Bence Jones protein < 4 g/24 h	
II	Not fitting stage I or III	0.6-1.2 (intermediate)
III	Hemoglobin < 8.5 g/dL	> 1.2 (high)
	Serum calcium level > 12 mg/dL	
	Multiple lytic bone lesions on x-ray	
	High M-component production rate:	
	IgG > 7 g/dL	
	IgA > 5 g/dL	
	Bence Jones protein > 12 g/24 h	

Subclassification	Criterion
A	Normal renal function (serum creatinine level < 2.0 mg/dL)
B	Abnormal renal function (serum creatinine level ≥ 2.0 mg/dL)

the kidneys, high levels are observed in patients with renal failure; in this setting, the interpretation of an elevated value is unclear.

ISS Recently, serum β2M and albumin have been used to develop the new three-stage ISS. Patients with serum β2M < 3.5 mg/L and serum albumin ≥ 3.5 g/dL are considered to have stage I disease, with the best survival, whereas patients with serum β2M ≥ 5.5 mg/L have stage III disease, with the worst prognosis. The other patients are considered to have stage II disease, with an intermediate prognosis. This prognostic model predicts for outcome following both high-dose therapy as well as treatment with novel agents. However, it lacks incorporation of the tumor biology-related factors such as cytogenetics and molecular markers.

LDH High LDH levels also have been associated with plasmablastic disease, extramedullary tumor, plasma cell leukemia, plasma cell hypodiploidy, drug resistance, and shortened survival.

Other indicators of shortened survival include elevated C-reactive protein, DNA hypodiploidy, high plasma cell labeling indices, and plasmablastic histology. Patients with DNA hypodiploidy are also less likely to respond to chemotherapy.

Treatment response criteria

Because the criteria for treatment response in patients with multiple myeloma have varied among institutions, response rates have been difficult to compare in the past. Bence Jones protein is reduced more rapidly in responders than is serum myeloma protein because of the rapid renal clearance of light chains.

The Center for International Bone Marrow Transplant Registry/European Bone Marrow Transplant Registry (CIBMTR/EBMTR) response criteria follow:

Complete response requires all of the following:

- No serum/urine M protein by immunofixation electrophoresis for ≥ 6 weeks
- < 5% plasma cells in bone marrow aspirate
- No increase in the size or number of lytic bone lesions
- Disappearance of soft-tissue plasmacytomas.

Partial response requires all of the following:

- > 50% reduction in serum M protein ≥ 6 weeks
- ≥ 90% reduction in 24-hr urinary light-chain excretion
- ≥ 50% reduction in soft-tissue plasmacytomas
- No increase in the size or number of lytic bone lesions.

Treatment

Exciting advances in the understanding of tumor biology and microenvironment–and their potential interaction–have helped to identify unique targets for rational therapeutic intervention to enhance outcome, which has not improved with conventional chemotherapy over the past 3 decades. Until recently, only 5% to 10% of patients with multiple myeloma lived longer than 10 years, and cure remains elusive.

NEWLY DIAGNOSED PATIENTS

Chemotherapy

Dexamethasone/thalidomide Thalidomide (Thalomid) has been employed alone and in combination with dexamethasone as initial therapy in newly diagnosed patients. When employed alone, response (50% reduction in paraprotein) was observed in 36% of patients; when it was used along with dexamethasone, the response rate was higher (72% and 64% in two studies), including a 16% complete response rate in one study. The results of a randomized Eastern Cooperative Oncology Group (ECOG) trial showed that the combination of thalidomide and dexamethasone was superior to dexamethasone alone (63%

TABLE 4: Proposed standard treatment of multiple myeloma

Disease or patient status	Treatment approach
Initial therapy	
Candidates for high-dose therapy	
Dexamethasone	40 mg on days 1-4, 9-12, and 17-20 every 35 days or on days 1-4 every 2 weeks
Dexamethasone/thalidomide	Dexamethasone as above or at a lower dose if clinically indicated with thalidomide (up to 200 mg/d)
VD	Bortezomib (1.3 mg/m^2) on days 1, 4, 8, 11 every 3 weeks Dexamethasone (40 mg) on day of and day after bortezomib
RD	Lenalidomide (25 mg PO) daily for 3 weeks out of 4 Dexamethasone (40 mg) once a week
Clinical trials	High-dose melphalan and SCT following induction therapy Bortezomib with dexamethasone Bortezomib with thalidomide and dexamethasone Lenalidomide and dexamethasone Bortezomib with liposomal doxorubicin Bortezomib with lenalidomide and dexamethasone
Noncandidates for high-dose therapy	
Above options or MP	MP with thalidomide Melphalan (8 mg/m^2/d PO) + prednisone (100 mg/d PO) on days 1-4 every 4-5 weeks
Clinical trials	Cyclophosphamide with bortezomib, lenalidomide, and dexamethasone MP with bortezomib
Relapsed myeloma	
Conventional chemotherapy	Bortezomib, lenalidomide, and dexamethasone Dexamethasone and thalidomide Alkylating-agent combination (MP, VBMCP) Cyclophosphamide, etoposide based therapy, DCEP
High-dose chemotherapy	Melphalan (200 mg/m^2) and autotransplant (if previously not transplanted) Mini-allogeneic transplant
Novel agents	Bortezomib (1.3 mg/m^2) on days 1, 4, 8, and 11 every 3 weeks with or without dexamethasone, liposomal doxorubicin, or thalidomide Bortezomib with cyclophosphamide Bortezomib with melphalan Lenalidomide with dexamethasone
Clinical trials	Lenalidomide with bortezomib and dexamethasone Melphalan, arsenic trioxide, ascorbic acid (MAC) Other phase II novel agents

DCEP = dexamethasone, cyclophosphamide, etoposide, and Platinol (cisplatin); MP = melphalan, prednisone; SCT = stem-cell transplantation; VAD = vincristine, Adriamycin (doxorubicin), dexamethasone; VBMCP = vincristine, BiCNU (carmustine), melphalan, cyclophosphamide, prednisone vs 41%; $P = .001$). This combination does not damage stem cells and allows adequate stem-cell collection. A definite increase in thrombotic episodes has been observed with this combination, prompting prophylactic administration of aspirin, coumadin, or low-molecular-weight heparin.

VAD or VDD (vincristine, liposomal doxorubicin [Doxil], and dexamethasone) regimens were widely used in the past as induction therapy before high-dose therapy. Use of this combination has decreased since the introduction of dexamethasone/thalidomide and other bortezomib and lenalidomide-based combinations due to the need for a central line, the inconvenience of IV administration, and attendant toxicities with VAD. Recent randomized trials have confirmed the inferiority of VAD when compared to both thalidomide and bortezomib-based regimens.

Pulse dexamethasone alone has also been used in older patients and patients who need vertebral radiotherapy for spinal cord compression or for painful vertebral compressions, as this approach avoids severe myelosuppression (Table 4).

MP The combination of melphalan (Alkeran) and prednisone has been used over the past 30 years, and other combinations of multiple alkylating agents have not been found to be superior to MP. A meta-analysis of 18 published randomized trials comparing MP with other combination chemotherapy regimens arrived at the same conclusion. Approximately 40% of patients respond to the MP regimen, with a median remission duration of 18 months and an overall median survival of 3 years. The MP regimen should be avoided in patients considered to be transplant candidates.

MP and thalidomide (MPT) In two large prospective, randomized trials in patients older than age 65, and a third randomized trial in patients over 75 years of age, MPT has been shown to be superior to MP for response rate as well as progression-free and overall survival. Side effects (including constipation, deep vein thrombosis [DVT], and peripheral neuropathy) were more commonly encountered with thalidomide but were found to be manageable. MPT offers a possible alternative for older people who generally are not candidates for high-dose therapy.

MP and Velcade (bortezomib; MPV) Bortezomib is a first-in-class, potent, selective, and reversible small-molecule inhibitor of the proteasome. The proteasome plays a key role in the degradation of ubiquinated proteins, which in turn have important functions in controlling tumor cell growth and survival both in vitro and in vivo. In a large international, randomized clinical trial in patients over age 65 who were not suitable for stem-cell transplantation, MPV was compared with MP. In this study MPV was shown to be superior to MP for response as well as survival end points. MPV induced complete remissions in one-third of the patients, with an overall response rate of 71% and a 2-year overall survival of > 80%. Such high complete responses were heretofore never seen in this population of patients, where one-third of the patients were over age 75 years. Adverse side effects such as peripheral neuropathy, asthenia, fatigue, diarrhea, and constipation were more frequently encountered on the bortezomib arm. Yet the treatment was well tolerated by most patients, with treatment discontinuation due to toxicity noted in only 14% of patients in both arms, and a treatment-related mortality of 1% (versus 2% in the MP group).

RD (lenalidomide [Revlimid], dexamethasone) and VD (bortezomib [Velcade], dexamethasone) combinations Combinations of novel agents with dexamethasone have now been extensively investigated to provide high response rates in newly diagnosed patients. In a pilot study of newly diagnosed patients, 4 courses of lenalidomide at 25 mg daily for 3 weeks out of 4 along with dexamethasone achieved a 91% overall response rate, with 18% complete response and 38% very good partial response.

Based on this study, a randomized study performed by ECOG compared lenalidomide with high-dose dexamethasone (40 mg/d on days 1 to 4, 9 to 12, and 17 to 20) versus lenalidomide with low-dose dexamethasone (40 mg once a week). In this study, the low-dose dexamethasone arm had significantly fewer toxicities than the high-dose dexamethasone arm, including a lower rate of early mortality (5% vs 0.5%, respectively) and reduced incidence of DVT (24% vs 9%, respectively). Interestingly, the low-dose dexamethasone arm had significantly superior overall survival compared with high-dose dexamethasone (1 year overall survival 96% vs 88%, respectively).

Bortezomib-containing regimens have also been evaluated in newly diagnosed patients. Using the combination of bortezomib and dexamethasone, Jagannath et al have reported a complete response rate of 18% and an overall response rate of 88% in a phase II study in newly diagnosed patients. In a randomized study in newly diagnosed patients, the IFM group has recently demonstrated a superior overall response rate and very good partial response rate (82% and 47%, respectively) with bortezomib and dexamethasone (n = 79) compared with VAD (n = 82); (63% and 19%, respectively; $P = .0001$). Currently, the combination of lenalidomide, bortezomib, and dexamethasone is under investigation in newly diagnosed patients.

High-dose therapy following induction therapy

High-dose therapy employed after induction therapy improves the response rate as well as event-free and overall survival. The impressive improvement in event-free (median, 28 vs 18 months) and overall survival (57 vs 42 months) reported in a randomized trial (IFM 90) has been confirmed by another large randomized trial (median overall survival, 54.8 vs 42.3 months; MRC VII). Most of these studies enrolled patients < 65 years old. Older individuals (< age 70) may tolerate high-dose therapy with peripheral stem-cell support well, without excess mortality. Moreover, outcome, in terms of event-free and overall survival, is comparable to that in matched cohorts < 65 years old, making older individuals (≥ 65 years old) also candidates for high-dose therapy. More recently, older patients (> age 70) receiving intermediate-dose melphalan (100 mg/m^2) with stem-cell support have been shown to have a better outcome than matched controls receiving conventional therapy.

A high-dose alkylating agent, most commonly melphalan at 200 mg/m^2 with peripheral blood stem-cell support, is a standard conditioning regimen. Addition of total-body irradiation (TBI) does not improve the outcome but increases morbidity and results in higher mortality. Interestingly, in a randomized study, Fermand et al have confirmed an equivalent survival benefit between up-front high-dose therapy versus high-dose therapy as a salvage regimen at relapse following initial induction therapy.

Tandem transplants Improved outcome reported after tandem transplants in large cohorts of patients in single-institution studies has been confirmed in a mature randomized study. Seven years after initiation of therapy, the event-free (42% vs 21%) and overall survival (20% vs 10%) rates were superior for patients receiving tandem transplants (IFM 94). Another randomized trial with a shorter follow-up has confirmed the superior event-free survival (median, 34 vs 25 months) for patients receiving tandem transplants. However, the added benefit of the second transplant was not seen in a subset of patients with a complete response or a very good partial response (> 90% paraprotein reduction) after the first transplant.

Radiotherapy

Higher doses of radiotherapy (40–50 Gy) are employed for local control and cure of solitary plasmacytoma involving bone and extramedullary sites. Lower doses (20–30 Gy) may be employed for palliation of local bone pain from tumor infiltration, pathologic fractures, and spinal cord compression. It should be emphasized that excellent pain relief may be obtained by prompt institution of high-dose corticosteroid therapy, especially in newly diagnosed patients.

Radiotherapy should be employed sparingly, as irradiation of multiple sites may impair stem-cell mobilization in patients who are candidates for high-dose therapy. Employment of high doses of radiation to the spine may preclude the subsequent use of TBI as a conditioning regimen for high-dose therapy.

REMISSION MAINTENANCE

Alkylating agents Maintenance therapy with alkylating agents has not prolonged survival, compared with no maintenance therapy. This approach is no longer recommended.

Steroids for maintenance Two large randomized trials have shown that glucocorticoid maintenance prolongs the duration of remission and improved life expectancy. The first trial by the Southwest Oncology Group (SWOG) used prednisone (50 mg) every other day, whereas the maintenance regimen in the National Cancer Institute (NCI)-Canada trial contained dexamethasone (40 mg) daily for 4 days every 4 weeks.

Thalidomide Patients responding to thalidomide and achieving maximal response have received lower-dose thalidomide (50–100 mg) with or without added dexamethasone (40 mg for 4 days every month) as maintenance therapy. In the MPT regimen, continued administration of thalidomide prolongs the duration of remission. The IFM 99-06 study evaluated maintenance therapy with thalidomide plus pamidronate compared with pamidronate alone compared with observation only following tandem autologous transplantation. Superior event-free survival (EFS) and overall survival were reported in the cohort receiving thalidomide plus pamidronate.

α-Interferon Twenty-four randomized trials have investigated α-interferon as maintenance therapy and reported no consistent significant benefit. A recent larger intergroup trial also reported no benefit of interferon maintenance therapy after conventional therapy and autotransplantation.

Novel agents Bortezomib is currently under study as a maintenance strategy. In the Assessment of Proteasome Inhibition for Extending Remissions (APEX) study, bortezomib administered weekly proved efficacious and was well tolerated in responding patients who had successfully completed initial treatment. Lenalidomide, a small-molecule thalidomide analog with immunomodulatory effects, is also under study as maintenance posttransplant, given at a low dose (10 mg/d) and then increased accordingly to a higher dose (15 mg/d).

REFRACTORY AND RELAPSED, REFRACTORY DISEASE

Approximately 10% to 15% of patients with newly diagnosed multiple myeloma are unresponsive to induction therapy. Moreover, virtually all patients who respond initially will relapse.

Conventional chemotherapy Alkylating agents, alone or in combination, have been effective in approximately one-third of patients with VAD-refractory disease. IV melphalan (70–100 mg/m^2) and the combination of high-dose cyclophosphamide and etoposide are two examples of such regimens (Table 4).

Thalidomide has an established role in therapy for refractory/relapsed multiple myeloma, with 30% of patients achieving at least 50% reduction in paraprotein levels. Remissions obtained are durable: In a large cohort of patients with multiple myeloma receiving thalidomide, 2-year EFS rates of ~25% have been observed. Initially, thalidomide was employed in a dose-escalating schedule, starting at 200 mg and achieving a maximal dose of 800 mg. Recently, lower doses have been employed in combination with steroids (Table 4).

High-dose chemotherapy High-dose melphalan and stem-cell rescue should be offered to patients who have deferred the transplant initially. A randomized trial on early versus late transplantation has shown that an equivalent survival is conferred on patients undergoing salvage compared to early transplantation.

Novel agents

Lenalidomide has greater potency than thalidomide in preclinical studies and is better tolerated, with less neurotoxicity, somnolence, and constipation.

Two large multicenter phase III trials of lenalidomide (25 mg daily for 3 weeks with 1 week off) with dexamethasone compared with dexamethasone and placebo in relapsed multiple myeloma have demonstrated a significant improvement in response rate (partial response, 59% vs 21%, respectively) and time to disease progression (11.1 vs 4.7 months, respectively) in the cohort receiving the lenalidomide combination in one study and almost identical results in the second study. Similar responses were seen in patients relapsing after prior bortezomib or thalidomide exposure. DVT was a significant complication of this combination, occurring in approximately 15% of patients.

Proteasome inhibition A large multi-institution phase II trial of the proteasome inhibitor bortezomib (given IV at a dose of 1.3 mg/m^2 on days 1, 4, 8, and 11 every 21 days) demonstrated remarkable activity in a heavily treated, relapsed and/or refractory patient population, including patients relapsing after transplantation or not responding to thalidomide, with durable responses in about 35% (with 10% complete response). Side effects related to the drug were predominantly gastrointestinal in nature, with neuropathy, fatigue, and reversible cytopenias also noted. Toxicities were generally manageable with supportive care and dose reduction. Patients who did not respond to bortezomib monotherapy (progressive disease after 2 cycles or stable disease after the first 4 cycles) were permitted to receive combination bortezomib and dexamethasone. Combination therapy induced additional responses in 18% of patients (13 of 74).

The results of a large, randomized phase III trial of bortezomib monotherapy compared with high-dose dexamethasone (APEX) enrolled 669 patients with relapsed multiple myeloma. This trial showed significant improvement in the median time to disease progression (6.5 vs 3.6 months, respectively; $P < .0001$) and median overall survival (29.8 vs 23.7 months, respectively; $P = .027$). Response rates to bortezomib as a single agent were impressive at 43%. The most commonly reported adverse events for bortezomib were gastrointestinal events, fatigue, pyrexia, and thrombocytopenia; for dexamethasone, they were fatigue, insomnia, and anemia. Neuropathy was also an issue with bortezomib but proved manageable with dose reduction and schedule change. DVT was very rare, and efficacy in patients with significant renal dysfunction was noted. Finally, encouraging responses were noted in patients with adverse cytogenetics as well as in patients with advanced bone disease.

Clinical studies are ongoing with bortezomib in combination with pegylated liposomal doxorubicin, thalidomide, melphalan, and lenalidomide and have shown impressive disease control in refractory myeloma. In a randomized phase III multicenter international study in relapsed refractory myeloma, the combination of bortezomib (1.3 mg/m^2 days 1, 4, 8, and 11) and pegylated liposomal doxorubicin (30 mg/m^2 on day 4) was reported to be superior to bortezomib alone in terms of both overall response (50% vs 42%, respectively; $P = .05$) and time to disease progression (9.3 months vs 6.5 months, respectively; $P < .0001$). When bortezomib (1.0 or 1.3 mg/m^2) was administered with thalidomide (in doses ranging from 50 to 200 mg starting at cycle 2), 86% of patients with relapsed or refractory disease achieved a complete or partial response. A phase I trial combining bortezomib with lenalidomide has recently been completed, and results have revealed less neuropathy than seen when bortezomib is used with thalidomide. Remarkable activity has been reported, with approximately 60% of patients achieving response despite having received multiple prior therapies, including both agents separately before study entry.

Allogeneic transplantation For younger patients with resistant relapse or poor-prognosis disease (ie, deletion of chromosome 13), allogeneic transplantation may be an important option. However, high treatment-related mortality (30%

TABLE 5: Supportive therapies for multiple myeloma

Problem	Therapy
Chronic anemia (especially with renal impairment)	Erythropoietin
Prolonged neutropenia with infection	G-CSF
Recurrent infections with IgG < 400 mg/dL	Gamma globulin
Osteoporosis	Bisphosphonates

G-CSF = granulocyte colony-stimulating factor; IgG = immunoglobulin G

to 50%) with myeloablative allogeneic transplantation has discouraged the use of allografts in early-phase myeloma. New nonmyeloablative transplantation procedures that reduce mortality and exploit a graft-versus-tumor effect are being studied. In one study, 34 patients, including patients with relapsed or refractory disease, received melphalan at 200 mg/m^2 with autografting and then (40 to 120 days later) received allograft after nonmyeloablative conditioning. Treatment-related mortality at day 100 was 6%, with 53% of patients achieving complete response. With a median follow-up of 328 days after allografting, the overall survival rate was 81%, but chronic graft-versus-host disease remains a major challenge, occurring in up to two-thirds of patients.

Supportive therapies

Various supportive therapies may be beneficial in patients with multiple myeloma (Table 5).

Chronic anemia Patients with chronic symptomatic anemia may benefit from a trial of epoetin alfa (Epogen, Procrit), 40,000 U given by SC injection once weekly. Darbepoetin alfa (Aranesp), dosed at 200 to 300 µg by SC injection every 2 to 3 weeks, is an alternative approach. Erythropoietic agents (ESAs) should not be used in patients with myeloma when the anticipated outcome is cure. See the chapter on hematopoietic growth factors for additional information about the use of ESAs in patients with cancer.

Infection Serious infection with encapsulated organisms is encountered by patients with myeloma due to their inability to mount successful antibody production (and lack of opsonization). Prompt institution of antibiotics is therefore recommended in the face of systemic infection. Antibiotic prophylaxis is also recommended whenever high-dose glucocorticoids are used for treatment. Patients with recurrent serious infections may benefit from monthly gamma globulin. Shingles is not uncommon in these patients, and prophylaxis following transplantation and during bortezomib therapy is advised.

Bone pain or imminent fracture Therapy with bisphosphonates, such as pamidronate, alendronate (Fosamax), or zoledronic acid (Zometa), may prevent or delay bone pain or recurrent or imminent pathologic fracture in patients with stage III disease and at least one bone lesion. Pamidronate administered over the long term (21 monthly treatments) to patients with stage III multiple myeloma with at least one lytic lesion has been shown to reduce skeletal events and decrease the need for irradiation. Moreover, patients without lytic lesions also show a decrease in bone mineral density, and this decrease persists despite chemotherapy. These patients may also benefit from therapy with pamidronate. Several clinical and preclinical studies suggest that pamidronate may have an antimyeloma effect.

Zoledronic acid, a more potent bisphosphonate, has comparable efficacy and safety to pamidronate in preventing skeletal lesions. The ease of administration of a 4-mg dose, which reduces the infusion time to 15 minutes compared with 2 hours for pamidronate, has led to approval of zoledronic acid by the US Food and Drug Administration (FDA) for prevention of bone-related complications in myeloma. Caution should be exercised with long-term use of bisphosphonates, as renal impairment and osteonecrosis of the jaw bones have been reported.

Percutaneous vertebroplasty provides pain relief that is not only rapid but sustained, and it also strengthens the vertebral bodies. Kyphoplasty is a safer procedure that involves insertion of a balloon followed by injection of polymethyl methacrylate, the principal component of bone cement, in the balloon. It is performed with the patient under local anesthesia. Transient worsening of pain and fever may occur and is responsive to nonsteroidal anti-inflammatory agents.

Smoldering myeloma

Smoldering myeloma or asymptomatic myeloma is characterized by the presence of monoclonal Ig > 3 g/dL and/or bone marrow plasmacytosis in excess of 10%. The diagnosis is often made by chance finding of an elevated serum protein level during a screening examination.

Laboratory features Features of low tumor mass are usually present, without renal disease, hypercalcemia, or lytic bone lesions (Table 2). Marrow plasma cytosis occurs in less than 30% of patients, and anemia, if present, is mild (hemoglobin value > 10.5 g/dL).

Treatment Chemotherapy should be withheld until there is clear disease progression or a risk of a complication. The role of bisphosphonates and thalidomide in this setting is under investigation. An MRI finding of multifocal plasmacytomas or FDG-PET/CT findings of multifocal osseous lesions would be considered as evidence of end-organ damage and would warrant initiation of systemic therapy.

Prognostic factors Smoldering myeloma generally progresses to multiple myeloma at the rate of 10% per year for the first 5 years, 3% per year for the next 5 years, and then 1% for the last 10 years. Risk factors for tumor progression include the serum level and isotype of the Ig, presence of Bence Jones proteinuria, excess free light chain in serum with abnormal free light-chain ratio, extent and pattern of bone marrow involvement, and reduction in uninvolved Ig.

OTHER PLASMA CELL DYSCRASIAS

Other plasma cell dyscrasias include MGUS, solitary plasmacytoma of bone (SPB), solitary extramedullary plasmacytoma, Waldenström's macroglobulinemia, amyloidosis, POEMS (polyneuropathy, organomegaly, endocrino-pathy, monoclonal gammopathy, and skin changes) syndrome, and heavy-chain diseases.

MGUS

MGUS occurs in 1% of normal individuals > 40 years old, and its frequency rises progressively with age.

Laboratory features Common laboratory features of MGUS are listed in Table 2.

Treatment Approximately 25% of patients with this disorder develop mul-tiple myeloma, macroglobulinemia, or non-Hodgkin lymphoma over 20 years. The initial concentration of serum monoclonal protein > 1.5 g/dL, non–IgG-type paraprotein, and abnormal serum free light-chain ratio are significant pre-dictors of disease progression at 20 years. The long period of stability supports annual monitoring with serum electrophoresis and blood counts and suggests that chemotherapy may be withheld until there is evidence of progression to myeloma.

SPB

Approximately 3% of patients with myeloma have SPB.

Laboratory features All patients have either no myeloma protein or very low levels in serum or urine (Table 2). MRI may reveal abnormalities not detected by bone survey and may upstage patients to multiple myeloma. Persistence of monoclonal protein for more than 1 year after irradiation predicts early disease progression to multiple myeloma.

Treatment of SPB consists of radiation therapy (at least 45 Gy). Multiple my-eloma becomes evident in most patients over time, so only 20% of patients remain free of disease for more than 10 years. The median time for disease progression is 2 to 3 years.

Solitary extramedullary plasmacytoma

In contrast to SPB, solitary extramedullary plasmacytoma is often truly local-ized and can be cured in up to 50% of patients with localized radiation therapy (45–50 Gy) and/or resection. Careful observation after treatment is nonetheless warranted.

Waldenström's macroglobulinemia

This uncommon disease is characterized by lymphoplasmacytic bone marrow and tissue infiltrate in addition to elevated IgM production. The mutation pat-tern analysis suggests that final transformation occurs in the postgerminal center IgM memory B cell. Corresponding with variation in cell morphology, there is variation in the immunophenotype. Mature plasma cells exhibit CD38 antigen; however, lymphoid cells are typically CD19, CD20, CD22, and FMC7 positive.

Waldenström's macroglobulinemia usually affects people in the fifth to seventh decades of life and can cause symptoms due to tumor infiltration (marrow, lymph nodes, and/or spleen), circulating IgM (hyperviscosity, cryoglobuline-mia, and/or cold agglutinin hemolytic anemia), and tissue deposition of IgM (neuropathy, glomerular disease, and/or amyloidosis). Neuropathy may be due to the IgM antibody reacting with myelin-associated glycoprotein.

Hyperviscosity syndrome With hyperviscosity syndrome, patients may have visual symptoms, dizziness, cardiopulmonary symptoms, decreased conscious-ness, and a bleeding diathesis.

Therapy for hyperviscosity consists of plasmapheresis followed by chemotherapy to control the malignant proliferation. Patients with poor performance status and elderly patients unable to tolerate chemotherapy may be maintained with periodic plasmapheresis.

Treatment Alkylating agents in combination with steroids or purine analogs remain the mainstay of therapy. Alkylating agents alone or in combination with steroids effect a 50% reduction in paraprotein in about half of patients, and the median survival time is around 5 years. The purine analogs fludarabine and cladribine (2-CdA) elicit a more rapid response than other agents, with a response rate of more than 75% observed in a small series of patients. Prelimi-nary results of a large, American multi-institution evaluation of fludarabine reported partial responses in only 33% of patients.

Purine analog therapy may result in significant myelosuppression in later cycles of therapy and prolonged immunosuppression with increased opportunistic infections. Purine analogs are effective salvage options in patients refractory to or relapsing following alkylator therapy. Patients refractory to one purine ana-log are rarely salvaged by a different purine analog. Patients with resistant re-lapse are less likely to benefit from purine analogs (response rate, 18%) and should be considered for more intensive intervention, including high-dose therapy.

Other treatment options Rituximab (Rituxan), an anti-CD20 monoclonal antibody, is effective in Waldenström's macroglobulinemia because the CD20 antigen is usually present on the lymphoid cell component of macroglobuline-mia. Preliminary results indicate that about 30% of previously treated patients (refractory or relapsing off therapy) may benefit from rituximab.

Striking activity of thalidomide in multiple myeloma has prompted its use in Waldenström's macroglobulinemia. In a series of 20 patients receiving thalido-mide, 25% achieved a 50% reduction in paraprotein. Higher doses of thalidomide were not well tolerated in an elderly cohort of patients. Interest-ingly, preliminary results of bortezomib-based therapy in relapsed Waldenström's macroglobulinemia have been promising.

High-dose therapy with autologous bone marrow or blood stem-cell rescue has been effective in achieving 50% reduction in paraprotein in almost all patients in small pilot trials.

Amyloidosis

Amyloidosis occurs in 10% of patients with multiple myeloma. This infiltrative process results from organ deposition of amyloid fibrils, which consist of the NH_2 terminal amino acid residues of the variable portion of the light-chain Ig molecule. The abnormal protein is produced by clonal plasma cells.

Clinical features include the nephrotic syndrome, cardiomyopathy, hepatomegaly, neuropathy, macroglossia, carpal tunnel syndrome, and periorbital purpura.

Laboratory features Serum and urine immunofixation studies show a monoclonal Ig in approximately 80% of patients. Measurement of serum free light chain may provide a marker to evaluate response to therapy. The light chain is more frequently of the λ than κ type. Diagnosis can be made by the presence of apple-green birefringence on polarized light examination of subcutaneous fat aspirates stained with Congo red. Elevated serum BNP levels may indicate cardiac involvement which in the majority of patients may be confirmed with echocardiography.

Treatment of AL (monoclonal protein–associated) amyloidosis Survival of patients with amyloidosis is variable. Patients with congestive heart failure have a median survival of only 4 months. Oral MP extends the median survival to 17 months, compared with 13 months in untreated patients. Complete hematologic response is rare; similarly, reversal of organ damage is uncommon.

In a large cohort of patients receiving high-dose melphalan with stem-cell support, a complete hematologic response was observed in 47% of patients with at least 1 year of follow-up. However, the transplant-related mortality is high with high-dose therapy (14% to 37%). Complete hematologic response was associated with improved clinical response (improved organ function) and survival. Complete hematologic response in the absence of cardiac involvement predicted excellent outcome (1-year survival, 91%). Preliminary studies have also shown encouraging results with bortezomib as well as lenalidomide.

Patients with the overlap syndrome of myeloma and AL amyloidosis should be treated aggressively for myeloma; response can be seen in terms of both myeloma and resolution of amyloid symptoms.

POEMS syndrome

Clinical features and course The POEMS syndrome is a rare plasma cell dyscrasia that presents with peripheral, usually sensorimotor, neuropathy; monoclonal gammopathy (IgA λ being more common); sclerotic bone lesions, noted in nearly all patients; and organomegaly, endocrinopathy, and skin changes.

Other features include hyperpigmentation, hypertrichosis, thickened skin, papilledema, lymphadenopathy, peripheral edema, hepatomegaly, splenomegaly, and hypothyroidism. Diabetes mellitus is not part of this syndrome.

Compared with patients with symptomatic myeloma, individuals with POEMS syndrome are younger (median age, 51 years) and live longer (median, 8 years). The clinical course is commonly characterized by progressive neuropathy.

Treatment Plasmapheresis does not appear to be of benefit in POEMS syndrome, and patients are often treated similarly to those with myeloma. Patients presenting with isolated sclerotic lesions may have substantial resolution of neuropathic symptoms after local therapy for plasmacytoma with surgery and/or radiotherapy. Autologous stem-cell transplantation has been pursued in selected patients and has been associated with prolonged progression-free survival.

Heavy-chain diseases

Heavy-chain diseases are rare plasma cell dyscrasias characterized by the production of heavy-chain Ig molecules that lack light chains (IgG, IgA, IgM).

α Heavy-chain disease results from lymphocyte and plasma cell infiltration of the mesenteric nodes and small bowel and has features of malabsorption, such as diarrhea, weight loss, abdominal pain, edema, and nail clubbing. The heavy-chain molecule may be detected in serum, jejunal secretions, and urine. There is an association with infection with *Campylobacter jejuni* and α heavy-chain disease. Large proportions of patients can benefit from antibiotic therapy directed at this infection.

γ Heavy-chain disease Patients with γ heavy-chain disease may present with fever, weakness, lymphadenopathy, hepatosplenomegaly, and involvement of Waldeyer's ring. Eosinophilia, leukopenia, and thrombocytopenia are common. Treatment with regimens similar to those used for non-Hodgkin lymphoma may be effective.

μ Heavy-chain disease is seen exclusively in patients with chronic lymphocytic leukemia (CLL). Vacuolated plasma cells are common in the marrow, and many patients have κ light chains in the urine. Therapy is similar to that used for CLL (see chapter 34).

SUGGESTED READING

ON MULTIPLE MYELOMA

Attal M, Harousseau JL, Facon T, et al: Single versus double autologous stem-cell transplantation for multiple myeloma. N Engl J Med 349:2495–2502, 2003.

Attal M, Harousseau JL, Leyvraz S, et al: Maintenance treatment with thalidomide after autologous transplantation for myeloma: Final analysis of a prospective random-ized study of the "Intergroupe Francophone du Myelome." Blood 106:1148, 2005.

Badros A, Barlogie B, Morris C, et al: High response rate in refractory and poor-risk multiple myeloma after allo-transplantation using a nonmyeloablative conditioning regi-men and donor lymphocyte infusions. Blood 97:2574–2579, 2001.

Barlogie B, Desikan R, Eddlemon P, et al: Extended survival in advanced and refrac-tory myeloma after single-agent thalidomide: Identification of prognostic factors in a phase II study of 169 patients. Blood 98:492–494, 2001.

Berenson JR, Crowley JJ, Grogan TM, et al: Maintenance therapy with alternate-day prednisone improves survival in multiple myeloma patients. Blood 99:3163–3168, 2002.

Dimopoulos M, Spencer A, Attal M, et al: Lenalidomide plus dexamethasone for relapsed or refractory multiple myeloma. N Engl J Med 357:2123–2132, 2007.

Facon T, Avet-Losieau H, Guillerm G, et al: Chromosome 13 abnormalities identi-fied by FISH analysis and serum β_2-microglobulin produce a powerful myeloma staging system for patients receiving high-dose therapy. Blood 97:1566–1571, 2001.

Fermand JP, Ravaud P, Chevret S, et al: High-dose therapy and autologous periph-eral blood stem cell transplantation in multiple myeloma: Up-front or rescue treatment? Results of a multicenter sequential randomized clinical trial. Blood 92:3131–3136, 1998.

Hideshima T, Richardson P, Chauhan D, et al: The proteasome inhibitor PS-341 inhibits growth, induces apoptosis, and overcomes drug resistance in human multiple myeloma cells. Cancer Res 61:3071–3076, 2001.

Jagannath S, Durie BG, Wolf J, et al: Bortezomib therapy alone and in combination with dexamethasone for previously untreated symptomatic multiple myeloma. Br J Haematol 129:776–783, 2005.

Kyle RA, Rajkumar SV: Multiple myeloma. N Engl J Med 351:1860–1873, 2004.

Munshi NC, Hideshima T, Carrasco D, et al: Identification of genes modulated in multiple myeloma using genetically identical twin samples. Blood 103:1799–1806, 2004.

Rajkumar SV, Blood E, Vesole D, et al: Phase III clinical trial of thalidomide plus dexamethasone compared with dexamethasone alone in newly diagnosed multiple my-eloma: A clinical trial coordinated by the Eastern Cooperative Oncology Group. J Clin Oncol 24:431–436, 2006.

Rajkumar SV, Hayman S, Lacy MQ, et al: Combination therapy with lenalidomide plus dexamethasone (Rev/Dex) for newly diagnosed myeloma. Blood 106:781, 2005.

Richardson PG, Sonneveld P, Schuster M, et al: Extended follow-up of a phase 3 trial in relapsed multiple myeloma: Final time-to-event results of the APEX trial. Blood 110:3557–3560, 2007.

Richardson PG, Sonneveld P, Schuster MW, et al, for the Assessment of Proteasome Inhibition for Extending Remissions (APEX) Investigators: Bortezomib or high-dose dexamethasone for relapsed multiple myeloma. N Engl J Med 352:2487–2498, 2005.

Rosen LS, Gordon D, Antonio BS, et al: Zoledronic acid vs pamidronate in the treatment of skeletal metastases in patients with breast cancer or osteolytic lesions of multiple myeloma: A phase III, double-blind, comparative trial. Cancer J 7:377–387, 2001.

San Miguel JF, Schlag R, Khuageva NK, et al: Bortezomib plus melphalan and prednisone for initial treatment of multiple myeloma. N Engl J Med 359:906–917, 2008.

Weber DM, Chen C, Niesvizky R, et al: Lenalidomide plus dexamethasone for relapsed multiple myeloma in North America. N Engl J Med 357:2133–2142, 2007.

ON OTHER PLASMA CELL DYSCRASIAS

Dhodapkar MV, Jacobson JL, Gertz MA, et al: Prognostic factors and response to fludarabine therapy in Waldenström's macroglobulinemia: Results of US intergroup trial (Southwest Oncology Group S9003). Blood 98:41–48, 2001.

Dimopoulos MA, Zomas A, Viniou NA, et al: Treatment of Waldenström's macroglobulinemia with thalidomide. J Clin Oncol 19:3596–3601, 2001.

Sanchorawala V, Wright DG, Seldin DC, et al: An overview of the use of high-dose melphalan with autologous stem-cell transplantation for the treatment of AL amyloidosis. Bone Marrow Transplant 28:637–642, 2001.

Weber D, Treon SP, Emmanouilides C, et al: Uniform response criteria in Waldenstrom's macroglobulinemia: Consensus panel recommendations for the Second International Workshop on Waldenstrom's macroglobulinemia. Semin Oncol 30:127–131, 2003.

CHAPTER 32

Acute leukemias

Margaret R. O'Donnell, MD

Hematopoietic malignancies account for 6% to 8% of new cancers diagnosed annually. In the year 2008, an estimated 44,270 new cases of leukemia were diagnosed, and 21,710 deaths were attributable to leukemias of all types. The total age-adjusted incidence of leukemia, including both acute and chronic forms, is 9.6 per 100,000 population; the incidence of acute lymphoblastic leukemia (ALL) is 1.5 per 100,000 and of acute myelogenous leukemia (AML) is 2.7 per 100,000 population.

Epidemiology

Gender The incidence of both ALL and AML is slightly higher in males than in females.

Age The age-specific incidence of AML is similar to that of other solid tumors in adults, with an exponential rise after age 40. With regard to ALL, 60% of cases are seen in children, with a peak incidence in the first 5 years of life and a subsequent drop in incidence until age 60, when a second peak emerges.

Race and ethnicity The incidence of acute leukemia is slightly higher in populations of European descent. Also, a report from the University of Southern California indicates that acute promyelocytic leukemia (APL) is more common in Hispanic populations than in other ethnic groups.

Etiology and risk factors

There is wide diversity in the behavior of the various subsets of acute leukemias. Thus, it is unlikely that there is one common etiology for these aberrant cellular proliferations. There are, however, some accepted risk factors for leukemogenesis.

Chemical exposure Increased incidence of AML and myelodysplasia (preleukemia) has been reported in persons with prolonged exposure to benzene and petroleum products. The interval between exposure and the onset of leukemia is long (10–30 years). Chromosomal damage is common.

Pesticide exposure also has been linked to some forms of AML. The incidence of AML is beginning to rise in developing countries, as industrialization and pollution increase.

Other environmental exposures Exposure to hair dyes, smoking, and non-ionic radiation may also increase the risk of leukemia.

Prior chemotherapy or irradiation Use of alkylating agents, such as cyclophosphamide and melphalan (Alkeran), in the treatment of lymphomas, myelomas, and breast and ovarian cancers has been associated with the development of AML, usually within 3 to 5 years of exposure and often preceded by a myelodysplastic phase. Cytogenetic abnormalities, particularly monosomy 5, 7, 11, and 17, are common. Concurrent radiation exposure slightly increases the risk of leukemogenesis posed by alkylating agents.

Topoisomerase II inhibitors (etoposide, teniposide [Vumon], doxorubicin and its derivatives, and mitoxantrone [Novantrone]), used to treat ALL, myeloma, testicular cancer, and sarcomas, as well as taxanes used to treat breast cancer, have also been implicated in leukemogenesis. These agents, in contrast to alkylators, are associated with a short latency period without antecedent myelodysplasia and with cytogenetic abnormalities involving chromosome 11q23 or 21q22 in the malignant clone.

Genetic disorders An increased incidence of AML is seen in patients with Down syndrome, Bloom syndrome, or Fanconi's anemia, as well as in individuals with ataxia-telangiectasia or Wiskott-Aldrich syndrome. In identical twins younger than age 10, if one child develops leukemia (usually ALL), there is a 20% chance that the other twin will develop leukemia within a year; subsequently, the risk falls off rapidly and joins that of nonidentical siblings, which is three to five times that of the general population.

Signs and symptoms

Effects on hematopoiesis Leukemia manifests symptomatically by its impact on normal hematopoiesis. Thus, easy fatigability, bruising, or bleeding from mucosal surfaces, fever, and persistent infection are all reflections of the anemia, thrombocytopenia, and decrease in functional neutrophils associated with marrow replacement by malignant cells. Bone pain is common in children with ALL (occurring in 40%–50%) but is less common in adults (5%–10%).

WBC count elevation and pancytopenia Whereas a marked elevation in WBC count is the classic hallmark of leukemia, pancytopenia is more common, particularly in patients of all ages with ALL or in elderly patients with AML, who may have had preexisting marrow dysfunction (myelodysplasia). Only 10% of newly diagnosed patients with either AML or ALL present with leukocyte counts > 100,000/μL. These patients, however, constitute a poor prognostic group and are at increased risk of CNS disease, tumor lysis syndrome, and leukostasis due to impedance of blood flow from intravascular clumping of blasts, which are "stickier" than mature myeloid or lymphoid cells.

Leukostasis may manifest as an alteration in mental status; intermittent or persistent cranial nerve palsies, particularly those involving extraocular muscles; priapism; dyspnea; or pleuritic chest pain, due to small leukemic emboli in the pulmonary vasculature.

Physical findings in AML are usually minimal. Pallor, increased ecchymoses or petechiae, retinal hemorrhage, gingival hypertrophy, and cutaneous involvement are more common with monocytic (M4 or M5) variants of AML than with other variants of AML.

Hepatosplenomegaly and lymphadenopathy Mild hepatosplenomegaly and lymphadenopathy are seen in many cases, particularly in childhood ALL. Massive hepatosplenomegaly occurs infrequently and should raise the suspicion of a leukemia evolving from a prior hematologic disorder, such as chronic myelogenous leukemia (CML) or myelodysplasia. Mediastinal adenopathy is seen in 80% of cases of T-cell ALL, is less common in other ALLs, and is rare in AML.

Visceral involvement is also rare, occurring as an initial manifestation of AML in < 5% of cases, but it may be more frequent during subsequent relapses. These focal collections of blasts, called chloromas or granulocytic sarcomas, can present as soft-tissue masses, infiltrative lesions of the small bowel and mesentery, or obstructing lesions of the hepatobiliary or genitourinary system.

CNS involvement is uncommon at presentation in adult AML (< 1%) and adult ALL (3%–5%). In most instances, CNS involvement is detected by screening lumbar puncture in high-risk patients who are asymptomatic at the time of the puncture. Symptoms, when they do occur, include headache, diplopia, cranial nerve palsies, radicular pain, and/or weakness in a particular nerve root distribution. CNS involvement usually is restricted to leptomeninges; parenchymal mass lesions are uncommon.

Testicular involvement Like the CNS, the testes appear to be a "sanctuary" for isolated relapses in pediatric but not adult ALL. Signs of testicular involvement include painless, asymmetric enlargement.

Metabolic effects of acute leukemia relate primarily to the rate of cell death.

Hyperuricemia with possible interstitial or ureteral obstruction is seen predominantly in AML with moderate leukocytosis; this condition may be exacerbated by a rapid response to chemotherapy and the "tumor lysis syndrome" (hyperuricemia with renal insufficiency, acidosis, hyperphosphatemia, and hypocalcemia), which may occur within the first 24 to 48 hours after initiating chemotherapy. To prevent this complication, all patients should receive allopurinol and urine alkalinization before marrow-ablative chemotherapy is initiated. In patients with a high tumor burden, renal insufficiency, or acidosis prior to initiation of chemotherapy, rasburicase (Elitek) may offer a more rapid treatment for hyperuricemia. (For a more detailed discussion of hyperuricemia and tumor lysis syndrome, see chapter 45.)

Coagulopathies can also complicate the hemostatic defects associated with thrombocytopenia. Disseminated intravascular coagulation (DIC) is most often seen in APL (French-American-British Cooperative group [FAB] subtype M3) due to release of procoagulants from the abnormal primary granules, which activate the coagulation cascade, leading to decreased factors II, V, VIII, and X, and fibrinogen, as well as rapid platelet consumption. Lysozyme released from monoblasts in M4 and M5 subtypes of AML can also trigger the clotting cascade. Finally, DIC can occur following asparaginase (Elspar) chemotherapy for ALL.

TABLE 1: WHO classification of AML

AMLs with recurrent cytogenetic translocations
> AML with t(8;21)(q22;q22), AML1(CBF-alpha)/ETO
> APL [APL with t(15;17),(q22;q11-12] and variants], PML/RAR-alpha (M₃)

APL [APL with t(15;17),(q22;q11-12] and variants], PML/RAR-alpha (M_3)
> AML with abnormal bone marrow eosinophils [inv(16)(p13;q22) or
> t(16;16)(p13;q11), CBFβ/MYH11X]
> AML with 11q23 (mixed-lineage leukemia) abnormalities

AML with multilineage dysplasia
> With prior myelodysplastic syndrome (MDS)
> Without prior MDS

AML and MDS, therapy-related
> Alkylating agent-related
> Epipodophyllotoxin-related (some may be lymphoid)
> Other types

AML not otherwise categorized
> AML minimally differentiated (M0)
> AML without maturation (M1)
> AML with maturation (M2)
> Acute myelomonocytic leukemia (M4)
> Acute monocytic leukemia (M5)
> Acute erythroid leukemia (M6)
> Acute megakaryocytic leukemia (M7)
> Acute basophilic leukemia
> Acute panmyelosis with myelofibrosis

Acute biphenotypic leukemias

AML = acute myelogenous leukemia; APL = acute promyelocytic leukemia; WHO = World Health
Organization
Vardiman JW, Harris NL, Brunning RD: Blood 100:2292–2302, 2002.

Diagnosis

Abnormalities on the CBC raise the possibility of leukemia. The diagnosis is substantiated pathologically by a bone marrow examination.

All patients should have cytochemistry, immunophenotyping by fluorescent-activated cell sorter (FACS) using monoclonal antibodies directed at leukemia-specific antigens and cytogenetic analysis of the marrow or peripheral blood blasts at diagnosis. Other tests used to evaluate metabolic abnormalities (electrolytes, creatinine, and liver function tests) and coagulopathies are also needed at diagnosis. A lumbar puncture should be performed at diagnosis in all pediatric patients with ALL and in all patients with neurologic symptoms regardless of age and pathology.

Pathology and cytogenetics

Acute leukemias comprise a group of clonal disorders of maturation at an early phase of hematopoietic differentiation. Morphology and cytochemical stains designed to detect intracellular myeloperoxidase or esterases have been the

TABLE 2: WHO classification of ALL

Precursor B-cell acute lymphoblastic leukemia (cytogenetic subgroups)
    t(9;22)(a34;q11); *BCR/ABL*
    t(v;11q23); *MLL* rearranged
    t(1;19)(q23;p13) *E2A/PBX1*
    t(12;21)(p12;q22) *ETV/CBF*-alpha

Precursor T-cell acute lymphoblastic leukemia

Burkitt-cell leukemia [t(8;14) or t(8;22)]

ALL = acute lymphoblastic leukemia; WHO = World Health Organization
Harris NL, Jaffe ES, Diebold J, et al: J Clin Oncol 17:3835–3849, 1999.

traditional methods used to classify acute leukemias into either myeloid or lymphoid derivations.

Coupling these traditional methods with cytogenetic analysis and highly specific monoclonal antibodies directed against cell-surface antigens has led to the detection of new prognostic factors and has provided an approach to detect minimal residual disease.

In 1997, a panel of hematopathologists met to update the FAB classification of hematologic malignancies, which was based on morphology and cytochemistry alone. They proposed a new classification, incorporating immunophenotyping, cytogenetics, and clinical disease features, which has been adopted by the World Health Organization (WHO; Tables 1 and 2).

Myeloid leukemias

The WHO classification retains the morphologic subgroups of the FAB system in the subgroup of "AML not otherwise categorized" but has created new categories that recognize the importance of certain cytogenetic translocations as predictors of response to therapy. In this category are AML with t(8;21)(q22;q22), AML with abnormal eosinophils and inv(16)(p13;q22) or t(16;16)(p13;q11), AML with 11q23 mixed-lineage leukemia abnormalities, and APL with t(15;17)(q22;q11-12) or variants (Table 1).

The WHO classification also attempts to deal with the evidence that, in many older patients, marrow dysfunction antedates the onset of acute leukemia. These myelodysplastic syndromes (MDSs) are characterized by ineffective hematopoietic production and disrupted maturation of one or more cell lines. These abnormalities are often accompanied by loss of chromosomal material, particularly loss of chromosomes –5 or –5q, –7 or –7q, and –3 or –20. As the bone marrow becomes more dysfunctional, increasing numbers of blasts are seen in the marrow.

In the FAB classification, the demarcation line between myelodysplasia and AML was 30% marrow blasts. However, patients with 20% to 29% blasts (previously classified as refractory anemia with excess blasts in transition [RAEB-t]) have a biologic behavior and poor survival similar to those of patients with

AML. WHO lowered the threshold for the diagnosis of AML to 20% marrow blasts and deleted the FAB category of RAEB-t. In addition, patients with 5% to 20% blasts who have t(15;17), t(18;21), or inv(16) are considered to have AML rather than MDS and should receive AML treatment.

The WHO system further subdivided the AML patients with dysplastic maturation into those with or without antecedent cytopenias (usually 3 months prior to diagnosis had been the arbitrary cutoff point) and those with a history of exposure to chemotherapy agents (alkylating agents, epipodophyllotoxins, or others). In 2003, the International Working Group for the Diagnosis and Standardization of Response Criteria accepted the WHO classification as the standard for AML diagnosis.

The genetic profile of malignant cells has been found to vary widely from normal, with many genes being either overexpressed or suppressed. DNA microarray techniques allow the simultaneous analysis of thousands of genes that are being studied in AML and ALL for their predictive ability to define cohorts of patients with similar outcomes; this process may in turn allow the selection of candidate genes that can be used as therapeutic targets in the future.

Lymphoblastic leukemias

Lymphoblastic leukemias can arise from either B-cell or T-cell progenitors that arrest at an early stage of maturation and then proliferate. Marrow involvement of > 25% lymphoblasts is used as the demarcation line between lymphoblastic lymphoma, in which the preponderance of tumor bulk is in nodal structures, and ALL. Approximately 75% of adult ALLs are B cell in derivation and 25% are T cell.

Precursor B-cell ALL Most B-cell leukemias are early or "pre-B" cell, expressing CD19 and CD10 (the common acute leukemia antigen [cALLa]) but lacking surface or cytoplasmic immunoglobulin; this group of early B-cell leukemias has a more favorable prognosis than that of B-cell leukemias in which the cells have a more mature phenotype. Chromosomal rearrangements juxtaposing an oncogene with a promoter region are often seen in this disease category (Table 2).

Mature B-cell ALL The more mature B-cell ALL, or Burkitt-cell leukemia, is associated with translocations of the c-*myc* gene on chromosome 8 and the immunoglobulin heavy-chain gene on chromosome 14q32 in 80% of cases or with the light-chain genes of chromosome 2p11 or 22q11 in the other 20%. Burkitt-cell leukemia has increased in frequency recently, as it is one of the lymphoproliferative disorders that occur in individuals infected with the human immunodeficiency virus (HIV); leukemia may appear early in the course of the HIV infection, before the onset of opportunistic infections or severe T-cell deficiency (see chapter 27).

A small fraction (2%) of patients with precursor B-cell ALL lack CD10 expression. Patients with CD10-negative disease have a high incidence of *MLL* gene expression (83%) and a very poor disease-free survival (DFS; 12%) at 2 years.

T-cell ALL is frequently associated with translocations of T-cell receptor genes on chromosome 14q11 or 7q34 with other gene partners. T-cell ALL had been associated with a poor prognosis when treated with conventional ALL regimens but now is associated with a better prognosis if treated with aggressive antimetabolite therapy. Precursor T-cell ALL has a poorer outcome.

Infection with human T-cell leukemia virus-1 (HTLV-1) should be looked for in patients with T-cell ALL presenting with hypercalcemia and lytic bone lesions. HTLV-1 infection is endemic in southern Japan, the southern Pacific basin, the Caribbean basin, and sub-Saharan Africa. High infection rates are also seen in parts of Iran, India, and Hawaii. Recent immigrants from endemic areas retain a risk of infection similar to that of their point of origin. However, fewer than 0.1% of persons carrying HTLV-1 will develop T-cell leukemia.

ALL with myeloid antigen expression vs undifferentiated leukemia

A subset of patients with leukemia exhibits features of both myeloid and lymphoid differentiation. These patients were originally classified as having mixed-lineage leukemia. Patients with a leukemic clone that expresses two or more ALL antigens and one myeloid antigen comprise 20% of adult ALL cases. Although expression of myeloid antigen is considered to be a poor-risk feature in children, it does not constitute a distinct poor-risk feature in adults.

Immunophenotyping has also helped define a group of patients with undifferentiated myeloid leukemia (M0) who previously were likely to be treated as if they had ALL. These leukemias have a primitive morphology and lack myeloperoxidase. On immunophenotyping, they express at least one early myeloid antigen, usually CD13 or CD33, and no T- or B-cell markers. Based on immunophenotyping, undifferentiated leukemias are now recommended to be treated in the same manner as myeloid malignancies.

ALL prognostic factors

Factors known to have an impact on the ability to achieve and maintain remission in ALL include age, lineage derivation, elevated WBC count, and cytogenetic abnormality. The cure rate for children aged 2 to 12 is over 80%; this 5-year DFS rate drops to 40% to 60% for younger adults and is less than 30% for adults over age 65. Poorer outcomes in adults have been attributed to a higher proportion of patients with poor-risk karyotypes, particularly t(9;22) or Philadelphia chromosome, as well as poorer tolerance to chemotherapy, especially L-asparaginase and high-dose methotrexate.

The recent 1,500 patient MRC XII/ECOG adult ALL trial reconfirmed that age (> 35 years), elevated WBC count, B-cell lineage, and karyotypic abnormalities are significant independent risk factors for DFS and overall survival (OS). In addition to the previously reported poor-risk karyotypes of t(9;22), t(4;11), and t(8;14), this trial also identified complex (75) abnormalities and low hypodiploid/near triploid as new poor-risk features.

Philadelphia chromosome The most common cytogenetic abnormality in ALL is the translocation of the *abl* gene from chromosome 9 to the breakpoint cluster region on chromosome 22, forming a new gene product (BCR-ABL) with tyrosine kinase activity. This translocation, referred to as the Philadelphia chromosome (Ph), is found in 95% of cases of CML and in 20% to 30% of newly diagnosed adults with ALL.

The fusion protein produced by the BCR-ABL translocation in Ph+ ALL (p190) differs from the product seen in CML (p210); the p190 product is a smaller protein than the p210 product and has higher tyrosine kinase activity. Use of polymerase chain reaction (PCR) techniques that target only the p210 product will significantly underestimate the incidence of Ph+ ALL. In a recent update of the German ALL trials, 37% of patients were Ph+, with 77% showing the p190 product versus 23% showing the p210 product.

Although patients with Ph+ ALL may attain a morphologic remission with conventional chemotherapy (82%), almost all such patients will have persistent molecular evidence of disease on PCR. Patients who do achieve a molecular remission have a longer duration of remission than those who continue to express p190 or p210 activity (30 vs 12 months).

Recently, GIMEMA, the Italian oncologic cooperative group, published outcomes data of a large trial of adult patients with ALL in which both cytogenetic data and molecular probes for specific gene products were combined to define prognostic groups. The molecular abnormalities that were evaluated were t(9;22) BCR-ABL, t(4;11)/ MLL-AFA, t(1;19) E$_2$A/PBX$_1$, 9p/p15-p16 deletions, and 6q deletions. Categories based primarily on classic karyotypes were normal, hyperdiploid, and miscellaneous structural abnormalities of uncertain significance.

The use of molecular probes was particularly informative in patients with failed karyotypic analysis or normal cytogenetics. The use of the BCR-ABL probe increased the number of cases with a t(9;22) abnormality from 64 to 104 (26% of patients in the trial); more than 50% of add(9p)/p15-p16 abnormalities were detected only by molecular testing. Patients with t(9;22), t(4;11), and t(1;19) had disease-free intervals of 0.4 to 0.6 years, whereas those with del(6q), hyperdiploid, or pseudodiploid karyotypes had intermediate DFS of 1.3 to 1.6 years; those with a normal karyotype or del(9p)/p15-p16 had better outcomes (2.9 and 4 years, respectively).

Other translocations Translocations involving the mixed-lineage leukemia gene at chromosome 11q23 are partnered with several other chromosomes, including 4q21, 9q22, and 19q13. Translocations involving chromosome 11q23 are frequently seen in secondary leukemias, particularly those arising after chemotherapy with etoposide or teniposide. Although most of these translocations are associated with AML, ALL has also arisen in this setting. All the 11q23 translocations, as well as the more common (1;19) translocation, are associated with poorer outcomes when compared with similar immunophenotypes coupled with normal cytogenetics.

Molecular techniques, such as PCR amplification of leukemia-specific sequences of RNA or DNA, have been used in research settings to reveal residual leukemia cells. These sensitive techniques can detect the persistence of cells with the leukemic phenotype at a sensitivity of 1 cell in 10^4 normal cells in patients who are deemed to be in CR by conventional techniques. In two pediatric studies, detection of leukemia-specific gene rearrangements (≥ 1 cell in 10^4 normal cells) 5–6 months after initiation of treatment was associated with a high relapse rate.

A confirmatory study in adults with standard-risk ALL using a combination of aberrant immunophenotyping and PCR amplification of T-cell receptor or immunoglobulin gene rearrangements was recently reported. Patients who had no detectable residual disease by day 11 from the start of induction therapy had a 3-year DFS rate of 92% compared with 65% for those with no residual disease by week 16. Patients who had detectable minimal residual disease beyond that point had a 3-year DFS of only 12%.

Time to remission and measurement of minimal residual disease have also been identified as prognostic factors in several pediatric trials. Molecular techniques such as PCR amplification of leukemia-specific sequences of RNA or DNA have been used to detect persistence of cells with the leukemic phenotype at a sensitivity of 1 cell in 10^4 normal cells. In two pediatric studies, the detection of 7 1×10^{-4} cells at 6 months post diagnosis was associated with a very high relapse rate.

Treatment strategy

Treatment for patients with ALL and AML can be subdivided into two or three phases. Induction chemotherapy is the initial treatment designed to clear the marrow of overt leukemia. This phase usually involves multiple drugs that cause pancytopenia for 2 to 3 weeks.

The purpose of consolidation therapy is to further reduce the residual leukemic burden in patients who are in morphologic remission. Molecular markers of residual disease can often be detected after induction chemotherapy, which indicates the need for further treatment. The intensity of consolidation therapy varies, depending on the risk of relapse (based primarily on cytogenetic risk groups) and patient age.

Maintenance chemotherapy using low-dose oral chemotherapy for 18 to 24 months has been shown to prolong relapse-free survival in pediatric patients with ALL and in adults with APL. Its value is less clear in adults with ALL; maintenance is rarely used in AML.

TREATMENT OF ALL

Induction therapy

The initial goal of therapy is to rapidly reduce the leukemic burden to a level undetectable by conventional methods of light microscopy and flow cytometry, a state that is deemed a complete remission (CR). Two standard induction regimens have been used in adults with ALL—the Hoelzer regimen, developed by the Berlin-Frankfurt-Munster (BFM) multicenter group, and the Larson regimen, developed by the Cancer and Leukemia Group B (CALGB).

TABLE 3: ALL induction and consolidation therapy

Induction	Consolidation	CNS prophylaxis	Maintenance
Berlin Franklin Munster (BFM) REGIMEN			
Phase I	**Phase I**[a]	**Weeks 5-8**	6-MP 60 mg/m² PO on weeks 10-18 and 29-130
VCR 2 mg IV on days 1, 8, 15, 22	VCR 2 mg IV on days 1, 8, 15, 22	MTX 10 mg IT on days 31, 38, 45, 52	MTX 20 mg PO or IV weekly on weeks 10-18 and 29-130
DNR 25 mg/m² IV on days 1, 8, 15, 22	Adria 25 mg/m² IV on days 1, 8, 15, 22	Cranial RT[b] 2,400 cGy (given along with phase II induction)	
PSE 60 mg/m² PO on days 1-28	Dex 10 mg/m² PO on days 1-28		
L-Asp 5,000 IU/m² IV on days 1-14			
Phase II	**Phase II**		
CTX 650 mg/m² IV on days 29, 43, 57 (maximum, 1,000 mg)	CTX 650 mg/m² IV on day 29		
Ara-C 75 mg/m² IV on days 31-34, 38-41, 45-48, 52-55	Ara-C 75 mg/m² IV on days 31-34, 38-41		
6-MP 60 mg/m² IV on days 29-57	6-TG 60 mg/m² PO on days 29-42		

Adria = Adriamycin (doxorubicin); ALL = acute lymphoblastic leukemia; Ara-C = cytarabine; BFM = Berlin-Frankfurt-Munster; CTX = cyclophosphamide; Dex = dexamethasone; DNR = daunorubicin; Dox = doxorubicin; L-Asp = L-asparaginase; 6-MP = mercaptopurine; MTX = methotrexate; PSE = prednisone; RT = radiation therapy; 6-TG = thioguanine; VCR = vincristine

a Begin week 20

b Cranial RT dose for prophylaxis is reduced to 1,800 cGy if patient is being considered for allogeneic BMT while in first complete remission

Induction and early intensification	CNS prophylaxis and interim maintenance	Late intensification	Prolonged maintenance
CALGB REGIMEN			

Induction and early intensification

CALGB REGIMEN

Course I: Induction (4 wk)

CTX	1,200 mg/m² IV on day 1[c]
DNR	45 mg/m² IV on days 1-3[c]
VCR	2 mg IV on days 1, 8, 15, 22
PSE	60 mg/m²/d PO/IV on days 1-21[c]
L-Asp	6,000 IU/m² SC on days 5, 8, 11, 15, 18, 22

Course II: Early intensification[d] (4 wk; repeat once)

MTX	15 mg IT on day 1
CTX	1,000 mg/m² IV on day 1
6-MP	60 mg/m²/d PO on days 1-14
Ara-C	75 mg/m²/d SC on days 1-4, 8-11
VCR	2 mg IV on days 15, 22
L-Asp	6,000 IU/m² SC on days 15, 18, 22, 25

CNS prophylaxis and interim maintenance

Course III: CNS prophylaxis and interim maintenance[e] (12 wk)

Cranial RT	2,400 cGy on days 1-12
MTX	15 mg IT on days 1, 8, 15, 22, 29
6-MP	60 mg/m²/d PO on days 1-70
MTX	20 mg/m² PO on days 36, 43, 50, 57, 64

Late intensification

Course IV: Late intensification[f] (8 wk)

Dox	30 mg/m² IV on days 1, 8, 15
VCR	2 mg IV on days 1, 8, 15
Dex	10 mg/m²/d PO on days 1-14
CTX	1,000 mg/m² IV on day 29
6-TG	60 mg/m²/d PO on days 29-42
Ara-C	75 mg/m²/d SC on days 29, 32, 36-39

Prolonged maintenance

Course V: Prolonged maintenance[g]

VCR	2 mg IV on day 1 of q4wk
PSE	60 mg/m²/d on days 1-5 of q4wk
MTX	20 mg/m² PO on days 1, 8, 15, 22
6-MP	80 mg/m²/d PO on days 1-28

[c] For patients > 60 years old, modify doses as follows: CTX, 800 mg/m² on day 1; DNR, 30 mg/m² on days 1-3; PSE, 60 mg/m² on days 1-7
[d] Weeks 5-12   [e] Weeks 13-25   [f] Begin week 26   [g] Until 24 months from diagnosis

TABLE 3: ALL induction and consolidation therapy (continued)

Induction/consolidation	Dosage
LINKER REGIMEN	
Induction 1A (DVPAsp)	
DNR	60 mg/m² IV on days 1-3 (and day 15 if day 14 bone marrow had residual leukemia)
VCR	1.4 mg/m² IV on days 1, 8, 15, and 22 (capped at 2.0 mg if age > 40 years)
PSE	60 mg/m² PO on days 1-28
Asparaginase	6,000 IU/m² SC on days 17-28 or peg L-asparaginase 2,000 IU/m² SC on day 15
Consolidation 1B, 2B (HDAC/etoposide)	
Ara-C	2,000 mg/m² IV over 2 h on days 1-4
Etoposide	500 mg/m² IV over 3 h on days 1-4
Consolidation 2A (DVPAsp)	
DNR	60 mg/m² IV on days 1-3
VCR	1.4 mg/m² IV on days 1, 8, and 15 (capped at 2.0 mg if age > 40 years)
PSE	60 mg/m² PO on days 1, 21
Asparaginase	6,000 IU/m² SC 6 doses over 2 weeks or peg L-asparaginase 2,000 IU/m² SC on day 15
Consolidation 1C, 2C, 3C (HDMTX/6-MP)	
MTX	220 mg/m² IV bolus, then 60 mg/m²/h × 36 h on days 1-2, 15-16
Leucovorin	50 mg/m² IV every 6 h for 3 doses, then oral leucovorin until methotrexate < 0.05 µmol/L
6-MP	75 mg/m² PO on days 1-28
Maintenance[h]	
MTX	20 mg/m² weekly
6-MP	75 mg/m² daily

DVPAsp = daunorubicin, vincristine, prednisone, and asparaginase; HDAC = high-dose cytarabine + Ara-C; HDMTX = high-dose methotrexate; 6-MP = mercaptopurine

[h]Beginning after hematologic recovery from cycle 3C and continuing until 30 months from complete response

TABLE 3: ALL induction and consolidation therapy *(continued)*

Induction/consolidation	Dosage
M. D. ANDERSON (HYPER-CVAD) REGIMEN	
CTX	300 mg/m² infused over 3 h q12h × 6 doses (days 1-3)
DOX	25 mg/m²/d continuous infusion over 24 h × 2 days to begin 12 h after last CTX dose (days 4 and 5)
VCR	1.4 mg/m² (max 2 mg) IV on days 4 and 11
DEX	40 mg/d days 1-4 and 11-14
Alternate q21 d with	
MTX	1 g/m² continuous infusion over 24 h (day 1)
Ara-C	3 g/m² over 2 h q12h × 4 doses (days 2 and 3)
Leucovorin rescue	50 mg PO at end of MTX infusion and then 25 mg PO q6h × 48 h
Methylprednisolone	50 mg IV twice daily (days 1–3)

All patients received a minimum of 4 doses of intrathecal methotrexate for CNS prophylaxis. All patients received maintenance therapy twice a year with 6-MP (150 mg/d), MTX (20 g/m² oral weekly), VCR (2 mg/month IV), and PSE (200 mg oral daily for 5 days along with VCR).

DVPAsp = daunorubicin, vincristine, prednisone, and asparaginase; HDAC = high-dose cytarabine (Ara-C) MTX = methotrexate; 6-MP = mercaptopurine

Along with the standard induction schemas, two newer regimens, the Hyper-CVAD (high-dose cytoxan, vincristine, adriamycin, dexamethasone) regimen from M. D. Anderson and the Linker regimen (2002 version), which have a similar induction drug dosing as the older regimens but include much higher doses of antimetabolites (cytarabine [Ara-C] and methotrexate) and etoposide for dose-dense consolidations, are outlined in Table 3 along with the standard induction schemas. Overall, CRs are obtained in 80% to 94% of adults younger than age 60 treated with any of these regimens.

The addition of an anthracycline to the standard pediatric leukemia induction regimen of vincristine, prednisone, and asparaginase increased the CR rate in adults from 50% to 60% to 70% to 85% in several series. In a recent CALGB study, the use of cytokines, ie, granulocyte colony-stimulating factor (G-CSF, filgrastim [Neupogen]), during induction in patients older than 60 years of age, reduced treatment-related mortality from 31% to 5% when compared with placebo-treated controls.

The US Food and Drug Administration (FDA) has approved pegaspargase (Oncaspar) as a component of a multiagent chemotherapy regimen for the first-line treatment of patients with ALL. The drug had originally been approved only for ALL patients who were allergic to native forms of asparaginase. A single dose of 2,000 IU/m^2 is now used to replace the multiple doses on the Linker regimen.

T-cell ALL There is evidence that patients with T-cell ALL may benefit from early treatment with Ara-C and cyclophosphamide. Pharmacologic studies show high levels of Ara-C triphosphate accumulation in T lymphoblasts and synergy between cyclophosphamide and Ara-C in cell lines of T-cell malignancies. T lymphocytes also have a lower expression of polyglutamate synthetase than pre-B blasts. Randomized trials in children with T-cell ALL showed that the use of high-dose methotrexate (up to 5 g/m^2) also improved outcome.

Mature B-cell ALL Patients with the more mature B-cell ALL (Burkitt-cell leukemia) experienced an improvement in survival when high doses of cyclophosphamide, methotrexate, and Ara-C were incorporated early in the treatment course. The probability of leukemia-free survival improved from 35% with standard ALL induction to 60% to 70% with these newer regimens.

Ph+ ALL

The development of imatinib (Gleevec), a selective BCR-ABL protein kinase inhibitor, provided a potent new agent in the treatment of Ph+ ALL. As a single agent, it produced CRs in 30% of patients with relapsed Ph+ disease. Several centers have reported improved remission rates of 90% to 95% when imatinib was added to initial induction therapy (usually in regimens lacking L-asparaginase) without additional toxicity. With continuation of imatinib through consolidation, 50% to 60% of patients will achieve a molecular remission by 60 days post induction. Patients who achieve a molecular remission and continue on imatinib therapy have an improved progression-free survival (PFS) of 40% to 50% at 1 to 2 years compared with < 25% at 1 year in the pre-imatinib era.

Consolidation therapy

The BFM, CALGB, Linker (2002), and Hyper-CVAD consolidation regimens for ALL are outlined in Table 3. As yet, no randomized trials have compared these regimens. However, in sequential studies from Memorial Sloan-Kettering Cancer Center, BFM group, and the Linker study, use of multiple cycles of non–cross-resistant drugs for 3 to 8 cycles after remission followed by maintenance with methotrexate and mercaptopurine (Purinethol) resulted in overall long-term DFS rates of 38% to 52%.

Long-term outcome data of 288 patients treated with Hyper-CVAD showed an 81% CR rate after cycle 1A and a 92% rate after receiving both cycles 1A and 1B (see Table 3); a 5% overall death rate during induction was noted, although treatment-related mortality reached 15% in patients older than age 60 despite the use of G-CSF. At a median follow-up of 63 months, the 5-year DFS was 38%, similar to that reported in the BFM and CALGB trials. In this series, adverse prognostic factors for DFS were age $\geq$ 45 years, poor performance status, WBC > 50,000/μL, Ph+ cytogenetics, more than 1 cycle to achieve a CR, or > 5% residual blasts at day 14. Patients with none or one of these factors had a 52% 5-year DFS rate, versus 37% for patients with two or three factors and only 10% for patients with at least four risk factors.

In the 2002 Linker trial, which intensifies the consolidation with alternating cycles of higher dose Ara-C (HDAC) and etoposide alternating with cycles of high-dose methotrexate, the 5-year relapse-free survival rate was 52% overall and 60% for patients with standard-risk features. Prognostic features that were associated with a poor outcome in this study included pre-B ALL with > 100,000/μL WBC count at diagnosis, cytogenetic abnormalities involving chromosome 11q23 or t(9;22), and time to remission > 30 days. Without either allogeneic or autologous transplantation, all high-risk patients relapsed within a short (1–9 month) time.

The French LALA-94 trial of 922 patients was designed to look at postremission therapy that was stratified by risk of relapse. The standard-risk patients who achieved CR with 1 cycle of induction therapy were randomized to receive either conventional cyclophosphamide, Ara-C, and mercaptopurine or early intensification with intermediate-dose Ara-C (1 g/m^2 × 8 doses) and mitoxantrone.

In this study, there was no difference in 5-year DFS (33% conventional vs 37% early intensification, with an OS at 5 years of 44%). High-risk patients included those with defined cytogenetic risks (excluding Ph+), WBC > 30,000/μL, and CNS disease at diagnosis or who required more than 35 days to achieve CR. Patients with a sibling donor received allogeneic transplant in CR, with the remainder randomized to receive either the early intensification chemotherapy or autologous transplant. The 5-year DFS was 45% for those receiving allogeneic transplant and 23% for those without a donor. There was no significant difference in OS with chemotherapy versus autologous transplant, but there was a different pattern of relapse, with fewer late relapses in the autologous patients.

High-risk patients Although the BFM regimen is now standard therapy for good-prognosis patients, high-risk patients are being selected for dose-intensive therapies, including HDAC and methotrexate or etoposide, high-dose methotrexate, and asparaginase.

For patients with Ph+ ALL, several centers have begun combining imatinib with induction and consolidation chemotherapy. In series from both Japan and the United States, the addition of imatinib during induction has resulted in a CR rate of 95% to 100% after 1 cycle of induction, and patients have achieved molecular remission documented by PCR in 50% to 60% of patients within 2 months.

Transplantation Recent series have reported a DFS rate of 55% to 68% for "high-risk" patients with ALL undergoing transplantation during first CR. When treated with conventional-dose chemotherapy prior to the discovery of imatinib, patients with Ph+ ALL had a DFS rate of < 10% regardless of other risk factors and a median time to relapse of 12 months. These patients should be referred for allogeneic or matched-unrelated donor (MUD) transplantation expeditiously upon attaining CR. Several centers are incorporating imatinib along with conventional consolidation chemotherapy in patients with Ph+ ALL to try to reduce the leukemic burden further before transplantation, primarily in patients awaiting an unrelated donor transplant. Trials using imatinib post allogeneic transplantation to reduce relapse rates are also in progress. (Strategies for the most effective use of the various transplant options are discussed in chapter 36.)

CNS prophylaxis

CNS relapse occurs at a much higher frequency in patients with ALL compared with those with AML. The rate of CNS relapse was 20% in the first year in a pediatric ALL trial in which the CNS therapy was attenuated to a subtherapeutic level.

Patients with ALL require preemptive therapy for occult CNS disease with either (1) intrathecal methotrexate and/or Ara-C combined with cranial irradiation or (2) high-dose systemic Ara-C or methotrexate combined with intrathecal therapy. Specific use of intrathecal liposomal Ara-C should not be used concomitantly with high-dose systemic chemotherapy such as cytarabine, methotrexate, or etoposide, which cross the blood-brain barrier due to a high risk (15% to 20%) of serious neurotoxicity (seizures, cauda equina syndrome, and encephalitis).

Maintenance therapy

Maintenance therapy with daily mercaptopurine and weekly methotrexate for 18 to 24 months beyond consolidation remains the standard of care for children with ALL. In adults, the benefit of maintenance therapy is less certain. In low-risk adults, who may have an outcome more similar to that in the pediatric population, maintenance therapy would appear to be justified (see Table 3 for maintenance regimens). In individuals who have mature B-cell ALL, it is unlikely that maintenance therapy has any effect. In other high-risk adult populations, more than half of patients relapse while on maintenance therapy, indicating the need for other strategies to eradicate minimal residual disease.

Treatment of relapse

Treatment of relapsed adult ALL is a major challenge. Since most protocols for initial treatment incorporate 6 to 11 agents with different cytotoxic mechanisms, a selection process for drug resistance has occurred. The overall remission rate for relapse therapy is 30% to 40%, with a median duration of remission of 6 months. In the MRC/ECOG trial, the 5-year overall survival for adults who relapsed was 7% in the absence of allogeneic transplant.

Salvage strategies include reinduction with the initial regimen in patients with late relapse or high-dose antimetabolites (Ara-C or methotrexate [see hyper-CVAD regimen, Table 3]) in those who relapse early. Recent experimental approaches include monoclonal antibodies directed against leukemia-specific antigens conjugated to either radionuclides or toxins, tyrosine kinase inhibitors, allogeneic or autologous transplantation, or new agents.

Clofarabine (Clolar) has been approved for treatment of relapsed refractory ALL in children. Of 61 patients, 12 achieved a CR, including children who had relapsed following allogeneic transplantation. The maximum tolerated dose was 52 mg/m^2 infused over 2 hours daily for 5 days. Significant toxic effects include febrile neutropenia, anorexia and nausea, capillary leak syndrome, hepatotoxicity, and skin rash.

In individuals with Ph+ ALL or CML in lymphoid blast crisis, imatinib (400–800 mg orally daily) can induce remissions in up to 30% of patients. These remissions are short-lived but may control the leukemia long enough for a donor to be identified, thus providing an option for an allogeneic transplant in second remission. Nilotinib (Tasigna), which has been recently approved by the FDA, is an imatinib analog with high binding affinity to BCR-ABL. It has been shown to overcome imatinib resistance in approximately 30% of Ph+ ALL patients.

Dasatinib (Sprycel), which is a kinase inhibitor of multiple targets including BCR-ABL, c-Kit, SRC, and PDGFR (platelet-derived growth factor) receptor can provide short-term salvage therapy for patients whose disease progresses while receiving combinations of imatinib and chemotherapy. Dasatinib has a higher propensity for complications related to serositis, with significant pleural and peritoneal effusion.

Nelarabine (Arranon) has also recently been approved for the treatment of T-cell lymphoblastic disease. In a recommended dose of 1,500 $mg/m2$ on days 1, 3, and 5, this agent has produced response rates of 30% to 50% in heavily pretreated patients. Vinorelbine has produced remission in 50% of adults with relapsed ALL in a small pilot study.

TREATMENT OF AML

Although the chemotherapeutic agents used in the initial therapy for AML have not changed much in the past 30 years, our knowledge of the biology of leukemia

TABLE 4: AML induction and consolidation therapy

Induction		Consolidation	
AML			
Ara-C	200 mg/m² IV as continuous infusion × 7 d	Ara-C[b]	3 g/m² q12h IV as 2- to 3-h infusion on days 1, 3, and 5; repeat q28d × 4 cycles
IDA[a]	12 mg/m² IV on days 1-3		
ALSG regimen			
Ara-C[b]	3 g/m² IV q12h as 2- to 3-h infusion on days 1, 3, 5, and 7 (8 doses)	Ara-C	100 mg/m² IV as continuous infusion × 5 d
Daun	45-60 mg/m² IV on days 1-3	Daun	50 mg/m² IV × 2 d
VP-16	75 mg/m² IV × 7 d	VP-16	75 mg/m² IV × 5 d

ALSG = Australian Leukemia Study Group; AML = acute myelogenous leukemia; Ara-C = cytarabine; Daun = daunorubicin; IDA = idarubicin; VP-16 = etoposide

[a] Idarubicin has been substituted for daunorubicin, 45 mg/m², which had been the prevalent anthracycline used in clinical trials prior to 1993. Mitoxantrone, 10 mg/m² × 5 days, has also been used as an alternative.

[b] For patients < 60 years of age

has increased. The identification of prognostic factors can provide more realistic expectations of response to standard treatment and can define the population for whom investigational therapy is appropriate early in the course of disease.

Prognostic factors Cytogenetic abnormalities are the major predictors of remission and risk of relapse for patients with AML. Patients with translocation of genetic material involving core binding regions [t(15;17), t(8;21) inv(16), or t(16;16)] have a good prognosis, with remission rates of 88% and 5-year DFS rates of 55% to 80%, whereas patients with loss of genetic material from chromosome 5 or 7 (−5 or −5q, −7 or −7q) and complex karyotypic abnormalities (defined as more than five abnormalities) have lower rates of CR (30% to 40%) and DFS (5%) at 5 years. Patients with either normal or intermediate cytogenetic abnormalities have a CR rate of 67% and a 5-year DFS rate of 25% to 30%, based on data from a large CALGB trial using HDAC-based consolidation.

Internal duplication of FLT_3 can be found in one-third of patients with normal cytogenetics or in patients with t(15;17) (APL) but is uncommon in either poor-risk karyotypes or non-APL translocations. This abnormality does not appear to have an impact on remission, but it is a predictor for relapse (74% relapse rate in patients with a normal karyotype with an isolated FLT_3 mutation vs 46% for patients with wild-type FLT_3).

Mutations of nucleophosmin protein (NPM1), which shuttle nucleic acids and proteins from the nucleus to the cytoplasm as well as binding *p53*, are also a commonly reported abnormality, prevalent (47%) in patients with a normal karyotype. Although there is frequent overlap with FLT_3 mutations, patients with an isolated NPM1 mutation and a normal karyotype have a 60% DFS versus 40% for those with either wild-type or mutations of both FLT_3 and NPM1 and 20% for those with an isolated FLT_3 mutation. In patients with otherwise favorable cytogenetic abnormalities [t(8;21) or inv(16)], the presence of c-Kit mutation increases the risk of relapse.

Poor-risk cytogenetics, antecedent MDS, and a high incidence of multidrug resistance (MDR-1) protein are found more commonly in patients older than age 60, which accounts for the lower CR rates (30% to 55%) seen in older individuals compared with their younger counterparts (60% to 80%). Many older patients with preexisting MDS may clear marrow blasts with antileukemic treatment but may still have impaired hematopoiesis and persistent cytopenias, since they may have no normal residual stem cells to repopulate the marrow.

Induction therapy

Ara-C and an anthracycline such as daunorubicin or idarubicin (Idamycin) have been the standard drugs used for AML induction chemotherapy for 30 years (Table 4). Depending on the prognostic groups, remission rates of 60% to 80% are seen in younger (< age 60) patients and of 35% to 55% in patients older than age 60. Other agents such as mitoxantrone and etoposide also have antileukemic activity, but no significant increase in remission rates or relapse-free survival has been seen when mitoxantrone was substituted for an anthracycline or etoposide was added to infusional Ara-C and daunorubicin. Mitoxantrone and etoposide were compared with Ara-C and daunorubicin as induction for patients older than age 55 in SWOG (Southwest Oncology Group) trials; CR rates were 44% for Ara-C and daunorubicin and 33% for mitoxantrone and etoposide, and median survival was 8 and 6 months, respectively. Older patients (> 65 years) with poor-risk cytogenetics have a CR rate of < 30% CR rate with standard induction chemotherapy, whereas those with a normal or favorable karyotype have CR rates of 45% to 50%. Therefore, in older patients, deferring treatment until prognostic cytogenetic information is available may identify patients who will benefit from novel approaches.

One strategy to improve remission rates in younger patients has been to use higher doses of Ara-C during induction. Both the Australian Leukemia Study Group (ALSG) and the SWOG compared standard Ara-C and daunorubicin (and etoposide in the ALSG trial) with HDAC in patients < 50 years (Table 4). The CR rates were 71% and 74% for standard versus high-dose therapy in the ALSG study and 55% versus 58% in the SWOG trial. In both studies, there was a significantly higher DFS for the high-dose arm at 5 years (48% versus 25% for ALSG and 33% versus 22% for SWOG) but no difference in OS due to increased early toxicity.

Subgroups of patients may benefit from HDAC. In the SWOG trial, patients with CD34+ blasts had a low CR rate of 36% with standard Ara-C but an equivalent rate to those with CD34– blasts (58%) when treated with HDAC. There was a strong correlation between CD34 positivity and MDR-1 expres-

TABLE 5: AML relapse therapy

Ara-C	2-3 g/m² IV q12h as 3-h infusion × 8 doses	plus	Mitox	12 mg/m² IV on days 1-3[a] or
			Daun	60 mg/m² IV on days 5 and 6 or
			VP-16	100 mg/m² IV daily × 5 d[a]
Ara-C	2 g/m²/d IV × 5 d	plus	FdURD	300 mg/m²/d × 5 d + G-CSF[a] ± Ida 10 mg/m²/d on days 1-3
Mitox	10 mg/m² IV	plus	VP-16	100 mg/m² IV as 2-h infusion daily × 5 d
Gemtuz	4-9 mg/m² on days 1 and 14			

AML = acute myelogenous leukemia; Ara-C = cytarabine; Daun = daunorubicin; FdURD = fludarabine: G-CSF = granulocyte colony-stimulating factor; Gemtuz = gemtuzumab ozogamicin; Ida = idarubicin; Mitox = mitoxantrone; VP-16 = etoposide

[a] Also used for relapsed acute lymphoblastic leukemia

sion in this cohort, leading to the inference that HDAC might help overcome drug resistance.

However, a recent 1,700-patient German trial showed no difference in DFS when 2 cycles of HDAC and mitoxantrone (HAM) were compared with 1 cycle of the standard Ara-C–containing regimen followed by HAM. The overall DFS was 40% for both arms in patients younger than age 60 and 29% for those older than age 60; 80% of young patients received both cycles, whereas only one-third of patients over 60 received cycle 2 irrespective of dose intensity of the initial cycle.

Gemtuzumab ozogamicin (Mylotarg), an anti-CD33 antibody conjugated to the drug calicheamicin, was originally approved for the treatment of relapsed AML in older patients. Currently, there are two clinical trials in Great Britain and the United States evaluating the addition of gemtuzumab ozogamicin to standard Ara-C and daunorubicin or fludarabine, idarubicin, Ara-C, and G-CSF. Preliminary reports from the British trial showed a CR rate of 86% in patients < 60 years old.

Gemtuzumab ozogamicin has also been used as a single agent for induction in patients > 61 years who were considered too frail for conventional therapy with Ara-C and daunorubicin. A CR rate of 26% was achieved in 7 patients aged 61 to 75 years; no benefit was seen in 22 patients older than age 75 due to high early mortality (7 of 22 patients).

Therapy-related AML has a particularly poor prognosis. At best, only 50% of patients will achieve a remission, usually of brief duration (median, 5 months), despite the use of aggressive drug combinations. Allogeneic or unrelated-donor transplants appear to offer the only curative option in these patients, achieving a 3-year DFS rate of 25% in two studies of allogeneic transplantation.

INITIAL TREATMENT OF AML IN OLDER PATIENTS

The majority of AML patients are over age 60. They constitute a group whose disease is often poorly responsive to conventional Ara-C and anthracycline-based chemotherapy; who often have poor marrow regenerative capacity due to preexisting myelodysplasia; and who have comorbid conditions that lead to excessive mortality (> 15% at day 30) compared with 3% to 5% for younger patients treated with the same regimen. Novel approaches have included trials of hypomethylating agents such as azacitadine; or decitabine (Dacogen) either alone or combined with histone deacetylators like valproic acid.

> Amonifide, a topoisomerase II inhibitor that is not affected by the MDR p- glycoprotein pump, combined with standard-infusion Ara-C produced a CR rate of 44% among 80 patients with secondary AML (either myelodysplastic syndrome or related to therapy). Remission rates were comparable in patients < 60 years old (42%) and in patients ≥ 60 years old (39%). Cytogenetic abnormalities remained prognostic, with a CR rate of 58% for patients with an intermediate-risk karyotype and a CR rate of 18% for those with a poor-risk karyotype (Erba HP, Rizzieri DA, O'Donnell MR, et al: J Clin Oncol 25[18s]:7065, 2007).

In a recent trial of decitabine (20 mg/m^2/d IV over 2 h daily x 10 days) alone or combined with valproic acid, Blum et al reported a 44% response rate in 25 patients with untreated or relapsed AML in patients over age 60. Similar results were reported from M.D. Anderson Cancer Center using a 5 day course of decitabine at 20 mg/m^2/d and valproic acid (50 mg/kg). Clinical trials are now in progress combining decitabine with a more potent histone deacetylating agent, vorinostat.

Farnesyl transferase inhibitors such as tipifarnib (Zarnestra) and tandutinib are being evaluated as initial therapy for patients over age 70 with newly diagnosed AML. The CR rate for tipifarnib as a single agent was 15% in several phase I/II trials. Cloretazine, a sulfonylhydrazine alkylating agent, showed a 28% CR rate overall and a 39% CR rate in patients without antecedent myelodysplasia in phase I/II trials for AML patients over age 60. However, treatment-related mortality with this agent was comparable (18%) to that of standard induction chemotherapy.

A trial of an intermediate dose of clofarabine (1 g/m^2/d x 5 days) produced CR rates of 60% in untreated AML patients aged 50 to 70, with an acceptable mortality of 7%. Median remission durations, however, were short (8 months).

GM-CSF An ECOG study showed that granulocyte-macrophage colony-stimulating factor (GM-CSF, sargramostim [Leukine]), used following completion of induction chemotherapy in older patients (55–70 years old), shortened the duration of neutropenia by 6 days and, thus, decreased treatment-related mortality, leading to both an improved CR rate and longer survival. The FDA approved GM-CSF for use in this setting. However, other trials using different cytokines in younger patients have not shown a survival benefit.

Consolidation therapy

Once remission of AML is attained, consolidation chemotherapy is required to achieve a durable remission or cure. Standard consolidation regimens are listed in Table 4.

Increased dose intensity In a CALGB study, 596 patients in CR were assigned to receive 4 courses of postremission Ara-C in one of three dosages: 100 mg/m^2 as a continuous infusion for 5 days, 400 mg/m^2 as a continuous infusion for 5 days, or 3 g/m^2 as a 3-hour infusion every 12 hours on days 1, 3, and 5. For patients ≤ 60 years old, the percentage of patients in CR at 4 years was significantly higher in the HDAC group (44%) than in either the 400-mg/m^2 or 100-mg/m^2 group (29% and 24%, respectively). For patients > 60 years old, consolidation dose intensity had no impact on DFS, with all groups plateauing at a rate of 16% by 2 years.

Other approaches to consolidation include 1 to 3 cycles of consolidation followed by autologous or allogeneic bone marrow transplantation. Both of these approaches also tend to be limited to patients < 60 years old and have produced long-term DFS rates of 45% to 60% in several studies. (See chapter 36 for a more detailed discussion of transplantation approaches.) Long-term DFS is strongly influenced by cytogenetic and molecular abnormalities present at diagnosis. Transplant options should be considered for patients with high-risk features while in first remission due to poor outcomes with conventional chemotherapy. Patients with t(8;21), inv(16), or isolated NPM1, mutations can expect a 60% relapse-free survival following 3 to 4 cycles of HDAC. Molecular mutations are being used to identify patients with normal karyotypes with a high risk (≥ 50%) of relapse for whom multiple cycles of HDAC consolidation will not be sufficient to prevent relapse.

CNS prophylaxis

Routine CNS prophylaxis is recommended only for adult patients with AML at high risk of CNS recurrence, ie, patients with a WBC count > 50,000/µL at presentation or those with myelomonocytic or monocytic AML (FAB M4 or M5). Patients receiving HDAC (≥ 7.2 g/m^2) for induction or consolidation therapy achieve therapeutic drug levels in the cerebrospinal fluid, obviating the need for intrathecal therapy. Patients given conventional Ara-C doses may be treated with intrathecal methotrexate (12 mg IT) or Ara-C (30 mg IT). Both agents can be combined with hydrocortisone (30 mg IT) for patients with active CNS disease.

TREATMENT OF REFRACTORY OR RELAPSED AML

Patients who do not respond to initial therapy or who relapse within 6 months of attaining CR, as well as those with antecedent myelodysplasia or therapy-related AML, are considered to have relatively resistant disease.

Efforts to overcome drug resistance have focused on (1) HDAC-containing regimens, (2) new agents, (3) targeted therapy using leukemia-specific monoclonal antibodies conjugated with radionuclides or toxins, and (4) nonchemotherapeutic agents to block the drug efflux pump associated with MDR-1 gene expression.

HDAC High doses of Ara-C (2–3 g/m^2 for 8–12 doses) paired with mitoxantrone, etoposide, methotrexate, or fludarabine have produced short-lived CRs in 40% to 60% of relapsed patients with AML (see Table 5 for dosage regimens). Response rates were higher in patients who had received standard-dose Ara-C for induction and who had subsequently relapsed than in those in whom induction therapy had failed. The median duration of remission was 4 to 6 months.

Combinations of mitoxantrone and etoposide have been reported to produce a 40% to 50% CR rate in patients who had relapsed or for whom standard-dose Ara-C and anthracycline had failed, again with a median duration of remission of 4 to 6 months. Combinations of intermediate-dose Ara-C (1 g/m^2/d for 6 days) with mitoxantrone and etoposide produced CR rates of 79% in relapsed patients and 46% in those who did not respond to induction therapy or had AML evolving from MDS, with a median CR duration of 8 months.

New agents Nucleoside analogs, such as cladribine (2-CdA) and fludarabine, showed activity in pediatric AML. A British trial reported a 61% CR rate for a combination of fludarabine, Ara-C, G-CSF, and idarubicin, with a median CR duration of 7 months. The combination of gemcitabine (Gemzar; 600 mg/m^2/hr, with infusion durations escalating from 6–12 hours) and mitoxantrone (12 mg/m^2/d × 3 days) produced 5 CRs and 6 partial remissions among 26 patients with relapsed or refractory AML. The maximum tolerated duration of gemcitabine infusion was 12 hours, with stomatitis and esophagitis being the nonhematologic toxicities in 50% of patients. Another nucleoside analog, clofarabine, showed a 16% remission rate in a phase I/II trial in patients with relapsed AML as a single agent and a 38% remission rate when combined with Ara-C (1 g/m^2).

As previously mentioned, another class of chemotherapeutic agents being evaluated are farnesyl transferase inhibitors, which target signal transduction pathways. One of these agents, tipifarnib, showed a 29% response rate as a single agent in patients with relapsed or refractory AML. Currently, SWOG is evaluating two different doses and schedules of this drug in patients at least 70 years old with newly diagnosed AML.

Temozolomide (Temodar), an oral alkylating agent currently approved for the treatment of astrocytoma, has been shown to have activity against myeloid malignancy, with a 20% clearance of marrow blasts in 18 patients with high-risk myeloid malignancy following a 7-day course of medication. Prolonged marrow aplasia was the dose-limiting toxicity.

Targeted therapy Gemtuzumab ozogamicin has been approved by the FDA for the treatment of relapsed AML in older patients (Table 5), as mentioned previously. Aggregate data from three trials involving 277 patients, with a median age of 61 years, showed a 26% CR rate, with a median remission duration of 6.4 months.

TABLE 6: APL induction and consolidation therapy

Induction	Consolidation		Maintenance
PETHEMA LPA 99 **(Sanz, et al)**			
ATRA 45 mg/m²/d PO daily in 2 divided doses until hematologic remission (max 90 days)	**Cycle 1** IDA ATRA	5 mg/m²/d IV days 1-4 45 mg/m²/d PO days 1-15 (for intermediate/high)	6-MP 50 mg/m²/d PO days 1-15 ATRA 45 mg/m²/d PO days 1-15 ⎫ MTX 15 mg/m² Im days 1, 8 and 15 ⎬ q 3m × 24 m
IDA 12 mg/m²/d IV days 2, 4, 6, 8 (omit day 8 if patient > age 70)	**Cycle 2** Mitox ATRA	10 mg/m²/d IV days 1-5 45 mg/m²/d PO day 1-15 (for intermediate/high)	
	Cycle 3 IDA	12 mg/m² day 1 IV + ATRA 45 mg/m² PO days 1-12	
French APL 2000 **(Ades, et al)**			
ATRA 45 mg/m²/d PO DNR 60 mg/m² IV days 1-3 Ara-C 200 mg/m² CI days 1-7	**Cycle 1** DNR Ara-C	60 mg/m² IV days 1-3 200 mg/m² CI days 1-7	Same as LPA 99
	Cycle 2 DNR Ara-C	45 mg/m² IV days 1-5 1 g/m² IV over 3 h q12h 8 doses (2 g for patient < 60 years with WBC > 10,000/µL prophylactically) For patients with WBC ≥ 10,000 all patients receive 5 doses of intrathecal Ara-C for CNS prophylaxis	

TABLE 6: APL induction and consolidation therapy *(continued)*

Induction	Consolidation		Maintenance
MDA (Estey, et al)			
ATRA 45 mg/m²/d PO in 2 divided doses; day 1– hematologic response	ATO	0.15 mg/kg IV M-F weeks 1–4, 9–12, 17–20, 25–28, 33–36, and 42–46	Treatment for differentiation syndrome Stop ATRA ± ATO Methylprednisolone 45–60 mg IV every day × 7
	ATRA	45 mg/m²/d PO × 7 days each month (weeks 1, 5, 9, 13, 17, 21, 25, 29, 33, 37, 42)	
ATO 0.15 mg/kg IV over 1 h daily; day 10–until CR (marrow every wk beginning d 25 until < 5% blasts and no abnormal promyelocytes; median time to CR day 28 (19–48)			
Gemtuzumab 9 mg/m² IV day 1 for high-risk patients			

ATO = arsenic trioxide; APL = acute promyelocytic leukemia; Ara-C = cytarabine; ATRA = all-*trans*-retinoic acid; CI = continuous infusion; CR = complete response; DNR = daunorubicin; IDA = idarubicin; Mitox = mitoxantrone; MTX = methotrexate; 6-TG = thioguanine; 6-MP = mercaptopurine; VP-16 = etoposide; WBC = white blood cell

Treatment-related toxicity was low; the only infusional side effects were fever/chills and slow platelet plus granulocyte recovery (≥ 5 weeks). No cardiac or cerebellar toxicities were reported. Liver function abnormalities were reported in 25% to 30% of patients. The median CR duration for responding patients was 9 months.

Transplantation Although none of the previous options currently offers more than a 10% to 15% chance of long-term DFS, they do provide temporary cytoreduction sufficient to permit further high-dose treatment strategies, such as bone marrow transplantation using sibling, unrelated donor, or purged autologous marrow. Allogeneic bone marrow transplantation achieves a 30% to 40% DFS rate at 5 years in patients transplanted during first relapse or second remission. Autologous bone marrow transplantation also has curative potential for patients beyond first CR, with most large series reporting DFS rates of 30% to 35% in selected patients (usually those with good-risk cytogenetics or initial CR duration longer than 1 year).

Reduced-intensity conditioning regimens are being explored as treatment options in older patients and in those with comorbidity that would otherwise preclude full-dose allogeneic transplantation. Preliminary results from several centers have shown 1- and 2-year disease-free survival rates of 50% for patients aged 55 to 70 years receiving reduced-intensity allogeneic transplantation for consolidation of first remission.

New methods of marrow purging and post-transplant immune stimulation also are being explored to decrease relapse-related mortality.

TREATMENT OF APL

APL represents a uniquely homogeneous subset of AML defined by its cytogenetic abnormality, t(15;17), which results in fusion of the retinoic acid receptor (RAR) α-gene on chromosome 17 with the promyelocytic leukemia (PML) gene on chromosome 15. This abnormality yields the PML/RAR α-fusion protein, detectable by PCR techniques, which is useful for both diagnosis and evaluation of minimal residual disease. Most patients (80%) with APL have characteristic hypergranular blasts; laboratory evidence of DIC is present in 70% to 90% of patients at diagnosis or shortly after. Hemorrhagic events contribute 10% to 15% excess mortality during induction chemotherapy for APL compared with other AML subtypes.

Because of the unique biology and specific clinical features of APL, induction and consolidation regimens for APL differ from strategies used for other FAB types.

Involvement of the RAR α– gene in the pathogenesis of APL suggested the use of retinoids as therapy. A study from Shanghai showed CR rates of 85% with single-agent all-*trans*-retinoic acid (ATRA, tretinoin, Vesanoid). ATRA offered the advantages of a shorter neutropenic period (2 weeks) and slightly faster resolution of DIC (4 vs 7 days), as compared with standard chemotherapy with Ara-C and daunorubicin. Normalization of marrow morphology and cytogenetics requires 30 to 60 days of ATRA.

Initial treatment options

Based on data from the Spanish PETHEMA Group trials, a stratification schema of risk of relapse was constructed using WBC and platelet counts at presentation. Patients with a WBC count < 10,000/μL and a platelet count > 40,000/mL have a DFS of 97%; those with a WBC < 10,000/μL and a platelet count < 40,000/mL have a DFS of 86%; those with a WBC count > 10,000/μL have a DFS of 78%.

The backbone of APL induction therapy includes an anthracycline and ATRA (Table 6). The French and North American APL trials have also included standard dose Ara-C as an integral part of induction and consolidation. All three groups report CR rates in excess of 90% in patients with initial WBC count < 10,000 /μL. In a recent comparison of the outcomes from the Spanish LAP 99 trial and the French APL 2000 trial, the CR rates and 3- year survival rates were similar for the low- and intermediate- risk groups with a lower rate of relapse (4% vs 14%) and fewer days in the hospital (50 vs 72 days) for the group that did not receive Ara-C. In patients with elevated WBC counts ≥ 10,000, Ara-C during induction significantly increased CR rates (95% versus 83%). Survival at 3 years was also higher for the group receiving Ara-C, (92% vs 81%), and relapse was lower, (9.9% vs 18.8%). In the LAP 99 trial, the use of ATRA along with anthracycline in consolidation significantly decreased the relapse rate among the low- and intermediate- risk groups.

The most recent North American Intergroup trial showed improved relapse-free survival when 2 cycles of arsenic trioxide (Trisenox) were used as the initial component of consolidation. All three groups were monitored for molecular remission at the end of consolidation and at frequent intervals during 2 years of maintenance chemotherapy. Relapse rates are lower than 5% for low-risk patients, and new trials will evaluate the need for maintenance therapy for this group.

Small single-institution series have reported favorable remission and DFS rates in patients induced with arsenic trioxide alone (86% CR) or combined with ATRA (95% for low- and intermediate-risk patients). High-risk patients had poorer response rates (75% CR) despite the addition of gemtuzumab ozogamicin (9 mg/m^2) on day 1 of induction therapy.

APL syndrome Approximately 25% of patients with APL develop "differentiation syndrome" (formerly known as ATRA syndrome). Symptoms of this syndrome are fever, respiratory distress with pulmonary infiltrates or pleural effusions, and cardiovascular collapse. Temporary pseudotumor cerebri is a fairly common (10%) side effect of ATRA. Although these symptoms most often correlate with leukocytosis (WBC count > 10,000/μL), many patients develop symptoms with WBC counts between 5,000/μL and 10,000/μL. The syndrome is seen in patients treated with arsenic trioxide as well as in those treated with ATRA.

Treatment of this syndrome involves prompt use of high-dose steroids, initiation of conventional Ara-C/daunorubicin chemotherapy to control leukocytosis, and temporary discontinuation of ATRA or arsenic trioxide.

Relapse therapy Arsenic trioxide is now the standard reinduction therapy for patients with APL who are refractory to, or have relapsed from, retinoid and anthracycline chemotherapy. As a single agent, arsenic trioxide has produced CR in 34 of 40 patients (85%) with relapsed APL, with 86% of patients achieving molecular remission. Relapsed patients who achieved a molecular remission with arsenic trioxide alone had a median relapse-free survival of 18 months; those who received arsenic trioxide followed by autologous transplantation have had relapse-free survivals in excess of 70% at 2 years. Allogeneic transplantation should be reserved for those who do not achieve a molecular remission.

Although liver toxicity was reported with the use of arsenic trioxide in the original Chinese studies, the most significant toxicities in the US multicenter trial were the "APL syndrome," ventricular arrhythmia in patients with prolongation of the AT/QTc interval on electrocardiogram, and peripheral neuropathy. It is important to monitor potassium, magnesium, and calcium levels closely, almost daily, during arsenic trioxide therapy; maintaining these levels near the upper range of normal is important in preventing arrhythmia.

Gemtuzumab ozogamacin is also an effective agent for patients with relapsed APL. In a small series, 91% of patients with a molecular relapse of APL achieved a molecular remission following two doses of gemtuzumab ozogamicin (6 mg/m^2).

Monitoring response to therapy Reverse-transcriptase (RT)- PCR for the PML/RAR α– fusion protein can be used to follow response to therapy. The marker clears slowly, with many patients still testing positive following induction therapy. However, patients with persistence of PML/RAR α– fusion protein at the end of consolidation therapy are at high risk of relapse, as are those with reemergence of the marker following a period without detectable protein. Salvage chemotherapy should be considered for patients with persistent or recurrent confirmed molecular relapse.

SUGGESTED READING

ON ALL

Bruggemann M, Ruff T, Florhr T, et al: Clinical significance of minimal residual disease quantification in adult patients with standard risk acute lymphoblastic leukemia. Blood 107:1116–1123, 2006.

DeAngelo DJ, Yu D, Johnson JL, et al: Nelarabine induces complete remissions in adults with relapsed or refractory T-lineage acute lymphoblastic leukemia or lymphoblastic lymphoma: Cancer and Leukemia Group B study 19801. Blood 109:5136–5142, 2007.

Jabbour E, O'Brien S, Kantarjian H, et al: Neurologic complications associated with intrathecal liposomal cytarabine given prophylactically in combination with high-dose methotrexate and cytarabine to patients with acute lymphocytic leukemia. Blood 109:3214–3218, 2007.

Kantarjian H, Thomas D, O'Brien S, et al: Long-term follow-up results of hyperfractionated cyclophosphamide, vincristine, doxorubicin, and dexamethasone (Hyper-CVAD), a dose-intensive regimen, in adult acute lymphocytic leukemia. Cancer 101:2788–2801, 2004.

Mancini M, Scappaticci D, Cimino G, et al: A comprehensive genetic classification of adult acute lymphoblastic leukemia (ALL): Analysis of the GIMEMA 0496 protocol. Blood 105:3434–3441, 2005.

Moorman AV, Harrison CJ, Buck GA, et al: Karyotype is an independent prognostic factor in adult acute lymphoblastic leukemia (ALL): Analysis of cytogenetic data from patients treated on the Medical Research Council (MRC) UKALLXII/Eastern Cooperative Oncology Group (ECOG) 2993 trial. Blood 109:3189–3197, 2007.

Rowe JM, Buck G, Burnett AK, et al: Induction therapy for adults with acute lymphoblastic leukemia: Results of more than 1,500 patients from the International ALL trial. Blood 106:3760–3767, 2005.

Yanada M, Takeuchi J, Sagiura I, et al: High remission rate and promising outcome by combinations of imatinib and chemotheraapy for newly diagnosed BCR/ABL positive acute lymphoblastic leukemia: A phase II study by the Japan Adult Leukemia Study Group. J Clin Oncol 24:460–466, 2006.

ON AML

Applebaum FR, Gundacker H, Head DR, et al: Age and acute myeloid leukemia. Blood 107:3481–3485, 2006.

Bachner T, Berdal WE, Schoch C, et al: Double induction containing either two or one course of high dose cytarabine plus mitoxantrone and post remission therapy with either autologous stem-cell transplantation or by prolonged maintenance for acute myeloid leukemia. J Clin Oncol 29:2480–2489, 2006.

Faderl S, Verstovsek S, Cortes J, et al: Clofarabine and cytarabine combination as induction therapy for acute myeloid leukemia (AML) in patients 50 years of age or older. Blood 108:45–51, 2006.

Verhaak R, Goudswaard C, von Putten W, et al: Mutations in nucleophosmin (NPM1) in acute myeloid leukemia (AML): Association with other gene abnormalities and previously established gene expression signatures and their favorable prognostic significance. Blood 106:3747–3756, 2005.

ON APL

Ades L, Sanz MA, Chevret S, et al: Treatment of newly diagnosed acute promyelocytic leukemia (APL): A comparison of French-Belgian-Swiss and PETHEMA results. Blood [Epub Nov 2007].

Estey E, Garcia-Manero G, Ferrajuli A, et al: Use of all trans-retinoic acid plus arsenic trioxide as an alternative to chemotherapy in untreated acute promyelocytic leukemia. Blood 107:3469–3473, 2006.

Sanz MA, Martin G, Gonzalez M, et al: Risk-adapted treatment of acute promyelocytic leukemia with all-trans-retinoic acid and anthracycline monochemotherapy: A multicenter study by the PETHEMA group. Blood 103:1237–1243, 2004.

CHAPTER 33

Chronic myeloid leukemia

Jorge E. Cortes, MD, Richard T. Silver, MD, and Hagop Kantarjian, MD

Chronic myeloid leukemia (CML) is a clonal myeloproliferative disorder resulting from the neoplastic transformation of the primitive hematopoietic stem
cell. The disease is monoclonal in origin, affecting myeloid, monocytic, erythroid, megakaryocytic, B-cell, and, sometimes, T-cell lineages. Bone marrow
stromal cells are not involved.

CML accounts for 15% of all leukemias in adults. Approximately 4,830 new
cases of CML will be diagnosed in 2008, and it is estimated that 450 patients
will die of CML this year. The incidence is 1.7 per 100,000 population. With
imatinib (Gleevec) therapy, the annual mortality may be reduced significantly
(less than 2%–3% per year).

Epidemiology

Gender The male-to-female ratio is 1.1–1.4:1.

Age According to SEER (Surveillance, Epidemiology, and End Results) and
MRC (Medical Research Council, UK) data, the median age of patients with
CML is 66 years. However, most patients who are admitted to medical therapy
studies are 50–60 years old, with a median age of ~53 years. Patients in bone
marrow transplantation (BMT) studies are even younger, with a median age of
~40 years. Age differences must be considered in all studies because this variable may affect results.

Etiology and risk factors

The etiology of CML is unclear. Some associations with genetic and environmental
factors have been reported, but in most cases, no such factors can be identified.

Genetic factors There is little evidence linking genetic factors to CML. Offspring of parents with CML do not have a higher incidence of CML than the
general population.

Environmental factors Nuclear and radiation exposures, including therapeutic radiation, have been associated with the development of CML. Exposure to
chemicals has not been consistently associated with greater risk.

TABLE 1: Criteria for accelerated-phase CML according to MDACC, IBMTR, and WHO

Characteristic	MDACC	IBMTR	WHO
Blasts	15%–29%	10%–29%	10%–19%[a]
Blasts + promyelocytes	≥ 30%	≥ 20%	NA
Basophils	≥ 20%	≥ 20%[b]	≥ 20%
Platelets	< 100	Unresponsive ↑ or persistent ↓	< 100 or > 1,000 unresponsive
Cytogenetics	CE	CE	CE not at diagnosis
WBC	NA	Difficult to control or doubling in < 5 days	NA
Anemia	NA	Unresponsive	NA
Splenomegaly	NA	Increasing	NA
Other	NA	Chloromas, myelofibrosis	Megakaryocyte proliferation, fibrosis

[a] Blast phase ≥ 20% blasts (≥ 30% for MDACC and IBMTR)
[b] Basophils + eosinophils
CE = clonal evolution; IBMTR = International Bone Marrow Transplant Registry; MDACC = M. D. Anderson Cancer Center; NA = not applicable; WHO = World Health Organization

Signs and symptoms

CML usually runs a biphasic or triphasic course. This process includes an initial chronic phase and a terminal blastic phase, which is preceded by an accelerated phase in 60%–80% of patients.

Chronic phase If untreated, chronic-phase CML is associated with a median survival of 3.5–5.0 years. During the chronic phase, CML is asymptomatic in 25%–60% of all cases and, in these cases, is discovered on a routine blood examination.

In symptomatic patients, the most common presenting signs and symptoms are fatigue, left upper quadrant pain or mass, weight loss, and palpable splenomegaly. Occasionally, patients with very high WBC counts may have manifestations of hyperviscosity, including priapism, tinnitus, stupor, visual changes from retinal hemorrhages, and cerebrovascular accidents.

Patients in chronic-phase CML do not have an increased risk for infection. Splenomegaly is documented in 30%–70% of patients. The liver is enlarged in 10%–20% of cases.

Accelerated phase This is an ill-defined transitional phase. The criteria (M. D. Anderson Cancer Center [MDACC]) used recently in all the studies with tyrosine kinase inhibitors include the presence of 15%–29% blasts, ≥ 30% blasts and promyelocytes, or ≥ 20% basophils in the peripheral blood or a platelet count < 100 × 10⁹/L unrelated to therapy. Cytogenetic clonal evolution is also a criterion for acceleration. Other classifications include more subjective criteria (Table 1). The classification used may affect the expected outcome for a group of patients defined as accelerated phase. With imatinib therapy, the estimated 4-year survival rate exceeds 50%. Thus, a new definition of accelerated phase (ie, predictive for short survival) needs to be developed.

The accelerated phase is frequently symptomatic, including the development of fever, night sweats, weight loss, and progressive splenomegaly.

Blastic phase The blastic phase morphologically resembles acute leukemia. Its diagnosis requires the presence of at least 30% of blasts in the bone marrow or peripheral blood. The World Health Organization has proposed to consider blast phase with ≥ 20% blasts, but this classification has not been validated, and recent evidence suggests that patients with 20% to 29% blasts have a significantly better prognosis than those with ≥ 30% blasts. In some patients, the blastic phase is characterized by extramedullary deposits of leukemic cells, most frequently in the CNS, lymph nodes, skin, or bones.

Patients in blastic phase usually die within 3–6 months. Approximately 70% of patients in blastic phase have a myeloid phenotype; 25%, lymphoid; and 5%, undifferentiated. Prognosis is slightly better for a lymphoid blastic phase than for myeloid or undifferentiated cases (median survival 9 vs 3 months).

Patients in blastic phase are more likely to experience symptoms, including weight loss, fever, night sweats, and bone pain. Symptoms of anemia, infectious complications, and bleeding are common. Subcutaneous nodules or hemorrhagic tender skin lesions, lymphadenopathy, and signs of CNS leukemia may also occur.

Laboratory features

Peripheral blood The most common feature of CML is an elevated WBC count, usually $> 25 \times 10^9$/L and frequently $> 100 \times 10^9$/L, occasionally with cyclic variations. The finding of unexplained, persistent leukocytosis (eg, $> 12–15 \times 10^9$/L) in the absence of infections or other causes of WBC count elevation should prompt a work-up for CML.

The WBC differential usually shows granulocytes in all stages of maturation, from blasts to mature, morphologically normal granulocytes. Basophils are elevated, but only 10%–15% of patients have ≥ 7% basophils in the peripheral blood. Frequently, eosinophils are also mildly increased. The absolute lymphocyte count is elevated at the expense of T lymphocytes.

The platelet count is elevated in 30%–50% of patients and is higher than $1,000 \times 10^9$/L in a small percentage of patients with CML. When thrombocytopenia occurs, it usually signals disease acceleration.

Some patients have mild anemia at diagnosis.

Neutrophil function is usually normal or only mildly impaired, but natural killer (NK) cell activity is impaired. Platelet function is frequently abnormal but usually has no clinical significance.

Bone marrow The bone marrow is hypercellular, with cellularity of 75%–90%. The myeloid-to-erythroid ratio is usually 10–30:1. All stages of maturation of the WBC series are usually seen, but the myelocyte predominates.

Megakaryocytes are increased in number early in the disease and may show dysplastic features. They are usually smaller than the typical normal megakaryocytes. Fibrosis may be evident at diagnosis but increases with disease progression and is usually an adverse prognostic finding.

Other laboratory findings Leukocyte alkaline phosphatase activity is reduced at diagnosis. Serum levels of vitamin B_{12} and transcobalamin are increased, sometimes up to 10 times normal values. Serum levels of uric acid and lactic dehydrogenase (LDH) are also frequently elevated.

Cytogenetic and molecular findings

Philadelphia chromosome CML is characterized by the Philadelphia (Ph) chromosome, which represents a balanced translocation between the long arms of chromosomes 9 and 22, t(9;22)(q34;q11.2). The c-*abl* proto-oncogene located in chromosome 9q34 encodes for a nonreceptor protein-tyrosine kinase expressed in most mammalian cells. In chromosome 22, the breakpoint occurs within the BCR gene and usually involves an area known as the major breakpoint cluster region (m-*bcr*), located either between exons b3 and b4 or between exons b2 and b3. Therefore, two different fusion genes can be formed, both of them joining exon 2 of *abl* with either exon 2 (b2a2) or exon 3 of *bcr* (b3a2). Among the 5% to 10% of patients who do not have the Ph chromosome detected by karyotyping, 30% to 40% have the molecular rearrangement identified by fluorescent in situ hybridization (FISH)/polymerase chain reaction (PCR). Those patients without this rearrangement are considered to have "atypical CML," a unique entity with different prognosis and treatment.

Upon translation, a new protein with a molecular weight of 210 kd (p210$^{BCR-ABL}$) is synthesized, which, compared with the normal c-*abl*, has markedly increased kinase activity and can transform transfected cells and induce leukemia in transgenic mice. Occasionally, the breakpoint can occur in other areas (m-*bcr* and μ-*bcr*), leading to different transcripts (eg, p190$^{BCR-ABL}$ and p230$^{BCR-ABL}$, respectively). The mechanism of oncogenesis of p210$^{BCR-ABL}$ is unclear, but, upon phosphorylation, it can activate several intracellular pathways, including *ras* and the MAP kinase pathway, the Jak-Stat pathway, the PI3 kinase pathway, and the *myc* pathway. Ultimately, this leads to altered adhesion to extracellular matrix and stroma, constitutive activation of mitogenic signals, and inhibition of apoptosis.

Staging and prognosis

Staging systems Several characteristics of CML affect the prognosis, including age; spleen size; WBC and platelet counts; and percentage of blasts, eosinophils, and basophils in the peripheral blood. Deletions of the derivative chromosome 9 are identified in 10% to 15% of patients and have been associated with an adverse prognosis with most treatment modalities. Imatinib may overcome the adverse prognosis associated with del der(9). These factors have been incorporated into several staging systems.

Sokal's classification A frequently used risk classification is Sokal's prognostic risk system. In this system, the hazard ratio function is derived from the following formula: $\lambda_i(+)/\lambda_0(t)$ = Exp 0.0116 (age − 43.4) + 0.0345 (spleen − 7.51) + 0.188 [(platelets/700)^2 − 0.563] + 0.0887 (blasts − 2.10).

This risk classification defines three prognostic groups with hazard ratios of < 0.8, 0.8.–1.2, and > 1.2 (ie, low-, intermediate-, and high-risk).

The Hasford classification has been suggested to separate more clearly and without overlap risk groups among patients treated with interferon therapy. The Hasford score is derived from the formula (0.6666 × age [0 when age < 50 years; 1, otherwise] + 0.0420 × spleen size [cm below costal margin] + 0.0584 × blasts [%] + 0.0413 × eosinophils [%] + 0.2039 × basophils [0 when basophils < 3%; 1, otherwise] + 1.0956 × platelet count [0 when platelet count < 1,500 × 10^9/L; 1, otherwise]) × 1000. Based on the score, patients can be classified into three risk groups: low (score ≤ 780), intermediate (score > 780 and ≤ 1480), and high (≥ 1480). This classification may be less predictive in the imatinib era.

Treatment

CHRONIC PHASE

Conventional chemotherapy
Busulfan (Busulfex, Myleran) and hydroxyurea were the chemotherapeutic agents used most frequently in CML until the development of imatinib. Busulfan is now rarely used.

Hydroxyurea is most frequently used to control the WBC while confirming the diagnosis of CML. The usual dose of hydroxyurea is 40 mg/kg/d. The dose is then adjusted individually to keep the WBC count in a range between 4 and 10 × 10^9/L.

Neither busulfan nor hydroxyurea significantly reduces the percentage of cells bearing the Ph chromosome, and, therefore, the risk of transformation to the blastic phase is unchanged. Their use should be limited to temporary control of hematologic manifestations before definitive therapy (eg, imatinib, stem-cell transplantation) is instituted. Once the diagnosis of CML is confirmed, imatinib should be initiated immediately. There is no need or benefit to initially "debulking" with hydroxyurea.

Interferon
Recombinant interferon (rIFN-α) can induce a complete hematologic response (Table 2) in 70%–80% of patients with CML, with some degree of suppression of Ph chromosome-positive cells (ie, cytogenetic response) in 40%–60% of patients, which is complete in up to 20%–25% of patients. Randomized studies have documented a survival advantage for patients treated with rIFN-α who achieved a major, and particularly a complete, cytogenetic response.

TABLE 2: Response definitions in CML

Response	Category	Criteria
Hematologic remission	Complete	Normalization of WBC counts to < 9 × 10⁹/L with normal differential; normalization of platelet counts to < 450 × 10⁹/L; disappearance of all signs and symptoms of disease
Cytogenetic response[b]	Complete[a]	No evidence of Ph chromosome-positive cells
	Partial[a]	5%–34% of metaphases Ph chromosome-positive cells
	Minor	35%–95% of metaphases Ph chromosome-positive cells
	None	Persistence of Ph chromosome in all analyzable cells

[a] Major cytogenetic response includes complete and partial cytogenetic responses.
[b] Response assessed on routine cytogenetic analysis with at least 20 metaphases counted.

Patients who achieve a complete cytogenetic response have a 10-year survival rate of 75% or more.

Interferon and cytarabine (Ara-C) The combination of IFN-α and low-dose Ara-C induced a higher (ie, 40%–50%) response rate compared with rIFN-α alone, and possibly a survival advantage.

Approximately 30% of those achieving complete cytogenetic remission with IFN-α may achieve a sustained molecular remission and are probably cured. Among the others, 40% to 60% remain free of disease after more than 10 years despite the presence of minimal residual disease. This has been called "operational cure."

Formulations of rIFN-α attached to polyethylene glycol (PEG-IFN) have a longer half-life that allows for weekly administration and may have decreased toxicity.

Imatinib is a potent inhibitor of the tyrosine kinase activity of BCR-ABL and a few other tyrosine kinases, such as PDGF-R (platelet-derived growth factor-receptor) and c-*kit*. It has demonstrated significant activity in patients with CML in all phases of the disease, whether they have received prior therapy or not. Among patients with chronic-phase CML for whom prior IFN-α therapy failed, 55%–85% of patients achieved a major cytogenetic remission, including 45%–80% with a complete cytogenetic remission. The estimated rate of survival free of transformation to accelerated with blast phase is 69% at 60 months. Among patients treated in early chronic-phase CML who had not received prior therapy, the rate of complete cytogenetic response is 82%, with an overall survival rate at 72 months of 93%, and event-free survival, 83%.

Overall and event-free survival with imatinib therapy is significantly better than what has been seen with other therapies. Thus, imatinib has become the standard therapy for CML (Figure 1). The proper management of patients receiving imatinib is important.

Dose The standard dose of imatinib is 400 mg daily for chronic phase and 600 mg for accelerated and blastic phases. Dose reductions may be needed in some patients because of toxicity, but doses less than 300 mg daily are not recommended. Available data from the phase I study show a clear decrease in the probability of response with doses lower than 300 mg daily. Several studies have suggested that starting therapy for patients in chronic phase with a higher dose of imatinib (600 or 800 mg daily) may improve the rate of complete cytogenetic and molecular responses and the event-free and progression-free survival with adequate tolerance. A randomized trial is currently ongoing to address whether the standard dose should be changed.

Toxicity Imatinib is well tolerated. However, a significant fraction of patients develop grade 1–2 adverse events, including nausea, peripheral or periorbital edema, muscle cramps, diarrhea, skin rashes, weight gain, and fatigue. These events frequently are minor and either do not require therapy or respond to adequate early intervention. Fluid retention responds to diuretics when indicated; diarrhea can be managed with loperamide or other agents; nausea usually responds to prochlorperazine, promethazine, or other agents; muscle cramps can be managed with tonic water or quinine; skin rash may be managed with antihistamines and/or corticosteroids (topical and/or systemic).

Myelosuppression is the most common grade 3–4 adverse event. Neutropenia can be seen in up to 45% of patients, thrombocytopenia in up to 25% of patients, and anemia in 10% of patients. Treatment is held for grade ≥ 3 neutropenia (neutrophil count $< 10^9/L$) or thrombocytopenia (platelet count $< 50 \times 10^9/L$) and restarted when counts recover above these levels. If the recovery takes longer than 2 weeks, the dose may be reduced. Treatment interruptions and dose reductions are not usually recommended for anemia. Myelosuppression is much more likely to occur during the first 2 to 3 months of therapy and is best managed

Early data from a phase III randomized, controlled clinical trial, Tyrosine Kinase Inhibitor Optimization and Selectivity Study (TOPS), show that responses occurred significantly faster with an 800 mg dose of imatinib in patients with newly diagnosed CML. The TOPS study was designed to evaluate the potential benefits of an 800 mg starting dose of imatinib across all risk categories of newly diagnosed, previously untreated patients with Philadelphia chromosome-positive chronic myeloid leukemia (Ph+ CML). Investigators reported that significantly more patients achieved a major molecular response (MMR) with the 800 mg dose than the 400 mg dose at 3, 6 and 9 months, although at 12 months the difference was not statistically significant (54% vs 46%). This trend toward improved time to MMR in the 800 mg vs 400 mg arms was most pronounced in the subset of patients with high-risk Sokal scores (41.1% vs 26.2%). The investigators added that further follow-up will be needed to assess what this rapid early response will mean in terms of long-term benefit. These data were presented at the recent Congress of the European Hematology Association (EHA), June 2008, in Copenhagen.

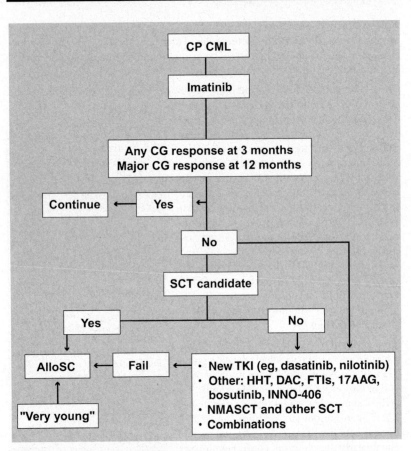

Figure 1: Treatment algorithm including imatinib for chronic-phase CML.

AlloSC = allogeneic stem–cell; CG = cytogenetic response; CP = chronic phase; DAC = decitabine; FTIs = farnesyl transferase inhibitors; HHT = homoharringtonine; NMASCT = nonmyeloablative allogeneic stem–cell transplantation; SCT = stem–cell transplantation; TKI = tyrosine kinase inhibitor

with treatment interruption and close monitoring. Hematopoietic growth factors (granulocyte colony-stimulating factor [G-CSF, filgrastim, Neupogen] and erythropoietin) have been used successfully to manage prolonged or recurrent myelosuppression but the long-term safety of this approach needs to be assessed.

Monitoring The treatment objective has evolved from hematologic responses (hydroxyurea) to cytogenetic responses (IFN-α), to molecular responses in the imatinib era. All patients have to be evaluated with cytogenetic analysis before the start of therapy, and a baseline quantitative PCR analysis is useful. Conventional cytogenetic analysis is important at baseline and for follow-up because it provides valuable information about the entire karyotype (ie, clonal evolution, cytogenetic abnormalities in Ph chromosome-negative cells) that cannot be obtained with FISH or PCR and has prognostic implications. A cytogenetic analysis every 3 to 6 months during the first year and every 6 to 12 months thereafter is recommended. Quantitative PCR is recommended every 3 to 6 months. It is inappropriate not to follow patients with cytogenetics and real-time PCR.

Duration of therapy At this time, the duration of therapy is unclear. A minority of patients have reached undetectable levels of disease by PCR, and few have discontinued therapy. This has usually resulted in relapse. Thus, until further evidence becomes available, patients should continue therapy indefinitely.

Allogeneic BMT

Allogeneic BMT is potentially curative in CML, although relapses and mortality from complications such as chronic graft-vs-host disease (GVHD) may occur many years after transplantation. Results are better for patients in the chronic phase than in either the accelerated or blastic phase. Long-term survival rates of 50%–80% and disease-free survival rates of 30%–70% can be achieved in the chronic phase. The role of BMT is now changing in view of the results obtained with imatinib.

Predictors of response Early BMT within the first 1–3 years after diagnosis may be associated with a better outcome than BMT later in the course of disease. Younger patients also have a better outcome than older patients, with those younger than age 20 to 30 having the best prognosis. The use of the European Bone Marrow Transplant (EBMT) score helps to separate those patients who may have a better outcome from those who will not.

The higher potency of the new tyrosine kinase inhibitors compared to imatinib and the significant clinical activity seen with these agents after imatinib failure has prompted investigation of these agents as first-line therapy for patients with CML in early chronic phase. In one study, 47 patients with previously untreated CML in chronic phase were treated with nilotinib 400 mg orally twice daily. Responses occurred very rapidly, with 100% of evaluable patients achieving a complete cytogenetic response by 6 months from the start of therapy. Major molecular response had been achieved by this time in 50% of patients. Treatment was well tolerated, with minimal extramedullary toxicity, and grade 3-4 neutropenia in 13% of patients and thrombocytopenia in 6% (*Cortes J, O'Brien S, Ferrajoli A, et al: J Clin Oncol [abstract] 26:376s, 2008*). In a similar study dasatinib was investigated in this patient population in two different schedules: 50 mg twice daily or 100 mg once daily. At 6 months from the start of therapy 94% of patients had achieved a complete cytogenetic response, and 23% a major molecular response. Treatment was well tolerated, with minimal grade 3 non-hematologic toxicity, and grade 3-4 thrombocytyopenia in 11% and neutropenia in 23% (*Borthakur G, Kantarjian HM, O'Brien S, et al: J Clin Oncol [abstract] 26:375s, 2008*). Randomized studies comparing these strategies to standard dose imatinib are ongoing.

Conditioning regimens, including total-body irradiation (TBI), have been traditionally used, but non–TBI-containing regimens (eg, with busulfan and cyclophosphamide [Cytoxan, Neosar]) have produced similar results. More recently, conditioning regimens using pharmacologic targeting of busulfan have been associated with decreased regimen-related toxicity while preserving the antileukemia effect.

Also, nonmyeloablative conditioning regimens frequently containing purine analogs (mini-BMT) have been tested recently to expand the use of transplants to older patients or to patients with medical conditions that preclude conventional BMT.

Graft-vs-host disease The major morbidity from BMT is GVHD. T-cell depletion of the graft can reduce the incidence of this complication but at the expense of higher relapse and graft failure rates. (For a full discussion of GVHD, see chapter 36.)

Alternatives to matched-related donors For patients who do not have a matched-related donor, matched unrelated donor (MUD) transplants are reasonable alternatives. The 9-year experience from the National Marrow Donor Program in 1,432 patients reported a 3-year survival rate of 37.5%. Early transplantation results in better outcome, with patients transplanted in chronic phase having a 3-year disease-free survival of 63%. The outcome of patients transplanted in accelerated, blastic, or second chronic phase is inferior.

Relapse after BMT Donor leukocyte infusions are the most effective strategy to treat patients who relapse after BMT. With this strategy, 70%–80% of patients can achieve a cytogenetic complete response; the best results are achieved when patients are treated during cytogenetic or molecular relapse. Imatinib has also been effective for patients who relapse after BMT. A complete hematologic response in > 70% of patients and a cytogenetic response in 58% have been reported, with the best responses obtained in patients relapsing in chronic phase.

Imatinib failure The most frequently identified mechanism of resistance to imatinib is the development of mutations at the Abl kinase domain. Mutations are identified in 40% to 60% of patients, with the most frequent occurring in the P-loop. Not all mutations confer the same level of resistance to imatinib, and some may be overcome by increased concentrations of imatinib. The most resistant mutation is T315I. Although P-loop mutations have been reported to be linked to a poor prognosis, this theory has not been confirmed in all studies and it is probably more appropriate to consider individual mutations rather than group them by location.

Changing therapy based on molecular responses cannot be justified in most instances at the present time. Even when patients who have not achieved a 3-log reduction in transcript levels after 12 months of therapy have an inferior prognosis compared with those with at least a 3-log reduction, they still have a 92% probability of disease progression-free survival at 3 years, and in most instances, this only represents a loss of cytogenetic response. If the proposed alternative treatment option has any significant risk of mortality, the risk may be unnecessary. The clinical significance of the presence of mutations in patients with an adequate response is still unclear. Thus, mutations should be investigated in patients with clinical evidence of failure. In this setting, a change of therapy is indicated whether a mutation is indicated or not, but in some instances specific mutations may guide the selection of therapy.

The European LeukemiaNet has established criteria for failure that have become standard (Table 3). These emphasize the response achieved and the time to such response. Patients who meet criteria for failure should be offered therapy with a second-generation tyrosine kinase inhibitor. For patients with suboptimal response there are no available data as to what the optimal management may be, although imatinib dose escalation is usually recommended. A second generation of tyrosine kinase inhibitors has been developed to overcome resistance to imatinib. Two of these agents have recently gained regulatory approval (dasatinib [Sprycel] and nilotinib [Tasigna], and others are being developed (Bosutinib, INNO-406). Nilotinib was designed based on the imatinib structure, with modifications to improve its binding to BCR-ABL and increase its selectivity; these modifications result in an agent at least one order of magnitude more potent than imatinib against BCR-ABL. Dasatinib is structurally unrelated to imatinib and, in contrast to it, can bind both the inactive and active configurations of BCR-ABL. In addition, dasatinib is a dual inhibitor that blocks Src as well as Abl and is two orders of magnitude more potent than imatinib. Both agents have been shown to inhibit both the wildtype BCR-ABL and nearly all of the clinically significant mutants of Bcr-Abl, except for T315I. The results from the initial clinical trials have been impressive.

Dasatinib and nilotinib have been approved for treatment of patients with resistance or intolerance to imatinib. Other agents have also shown activity in this setting and may have unique properties. Bosutinib is an inhibitor of Bcr-Abl and Src family of kinases, but in contrast to imatinib, nilotinib and dasatinib, it has no effect against PDGFR and c-Kit. This increased selectivity could offer an improved toxicity profile. Bosutinib has been investigated in patients with CML who have failed other agents. Among those resistant to imatinib, 40% have achieved a major cytogenetic response after median follow up of only 6 months, with major molecular response in 35%. No pleural effusions have been reported and grade 3-4 thrombocytopenia has been reported in 19% and neutropenia in 10% (Bruemmendorf TH, Cervantes F, Kim D, et al: J Clin Oncol [abstract] 26:384s, 2008). INNO-406 inhibits Bcr-Abl and Lyn, and crosses the blood-brain barrier. In a study for patients who had failed at least imatinib (most had failed also nilotinib and or dasatinib), 3 of 46 patients achieved a complete cytogenetic response. (Pinilla-Ibarz J, Kantarjian HM, Cortes JE, et al: J Clin Oncol [abstract] 26:376s, 2008).

Dasatinib The initial phase II trials used a dose of 70 mg twice daily. Significant clinical activity was seen in patients in all stages of the disease after imatinib resistance or intolerance, with complete cytogenetic responses in 53% in chronic phase, 33% in accelerated phase, 27% in myeloid blast phase, and 46% in lymphoid blast phase. Duration of response correlates with the stage of the disease, with progression free-survival of 80% at 24 months for those in chronic phase, and 46% in accelerated phase. In contrast, the median progression-free survival was 5.6 and 3.1 months, respectively, for those in myeloid and lymphoid blast phase. Some of the most significant adverse events include myelosuppression (grade 3-4 neutropenia and thrombocytopenia in nearly 50% each), pleural effusion, and gastrointestinal hemorrhage (particularly in the advanced stages). Alternative schedules may improve the toxicity profile. In a randomized study, dasatinib administered as 100 mg once daily was associated

None of the currently available kinase inhibitors has significant activity against T315I. Homoharringtonine (omacetaxine) has been shown to have pre-clinical activity against cells carrying this mutation. In a phase II study of patients with CML resistant to imatinib and T315I mutation, hematologic responses have been reported in 64% of patients treated in chronic phase (complete hematologic response in 45%), 100% of those in accelerated phase, and 34% of patients in blast phase. Cytogenetic responses occurred in 27% of patients treated in chronic phase and 25% of those in accelerated phase. T315I transcripts became undetectable in 50% of all patients. Thus, homoharringtonine offers a good treatment option for patients with this mutation *(Benichou A, Khoury HJ, Corm S, et al: J Clin Oncol [abstract] 26:377s, 2008).*

with significantly less myelosupression and pleural effusion compared to 70 mg twice daily (and to 50 mg twice daily or 140 mg once daily). The response to therapy was identical, with a trend toward improved progression-free survival with the 100 mg once daily schedule. Dasatinib is approved for treatment of patents with CML in all phases of the disease who have experienced resistance or intolerance to imatinib. The standard dose for patients in chronic phase is 100 mg once daily, and 70 mg twice daily for patients in advanced stages.

Nilotinib Significant activity has been documented in patients treated after imatinib failure with nilotinib 400 mg twice daily in phase II studies. Rates of CCgR for patients treated in chronic phase after imatinib resistance or intolerance were 42% and for those treated in accelerated phase 19%. Responses have been durable with a sustained MCyR at 18 months in 84% of patients treated in chronic phase. In accelerated phase progression-free survival is 57% at 12 months. The most significant toxicities reported have been myelosuppression (grade 3-4 neutropenia or thrombocytopenia in approximately 30%, each), and biochemical abnormalities (elevation of indirect bilirubin, lipase, and glucose) that have been usually transient and asymptomatic. There is also the potential for QTc prolongation (a class effect for all tyrosine kinase inhibitors), although less than 3% of patients have had significant prolongation, most frequently asymptomatic. Nilotinib is currently approved for treatment of patients in chronic or accelerated phase of the disease who have experienced resistance or intolerance to imatinib, and the standard dose is 400 mg twice daily. Nilotinib should be taken on an empty stomach as food may significantly increase the absorption.

Other agents Other investigational agents are being developed for patients who fail imatinib therapy. Bosutinib is another Src and Abl inhibitor with activity against most mutants of BCR-ABL. Early results auggest significant activity among patients who fail imatinib therapy. Bosutinib has minimal or no activity against PDGF-R and *c-kit*, which could lead to decreased toxicity (eg, pleural effusions and myelosuppression). INNO-406 has activity against Lyn and Abl and has also shown activity in patients who have failed imatinib and other tyrosine kinase inhibitors. Several agents are being developed to treat patients with the T315I mutation that is resistant to all available agents. These include homoharringtonine, MK-0457, XL-228, PHA-739358, DCC-2036, and AP24534. Early results from these trials suggest activity in some patients.

TABLE 3: European LeukemiaNet Criteria for failure

Time (mo)	Response Failure	Suboptimal
3	No HR	No CHR
6	No CHR 100% Ph+	≥ 35% Ph+
12	≥ 35% Ph+	≥ 5% Ph+
18	≥ 5% Ph+	No MMR (< 3-log ⇓ BCR-ABL/ABL)
Any	Loss of CHR Loss of CCgR Mutation	Clonal evolution Loss of MMR Mutation

CCgR = complete cytogenetic response; CHR = complete hematologic response; HR = hematologic response; MMR =major molecular response; Ph+ = Philadelphia chromosome positive

Treatment recommendations

The long-term results of imatinib are excellent with an overall survival of greater than 90% at 6 years. Thus, all patients in chronic phase should be offered standard-dose imatinib as initial therapy. Patients should be followed closely to determine that the expected results are met at the specified times (Table 3). If this is the case, treatment should continue uninterrupted indefinitely. For patients with suboptimal response, a dose escalation is recommended. For patients with failure to respond to imatinib, a change in therapy should be considered to one of the second-generation tyrosine kinase inhibitors.

Allogeneic stem cell transplant The role of transplant in CML has changed and nowadays it is considered mostly a second-line treatment option. For patients who fail imatinib therapy, transplant should be considered, although an initial trial with a second-generation tyrosine kinase inhibitor should be considered. Adequate response at early time points is important, particularly for young patients with a transplant option. If there is no cytogenetic response at 6 months or no major cytogenetic response by 12 months, transplant should be considered in such patients.

ACCELERATED AND BLASTIC PHASES
Imatinib

Imatinib is also effective for patients with CML in transformation. Seventy-one percent of patients in accelerated phase treated with 600 mg/d of imatinib had a hematologic response. The major cytogenetic response rate was 24%, with a time to disease progression of 12 months at 67%. These results are significantly superior to those with 400 mg/d, making 600 mg/d the standard dose in accelerated phase. In blast phase, 52% of patients achieved a hematologic remission and 31% a sustained remission lasting at least 4 weeks with imatinib. However, the median response duration is only 10 months, even when considering only patients with sustained remission (ie, lasting at least 4 weeks). Patients with clonal evolution have a lower probability of response and shorter survival than patients without clonal evolution when treated with imatinib.

Nilotinib and dasatinib also have significant clinical activity in patients with advanced stage disease. They should be considered for patients who have failed prior therapy, including imatinib.

BMT

Compared with those results in patients in chronic phase, results with allogeneic BMT are worse in patients in accelerated or blastic phase, with 4-year survival rates of only 10%–30%. Patients in accelerated phase (determined on the basis of clonal evolution only) who undergo BMT < 1 year after diagnosis have a 4-year probability of survival of 74%. Patients in blast phase who respond to therapy with a second-generation tyrosine kinase inhibitor should be offered a BMT in second chronic phase if an adequate donor is available.

SUGGESTED READING

Apperley JF: Part I: Mechanisms of resistance to imatinib in chronic myeloid leukaemia. Lancet Oncol 8:1018–1029, 2007.

Apperley JF: Part II: Management of resistance to imatinib in chronic myeloid leukaemia. Lancet Oncol 8:1116–1128, 2007.

Baccarani M, Saglio G, Goldman J, et al: Evolving concepts in the management of chronic myeloid leukemia: Recommendations from an expert panel on behalf of the European LeukemiaNet. Blood 108:1809–1820, 2006.

Bocchia M, Gentili S, Abruzzese E, et al: Effect of a p210 multipeptide vaccine associated with imatinib or interferon in patients with chronic myeloid leukaemia and peristent residual disease: A multicentre observational trial. Lancet 365:657–662, 2005.

Cortes J, Jabbour E, Kantarjian H, et al: Dynamics of BCR-ABL kinase domain mutations in chronic myeloid leukemia after sequential treatment with multiple tyrosine kinase inhibitors. Blood 110:4005–4011, 2007.

Cortes J, Rousselot P, Kim DW, et al: Dasatinib induces complete hematologic and cytogenetic responses in patients with imatinib-resistant or -intolerant chronic myeloid leukemia in blast crisis. Blood 109:3207–3213, 2007.

Cortes J, Talpaz M, O'Brien S, et al: Molecular responses in patients with chronic myelogenous leukemia in chronic phase treated with imatinib mesylate. Clin Cancer Res 11:3425–3432, 2005.

Druker BJ, Guilhot F, O'Brien SG, et al: Five-year follow-up of patients receiving imatinib for chronic myeloid leukemia. N Engl J Med 355:2408–2417, 2006.

Guilhot F, Apperley J, Kim DW, et al: Dasatinib induces significant hematologic and cytogenetic responses in patients with imatinib-resistant or -intolerant chronic myeloid leukemia in accelerated phase. Blood 109:4143–4150, 2007.

Hochhaus A, Kantarjian HM, Baccarani M, et al: Dasatinib induces notable hematologic and cytogenetic responses in chronic-phase chronic myeloid leukemia after failure of imatinib therapy. Blood 109:2303–2309, 2007.

Kantarjian H, Pasquini R, Hamerschlak N, et al: Dasatinib or high-dose imatinib for chronic-phase chronic myeloid leukemia after failure of first-line imatinib: A randomized phase 2 trial. Blood 109:5143–5150, 2007.

Kantarjian H, Schiffer C, Jones D, Cortes J: Monitoring the response and course of chronic myeloid leukemia in the modern era of BCR-ABL tyrosine kinase inhibitors: Practical advice on the use and interpretation of monitoring methods. Blood 111:1774–1780, 2008.

Kantarjian HM, Giles F, Gattermann N, et al: Nilotinib (formerly AMN107), a highly selective BCR-ABL tyrosine kinase inhibitor, is effective in patients with Philadelphia chromosome-positive chronic myelogenous leukemia in chronic phase following imatinib resistance and intolerance. Blood 110:3540–3546, 2007.

Kantarjian H, Talpaz M, O'Brien S, et al: Survival benefit with imatinib mesylate therapy in patients with accelerated-phase chronic myelogenous leukemia: Comparison with historic experience. Cancer 103:2099–2108, 2005.

le Coutre P, Ottmann OG, Giles F, et al: Nilotinib (formerly AMN107), a highly selective BCR-ABL tyrosine kinase inhibitor, is active in patients with imatinib-resistant or -intolerant accelerated-phase chronic myelogenous leukemia. Blood 111:1834–1839, 2008.

Quintas-Cardama A, Kantarjian H, Cortes J: Flying under the radar: The new wave of BCR-ABL inhibitors. Nat Rev Drug Discov 6:834–848, 2007.

Quintas-Cardama A, Kantarjian H, O'Brien S, et al: Pleural effusion in patients with chronic myelogenous leukemia treated with dasatinib after imatinib failure. J Clin Oncol 25:3908–3914, 2007.

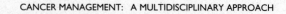

CHAPTER 34

Chronic lymphocytic leukemia

William G. Wierda, MD, PhD, Nicole Lamanna, MD, and Mark A. Weiss, MD

Chronic lymphocytic leukemia (CLL) is a clonal malignancy that results from expansion of the mature lymphocyte compartment. This expansion is a consequence of prolonged cell survival, despite a varied cell. The affected lymphocytes are of B-cell lineage in 95% of cases, and the remaining cases involve T lymphocytes, representing a distinct disorder.

CLL is the most common leukemia in adults in Western countries, accounting for approximately 25% to 30% of all leukemias. The proportion of cases diagnosed with the early stages of the disease (Rai stage 0) has risen from 10% to 50%, probably because of earlier diagnosis (routine automated blood counts).

Epidemiology

The incidence of CLL in the general population is 3.9:100,000 population, with an estimated death rate of 1.1:100,000 population. It was estimated that there were 15,340 patients diagnosed with CLL in 2007.

Gender The male-to-female ratio is 2:1. There is little change with age, as the male-to-female ratio is 2.1:1.0 for patients < 65 years old, compared with 1.9:1.0 for those ≥ 65 years old.

Age The median age at diagnosis is 72 years, and CLL is rarely seen before the age of 35 years. Less than 3% of all cases are younger than 45 years at the time of diagnosis.

Race In the American population, the incidence of CLL is similar in different races. However, the incidence is much lower in Asia (Japan, Korea, and China), Latin America, and Africa than in the United States and Western Europe.

Etiology and risk factors

The etiology of CLL is unclear. However, some factors associated with CLL have been identified.

Genetic factors There is a high familial risk for CLL, with family members of CLL patients having a twofold to sevenfold higher risk of developing the disease. CLL with a familial association tends to occur in younger individuals with subsequent generations, perhaps because of increased screening. Association

CLL

with certain human lymphocyte antigen (HLA) patterns has not been consistent.

Environmental factors There is no documented association of CLL with exposure to radiation, alkylating agents, or known leukemogenic chemicals. However, exposure to some chemicals used in agriculture may increase the risk of developing CLL.

Viral infections Associations between CLL and several viruses, including human T-cell lymphotrophic viruses I and II (HTLV-I and HTLV-II) and Epstein-Barr virus (EBV), have been suggested. However, no conclusive evidence of a causal relationship exists. Adult T-cell leukemia/lymphoma, a T-cell disorder that can resemble CLL, is caused by HTLV-I.

Monoclonal B lymphocytosis In one study, 3.8% of unselected healthy individuals older than age 65 in the general population had monoclonal (by light chain analysis) $CD5^+/19^+/23^+$ B cells. These asymptomatic individuals did not have lymphocytosis or clinical evidence of disease and did not fulfill diagnostic criteria for CLL. Whether or not these individuals will eventually develop diagnostic criteria or symptomatic disease is unknown. Nevertheless, this finding indicates that the incidence of a monoclonal lymphoproliferative process is potentially much more common in the aging population than previously appreciated.

Signs and symptoms

In the majority of patients, CLL is asymptomatic at diagnosis and is discovered on a routine blood examination. When symptoms are present, they are nonspecific and include fatigue, weakness, and malaise and, in fact, may not even be attributable to CLL.

Constitutional B symptoms (ie, fever, weight loss, and night sweats) are not common at diagnosis but may signal disease transformation. Patients frequently notice enlarged lymph nodes or abdominal discomfort and early satiety related to splenomegaly.

Patients with CLL have an increased susceptibility to infections, which may be the presenting complaint.

Lymphadenopathy is common at diagnosis. Lymph nodes are usually symmetrical, mobile, and nontender.

Splenomegaly and hepatomegaly The spleen and, less frequently, the liver may be enlarged. Splenomegaly may be massive in advanced cases. Only occasionally is splenomegaly found in the absence of lymphadenopathy, but recognition of such patients may identify a group that may benefit from splenectomy.

Other organs In advanced disease, other organs may be involved, including the GI mucosa, prostate, lungs, pleura, and bones. Rarely is such involvement clinically important unless (Richter's) transformation has occurred.

TABLE 1: Diagnostic criteria for CLL according to the National Cancer Institute (NCI) and International Workshop on CLL (IWCLL)

Cells	NCI	IWCLL
Lymphocytes	$\geq 5 \times 10^9/L + \geq 1$ B-cell marker (CD19, CD20, CD23) + CD5, monoclonal	$\geq 10 \times 10^9/L +$ B-cell phenotype or bone marrow involvement
Atypical cells (eg, prolymphocytes)	< 55%	Not stated
Bone marrow lymphocytes	$\geq 30\%$	> 30%

Laboratory features

Peripheral blood The most consistent feature of CLL lymphocytosis, with median values of $30–50 \times 10^9/L$. The lymphocytes are small and mature-appearing, with little cytoplasm and clumped chromatin. A few larger nucleolated cells, which represent prolymphocytes, usually constitute < 10% of the total lymphocytes. Diagnostic criteria for CLL defined by the National Cancer Institute (NCI) and International Workshop on CLL (IWCLL) are presented in Table 1.

A positive Coombs' test is seen in as many as 30% of patients at some time during the disease course, although it is uncommon (< 5%) during early stages. Autoimmune phenomena are relatively frequent, with hemolytic anemia (lifetime risk, approximately 10% to 20%) and thrombocytopenia (lifetime risk, approximately 5% to 10%) occurring most commonly. Autoimmune neutropenia and other autoimmune sequelae are infrequent but more common than in the general population.

Bone marrow The bone marrow is usually hypercellular but can be normocellular. The most characteristic feature is the presence of at least 30% mature lymphocytes. The lymphocyte infiltration can be interstitial, nodular, mixed interstitial and nodular, or diffuse. Diffuse lymphocyte infiltration is associated with a poor prognosis.

Other laboratory findings Progressive hypogammaglobulinemia is seen in > 50% of patients with CLL, usually affecting IgA first, followed by IgM and IgG. However, 5% to 10% of patients may have a small monoclonal peak. Paraproteinemia is more common at disease transformation.

Elevated serum levels of B_2-microglobulin ($\beta2M$) have been associated with a poor prognosis. Elevation of serum lactate dehydrogenase (LDH) levels is found in < 10% of patients at diagnosis and may indicate autoimmune hemolytic anemia or (Richter's) transformation to large-cell lymphoma (LCL).

Immunophenotyping More than 95% of all cases of CLL have a B-cell phenotype with monoclonality by light chain restriction. In these patients, CD19 and/or CD20 are essentially always coexpressed with CD5, which normally is expressed on T cells and a subset of normal B cells. Other markers, such as CD21 and CD22, may also be expressed. Expression of CD23 helps to differentiate CLL from mantle cell lymphoma, in which cells coexpress CD19 and CD5 but lack CD23. Furthermore, the monoclonal antibody FMC7 (which recognizes an epitope on CD20) rarely reacts with CLL cells but frequently binds the cells of patients with mantle cell lymphoma.

Expression of surface immunoglobulin is usually weak and is lower than in normal B lymphocytes or most other B-cell lymphomas. Expression of CD38 on the surface of CLL cells portends a worse prognosis than that for patients whose cells do not express CD38.

Cytogenetic and molecular findings

Chromosomal abnormalities

A number of recurrent cytogenetic abnormalities have been identified in CLL. Most have not been associated with a specific gene defect or abnormality; however, their detection is prognostically important, and work continues toward identifying the associated gene or genes.

Chromosomal abnormalities occur in 50% to 65% of CLL patients with analyzable metaphases. Because of the low mitotic rate in CLL, traditional karyotypic methods frequently fail. Fluorescent in situ hybridization (FISH) has increased the detection of clonal genetic abnormalities in CLL patients. In a landmark study, Dohner et al evaluated 325 patients with CLL. Using a variety of fluorescent probes, they identified chromosomal aberrations in 82%. Among these findings was the recognition that some subtypes (17p del and 11q del) had markedly shorter time to initiate chemotherapy and shorter overall survival than did other types. In this study, the most frequent change was a deletion in 13q14 (55% of patients). Other typical abnormalities included deletion 11q22–23 (18%), trisomy 12q13 (16%), and deletion 17p13 (7%).

These genetic abnormalities help explain some of the clinical variations seen in CLL. For example, patients with 13q deletions tend to have modest or absent lymphadenopathy, whereas patients with deletion 11q frequently have bulky adenopathy.

Disease progression also is heavily influenced by the underlying genetic abnormality. Time from diagnosis to treatment averaged only 9 months for patients with 17p abnormalities, compared with 92 months for patients with 13q deletions.

Prognostic importance These chromosomal abnormalities were potent predictors of outcome with the following median survivals: deletion 17p, 32 months; deletion 11q, 79 months; trisomy 12, 114 months; and deletion 13q, 133 months.

Molecular abnormalities

No single gene has been implicated in the pathogenesis of CLL. However, several genetic abnormalities have biologic and/or prognostic implications.

The *p53* gene is located on the short arm of chromosome 17 and is deleted in the leukemia clone of up to 10% of patients with CLL. Mutations of *p53* occur in a similar proportion of CLL cases, usually in association with *p53* deletion in the other *p53* allele. The 17p deletion involving *p53* is considered the most significant negative cytogenetic prognostic factor in CLL. The p53 protein normally responds to DNA damage by inducing cell cycle arrest and facilitating DNA repair. It can also induce apoptosis in cells with damaged DNA and in this way mediates the cytotoxicity of many anticancer agents. Resistance to treatment is a particular characteristic of p53 deletion and has been observed for agents including purine analogs.

Further investigation of the common 13q deletion has revealed the detection of specific micro-RNA genomic sequence abnormalities expressed in patients with CLL. Further analysis suggests a micro-RNA signature profile may be associated with Zap-70 expression and mutational status of IgVH as well as disease progression *(Calin GA, Ferracin M, Cimmino A, et al: N Engl J Med 353:1793-1801, 2005).* Though the exact significance of this finding is not known with certainty, the specific micro-RNA signature may be relevant to the pathogenesis of CLL. In addition, germline mutations affecting these micro-RNAs may be a predisposing factor in familial CLL.

Overexpression of *bcl-2* Abnormalities of the long arm of chromosome 14 frequently involve region 14q32, the site encoding for the immunoglobulin heavy-chain gene. However, gene translocations such as t(11;14)(q13;q32) and t(14;18)(q32;q21), which juxtapose genes *bcl-1* and *bcl-2* to the heavy-chain immunoglobulin gene, are relatively uncommon and should prompt consideration of alternative diagnoses (mantle cell or follicular lymphoma). Nevertheless, increased expression of *bcl-2* mRNA and protein is common in CLL. Since overexpression of *bcl-2* inhibits apoptosis, it is possible that this gene participates in the pathogenesis of CLL.

Staging and prognosis

Staging systems Two staging systems of CLL are commonly used: one proposed and later modified by Rai and the other proposed by Binet (Table 2). Both systems include three categories of low, intermediate, and high risk, with median survival durations of approximately 10, 6, and 2 years, respectively.

Other prognostic factors Stage of disease has been considered the main prognostic indicator for CLL. However, other factors have prognostic implications, such as chromosomal aberrations, serum level of β2M, pattern of bone marrow infiltration, the lymphocyte doubling time, and serum levels of soluble CD23.

Somatic hypermutation (SHM) normally occurs in germinal centers of lymphoid tissues and is a process that introduces mutations in the variable region of immunoglobulin genes. It is responsible for affinity maturation, the process of producing B cells with high-affinity antibody. CLL can be divided into two

TABLE 2: Staging systems for CLL

RAI SYSTEM

Rai stage	Modified Rai stage (risk)	Clinical characteristics	Median survival (yr)
0	Low	Lymphocytosis in peripheral blood and bone marrow only	> 10
I	Intermediate	Lymphocytosis and enlarged lymph nodes	6
II		Lymphocytosis and enlarged spleen and/or liver	
III	High	Lymphocytosis and anemia (hemoglobin < 11 g/dL)	2
IV		Lymphocytosis and thrombocytopenia (platelets < 100 × 10^9/L)	

BINET SYSTEM

Binet stage	Clinical characteristics	Median survival (yr)
A	Hemoglobin level ≥10 g/dL, platelet count ≥100 × 10^9/L, and < 3 areas involved	> 7
B	Hemoglobin level ≥10 g/dL, platelet count ≥100 × 10^9/L, and ≥ 3 areas involved	< 5
C	Hemoglobin level < 10 g/dL, platelet count < 100 x 10^9/L, or both (independent of areas involved)	< 2

distinct prognostic groups based on the extent to which the expressed immunoglobulin heavy chain variable (IgV_H) gene has undergone SHM. CLL cases with an IgV_H gene with < 98% homology to germline are considered mutated and those with an IgV_H gene with ≥ 98% homology to germline are considered unmutated.

CLL cases with an unmutated IgV_H gene generally have rapid progression and an unfavorable prognosis, whereas CLL cases with a mutated IgV_H gene generally have slowly progressive disease and a favorable prognosis. Patients with unmutated IgV_H genes have a median survival of 8 years, compared with 24 years for those with mutated IgV_H genes. The biologic differences between these groups are also reflected in the association of unmutated IgV_H genes with other poor prognostic features, such as expression of CD38, and unfavorable cytogenetic abnormalities. These results need to be interpreted carefully in light of the fact that the study population was not representative of the epidemiology of CLL, where the median survival for all patients is approximately 5 years.

The immunoglobulins expressed by CLL cells can be polyreactive autoantibodies. It follows that the cell that gives rise to the CLL B cell may experience

TABLE 3: Suggested indications for therapy for early-stage CLL

Progressive disease-related symptoms (eg, fever, night sweats, weight loss)

Bone marrow involvement with progressive anemia and thrombocytopenia

Progressive or painful splenomegaly

Progressive or bulky lymphadenopathy

Rapidly increasing lymphocytosis

Autoimmune hemolytic anemia or thrombocytopenia

persistent antigen stimulation, which contributes to malignant transformation. The role of antigen selection is implicated by the overrepresentation of certain IgV_H genes in CLL. In addition, there is also a biased distribution of these genes between the mutated and unmutated subgroups. The VH3 and VH4 families of genes are frequently found in the subgroup with mutated IgV_H genes, whereas the VH1 family, particularly VH1-69, is more common in the subgroup with unmutated IgV_H genes. Specific genes, such as VH3-21, have also been associated with a poor prognosis, independent of IgV_H mutation status.

ZAP-70 encodes a protein tyrosine kinase normally expressed by T cells and involved in intracellular signaling initiated by T-cell receptor ligation. Expression of ZAP-70 by CLL B cells (> 20% of CLL are cells ZAP-70 positive) is associated with unmutated IgV_H genes, shorter time to initial treatment, and inferior survival compared with ZAP-70 negative (< 20% cases). Detection of ZAP-70 protein by flow cytometry or immunohistochemistry may provide a useful prognostic marker for patients with CLL.

Treatment

TREATMENT RECOMMENDATIONS

Traditionally, the initial therapy for CLL has been chlorambucil (Leukeran) with or without prednisone. However, accumulating data suggest that fludarabine has significantly greater activity than these agents. This agent produces higher overall and complete remission (CR) rates and provides a longer remission duration than chlorambucil. Newer data suggest that combination chemotherapy, particularly a nucleoside analog combined with an alkylating agent, produces higher response rates, and the addition of monoclonal antibodies to such regimens appears to increase the CR rates. However, to date, a survival advantage has not been demonstrated for administering these regimens as initial therapy.

TABLE 4: Response criteria in CLL according to the IWCLL

Complete response

Resolution of lymphadenopathy, splenomegaly, hepatomegaly, and constitutional symptoms

Normalization of blood counts:

      Neutrophils > 1.5×10^9/L

      Platelets > 100×10^9/L

      Lymphocytes < 4×10^9/L

Normalization of bone marrow

      < 30% lymphocytes[a]

      Nodular or focal infiltrates[b]

Partial response

Downstaging (from Binet stages C to A or B and from B to A)[b]

      or

> 50% decrease in absolute lymphocyte count, splenomegaly, lymphadenopathy, hepatomegaly

      Neutrophils ≥ 1.5×10^9/L

      Platelets ≥ 100×10^9/L

      Hemoglobin > 11 g/dL

      > 50% improvement in peripheral blood counts[a]

[a] National Cancer Institute (NCI) criteria; [b] International Workshop on CLL (IWCLL) criteria

---

There have been three prospective clinical trials for chemotherapy-naive patients with CLL that randomized patients to receive monotherapy with fludarabine or combination therapy with fludarabine and cyclophosphamide. All three studies reported an increased frequency of complete and overall response rates and a longer PFS with fludarabine and cyclophosphamide combination therapy compared with monotherapy. These studies included the Eastern Cooperative Oncology Group (ECOG) 2997, British MRC CLL 4 trial, and German CLL Study Group CLL 4 trials. Despite improvements in OR, CR, and PFS, none of these studies demonstrated a survival advantage for patients receiving combination therapy.

The development of nonmyeloablative transplants has provided the possibility of allogeneic transplantation for CLL, where the median age of patients is near 70, but this new technique should only be performed in the context of a clinical trial. An effort should be made to enroll patients in clinical trials that offer them the possibility of receiving some of the new alternatives, which may eventually achieve the goal of curing CLL.

EARLY-STAGE DISEASE

Since patients with early-stage CLL have a good long-term prognosis, and early therapy has not changed the outcome of the disease, patients in the early stages should not be treated unless specific indications exist (Table 3). Randomized trials comparing chlorambucil versus no therapy have documented no advantage for patients with early-stage CLL who received immediate therapy with

Patient characteristic	Response rate		
	Fludarabine	**CAP**	**CHOP**
Response	71%	58%	72%
Complete response	8%	2%	9%
Median survival	69 months	70 months	67 months

CAP = cyclophosphamide, Adriamycin (doxorubicin), and prednisone; CHOP = cyclophosphamide, low-dose doxorubicin, vincristine (Oncovin), and prednisone

chlorambucil. New alternatives for treatment of high-risk early-stage CLL (ZAP-70–positive, unmutated IgH status) are being investigated (eg, monoclonal antibodies).

CONVENTIONAL CHEMOTHERAPY

Single-agent chemotherapy

Chlorambucil Historically, the initial agent used for CLL has been chlorambucil, given as either 0.1 mg/kg daily or 20 to 40 mg/m² every 2 to 4 weeks. Therapy is continued until the signs or symptoms requiring therapy are controlled.

Chlorambucil is frequently combined with oral prednisone (30 to 100 mg/m²/d), although there is no clear evidence that the combination improves responses or overall survival over chlorambucil alone. Prednisone is of value, however, in the management of autoimmune cytopenias.

Cyclophosphamide is an alternative to chlorambucil. The usual dose is 0.5 to 1 g/m² every 3 to 4 weeks alone or together with vincristine and steroids (eg, COP [cyclophosphamide, vincristine (Oncovin), and prednisone] regimen).

Combination chemotherapy

COP and CHOP Various drug combinations have been used in CLL, mostly in patients with advanced-stage disease. The most frequently employed combinations have been COP and these three drugs plus doxorubicin

In March 2008, the US Food and Drug Administration approved bendamustine (Treanda) for treatment of chronic lymphocytic leukemia (CLL). In a randomized, multicenter study of 301 treatment-naïve patients with CLL, those treated with bendamustine had a significantly higher overall response than those treated with chlorambucil (59% vs 26%; P < .0001). Eight percent of the bendamustine group had a complete response, compared with less than 1% of the chlorambucil group. In addition, patients who received bendamustine had a longer progression-free survival than those who received chlorambucil (18 months vs 6 months; hazard ratio = 0.27; P < .001). The most common adverse events in the trial were myelosuppression, fever, nausea, and vomiting (Treanda [package insert]. Frazer, PA: Cephalon, Inc.; 2008).

(CHOP). The dose of doxorubicin used is usually low (25 mg/m²). A higher dose of doxorubicin (50 mg/m²) has been employed in some regimens, such as CAP (cyclophosphamide, doxorubicin [Adriamycin], and prednisone).

Response rates have been 40% to 85% with these combinations. In randomized studies, COP was no better than chlorambucil plus prednisone. Although CHOP initially achieved better survival than COP (in patients with Binet stage C disease) or chlorambucil plus prednisone, longer follow-up has not confirmed this survival advantage.

Nucleoside analogs

Fludarabine, now frequently the drug of choice for treating CLL, has been demonstrated to be more effective than chlorambucil for the treatment of CLL. When given to previously treated patients at a dose of 25–30 mg/m²/d for 5 days every 3 to 4 weeks, this nucleoside analog produced responses in 20% to 50% of patients, with 5% to 15% of patients achieving CR and an additional 5% to 20% achieving a "nodular partial response (PR)," ie, a CR but with the presence of lymphoid nodules in the bone marrow (Table 4). In previously untreated patients, the response rate was 63% to 80%, with 8% to 35% of patients achieving a CR.

The addition of prednisone or chlorambucil to fludarabine therapy did not improve the response rate and is associated with an increased incidence of opportunistic infections and other toxicities. A large randomized study comparing fludarabine, CAP, and CHOP demonstrated an increased response rate with fludarabine but no difference in survival (Table 5). Randomized trials of fludarabine versus chlorambucil in previously untreated patients showed improvements in response rate (overall and CR), duration of response, and disease progression-free survival with fludarabine but no survival advantage.

Other nucleoside analogs Cladribine (2-chlorodeoxyadenosine, 2-CdA) is also active in CLL when given at doses of 0.1 mg/kg/d (or 4 mg/m²/d) for 7 days. At therapeutic doses, this agent appears to be associated with more myelosuppression, particularly thrombocytopenia, than fludarabine. This finding limits its utility in treating CLL, but a direct comparison with fludarabine has not been reported.

The third purine analog active against CLL is pentostatin (Nipent). Previously, toxicity limited its use as an antineoplastic agent. More recently, the recognition that safe use of this drug requires concomitant hydration and close attention to renal function (it is both toxic to and cleared by the kidneys) has renewed interest in clinical evaluation with this agent. The group at Memorial Sloan-Kettering Cancer Center has studied pentostatin combined with cyclophosphamide and demonstrated responses in > 70% of previously treated patients (including those whose disease is refractory to fludarabine) with acceptable toxicity.

NEW APPROACHES

Combination chemotherapy The combination of fludarabine, cyclophosphamide, and rituximab (Rituxan) has been studied by the group at M. D.

Anderson. In 224 previously untreated patients, the overall response rate was 95%, with 70% achieving a CR and two-thirds of patients achieving a flow CR.

Using a sequential approach with these two agents, the group at Memorial Sloan-Kettering Cancer Center has shown that consolidation therapy with high-dose cyclophosphamide with and without rituximab markedly improves the frequency of a CR over fludarabine alone.

Data suggest that the addition of a monoclonal antibody to fludarabine-based therapy may markedly improve CR rates in this disease. A study conducted by the Cancer and Leukemia Group B (CALGB) randomized patients with previously untreated CLL to receive fludarabine or a combination of fludarabine and the anti-CD20 antibody rituximab at standard doses. Patients in both arms subsequently received a consolidation course of rituximab for 4 weeks.

Building on the positive results of combination pentostatin, cyclophosphamide, and rituximab (PCR) in previously treated patients, Kay et al reported on the use of this regimen in patients with untreated CLL. Responses occurred in 91% of patients, with 63% achieving a CR or nodular response. More importantly, a subset analysis demonstrated that PCR treatment was equally effective in patients over the age of 70 as in younger individuals (Kay NE, Geyer SM, Call TG, et al: Blood 109:405-411, 2007).

Overall response rates were high in both arms, but there was a significantly higher CR rate (33%) in the concurrent arm than in the arm with fludarabine alone (15%); however, both groups experienced similar response durations and overall survival. The CR rate increased in both groups after consolidation therapy with rituximab. This study illustrated the fact that adding rituximab to fludarabine increases the frequency of a CR both when administered concomitantly and sequentially.

Elter et al reported on the use of fludarabine in combination with alemtuzumab (Campath), a humanized monoclonal antibody targeting the panlymphocyte antigen CD52, in 36 patients with relapsed or refractory disease. The overall frequency of response was 83%, with 11 complete responses.

Monoclonal antibody–targeted therapy Monoclonal antibodies have been used in patients with CLL to exploit antibody-mediated cytotoxicity. Alemtuzumab has been approved by the US Food and Drug Administration (FDA) for the treatment of refractory CLL. In a pivotal trial in patients with fludarabine-refractory disease, alemtuzumab resulted in an overall response rate of 33%.

Rituximab also has been investigated and is active both as a single agent and in combination with chemotherapy. Because of rituximab's efficacy without significant toxicity, it is assuming a greater role in the treatment of patients with CLL.

The combination of alemtuzumab and rituximab has been evaluated in patients with relapsed or refractory lymphoid malignancies. Alemtuzumab was given twice weekly at 30 mg IV for 4 weeks. Rituximab (375 mg/m²) was given concurrently weekly for the 4 weeks. Responses were reported for 48 patients, 32 with CLL, 9 with CLL/PLL (prolymphocytic leukemia), 1 with PLL, 4 with mantle cell lymphoma, and 2 with Richter's transformation. The overall response rate was 52%; CR was noted in 8%, nodular PR in 4%, and PR in 40% of treated patients. Toxicities included infusion-related reactions. Infections occurred in 52% of patients with cytomegalovirus reactivation occurring in 27% of patients. Overall, this was a well-tolerated combination for relapsed patients with CLL.

Achieving minimal residual disease-free status The current formal criteria to assess response are based on physical examination, blood counts, and microscopic evaluation of bone marrow (Table 4). Minimal residual disease (MRD) can be evaluated by more sensitive methods such as polymerase chain reaction (PCR) for the IgV_H gene or 4-color flow cytometry. In a study of 91 previously treated patients who received alemtuzumab (30 mg thrice weekly for up to 16 weeks), 36% achieved CR, and the overall response rate was 54%. Of the 91 patients, 18 achieved MRD-free status by flow-cytometry evaluation of their bone marrow. Survival was significantly longer for patients who achieved MRD-free status. Overall survival for the 18 patients with MRD-free remission was 84% at 5 years.

For patients who have residual disease after purine analog–based therapy, the marrow has been the major site of involvement. Elimination of residual disease, particularly in the marrow, may improve treatment outcome. Because of the significant activity of alemtuzumab at clearing blood and marrow of disease, its ability to eliminate residual disease after chemotherapy is under investigation.

Stem-cell transplantation

Both allogeneic and autologous stem-cell transplantations (SCTs) have been tested in patients with CLL.

Allogeneic SCT is a viable option for younger patients with CLL, particularly if they have not responded to alkylating agents and/or nucleoside analogs and are in an advanced stage of disease. The series reported to date, including a majority of patients with advanced refractory disease, has documented a CR rate in excess of 70%. The response is sustained in most patients, although reported follow-up is typically short. SCT using nonablative conditioning regimens has produced encouraging results and should be considered in the setting of a clinical trial, particularly for patients > 60 years.

Autologous SCT Since the median age of patients with CLL is usually higher than the age considered acceptable for allogeneic SCT, autologous transplants using purged marrow have also been investigated. In general, results have been disappointing, with the best results seen in patients with responsive disease and low tumor burdens—a group that might have fared well without a transplant.

Splenectomy

Splenectomy may be beneficial for patients in whom hypersplenism is the cause of cytopenias (particularly in patients without significant lymphadenopathy) or for palliation when splenomegaly is symptomatic and refractory to chemotherapy. Cytopenias frequently respond to splenectomy. Perioperative mortality varies widely and is largely related to the experience of the surgeon in performing splenectomy in these patients. In experienced hands, splenectomy can be performed with minimal mortality, even in patients with end-stage disease.

Complications

Infections Patients with CLL are prone to multiple infections, and infectious complications are a leading cause of death in patients with CLL. Hypogammaglobulinemia plays a central role in the predisposition of patients to this problem, and prophylactic IV administration of immunoglobulin preparations may reduce the incidence of infections. Cytotoxic therapy further weakens the immune system and may increase the risk of opportunistic infections.

Autoimmune cytopenias frequently complicate CLL and may be precipitated or aggravated by therapy (eg, fludarabine) for CLL. Autoimmune hemolytic anemia can be treated successfully with prednisone in the majority of patients. Combinations of cyclophosphamide with rituximab are beneficial in cases refractory to prednisone, splenectomy, or cyclosporine. Similar approaches may be useful for autoimmune thrombocytopenia. In a study from M. D. Anderson Cancer Center, 31 patients with CLL and autoimmune anemia or thrombocytopenia received cyclosporine (300 mg/day). Sixty-three percent of patients responded, with a median duration of response of 10 months. No grade 3/4 toxicity was seen.

Pure red cell aplasia and the less commonly amegakaryocytic thrombocytopenia are infrequent complications of CLL, which are mediated by immune mechanisms. Therapy with cyclosporine (3 to 6 mg/kg/d) is frequently effective.

TRANSFORMATION

LCL CLL transforms into LCL in 3% to 10% of patients. This phenomenon, known as Richter's transformation, has an aggressive presentation with fever and other B symptoms and progressive lymphadenopathy. Extranodal involvement occurs in approximately 40% of patients. Paraproteinemia, hypercalcemia, and a sharp rise in serum LDH levels can be frequently seen.

The prognosis of patients whose disease progresses to LCL is variable and depends in part on the degree of prior treatment used for the underlying CLL. In treatment-naive patients with LCL, standard therapy with CHOP and rituximab may offer long-term control of the transformed component. In patients who have had significant prior therapy, the disease is often refractory, and combination chemotherapy including SCT is frequently ineffective.

PLL More rarely, CLL can transform into PLL, characterized by a > 55% increase in prolymphocytes. The transformation is frequently accompanied by progression of splenomegaly, cytopenias, and refractoriness to therapy.

Other diseases Anecdotal cases of CLL evolving into acute lymphocytic leukemia, myeloma, low-grade lymphoma, and Hodgkin lymphoma have been reported. The rarity of these reports makes a true causal connection less likely.

HAIRY-CELL LEUKEMIA

Hairy-cell leukemia (HCL) is an infrequent B-cell malignancy usually associated with pancytopenia and splenomegaly. About 600 cases are reported yearly in the United States. Despite its relative rarity, there are a disproportionate number of highly effective therapies available.

Epidemiology and etiology

The male-to-female ratio of HCL is 4:1. The median age at presentation is 50 years. The etiology is unknown.

Differential diagnosis

HCL can be confused with malignant lymphomas, splenic lymphoma with villous lymphocytes (SLVLs), CLL, other non-Hodgkin's lymphomas in leukemic phase, and occasionally even myelodysplastic syndromes.

Treatment

The indications for treatment of HCL are an absolute neutrophil count (ANC) < 1,000/μL, platelet count < 100 × 10³/μL, or hemoglobin level < 10 g/dL; leukemic phase of HCL; symptomatic splenomegaly; recurrent infections; or autoimmune complications.

Response criteria The criteria for a CR are normalization of the complete blood cell (CBC) count, with ANC > 1,500/μL, platelet count > 100,000/μL, and hemoglobin level > 12 g/dL; regression of organomegaly to normal; and bone marrow and peripheral blood free of hairy cells. PRs require reduction of the hairy cells in the bone marrow to < 50%, < 5% hairy cells in peripheral blood, > 50% reduction in organomegaly, and normalization of the CBC count.

Splenectomy is reserved for patients with splenic rupture, infarcts, a massively enlarged spleen, severe hypersplenism, or failure to respond to systemic chemotherapy.

Interferon-α (IFN-α), at a dose of 3 mU/d administered by IM or SC injection for 6 months followed by 3 mU/d three times weekly for 12 or 24 months, induces a CR in 8% to 10% of patients and a PR in 74%. The median time to response was 6 months in patients achieving a PR and 14 months in those achieving a CR. Patients frequently relapse between 12 and 24 months after discontinuation of therapy. The superiority of purine analog therapy (discussed later) has essentially led most clinicians to abandon the use of IFN for this disease.

Purine analogs The recommended dose of pentostatin is 4 mg/m^2 by IV bolus every other week until a CR is obtained. Usually, patients require a median of 8 courses (range, 4–15). The CR rate varies between 59% and 89% in different studies, and the PR rate varies between 4% and 37%. Responses can last for many years, and patients who relapse often respond to retreatment with pentostatin. In an update of a large randomized trial comparing pentostatin and IFN-α, Flinn et al reported that in 241 patients with HCL treated with pentostatin, the 10-year overall survival rate was 81%, with only two deaths (1%) attributable to HCL.

Cladribine shows activity in treating HCL similar to that of pentostatin. Due to this finding and the fact that cladribine is given as 1 cycle of a 7-day continuous infusion or a 5-day bolus, this agent usually is the preferred treatment of this disorder. Piro et al treated 144 HCL patients with cladribine, 0.1 mg/kg/d by continuous IV infusion for 7 days. A total response rate of 97% was obtained, with 85% CRs and 12% PRs. Response was independent of previous treatment with IFN or splenectomy, and three patients whose disease was refractory to pentostatin responded to cladribine. Recovery of CBC counts occurred on average by day 61 (range, 11–268 days).

The largest series reporting long-term follow-up results on patients with HCL treated with cladribine was from the Scripps group. A total of 349 patients, with a median duration of response follow-up of 59 months, were evaluated. Twenty-six percent had relapsed at a median of 29 months, but most of them were patients who had achieved only a PR. The time-to-treatment failure rate at 48 months was only 16% in complete responders.

Else et al reported on a large series of 219 patients with HCL, comparing their experience with pentostatin and cladribine. Treatment results were similar in terms of frequency of CR, relapse, and overall survival. Though the results are excellent, with more than 95% of patients alive at 10 years, the disease-free survival curves do not plateau, indicating these drugs are not curative in HCL.

Immunotoxin The NCI evaluated a recombinant immunotoxin containing an anti-CD22 variable domain fused to a truncated Pseudomonas exotoxin; it was given by IV infusion every other day for a total of three doses. Sixteen patients whose disease was resistant to cladribine were treated; 2 achieved a PR and 11 achieved a CR. Of the 11 patients, 3 who had a CR relapsed and were retreated; all of these patients achieved a second CR.

SUGGESTED READING

Byrd JC, Peterson BL, Morrison VA, et al: Randomized phase II study of fludarabine with concurrent vs sequential treatment with rituximab in symptomatic, untreated patients with B-cell chronic lymphocytic leukemia: Results from Cancer and Leukemia Group B 9712 (CALGB 9712). Blood 101:6–14, 2003.

Calin GA, Ferracin M, Cimmino A, et al: A MicroRNA signature associated with prognosis and progression in chronic lymphocytic leukemia. N Engl J Med 353:1793–1801, 2005.

Catovsky D, Richards S, Matutes E, et al: Assessment of fludarabine plus cyclophosphamide for patients with chronic lymphocytic leukaemia (the LRF CLL4 Trial): A randomised controlled trial. Lancet 370:230–239, 2007.

Crespo M, Bosch F, Villamor N, et al: ZAP-70 expression as a surrogate for immunoglobulin-variable-region mutations in chronic lymphocytic leukemia. N Engl J Med 348:1764–1775, 2003.

Damle RN, Wasil T, Fais F, et al: Ig V gene mutation status and CD38 expression as novel prognostic indicators in chronic lymphocytic leukemia. Blood 94:1840–1847, 1999.

Eichhorst BF, Busch R, Hopfinger G, et al: Fludarabine plus cyclophosphamide versus fludarabine alone in first-line therapy of younger patients with chronic lymphocytic leukemia. Blood: 107:885–891, 2006.

Else M, Ruchlemer R, Osuji N, et al: Long remissions in hairy cell leukemia with purine analogs. Cancer 104:2442–2448, 2005.

Flinn IW, Neuberg DS, Grever MR, et al: Phase III trial of fludarabine plus cyclophosphamide compared with fludarabine for patients with previously untreated chronic lymphocytic leukemia: US Intergroup Trial E2997. J Clin Oncol 25:793–798, 2007.

Hamblin TJ, Davis Z, Gardiner A, et al: Unmutated Ig V(H) genes are associated with a more aggressive form of chronic lymphocytic leukemia. Blood 94:1848–1854, 1999.

Hillmen P, Skotnicki AB, Robak T, et al: Alemtuzumab compared with chlorambucil as first-line therapy for chronic lymphocytic leukemia. J Clin Oncol 25:5616–5623, 2007.

Kay NE, Geyer SM, Call TG, et al: Combination chemoimmunotherapy with pentostatin, cyclophosphamide, and rituximab shows significant clinical activity with low accompanying toxicity in previously untreated B chronic lymphocytic leukemia. Blood 109:405–411, 2007.

Keating MJ, O'Brien S, Albitar M, et al: Early results of a chemoimmunotherapy regimen of fludarabine, cyclophosphamide, and rituximab as intital therapy for chronic lymphocytic leukemia. J Clin Oncol 23:4079–4088, 2005.

Lamanna N, Kalaycio M, Maslak P, et al: Pentostatin, cyclophosphamide, and rituximab is an active, well-tolerated regimen for patients with previously treated chronic lymphocytic leukemia. J Clin Oncol 24:1575–1581, 2006.

Lundin J, Kimby E, Bjorkholm M, et al: Phase II trial of subcutaneous anti-CD52 monoclonal antibody alemtuzumab (Campath-1H) as first-line treatment for patients with B-cell chronic lymphocytic leukemia (B-CLL). Blood 100:768–773, 2002.

Moreton P, Kennedy B, Lucas G, et al: Eradication of minimal residual disease in B-cell chronic lymphocytic leukemia after alemtuzumab therapy is associated with prolonged survival. J Clin Oncol 23:2971–2979, 2005.

Rai KR, Peterson BL, Appelbaum FR, et al: Fludarabine compared with chlorambucil as primary therapy for chronic lymphocytic leukemia. N Engl J Med 343:1750–1757, 2000.

Schetelig J, Thiede C, Bornhauser M, et al: Evidence of a graft-versus-leukemia effect in chronic lymphocytic leukemia after reduced-intensity conditioning and allogeneic stem-cell transplantation: The Cooperative German Transplant Study Group. J Clin Oncol 21:2747–2753, 2003.

Wierda W, O'Brien S, Wen S, et al: Chemoimmunotherapy with fludarabine, cyclophosphamide, and rituximab for relapsed and refractory chronic lymphocytic leukemia. J Clin Oncol 23:4070–4078, 2005.

CHAPTER 35

Myelodysplastic syndromes

Guillermo Garcia-Manero, MD, Alan List, MD, Hagop Kantarjian, MD, and Jorge E. Cortes, MD

Myelodysplastic syndromes (MDS) are a group of hematologic malignancies of the pluripotent hematopoietic stem cells. These disorders are characterized by ineffective hematopoiesis, including abnormalities in proliferation, differentiation, and apoptosis. The overall clinical result is peripheral cytopenias in the setting of a normocellular or hypercellular bone marrow and a high incidence of transformation to acute leukemia.

The incidence of MDS approximates 2 cases per 100,000 population per year, with 30 cases per 100,000 population per year in patients > 70 years old. It is estimated that approximately 15,000 to 20,000 new cases are diagnosed annually in the United States. Unfortunately, there are no accurate statistics on the actual incidence of MDS.

Epidemiology

Gender The overall incidence of MDS is slightly higher in males than in females (1.5 to 2.0:1).

Age The incidence of MDS increases with age, with a median age at diagnosis of about 70 years. MDS is rare in children; childhood cases are more frequently associated with monosomy of chromosome 7.

Etiology and risk factors

MDS is a clonal disorder of bone marrow stem cells. The vast majority of cases (80% to 90%) occur de novo, whereas 10% to 20% of cases are secondary. The etiology of de novo MDS is unclear. Exposure to radiation and/or cytotoxic agents is a recognized etiologic factor in secondary disease forms. Cumulative exposure to environmental toxins, genetic differences in leukemogen susceptibility and metabolism, and genomic senescence may contribute to disease pathogenesis in de novo cases.

Genetic factors It has been suggested that a genetic change causes an irreversible alteration in the structure and function of the stem cell, with disruption of a multistep process involving control of cell proliferation, maturation, and in-

MDS

teractions with growth factors; mutations of tumor-suppressor genes and proto-oncogenes; and deregulation of apoptosis.

Constitutional childhood disorders, such as Fanconi's anemia, Shwachman-Diamond syndrome, Down's syndrome, neurofibromatosis, and mitochondrial cytopathies, have been associated with MDS and monosomy of chromosome 7.

Environmental factors Exposure to benzene and its derivatives may result in karyotypic abnormalities often seen in MDS and acute myelogenous leukemia (AML). Persons chronically exposed to insecticides and pesticides may have a higher incidence of MDS than the general population.

An increased incidence of MDS has been reported among smokers and ex-smokers, possibly linked to associated exposures to polycyclic hydrocarbons and radioactive polodium present in tobacco smoke.

An association of MDS with magnetic fields, alcohol, or occupational exposure to other chemicals has not been demonstrated.

Antineoplastic drugs Therapy-related myelodysplasia and therapy-related AML are recognized long-term complications of chemotherapy and radiotherapy. Therapy-related MDS usually develops 3 to 7 years after exposure to chemotherapy and is most frequently related to complete or partial loss of chromosomes 5 or 7 in patients previously treated with alkylating agents. Approximately 80% of cases of AML occurring after exposure to antineoplastic drugs, particularly alkylating agents, are preceded by MDS.

More than 85% of patients who develop chemotherapy-related leukemia or MDS have been exposed to alkylating agents. Patients exposed to nitrosoureas have a relative risk of developing MDS or AML of 14.4 and a 6-year actuarial risk of 4%. The mean cumulative risk of leukemia in patients exposed to epipodophyllotoxins (eg, etoposide and teniposide [Vumon]) is about 5% at 5 years. Most of these therapy-related leukemias are not preceded by a dysplastic phase and are associated with abnormalities in chromosome 11q23.

Autologous bone marrow transplantation (BMT) has also been associated with a 5-year actuarial risk of MDS of 15% (95% confidence interval, 3.4–16.6). Fluorescent in situ hybridization (FISH) analyses of pretreatment bone marrow specimens for informative cytogenetic markers indicate that these secondary myeloid malignancies derive from clones demonstrable before the transplant procedure. Prior therapy with fludarabine, older age, low CD34+ dose, and prolonged platelet reconstitution have been associated with the development of MDS or AML in patients with lymphoid malignancies after autologous stem-cell transplantation (SCT).

TABLE 1: Main features of MDS according to the FAB classification

FAB subgroup	BM blasts (%)	Ringed sideroblasts (%)	PB monocytes (× 10⁹/L)	Chromosomal abnormalities (%)	Frequently associated karyotype	Rate of leukemic progression (%)	Median survival (mo)
RA	< 5	< 15	< 1	30	5q-, -7, +8, 20q-	12	32
RARS	< 5	≥ 15	< 1	20	+8, 5q-, 20q-	8	42
RAEB	5-20	Variable	< 1	45	-7, 7q-, -5, 5q-, +8	44	12
RAEB-t	21-30	Variable	Variable	60	-7, 7q-, -5, 5q-, +8	66	5
CMML	1-20	Variable	≥ 1	30	-7, +8, t(5;12), 7q-, 12q-	14	20

BM = bone marrow; CMML = chronic myelomonocytic leukemia; FAB = French-American-British; MDS = myelodysplastic syndromes; PB = peripheral blood; RA = refractory anemia; RAEB = refractory anemia with excess blasts; RAEB-t = refractory anemia with excess blasts in transformation; RARS = refractory anemia with ringed sideroblasts

Classification

In 1982, the French-American-British (FAB) group proposed a classification system for MDS that consists of five subgroups, based on the percentage of blast cells in the peripheral blood and bone marrow, the presence of ringed sideroblasts in the bone marrow, and the monocyte count in the peripheral blood (Table 1). The five subgroups are:

- refractory anemia (RA)
- refractory anemia with ringed sideroblasts (RARS)
- refractory anemia with excess blasts (RAEB)
- refractory anemia with excess blasts in transformation (RAEB-t)
- chronic myelomonocytic leukemia (CMML).

The presence of Auer rods in granulocyte precursors classifies a patient as having RAEB-t, even if blasts comprise < 20% of bone marrow cells. The presence of > 30% blast cells in the bone marrow or peripheral blood establishes the diagnosis of AML rather than MDS.

More recently, the World Health Organization (WHO) has proposed a modified classification of hematologic malignancies (Table 2). The following changes were proposed, based on the effect of cytogenetics and the number of dysplastic lineages on clinical behavior:

- The FAB classification of RAEB-t is eliminated.
- The blast percentage that defines AML is changed to ≥ 20%.
- RA and RARS are defined by dysplasia restricted to the erythroid lineage either with or without ringed sideroblasts, respectively.
- The presence of dysplasia in erythroid and nonerythroid lineages (multilineage dysplasia with or without ringed sideroblasts) and 5q-syndrome are regarded as separate entities of MDS.
- RAEB is divided into two categories distinguished by marrow blast percentage (ie, RAEB-1: 5% to 9%; RAEB-2: 10% to 19%) or the presence of Auer rods (RAEB-2).
- A category is added to include unclassifiable MDS defined by nonerythroid dysplasia.
- CMML is included in a separate category of myelodysplastic/myeloproliferative diseases that also includes atypical CML and juvenile myelomonocytic leukemia. CMML is further classified into CMML-1 (≤ 9% blasts), CMML-2 (10% to 19% blasts), and CMML-Eos (eosinophils ≥ 1,500/µL).

This proposal represents a step ahead, but there are some aspects that still need to be addressed. For example, some biologic features that have been associated with MDS, such as the presence of spontaneous apoptosis, increased angiogenesis, and infrequent FLT$_3$ mutations, may define better specific subsets, and the WHO classification does not incorporate unfavorable cytogenetic patterns.

TABLE 2: Criteria for myelodysplastic syndromes (MDS) according to the WHO classification

Disease	Blood findings	Bone marrow findings
Refractory anemia (RA)	Anemia No or rare blasts	Erythroid dysplasia *only* < 5% blasts < 15% ringed sideroblasts
Refractory anemia with ringed sideroblasts (RARS)	Anemia No blasts	Erythroid dysplasia *only* ≥ 15% ringed sideroblasts < 5% blasts
Refractory cytopenias with multilineage dysplasia (RCMD)	Cytopenias (bicytopenia or pancytopenia) No or rare blasts No Auer rods < 1 × 10^9/L monocytes	Dysplasia in ≥ 10% of cells in 2 or more myeloid cell lines, including erythroids < 5% blasts in marrow No Auer rods < 15% ringed sideroblasts
RCMD and ringed sideroblasts (RCMD-RS)	Cytopenias (bicytopenia or pancytopenia) No or rare blasts No Auer rods < 1 × 10^9/L monocytes	Dysplasia in ≥ 10% of cells in 2 or more myeloid cell lines ≥ 15% ringed sideroblasts < 5% blasts No Auer rods
Refractory anemia with excess blasts-1 (RAEB-1)	Cytopenias < 5% blasts No Auer rods < 1 × 10^9/L monocytes	Unilineage or multilineage dysplasia 5%-9% blasts No Auer rods
Refractory anemia with with excess blasts-2 (RAEB-2)	Cytopenias 5%-19% blasts Auer rods ± < 1 × 10^9/L monocytes	Unilineage or multilineage dysplasia 10%-19% blasts Auer rods ±
Myelodysplastic syndrome, unclassified (MDS-U)	Cytopenias No or rare blasts No Auer rods	Unilineage dysplasia in granulocytes or megakaryocytes < 5% blasts No Auer rods
MDS associated with isolated del(5q)	Anemia < 5% blasts Platelets normal or increased	Normal to increased megakaryocytes with hypolobulated nuclei < 5% blasts No Auer rods Isolated del(5q31.1)

WHO = World Health Organization

Signs and symptoms

Nearly 50% of patients with MDS are asymptomatic at the time of initial diagnosis. Signs and symptoms relate to hematopoietic failure, leading to anemia, thrombocytopenia, or leukopenia.

Symptoms related to anemia may range from fatigue to exertional dyspnea that may exacerbate angina or cause congestive heart failure.

Infection Approximately one-third of patients report recurrent localized or systemic infections as a result of granulocytopenia or dysfunctional granulocytes and monocytes.

Bleeding manifestations, such as petechiae or gross hemorrhage, can occur with thrombocytopenia or platelet dysfunction. However, < 10% of patients present with serious bleeding.

Organomegaly and lymphadenopathy Splenomegaly and/or hepatomegaly may be found in 5% to 25% of patients. A large spleen is more frequently seen in CMML.

Acute neutrophilic dermatosis (Sweet's syndrome) and pyoderma gangrenosum may be observed, particularly in patients with CMML or advanced MDS.

Paraneoplastic syndromes Diabetes insipidus, vasculitis, and other rare paraneoplastic syndromes have been described in patients with MDS.

Laboratory features

Peripheral blood

Anemia is the most frequent abnormality in MDS, with > 80% of patients presenting with hemoglobin concentrations < 10 g/dL. The anemia is usually normocytic or macrocytic, but the mean corpuscular volume rarely exceeds 120 μm^3.

Other RBC abnormalities Hypochromic changes and red-shape abnormalities are frequent, including poikilocytosis, anisocytosis, elliptocytosis, macro-ovalocytosis, and sometimes stomatocytes. Stippled and nucleated RBCs can be observed in 10% of cases. Reticulocyte counts are usually reduced.

WBC abnormalities The peripheral WBC count may be normal or low in MDS but is frequently elevated in CMML. The proportion of monocytes may be increased, and a circulating monocyte count of $\geq 1 \times 10^9$/L defines CMML.

Neutropenia is seen in about 50% of patients with MDS at diagnosis, often associated with pseudo–Pelger-Huët anomaly (neutrophils have a condensed chromatin and unilobed or bilobed nuclei with a pince-nez shape), ring-shaped nuclei, hypogranulation, and hypolobulation or other signs of dysgranulopoiesis.

Granulocytes frequently disclose reduced myeloperoxidase activity, increased α-naphthyl acetate esterase activity, and other functional abnormalities.

Chemotactic and bactericidal capability is impaired, which can potentiate the risk of infection, even in the presence of normal WBC counts.

Patients frequently have a decreased number of natural killer cells and helper T lymphocytes.

Platelet abnormalities Thrombocytopenia is present at diagnosis in approximately 30% of patients.

Platelets may be abnormally large; have poor granulation; or have large, fused central granules.

Decreased platelet aggregation is observed when platelets of patients with MDS are challenged with collagen or epinephrine.

Thrombocytosis may be seen in association with the 5q- syndrome.

Bone marrow

Bone marrow aspiration and biopsy should be performed in every patient suspected of having MDS or unexplained persistent cytopenias. The bone marrow is normocellular or hypercellular in 85% to 90% of patients with MDS but may be hypocellular for the patients' age in as many as 10% to 15%.

Trilineage dyspoiesis The main morphologic feature of MDS is hematopoietic dyspoiesis, although myelodysplastic features do not always involve all three lineages. Cytologic dysplasia must be detected in ≥ 10% of the affected lineages.

Dyserythropoiesis Erythroblasts usually have a megaloblastoid appearance. Iron may be abnormally deposited in mitochondria and is easily stained with Prussian blue, producing a ring-shaped staining pattern around the nucleus. Pathologic sideroblasts have five or more granules/cell.

Dysgranulopoiesis The characteristic findings in dysgranulopoiesis are hypogranulation and hyposegmentation with nuclear morphologic abnormalities.

Excess bone marrow blasts Bone marrow blasts > 5% but < 30% are seen in 30% to 50% of patients with MDS; in the context of myelodysplasia, this finding is a feature of MDS.

The FAB group distinguishes three types of blasts on the basis of the maturation as assessed by morphology. Type I blasts have an uncondensed nuclear chromatin, one to three nucleoli, and basophilic cytoplasm without a Golgi zone. Cytoplasmic granules and Auer rods are absent. In type II blasts, the nuclear/cytoplasm ratio is lower than in type I blasts, and few primary granules are seen. Type III blasts have 20 or more azurophilic granules without a Golgi zone.

Dysmegakaryocytopoiesis At least 10 megakaryocytes should be evaluated. Micromegakaryocytes are small cells with a diameter two times smaller than the normal megakaryocyte (< 80 μm). Multiple, dispersed, small nuclei or mononucleated forms, as well as hypogranulated megakaryocytes, also can be found.

Other abnormalities An increase in reticulin and collagen fibers in the bone marrow may be seen in some patients.

Angiogenesis Increased marrow vascularity and increased levels of angiogenic cytokines such as vascular endothelial growth factor (VEGF) and basic fibroblast growth factor (bFGF) have been described in patients with MDS.

Other laboratory findings

Serum iron, transferrin, and ferritin levels may be elevated. As a result of ineffective hematopoiesis, lactic dehydrogenase (LDH) and uric acid concentrations are frequently increased. Monoclonal gammopathy, polyclonal hypergammaglobulinemia, and hypogammaglobulinemia are found occasionally but may be detected in up to 15% of patients with CMML.

Cytogenetic and molecular findings

Chromosomal abnormalities

Clonal cytogenetic abnormalities are found at diagnosis in 50% to 60% of patients with de novo MDS and 75% to 85% of those with secondary MDS or AML. An interesting feature that distinguishes MDS from AML is the high incidence of complete or partial chromosomal loss or, less frequently, chromosomal gain and the relative rarity of translocations. Among the translocations, unbalanced translocations leading to a loss of chromosomal material are most frequent.

Common cytogenetic abnormalities are listed in Table 1. None of them is specific for MDS, since all can be found in other myeloid disorders.

Some of the most frequent abnormalities are interstitial deletion of the long arm of chromosome 5 (5q-), monosomy of chromosome 7, trisomy of chromosome 8, 20q-, and loss of the Y chromosome. "Complex" cytogenetic abnormalities involving three or more chromosomes occur in approximately 15% of de novo MDS cases and 50% of secondary MDS cases.

Therapy-related MDS Loss of chromosome 7 and/or 7q- has been reported in as many as 50% of patients previously exposed to chemotherapy for other malignancies, most frequently in association with prolonged use of alkylating agents. Other abnormalities commonly associated with prior exposure to alkylating agents include -5 and/or del(5q) in 25% of cases and involvement of chromosomes 17p and 21 in 10% to 15%. Complex chromosomal abnormalities may be found in nearly 50% of patients.

Cytogenetics and FAB classification

RA and RARS Approximately 15% to 30% of patients with RA and RARS have abnormal karyotypes. The most frequent abnormality in patients with RA is 5q, whereas the most common abnormalities in patients with RARS are 5q-, +8, and 20q- (each occurring in 20% of patients).

RAEB and RAEB-t Nearly 60% of patients with RAEB and RAEB-t have cytogenetic abnormalities, with 5q-, -7, 7q-, and +8 being the most frequent.

CMML Chromosomal abnormalities are found in 25% to 30% of patients with CMML; the predominant abnormalities include -7, 7q-, +8, 12q-, and t(5;12). Interestingly, 5q- is seen in < 1% of cases of CMML.

Monosomy of chromosome 7 is found in up to 25% of children with MDS, most frequently as an isolated abnormality. In contrast, older patients most often have monosomy of chromosome 7 associated with other chromosomal abnormalities.

5q- syndrome

The isolated interstitial deletion characteristic of the 5q- syndrome involves a variable segment length that includes the critical deleted region at 5q31, a region known to contain genes coding for granulocyte-macrophage colony-stimulating factor (GM-CSF), macrophage colony-stimulating factor (M-CSF), interleukin (IL)-3, IL-4, IL-5, IL-9, IL-12, M-CSF receptor, platelet-derived growth factor receptor-beta, interferon-regulatory factor-1 (IRF-1), endothelial cell growth factor, glucocorticoid receptor, and early growth response gene-1 (EGR-1). However, the critical gene deletion involved in this syndrome may be a ribosomal protein processing gene, RPS14, haploinsufficiency which limits erythroid differentiation and survival in laboratory models.

Clinical features This syndrome has characteristic clinical features, including older age, female predominance, diagnosis of RA without excess (< 5%) blasts in 75% of cases, macrocytosis with severe anemia, erythroblastopenia, normal leukocyte counts, normal or increased platelet counts, and hypolobulated megakaryocytes in the bone marrow.

Progression to AML is infrequent (< 20%), and the prognosis is usually good. However, not every patient with del(5q) has this syndrome and its associated good prognosis. Additional cytogenetic abnormalities or the presence of ≥ 5% blasts in the peripheral blood or bone marrow is inconsistent with this diagnosis.

Molecular findings

The *ras* family of genes is most frequently altered in MDS, although other abnormalities involving NF1, FMS, *p53*, TEL, EVI, AXL, TEC, HCK, c-*mpl*, and other genes have also been described.

Mutations in *ras* Mutations in the *ras* family occur in approximately 20% to 40% of patients with MDS but are most frequently found in those with CMML. Mutations in *ras* are more common in codons 12, 13, and 61. Mutations in N-*ras* are more common than those in K-*ras* or H-*ras*.

A difference in the surface expression of phosphatidylserine (a marker of apoptosis) on cell membranes among de novo AML, MDS, and secondary AML and normal bone marrow cells has been found (increased in MDS and secondary AML). Epigenetic silencing of the *p15* tumor-suppressor gene by promoter hypermethylation occurs particularly among patients with high-risk MDS and is associated with a poor prognosis. FLT_3 mutations or internal tandem duplications occur much less frequently in MDS (usually < 5%) than in AML.

TABLE 3: International Prognostic Scoring System (IPSS) for MDS

Characteristic	Value	Score
Bone marrow blasts (%)	< 5	0
	5-10	0.5
	11-20	1.5
	21-30	2.0
Karyotype[a]	Good	0
	Intermediate	0.5
	Poor	1.0
Cytopenias	0-1	0
	2-3	0.5

Risk group	Sum of score
Low	0
Intermediate 1	0.5-1.0
Intermediate 2	1.5-2.0
High	≥ 2.5

[a] Good = diploid, -y, del(5q), del(20 q); Poor = chromosome 7 abnormalities or complex (≥ 3) abnormalities; Intermediate = all others

Staging and prognosis

Prognostic factors

FAB and WHO classifications The FAB classification has a long history of use to evaluate survival and risk for AML transformation (Table 1). The WHO classification has similar prognostic implications, based primarily upon the prognostic impact of blast percentage and the number of dysplastic lineages.

Cytogenetics Patients with complex karyotypes and abnormalities in chromosome 7 have a poor prognosis, whereas those with a normal karyotype, -Y, 5q-, or 20q- have a favorable prognosis.

Peripheral cytopenias (hemoglobin level < 10 g/dL, absolute neutrophil count [ANC] < 1.8×10^9/L, and platelet count < 100×10^9/L) have a cumulative adverse effect on prognosis.

Other prognostic factors Other parameters associated with a poor outcome include CD34 cell expression, high serum LDH levels, expression of the c-*mpl* gene, *ras* mutations, *p*-glycoprotein (Pgp) expression, *p15* inactivation, and *p53* mutations. However, it is unclear whether these factors have independent prognostic value.

International Prognostic Scoring System (IPSS)

An International MDS Risk Analysis Workshop has proposed a system that combines clinical, morphologic, and cytogenetic data to generate a consensus prognostic system.

By multivariate analysis, the most significant independent variables were percentage of bone marrow blasts, cytogenetics, and number of cytopenias (Table 3). It is important to keep in mind, however, that other variables (eg, age and prior therapy) not included in this system may alter the prognosis and influence the results of therapy among patients in similar IPSS groups. Still, this may be the most valuable risk classification for treatment planning.

Other scoring systems

The IPSS and WHO classifications have limitations in assessing the risk of patients with MDS: excess weight toward percentage of blasts, lack of discrimination of patients with lower-risk disease, and other clinical characteristics. Recently, several newer models have been developed to address these issues such as the WHO classification-based prognostic scoring system (WPSS) and the M. D. Anderson low-risk model.

Histone deacetylase (HDAC) inhibitors are being investigated in patients with MDS. Valproic acid has been reported to induce the differentiation of several tumor cell lines, and this effect has been presumed to be related to its ability to inhibit HDAC. In a recent study, 18 patients with MDS were treated with valproic acid alone (n = 18) or in combination with all-*trans*-retinoic acid (ATRA; n = 5). Eight patients (44%) responded to valproic acid alone (most hematologic improvement), with a median duration of response of 4 months. None of the patients treated with valproic acid and ATRA from the beginning responded, but two of five who lost their response to valproic acid alone responded again to the combination (Kuendgen A, Strupp C, Aivado M, et al: Blood 104:1266-1269, 2004). Studies are ongoing with more potent HDAC inhibitors such as vorinostat (Zolinza), LBH589, and MGCD0103.

Deferasirox (Exjade, ICL670) is an orally available iron-chelating agent shown to be effective in patients requiring frequent transfusion, including those with MDS. In 184 patients with transfusion-dependent anemia, including 47 with MDS, the mean (± SD) decrease in ferritin levels after administration of deferasirox was 268 ± 2053 ng/mL, with a mean decrease in liver iron concentration of 5.7 ± 6.3 mg Fe/g dw (Greenberg P, Dine G, Ganser A, et al: Blood 106:757a, 2005). Also, daily doses of 20–30 mg/kg of deferasirox induced iron balance or net negative iron balance was achieved in regularly transfused patients, including patients with MDS (Porter J, Borgna-Pignatti C, Baccarani M, et al: Blood 106:755a, 2005). For NCCN guidelines on use of deferasirox, see http://www.nccn.org/professionals/physician_gls/PDF/mds.pdf.

Treatment

The treatment of MDS is dictated by the risks imposed by the disease, age, and patient preference. Suggested guidelines are outlined in Table 4 and discussed below.

Supportive care

The use of transfusions affords temporary benefits and is an alternative that can be considered in patients with lower risk MDS or that otherwise can be used in conjunction with more definitive therapy. To delay or prevent end-organ complications, chelation therapy

TABLE 4: Suggested approach to the treatment of MDS

IPSS risk group	Treatment
Low, intermediate 1	Observation (particularly if mild cytopenia) Supportive care (transfusions, hematopoietic growth factors, iron chelation) Lenalidomide (for patients with 5q- abnormalities) Hypomethylating agents (azacitidine, decitabine) New (investigational) approaches, such as arsenic trioxide, farnesyl transferase inhibitors, histone deacetylase (HDAC) inhibitors, thalidomide, ATG (particularly if hypoplastic and low platelet count)
High, intermediate 2	Hypomethylating agents (azacitidine, decitabine) SCT (particularly for young patients with HLA-identical siblings; front-line vs in remission?) New (investigational) agents, such as topoisomerase inhibitors (topotecan, rubitecan), farnesyl transferase inhibitors, HDAC inhibitors, combination of hypomethylating agents and HDAC inhibitors

ATG = antithymocyte globulin; HLA = human lymphocyte antigen; IPSS = International Prognostic Scoring System; MDS = myelodysplastic syndromes; SCT = stem-cell transplantation

should be considered when RBC transfusions exceed 25 U or ferritin levels > 1,000 to 2,500 ng/mL.

Cytokines

Recent reports suggest that the use of chelation or growth factors may be associated with improved survival.

G-CSF and GM-CSF Granulocyte colony-stimulating factor (G-CSF, filgrastim, [Neupogen] or GM-CSF may improve neutropenia and decrease infections in up to 70% of patients with MDS, but the effect is usually transient. No increase in the probability of developing AML has been demonstrated with extended use of these cytokines.

Other alternatives

Antithymocyte globulin (ATG [Atgam]) has been associated with response (defined as independence from transfusions) in 34% of patients, which was sustained for a median of 36 months in 81% of them. Also, 48% had sustained platelet improvement and 55% had an increase in neutrophils. Younger patients and those with low platelet counts are more likely to respond than older patients and those with higher platelet counts.

A simple method for predicting response to immunosuppressive therapy in MDS has been proposed. It is based on the age of the patient, the duration of RBC transfusion dependence, and the HLA (human lymphocyte antigen)-DR15 status. Younger patients with a shorter duration of transfusion requirements have a higher predicted probability of response (40% to 100%), particularly when their status is positive for HLA-DR15. These data have not been confirmed and ATG should be reserved for patients with hypoplastic MDS.

Cyclosporine significantly increases cell colony growth in laboratory studies of hypoplastic RA. Responses have been reported in a limited number of patients.

Lenalidomide Lenalidomide (Revlimid) is a thalidomide analog that belongs to the immunomodulatory family of drugs. Lenalidomide has numerous properties that make it attractive for the management of neoplastic and inflammatory conditions, including the inhibition of production of cytokines such as tumor necrosis factor-α (TNF-α) and IL-1, IL-6, IL-10, and IL-12. Lenalidomide is markedly more potent than thalidomide (Thalomid) in inhibiting the secretion of TNF-α. In addition, lenalidomide may potentiate EPO-induced signaling in erythroid progenitors and stimulate stem-cell differentiation to erythroid cells.

Lenalidomide has been recently approved for the treatment of patients with MDS with abnormalities in the long arm of chromosome 5 (5q- abnormalities), whether they are isolated or present together with other cytogenetic abnormalities. In a study of patients with transfusion-dependent MDS with 5q- abnormalities, 75% of patients responded, with 66% of the total population becoming transfusion independent. The response rate was similar regardless of whether the cytogenetic abnormality was isolated or seen in conjunction with other cytogenetic abnormalities, and more than half of the responses were durable for more than 1 year. In addition, a cytogenetic response was observed in 70% of patients. Lenalidomide has also been investigated for patients with MDS without 5q- abnormalities. Erythroid responses were seen in over 40%, with 27% of the total population becoming transfusion independent.

Azacitidine (Vidaza) and 5-Aza-2'-deoxycytidine (Dacogen, DAC, decitabine) are hypomethylating agents that have shown activity in MDS. In a randomized trial, 191 patients with MDS (63% RAEB

In a study of 92 patients with MDS, three different schedules of decitabine (Dacogen) were investigated: 20 mg/m^2 IV over 1 hour daily for 5 days, 10 mg/m^2 IV over 1 hour daily for 10 days, or 10 mg/m^2 SQ twice daily for 5 days. The overall response rate was 76%, with the complete response rate being 36%. The complete response rate by schedule was 41%, 28%, and 24%, respectively. Compared with a historic control treated with intensive chemotherapy, those treated with decitabine had a lower induction mortality (15% vs 21%) and improved overall survival. These results suggest that decitabine is an effective agent for the management of patients with MDS (Kantarjian H, O'Brien S, Giles F, et al: Blood [abstract]106:708a, 2005). A recent multicenter report of this schedule of decitabine (ADOPT trial) indicated a complete response rate of 15% and a partial response rate of 15% (Steensma DP, Baer MR, Slack JL, et al: Blood 110:434a [abstract 1450], 2007).

or RAEB-t) were treated with azacitidine or supportive care. Responses were observed in 60% of those treated with azacitidine (complete response [CR]: 6%; partial response [PR]: 10%; hematologic improvement: 47%) compared with 5% with supportive care. There was a significant improvement in probability of transformation to AML and overall survival when the confounding effect of early crossover to azacitidine was eliminated.

Azacitidine is approved by the US Food and Drug Administration for the treatment of patients with all types of MDS. The standard dose is 75 mg/m^2/d subcutaneously for 7 days every 4 weeks for as long as the patient benefits. Responses occur after a median of 3 to 4 cycles, so it is recommended to continue therapy for at least 4 to 6 cycles, unless there is significant toxicity or progression of disease. The dose may be increased to 100 mg/m^2/d after 2 cycles if no improvement has occurred. Myelosuppression may occur but is not a reason to discontinue therapy. Rather, patients should be supported during myelosuppression and should continue therapy to give them the best opportunity of response. In a post-approval phase III trial, treatment with azacitidine significantly improved survival by a median of 29 months (median survival, 24.5 months vs 15 months) compared with a conventional care arm that included supportive care, low-dose cytarabine, and conventional leukemia induction and consolidation therapy.

Decitabine is approved by the FDA for the treatment of patients with all types of MDS. In a multicenter phase II study, 66 patients (73% RAEB or RAEB-t) were treated with decitabine. The overall response rate was 49% (CR: 20%; PR: 4%; improvement: 24%). The actuarial median response duration was 31 weeks, and median survival was 22 months. In addition, 31% of patients with cytogenetic abnormalities presented before treatment achieved a cytogenetic response. Cytogenetic response conferred a survival advantage to these patients.

A report of a randomized phase III study of azacitidine (n = 179) versus conventional care (n = 179); (supportive care, low-dose cytarabine or "7 + 3" induction chemotherapy) was presented at ASH 2007. It demonstrated that treatment with 5-azacitidine was associated with a significant improvement in overall survival (hazard ratio 0.58; P = .0001), translating into a doubling of survival at 24 months. The median number of courses of azacitidine administered was 9 and the overall response rate was 78% (complete response 17%, partial response 12%, and complete response [HI] 49%) (Fenaux P, Mufti GJ, Santini V, et al: Blood 110:250a [abstract 817], 2007).

Recently, several studies combining decitabine or azacitidine with valproic acid (a histone deacetylase [HDAC] inhibitor) have shown success in MDS and AML.

Steroids, androgens, and pyridoxine are rarely effective, although they are often used clinically.

Chemotherapy

The rationale for this strategy stems from the concepts that MDS is a clonal disorder and that MDS and AML are overlapping illnesses with an arbitrary frontier defined by the WHO and FAB classifications (ie, a 20% to 30% blast threshold).

The Cancer and Leukemia Group B (CALGB) treated 874 patients with AML and 33 patients with MDS with AML-like chemotherapy. The CR rate was 79% for patients with MDS versus 68% for patients with AML ($P= .37$), median CR duration was 11 versus 15 months ($P= .28$), and median survival was 13 versus 16 months. The authors concluded that the FAB distinction between MDS (RAEB and RAEB-t) and AML has minimal therapeutic implications.

Estey et al treated 372 patients with AML, 52 with RAEB, and 106 with RAEB-t with AML-type chemotherapy. CR rates were 62% for patients with RAEB, 66% for those with RAEB-t, and 66% for those with AML ($P= .79$). Event-free survival was significantly better for patients with AML/RAEB-t than for patients with RAEB. However, when cytogenetics and other prognostic variables were considered in a multivariate analysis, no difference in outcome could be identified among FAB subgroups.

These findings suggest that the prognosis is determined more by cytogenetics and other prognostic features than by the percentage of blasts or FAB classification. However, this finding does not necessarily mean that MDS and AML are biologically equivalent entities.

Combination regimens Different combination chemotherapy regimens have been investigated. The combination of cytarabine (Ara-C) and anthracycline is the cornerstone of intensive chemotherapy, leading to CRs in 40% to 60% of patients. However, despite the fact that cytogenetic remissions frequently accompany hematologic CRs, the median remission duration and survival times are brief, rarely exceeding 1 year. The death rate during induction therapy is 5% to 20%.

Myeloblasts in RAEB-t and secondary AML commonly express the multidrug exporter Pgp, which extrudes anthracyclines and limits their activity. A randomized, controlled trial performed by the Southwest Oncology Group (SWOG) reported a twofold improvement in survival for patients treated with an anthracycline- and Ara-C–containing induction and consolidation regimens with the Pgp antagonist cyclosporine added.

It is possible that certain chemotherapeutic agents may be particularly useful in MDS.

SCT

Allogeneic SCT can be of benefit in a subset of patients with MDS. However, most series have concentrated on younger patients, who constitute a minority of patients with MDS and frequently have favorable cytogenetics and therefore a better prognosis. The best results to date have been reported in patients with a better prognosis (ie, those with

Stem-cell transplantation is a treatment option for some patients with MDS, although its timing remains controversial. An International Bone Marrow Transplant Registry analysis used a Markov model to examine three transplantation strategies for newly diagnosed MDS: transplantation at the time of diagnosis, transplantation at the time of progression to leukemia, and transplantation at an interval from diagnosis but prior to leukemic progression. Although transplantation at diagnosis may be superior for patients with intermediate-2 and high-risk IPSS (International Prognostic Scoring System) scores, delayed transplantation was associated with improved life expectancy (*Cutler CS, Lee SJ, Greenberg P, et al: Blood* 104:579-585, 2004).

RA/RARS). In most series, allogeneic SCT is associated with a long-term remission rate of approximately 40%, a 30% relapse rate, and a 30% rate of transplant-related death.

The timing of transplantation remains controversial. Runde et al reported on a group of 131 patients (median age, 33 years; range, 2 to 55 years) who underwent allogeneic SCT as front-line therapy without prior induction chemotherapy. The 5-year disease-free survival rate was 34%, overall survival rate was 41%, and transplant-related mortality was 38%. The actuarial probability of relapse at 5 years was 39%, with better results observed in the RA/RARS subgroup.

Patients with adverse cytogenetics have a poor outcome with other treatment modalities, and SCT can be considered for such patients during first CR. However, the long-term outcome for these patients after SCT has not proved to be superior to that after any other approach, although the procedure may prove to be curative in a small percentage of patients. SCT should be considered particularly in the setting of a clinical trial.

New applications for allogeneic SCT (eg, nonmyeloablative) to make this option available to the typical patient with MDS (who is frequently older and has other associated medical problems), as well as for matched-unrelated donor SCT, should be investigated further.

Autologous SCT In the majority of patients with MDS, lymphocytes do not appear to be part of the clone, suggesting the presence of normal nonclonal stem cells. De Witte et al described 79 patients with MDS or secondary AML who underwent autologous SCT during first CR. The 2-year survival, disease-free survival, and relapse rates were 39%, 34%, and 64%, respectively. The 2-year survival rate for the MDS group was 40%, and treatment-related mortality was 9%. The best outcome was seen among patients with RA/RARS.

In a study reported by investigators at M. D. Anderson Comprehensive Cancer Center, 14 patients with MDS were treated with decitabine following azacitidine failure, lack of response, or intolerance. Complete remission was achieved with decitabine in 3 patients, and hematologic improvement was seen in 1 patient; there was an overall response rate of 28%. Among patients who responded to decitabine, treatment with azacitidine had been stopped for disease progression in one patient, no response in two patients, and severe skin toxicity in a fourth patient. The authors reported that grade 3-4 toxicity from decitabine was minimal and concluded that decitabine may produce clinically significant responses in some patients following azacitidine-failure *(Borthakur G, Ahdab SE, Ravandi F, et al: Leuk Lymphoma 49:690-695, 2008).*

Treatment recommendations

Treatment of patients with MDS is an evolving and controversial issue, and enrollment in a clinical trial should be encouraged. Treatment can be considered according to the IPSS.

Patients with low or intermediate-1 IPSS scores can frequently be treated with supportive measures. Agents such as ATG and cyclosporine could be used alone or in combination. Patients with 5q- benefit from lenalidomide, particularly in terms of erythroid response, and this should be considered the treatment of choice. Some patients with MDS without the 5q- abnormality may also benefit from lenalidomide, but its use in this setting is still being investigated. Azacitidine should be considered for all patients in view of its effect on survival. Decitabine is another good option recently approved for patients with MDS.

Patients with high or intermediate-2 IPSS scores have significant risk of mortality from cytopenias or AML evolution. They should be considered for treatment options with the intention to cure, extend survival, or delay the progression of AML. In view of the survival effect of azacitidine, it should be considered as first-line therapy for patients with higher-risk disease. The results of a similar survival study with decitabine will be reported in the near future. Intensive chemotherapy should be reserved for younger patients with good prognostic features (diploid cytogenetics). Lenalidomide has no role yet in this patient population.

SCT is an alternative for younger patients with higher-risk MDS and an HLA-identical donor, particularly patients with adverse cytogenetic abnormalities. However, the best results to date have been reported in patients with a better prognosis (ie, younger patients and those with RA/RARS). Therefore, allogeneic transplantation and other transplant alternatives should be considered preferentially in a research setting (eg, mixed-unrelated donor and minitransplants) or in patients who have failed to respond to other therapies.

SUGGESTED READING

Fenaux P, Mufti GJ, Santini V, et al: Azacitidine (AZA) treatment prolongs overall survival (OS) in higher-risk MDS patients compared with conventional care regimens (CCR): Results of the AZA-001 phase III study (abstract). Blood 110:817, 2007.

Garcia-Manero G, Kantarjian HM, Sanchez-Gonzalez B, et al: Phase 1/2 study of the combination of 5-aza-2'-deoxycytidine with valproic acid in patients with leukemia. Blood 108:3271–3279, 2006.

Garcia-Manero G, Shan J, Faderl S, et al: A prognostic score for patients with lower risk myelodysplastic syndrome. Leukemia 22:538–543, 2008.

Garcia-Manero G, Yang H, Bueso-Ramos C, et al: Phase I study of the histone deacetylase inhibitor vorinostat (suberoylanilide hydroxamic acid, SAHA) in patients with advanced leukemias and myelodysplastic syndromes. Blood 111:1060–1066, 2007.

Greenberg P, Cox C, LeBeau MM, et al: International scoring system for evaluating prognosis in myelodysplastic syndromes. Blood 89:2079–2088, 1997.

Kantarjian H, Issa JP, Rosenfeld CS, et al: Decitabine improves patient outcomes in myelodysplastic syndromes: Results of a phase III randomized study. Cancer 106:1794–1803, 2006.

Kantarjian H, Oki Y, Garcia-Manero G, et al: Results of a randomized study of 3 schedules of low-dose decitabine in higher-risk myelodysplastic syndrome and chronic myelomonocytic leukemia. Blood 109:52–57, 2007.

List A, Dewald G, Bennett J, et al: Lenalidomide in the myelodysplastic syndrome with chromosome 5q deletion. N Engl J Med 355:1456–1465, 2006.

Malcovati L, Germing U, Kuendgen A, et al: Time-dependent prognostic scoring system for predicting survival and leukemic evolution in myelodysplastic syndromes. J Clin Oncol 25:3503–3510, 2007.

Silverman LR, Demakos EP, Peterson BL, et al: Randomized controlled trial of azacitidine in patients with the myelodysplastic syndrome: A study of the cancer and leukemia group B. J Clin Oncol 20:2429–2440, 2002.

Soriano AO, Yang H, Faderl S, et al: Safety and clinical activity of the combination of 5-azacytidine, valproic acid, and all-trans retinoic acid in acute myeloid leukemia and myelodysplastic syndrome. Blood 110:2302–2308, 2007.

Steensma DP, Baer MR, Slack JL, et al: Preliminary results of a phase II study of decitabine administered daily for 5 days every 4 weeks to adults with myelodysplastic syndrome (MDS). Blood 110:1450, 2007.

CHAPTER 36

Hematopoietic cell transplantation

Stephen J. Forman, MD

Hematopoietic cell transplantation (HCT) is the IV infusion of hematopoietic progenitor cells designed to establish marrow and immune function in patients with a variety of acquired and inherited malignant and nonmalignant disorders. They include hematologic malignancies (eg, leukemia, lymphoma, and myeloma), nonmalignant acquired bone marrow disorders (aplastic anemia), and genetic diseases associated with abnormal hematopoiesis and function (thalassemia, sickle cell anemia, and severe combined immunodeficiency). HCT also is used in the support of patients undergoing high-dose chemotherapy for the treatment of solid tumors for which hematologic toxicity would otherwise limit drug administration (eg, breast, germ-cell, and ovarian cancers).

Types of transplantation

Since the advent of HCT in the 1960s, several different methods of transplantation have evolved. At present, the hematopoietic cells used for HCT are obtained from either bone marrow or peripheral blood. The decision to use a certain type of HCT is dictated by the patient's disease and condition and the availability of a donor. In some cases, more than one approach is possible. Table 1 summarizes the advantages and disadvantages of each stem-cell source.

Allogeneic BMT, matched related This method involves procurement of bone marrow from a human leukocyte antigen (HLA)-identical sibling of the patient. In some cases, a partially matched sibling or family donor (one antigen mismatch) can be used for bone marrow transplantation (BMT).

Allogeneic BMT, matched unrelated Given that there are a limited number of alleles of the HLA system, typing of large numbers of individuals has led to the observation that full matches for patients exist in the general population. Tissue typing is performed on the patient's blood, and a search of the computer files of various international registries is made to determine whether a patient has a match with an unrelated individual.

Haploidentical transplantation involves the transplantation of large numbers of T-cell–depleted stem cells from a donor, usually a sibling or a parent, who is half matched to the patient. Although these are the most difficult transplantations to perform successfully, there is great interest in this approach because most patients will have a donor in their family who is at least a 50% HLA match. Although most transplants will engraft and few patients will have significant graft-versus-host disease (GVHD), the relapse rate is high and the process of immune reconstitution is slow, with patients often having troublesome infections for a long time after transplantation.

Autologous BMT This form of transplantation entails the use of the patient's own bone marrow, which is harvested and then cryopreserved prior to administration of chemotherapy and/or high-dose radiation therapy. Following completion of therapy, the marrow cells are then thawed and reinfused into the patient to reestablish hematopoiesis.

Autologous peripheral blood stem-cell transplantation With the recognition that the marrow stem cells circulate in the peripheral blood, methods have been devised to augment the number of these cells in the patient's circulation. The blood is then collected on a cell separator and frozen, similar to autologous marrow, to be utilized after high-dose chemotherapy and/or radiation therapy. This is now the most common source of stem cells used in the autologous setting.

Syngeneic transplantation In this form of transplantation, marrow or peripheral blood stem cells are procured from an individual who is a genetic identical twin to the patient.

Donor leukocyte infusion This method involves the infusion of mononuclear cells from the marrow donor into the recipient to treat relapse after transplantation. The cells can mediate an antitumor effect, known as a graft-versus-tumor effect (often in association with concomitant GVHD), and can achieve remission of the malignancy.

Nonmyeloablative or reduced-intensity transplantation This approach uses lower doses of chemotherapy, with or without total-body irradiation (TBI) and immunosuppression, to facilitate engraftment of donor stem cells. Donor stem cells obtained from either the peripheral blood or marrow are then infused into the patient, leading to hematopoietic engraftment. The major therapeutic effect that results from this type of transplantation is a graft-versus-tumor effect, as the nonmyeloablative regimen has limited long-term antitumor efficacy. Some disorders such as chronic myelogenous leukemia (CML), acute myelogenous leukemia (AML), low-grade lymphoma, and multiple myeloma are particularly sensitive to this approach. This type of transplant allows older patients to undergo the procedure, as the transplant-related mortality is greatly reduced with this approach.

Cord blood transplantation The blood in the umbilical cord of newborn babies contains large numbers of stem cells, which have been shown to be capable of long-term engraftment in children and some adults after transplantation. Similar to unrelated-donor registries, cord blood banks have been developed to store cord blood cells that can be utilized for unrelated-donor transplantation. Given the immunologic immaturity of cord blood cells, these transplants can be accomplished even when there are disparities (mismatching) in the HLA typing between the donor and recipient. Cord blood transplants are generally used in situations where an adult unrelated donor cannot be identified through the international registries.

TABLE 1: Stem-cell sources for allogeneic BMT

Type	Advantages	Disadvantages
Allogeneic		
Sibling donor 6/6 HLA match or 5/6	Match able to be identified rapidly (2 weeks)	GVHD (25%-40%) for non–T-cell-depleted marrow grafts
	Low rate of graft rejection (2%-5%)	Only 30% of patients will have sibling donor
Matched unrelated donor	Extends donor availability (60%-70% of patients will have potential match)	Takes time to find donor (6 weeks to > 6 months)
	Greater graft-versus-tumor effect	Higher graft failure rates (5%-10%)
		Higher GVHD rates (50%-60%)
Umbilical cord donor	Lesser degrees of match can be used	Limited number of cells (reduced applicability to large recipient)
		Slower engraftment
	Much lower rate of GVHD (10%-20%) despite one and two antigen mismatches	Higher rate of graft failure (10%)
		No chance for second infusion for graft failure or DLI for relapse
Haploidentical family donor	Almost all patients have a sibling, parent, or child who is haploidentical. These donors can be used if patients have relapsed or there is refractory disease and no better donor has been identified	Needs much more profound immunosuppression (T-cell depletion of donor product included) to achieve engraftment
		High risk of infectious complications
		Graft failure rate of 10%-15%
Syngeneic Identical twin	No need for immunosuppression	No graft-versus-tumor effect
	No GVHD	

BMT = bone marrow transplantation; DLI = donor lymphocyte infusion; GVHD = graft-versus-host disease

Allogeneic transplantation

HLA typing

Finding a related donor As noted previously, matched related allogeneic BMT involves a donor who is an HLA-matched sibling of the recipient. The formula for calculating the chances of a particular person having an HLA-matched sibling is $1 - (0.75)^N$, where N denotes the number of potential sibling donors. In general, a patient with one sibling has a 25% chance of having a match. The average American family size usually limits the success of finding a family donor to approximately 30% of patients.

HLA typing is performed on blood samples obtained from the patient and potential donor. Serologic methods have been used to detect the identity of the class I and II antigens; molecular methods are now utilized for more refined matching of both classes. A match is noted when the major class I antigens (A and B loci), as well as class II antigens (DR), are the same as those of the donor. Each sibling receives one set of antigens (A, B, DR) from each parent (chromosome 6). Genotypic identity can be confirmed by testing the parents and determining the inheritance of each set of antigens.

Finding an unrelated donor In cases in which the patient needs an allogeneic transplant and a donor cannot be found within the family, the identification of a matched-unrelated donor is accomplished by searching the computer files of the National Marrow Donor Program, as well as other international registries. As there are multiple alleles of any given HLA locus, serologic identity does not necessarily imply genotypic identity, such as is the case among sibling donor-recipient pairs. The development of oligonucleotide probes has greatly increased the precision of HLA typing and has allowed for more specific selection of bone marrow donors by matching molecular alleles of the class I and II antigens.

Advantages and disadvantages

The major advantages of an allogeneic graft include the absence of malignant cells contaminating the graft; the potential for an immunologic anticancer graft-versus-tumor effect; and the ability to treat malignant and nonmalignant disorders of the bone marrow, including genetic and immunologic diseases.

The disadvantages of an allogeneic transplant include the difficulty in finding an appropriate HLA-matched donor and the development of GVHD after BMT, which contributes to the morbidity and mortality of the procedure.

Autologous transplantation

Advantages and disadvantages

In autologous transplantation, the reinfused stem cells come from either the patient's own bone marrow or peripheral blood. These cells do not cause GVHD, and, thus, autologous transplantation is associated with less morbidity and mortality than allogeneic BMT and increases the number of patients who can undergo the procedure, as well as the upper age limit.

The disadvantages of autologous BMT include the likelihood of tumor cell contamination within the graft in many diseases, which can cause relapse; the lack of a significant therapeutic graft-versus-tumor effect; and the limited ability to use autologous stem cells in the treatment of patients not in remission or with inherited nonmalignant lymphohematopoietic diseases. Table 2 summarizes the advantages and disadvantages of these two approaches.

TABLE 2: Comparison of allogeneic versus autologous stem-cell transplantation

Allogeneic

Advantages

No tumor contamination of the graft and no prior marrow injury from chemotherapy (less risk of later myelodysplasia)

Graft-versus-tumor effect

Can be used for patients with marrow involvement by tumor or with bone marrow dysfunction, such as aplastic anemia, hemoglobinopathies, or prior pelvic irradiation

Disadvantages

Dose-intensive regimen limited by toxicity (usually limited to patients < age 55)

Takes time to identify donor if no sibling donor available/limited availability of donor for some ethnic groups

Higher early treatment-related mortality from graft-versus-host disease and infectious complications (20%-40% depending on age and donor source)

Autologous

Advantages

No need to identify donor if peripheral blood marrow uninvolved by tumor at the time of collection

No immunosuppression = less risk of infections

No graft-versus-host disease

Dose-intensive therapy can be used for older patients (usually up to age 70)

Low early treatment-related mortality (2%-5%)

Disadvantages

Not feasible if peripheral blood stem cells/marrow involved

Possible marrow injury leading to late myelodysplasia (either from prior chemotherapy or transplant regimen)

No graft-versus-tumor effect

Not all patients can be mobilized to give adequate cell doses for reconstitution

Modifications of the stem-cell graft

The disadvantages of both allogeneic and autologous transplantations have led to the development of modifications of the stem-cell graft.

Removing T cells from donor marrow With regard to allogeneic BMT, it is known that contaminating T cells from the donor mediate the onset and persistence of acute and chronic GVHD. T cells have been removed from the donor marrow to prevent the development of severe GVHD. However, this approach has increased the incidence of both graft rejection and relapse of malignancy. Some investigators are exploring planned return of donor T cells after hematopoietic recovery to help prevent relapse.

Primed peripheral blood stem cells from marrow donors have reduced transplant-related complications without a substantial increase in acute GVHD. Thus far, the data show that this approach induces more rapid engraftment. Most studies have reported an increase in chronic GVHD.

Eliminating tumor cells from autologous grafts Although autologous peripheral blood stem-cell transplantation has led to more rapid restoration of hematopoiesis, it is associated with a higher relapse rate than is allogeneic BMT. Attempts to deplete the autologous graft of tumor cells have included in vitro purging with monoclonal antibodies and/or chemotherapeutic agents and the enrichment of stem cells over various separation columns.

Post-transplantation immunomodulation For patients undergoing autologous transplantation, several post-transplantation immunomodulating strategies, such as rituximab (Rituxan) after autologous transplantation for B-cell lymphoma, are being tested to determine whether they will decrease relapse by augmenting immunologic antitumor responses following transplantation. In some diseases such as myeloma, post-transplant treatment with medication such as dexamethasone and with thalidomide (Thalomid) helps prolong remission.

Collection of the graft

Allogeneic bone marrow cells Current techniques for harvesting bone marrow involve repeated aspirations from the posterior iliac crests, designed to obtain adequate numbers of cells that can lead to hematopoiesis. While the donor is under general or spinal anesthesia, between 1 to 3×10^8 cells/kg of the recipient's body weight are procured. The procedure has no long-term side effects and poses little risk if care is taken to ensure that the donor has no confounding medical conditions. In most cases of ABO incompatibility, the marrow can be treated to remove RBCs to prevent lysis after infusion.

Autologous peripheral stem cells Collection of circulating peripheral blood progenitor cells is performed via an apheresis technique. Although this procedure can be accomplished in an individual with a baseline blood count, the number of cells and the efficiency of collection are increased if the cells are procured during WBC recovery following chemotherapy or after the administration of hematopoietic growth factors.

Although busulfan-based regimens are the most commonly used worldwide for allogeneic transplantation, the oral administration of busulfan (Myleran) leads to unpredictable absorption, which has been correlated with relapse (low absorption) and increased toxicity (increased absorption). Recent studies with an intravenous formulation of the drug have shown much more predictable pharmacokinetics, less toxicity, and good survival when utilized in the transplantation regimen.

The most effective strategy appears to be the collection of cells after both chemotherapy and administration of growth factors. In most circumstances, adequate numbers of cells can be collected utilizing granulocyte colony-stimulating factor (G-CSF, filgrastim [Neupogen]) to prime the patient prior to one to three apheresis procedures.

Currently, the adequacy of the number of

hematopoietic stem cells is assessed by determining the number of cells that have the CD34 antigen (stem-cell) marker. Usually, a minimum of 2×10^6 CD34 cells/kg of body weight is required to ensure engraftment.

The use of autologous stem cells continues to undergo refinement. Approaches under study include ex vivo expansion to augment the number of progenitor cells, as well as techniques that separate hematopoietic cells from any potential contaminating tumor cells. In addition, hematopoietic stem cells are the usual targets of marrow-based gene therapy utilizing viral vectors for transduction of cells prior to cryopreservation.

Indications for transplantation

The expanded methods of stem-cell transplantation have complicated the choice for patients and their physicians among the different types of transplantation in some instances. Therefore, the decision requires evaluation of the patient and the disease involved. In general, for disorders that require replacement of an abnormally functioning hematopoietic system, such as thalassemia and aplastic anemia, an allogeneic transplantation is performed. However, as genetic therapy for hematopoietic stem cells becomes more of a reality, even patients with these diseases may be candidates for autologous transplantation after gene modification (adenosine deaminase deficiency, chronic granulomatous disease).

Hematologic malignancies The most common use of allogeneic BMT has been for the eradication of hematologic malignancies, such as leukemia and non-Hodgkin lymphoma. For some disorders (aplastic anemia, myelodysplasia, leukemia in relapse, and CML), allogeneic transplantation is the only significant therapeutic option, whereas for other diseases (AML in remission, lymphoma, Hodgkin lymphoma, and multiple myeloma), either autologous or allogeneic marrow grafting may be possible.

Nonmyeloablative or reduced-intensity transplantation approaches are being studied worldwide, which has facilitated transplantation for many people who otherwise would not have been candidates due to concomitant medical problems or older age. The results indicate that slower growing malignancies are the most responsive. Thus, patients with low-grade lymphoma, AML, myeloma, myelodysplasia, and CML are probably good candidates for this type of allogeneic transplantation, whereas those with advanced disease such as leukemia in relapse or high-grade lymphoma benefit less, as the allogeneic antitumor effect requires time to develop and achieve remission of the disease. Table 3 shows the relative sensitivity of different hematologic malignancies to a graft-versus-malignancy effect that could be mediated by a nonmyeloablative transplant.

Solid tumors In general, only autologous transplantation is utilized for some solid tumors, such as breast, germ-cell, and ovarian cancers. Studies and longer follow-up of recently completed trials continue to determine whether there is a benefit to the use of transplant-based approaches in the treatment of high-risk (stages II, IIIA, IIIB) breast cancer. Allogeneic transplant studies in patients

TABLE 3: Disease sensitivity to a graft-versus-malignancy effect

Most sensitive

Chronic myelogenous leukemia
Low-grade lymphoma
Mantle cell lymphoma
Chronic lymphocytic leukemia

Intermediately sensitive

Acute myelogenous leukemia
Intermediate-grade lymphoma
Multiple myeloma

Least sensitive

Acute lymphoblastic leukemia
High-grade lymphoma
Hodgkin lymphoma (?)
Renal cell carcinoma

---

with renal cell cancer suggest that a graft-versus-tumor effect can be elicited against this tumor as well.

Timing of transplantation

The Goldie-Coldman model proposes that the probability that a tumor contains treatment-resistant cells is a function of its size and inherent mutation rate. This finding suggests that the likelihood of cure is greatest when marrow transplantation is performed early in the natural history of an inherently chemosensitive tumor. Studies to date indicate that patients undergoing transplantation late in their disease course have inferior disease-free survival, compared with those who undergo transplantation early.

Phases of transplantation

PREPARATIVE PHASE

In the first phase of marrow transplantation, the preparative phase, patients receive high-dose chemotherapy and/or radiation therapy (sometimes referred to as a conditioning regimen).

Allogeneic transplantation The conditioning regimen used in the allogeneic setting has both a therapeutic component designed to eliminate tumor cells and an immunosuppressive component to prevent host immune responses from rejecting the transplanted donor graft. The doses of radiation therapy and chemotherapy employed take advantage of the steep dose-response curve that exists for many malignancies. The doses have been established based on the limitations of other nonhematopoietic organs, such as the liver and lungs.

TABLE 4: Acute and long-term toxicities of common preparative agents used for BMT

Agent	Acute toxicity	Long-term toxicity
Total-body irradiation	Nausea, vomiting, enteritis, mucositis	Cataracts, sterility, pneumonitis, myelodysplasia
Cyclophosphamide	Nausea, vomiting, hemorrhagic cystitis, cardiac toxicity	Sterility, leukemia
Etoposide	Skin rash, hypotension, acidosis, mucositis	Leukemia
Carmustine	Seizures, nausea, vomiting, headaches	Interstitial pneumonitis
Busulfan	Seizures, nausea, vomiting, veno-occlusive disease	Alopecia, pulmonary fibrosis
Cisplatin	Renal impairment, hearing loss, tinnitus	Hearing loss, tinnitus, neuropathy
Thiotepa	Nausea, vomiting, CNS changes, veno-occlusive disease	—
Paclitaxel	Allergic reactions	Neuropathy
Fludarabine	Hemolytic anemia, CNS changes	Prolonged immune suppression, EBV-related lympho-proliferative disorder
Melphalan	Nausea, pulmonary toxicity	Peripheral neuropathy

BMT = bone marrow transplantation; EBV = Epstein-Barr virus

Typically, preparative regimens for full allogeneic BMT consist of TBI and/or chemotherapeutic agents (cyclophosphamide, busulfan [Busulfex, Myleran], and etoposide). The most commonly used regimens are (1) TBI (1,200–1,400 cGy administered in multiple fractions over a period of days) and cyclophosphamide (60 mg/kg for 2 days); (2) fractionated TBI and etoposide (60 mg/kg); and (3) busulfan (16 mg/kg over 4 days) and cyclophosphamide (60 mg/kg for 2 days).

Autologous transplantation For patients undergoing autologous transplantation, stem cells are reinfused following high-dose therapy to reestablish hematopoiesis as rapidly as possible. The regimens used for autologous BMT depend on the disease being treated. High-dose melphalan (Alkeran; 200 mg / m^2) is the most commonly used regimen for myeloma and BEAM (BiCNU [carmustine], etoposide, cytosine arabinoside, and melphalan) or CBV (cyclophosphamide, BiCNU [carmustine], and etoposide) are the two most commonly used regimens for lymphoma.

Toxicities of preparative regimens The acute toxicities of irradiation and chemotherapy include nausea and vomiting, which can be managed by prophylactic use of antiemetics, particularly serotonin antagonists. Busulfan can cause seizures; prophylactic phenytoin is effective in preventing this complication. Both cyclophosphamide and etoposide require forced hydration to reduce toxicities. Table 4 lists the acute and long-term toxicities of the major agents used in BMT preparative regimens.

TRANSPLANT PHASE

After completion of the preparative regimen, there is a day or more wait before reinfusion of marrow or peripheral blood stem cells. This delay allows for elimination of any active drug metabolites so that the reinfused cells are not injured by any remaining drug.

Minimal toxicities are associated with the infusion. They include headache, nausea, and dizziness. Dizziness is related more to the cryoprotectant dimethyl sulfoxide (DMSO) used to store cells from most patients undergoing autologous transplantation.

SUPPORTIVE CARE PHASE

Following administration of the preparative regimen and during and after marrow transplantation, all patients require strict attention to infectious disease-related complications secondary to neutropenia. The duration of neutropenia following transplantation increases the risk of complicating infections. Patients undergoing full allogeneic transplantation usually require more stringent isolation, whereas patients undergoing autologous transplantation need less rigorous protection. With the availability of more effective antiemetics (eg, ondansetron and granisetron), portions of the transplantation can now be performed in the outpatient setting.

Following allogeneic transplantation, various complications may develop that require treatment. For some complications, prophylactic measures can be instituted to prevent their occurrence.

Neutropenic sepsis

Nearly all patients undergoing transplantation will develop fever, often with positive blood cultures, within 7 days of becoming neutropenic. Sepsis usually is caused by enteric bacteria or those found on the skin, and antibiotic choices are based on initial assessment and the results of blood cultures. The antibiotics chosen are continued until the neutrophil count begins to rise (> 500 k/µL). Most patients undergoing allogeneic transplantation usually receive bowel decontamination (eg, with a fluoroquinolone, such as levofloxacin [Levaquin], 500 mg/d PO) in the post-transplantation phase to reduce the risk of serious infection during neutropenia.

Prevention of fungal infections For patients who are expected to have prolonged neutropenia, various methods of antifungal prophylaxis are used, including PO fluconazole (Diflucan; 200 mg bid) or voriconazole (Vfend; 200 mg IV or PO bid). The use of liposomal amphotericin B (AmBisome or Abelcet) or caspofungin (Cancidas) formulations has improved safety and lowered toxicity of antifungal therapy and is particularly worthwhile in patients with renal compromise.

Mucositis, nausea, and anorexia

Regimen-related toxicity often results in severe oral mucositis, nausea, and anorexia. Patients often require supplemental parenteral nutrition to maintain adequate caloric intake during this period. Because of the mucositis, enteral feedings are usually not employed, and total parenteral nutrition is maintained until patients are able to eat. Studies are exploring novel agents that could prevent severe mucositis or accelerate healing with keratinocyte growth factor (KGF), which has been shown to decrease this complication following TBI-based autologous transplant regimens.

Oral HSV reactivation

Nearly all patients who are seropositive for herpes simplex virus (HSV) will have a reactivation of the virus, which can accentuate the pain and oral discomfort following BMT. To prevent this problem, most transplant programs utilize acyclovir at a dose of 250 mg/m^2 tid during the neutropenic phase.

Transfusion

All patients will require both RBCs and platelets in proportion to the duration of the pancytopenia. Platelets are kept over $10,000$ to $20,000/\mu L$ because of complicating bleeding from mucositis, although, in some instances, a lower threshold is feasible. Patients no longer receive granulocyte transfusions unless they have uncontrolled sepsis with positive blood cultures. For patients who are negative for cytomegalovirus (CMV) and who have a CMV-negative donor, CMV-negative cell support is generally provided (see section on "CMV infection").

All blood products are irradiated to prevent engraftment of lymphoid cells and are often filtered to reduce CMV or alloimmunization and febrile reactions. Most patients receive single-donor platelet pheresis products, which may need to be HLA-matched if patients show evidence of refractoriness to the transfusion (ie, if platelet levels fail to rise after transfusion).

Sinusoidal obstruction syndrome (veno-occlusive disease)

In the first few weeks after BMT, sinusoidal obstruction syndrome, characterized by hepatomegaly, jaundice, and fluid retention, develops in 5% to 20% of patients. It is caused by damaged endothelial cells, sinusoids, and hepatocytes and is related to the intensity of the cytoreductive therapeutic regimen.

The diagnosis of sinusoidal obstruction syndrome is usually made on clinical grounds, based on the occurrence (usually within 8 to 10 days after starting the cytoreductive regimen) of the triad of hepatomegaly, weight gain, and jaundice. Patients also exhibit renal sodium retention, and the prognosis is related to the degree of liver and kidney dysfunction and the level of bilirubin. The use of regimens that contain busulfan has been associated with the highest incidence of veno-occlusive disease, which has decreased with targeted oral or intravenous busulfan dosing.

TABLE 5: Clinical classification of acute GVHD according to organ injury

Stage key	0	1	2	3	4
Skin	No rash	Maculopapular rash, less than 25% of body surface	Maculopapular rash, 25%-50% of body surface	Rash on greater than 50% of body surface or generalized erythroderma	Generalized or erythroderma with bullous formation and/or desquamation
Lower GI (diarrhea)	Less than or equal to 500 mL/d or less than 280 mL/m²	Greater than 500 but ≤ 1,000 mL/d or 280 to 555 mL/m²	Greater than 1,000 but ≤ 1,500 mL/d or 556 to 833 mL/m²	> 1,500 mL/d or > 833 mL/m²	Severe abdominal pain with or without ileus or stool with frank blood or melena
Upper GI	No protracted nausea and vomiting	Persistent nausea, vomiting, or anorexia plus biopsy showing GVHD of the stomach or duodenum			
Liver (total bilirubin)	Less than 2.0 mg/dL	2.0-3.0 mg/dL	3.1-6.0 mg/dL	6.1-15.0 mg/dL	> 15 mg/dL

Overall clinical grading of severity of acute GVHD–1994 Keystone Consensus Criteria

Grade	Skin		Liver		Gut	Karnofsky performance scale (KPS)
I	1-2	&	0	&	0	
II	3	or	1	or	1	
III	0-4	or	2-3	or	2-4	
IV	4	or	4	or	0-4	or	KPS score ≤ 30 or decrease ≥ 40% from baseline KPS score

GVHD = graft-versus-host disease

TABLE 6: Prophylaxis of acute graft-versus-host disease

Day	Cyclosporine	Methotrexate
−2	5 mg/kg IV daily	
+1	5 mg/kg IV daily	15 mg/m^2 IV single dose
+3	5 mg/kg IV daily	10 mg/m^2 IV single dose
+4	3 mg/kg IV daily	
+6	3 mg/kg IV daily	10 mg/m^2 IV single dose
+11	3 mg/kg IV daily	10 mg/m^2 IV single dose
+15	2.75 mg/kg IV daily	
+36	10 mg/kg PO daily	
+84	8 mg/kg PO daily	
+98	6 mg/kg PO daily	
+120	4 mg/kg PO daily	
+180	off	

Treatment Once veno-occlusive disease has occurred, treatment is primarily supportive, consisting of careful management of fluid overload, kidney dysfunction, and other attendant complications. In few cases, the early use of thrombolytic agents can reverse established veno-occlusive disease. Based on early phase II studies, defibrotide is now being tested in phase III trials as an agent that can help reverse the syndrome.

Acute GVHD

GVHD is a clinical syndrome that results from the infusion of immuno-competent lymphocytes accompanying the marrow graft that are capable of recognizing minor HLA-related antigens in the host and initiating an immunologic reaction. This syndrome may arise after allogeneic transplantation or rarely after transfusion of cellular blood products in patients who are immunodeficient and share HLA loci that allow engraftment of transfused cells. For unknown reasons, the primary organs affected by acute GVHD are the skin, liver, and GI tract.

The syndrome usually occurs within 15 to 60 days after transplantation and can vary in severity. Table 5 shows a commonly used grading system for GVHD. This system has both therapeutic and prognostic importance.

Prophylaxis All patients undergoing non–T-cell-depleted transplantation require some form of GVHD prophylaxis. The most common regimens involve a combination of methotrexate and cyclosporine or tacrolimus [Prograf]. The combination of tacrolimus and sirolimus (Rapamune) has been studied and appears to be an effective approach for the prevention of GVHD. These medications, in the absence of GVHD, are tapered over 6 to 12 months after BMT. Table 6 shows a common regimen used to prevent GVHD after an allogeneic sibling transplantation. The regimens of sirolimus and tacrolimus are tapered in a similar manner. Side effects of tacrolimus and cyclosporine include renal toxicity, hypertension, magnesium wasting, seizures, and microangiopathy. Sirolimus, an oral agent, can cause hemolytic uremic syndrome in association with tacrolimus and requires careful dose and drug level monitoring. It can also raise blood triglyceride levels.

Treatment Despite prophylaxis, many allogeneic transplant recipients still develop some degree of GVHD and require increasing doses of prednisone (1–2 mg/kg/d). For patients who do not respond to steroids, antithymocyte globulin (Atgam; 10 mg/kg/d for 5–10 days) has been used. Daclizumab (Zenapax; 1 mg/kg on days 1, 4, 8, 15, and 22), pentostatin (Nipent), and etanercept (Enbrel) are likely more effective agents than antithymocyte globulin.

Chronic GVHD

Chronic GVHD may occur within 3 to 6 months in patients who have undergone allogeneic BMT. It is often preceded by acute GVHD, which may or may not have resolved. Although chronic GVHD is also related to infusion of T cells with the marrow graft, it resembles other autoimmune connective tissue diseases, such as scleroderma, Sjögren's syndrome, biliary cirrhosis, and bronchiolitis obliterans. Patients with chronic GVHD often have accompanying cytopenias and immune deficiency as well as abnormalities of the oral mucosa, conjunctiva, and gastrointestinal tract.

Treatment Chronic GVHD is generally treated with prolonged courses of steroids, cyclosporine, tacrolimus, and, occasionally, azathioprine and other modalities, such as psoralen-ultraviolet A light (PUVA) for skin and mouth GVHD. Thalidomide, mycophenolate mofetil (CellCept), sirolimus, and photopheresis have also been employed, with varying response rates. Like that for acute GVHD, the prognosis for chronic GVHD is related to the extent of organ compromise and response to treatment.

GVHD and relapse Although, in general, GVHD has contributed to significant morbidity and mortality in patients undergoing allogeneic BMT, it is also associated with reduced relapse rates, primarily in patients with hematologic malignancies.

Late infections

Late infections after BMT are caused by impaired cellular and humoral immunity. The most common late pathogens include *Pneumocystis carinii*, varicella zoster, and encapsulated bacteria.

Pneumocystis prophylaxis All patients undergoing allogeneic transplantation require prophylaxis against *P carinii*. This can be accomplished with one double-strength trimethoprim-sulfamethoxazole tablet bid twice a week once hematopoiesis has been restored. Alternatively, atovaquone (Mepron; 750 mg bid) has been utilized.

Treatment of herpes zoster Approximately 40% of patients will develop herpes zoster (either dermatomal or disseminated), which is often treated with oral or IV acyclovir. A patient may complain of severe localized pain for several days before the rash develops. The use of valacyclovir (Valtrex) for 1 year after BMT can reduce or delay the risk of reactivation of herpes zoster after allogeneic BMT.

Bacterial prophylaxis Many patients with chronic GVHD develop an accompanying severe immunodeficiency syndrome that leaves them susceptible to infection with encapsulated bacteria, primarily in the sinuses and lungs. In some cases, prolonged prophylaxis with trimethoprim-sulfamethoxazole or penicillin is necessary, as well as immunoglobulin replacement.

CMV infection

Historically, CMV interstitial pneumonia has been responsible for approximately 15% to 20% of patient deaths following allogeneic BMT. CMV pneumonia occurs 7 to 10 weeks after BMT and is due to reactivation of latent CMV or is acquired from donor marrow or transfusions. Active CMV infection, GVHD, and the inability to develop a virus-specific immune response that limits viral infection are risk factors for CMV pneumonia.

Diagnosis Infection is diagnosed by the combination of an abnormal chest x-ray, hypoxemia, and the detection of CMV in bronchoalveolar lavage or lung biopsy specimens, as well as the absence of other pathogens.

Treatment The only consistent treatment has been the combination of ganciclovir, 5 mg/kg bid for 3 weeks, and IV immunoglobulin, given every other day. Although the reason for the synergy between these agents is unclear, neither one alone is effective in reversing pneumonia once it has developed.

Prevention in CMV-seronegative patients The most successful means of preventing CMV infection in CMV-seronegative patients who have a seronegative donor is to limit their exposure to the virus by providing CMV-negative blood and platelet support. As most patients who undergo marrow transplantation are CMV-seropositive, this strategy has limited application. However, the presence of leukocytes in blood products increases the transmission of CMV. Thus, the use of CMV-seronegative blood products in CMV-seronegative recipients decreases the incidence of primary CMV infection. Also, CMV status should be determined in all patients prior to BMT to plan for post-transplantation transfusion strategies.

Prevention in CMV-seropositive patients The most effective strategy for preventing reactivation of CMV infection in patients who are CMV-seropositive is the preemptive use of ganciclovir, either prophylactically in all CMV-seropositive patients or at the first sign of CMV after transplantation (as indicated by blood culture, shell viral culture, or antigen or polymerase chain reaction [PCR] detection of the virus). The timing and duration of prophylaxis are somewhat controversial.

Ganciclovir has been the most effective agent for both strategies, as it significantly reduces both viral reactivation and associated disease. However, if one waits until after viral reactivation to initiate ganciclovir therapy, there are some patients who will not benefit from a prophylactic strategy, namely those in whom reactivation occurs simultaneously with disease. Ganciclovir has many side effects, including neutropenia and elevated creatinine levels, and thus exposes a large number of patients to potential toxicity.

The required duration of ganciclovir treatment is also unclear, but it appears that several weeks is necessary to protect the patient from viral reactivation and the development of pneumonitis within the first 3 months after BMT. Monitoring for CMV of all patients after completion of antiviral therapy is necessary, as some patients, particularly those with GVHD, are at risk for infection due to an inadequate immune response against CMV. Some patients have developed late CMV pneumonia after drug discontinuation, which is probably related to ganciclovir inhibition of the development of CMV-specific cytolytic T cells. Nevertheless, the use of ganciclovir has reduced the problems related to CMV pneumonia and should be a part of every management strategy for preventing complications following allogeneic transplantation. Currently, newer antiviral drugs such as miribavir are being tested and appear to have good antiviral activity with less toxicity.

Other post-transplantation therapies

Growth factors have found their most significant use in the acceleration of hematopoietic recovery after autologous reinfusion of stem cells. Clinical trials in allogeneic transplantation have not yet shown an advantage to their use, probably due to the immunosuppressive medications such as methotrexate used to prevent GVHD. Studies do support the use of G-CSF or granulocyte-macrophage colony-stimulating factor (GM-CSF); sargramostin [Leukine, Prokine] after autologous marrow transplantation, although the impact of these growth factors on acceleration of hematopoietic recovery, beyond that achieved with the use of primed autologous stem cells, is not clear.

Epoetin alfa (Epogen, Procrit) or darbepoetin alfa (Aranesp) is sometimes used effectively in patients who have persistent anemia after transplantation.

Management of relapse

Despite the intensity of the preparative regimen, some patients relapse after allogeneic BMT. For patients with CML, withdrawal of immunosuppression to allow for an augmented graft-versus-tumor effect sometimes leads to remission. Other patients with CML may respond to post-transplantation interferon or reintroduction of drugs such as imatinib (Gleevec), which appears to be a useful approach. Intriguingly, infusion of donor lymphoid cells in patients with CML is an effective means of inducing hematologic and cytogenetic responses in those who have relapsed after transplantation; this approach has led to complete and durable remissions.

Some patients with AML have responded to either infusion of donor stem cells or the combination of chemotherapy and donor stem cells. Patients with acute lymphoblastic leukemia have had the lowest response rate to this strategy. Patients who develop myelodysplasia after autologous transplantation can sometimes be treated with reduced-intensity allogeneic transplant to restore normal hematopoiesis and cure the myelodysplastic syndrome.

Long-term problems

For patients undergoing autologous stem-cell transplantation, the major long-term problem is the risk of relapse and myelodysplasia, but changes in libido, sexual dysfunction, and infertility also should be addressed to help patients achieve good long-term quality of life. Patients undergoing allogeneic transplantation also have similar long-term issues but also have major long-term effects related to chronic GVHD and the complications related to immunosuppression, especially infection. In addition, patients undergoing allogeneic transplantation are at higher risk for second malignancies, and thus aggressive screening studies should be part of the care of all long-term survivors of transplantation.

Second malignancy after hematopoietic cell transplantation

Patients undergoing transplantation are at risk for developing a second cancer. For those undergoing autologous transplantation, particularly for treatment of lymphoma and Hodgkin lymphoma, the most common cancer is myelodysplasia/AML, which occurs in up to 10% of patients, usually within 3 to 7 years after transplantation.

Risk factors for the development of myelodysplasia/AML after transplantation include the number of prior chemotherapy and radiation therapy treatments, specific drugs such as alkylating agents or topoisomerase inhibitors, difficulty in mobilizing stem cells, persistent cytopenias after transplantation, and use of TBI in the transplant preparative regimen. All patients should undergo cytogenetic screening of the marrow prior to stem-cell collection and should be followed for this complication after recovery from transplantation.

Patients undergoing either autologous or allogeneic transplantation are also at risk for the development of solid tumors, up to 20 years after transplantation. The risk is greater in patients receiving an allogeneic transplant. The most common tumors are related to the skin, but both common (breast, lung, and colon) and less common (sarcoma) tumors have been seen. As part of their long-term follow-up, all patients require screening for this complication to diagnose the cancer in its earliest stage.

SUGGESTED READING

Antin JH, Kim HT, Cutler C, et al: Sirolimus, tacrolimus, and low-dose methotrexate for graft-versus-host disease prophylaxis in mismatched related donor or unrelated donor transplantation. Blood 102:1601–1605, 2003.

Arvin AM: Varicella-zoster virus: Pathogenesis, immunity, and clinical management in hematopoietic cell transplant recipients. Biol Blood Marrow Transplant 6:219–230, 2000.

Attal M, Harousseau JL, Facon T, et al: Single versus double autologous stem-cell transplantation for multiple myeloma. N Engl J Med 349:2495–2502, 2003.

Bethge WA, Hegenbart U, Stuart MJ, et al: Adoptive immunotherapy with donor lymphocyte infusions after allogeneic hematopoietic cell transplantation following nonmyeloablative conditioning. Blood 103:790–795, 2004.

Blume KG, Forman SJ, Appelbaum FR (eds): Hematopoietic Cell Transplantation, 2nd ed. Malden, Massachusetts, Blackwell Science, 2004.

Cutler C, Kim HT, Hochberg E, et al: Sirolimus and tacrolimus without methotrexate as graft-versus-host disease prophylaxis after matched related donor peripheral blood stem cell transplantation. Biol Blood Marrow Transplant 10:328–336, 2004.

de Lima M, Giralt S: Allogeneic transplantation for the elderly patient with acute myelogenous leukemia or myelodysplastic syndrome. Semin Hematol 43:107–117, 2006.

Deeg HJ, Gooley TA, Flowers ME, et al: Allogeneic hematopoietic stem cell transplantation for myelofibrosis. Blood 102:3912–3918, 2003.

Fung HC, Cohen S, Rodriguez R, et al: Reduced-intensity allogeneic stem cell transplantation for patients whose prior autologous stem cell transplantation for hematologic malignancy failed. Biol Blood Marrow Transplant 9:649–656, 2003.

Gopal AK, Gooley TA, Maloney DG, et al: High-dose radioimmunotherapy versus conventional high-dose therapy and autologous hematopoietic stem cell transplantation for relapsed follicular non-Hodgkin lymphoma: A multivariable cohort analysis. Blood 102:2351–2357, 2003.

Harousseau JL, Moreau P: Evolving role of stem cell transplantation in multiple myeloma. Clin Lymphoma Myeloma 6:89–95, 2005.

Hertzberg M, Grigg A, Gottlieb D, et al: Reduced-intensity allogeneic haemopoietic stem cell transplantation induces durable responses in patients with chronic B-lymphoproliferative disorders. Bone Marrow Transplant 37:923–928, 2006.

Laughlin MJ, Eapen M, Rubinstein P, et al: Outcomes after transplantation of cord blood or bone marrow from unrelated donors in adults with leukemia. N Engl J Med 351:2265–2275, 2004.

Lavoie JC, Connors JM, Phillips GL, et al: High-dose chemotherapy and autologous stem cell transplantation for primary refractory or relapsed Hodgkin lymphoma: Long-term outcome in the first 100 patients treated in Vancouver. Blood 106:1473–1478, 2005.

Ljungman P, Urbano-Ispizua A, Cavazzana-Calvo M, et al: Allogeneic and autologous transplantation for haematological diseases, solid tumours, and immune disorders: Definitions and current practice in Europe. Bone Marrow Transplant 37:439–449, 2006.

Maloney DG, Molina AJ, Sahebi F, et al: Allografting with nonmyeloablative conditioning following cytoreductive autografts for the treatment of patients with multiple myeloma. Blood 102:3447–3454, 2003.

McSweeney PA, Niederwieser D, Shizuru JA, et al: Hematopoietic cell transplantation in older patients with hematologic malignancies: Replacing high-dose cytotoxic therapy with graft-vs-tumor effects. Blood 97:3390–3400, 2001.

Nademanee A, Forman S, Molina A, et al: A phase 1/2 trial of high-dose yttrium-90-ibritumomab tiuxetan in combination with high-dose etoposide and cyclophosphamide followed by autologous stem cell transplantation in patients with poor-risk or relapsed non-Hodgkin lymphoma. Blood 106:2896–2902, 2005.

Richardson PG, Murakami C, Jin Z, et al: Multi-institutional use of defibrotide in 88 patients after stem cell transplantation with severe veno-occlusive disease and multisystem organ failure: Response without significant toxicity in a high-risk population and factors predictive of outcome. Blood 100:4337–4343, 2002.

Syrjala KL, Langer SL, Abrams JR, et al: Late effects of hematopoietic cell transplantation among 10-year adult survivors compared with case-matched controls. J Clin Oncol 23:6596–6606, 2005.

Tauro S, Craddock C, Peggs K, et al: Allogeneic stem-cell transplantation using a reduced-intensity conditioning regimen has the capacity to produce durable remissions and long-term disease-free survival in patients with high-risk acute myeloid leukemia and myelodysplasia. J Clin Oncol 23:9387–9393, 2005.

Van Besien K: The evolving role of autologous and allogeneic stem cell transplantation in follicular lymphoma. Blood Rev 20:235–244, 2006.

Zaia JA: Prevention of cytomegalovirus disease in hematopoietic stem cell transplantation. Clin Infect Dis 35:999–1004, 2002.

CHAPTER 37

Pain management

Sharon M. Weinstein, MD, Penny R. Anderson, MD, Alan W. Yasko, MD, and Lawrence Driver, MD

Most patients with advanced cancer and up to 60% of patients with any stage of the disease experience significant pain. The World Health Organization (WHO) estimates that 25% of all cancer patients die with unrelieved pain.

The cause of cancer pain should be treated whenever possible. By doing so, one can frequently achieve rapid, lasting pain relief and may prevent the problems associated with untreated progressive disease, such as spinal cord compression and pathologic fracture. Also, the need for pain medications may be diminished, thus reducing side effects and drug interactions.

In most cancer patients, pain can be relieved adequately, and yet it is undertreated for a multitude of reasons. The problem is not trivial, as unrelieved pain is known to be a risk factor for suicide in cancer patients. Current efforts are being directed toward standardizing pain treatment and separating issues of pain treatment from those of substance abuse.

The effective management of cancer patients with pain is best accomplished with coordination of the services of multidisciplinary professionals, community volunteers, and the family.

Pathophysiology

Pathophysiologic classification of pain forms the basis for therapeutic choices. Pain states may be broadly divided into those associated with ongoing tissue damage (nociceptive) and those resulting from nervous system dysfunction in the absence of ongoing tissue damage (non-nociceptive or neuropathic).

Damage to the nervous system may result in pain in an area of altered sensation. Such pain is typically described as burning or lancinating. Patients may report bizarre complaints, such as painful numbness, itching, or crawling sensations. The postamputation phenomenon of phantom pain (pain referred to the lost body part) may be disabling.

Psychological factors Psychological factors may affect the reporting of pain. Chronic unrelieved pain has psychological consequences, but this does not support a psychiatric basis for the pain complaint. "Psychogenic pain" or somatoform pain disorder is rare in cancer patients.

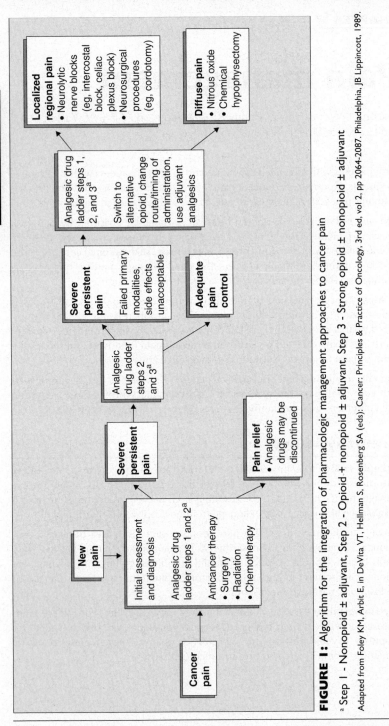

FIGURE 1: Algorithm for the integration of pharmacologic management approaches to cancer pain

[a] Step 1 - Nonopioid ± adjuvant, Step 2 - Opioid + nonopioid ± adjuvant, Step 3 - Strong opioid + nonopioid ± adjuvant

Adapted from Foley KM, Arbit E, in DeVita VT, Hellman S, Rosenberg SA (eds): Cancer: Principles & Practice of Oncology, 3rd ed, vol 2, pp 2064-2087. Philadelphia, JB Lippincott, 1989.

Pain syndromes

Cancer pain syndromes vary by tumor type and are related to patterns of tumor growth and metastasis. Pain may also be related to antineoplastic therapy or may be unrelated to either the neoplasm or its treatment.

Elements of management

Elements of cancer pain management include a proper medical evaluation, psychosocial assessment, formulation of the pain "diagnosis," and consideration of pharmacologic and nonpharmacologic treatments. Ongoing care is needed to monitor the efficacy of analgesics and the evolution of different symptoms during treatment or disease progression.

The steps in medical decision-making are to:

- determine whether primary antineoplastic therapy is indicated for palliation
- tailor pharmacologic analgesic therapy to individual needs
- consider concurrent nonpharmacologic analgesic methods
- monitor response and modify treatment accordingly (Figure 1).

The patient is the focus of care, although family members and others often participate in treatment decisions and require emotional support.

Medical evaluation

Pain history The medical evaluation should begin with a thorough history. As there are no objective means with which to verify the presence of pain, one must believe a patient's complaint. The physiologic signs of acute pain—elevated blood pressure and pulse rate—are unreliable in subacute or chronic pain.

Most cancer patients report more than one site of pain. A detailed history of each type of pain should be elicited (Table 1). As the chief complaint resolves, what was initially a secondary problem may require attention.

Pain rating scales should be used to establish a baseline against which the success of treatment may be judged (Figure 2). Behavioral observations may be used to assess patients who are unable to communicate. Although there are standardized tools for preverbal children, they are not available for impaired adults. Thus, it is sometimes necessary to treat pain presumptively.

Physical examination includes careful neurologic testing, especially if neuropathic pain is suspected. Pain in an area of reduced sensation, allodynia (ie, when normal stimuli are reported as painful), and hyperpathia or summation of painful stimuli indicate a neuropathic process. The assessment should evaluate the putative mechanisms that may underlie the pain.

Review of disease extent and current conditions The extent of disease and current medical conditions must be determined.

TABLE 1: Features of the pain history—"PQRST"

P	Provocative factors, palliative factors
Q	Quality (characteristics)
R	Region, pattern of radiation, referral
S	Severity, intensity (use pain rating scales [Figure 2])
T	Temporal factors: onset, duration, time to maximum intensity, frequency, daily variation

Diagnostic tests should be reviewed and supplemented as necessary.

Treatment and drug history Cancer treatment and prior analgesic interventions, along with their outcomes, should be recorded. Psychological dependency on any drug, including alcohol, must be identified.

Psychosocial assessment

To establish trust, the evaluating clinician should explore with the patient the significance of the pain complaint. The impact of pain and other symptoms on functional status must be understood to establish treatment goals. Suffering may be attributable to many factors besides physical complaints. The clinician should ask about such psychological factors as financial worries, loss of independence, family problems, social isolation, and fear of death. Often, cancer patients meet diagnostic criteria for the psychiatric diagnosis of adjustment disorder with anxiety and/or depressed mood.

FIGURE 2: Pain rating scales used to establish a baseline against which treatment results are judged; the numeric scale is also administered verbally.

Patient subgroups

To help define therapeutic goals, the patient's age and prognosis may be considered. Adjustments in drug doses are usually needed for elderly patients, who are more sensitive to analgesics and their side effects. Adolescents may require relatively larger doses of opioids. Pain in children is underreported and should be specifically elicited using age-appropriate assessment tools.

Pharmacologic treatment

The WHO has devised a three-step analgesic ladder outlining the use of nonopioid analgesics, opioid analgesics, and adjuvant medications for progressively severe pain. According to this schema, a nonopioid analgesic, with or without an adjuvant agent, should be tried first (step 1). If pain persists or increases on this regimen, the patient should be switched to an opioid plus a nonopioid agent, with or without an adjuvant medication (step 2). If pain continues or intensifies despite this change in therapy, a more potent dose of opioid analgesic should be prescribed, with or without a nonopioid and/or an adjuvant agent (step 3).

Nonopioid analgesics

Nonopioid analgesics are associated with ceiling effects, and exceeding the maximum dose ranges can result in organ toxicity. Potential side effects, such as hematologic, renal, and GI reactions, may be of clinical concern in cancer patients (Table 2). Cyclo-oxygenase-2 (COX-2) inhibitors are many times more potent against COX-2 than COX-1. Clinicians are advised to watch the emerging literature regarding the safety of these agents.

Opioid analgesics

General guidelines for the use of opioid therapy are outlined in Table 3.

Dosage Opioid agonists do not exhibit ceiling effects. Dosing is guided by efficacy and limited by side effects (Table 4). Dosages of tablets combining a nonsteroidal anti-inflammatory drug (NSAID) or acetaminophen and an opioid are limited according to the nonopioid component.

Routes of administration The oral route should be used when possible, though some patients may express a preference for an alternative route. If so, or if the oral route is not feasible or systemic side effects are uncontrollable, alternative routes are indicated, such as transdermal, transmucosal, rectal, and neuraxial infusion. Such alternative routes of administration of certain opioid agonists (see Table 5) may improve patients' quality of life and may be particularly useful for treating certain types of cancer pain.

Side effects of opioids can usually be anticipated and treated. In particular, with regular opioid dosing, laxatives should be prescribed for constipation.

Physical dependence and tolerance to some effects develop with chronic opioid use. Tolerance to respiratory depression, sedation, and nausea is likely to de-

TABLE 2: Nonopioid analgesics and NSAIDs useful for treating cancer pain

Generic name (usual dosage range)	Maximum dose/day	Adverse effects/ comments
Acetaminophen (325-975 mg q4-6h)	4,000 mg	Hepatic and renal impairment
Acetylsalicylic acid (aspirin, ASA) (325-975 mg q4-6h)	4,000 mg	Dyspepsia and GI ulceration, antiplatelet effect, bleeding
Celecoxib	400 mg	[a]
Choline magnesium trisalicylate (500-1,500 mg q8-12h)	4,500 mg	Dyspepsia, reduced antiplatelet effect, hypermagnesemia in renal failure
Choline salicylate (435-870 mg q3-4h)	5,220 mg	Dyspepsia, reduced antiplatelet effect
Magnesium salicylate (300-600 mg q4h)	4,800 mg	Same as choline salicylate
Salsalate (1,000-1,500 mg q8-12h)	4,000 mg	Same as choline salicylate
Sodium salicylate (325-650 mg q3-4h)	5,200 mg	Same as choline salicylate
Ibuprofen (200-800 mg q4-6h)	2,400 mg	[b]Dermatitis +
Ketoprofen (25-75 mg q6-8h)	300 mg	[b]Headache +++
Ketorolac tromethamine (oral: 10 mg q4-6h; parenteral: 60 mg, then 15-30 mg q6h)	Oral: 40 mg Parenteral: 120 mg	[b]Limit duration of therapy; headache +++, GI bleeding [b]Limit therapy to 5 days; headache +++, GI bleeding
Meclofenamate sodium (50-100 mg q4-6h)	400 mg	[b]Headache +, dermatitis +
Mefenamic acid (250 mg q6h)	1,000 mg	[b]Limit therapy to 7 days
Naproxen sodium (220-550 mg q8-12h)	1,375 mg	[b]Headache +
Naproxen (250-500 mg q8-12h)	1,500 mg	[b]Headache +

[a] Monitor emerging literature regarding safety concerns.

[b] Minor adverse reactions include dyspepsia, heartburn, nausea, vomiting, anorexia, diarrhea, constipation, flatulence, bloating, epigastric pain, abdominal pain, dizziness, and drowsiness. Major adverse reactions that may appear at any time include renal failure, hepatic dysfunction, bleeding, and gastric ulceration.

+ Each plus sign represents a 5% incidence of the reported adverse effect.

Adapted with permission from American Pain Society: Principles of Analgesic Use in the Treatment of Acute Pain and Cancer Pain, 5th ed. Skokie, Illinois, American Pain Society, 2003.

NSAIDs = nonsteroidal anti-inflammatory drugs

TABLE 3: Guidelines for the use of opioid analgesics

Start with an analgesic with the potential to provide relief

Know the essential pharmacology of the analgesic:

    Analgesic type

    Pharmacokinetics

    Influences of coadministered drugs, disease, or age on analgesic disposition and response

    Equianalgesic starting dose for the drug and route to be used

    Route of administration and a dosage form to fit the patient's needs

Individualize/titrate the dosage

Administer analgesics regularly after the initial dose titration

Provide for breakthrough pain

Use drug combinations that enhance analgesia

Recognize and treat side effects

Make conversions from one route to another or from one agent to another using known equianalgesic doses

Manage physical dependence (ie, prevent withdrawal)

Adapted with permission from Inturrisi C: Cancer 63(suppl):2308–2320, 1989.

TABLE 4: Opioid agonist analgesics for mild to moderate pain

Drug	Equianalgesic dose to 650 mg of aspirin[a]	Dose interval	Half-life (h)	Comments
Codeine	32-65 mg	q4-6h	2-3	[b,c]
Hydrocodone	—	q3-4h	4	[b]
Oxycodone	2.5 mg	q3-6h	—	[b]

[a] The equianalgesic dose should not be interpreted as the starting, standard, or maximum dose but rather as a guide for switching drugs or changing routes of administration.

[b] Doses of products containing aspirin or acetaminophen should be monitored for safety.

[c] Doses above 65 mg provide diminished incremental analgesia with increasing doses, but side effects may worsen.

Adapted with permission from American Pain Society: Principles of Analgesic Use in the Treatment of Acute Pain and Cancer Pain, 3rd ed. Skokie, Illinois, American Pain Society, 1992.

TABLE 5: Opioid agonist analgesics for severe pain

Drug	Equianalgesic dose to 10 mg of IV morphine		Half-life	Comments
	Oral	Parenteral	(h)	
Fentanyl, oral transmucosal	a	NA	a	For breakthrough cancer pain
Fentanyl, transdermal	NA	NA	—	b, c Patch sizes of 12, 25, 50, 75, 100 µg/h; slow onset to effect, necessitating "breakthrough" analgesics
Hydromorphone	4 mg	1.5 mg	2-3	b
Levorphanol	4 mg	2 mg	12-16	b
Methadone	20 mg	10 mg	15-36	b,d Risk of delayed toxicity due to accumulation; reduce dose or lengthen dose interval if over-sedation occurs after 4-5 days; may schedule as prn initially
Morphine sulfate, controlled release	30 mg	NA	3	b Mg-for-mg conversion from immediate-release form; do not crush or chew tablets
Morphine sulfate, immediate release	30 mg	10 mg	3	b

velop. Tolerance to analgesia is not a major clinical problem and can usually be managed by changing the dose or substituting another agent.

Most current definitions of addiction imply a behavioral syndrome of compulsive, harmful use but do not require the existence of physical dependence or tolerance. Aberrant drug-taking is not likely to occur in patients without a history of substance abuse.

Precautions during chronic therapy During chronic opioid therapy, certain precautions should be observed:

- Normeperidine is a toxic metabolite of meperidine that accumulates with repetitive dosing; thus, use of meperidine for chronic pain should be limited. Propoxyphene is also relatively contraindicated due to accumulation of norpropoxyphene.

Drug	Equianalgesic dose to 10 mg of IV morphine		Half-life (h)	Comments
	Oral	Parenteral		
Oxycodone, controlled release	15 mg	NA	—	b, e
Oxycodone, immediate release	15 mg	NA	2-3	b
Oxymorphone	10 mg	1 mg	2-3	b
Oxymorphone, controlled release	10 mg	NA	—	

Adapted with permission from American Pain Society: Principles of Analgesic Use in the Treatment of Acute Pain and Cancer Pain, 5th ed. Skokie, Illinois, American Pain Society, 2003.

NA = not available

a See package insert for dosing instructions.

b Common side effects include constipation, nausea, and sedation. Uncommon side effects include itching, dry mouth, and urinary retention. Rare side effects are hypotension and inappropriate antidiuretic hormone secretion.

c Patch duration = 72 hours but may be 48 hours for some patients.

Equianalgesic conversion for fentanyl:

Parenteral morphine dose (mg/24 h)	Transdermal fentanyl (µg/h)
8-22	25
23-37	50
38-52	75
53-67	100
68-82	125
83-97	150

d Consult pain expert if converting to/from methadone in high-dose patients. Unique cardiac toxicity. See FDA warnings.

e Available alone and in combination with aspirin or acetaminophen; at higher doses, use as a single agent.

- Placebo use is discouraged, as it does not help distinguish the pathophysiology of pain.

- Physical withdrawal symptoms can be avoided by tapering doses.

- A change in mental status should not be attributed to opioid therapy until medical and neurologic factors have been fully evaluated.

- Mixed agonist-antagonist drugs and partial agonist drugs are not recommended for cancer pain.

Adjuvant medications Neuropathic pain may be less responsive to standard analgesics alone. Adjuvants, such as antidepressants, anticonvulsants, benzodiazepines, local anesthetics, neuroleptics, psychostimulants, antihistamines, corticosteroids, levodopa, calcitonin, and bisphosphonates, are useful for particular indications (Table 6). These agents may be administered via oral and other

TABLE 6: Adjuvant drug therapy for cancer pain

Antidepressants

Anticonvulsants

Anxiolytics

Muscle relaxants

Topical local anesthetics and other agents

Amphetamines

Phenothiazines

Bisphosphonates

Corticosteroids

---

routes. Topical local anesthetic, NSAID and other preparations (Table 7), and neurolytic blocks (Table 8) should also be considered.

Surgery for bone metastasis

Surgical intervention is warranted for bone metastases to stabilize a pathologic fracture or preempt an impending fracture. The objectives of surgery are to palliate pain, reduce patient anxiety, improve patient mobility and function, facilitate nursing care, and control local tumor when nonsurgical therapies fail. In general, surgery involves excision of all gross tumor followed by stabilization of the bone, prior to or after fracture, by means of an internal fixation or prosthetic device.

Indications

No strict criteria have been established for surgical treatment. Clinical parameters, such as the patient's general medical condition, performance status, nature of the primary tumor, effectiveness of other therapies, extent of extraskeletal disease, and degree of osseous involvement, as well as the patient's life expectancy, must be considered before surgery.

> There are no clearly defined criteria for the presence of an impending fracture of a long bone. Current guidelines, derived from retrospective clinical studies, include lytic lesions > 2.5 cm in diameter, cortical destruction > 50%, and pain despite local irradiation. In the proximal femur, an avulsion fracture of the lesser trochanter places the hip at high risk for fracture, and operative intervention should be considered.

Fracture and long bone pain In general, the presence of a pathologic fracture, an impending fracture, or a painful lesion in a long bone despite radiotherapy should be considered indications for surgery. A pathologic fracture can result from structural insufficiency and can develop in the absence of viable tumor following treatment with irradiation and/or systemic therapy.

TABLE 7: Anesthetic/neurosurgical approaches for controlling cancer pain

Procedure	Usual indication(s)	Examples
Local anesthetic blocks with or without steroids	Diagnostic blocks Prognostic blocks Acute pain, muscle spasm Premorbid chronic pain Postsurgical syndromes Herpes zoster	Trigger point injection Intercostal block Epidural steroids
Neurolytic/neuroablative blocks and ablative neurosurgery	Localized refractory pain that is expected to persist, usually in the presence of a short life expectancy; pain localized to a region that is associated with a low risk of neurologic complications	Alcohol celiac plexus block Phenol intercostal block Percutaneous cordotomy Midline myelotomy
Spinal analgesics	Refractory pain, usually in the lower body but may be widespread or diffuse	Externalized epidural catheter Intrathecal catheter with fully implanted pump

TABLE 8: Neurolytic procedures[a] that may be considered early in certain pain situations

Procedure	Indication
Celiac plexus neurolysis	Abdominal pain, back pain
Superior hypogastric plexus neurolysis	Pelvic pain
Phenol saddle block	Perineal pain with urinary diversion
Thoracic subarachnoid neurolysis	Focal chest wall pain
Intercostal neurolysis	Focal chest wall pain
Lumbar subarachnoid neurolysis	Unilateral leg pain

[a] The risk-benefit ratio of these procedures in the specified settings is sufficiently favorable and well established to warrant early consideration.

Other considerations Patients deemed to be candidates for surgery should have an expected longevity of > 1 month. All patients should be medically able to withstand the planned surgical procedure. The surgical goals should be achievable with reasonable certainty, and the potential benefits should outweigh the operative risks. All surgical interventions should be performed with the intent to provide benefit that will outlast the patient's anticipated survival.

Lesion site Major long bones (femur, tibia, and humerus), the vertebrae, and periacetabular regions demand specific attention, as optimal patient function and mobility are predicated on a stable, painless extremity. Osseous destruction sufficient to compromise the mechanical integrity of these bones should be addressed surgically. Lesions in the weight-bearing bones of the lower extremity (femur and tibia) are particularly vulnerable to fracture.

Lesions in the humerus should be treated surgically when the upper extremities serve a weight-bearing function (eg, assisted ambulation using a walker, crutches, or cane). Early surgical intervention, aggressive rehabilitation, and vigilant postoperative surveillance may optimize patient outcome.

Role of radiation therapy

Cancer pain can often be relieved by radiation therapy delivered by localized external-beam irradiation (also known as involved-field irradiation), wide-field external-beam irradiation (eg, hemibody irradiation [HBI]), or systemic treatment with radioactive isotopes (eg, strontium-89 chloride [Metastron], samarium SM 153 lexidronam [Quadramet], phosphorus-32, and iridium-131). Because the most common cause of cancer pain is bone metastasis, this discussion will focus on the use of irradiation in its treatment. Other examples of cancer pain due to primary or metastatic cancer that are amenable to irradiation include headache from CNS involvement, pain due to localized neural involvement (eg, brachial plexus or sciatic nerve), visceral pain (eg, liver or adrenal), pain due to effusions (eg, pericardial or pleural), and pain due to obstruction (eg, urethral, esophageal).

Systemic radiotherapy

Strontium-89 is a systemic radionuclide that has clinical efficacy in the palliation of pain from bone metastases. Reduction of pain due to bone metastases has been observed most frequently in patients with metastases from prostate cancer.

The primary toxicity of strontium-89 is myelosuppression, particularly thrombocytopenia. Therefore, it should not be administered to patients with thrombocytopenia or significant bone marrow suppression. Strontium-89 levels in bone are regulated much like calcium, and strontium-89 has less hematologic toxicity than phosphorus-32.

Samarium-153 is a β-emitting radioisotope that is bound to a phosphonate that preferentially localizes in active bone, specifically in sites of metastatic disease. Mild-to-moderate myelosuppression was noted in the samarium-153 group, yet a potential advantage of samarium-153 over strontium-89 is the decreased incidence and severity of hematologic toxicity noted with samarium-153.

Physical treatments

Cancer patients may benefit from formal rehabilitation, evaluation, and treatment. Physical modalities, such as massage, ultrasonography, hydrotherapy, transcutaneous electrical nerve stimulation (TENS), electroacupuncture, and trigger-point manipulation, are indicated for musculoskeletal pain. Also, any of these techniques may enhance exercise tolerance in a patient undergoing rehabilitation. Skillful soft-tissue manipulation is probably underutilized. Electrical stimulation may also be applied to the peripheral nerves, spinal cord, and even deep brain structures.

Management of psychological, sociocultural, and spiritual factors

The appropriate treatment of cancer pain must extend beyond the physical complaint. Psychological, sociocultural, and spiritual factors significantly affect the patient's quality of life. Thus, the clinician must always care for the whole person. A multifactorial approach to pain management recognizes the complexity of the human being, especially one with a terminal illness.

Although the physician's initial therapeutic goal is to cure the disease, cancer is often incurable. Caring entails recognizing the whole person as a physical, intellectual, social, emotional, and spiritual being. Empathic caring helps the patient perceive the value in life despite the gravity of the situation.

Psychological factors, such as anxiety and depression, must be thoroughly addressed, as revealed by emerging evidence from the disciplines of psychooncology and psychoneuroimmunology. Attitude and state of mind affect the individual's perception of pain and response to it in myriad ways and may affect the duration of survival.

A detailed discussion of pharmacologic and nonpharmacologic approaches to anxiety and depression in cancer patients may be found in chapter 39. In addition, patients may regain a much needed sense of control by using psychological techniques, such as imagery, hypnosis, relaxation, biofeedback, and other cognitive or behavioral methods.

Sociocultural influences affect the patient's experience and expression of pain. This is especially true for the patient whose cancer does not respond to therapy and progresses to end-stage disease.

Pain may be an unwelcome reminder of the presence and progression of cancer. Concomitant fear, anger, frustration, disappointment, and other negative emotions may hold the patient hostage to physical pain.

Existential distress may bridge an undesirable transition from hopeful coping with pain to hopeless suffering from it. As patients are confronted with personal mortality, the limits of their life spans move from an abstract concept to a real issue. Self-image changes, and patients may develop emotional and psychic turmoil, which may compromise their medical condition and treatment.

Achieving relief of psychic suffering may enable the patient to transcend physical pain, enhancing the effects of pain medications and other treatments. Prayer, meditation, counseling, clergy visits, and support groups may all be beneficial. Relieving suffering means allowing the patient and family to realize improved quality of life and even find contentment or peace in the face of failing health and imminent death. Palliative care of the family includes bereavement counseling in anticipation of and after the loss of a loved one.

Ongoing care

The goals of pain management must be frequently reviewed and integrated into the overall management plan. Communication among the professional staff, patient, and family is essential. A sensitive, frank discussion with the patient regarding his or her wishes should guide medical decision-making during all phases of the illness.

SUGGESTED READING

ON CANCER PAIN MANAGEMENT

American Pain Society: Principles of Analgesic Use in the Treatment of Acute Pain and Cancer Pain, 5th ed. Skokie, Illinois, American Pain Society, 2003.

Breitbart W: Suicide, in Holland J, Rowland J (eds): Handbook of Psychooncology. New York, Oxford University Press, 1999.

Chochinov HM, Breitbart W (eds): Ethical and Spiritual Issues: Handbook of Psychiatry in Palliative Medicine, Part VI, pp 337–396. New York, Oxford University Press, 2000.

Doyle D, Hanks G, Cherny NI, et al (eds): Oxford Textbook of Palliative Medicine, 3nd ed. New York, Oxford University Press, 2005.

World Health Organization: Cancer Pain Relief and Palliative Care in Children. Geneva, Switzerland, World Health Organization, 1998.

ON ANESTHETIC AND SURGICAL APPROACHES

Weinstein SM: Management of spinal cord and cauda equina compression, in Berger A, Levy MH, Portenoy RK, Weissman DE (eds): Principles and Practice of Palliative Care and Supportive Oncology, 3rd ed. Philadelphia, JB Lippincott, 2006.

ON RADIATION THERAPY IN CANCER PAIN MANAGEMENT

Gaze MN, Kelly CG, Kerr GR, et al: Pain relief and quality of life following radiotherapy for bone metastases: A randomized trial of two fractionation schedules. Radiother Oncol 45:109–116, 1997.

Rose CM, Kagan AR: The final report of the expert panel for the radiation oncology bone metastasis work group of the American College of Radiology. Int J Radiat Oncol Biol Phys 40:1117–1124, 1998.

CHAPTER 38

Management of nausea and vomiting

Steven M. Grunberg, MD, Madhuri Vithala, MD, and Richard Gralla, MD

Although marked progress in controlling chemotherapy-induced emesis has occurred over the past 10 to 20 years, nausea and vomiting remain among the most distressing side effects of cancer chemotherapy. With the increased use of chemotherapy in primary and adjuvant treatment settings, the need for improved control of emesis remains an important consideration in both medical oncology and supportive care.

Over the past few years, several major oncology groups have published consensus reports or guidelines on the prevention of chemotherapy-induced emesis. However, the introduction of several new agents may change these paradigms. In addition, an understanding of the neuropharmacology of this problem is useful in planning patient care.

Pathophysiology of emesis

Although the mechanism by which cancer chemotherapy induces emesis is still not completely understood, a physiologic basis for our current understanding of this complex problem has now emerged.

Stimulation of neurotransmitter receptors

The emetic reflex arc is activated by stimulation of receptors in the CNS and/or GI tract. These receptor areas relay information to the vomiting center in the medulla, which then coordinates the act of vomiting. The chemoreceptor trigger zone (CTZ), also located in the medulla, serves as a "chemosensor" and is exposed to blood and CSF. These areas are rich in a variety of neurotransmitter receptors.

Dopamine For many years, the dopamine receptors were the main focus of interest in antiemetic research. Available antiemetics, such as phenothiazines (chlorpromazine and prochlorperazine) and substituted benzamides (metoclopramide), were known to affect these receptors, as were butyrophenones (haloperidol and droperidol).

Serotonin The role of the neurotransmitter serotonin (5-hydroxytryptamine [5-HT]) has also been elucidated. The improved antiemetic activity of higher doses of metoclopramide was not explained by its dopamine-binding properties but by the fact that it also affects serotonin receptors. This led to the development of several highly specific compounds that interact solely with serotonin receptors, specifically the type 3, or 5-HT$_3$, receptor subtype. Four compounds (ondansetron, granisetron, dolasetron [Anzemet], palonosetron [Aloxi]) from this family are currently available in the United States. The 5-HT$_3$ receptor, which is found in both the GI tract and CNS, is an important mediator of the emetic reflex arc. Recent work has suggested that mutation of the 5-HT$_{3B}$ receptor subunit may affect antiemetic efficacy.

Substance P Tachykinins, such as substance P, play an important role in emesis, as well as in pain and a variety of inflammatory conditions. These neurotransmitters are 11–amino acid molecules that bind to specific receptors. Substance P binds to the neurokinin type 1, or NK$_1$, receptor.

Several NK$_1$ receptor antagonists have been synthesized and used both preclinically and in clinical trials in patients receiving cancer chemotherapy. Results indicate that these agents are effective against a broad range of causes of emesis, particularly delayed emesis. One member of this family, aprepitant (Emend), has been approved for clinical use.

Emetic problems

Emesis related to chemotherapy

Both nausea and vomiting are seen in patients receiving cancer chemotherapy. Nausea occurs at a higher frequency than vomiting and is more difficult to control. The control of vomiting is strongly correlated with the control of nausea, although some patients experience nausea without vomiting.

The three most common emetic patterns in patients receiving chemotherapy are outlined below.

Acute chemotherapy-induced emesis is defined as nausea or vomiting that occurs within the initial 24 hours of chemotherapy administration. The time of greatest risk is from 1 to 6 hours after chemotherapy with most agents.

Delayed emesis is emesis that begins ≥ 24 hours after chemotherapy. Delayed emesis is particularly likely to occur in patients who have received cisplatin, carboplatin, or cyclophosphamide. Recent data indicate that this problem may begin somewhat earlier than 24 hours in some patients.

Anticipatory emesis is defined as a conditioned vomiting response following inadequate antiemetic protection with prior courses of chemotherapy.

Emesis unrelated to chemotherapy

Patients receiving anticancer drugs may also develop emesis for other reasons. Emesis can be induced by concomitant medications (such as analgesics, anti-infectives, or bronchodilators) or by tumor-related complications (such as intestinal obstruction or brain metastases). In these instances, adjustment of medication or treatment of tumor-related complications is more important than selecting an antiemetic agent.

Patient characteristics and emesis

History of poor emetic control Poor control of emesis with past courses of chemotherapy predisposes a patient to unsatisfactory antiemetic results with any subsequent treatment, regardless of the emetic stimulus or antiemetic employed. Both delayed and conditioned anticipatory emesis are more likely to occur in these patients, and there is likely to be greater difficulty in controlling acute emesis.

History of alcohol intake Emesis is easier to control in patients with a history of chronic, high alcohol intake (> 100 g/d of alcohol [approximately five alcohol units or drinks]). In a prospective evaluation of 52 patients receiving high-dose cisplatin and an effective combination antiemetic regimen, 93% of those with a history of high alcohol intake had no emesis, as opposed to 61% of those without such a history. This difference in emesis control is independent of the patient's current alcohol intake.

Age Most trials have found that it is easier to control emesis in older patients than in younger ones. Younger patients have a predilection for developing acute dystonic reactions when dopamine-blocking antiemetics are administered (see section on "Antiemetic agents for high-emetic-risk chemotherapy"). Younger patients also have a greater tendency to develop anticipatory emesis than do older patients.

Gender It is more difficult to control emesis in women than in men given the same chemotherapy and antiemetic regimen.

Motion sickness Patients with a history of motion sickness are more likely to develop chemotherapy-induced nausea and vomiting than are those without such a history.

The above predisposing factors appear to be additive. One can identify patients at particularly high risk of emesis, such as younger women without a history of high alcohol intake. Awareness of these factors is helpful in monitoring individual patients and interpreting the results of clinical trials.

Chemotherapeutic agents and emesis

Emetic potential The most accurate predictor of the risk of emesis is the chemotherapeutic agent that a patient is receiving. Several different classifications of commonly used chemotherapy agents have been devised. Table 1 is based on the consensus report of the Multinational Association of Supportive Care in Cancer (MASCC) as updated in June 2004.

The emetic potential of a chemotherapeutic combination is determined by identifying the most emetic agent in the combination. Other agents in a combination may also increase the risk.

In general, agents that have the highest *incidence* of emesis also induce the most *severe* emesis. Differences occur among patients and even between identical treatment courses in the same patient. The dose, route, and schedule of administration of the chemotherapeutic agent can affect the incidence of nausea and vomiting.

TABLE 1: Emetic potential of chemotherapy agents

Level	Frequency of emesis (%)[a]	Agent
High	> 90	Carmustine
		Cisplatin
		Cyclophosphamide ($\geq$ 1,500 mg/m^2)
		Dacarbazine
		Hexamethylmelamine
		Mechlorethamine
		Procarbazine
		Streptozocin
Moderate	30-90	Carboplatin
		Cyclophosphamide (< 1,500 mg/m^2)
		Cytarabine (> 1,000 mg/m^2)
		Daunorubicin
		Doxorubicin
		Epirubicin
		Idarubicin
		Ifosfamide
		Irinotecan
		Oxaliplatin
		Temozolomide
Low	10-30	Capecitabine
		Cytarabine ($\leq$ 100 mg/m^2)
		Docetaxel
		Etoposide
		Fluorouracil
		Gemcitabine
		Methotrexate (> 50 mg/m^2)
		Mitomycin
		Mitoxantrone
		Paclitaxel
		Pemetrexed
		Topotecan
Minimal	< 10	Bleomycin
		Busulfan
		Chlorambucil
		2-Chlorodeoxyadenosine
		Fludarabine
		Hydroxyurea
		Melphalan
		Thioguanine
		Vinblastine
		Vincristine
		Vinorelbine

[a] Proportion of patients experiencing emesis in the absence of effective antiemetic prophylaxis

Time of onset of emesis In patients receiving initial chemotherapy of high emetic risk, nausea or vomiting typically begins between 1-2 hours after chemotherapy. Cyclophosphamide and carboplatin may be associated with a late onset of emesis (ie, 8-18 hours following chemotherapy administration).

Antiemetic agents for high–emetic-risk chemotherapy

Careful antiemetic research has shown that numerous agents are safe and effective. Dosage and administration schedules for some of these agents are given in Table 2. Antiemetic therapy is commonly administered either orally or intravenously.

Among the best studied agents are ondansetron, granisetron, dolasetron (Anzemet), palonosetron (Aloxi), metoclopramide, haloperidol, dexamethasone, aprepitant, lorazepam, dronabinol (Marinol), prochlorperazine, and chlorpromazine.

The combination of a single prechemotherapy dose of a 5-HT$_3$ antagonist and dexamethasone is the most commonly used therapy to prevent emesis in patients receiving chemotherapy of high emetic risk (both cisplatin and noncisplatin) as listed in Table 1. Addition of aprepitant may increase the rate of antiemetic protection.

Serotonin antagonists: Ondansetron, granisetron, dolasetron, and palonosetron

Ondansetron, granisetron, dolasetron, and palonosetron are highly selective 5-HT$_3$ receptor antagonists. All are effective in controlling emesis induced by a variety of chemotherapeutic agents. Oral and IV routes of administration available for ondansetron, granisetron, and dolasetron are equally effective, as demonstrated in large randomized trials. Granisetron is also now available as a patch (Sancuso). Single-dose regimens given before chemotherapy are as effective as more cumbersome multiple- or continuous-dose regimens. Alternative formulations of granisetron for transdermal administration are also under development.

All four serotonin receptor antagonists are similar with regard to efficacy and side effects, although palonosetron has a significantly longer half-life of approximately 40 hours. Choice of one agent over another may therefore reflect economic or convenience factors as well as therapeutic index. Doses of these agents are given in Table 2.

Side effects Ondansetron, granisetron, dolasetron, and palonosetron have all demonstrated excellent safety characteristics over a large dosing range. Toxicities have been minor and have included headache, mild transient elevation of hepatic enzyme levels, constipation, and, with some agents, minor prolongation of cardiac conduction intervals.

TABLE 2: Dosage and administration schedules of antiemetic agents for acute emesis for chemotherapy of high emetic risk

Antiemetic agent	Dosage[a]	
	Oral	Intravenous
Dolasetron	100 mg once	100 mg (1.8 mg/kg) once
Granisetron	1 or 2 mg once	1 mg (0.01 mg/kg) once
Ondansetron	16-24 mg once or 8 mg bid	8 mg (0.15 mg/kg) once
Palonosetron	In development	0.25 mg once
Dexamethasone	20 mg once	20 mg once over 5 min
Metoclopramide	Not recommended	2-3 mg/kg q2h
Haloperidol	1-2 mg q4-6h	1-3 mg q4-6h
Dronabinol	5 mg/m^2 q4h	Not available
Nabilone	1-2 mg bid	Not available
Prochlorperazine	Not recommended	10-20 mg q3-4h
Lorazepam[b]	0.5-2.0 mg	0.5-2.0 mg q4-6h
Aprepitant	125 mg	Not available

[a] All agents are to be administered prior to chemotherapy, usually 30 minutes beforehand, although the serotonin antagonists can be effective if administered as late as immediately before the start of chemotherapy. Recommended dosages have been found to be effective in clinical trials and may vary from those given in package inserts.

[b] Lorazepam is indicated only as an adjunct to antiemetics in this setting.

Dystonic reactions and akathisia (restlessness), which may be treatment-limiting with antiemetic agents known to block dopamine receptors, are not seen with serotonin antagonists, even when given on consecutive days. This finding is of particular importance for younger patients, in that several regimens used to treat malignancies in this age group utilize a schedule of daily chemotherapy.

Efficacy The serotonin antagonists have been reported to achieve complete control of emesis in 30%-50% of patients receiving cisplatin. These agents have also proved to be at least as effective against all other chemotherapeutic agents, with complete control rates of about 70%.

Many trials have examined the benefit of adding corticosteroids to a serotonin antagonist. Typically, the complete control of emesis is improved by 10%-20% in patients receiving highly emetic chemotherapy. Both the American Society of Clinical Oncology (ASCO) and MASCC guidelines recommend that a corticosteroid be added whenever a serotonin antagonist is indicated (ie, in all patients receiving chemotherapy of high emetic risk).

Dexamethasone

The antiemetic mechanism of action of dexamethasone remains unclear. Several randomized trials and a meta-analysis have all confirmed its effectiveness in controlling emesis and its safety. Other corticosteroids are also effective; however, dexamethasone is the most widely studied steroid and is available in oral and parenteral dosage forms as an inexpensive generic product. Dexamethasone is an excellent agent for use in combination antiemetic regimens and as a single agent for patients receiving chemotherapy of low emetic risk (< 30% incidence).

Dose Dexamethasone doses have generally ranged from 4 to 20 mg/d. In a randomized trial in patients receiving chemotherapy of high emetic risk, a single 20-mg dose was superior in completely controlling both nausea and vomiting. Thus, the 20-mg dose is recommended in this setting. For patients receiving chemotherapy of moderate emetic risk, a single 8-mg dose may be sufficient.

Side effects Toxicities associated with short courses of dexamethasone used for antiemetic therapy have been mild and generally consist of insomnia and mild epigastric burning. Care using this agent in patients with diabetes is particularly warranted.

Metoclopramide

Metoclopramide has proved to be safe and effective when given in high IV doses. Metoclopramide was thought to function as an antiemetic through blockade of dopamine receptors. However, high concentrations of this agent effectively block $5\text{-}HT_3$ receptors as well.

Efficacy High-dose metoclopramide is a second-choice agent, after the serotonin antagonists, in patients receiving cisplatin.

Side effects Commonly observed side effects with metoclopramide include mild sedation, dystonic reactions, akathisia, anxiety, and depression. Dystonic reactions are age-related and route-related. In a report summarizing the experience of nearly 500 patients receiving metoclopramide, the incidence of trismus or torticollis was only 2% in those older than age 30; in contrast, a 27% occurrence was reported in younger patients. Also, such reactions are more common when metoclopramide is administered by the oral route or is given over several consecutive days.

Acute dystonic reactions are not allergic in nature. In general, dystonic reactions and akathisia can be prevented or easily controlled by administering diphenhydramine, benztropine (Cogentin), or a benzodiazepine. These reactions should not be viewed as a contraindication to further use of dopamine-blocking drugs.

Haloperidol

Haloperidol exerts its antiemetic action through dopaminergic blockade. A formal study comparing haloperidol with metoclopramide in patients receiving cisplatin found both agents to be effective, although metoclopramide afforded better emetic control.

Dose Haloperidol doses of 1-3 mg given IV q4-6h have been used.

Side effects Toxicities of haloperidol include sedation, dystonic reactions, akathisia, and occasional hypotension.

Benzodiazepines

Although lorazepam and other benzodiazepines are potent anxiolytic agents that can be useful additions to antiemetic therapy, they should not be used as single agents for chemotherapy-induced emesis. Lorazepam has been shown to achieve a high degree of patient acceptance and subjective benefit but only minor objective antiemetic activity. However, the anxiolytic properties of benzodiazepines may be particularly useful in the treatment of anticipatory nausea and vomiting.

Dose Lorazepam is usually given in doses of 0.5-1.5 mg/m^2 IV or 1-2 mg PO. These doses, especially the higher IV administrations, can be associated with marked sedation lasting for several hours.

Cannabinoids

Many trials have tested the antiemetic effects of dronabinol (delta-9-tetrahydrocannabinol [THC]), a component of marijuana. Dronabinol has modest antiemetic activity, similar to that seen with oral prochlorperazine.

Semisynthetic cannabinoids (such as nabilone) have been tested but appear to have no clear advantage over dronabinol. The modest antiemetic activity and significant toxicity of cannabinoids make them a second choice for the control of chemotherapy-related emesis.

Dose Dronabinol has been tried in many doses and schedules. The most useful doses have ranged from 5 to 10 mg/m^2 PO q3-4h. The usual dose of nabilone is 1 to 2 mg PO bid.

Side effects are frequently associated with cannabinoids and are particularly bothersome in older adults. They include dry mouth, sedation, orthostatic hypotension, ataxia, dizziness, euphoria, and dysphoria.

Phenothiazines

Although phenothiazines were the first effective antiemetics, the results of antiemetic trials with this class of agents against highly emetogenic chemotherapy have been poor. Randomized trials have found standard-dose prochlorperazine, given orally or intramuscularly, to be less effective than metoclopramide or dexamethasone and equivalent to or less effective than dronabinol. IV administration is more effective than oral administration but can rarely cause profound hypotension (unlike serotonin antagonists or metoclopramide). Phenothiazines are seldom used as first-line antiemetic agents for highly or moderately emetogenic chemotherapy.

Side effects of phenothiazines include sedation, akathisia, hypotension, and dystonic reactions.

TABLE 3: Antiemetic regimens for acute emesis by emetic risk

Risk level	Recommended antiemetic regimen[a]
High (cisplatin)	Serotonin antagonist
	plus
	Dexamethasone (12 mg)
	plus
	Aprepitant (125 mg)
High/moderate	Serotonin antagonist
	plus
	Dexamethasone (20 mg)
Low	Single agent, such as a corticosteroid or serotonin antagonist
Minimal	No preventive agent is recommended for general use

[a] See Table 2 for doses.

NK₁ antagonists

Aprepitant is the first NK_1 antagonist antiemetic. NK_1 antagonists have demonstrated activity against a wide range of emetogenic stimuli. Although less effective than serotonin antagonists as single agents against acute emesis, NK_1 antagonists have shown superior activity against delayed emesis, suggesting the value of combination therapy.

In a multicenter, randomized, double-blind, phase III trial, 866 breast cancer patients being treated with cyclophosphamide with or without doxorubicin or epirubicin (Ellence) were randomized to receive either a regimen of aprepitant (125 mg), ondansetron (8 mg bid), and dexamethasone (12 mg) on day 1 with aprepitant (80 mg qd) on days 2 to 3 or a standard regimen of ondansetron (8 mg bid) on days 1 to 3 and dexamethasone (20 mg) on day 1. Of the 857 evaluable patients, 50.8% in the aprepitant arm, versus 42.5% ($P = .015$) in the standard regimen arm, achieved a complete response. In addition, more patients in the aprepitant arm achieved a complete response during both acute (75.7% vs 69.0%; $P = .034$) and delayed (55.4% vs 49.1%; $P = .064$) phases. Both treatments were generally well tolerated.

Combination antiemetic regimens

Table 3 summarizes recommended antiemetic regimens, according to the emetic potential of the chemotherapy regimen.

Serotonin antagonist plus dexamethasone Combinations of a 5-HT$_3$ antagonist and dexamethasone form the basis of the most effective regimens for controlling acute chemotherapy-induced emesis. Use of these two agents combined has proved to be more effective than either agent alone. Addition of an NK$_1$ antagonist (aprepitant) results in increased activity against acute cisplatin-induced emesis. However, inhibition by aprepitant of the CYP3A4 metabolic pathway may require a decrease in the dose of concomitantly administered dexamethasone.

Treatment of emesis

ACUTE EMESIS

A management strategy to prevent acute chemotherapy-induced emesis is outlined in Table 3. All patients should receive education and reassurance, as well as antiemetics tailored to the chemotherapy regimen. For regimens that commonly cause emesis (> 30%), antiemetic combinations are recommended; for regimens of low risk (10%-30% incidence), a single agent will usually suffice. As stated in Table 3, chemotherapy of minimal risk typically does not require preventive treatment.

DELAYED EMESIS

Delayed emesis is defined as nausea or vomiting beginning or persisting ≥ 24 hours after chemotherapy administration. The pathophysiology of this problem is unclear, but it is particularly common after high-dose cisplatin (≥ 50 mg/m^2), carboplatin (≥ 300 mg/m^2), cyclophosphamide (≥ 600 mg/m^2), or doxorubicin (≥ 50 mg/m^2).

In one natural history study, 89% of patients experienced some delayed emesis from 24 to 120 hours after receiving high-dose cisplatin, with a peak incidence occurring between 48 and 72 hours. With anthracyclines or cyclophosphamide, the rate of delayed emesis without preventive antiemetics is about 30%.

Some observations suggest that delayed emesis may begin earlier. When combination antiemetic regimens for acute emesis "fail," the initial emetic episode is often at 17 to 23 hours following chemotherapy. In some trials, antiemetics to prevent delayed emesis have been initiated at 16 to 17 hours.

Treatment options The combination of oral dexamethasone and metoclopramide has been found to be superior to dexamethasone alone or placebo in a double-blind, randomized trial. The combination of dexamethasone and aprepitant has also demonstrated efficacy. The recommended doses and schedules for the prevention of delayed emesis are given in Table 4.

ANTICIPATORY EMESIS

This problem is defined as nausea or vomiting beginning before the administration of chemotherapy in patients with poor emetic control during previous chemotherapy. As this problem is a conditioned response, the hospital environment or other treatment-related associations may trigger the onset

TABLE 4: Treatment regimens for delayed emesis

Risk level	Duration	Agent	Dose and schedule
High	Days 2-4	Aprepitant *plus*	80 mg PO qd x 2
		Dexamethasone	8 mg PO qd x 3
		Serotonin antagonist	
		Ondansetron	8 mg PO bid
		Dolasetron	100 mg PO bid
		Granisetron	1 mg PO bid
		Palonosetron[a] *plus*	0.25 mg IV day 1 only
		Dexamethasone	8 mg PO bid
		Metoclopramide *plus*	30-40 mg PO bid
		Dexamethasone	8 mg PO bid
Moderate	Days 2-3	Serotonin antagonist or dexamethasone or metoclopramide as single agent or in combination at dose and schedule above	
Low		No preventive regimen is recommended for general use	
Minimal		No preventive regimen is recommended for general use	

[a] Palonosetron has only been studied when given on day 1 with a single dose of dexamethasone (20 mg IV)

of emesis unrelated to chemotherapy. Strong emetic stimuli combined with poor emetic control increase the likelihood that anticipatory emesis will occur.

Treatment approach Behavioral therapy involving systematic desensitization can be helpful in managing anticipatory emesis. Also, benzodiazepines appear to be useful. However, the best approach to anticipatory emesis is prevention, which underscores the need to provide the most effective and appropriate antiemetic regimens with the initial course of emesis-producing chemotherapy.

SUGGESTED READING

Gralla R, Lichinitser M, Van Der Vegt S, et al: Palonosetron improves prevention of chemotherapy-induced nausea and vomiting following moderately emetogenic chemotherapy: Results of a double-blind randomized phase III trial comparing single doses of palonosetron with ondansetron. Ann Oncol 14:1570–1577, 2003.

Italian Group for Antiemetic Research: Dexamethasone, granisetron, or both for the prevention of nausea and vomiting during chemotherapy for cancer. N Engl J Med 332:1–5, 1995.

Koeller JM, Aapro MS, Gralla RJ, et al: Antiemetic guidelines: Creating a more practical treatment approach. Support Care Cancer 10:519–522, 2002.

Kris MG, Gralla RJ, Clark RA, et al: Incidence, course, and severity of delayed nausea and vomiting following the administration of high-dose cisplatin. J Clin Oncol 3:1379–1384, 1985.

Poli-Bigelli S, Rodrigues-Pereira J, Carides AD, et al: Addition of the neurokinin 1 receptor antagonist aprepitant to standard antiemetic therapy improves control of chemotherapy-induced nausea and vomiting: Results from a randomized, double-blind, placebo-controlled trial in Latin America. Cancer 97:3090–3098, 2003.

Tremblay PB, Kaiser R, Sezer O, et al: Variations in the 5-hydroxytryptamine type 3B receptor gene as predictors of the efficacy of antiemetic treatment in cancer patients. J Clin Oncol 21:2147–2155, 2003.

Warr DG, Hesketh PJ, Gralla RJ, et al: Efficacy and tolerability of aprepitant for the prevention of chemotherapy-induced nausea and vomiting in patients with breast cancer after moderately emetogenic chemotherapy. J Clin Oncol 23:2822–2830, 2005.

CHAPTER 39

Depression, anxiety, and delirium

Ilana Braun, MD, and Alan Valentine, MD

Although many cancer patients cope well with their disease, psychiatric disorders occur in almost 50% of patients in the setting of malignancy. Untreated psychological and neuropsychiatric disorders can compromise quality of life as well as treatment compliance. Three behavioral syndromes that are often encountered in clinical practice will be discussed here: depression, anxiety, and delirium.

Depression

Sadness exists on a continuum, ranging from an emotion common in daily life to a syndrome of severe physical and psychological symptoms consistent with a defined psychiatric disorder (Major Depressive Disorder). Several studies of cancer inpatients report Major Depression prevalence rates of 25% to 42%.

SIGNS AND SYMPTOMS/DIAGNOSIS

Patients with depressive syndromes may experience an array of psychological and somatic symptoms.

Psychological symptoms include dysphoria (sadness), anhedonia (pervasive loss of pleasure in activities), feelings of guilt or low self-esteem, and thoughts of death or suicide.

Somatic symptoms include sleep disturbance (ie, sleeping too much or too little), change in appetite, fatigue, diminished concentration, and psychomotor agitation or withdrawal.

Focus of diagnostic evaluation Although the diagnosis of Major Depressive Disorder requires that greater than half of these symptoms (including dysphoria or anhedonia) be present for at least 2 weeks, patients who do not meet these criteria may be in significant distress, and may be described as having an Adjustment Disorder. In medically ill patients, diagnosis is complicated by the fact that somatic symptoms may also arise as a result of disease and treatment. For this reason, when evaluating the depressed cancer patient, special attention should be paid to those psychological symptoms that are less likely to be directly related to somatic disease or treatment.

ETIOLOGY

Psychological causes

Major depressive disorder is common in the general population (point prevalence, ~6%) and is a recurrent disease. Patients with a history of mood disorder are at risk for relapse in the face of a cancer diagnosis. In the setting of malignancy, obvious stressors include news of initial diagnosis, treatment failure, or disease progression. Patients may also confront more subtle stressors, including loss of independence, financial woes, diminished body image, family strain, and existential angst.

Disease- and treatment-related causes

Presenting symptom of malignancy Depression may be a presenting symptom of some primary malignancies, most notably pancreatic carcinoma. Primary and metastatic brain tumors can cause frontal lobe disinhibition syndromes or personality changes that mimic depression and other psychiatric disorders.

Drugs Many drugs used in general medical practice are associated with psychiatric syndromes. The most common of these drugs are β-blockers, antihypertensives, barbiturates, opioids, and benzodiazepines. Many primary and supportive therapies for cancer are also commonly associated with depression. They include corticosteroids (also possibly associated with mania), cytokines (especially interferon-alfa and interleukin-2), whole-brain radiation therapy, and chemotherapeutic agents, including procarbazine (Matulane). Patients treated with tamoxifen may complain of depression or "chemo brain." The latter term usually refers to cognitive slowing. Treatment of tamoxifen-related depression raises particular challenges. Recent evidence suggests that many antidepressants used to treat these symptoms inhibit tamoxifen's anticancer effect through P450 interactions.

MANAGEMENT

Management of depressive syndromes begins with accurate diagnosis. Clinicians should assess for somatic and psychological symptoms of the syndrome and should always ask about suicidal thoughts or intent. In addition to medication, laboratory assessments should be reviewed, as metabolic disarray, anemia, low B_{12} levels, and thyroid dysfunction can all contribute to the development of depressive symptoms. Once depression is diagnosed, treatment involves antidepressant medication, sleep aids, when possible, removal of exacerbating agents, and psychotherapy.

In cancer patients, diagnosis and treatment of depression require a high index of suspicion and regular, careful follow-up. Ideally, only patients with clinically significant or progressive symptoms are offered antidepressant therapy. When the diagnosis of depression is in doubt, however, it may be best to seek psychiatric consultation.

Antidepressants

Selected antidepressants used in cancer patients are listed in Table 1. No antidepressant has been shown to be more effective than any other in the cancer setting. Often, the choice of an antidepressant is based on side-effect profile.

In the general population, antidepressants often take at least 2 weeks or longer to produce initial relief of symptoms. As a general rule, antidepressant therapy should continue for 4 to 6 months after symptoms stabilize.

Selective serotonin reuptake inhibitors (SSRIs), such as citalopram (Celexa), escitalopram (Lexapro), fluoxetine (Prozac, Sarafem), paroxetine, and sertraline

TABLE 1: Selected antidepressants used in cancer patients

Drug	Starting dose	Maintenance dose	Comments
Selective serotonin reuptake inhibitors			
Citalopram	10-20 mg qd	20-40 mg/d	Usually well tolerated; possible nausea, sexual dysfunction
Escitalopram	5-10 mg qd	10-20 mg/d	Usually well tolerated; possible nausea, sexual dysfunction
Fluoxetine	10-20 mg qd	20-60 mg/d	Long half-life; possible nausea, sexual dysfunction
Paroxetine	10-20 mg qd	20-60 mg/d	Possible nausea, sexual dysfunction, sedation
Sertraline	25-50 mg qd	50-200 mg/d	Usually well tolerated; possible nausea, sexual dysfunction
Other agents			
Bupropion	100 mg qAM - 100 mg bid	200-300 mg/d	Activating; few reports of sexual dysfunction; risk of seizures in predisposed patients
Duloxetine	20-30 mg	60 mg/d	May increase blood pressure; possible efficacy for neuropathic pain
Methylphenidate	2.5 mg qAM	10-60 mg/d	Activating; rapid effect possible; monitor blood pressure
Mirtazapine	7.5-15 mg qhs	15-45 mg qhs	Sleep aid and appetite-stimulant
Venlafaxine	18.75-37.5 mg qd	75-375 mg/d	May increase blood pressure; may be useful for neuropathic pain, hot flashes

(Zoloft), are often used in patients with cancer because of their benign side-effect profile. In particular, their lack of anticholinergic and α-adrenergic–blocking properties makes them attractive options for patients with a serious medical illness. SSRIs are rarely lethal in overdose, making them a reasonably safe choice in the treatment of patients experiencing suicidal ideations.

Side effects Common side effects of SSRIs include mild nausea, which tends to improve with continued use; reduced appetite; sexual dysfunction, including decreased libido, impotence, and anorgasmia; jitteriness; and insomnia. Paroxetine, in particular, may cause sedation; other side effects include dry mouth, rash, and weight gain.

Dosage In ambulatory patients with normal metabolic function, SSRIs can be started at the same doses used in general psychiatry (10 mg once daily for escitalopram; 20 mg once daily for citalopram, fluoxetine, and paroxetine; 50 mg once daily for sertraline). These doses can be increased if there is no response within 2 to 3 weeks.

Hospitalized or elderly patients, those with compromised renal or hepatic function, and those receiving highly emetogenic treatments should be started at one-half or even one-quarter of these starting doses, which can then be increased if tolerated.

Atypical and newer antidepressants Bupropion (Wellbutrin) is a well-tolerated medication that works to increase norepinephrine levels in the brain. In addition to its antidepressant effects, bupropion is activating and may help to improve attention. Unlike SSRIs, it is rarely associated with sexual dysfunction. A note of caution, however, is that bupropian lowers the seizure threshold and should not be used in patients with a history of seizures.

Venlafaxine (Effexor), mirtazapine (Remeron), and duloxetine (Cymbalta) are newer agents with selective effects on serotonin and norepinephrine metabolism. They should be started at low doses in order to establish tolerability. Venlafaxine may be quite effective against treatment-induced hot flashes. It tends to have an intense discontinuation syndrome, and patients should be titrated off slowly. Mirtazapine has sedative, appetite-stimulating, and antiemetic effects, which can all be useful in selected cases. Duloxetine is approved for treatment of diabetic neuropathy and may have applications in the depressed cancer patient with neuropathic pain.

Psychostimulants

Psychostimulants that have direct or indirect dopamine-agonistic properties, such as methylphenidate, have established role in the treatment of depression in the medically ill. Psychostimulants are activating agents useful in patients with psychomotor retardation, deconditioning, or apathy states associated with depression, as well as in those with CNS disease or treatment side effects.

The antidepressant effects of psychostimulants may be seen more quickly than those of first-line antidepressants. Improvements in mood, physical activity, well-being, and appetite are sometimes observed within 24 to 48 hours of the initiation of psychostimulant treatment.

Side effects Like other activating agents, psychostimulants may cause insomnia, decreased appetite, GI upset, anxiety, palpitations, and even arrhythmia. Pulses should be monitored with their use.

Dosage Initial dosing should be conservative (ie, 2.5–5 mg/d, the latter in divided doses) for methylphenidate. If tolerated, stimulant doses can be increased until a therapeutic effect is achieved or side effects develop. To prevent insomnia, afternoon doses should not be administered after 2 PM.

Psychotherapy

Although antidepressants alone are effective in the treatment of depression, they are often synergistic with psychotherapy. Talk therapy may provide patients with basic support and encouragement during cancer treatment. Cognitive-behavioral therapy may help them tackle fundamental misperceptions about themselves and their disease and to develop new coping skills.

Anxiety

Like depression, "anxiety" refers to both a subjective emotion and a constellation of signs and symptoms that can be of physical or psychological origin.

Especially in seriously ill patients, subjective anxiety may be the first sign of a serious or catastrophic physiologic derangement (ie, sepsis or pulmonary embolus). It is also common at disease milestones, especially at initial diagnosis, time of recurrence, and progression to the terminal phase. In patients whose disease is stable or in remission, anxiety frequently occurs in conjunction with routine reevaluation.

SIGNS AND SYMPTOMS/DIAGNOSIS

Psychological symptoms Patients with anxiety typically report worry, irritability, insomnia, and even depression, as there is considerable overlap between the two syndromes. They may appear hypervigilant or emotionally labile, crying unexpectedly or growing suddenly enraged. Typically, their thought processes are ruminative.

If anxiety proceeds to panic, patients may report time-limited feelings of impending doom, suffocation, or annihilation. Occasionally, distress is so intense that patients experience suicidal thoughts.

Physical symptoms A variety of somatic symptoms can be associated with anxiety. Cardiovascular signs and symptoms include palpitations and tachycardia, as well as subjective chest tightness or even pain. Respiratory symptoms include dyspnea, hyperventilation, and, as a result, light-headedness and dizziness. GI symptoms are common and include difficulty swallowing, abdominal cramping, nausea, diarrhea, and constipation. Patients may become diaphoretic. Preexisting pain may be aggravated.

ETIOLOGY

Psychological causes

Generalized anxiety disorder, panic disorder, and specific phobias (ie, to blood, needles, and even hospitals) are relatively common in the general population. Affected individuals are at risk for exacerbations of their anxiety disorders in the setting of cancer treatment. The stress associated with a cancer diagnosis can also trigger the onset of an anxiety disorder in a patient without a premorbid psychiatric diagnosis.

Cancer patients fear pain, suffering, disfigurement, and even death. Their concerns frequently center on loss of control or independence, strained finances, and family dynamics. Unpleasant procedures or medications can trigger anxiety, and this response can become conditioned, as in the case of anticipatory nausea. Even patients in the surveillance stage of treatment may find themselves suffering with considerable anxiety. In the absence of active treatment, these individuals become ruminative and fearful as they "wait for the other shoe to drop." Anxiety of this type often peaks in anticipation of follow-up appointments.

Disease and treatment-related causes

Life-threatening causes of anxiety include hypoxia, (secondary to pulmonary edema, pulmonary embolus or sepsis). Other possible medical etiologies include severe anemia, electrolyte disturbances, endocrine disorders such as hyperthyroidism, hypercalcemia, hyperadrenalism, pain syndromes, and the presence of hormone-secreting neoplasms, such as pheochromocytomas.

Cancer-related medications can also cause or exacerbate anxiety. Frequent offending agents include corticosteroids, which can trigger nervousness, agitation, and even frank mania, and antiemetics, including promethazine, and metoclopramide, which can produce akathisia, a subjective sense of restlessness. Other medications such as anticholinergics (ie, benztropine [Cogentin]), opioids, and benzodiazepines can produce paradoxical reactions including anxiety states. These paradoxical reactions occur more frequently in geriatric and in CNS-impaired populations. Finally, drug toxicity (ie, from immunosuppressants, bronchodilators, or psychostimulants) and drug withdrawal states (ie, from opioids, benzodiazepines, and alcohol) can also trigger significant anxiety.

MANAGEMENT

Initial approaches to anxious patients vary with the severity of the symptom and the medical status of the patient. In all cases, medical underpinnings for anxiety should be considered and corrected when possible.

Psychotherapy

Talk therapy for anxious patients is universally appropriate. This intervention can take several forms. Supportive psychotherapy may enable an anxious patient to ventilate emotion in a safe setting. Cognitive-behavioral therapy may aid a patient in developing new coping skills through relaxation therapy, guided imagery training, or through a careful review of the patient's core beliefs and the behaviors that help to trigger the emotion.

MEDICATIONS

The pharmacologic mainstay of anxiety disorders is antidepressant medication. These agents may take 4 to 6 weeks for maximal effect but promise long-lasting symptom amelioration once fully active. Currently, escitalopram, paroxetine, and venlafaxine have FDA (US Food and Drug Administration) indications for the management of generalized anxiety disorder. Most SSRIs have been used successfully in the treatment of panic disorder. Typical dose ranges for these agents follow: paroxetine, 20 to 60 mg/d; escitalopram, 10 to 20 mg/d; sertraline, 50 to 200 mg/d; and extended-release venlafaxine, 75 to 375 mg/d (see Table 1).

Benzodiazepines Because of the delayed onset of antidepressant action, benzodiazepines are often useful adjuncts to initial treatment. These medications have variable hypnotic, antiemetic, and muscle-relaxant effects useful in other aspects of supportive cancer care. Caution is required when using these agents in the settings of serious illness (because of the risk of additive sedation with other medications), advanced age, or CNS impairment (because of the risk of disinhibition or delirium). Benzodiazepines commonly used to treat anxiety in cancer patients are listed in Table 2.

Short-acting benzodiazepines, such as lorazepam and alprazolam, have a rapid onset but relatively short duration of action, making them useful for treating intermittent paroxysmal anxiety or panic attacks. For the same reason, they are also useful in patients with severe medical illness. Typical doses are lorazepam 0.5 to 1.0 mg PO (by mouth)/IM (intramuscular)/IV (intravenous) every 4 to 12 hours or alprazolam 0.25 to 0.5 mg PO every 6 to 8 hours as needed. For patients with persistent anxiety, these medications can be given on a regular schedule. Lorazepam's lack of active metabolites makes it a good choice in patients with hepatic or renal compromise.

Withdrawal develops more rapidly to short-acting benzodiazepines than to their longer-acting counterparts. Therefore, if short-acting agents are used for any length of time, they should be discontinued gradually.

Longer-acting benzodiazepines, such as diazepam and clonazepam, are useful for persistent anxiety. Their longer duration of action is such that they do not "wear off" quickly and leave patients unprotected.

Clonazepam is typically given at a dose of 0.25 to 1.0 mg every 8 to 24 hours and diazepam at a dose of 2 to 10 mg every 6 to 24 hours. These drugs have multiple active metabolites that can adversely affect the elderly and patients with renal or hepatic impairment. In such patients, it is best to avoid these medications if at all possible.

TABLE 2: Selected benzodiazepines used to treat anxiety in cancer patients

Drug	Dose range (prn or scheduled)	Comments
Lorazepam	0.5-2.0 mg PO/IM/IVP/IVPB q6-12h	Versatile; can be administered via continuous infusion in rare cases; approved for chemotherapy-related nausea and vomiting
Alprazolam	0.25-1.0 mg PO q8-24h	Potent, rapid onset and cessation of effects; interdose withdrawal lessened with extended-release formulation
Diazepam	2-10 mg PO/IV q6-24h	Useful for general/persistent anxiety but problematic in elderly or seriously ill patients
Clonazepam	0.25-1.0 mg PO q8-24h	Long half-life; useful for general/ persistent anxiety

PO = by mouth; IM = intramuscular; IVP = IV push; IVPB = IV piggyback

Other medications At low doses, antipsychotic medications, such as haloperidol (Haldol), olanzapine (Zyprexa), quetiapine (Seroquel), and risperidone (Risperdal), may be used as anxiolytics. These agents are most appropriate for patients with a history of, or at high risk for, adverse reactions to benzodiazepines.

Delirium

Delirium is a syndrome of diffuse brain dysfunction incited, typically acutely, by aspects of medical illness or treatment. In some surveys, 15%–30% of cancer inpatients and up to 85% of those who are terminally ill experience the syndrome. Its presence is linked to increased length of hospital stays, morbidity, and mortality. For this reason, accurate diagnosis and identification of causes are critical. With neutralization of inciting factors, many cases of delirium are reversible.

SIGNS AND SYMPTOMS

Waxing and waning impairments in attention, orientation, and memory are the hallmarks of the syndrome. Other features that occur more variably include disturbances in affect, mood, sleep pattern, level of agitation, insight, and perception; a delirious patient may, for instance, experience an altered sense of reality, whether in the form of an illusion or a hallucination. The presence of several of these signs and symptoms or history or an exam should raise the specter of the diagnosis.

Distractibility is the sine qua non of the syndrome. Delirious patients perform poorly on tasks requiring concentration. They may have trouble naming the months of the year in reverse, counting backward by 7's from 100, or drawing a clock face set to a particular hour. Memory impairment is also prominent. Delirious patients often encounter difficulty encoding new information, for instance, registering three new words if specifically asked to remember them or recalling them after 5 minutes. They may also have difficulty with biographical information, such as their phone number or the ages of their children. Not infrequently, delirious patients prove to be amnestic to their delirious episodes. They are typically disoriented to time and place but rarely to person. These deficits wax and wane, and the presence of lucid intervals may seem to discount the diagnosis. For this reason, serial examinations are useful.

ETIOLOGY

Organic disturbances that can produce a state of delirium are multifold and range from primary intracranial abnormalities such as tumors to systemic diseases that secondarily affect the brain to substance intoxication or substance withdrawal. Life-threatening causes that are potentially reversible include substance withdrawal (including from alcohol, prescription drugs, and illicit drugs), hypertensive encephalopathy, Wernicke's encephalopathy, hypoxia, hypoglycemia, intracranial bleeding, meningitis, encephalitis, and poisoning. Another potentially reversible cause is substance intoxication. Many medications used commonly in the context of cancer can trigger delirium. They include benzodiazepines, opioids, anticholinergic medications, corticosteroids, and chemotherapeutics.

MANAGEMENT

Treatment

The management of delirium centers on identifying and addressing the causative medical factors. Work-up should explore potential infectious, metabolic, neurologic, and biochemical causes. Imaging of the head may be indicated. In more than half of delirium cases, no definitive etiology can be identified. In these instances, care is supportive.

Behavioral management

Delirious patients should be managed in a setting of moderate stimulation. As much as possible, they should be provided with appropriate environmental cues: lights should be shut off during the night; they should be frequently reminded of the day and date, and, if possible, should be surrounded by family and other familiar faces. Their safety must be guarded, and close observation may be required. Some afflicted patients may lie listlessly, whereas others may become agitated and even violent. In these instances, chemical and even physical restraints may be required.

TABLE 3: Selected medications used to treat delirium in cancer patients

Drug	Dose range (in divided doses)	Comments
Antipsychotics		
Haloperidol	0.5-50 mg PO/d or IM/d; 0.5-20 IV/d	IV route twice as potent as PO route and has fewer side effects
Risperidone	0.5-6 mg PO/d	Comes in an orally disintegrating tablet that is easily swallowed
Olanzapine	2.5-20 mg PO/d or IM/d	Zydis formulation is an orally disintegrating tablet that is easily swallowed
Quetiapine	12.5-750 mg PO/d	Very sedating, especially attractive option for sleep-deprived patients

PO = by mouth; IM = intramuscular; IV = intravenous

MEDICATIONS

Antipsychotics

If more conservative measures are ineffective, pharmacotherapy may be required to manage the behavioral disturbances associated with delirium. Antipsychotic medications may help to treat sensory misperceptions, as well as provide a degree of anxiolysis. Table 3 lists selected drugs often used to treat delirium in cancer patients. Because of a growing understanding of the health risks associated with use of these drugs (ranging from extrapyramidal symptoms to hyperglycemia, stroke, and increased risk of death in the elderly), antipsychotics should be reserved for use in patients with hyperactivity, for instance those who pull out blood access lines or those who wander.

Haloperidol is a potent antipsychotic that may be administered PO, IM, or IV. The IV formulation is twice as potent as the PO preparation.

Side effects Haloperidol is usually well tolerated, although it does carry a risk of akathisia and Parkinsonian side effects. The risk of these adverse reactions can be minimized by IV administration.

Dosage Elderly patients or patients with end-stage disease usually require very modest doses (0.5 to 1.0 mg PO or IV at night or twice daily) to control delirium. Especially in hyperactive delirium, higher and more frequent dosing is usually required (ie, 2 to 5 mg IV every 6 hours). In unusual cases, total doses of ≥ 50 mg/d may be administered via continuous infusion.

Risperidone is given orally. At doses of 0.5 to 3.0 mg once or twice daily, it is useful in managing delirium or delusional symptoms, especially in elderly patients, in whom it may have fewer adverse effects than oral haloperidol.

Olanzapine has been shown to be effective in the management of delirious cancer patients and is available for administration PO or IM in cases of severe agitation. The Zydis formulation of olanzapine is an orally disintegrating tablet that easily dissolves in the mouth and may be useful for some agitated patients and for those with swallowing difficulties.

Quetiapine is fairly sedating and is an attractive option for treatment of low-intensity delirium, especially when given at night to control behavior and promote sleep.

SUGGESTED READING

ON DEPRESSION

Jacobsen PB, Donovan KA, Weitzner MA: Distinguishing fatigue and depression in patients with cancer. Semin Clin Neuropsychiatry 8:229–240, 2003.

Spiegel D, Giese-Davis J: Depression and cancer: Mechanisms and disease progression. Biol Psychiatry 54:269–282, 2003.

Trask PC: Assessment of depression in cancer patients. J Natl Cancer Inst 32:80–92, 2004.

ON ANXIETY

Stark D, Kiely M, Smith A, et al: Anxiety disorders in cancer patients: Their nature, associations, and relation to quality of life. J Clin Oncol 20:3137–3148, 2002.

ON DELIRIUM

Centeno C, Sanz A, Bruera E: Delirium in advanced cancer patients. Palliat Med 18:184–194, 2004.

Fann JR, Sullivan AK: Delirium in the course of cancer treatment. Semin Clin Neuropsychiatry 8:217–228, 2003.

Gaudreau J-D, Gagnon P, Harel F, et al: Psychoactive medications and risk of delirium in hospitalized cancer patients. J Clin Oncol 23:6712–6718, 2005.

ON PSYCHOTROPIC DRUGS

Buclin T, Mazzocato C, Berney A, et al: Psychopharmacology in supportive care of cancer: A review for the clinician, IV. Other psychotropic agents. Support Care Cancer 9:213–222, 2001.

Fisch MJ, Kim HF: Use of atypical antipsychotic agents for symptom control in patients with advanced cancer. J Support Oncol 2:447–452, 2004.

Jin Y, Desta Z, Stearns V, et al: CYP2D6 genotype, antidepressant use, and tamoxifen metabolism during adjuvant breast cancer treatment. J Natl Cancer Inst 97:30–39, 2005.

Joshi N, Breitbart WS: Psychopharmacologic management during cancer treatment. Semin Clin Neuropsychiatry 8:241–252, 2003.

CHAPTER 40

Hematopoietic growth factors

Sally Yowell Barbour, PHARMD, and Jeffrey Crawford, MD

For years, chemotherapy-associated myelosuppression has represented a major limitation to a patient's tolerance of anticancer therapy. In addition, the clinical consequences of chemotherapy-induced myelosuppression (such as febrile neutropenia, dose reductions, or lengthy dose delays) may have had significant negative effects on quality of life or even response to treatment.

Before the widespread availability of agents to stimulate host hematopoiesis, administration of antibiotics, transfusion of blood products, and reductions or delays in chemotherapy dose have been the major means of combating the myelotoxicity of chemotherapy. It is now possible to stimulate clinically relevant production of several formed elements of the blood: neutrophils, erythrocytes, and platelets.

This chapter summarizes data supporting the clinical activity of several hematopoietic growth factors. A thorough knowledge of these data will help clinicians to make judicious, informed decisions about how to use these agents most responsibly.

Hematopoietic growth factors

Over the past several years, a great deal of progress has been made in understanding the process of hematopoiesis by which mature cellular elements of blood are formed. Hematopoietic growth factors are a family of regulatory molecules that play important roles in the growth, survival, and differentiation of blood progenitor cells, as well as in the functional activation of mature cells.

Table 1 lists the recombinant human hematopoietic growth factors (also known as hematopoietic cytokines) that have been approved by the US Food and Drug Administration (FDA) for clinical use: granulocyte colony-stimulating factor (G-CSF, filgrastim [Neupogen]); pegfilgrastim [Neulasta]; yeast-derived granulocyte-macrophage colony-stimulating factor (GM-CSF, sargramostim [Leukine, Prokine]); recombinant human erythropoietin (epoetin alfa, EPO [Epogen, Procrit]); darbepoetin alfa (Aranesp); and interleukin-11 (IL-11, oprelvekin [Neumega]). In addition, several other hematopoietic cytokines are under clinical development.

The commercial availability of these recombinant human hematopoietic growth factors has led to their wide clinical application in oncology practice. However,

GROWTH FACTORS

TABLE 1: FDA-approved indications for hematopoietic growth factors/cytokines

Growth factor/ cytokine	Generic name	Trade name(s)	Distributor(s)/ manufacturer(s)	Indication(s)
G-CSF	Filgrastim Pegfilgrastim	Neupogen Neulasta	Amgen Amgen	Cancer patients receiving myelosuppressive chemotherapy
				Patients with nonmyeloid malignancy following BMT
				For mobilization of PBPCs
				Patients with severe chronic neutropenia
				Following induction chemotherapy in AML
GM-CSF	Sargramostim	Leukine Prokine	Immunex	Following autologous BMT, BMT engraftment delay, or failure
				Following induction chemotherapy in older patients with AML
				Allogeneic BMT For mobilization of PBPCs and for use after PBPC transplantation
EPO[a]	Epoetin alfa	Epogen Procrit	Amgen Ortho Biotech	Anemia in chronic renal failure (predialysis or dialysis)
				Anemia in zidovudine-treated HIV-infected patients
				Anemia in patients with nonmyeloid malignancy receiving chemotherapy
				Anemia in patients scheduled for elective, noncardiac, nonvascular surgery
	Darbepoetin alfa	Aranesp	Amgen	Anemia in chronic renal failure patients
				Anemia in patients with nonmyeloid malignancy receiving chemotherapy
IL-11	Oprelvekin	Neumega	Genetics Institute	Following myelosuppressive chemotherapy in patients with nonmyeloid malignancy who are at high risk for severe thrombocytopenia

[a] FDA letter issued July 30, 2008, to provide new safety information about erythropoiesis-stimulating agents, including "ESAs are not indicated in patients receiving myelosuppressive therapy when the anticipated outcome is cure." See box on opposite page.

AML = acute myelogenous leukemia; BMT = bone marrow transplantation; PBPC = peripheral blood progenitor cell the substantial costs of colony-stimulating factor utilization as supportive care for patients receiving myelosuppressive chemotherapy make it imperative to identify the optimal settings in which their use can make a significant difference in patient outcomes.

This chapter discusses the appropriate uses of only the FDA-approved hematopoietic growth factors/cytokines: G-CSF, GM-CSF, EPO, darbepoetin alfa, and IL-11. For a more detailed review of recommendations for the use of myeloid CSFs, readers are referred to the evidence-based, clinical practice guidelines developed in 1994 (last updated in 2007) by the American Society of Clinical Oncology (ASCO). The ASCO guidelines were formulated to encourage reasonable use of CSFs when their efficacy has been well documented but to discourage excess use when marginal benefit is anticipated. These clinical practice guidelines have been published and are most easily accessed at the official web site of ASCO (www.asco.org). In addition, the National Comprehensive Cancer Network (NCCN; www.nccn.org) has published guidelines on the use of colony-stimulating factors, which are updated annually.

Strengthened Oncology Safety Information and New Medication Guide and Patient Instructions for Erythropoietic Stimulating Agents (ESAs)

FDA issued a letter to the manufacturers of Epogen/Procrit (epoetin alfa) and Aranesp (darbepoetin alfa) on July 30, 2008 of its decision to require additional safety-related changes to the labeling for these products. On August 6, 2008, the Epogen/Procrit and Aranesp labeling was revised to strengthen the safety information for healthcare professionals and patients.

Prescribing information for Epogen/Procrit and Aranesp information has been revised as follows:

Cancer

· Therapy should not be initiated at hemoglobin levels ≥ 10 g/dL.

· ESAs shortened overall survival and/or increased the risk of tumor progression or recurrence in some clinical studies in patients with breast, non–small-cell lung, head and neck, lymphoid, and cervical cancers.

· To decrease these risks, as well as the risk of serious cardio- and thrombovascular events, use the lowest dose needed to avoid red blood cell transfusion.

· Use ESAs only for treatment of anemia due to concomitant myelosuppressive chemotherapy.

· ESAs are not indicated for patients receiving myelosuppressive therapy when the anticipated outcome is cure.

· Discontinue following the completion of a chemotherapy course.

Note: Important changes have also been made to labeling of these drugs to ensure use of the lowest dose needed to avoid transfusion and to discontinue treatment with ESAs if after 8 weeks of therapy there is no response as measured by hemoglobin levels or if transfusions are still required.

For the latest information about ESAs, go to: www.fda.gov/CDER/DRUG/infopage/RHE/default.htm.

Myeloid growth factors

Three myeloid growth factors are currently licensed for clinical use in the United States: G-CSF, pegfilgrastim, and GM-CSF.

G-CSF (filgrastim) is lineage-specific for the production of functionally active neutrophils. G-CSF has been extensively evaluated in several clinical scenarios.

G-CSF was first approved in 1991 for clinical use to reduce the incidence of febrile neutropenia in cancer patients receiving myelosuppressive chemotherapy.

This broad initial indication has since been expanded even further to include many other areas of oncologic practice, such as stimulation of neutrophil recovery following high-dose chemotherapy with stem-cell support. In addition, G-CSF is indicated to increase neutrophil production in endogenous myeloid disorders, such as congenital neutropenic states.

Pegylated G-CSF (pegfilgrastim) When polyethylene glycol was attached to the protein backbone of filgrastim, a new molecule (pegfilgrastim) with a longer half-life than the standard human G-CSF was created. Pegfilgrastim was approved in 2002 to reduce febrile neutropenia. It has been studied and shown to be equally efficacious as filgrastim, with the advantage of once-per-cycle dosing and self-regulating features of clearance of the drug during neutrophil recovery. Findings have suggested that pegfilgrastim is more effective than G-CSF in preventing febrile neutropenia, but further study is required. The use of pegfilgrastim in cycles < 3 weeks has not been approved; however, it has been studied in 2-week regimens and appears to be safe and effective. In addition, pegfilgrastim is not currently approved in bone marrow transplantation (BMT) or in pediatrics, but studies are under way.

GM-CSF (sargramostim), primarily a myeloid lineage-specific growth factor, stimulates the production of neutrophils, monocytes, and eosinophils. It has been extensively evaluated and received a more narrow FDA approval in 1991 for clinical use in patients with nonmyeloid malignancies undergoing autologous BMT. Since that initial indication, GM-CSF has also been approved for an expanded range of conditions, such as mitigation of myelotoxicity in patients with leukemia who are undergoing induction chemotherapy.

To date, no large-scale randomized trials have directly compared the efficacy of sargramostim with that of either filgrastim or pegfilgrastim in the same clinical setting. Future comparative trials may help to determine the optimal clinical utility of these CSFs in different clinical situations.

INDICATIONS

Uses to support chemotherapy

CSFs have been used to support both conventional and intensified doses of chemotherapy. The use of CSFs in this setting can be defined as prophylactic or therapeutic.

Prophylactic use is defined as the administration of a growth factor to prevent febrile neutropenia. "Primary prophylaxis" denotes the use of CSFs following the first cycle of multicourse chemotherapy *prior to* any occurrence of febrile neutropenia. The term "secondary prophylaxis" is reserved for the use of CSFs to prevent a subsequent episode of febrile neutropenia in a patient who has already experienced infectious complications in a previous chemotherapy cycle.

Primary prophylaxis G-CSF has been evaluated in at least three major randomized clinical trials in cancer patients receiving chemotherapy. The use of G-CSF as primary prophylaxis reduced the incidence of febrile neutropenia by approximately 50% in these trials, in which the incidence of febrile neutropenia in the control group was high (≥ 40%). More recently studies have evaluated the value of CSFs in patients receiving less myelosuppressive (~20%) regimens.

Vogel and colleagues evaluated a single dose of pegfilgrastim versus placebo 24 hours after chemotherapy in 950 patients with breast cancer receiving docetaxel (Taxotere; 100 mg/m^2). This regimen was specifically chosen to try to assess the potential benefit of growth factor in a setting associated with approximately a 20% risk of febrile neutropenia. The placebo group experienced a 17% incidence of febrile neutropenia, compared with a 1% incidence in the pegfilgrastim group. The results from this study and other abstracts presented over the past several years suggest a benefit to pegfilgrastim at least as great or greater than that seen in the previous clinical trials that evaluated filgrastim in treatment settings where the risk of febrile neutropenia was higher. The results of this study were pivotal in the new labeling of pegfilgrastim and recommendations for prophylactic use with regimens associated with a 17% risk of febrile neutropenia. Furthermore, pharmacoeconomic sensitivity analyses have suggested that CSF use may be cost-effective if the anticipated risk of febrile neutropenia is > 20%.

A recent update of the ASCO guidelines established the threshold for use of prophylactic growth factor at 20%. In addition, the NCCN guidelines have recommended CSFs be used in regimens with a 20% risk of neutropenic fever (Table 2). In addition, certain patient risk factors for neutropenia have been identified and should be considered in conjunction with the chemotherapy regimen (Table 3).

Secondary prophylaxis Available data indicate that the use of CSFs as secondary prophylaxis in patients who have had a prior episode of febrile neutropenia can decrease the likelihood of febrile neutropenia in subsequent cycles of chemotherapy. It is important to recognize that this conclusion has never been specifically proven in any randomized clinical trial. Rather, it has been derived from analyses of subsets of patients who crossed over from the placebo arms of the initial randomized clinical trials, as well as large clinical experience.

Thus, in clinical settings where maintenance of chemotherapy dose appears to be important, secondary prophylaxis with CSFs to prevent new episodes of neutropenic fever is appropriate. CSF support can also be considered to maintain standard-dose delivery of chemotherapy when the maintenance of dose may impact outcome.

Therapeutic use is defined as the administration of a growth factor at the time when neutropenia or neutropenic fever is documented in a patient who had not been receiving CSFs previously.

Clinical trials do not support the routine use of CSFs as an adjunct to antibiotics in the treatment of all patients with uncomplicated febrile neutropenia. However, in certain high-risk patients who have features predictive of poor outcome (eg, sepsis syndrome, pneumonia, fungal infection), use of a CSF with antibiotics may be justified. To conduct appropriate clinical trials to test the

TABLE 2: Chemotherapy regimens with a 20% risk of neutropenic fever

Cancer type	Regimen
Bladder	TC, MVAC
Breast	AC → T, AT, TAC
NHL	VAPEC-B
Ovarian	Topotecan, paclitaxel, docetaxel
Sarcoma	MAID
SCLC	CAE, topotecan
Testicular	VIP

AC → T = Adriamycin (doxorubicin]) cyclophosphamide, Taxotere (docetaxel); AT = Adriamycin (doxorubicin), Taxol (paclitaxel); CAE = cyclophosphamide, Adriamycin (doxorubicin), etoposide; NHL = non-Hodgkin lymphoma; MAID = mesna, Adriamycin (doxorubicin), ifosfamide, dacarbazine; MVAC = methotrexate, vinblastine, Adriamycin (doxorubicin) cisplatin; SCLC = small-cell lung cancer; TAC = Taxotere (docetaxel), Adriamycin (doxorubicin), cyclophosphamide; TC = Taxol (paclitaxel), cisplatin; VAPEC-B = vincristine, Adriamycin (doxorubicin), prednisolone, etoposide, cyclophosphamide, bleomycin; VIP = vinblastine, ifosfamide, Platinol (cisplatin)
Adapted from NCCN Myeloid Growth Factors in Cancer Treatment, v.1.2008 (www.nccn.com)

hypothesis that CSF support may improve the outcomes of subsets of patients, selection of patients based on risk-stratification criteria that have been validated to predict poor outcomes or delayed recovery from neutropenia will be critical. Certain trials performed with more selective entry criteria (such as absolute neutrophil count [ANC] < 100 cells/µL) have, in fact, shown statistically significant benefits from the use of CSFs as an adjunct to antibiotics in these high-risk patients with febrile neutropenia. Continued analyses of these data and the performance of larger scale, confirmatory studies are needed to further assess the therapeutic use of CSFs.

There are no indications for CSF use to treat uncomplicated neutropenia without fever. A large-scale randomized clinical trial noted no difference in patients who had CSF support in whom afebrile neutropenia was detected versus those patients whose hematologic status was allowed to recover spontaneously without CSF support. Thus, low neutrophil counts alone do not represent a reason to prescribe CSF support. One effective way to use CSFs is prophylactically, 24 hours after chemotherapy is completed.

Use to increase dose intensity of chemotherapy

The available evidence indicates that CSF use can permit chemotherapy dose maintenance or allow modest increases in dose intensity in clinical scenarios where the main toxicity is neutropenia. Recently, delivery of dose-dense chemotherapy every 2 weeks with G-CSF support has improved survival compared with standard every-3-week dosing in women with breast cancer receiving adjuvant cyclophosphamide and doxorubicin, followed by paclitaxel. This

TABLE 3: Selected risk factors for neutropenia

Treatment related
History of severe neutropenia with similar chemotherapy
Planned relative dose intensity > 80%
Preexisting neutropenia (absolute neutrophil count < 1,000 cells/µL)
Extensive prior chemotherapy

Patient related
Poor performance status (Eastern Cooperative Oncology Report [ECOG] > 2)
Poor nutritional status (eg, low albumin level)
Age > 65 years
Female gender
Decreased immune function

Cancer related
Bone marrow involvement with tumor
Elevated lactic dehydrogenase level (lymphoma)

Conditions associated with increased risk of serious infection
Open wounds
Active tissue infection

Comorbidities
Chronic obstructive pulmonary disease
Cardiovascular disease
Diabetes mellitus
Low baseline hemoglobin level
Liver disease (elevated levels of bilirubin, alkaline phosphatase)

Adapted from NCCN Myeloid Growth Factors in Cancer Treatment, v.1.2008 (www.nccn.com)

promising dose-dense approach warrants study in other settings. Outside this setting of dose-dense adjuvant chemotherapy, the study of dose density/intensity should be limited to clinical trials.

Meanwhile, in patients with potentially curable disease for which chemotherapy dose delivery may be critical, the use of CSF support to maintain dose intensity may be appropriate. In settings where dose is not a critical determinant of outcomes, modification of chemotherapy dose and implementation of reasonable supportive care measures remain sound alternatives.

Use following stem-cell transplantation

Autologous stem-cell and/or BMT High-dose chemotherapy with autologous hematopoietic stem-cell support has been used in the treatment of several malignancies, based on the notion that dose intensity may be an important determinant of response in chemosensitive malignancies. The prolonged period of myelosuppression following such cell-supported high-dose therapy, with its attendant increased risk of infectious and bleeding complications, has been deemed justifiable in such diseases as Hodgkin lymphoma, other lymphomas, multiple myeloma, high-risk or relapsed germ-cell cancers, and sarcomas, for which other less toxic therapeutic options yield suboptimal outcomes.

Several randomized trials have documented that CSFs can effectively reduce the duration of neutropenia, infectious complications, and hospitalization in patients who are receiving high-dose cytotoxic treatment with autologous BMT. GM-CSF was the first hematopoietic growth factor evaluated and approved for clinical use in this setting. G-CSF has subsequently been approved for this indication as well. Pegfilgrastim is under study.

Allogeneic BMT Similar beneficial effects of CSFs have been seen following allogeneic BMT, and the routine use of hematopoietic growth factors is appropriate in this setting. There has been no evidence of any increase in graft-versus-host disease, graft rejection, or relapse with the use of CSFs.

Delayed or inadequate neutrophil engraftment CSFs can also be useful in patients who have delayed or inadequate neutrophil engraftment following progenitor cell transplantation.

Mobilization of peripheral blood progenitor cells

CSFs have been used successfully to enhance mobilization of peripheral blood progenitor cells (PBPCs) into the peripheral blood. Available data suggest that mobilization of PBPCs may decrease the costs of harvesting cells and post-transplantation supportive care. Reinfusion of mobilized PBPCs following high-dose chemotherapy results in more rapid hematopoietic recovery than does autologous BMT. CSFs have also been utilized to mobilize donor PBPCs for allogeneic transplantation.

Administration of CSFs can enhance hematopoietic recovery following PBPC transplantation.

Use in myeloid malignancies

Acute myelogenous leukemia Since myeloid leukemia cells express receptors for CSFs, there has been a concern that leukemia cells might be stimulated after chemotherapy. However, given the high incidence of infectious complications following induction therapy for acute myelogenous leukemia (AML), especially in older patients, studies have evaluated CSFs in this setting. Data from several such studies demonstrate that CSFs, when given after the completion of induction chemotherapy, can shorten the duration of neutropenia and may reduce infectious complications. There does not appear to be any detrimental effect, on either response rate or regrowth of leukemia, by CSF administration following induction therapy.

GM-CSF has been approved for use in patients with AML (≥ 55 years old) following induction therapy to shorten the time to neutrophil recovery and to reduce severe, life-threatening infections. Clinical data on the use of CSFs in younger patients (< 55 years old) are currently limited. G-CSF has also proved to be effective in mitigating the myelotoxicity of leukemia therapy without increasing the risk of leukemic relapse or impairing response rates.

Myelodysplastic syndrome Patients with myelodysplastic syndrome (MDS) are prone to infections related to neutropenia and functional abnormalities of mature neutrophils. Although no data supporting the safety of long-term CSF use are available, short-term use of CSFs may be appropriate in severely neutropenic patients who experience recurrent infections. CSFs have not been shown to have a significant impact on clinical outcomes in patients with MDS or other marrow dysfunction states overall, perhaps reflecting abnormalities in the underlying stem-cell pool, which is unable to respond optimally to pharmacologic doses of CSFs.

Severe chronic neutropenia (ie, an ANC < 500 cells/µL) resulting from congenital, cyclic, or idiopathic neutropenia is often associated with recurrent infections. G-CSF is effective in normalizing neutrophil levels and significantly reducing the incidence of infections in > 90% of patients with these conditions.

TOXICITY

G-CSF (filgrastim and pegfilgrastim)

G-CSF has been a remarkably well-tolerated growth factor overall, based on extensive clinical experience with this cytokine over the past decade.

Bone pain The predominant side effect observed with the use of filgrastim and pegfilgrastim is mild to moderate bone pain, which typically occurs in the lower back, pelvis, or sternum in about one-third of patients. Bone pain is usually seen at the initiation of G-CSF therapy or at the very beginning of neutrophil recovery. In randomized studies, no difference in the incidence, severity, or duration of bone pain was noted between filgrastim and pegfilgrastim.

Uncommon side effects Other uncommon side effects include exacerbation of preexisting psoriasis, Sweet's syndrome (neutrophilic dermatitis), and cutaneous vasculitis. Chronic administration of G-CSF to patients with congenital or idiopathic neutropenia has been associated with splenomegaly.

Laboratory abnormalities observed with the rise in WBC count that occurs during G-CSF administration include elevations in serum lactic dehydrogenase (LDH), uric acid, and alkaline phosphatase levels. Finally, a modest decrease in platelet count without significant clinical sequelae has been reported occasionally with G-CSF use. Antibody formation to either preparation with resultant neutropenia has not been seen in large clinical trials.

GM-CSF

Yeast-derived GM-CSF is generally well tolerated at recommended doses. In the transplant setting, no excessive toxicity is seen in patients treated with this form of GM-CSF, as compared with controls.

Constitutional symptoms In phase I/II trials in other settings, the most commonly reported side effects of GM-CSF have included constitutional symptoms, such as fever, bone pain, myalgia, headaches, and chills. These side effects have been dose- and schedule-dependent and are seen more frequently when GM-CSF is administered at higher doses and by continuous IV infusion than when given at recommended doses by the SC route.

Uncommon side effects Other less frequently observed side effects of GM-CSF include diarrhea, anorexia, facial flushing, dyspnea, and edema. Other side effects that have been reported with *Escherichia coli*-derived GM-CSF, such as the first-dose phenomenon and capillary leak syndrome, have rarely been observed with sargramostim.

Laboratory abnormalities, such as elevation of LDH, uric acid, and alkaline phosphatase levels; decreases in serum cholesterol and albumin; and occasional thrombocytopenia, have been reported with GM-CSF.

DOSE, ROUTE, AND SCHEDULE OF ADMINISTRATION

Recommended doses The recommended dose of filgrastim (recombinant human G-CSF) is 5 µg/kg/d. This dose is clinically well tolerated and is effective in reducing the duration of neutropenia. The dose should begin 24 hours after chemotherapy and continue until the ANC is > 10,000 cells/µL. However, in clinical practice, dosing is commonly stopped when adequate neutrophil recovery has occurred.

G-CSF is used at a higher dose (10 µg/kg/d) for mobilization of progenitor cells and following BMT. Outside the context of stem-cell mobilization and transplantation, however, there are no data indicating that doses in excess of 5 µg/kg/d are indicated.

Pegfilgrastim is given as a fixed 6-mg dose. This dose has been shown to be effective regardless of age and weight in adults. It is given only once per cycle 24 hours after chemotherapy. For patients who develop febrile neutropenia after administration of pegfilgrastim, further dosing with daily filgrastim is not beneficial and is not recommended.

The recommended dose of sargramostim (yeast-derived GM-CSF) following autologous BMT is 250 µg/m^2/d given by a 2-hour IV infusion. In phase I/II studies in the chemotherapy setting, activity has been observed at doses ranging from 250 to 750 µg/m^2/d. In patients with MDS, neutrophil responses have been seen at much lower doses (30 to ≤ 250 µg/m^2/d).

Although recommended doses in patients receiving chemotherapy are 5 µg/kg/d for G-CSF and 250 µg/m^2/d for GM-CSF, rounding these doses to the nearest vial size is appropriate for cost savings and convenience. In patients with MDS, the dose can be titrated to the smallest effective level to avoid untoward side effects.

Route of administration The SC route is the preferred route of administering filgrastim, pegfilgrastim, and sargramostim, for convenience. However, IV infusion is an acceptable route for filgrastim and sargramostim, if clinically indicated.

Timing of administration To obtain the greatest benefit from CSFs, the appropriate timing of administration is 24 to 48 hours following the completion of chemotherapy. CSF therapy should be continued until neutrophil recovery is adequate. The discontinuation of CSF therapy after neutrophil recovery is sometimes followed by a decline in ANC, especially in patients with compromised bone marrow reserve. This fall in neutrophil count can be precipitous with G-CSF and appears to be somewhat less pronounced following discontinuation of GM-CSF. Therefore, blood counts should be checked before initiating the next cycle of chemotherapy.

Initiation of the next cycle of chemotherapy is not recommended for at least 24 hours after the completion of CSF therapy because of the potential concern that progenitor cells, which are rapidly dividing following CSF administration, may be sensitized to chemotherapy. Future trials should help to determine the optimal interval that should be allowed between CSF discontinuation and initiation of the next chemotherapy cycle. There remains some theoretic concern that serial exposure of cycling progenitor cells to chemotherapy may accelerate cumulative marrow damage.

Because of the same concern, concurrent administration of CSFs with chemotherapy or radiotherapy is not recommended outside the context of clinical trials. Same-day dosing of pegfilgrastim with chemotherapy has been studied in a variety of tumor types and regimens. To date, these trials have shown that pegfilgrastim is not as effective when administered concurrently with chemotherapy. Therefore, this dosing strategy is not recommended. Trials using GM-CSF concurrently with radiotherapy to the chest area have shown excessive hematologic toxicity, especially thrombocytopenia. It has been speculated that CSF-mobilized progenitor cells in the great vessels may be sensitized to radiation delivered to the chest.

EPO

EPO, an RBC lineage-specific glycoprotein hormone, was the first hematopoietic growth factor to become commercially available for clinical use in the United States. Recombinant human EPO has been approved for the treatment of anemia of chronic renal failure in predialysis or dialysis patients; anemia associated with zidovudine (Retrovir) therapy in patients infected with human immunodeficiency virus (HIV); anemia in cancer patients receiving chemotherapy in nonmyeloid malignancies; and anemia in patients scheduled for elective, noncardiac, nonvascular surgery. (See new safety information box earlier in chapter).

In 2001, darbepoetin alfa was approved by the FDA to allow a new option of treatment of anemia associated with chronic renal failure. Darbepoetin alfa is approved by the FDA for the treatment of chemotherapy-induced anemia in patients with nonmyeloid malignancies. Darbepoetin alfa is a hyperglycosylated molecule based on the protein backbone structure of human EPO. The increased level of glycosylation allows a longer duration of the drug in the circulation after administration (with an up to three times longer half-life than EPO).

CHEMOTHERAPY-INDUCED ANEMIA

The anemia caused by chemotherapy is due mainly to drug effects on bone marrow precursor cells and is proportional to chemotherapy dose intensity. In addition, with platinum agents, anemia may be related to renal effects of these drugs on the production of EPO. Based on these observations, multicenter trials in the United States and Europe have examined the efficacy of recombinant human EPO in correcting the anemia of cancer caused by chemotherapy.

DOSE AND SCHEDULE OF ADMINISTRATION

The original FDA-approved recommended initial dose of EPO in cancer patients is 150 units/kg SC 3 times a week. This dose can be increased to 300 units/kg 3 times weekly if an adequate response (ie, a decrease in transfusion requirements or a rise in hemoglobin value [≥ 1 g/dL]) does not occur after 4 weeks of therapy. However, very few oncologists use the thrice-weekly regimen of EPO dosing anymore. A more common practice, based on data from several clinical trials and the recently FDA-approved dose, is to administer EPO at a dose of 40,000 units SC *once weekly*, with an increase to 60,000 units once weekly if there is no adequate response after 4 weeks. This dose is well tolerated and appears to be equivalent in clinical effectiveness to three-times-weekly dosing while increasing patient convenience. EPO is approved by the FDA for once-weekly administration in the surgical population. A recent pharmacokinetic/pharmacodynamic study in healthy volunteers demonstrated that once-weekly EPO doses of 600 units/kg resulted in similar increases in hemoglobin value as did 150 units/kg 3 times weekly.

Darbepoetin alfa has a longer half-life than EPO and requires less frequent dosing. The current FDA-approved recommended initial dose of darbepoetin alfa in cancer patients is 2.25 µg/kg SC once a week or 500 µg once every 3 weeks. The weekly dose can be increased to 4.5 µg/kg once a week at 6 weeks if hemoglobin values increase less than 1 g/dL. No dose increase is recommended for the 500-µg-every-3-weeks regimen. Other commonly used dosing regimens of darbepoetin alfa are 200 µg every 2 weeks or 300 µg every 3 weeks, with an increase to 300 µg every 2 weeks at 6 weeks or 500 µg every 3 weeks, respectively, if hemoglobin values increase less than 1 g/dL. Additional dosing schedules have been studied (ie., loading doses, etc.) with both agents.

A patient who does not respond after 8 weeks of therapy (despite a dose increase) is unlikely to respond to higher doses, and erythropoietic therapy should be stopped. The dose of EPO/darbepoetin alfa should be reduced appropriately (25%–40%) if there is a rapid rise in hemoglobin value (ie, > 1 g/dL after 2 weeks) or if hemoglobin values are 12 g/dL or higher and should be titrated to maintain the desired hemogloblin value (10–12 g/dL). In patients treated with 500 µg every 3 weeks, once hemoglobin levels reach 11 g/dL, the dose should be reduced to 300 µg every 3 weeks. If response is suboptimal, the clinician should consider rechecking levels of nutritional cofactors (eg, iron, total iron-binding capacity, ferritin) or evaluate other reasons for lack of response (eg, underlying infection, inflammatory process, occult blood loss, other vitamin deficiencies). Patients (especially premenopausal women) may require supplemental iron to avoid depletion of marginal iron stores and to adequately support erythropoiesis stimulated by EPO. Recent data support the use of intravenous iron products for supplementation, as oral agents are relatively ineffective and often poorly tolerated.

EMERGING SAFETY ISSUES

Recent reports of four new studies in patients with cancer found a higher chance of serious and life-threatening side effects and/or death with the use of erythropoiesis-stimulating agents (ESAs). These research studies evaluated unapproved dosing regimens; a patient population for which ESAs are not approved (patients not receiving concurrent chemotherapy); had target hemoglobin levels up to 15.5 g/dL; or focused on a new, unapproved ESA. Based on these data, the FDA issued a black box warning and updated the package labeling on all ESA products. Further, the prescribing information has been revised to clarify the FDA-approved conditions for use of erythropoiesis-stimulating agents (ESAs) in patients with cancer and revised directions for dosing to state the hemoglobin level (≥ 10 g/dL) at which treatment with an ESA should not be initiated. The new label states that ESAs are not indicated for patients receiving myelosuppressive therapy when the anticipated outcome is cure. In addition, the Center for Medicare Services (CMS) issued further restrictions on the use of these agents in oncology patients with Medicare. For more information and the most up-to-date announcements regarding use of ESAs in patients with cancer, see the box on safety earlier in this chapter and go to **www.fda.gov/cder/drug/infopage/RHE/default.htm**.

Cytokines with thrombopoietic activity

Although G-CSF and GM-CSF have significantly reduced neutropenia in patients receiving chemotherapy, thrombocytopenia still remains a frequent dose-limiting toxicity of several chemotherapeutic regimens. Several hematopoietic cytokines with thrombopoietic activity have been evaluated in clinical trials. They include IL-1, IL-3, IL-6, IL-11, thrombopoietin (TPO), megakaryocyte growth and development factor (MGDF), and hybrid/synthetic cytokines, such as PIXY321 (a GM-CSF/IL-3 fusion protein) or SC71858 (promegapoietin, a synthetic cytokine comprising mutated versions of IL-3 and TPO).

Most of these cytokines have shown modest thrombopoietic activity and have the potential to induce nonspecific biologic activities, including some undesirable effects. To date, IL-11 is the only thrombopoietic cytokine that has received FDA approval for clinical use.

IL-11

IL-11 is a pleiotropic cytokine with thrombopoietic activity. In vitro, IL-11 acts synergistically with other hematopoietic growth factors, such as TPO, IL-3, and stem-cell factor (c-*kit* ligand), to promote the proliferation of hematopoietic progenitor cells and to induce maturation of megakaryocytes.

IL-11 was approved by the FDA to prevent severe thrombocytopenia and to reduce the need for platelet transfusions following myelosuppressive chemotherapy in patients with nonmyeloid malignancies who are at risk of severe thrombocytopenia based on the results of a randomized clinical trial of IL-11 in cancer patients who required at least one platelet transfusion after a chemotherapy cycle. In this trial, the use of IL-11 as secondary prophylaxis reduced the need for platelet transfusions in a subsequent cycle of chemotherapy.

However, it should be recognized that severe thrombocytopenia requiring platelet transfusions is an uncommon, acute problem with initiation of standard-dose chemotherapy. Nonetheless, thrombocytopenia can represent a cumulative problem with the many chemotherapeutic regimens often used to treat solid tumors, especially in patients with more heavily pretreated marrows.

Major bleeding is a rare complication related to chemotherapy-induced thrombocytopenia. Therefore, the appropriate use of thrombopoietic agents will require careful attention to several endpoints, including the need for platelet transfusions, ability to deliver chemotherapy without treatment-limiting thrombocytopenia, the safety profile of the thrombopoietic agent, and the associated health care costs.

Dose and schedule of administration The recommended dose of IL-11 for prophylaxis in adults is 50 μg/kg SC once daily. Therapy is started from 6 to 24 hours after the completion of chemotherapy and is continued until the postnadir platelet count is ≥ 50,000 cells/μL. Dosing beyond 21 days per treatment cycle is not recommended.

Adverse reactions Patients treated with IL-11 commonly experience mild to moderate fluid retention, as manifested by peripheral edema and/or dyspnea. In some patients, preexisting pleural effusions have increased during IL-11 administration. Therefore, patients with a history of pleural or pericardial effusions or ascites should be carefully monitored during IL-11 therapy. In addition, fluids and electrolytes should be monitored carefully in patients requiring the use of a diuretic.

Moderate decreases in hemoglobin values (thought to be related to dilutional anemia) have also been observed in patients receiving IL-11. The fluid retention and anemia are reversible within several days after IL-11 is discontinued.

IL-11 should be used with caution in patients with a history of cardiac arrhythmia, since palpitations, tachycardia, and atrial arrhythmia (atrial fibrillation or flutter) have been reported in some patients receiving this agent.

TPO

TPO is a lineage-dominant hematopoietic cytokine that regulates proliferation and maturation of cells of the megakaryocyte/platelet lineage. Preclinical studies have clearly shown that TPO cells are the key regulators of megakaryocyte mass and platelet production. Mice with induced genetic defects in TPO or its receptor, c-*mpl,* have > 90% loss of platelet production capacity.

The results of initial clinical trials of TPO are encouraging and suggest an important role for this agent in the treatment of cancer patients undergoing myelosuppressive treatment. No recombinant version of TPO has yet been approved by the FDA, showing the difficulty in developing thrombopoietic growth factors.

Development of TPO and related molecules has been complicated by the development of antibodies directed against some—but not all—of the recombinant human versions of this molecule. Clinical development of MGDF, a highly truncated recombinant version of TPO, was halted due to the occurrence of neutralizing antibodies directed against TPO. These potentially dangerous antibodies could prolong thrombocytopenia. However, similar antibodies have not been detected with the full-length version of recombinant human TPO. For that reason, further clinical trials of TPO continue. This promising agent does not produce the edema or other nonspecific side effects that occur with IL-11, and, thus, further data from larger trials of TPO are awaited.

SUGGESTED READING

Auerbach M, Ballard H, Trout JR, et al: Intravenous iron optimizes the response to recombinant human erythropoietin in cancer patients with chemotherapy-related anemia: A multicenter, open-label, randomized trial. J Clin Oncol 22:1301–1307, 2005.

Bennett CL, Luminari S, Nissenson AR, et al: Pure red-cell aplasia and epoetin therapy. N Engl J Med 351:1403–1408, 2004.

Citron ML, Berry DA, Cirrincione C, et al: Randomized trial of dose-dense versus conventionally scheduled and sequential versus concurrent combination chemotherapy as postoperative adjuvant treatment of node-positive primary breast cancer: First report of Intergroup Trial C9741/Cancer and Leukemia Group B trial 9741. J Clin Oncol 21:1431–1439, 2003.

Crawford J, Cella D, Cleeland CS, et al: Relationship between changes in hemoglobin level and quality of life during chemotherapy in anemic cancer patients receiving epoetin alfa therapy. Cancer 95:888–895, 2002.

Holmes FA, O'Shaughnessy JA, Vukelja S, et al: Blinded, randomized, multicenter study to evaluate single administration pegfilgrastim once per cycle versus daily filgrastim as an adjunct to chemotherapy in patients with high-risk stage II or stage III/IV breast cancer. J Clin Oncol 20:727–731, 2002.

Kuderer NM, Dale DC, Crawford J, et al: Impact of primary prophylaxis with granulocyte colony-stimulating factor on febrile neutropenia and mortality in adult cancer patients receiving chemotherapy: A systematic review. J Clin Oncol 25:3158–3167, 2007.

Rossert J, Casadevall N, Eckardt KU: Anti-erythropoietin antibodies and pure red cell aplasia. J Am Soc Nephrol 15:398–406, 2004.

Smith TJ, Khatcheressian J, Lyman GH, et al: 2006 update of recommendations for the use of white blood cell growth factors: An evidence-based clinical practice guideline. J Clin Oncol 24:3187–3205, 2006.

Vogel CL, Wojtukiewicz MZ, Carroll RR, et al: First and subsequent cycle use of pegfilgrastim prevents febrile neutropenia in patients with breast cancer: A multicenter, double-blind, placebo-controlled phase III study. J Clin Oncol 23:1178–1184, 2005.

CHAPTER 41

Fatigue and dyspnea

Sriram Yennurajalingam, MD, and Eduardo Bruera, MD

Fatigue and dyspnea are two of the most common symptoms associated with advanced cancer. Fatigue is also commonly associated with cancer treatment and occurs in up to 90% of patients undergoing chemotherapy. Both symptoms have many possible underlying causes. In most patients, the etiology of fatigue or dyspnea is multifactorial, with many contributing interrelated abnormalities. In one study of patients with advanced cancer, fatigue was found to be significantly correlated with the intensity of dyspnea. This chapter will discuss the mechanisms, clinical features, assessment, and management of both of these troublesome and often undertreated symptoms in cancer patients.

Fatigue

Cancer-related fatigue is defined by the National Comprehensive Cancer Network (NCCN) as "a distressing, persistent, subjective sense of tiredness or exhaustion related to cancer or cancer treatment that is not proportional to recent activity and interferes with usual functioning." In cancer patients, fatigue is often severe; has a marked anticipatory component; and results in lack of energy, malaise, lethargy, and diminished mental functioning that profoundly impairs quality of life. It may be present early in the course of the illness, may be exacerbated by treatments, and is present in almost all patients with advanced cancer.

Fatigue is sometimes referred to as asthenia, tiredness, lack of energy, weakness, and exhaustion. Not all these terms have the same meaning to all patient populations. Moreover, different studies of fatigue and asthenia have looked at different outcomes, ranging from physical performance to the purely subjective sensation.

MECHANISM

The mechanisms of cancer-related fatigue are not well understood. Substances produced by the tumor are postulated to induce fatigue. Blood from a fatigued subject when injected into a rested subject has produced manifestations of fatigue. The host production of cytokines in response to the tumor can also have a direct fatigue-inducing effect. Muscular or neuromuscular junction abnormalities are a possible cause of chemotherapy- or radiotherapy-induced fatigue. In summary, fatigue is the result of many syndromes—not just one. Multiple mechanisms are involved in causing fatigue in most patients with advanced cancer.

CLINICAL FEATURES

The causes of fatigue in an individual patient are often multiple with many interrelated factors. Figure 1 summarizes the main contributors to fatigue in cancer patients.

Cachexia Cancer cachexia results from a complex interaction of host and tumor products. Host cytokines such as tumor necrosis factor, interleukin-1 (IL-1), and IL-6 are capable of causing decreased food intake, loss of body weight, a decrease in synthesis of both lipids and proteins, and increased lipolysis. Tumors are also capable of producing lipolytic factors (lipolytic factor, toxohormone L-2) and proteolytic by-products (proteolysis-inducing factor). The metabolic abnormalities involved in the production of cachexia and the loss of muscle mass resulting from progressive cachexia may cause profound weakness and fatigue. However, many abnormalities described in Figure 1 are capable of causing profound fatigue in the absence of significant weight loss.

Immobility has been shown to cause deconditioning and decreased endurance to both exercise and normal activities of daily living. On the other hand, over-exertion is a frequent cause of fatigue in noncancer patients. It should also be considered in younger cancer patients who are undergoing aggressive antine-oplastic treatments such as radiation therapy and chemotherapy and who are nevertheless trying to maintain their social and professional activities.

Psychological distress In patients without cancer who present with fatigue, the final diagnosis is psychological in almost 75% of patients (depression, anxiety, and other psychological disorders). The frequency of major psychiatric disorders in cancer patients is low. However, symptoms of psychological distress or adjustment disorders with depressive or anxious moods are much more frequent. Patients with an adjustment disorder or a major depressive disorder can have fatigue as their most prevalent symptom.

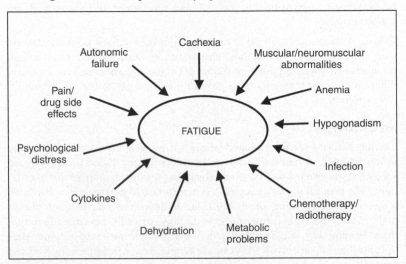

FIGURE 1: Contributors to fatigue in cancer patients

Anemia related to advanced cancer or chemotherapy has been associated with fatigue, and its treatment results in improvement of fatigue and quality of life in these patients. In terminally ill patients with advanced cancer, treatment of anemia may not resolve the symptom adequately due to the multifactorial nature of the etiology of fatigue. It may be the result of the more intense nature of the other contributory factors.

Autonomic failure Autonomic insufficiency is a frequent complication of advanced cancer. Autonomic failure has also been documented in patients with a subset of severe chronic fatigue syndrome. Although the association between fatigue and autonomic dysfunction has not been established in cancer patients, it should be suspected in patients with severe postural hypotension or other signs of autonomic failure.

Hypogonadism Research has shown that both intrathecal and systemic opioid therapies, as well as cachexia and some antineoplastic therapies, can result in hypogonadotropic hypogonadism. This condition can lead to fatigue, depression, and reduced libido.

Chemotherapy These treatments are common causes of fatigue in cancer patients. Chemotherapy and radiotherapy for malignancy cause a specific fatigue syndrome. Combined therapy with the two modalities appears to cause worse fatigue than either modality given alone. The pattern of fatigue reported by patients with cancer who receive myelosuppressive chemotherapy is cyclical. It begins within the first few days after therapy is started, peaks around the time of the white blood cell nadir, and diminishes in the week thereafter, only to recur again with the next cycle of chemotherapy. Fatigue tends to worsen with subsequent cycles of chemotherapy, which suggests a cumulative dose-related toxic effect. Compared with women with no history of cancer, former patients with breast cancer who had received adjuvant chemotherapy reported more fatigue and worse quality of life due to this symptom. Similar results have been noted in breast cancer patients who have been treated with high-dose chemotherapy and autologous stem-cell support and in patients treated for lymphoma.

Radiotherapy Radiation therapy tends to cause a different pattern of fatigue. It is often described as a "wave" that starts abruptly within a few hours after treatment and subsides shortly thereafter. Fatigue has been noted to decrease in the first 2 weeks after localized treatment for breast cancer but then to increase as radiation therapy persists into week 4. It then decreases again 3 weeks after radiation therapy ceases. The mechanism for fatigue in these situations is not well understood.

Surgery is another common cause of fatigue in patients with cancer. In addition, commonly used medications such as opioids and hypnotics may cause sedation and fatigue.

Other Comorbid conditions not necessarily related to cancer, such as renal failure or congestive heart failure, may coexist and contribute to the problem. Other conditions include the chronic stress response (possibly mediated through hypothalamic-pituitary axis), disrupted sleep or circadian rhythms, and

TABLE 1: Assessment of fatigue

Functional capacity
> Treadmill performance (time, speed)
> Number of errors (eg, driving, pilots)

Task-related fatigue (eg, treadmill, driving)
> VAS (visual analog scales), numerical scale
> Pearson and Byars Fatigue Feeling Checklist

Performance status
> ECOG (Eastern Cooperative Oncology Group)
> Karnofsky performance status
> Edmonton Functional Assessment Tool (EFAT)

Subjective assessment of fatigue
> VAS, numerical scale
> Brief Fatigue Inventory
> Piper Fatigue Self-Report Scale

hormonal changes (eg, premature menopause and androgen blockade secondary to cancer treatment).

ASSESSMENT

Since fatigue is essentially a subjective sensation, it is by nature difficult to assess. There is agreement that self-assessment should be the "gold standard." Due to the complex nature of the symptoms of fatigue, an effort to identify a set of diagnostic criteria similar to those for depression has been attempted. This syndromal approach has been useful to assess the presence or absence of the clinical syndrome of fatigue.

Table 1 summarizes the four most common measurable indices to assess fatigue. The first category in Table 1 looks at the objective function that the patient is capable of performing when subjected to a standard task. These functional tasks have limited value in cancer care, however, as they are very difficult for the advanced cancer patient to perform.

The second category in Table 1 attempts to assess the subjective effects of standard tasks.

The third category in Table 1 has been the most commonly used in oncology. The two most common scales (ECOG [Eastern Cooperative Oncology Group] and Karnofsky performance status) consist of a physician's rating of the patient's functional capabilities after a regular medical consultation. A physiotherapist performs the Edmonton Functional Assessment Tool and attempts to determine the functional status, as well as all the obstacles to clinical performance in these patients.

FIGURE 2: Therapeutic approach to managing fatigue

The fourth category in Table 1 is the most relevant for both clinical management and clinical trials in fatigue. Visual analog scales (VAS), numerical scales, the Brief Fatigue Inventory, and the Piper Fatigue Self-Report Scale have been validated. In addition, there are validated functional assessments in most quality-of-life questionnaires.

In addition to the assessment of the intensity of fatigue, the clinical assessment of these patients requires clinicians to determine the impact of all factors on the presence of fatigue.

MANAGEMENT

To treat fatigue optimally, it is vital to identify and prioritize the different underlying factors in each individual patient. A thorough history, including recent treatment history, physical examination, and medication review, in addition to simple laboratory investigations will help identify possible underlying causes. Figure 2 outlines a therapeutic approach to fatigue management in cancer patients. Whenever possible, an attempt should be made to treat these contributing factors. It is impossible to be certain whether one of these identified problems is a major contributor to fatigue or is simply a coexisting problem in a given patient. Therefore, it is of great importance to measure the intensity of fatigue and the patient's performance before and after treating any contributing factor. If the level of fatigue does not improve after correction of these abnormalities, it is clear then that further treatment will not result in improvement in the future.

In patients with cancer treatment-related fatigue, it is important to exclude specific causes, such as hypothyroidism, hypogonadism, and anemia, and to consider other potential adverse effects of treatment. If specific problems are identified, they should be appropriately managed. For instance, patients with anemia may experience symptomatic improvement with the administration of erythropoietic therapy (epoetin alfa [Epogen, Procrit] and darbepoetin alfa [Aranesp]) at the dose and frequency interval that best fit the patient's need. Epoetin alfa may be administered weekly by subcutaneous injection; darbepoetin alfa has a longer half-life, requiring less frequent dosing. Dosages and schedules of both agents may be increased if necessary. (See section on "Dose and schedule of administration" in chapter 40 for specific information about dosages and schedules.)

In most patients, there will be no identified reversible causes. A number of effective pharmacologic and nonpharmacologic symptomatic treatments are available for these patients.

Pharmacologic treatments

Corticosteroids There is substantial evidence that corticosteroids can reduce fatigue and other symptoms in cancer patients. They are probably best retained for short-term use. Their beneficial effects generally last between 2 and 4 weeks, and longer term use carries the risk of serious adverse effects. Most studies have used the equivalent of 40 mg/d of prednisone.

Progestational agents In recent studies of terminally ill patients, megestrol (60–480 mg/d) has been shown to have a rapid (less than 1 week) beneficial effect on appetite, fatigue, and general well-being.

Psychostimulants Psychostimulants (eg, methylphenidate, 5–10 mg in the morning and at noon or 5 mg as needed) may be of use in treating fatigue in patients with advanced cancer. The safety and efficacy of long-term use of methylphenidate for fatigue have not been established.

A National Cancer Institute-sponsored trial on the use of modafinil (Provigil) for treatment of cancer-related fatigue is under way. In addition, dexmethylphenidate (D-MPH, Focalin) has been found to be more effective than placebo in the treatment of fatigue and impaired memory after chemotherapy in adults with cancer in a randomized phase III trial.

In addition to these agents, a number of other drugs have been tried in preliminary studies in patients with fatigue. Early positive results have been observed with both thalidomide (Thalomid) and fish oils. In addition, there are donezepil for fatigue associated with opioid sedation and midodrine (ProAmatine) in cases of autonomic failure.

In a recent double-blind, randomized controlled trial by the North Central Cancer Treatment Group (NCCTG), 282 patients with cancer reported improvement of cancer- related fatigue on treatment with American ginseng (*Panax quinquefolius*) versus placebo.

In a randomized controlled study of 142 patients with advanced cancer conducted by Bruera et al, donepezil was not significantly superior to placebo in the treatment of cancer-related fatigue.

Nonpharmacologic treatment

Physiotherapy and occupational therapy Physiotherapy may encourage increased activity where appropriate and provide active range of motion to prevent painful tendon retraction. Recent evidence suggests that aerobic exercise may reduce fatigue during chemotherapy. Assessment of the home environment by

FIGURE 3: Mechanisms of dyspnea

an occupational therapist can be useful. The provision of ramps, walkers, wheelchairs, elevated toilets, and hospital beds may allow the patient to remain at home in a safe environment. Education regarding the pattern of fatigue during treatment has been helpful. Counseling for stress management, depression, and anxiety may reduce distress and fatigue as well as improve mood.

Dyspnea

Dyspnea has been defined as an uncomfortable awareness of breathing. It is a subjective sensation and does not necessarily correlate with clinical findings in a given patient. It occurs in up to 75% of patients with advanced cancer, and good symptom control is less frequently achieved, even by experienced palliative care teams, than with other symptoms of terminal cancer such as pain or nausea.

MECHANISMS

The pathophysiology of dyspnea is complex and has not been completely elucidated. The respiratory center in the medulla controls breathing, but dyspnea is the result of cortical stimulation. Abnormalities of blood gases detected by both lung and central chemoreceptors and stimulation of lung and respiratory muscle mechanoreceptors stimulate the respiratory center. Mechanoreceptors respond to stretch and irritants and also have a demonstrated effect on the brain cortex, causing dyspnea. In addition, it is possible that both the chemoreceptors and the medullary respiratory center stimulate the cerebral cortex, directly contributing to the sensation of dyspnea. Figure 3 summarizes the mechanisms of dyspnea.

TABLE 2: Management of specific causes of dyspnea in cancer patients

Cause	Treatment
Airway obstruction by tumor	Corticosteroids (eg, dexamethasone 6-8 mg qid), radiation therapy
Pleural or pericardial effusion	Drain if effusion is significant
Pneumonia	Antibiotics (oral route preferred)
Carcinomatous lymphangitis	Corticosteroids (eg, dexamethasone 6-8 mg qid)
Congestive heart failure	Diuretic therapy (eg, furosemide 10-20 mg IV/SC) and angiotensin-converting enzyme (ACE) inhibitors
Underlying asthma, COPD	Optimize bronchodilators, corticosteroids if required
Anemia	Transfuse packed red blood cells, erythropoietic therapy

COPD = chronic obstructive pulmonary disease, IV = intravenous; SC = subcutaneous

CLINICAL FEATURES

There are many causes of dyspnea in patients with advanced cancer, such as pulmonary embolism, lung metastasis, pleural effusion, congestive heart failure, anemia, psychological distress, pneumonia, muscle weakness, and preexisting pulmonary disease.

Direct tumor effects Dyspnea may be the result of direct primary or metastatic tumor effects such as airway obstruction, atelectasis, parenchymal lung involvement, phrenic nerve palsy, carcinomatous lymphangitis, or superior vena caval obstruction.

Indirect tumor effects Indirect cancer effects include pneumonia, anemia, pleural effusion, and pulmonary embolism. Cardiac complications of cancer such as congestive heart failure, pericarditis, or pericardial effusion may contribute to the problem. Intra-abdominal disorders such as gross ascites or hepatomegaly may cause elevation of the diaphragm and may interfere with respiratory function. Generalized muscle weakness due to cachexia or fatigue may exacerbate breathlessness. Preexisting lung diseases including asthma or chronic obstructive pulmonary disease (COPD) may contribute to the problem.

Treatment side effects Contributing treatment side effects include pneumonitis or fibrosis following chemotherapy or radiotherapy.

Psychological conditions Anxiety, depression, or somatization will alter a patient's perception of dyspnea. Anxiety has been found to be an independent correlate with the intensity of dyspnea in cancer patients with moderate to severe dyspnea. Any of these factors may occur in isolation or in combination, and care is needed during assessment, as there are often many contributors in an individual patient.

ASSESSMENT

Dyspnea is a subjective sensation, and researchers have found much variability in the expression of dyspnea in individuals with similar levels of functional abnormalities. In addition, patients' perception of dyspnea can be influenced by their beliefs and intrapsychic and cultural factors. The presence or absence of physical signs such as tachypnea, wheezing, or use of accessory muscles is not a reliable indicator of the degree of distress felt by patients. The intensity of dyspnea can be easily assessed using verbal, numeric, or visual analog scales similar to those used in pain or nausea. A descriptive study by Henoch et al examined dyspnea in correlation with other symptoms, as well as personal and health factors in 105 patients with advanced lung cancer. More than 50% of patients had perceived dyspnea. The intensity of dyspnea and the occurrence of activity-related dyspnea correlated with the presence of anxiety, depression, fatigue, and cough. A lower coping capacity was associated with a greater likelihood of dyspnea.

Recently, maximal inspiratory pressure has been found to be an independent correlate of the intensity of dyspnea. Physical examination, chest x-ray, and pulse oximetry should be performed. Other investigations such as complete blood count, echocardiography, or pulmonary function tests may be indicated.

MANAGEMENT

Specific causes

Underlying specific causes will require treatment as indicated in Table 2.

Symptomatic management

The three modalities of symptomatic treatment in cancer-related dyspnea are oxygen therapy, drug therapy, and counseling.

Oxygen therapy In hypoxemic cancer patients with dyspnea, oxygen has been shown to provide significant symptomatic relief. Oxygen can be administered by nasal cannula at 2–6 L/min or by mask and titrated to maintain an O_2 saturation at > 90%. Care must be taken in patients with COPD. Oxygen is not useful in patients with dyspnea and an O_2 saturation > 90%.

Drug therapy There is substantial evidence that systemic opioids have a beneficial effect on cancer-related dyspnea. This is possible without inducing respiratory depression. The optimal type, dose, and mode of administration have not been determined. If the patient is already on opioids, the breakthrough dose can be used to manage dyspnea as well as pain. If not, morphine can be started at 5–10 mg PO (or 2.5–5.0 mg SC) q4h with additional prn doses of 2.5–5.0 mg PO (or 2.5 mg SC) every hour for breakthrough dyspnea. Nebulized opiates are not recommended, as there is insufficient evidence to support their use.

Benzodiazepines have not been found to be effective in the general management of dyspnea, but they may be useful for treatment of episodes associated with anxiety attacks. Regular use of benzodiazepines should be avoided where possible to limit side effects such as confusion or falls.

A number of conditions that cause dyspnea in cancer patients respond to corticosteroid medication, including superior vena caval obstruction, carcinomatous lymphangitis, and COPD. However, corticosteroids may adversely affect muscle function, and the diaphragm may be more susceptible than other muscles. This may be of importance because of the frequency of muscle weakness and fatigue in patients with advanced cancer.

Counseling Dyspnea is a variable symptom and is exacerbated by physical activities. Patients and families should be educated so they can identify factors likely to worsen dyspnea. Devices such as bathroom aids and wheelchairs can help reduce physical activity, and the addition of portable oxygen can enable the patient to remain active and autonomous. Medication used for symptomatic relief such as opioids can be administered 30–45 minutes prior to dyspnea-causing maneuvers. The family should be educated that dyspnea is subjective and that tachypnea and use of accessory muscles do not necessarily indicate that the patient is suffering. The aim of treatment is to relieve the patient's subjective dyspnea, not to abate physical signs of respiratory distress.

SUGGESTED READING

ON FATIGUE

Bruera E, Driver L, Barnes EA, et al: Patient-controlled methylphenidate for the management of fatigue in patients with advanced cancer: A preliminary report. J Clin Oncol 21:4439–4443, 2003.

Bruera E, El Osta B, Valero V, et al: Donepezil for cancer fatigue: A double-blind, randomized, placebo-controlled trial. J Clin Oncol. 25:3475–3481, 2007

Bruera E, Strasser F, Shen L, et al: The effect of donezepil on sedation and other symptoms in patients receiving opioids for cancer pain: A pilot study. J Pain Symptom Manage 26:1049–1054, 2003.

Cleary J: The reversible causes of asthenia in cancer patients, in Portenoy R, Bruera E (eds): Topics in Palliative Care, vol 2, pp 183–202. New York, Oxford University Press, 1998.

Dimeo F, Stieglitz R, Novelli-Fischer U, et al: Effects of physical activity on the fatigue and psychological status of cancer patients during chemotherapy. Cancer 85:2273–2277, 1999.

Hann DM, Garovoy N, Finkelstein B, et al: Fatigue and quality of life in breast cancer patients undergoing autologous stem-cell transplantation: A longitudinal comparative study. J Pain Symptom Manage 17:311–319, 1999.

Henoch I, Bergman B, Gustafsson M, et al: Dyspnea experience in patients with lung cancer in palliative care. Eur J Oncol Nurs. 2007 Nov 16 [Epub ahead of print].

Howell SJ, Radford JA, Adams JE, et al: Randomized placebo-controlled trial of testosterone replacement in men with mild Leydig cell insufficiency following cytotoxic chemotherapy. Clin Endocrinol 55:315–324, 2001.

Munch TN, Zhang T, Willey J, et al: The association between anemia and fatigue in patients with advanced cancer receiving palliative care. J Palliat Med 8:1144–1149, 2005.

Neuenschwander H, Bruera E: Pathophysiology of cancer asthenia, in Portenoy R, Bruera E (eds): Topics in Palliative Care, vol 2, pp 171–181. New York, Oxford University Press, 1998.

Reddy S, Elsayem A, Palmer L, et al: The characteristics and correlates of dyspnea in advanced cancer patients [abstract]. J Clin Oncol 23(suppl):733s, 2005.

Sadler IJ, Jacobsen PB, Booth-Jones M, et al: Preliminary evaluation of a clinical syndrome approach to assessing cancer-related fatigue. J Pain Symptom Manage 23:406–416, 2002.

Seidenfeld J, Piper M, Flamm C, et al: Epoetin treatment of anemia associated with cancer therapy: A systematic review and meta-analysis of controlled clinical trials. J Natl Cancer Inst 93:1204–1214, 2001.

ON DYSPNEA

Allard P, Lamontagne C, Bernard P, et al: How effective are supplementary doses of opioids for dyspnea in terminally ill cancer patients? A randomized continuous sequential clinical trial. J Pain Symptom Manage 17:256–265, 1999.

Bruera E, Schmitz B, Pither J, et al: The frequency and correlates of dyspnea in patients with advanced cancer. J Pain Symptom Manage 19:357–362, 2000.

Mancini I, Body JJ: Assessment of dyspnea in advanced cancer patients. Support Care Cancer 7:229–232, 1999.

Ripamonti C, Fulfaro F, Bruera E: Dyspnea in patients with advanced cancer: Incidence, causes, and treatments. Cancer Treat Rev 42:60–80, 1998.

CHAPTER 42

Anorexia and cachexia

Charles Loprinzi, MD, and Aminah Jatoi, MD

Many patients with advanced cancer undergo a wasting syndrome associated with cancer anorexia/cachexia and asthenia. In a study that looked at symptoms in cancer patients being entered on a palliative care service, anorexia/cachexia and asthenia were more common problems than were pain or dyspnea. Patients who exhibit such symptoms generally have a short survival, respond poorly to cytotoxic agents, and suffer from increased toxicity from these agents.

In addition, cancer anorexia/cachexia is oftentimes associated with weakness, fatigue, and a poor quality of life. This problem not only affects the patient but also frequently has an impact on family members, as the patient is no longer able to participate fully in eating as a social activity.

Diagnostic criteria

Although some authors have tried to define criteria for diagnosing cancer cachexia, in general, it is not difficult to identify affected patients. In North Central Cancer Treatment Group (NCCTG) research trials involving more than 2,500 patients, simple criteria for anorexia/cachexia have been used:

- a 5-lb weight loss in the preceding 2 months and/or an estimated daily caloric intake of < 20 calories/kg
- a desire by the patient to increase his or her appetite and gain weight
- the physician's opinion that weight gain would be beneficial for the patient.

Management

Nutritional counseling

Nutritional counseling, as provided by written materials, dietitians, physicians, and nurses, has been recommended, although its value has not been well demonstrated. Recommendations typically include eating frequent, small meals (as opposed to large meals), consuming larger quantities of food in the morning than in the evening, and avoiding spicy foods. Patients may do better if they are not exposed to the aroma of cooking. Although the benefits of such nutritional counseling are clearly limited, it does appear reasonable to provide.

Recent trials have led to further interest in studying dietary counseling. Ravasco and others observed improvements in treatment-related side effects and qual-

A recent placebo-controlled trial from the North Central Cancer Treatment Group showed that etanercept, a tumor necrosis factor alpha inhibitor, did not appear to be effective in the treatment of the cancer anorexia/weight loss syndrome (Jatoi A, Dakhil SR, Nguyen PL, et al: Cancer 110:1396-1403, 2007).

ity of life among colorectal cancer patients who had received dietary counseling as part of a randomized controlled trial. Similar findings from this same group were observed among head and neck cancer patients. These findings require confirmation.

Appetite stimulants

Corticosteroids were the first agents to undergo placebo-controlled, double-blind evaluation for possible use in cancer cachexia. The first such trial, conducted in the 1970s by Moertel and colleagues at the Mayo Clinic, demonstrated that corticosteroids can stimulate appetite in patients with advanced, incurable cancer. Several subsequent placebo-controlled trials, using various steroid preparations and doses, have confirmed these results.

Dexamethasone (3 to 8 mg/d) is a reasonable option for clinical use. Known detriments to corticosteroid use include the well-known toxicities associated with chronic administration, including myopathy, peptic ulcer disease, infection, and adrenal suppression. Many patients with advanced cancer anorexia and cachexia, however, do not survive long enough to suffer from these toxicities.

Progestational agents Several placebo-controlled, double-blind clinical trials have demonstrated that progestational agents, such as megestrol and medroxyprogesterone, can lead to appetite stimulation and weight gain in patients with anorexia and cachexia. These trials also demonstrated that the effect of these drugs is seen in a matter of days and that they are effective antiemetics.

Although high doses of progestational agents can cause adrenal suppression because of their mild corticosteroid-type activity (a phenomenon not well understood by many clinicians), they do not appear to cause many of the side effects attributable to classic corticosteroids (such as peptic ulcer disease, myopathy, and opportunistic infections). In lieu of this adrenal suppression, however, stress doses of corticosteroids may be necessary in patients with trauma or infection or in surgical patients while on progestational agents. On the other hand, progestational agents increase the risk of thromboembolic phenomena–a side effect that is not seen with classic corticosteroids.

A dose-response study with megestrol demonstrated a positive correlation between appetite stimulation and increased megestrol doses, as doses ranged from 160 to 800 mg/d. Nonetheless, given that appetite stimulation has been demonstrated with megestrol acetate doses as low as 240 mg/d, much lower doses are used by many physicians, based primarily on cost considerations.

In the United States, a liquid formulation of megestrol is considerably less expensive than the tablet form, and, milligram for milligram, the liquid preparation is more bioavailable. It is reasonable to start with 400 mg/d of liquid megestrol, titrating this dose upward (maximum, 800 mg/d) or downward based

ANOREXIA

on clinical response or the emergence of side effects.

A randomized, prospective clinical trial comparing the utility of megestrol (800 mg/d) with dexamethasone (0.75 mg qid) demonstrated similar effects of these medications on patients' appetites but different toxicity profiles. Whereas megestrol was associated with a higher incidence of thromboembolic phenomena, dexamethasone was associated with more myopathy, cushingoid body changes, and peptic ulcers.

Other agents Various other drugs have been evaluated definitively for the treatment of cancer anorexia and cachexia and have demonstrated little or no benefit. These drugs include fluoxymesterone (Halotestin), pentoxifylline, hydrazine sulfate, dronabinol (Marinol), cyproheptadine, and eicosapentaenoic acid (EPA). Of note, however, the antiserotonergic drug cyproheptadine does appear to be a relatively strong appetite stimulant in patients with the carcinoid syndrome, presumably because it directly counteracts the large amounts of serotonin secreted in these patients.

EPA has been tested extensively for cancer anorexia and cachexia. Although preliminary studies had claimed improvement in appetite, body composition, and survival with EPA, these favorable findings have not been borne out in subsequent phase III trials. A total of three recently completed phase III trials have shown that EPA does relatively little for cancer anorexia and cachexia when tested in the setting of either EPA versus placebo or EPA versus megestrol.

A number of other drugs have been evaluated in a pilot fashion for the treatment of cancer anorexia and cachexia. They include branched-chain amino acids, thalidomide (Thalomid), metoclopramide, oxandrolone (Oxandrin), and adenosine triphosphate. It is hoped that new information will be available in the near future to shed light on the possible therapeutic roles of these agents.

Enteral or parenteral nutrition

Despite the demonstrated efficacy of corticosteroids and progestational agents in patients with cancer anorexia and cachexia, these drugs do not have a major long-term impact on the vast majority of such patients. Consequently, other treatment approaches, such as enteral or parenteral nutritional methods, have been studied extensively. Several randomized trials failed to demonstrate that these nutritional approaches improve either quantity or quality of life. As a result, experts generally agree that the routine use of parenteral or enteral nutrition cannot be justified in patients with advanced cancer anorexia and cachexia.

There are, however, relatively rare circumstances in which parenteral nutrition may play a role in patients with advanced cancer. Such circumstances have been documented by case reports and small case series of patients and have included patients with GI insufficiency due to surgery, radiation therapy, or abdominal carcinomatosis (without impending failure of other organs). The decision to initiate parenteral nutrition under these circumstances typically requires a multidisciplinary approach with extensive discussions between healthcare providers and family members.

Prophylactic therapy

Given the positive impact of corticosteroids and progestational agents on cancer anorexia and cachexia and the fact that many patients with advanced cancer die with, and/or of, inanition, the potential prophylactic use of these agents was evaluated. A double-blind trial was conducted in which patients with newly diagnosed extensive-stage small-cell lung cancer were randomized to receive megestrol or placebo along with standard chemoradiation therapy. This trial was unable to demonstrate any beneficial effect of megestrol on treatment response, quality of life, or survival.

Thus, patients should not be treated prophylactically for cancer anorexia and cachexia outside a clinical trial. Rather, such treatment should be reserved for patients in whom anorexia and cachexia are patient-determined, symptomatic clinical problems.

Nutrition as it relates to end-of-life care

Anorexia and cachexia are major problems for many oncology patients as they approach the final stage of life. Family members are generally more distressed than the patients if/when appetite stimulants do not provide relief. Questions commonly arise about giving enteral or parenteral nutrition or "forcing" patients to consume more calories in the belief that they would feel better, get stronger, and live longer. A small measure of appropriate education, noting that the intake of more calories does not appear to have a clinical benefit, provides substantial relief. It is worthwhile to note that patients randomized to receive total parenteral nutrition or appetite stimulants (such as megestrol) do not live any longer than do control patients and that "force-feeding" is not in the patients' best interests.

SUGGESTED READING

Jatoi A, Dakhil SR, Nguyen PL, et al: A placebo-controlled double blind trial of etanercept for the cancer anorexia/weight loss syndrome: Results from N00C1 from the North Central Cancer Treatment Group. Cancer 110:1396–1403, 2007.

Jatoi A, Rowland K, Loprinzi CL, et al: An eicosapentaenoic acid supplement versus megestrol acetate versus both for patients with cancer-associated wasting: A North Central Cancer Treatment Group and National Cancer Institute of Canada collaborative effort. J Clin Oncol 22:2469–2476, 2004.

Jatoi A, Windschitl HE, Loprinzi CL, et al: Dronabinol vs megestrol acetate vs both for cancer-associated anorexia: A North Central Cancer Treatment Group Study. J Clin Oncol 20:567–573, 2002.

Loprinzi CL, Kugler JW, Sloan JA, et al: Randomized comparison of megestrol acetate versus dexamethasone versus fluoxymesterone for the treatment of cancer anorexia/cachexia. J Clin Oncol 17:3299–3306, 1999.

Mann M, Koller E, Murgo A, et al: Glucocorticoid-like activity of megestrol. Arch Intern Med 157:1651–1656, 1997.

Moertel CG, Schutt AJ, Reitemeier RJ, et al: Corticosteroid therapy of preterminal gastrointestinal cancer. Cancer 33:1607–1609, 1974.

Ravasco P, Monteiro-Grillo I, Marques Vidal P, et al: Impact of nutrition on outcome: A prospective randomized controlled trial in patients with head and neck cancer undergoing radiotherapy. Head Neck 27:659–668, 2005.

Ravasco P, Monteiro-Grillo I, Vidal PM, et al: Dietary counseling improves patient outcomes: A prospective, randomized controlled trial in colorectal cancer patients undergoing radiotherapy. J Clin Oncol 23:1431–1438, 2005.

Rock CL: Dietary counseling is beneficial for the patient with cancer. J Clin Oncol 23:1348–1349, 2005.

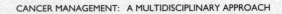

CHAPTER 43

Long-term venous access

Stephen P. Povoski, MD

The use of multidrug chemotherapy and bone marrow transplantation in cancer treatment has made the utilization of reliable, long-term venous access (LTVA) an essential component of cancer therapy. The placement of LTVA devices not only permits the delivery of these complex therapeutic regimens but also drastically improves patients' quality of life.

Indications

No definitive guidelines are available for utilization of central venous access. There are several important factors to consider when deciding upon LTVA device placement:

- the frequency and duration of therapy
- the frequency of blood draws
- the nature of therapy (eg, delivering vesicating agents into a central vein decreases the risk of extravasation)
- the need for supportive therapies (eg, total parenteral nutrition or systemic antibiotics)
- the need for stem-cell collection, plasmapheresis, and bone marrow reinfusion
- patient preference.

Patient selection

LTVA should always be considered an elective procedure. Therefore, before an LTVA device is placed, the patient should have recovered from acute infections and the treatment of complications. If there is an absolute need for immediate central venous access before such times, a temporary percutaneous central venous access catheter can be placed. A history of vascular access catheter insertion, deep venous thrombosis of an upper extremity or central vein, thoracic surgery, neck surgery, irradiation, or mediastinal and thoracic disease should alert the surgeon to possible changes in normal venous drainage. Always assess and correct the volume status of the patient (if possible) before attempting the elective placement of an LTVA device.

Physical examination, documenting the integrity of the skin, changes in the skin secondary to previous surgical treatment and reconstruction, sites of previous central venous access catheter insertions, evidence of venous obstruction (presence of venous collaterals in the skin of the chest, unilateral arm swelling, or superior vena cava syndrome), and pulmonary reserve, should be performed in every patient. If there is any evidence of venous obstruction or a history of multiple central venous access catheters, the physical examination should be complemented with a formal venous imaging study.

Duplex Doppler ultrasonography can visualize the patency and flow of the neck and arm veins. Intrathoracic veins and the right atrium are not well visualized by duplex Doppler ultrasonography but are better visualized with transesophageal echocardiography. This can be utilized preoperatively or intraoperatively.

CT and MRI are useful for documenting the presence of thrombosis and the patency of major intrathoracic veins.

Venography is still the gold standard for studying venous anatomy. Venography should be performed whenever the clinical situation warrants it and noninvasive venous imaging studies fail to provide a definitive diagnosis. This can be utilized preoperatively or intraoperatively.

Chest radiography can disclose important information (such as the presence of pleural effusions, lung metastases, mediastinal adenopathy, and mediastinal tumors) that can modify selection of a site for LTVA placement.

Contraindications and precautions

Neutropenia A neutrophil count < 1,000/μL is a relative contraindication to the placement of an LTVA device, since patients with neutropenia may have a higher incidence of septic episodes. The use of prophylactic antibiotics may reduce the incidence of infection in patients with a low absolute neutrophil count (ANC).

Thrombocytopenia and platelet dysfunction are frequently encountered in the cancer patient. Preoperative platelet transfusion to approximately 50,000/μL may allow the catheter to be safely placed with a reduction in the risk of bleeding complications. In those patients with thrombocytopenia refractory to platelet transfusions, venous cutdown may be a safer approach for catheter placement.

Clotting factor abnormalities Many cancer patients have abnormalities in their clotting factors secondary to malnutrition or chemotherapy. Correction with vitamin K or fresh frozen plasma may be necessary.

Active infection The presence of an active infection represents an absolute contraindication to the placement of an LTVA device. In those patients with an active infection who require long-term antibiotic treatment, a temporary central venous access catheter or a peripherally inserted central venous catheter is preferable.

LTVA device selection

Two types of LTVA devices are available. There are tunneled external catheters that have skin surface access (Hickman, Broviac, Groshong, Quinton). Likewise, there are subcutaneous implanted ports (Port-A-Cath, Infusaport). Both types of central venous access devices are available with different lumen diameters and numbers. Peripherally placed central venous access devices, such as the PAS (peripherally accessed system) port or PICC (peripherally inserted central catheter), have become popular because of their ease of placement. PICC devices can be placed by specially trained nursing personnel. Important differences between tunneled external catheters and subcutaneous implanted ports are outlined in Table 1.

General considerations An important general consideration in the selection of an appropriate LTVA device is that the infusion flow resistance depends on the catheter length and lumen diameter. Likewise, catheters with a split valve at the tip (Groshong catheter) are less reliable for blood drawing.

Frequency of device access Subcutaneous implanted ports are preferred in patients who require intermittent device access for treatment or blood drawing. Tunneled external catheters are preferred in patients who require continuous or frequent device access for treatment, blood drawing, or delivery of supportive therapies (parenteral nutrition, blood product transfusion, pain medication) or who are receiving therapy that would be potentially toxic if extravasated into the subcutaneous tissue. Peripherally placed devices are used mainly in patients who require single, continuous, infusional therapy (systemic antibiotics, hydration, pain medication), as is seen frequently for palliation.

TABLE 1: Differences between tunneled external catheters and subcutaneous implanted ports

Characteristic	Tunneled external catheters	Subcutaneous implanted ports
Lumen	Single, dual, and triple lumen	Single and dual lumen only
Maintenance	Usually daily; requires patient training	Monthly; no patient training required
Activity	Some restrictions (eg, swimming)	No restrictions
Blood draw	Very reliable	Moderately reliable
Cost	Higher maintenance cost	Higher initial cost
Access	External	Percutaneous Huber needle
Flow	Determined by the lumen diameter gauge	termined by the Huber needle gauge
Complication rate (for infections)	Higher	Lower
Removal	Can usually be done in the office or at the bedside	May require a second surgical procure

Number of lumens The choice of the number of lumens should be based on the intensity and complexity of the therapy.

Specially designed catheters There are specially designed catheters for hemodialysis or apheresis treatment. These catheters are shorter in length and have a lumen that is larger in diameter and is staggered at the tip to prevent recirculation. These catheters have a higher incidence of kinking, and, thus, care should be taken to avoid sharp angles at the skin exit site. In patients who already have an LTVA device in place and require short-term access for apheresis or stem-cell collection, consideration should be given to placing a temporary percutaneous hemodialysis or apheresis catheter rather than replacing the existing LTVA device.

Insertion technique

Placement of LTVA devices is best performed in a surgical suite or an appropriate interventional radiology suite to minimize the incidence of infections. Most procedures are performed on an outpatient basis or immediately prior to a scheduled admission. Local anesthesia and short-acting barbiturates and sedatives are safe and provide excellent patient comfort and sedation. The use of intraoperative fluoroscopy is strongly recommended to document appropriate device placement and to prevent potential complications.

The most common technique used in LTVA device placement is the percutaneous method of Seldinger, using the subclavian or internal jugular vein. Alternatively, a venous cutdown of the cephalic, external jugular, internal jugular, or saphenous vein can provide appropriate access for central venous device placement. The use of a venous cutdown approach (instead of a percutaneous venipuncture approach) for LTVA device placement can essentially eliminate the risk of significant perioperative complications, such as pneumothorax or injury to major vascular structures.

Placement of tunneled external catheters

For the percutaneous approach, the patient is placed supine and in the Trendelenburg position. Patients who cannot tolerate the Trendelenburg position frequently can have their device placed through a venous cutdown approach. A rolled sheet placed vertically in the small of the back is preferred by some to rotate the tips of the shoulders posteriorly. The region of the anterior chest, neck, and shoulders is prepared and draped in a sterilized fashion. The skin overlying the anticipated venipuncture site is infiltrated with a local anesthetic.

Vein penetration The venipuncture needle is carefully and slowly advanced, bevel up, into the vein, while the attached syringe is aspirated (without Luerlock). If the vein is unable to be accessed after multiple attempts with the venipuncture needle, the contralateral side should not be approached during the same session without documenting the absence of complications.

Guidewire placement Once easy flow of blood into the syringe confirms vein penetration, the bevel is rotated downward, the syringe is disconnected without allowing introduction of air through the venipuncture needle, and a flexible J guidewire is advanced through the venipuncture needle.

Fluoroscopy should be used to confirm the placement of the tip of the guidewire within the right atrium. Atrial arrhythmia may be seen when the guidewire is advanced into the right atrium. If pulsatile blood flow is noted upon introducing the venipuncture needle (indicating an arterial puncture), the venipuncture needle should be withdrawn and local pressure applied for 5-10 minutes (see section on "Complications"). Resistance to the advancement of the guidewire is usually due to misdirection of the guidewire into a secondary vein or migration of the guidewire outside the vein. Fluoroscopy will confirm the guidewire's position. If the guidewire is suspected to be outside the vein, the venipuncture needle and the guidewire should be removed together, as a unit, to prevent shearing of the guidewire. If the guidewire is suspected to be in the wrong vein tributary, the venipuncture needle can be removed and a 16-gauge angiocatheter can be placed over the guidewire prior to readjusting the position of the guidewire.

Catheter placement The anticipated skin exit site and subcutaneous tunnel for the external catheter are infiltrated with a local anesthetic. The catheter is then advanced along the subcutaneous tunnel from the anticipated skin exit site to the venipuncture site. The catheter is measured and custom cut to reach the junction between the superior vena cava and right atrium (approximately at the fourth anterior intercostal space). The catheter cuff is positioned midway in the subcutaneous tunnel.

The dilator and peel-away introducer sheath are slowly and carefully advanced over the guidewire under fluoroscopy. The guidewire is gently and slightly withdrawn and advanced while the dilator and peel-away introducer sheath are advanced over the guidewire to confirm that they are indeed threading over the guidewire and that the guidewire has not migrated outside the vessel. The dilator and guidewire are then withdrawn from the peel-away introducer sheath. The catheter is then advanced through the peel-away introducer sheath and the tip of the catheter is advanced to the junction of the superior vena cava and right atrium.

Difficulties in advancing the catheter through the peel-away introducer sheath usually imply that the peel-away introducer sheath is bent. This occurs most frequently during the subclavian vein approach if the venipuncture is attempted too medially and through the costoclavicular ligament. If the catheter cannot be advanced through the peel-away introducer sheath, repeat venipuncture in a more lateral position may be necessary. The catheter should never be handled with sharp instruments. Only nontoothed forceps should be used, if needed.

Confirmation of catheter position Prior to removal of the peel-away introducer sheath, the catheter position should be confirmed by fluoroscopy. Failure to position the fluoroscopic beam perpendicular to the patient will give a false impression of the catheter's position.

At the completion of catheter placement, the entire catheter should be examined with fluoroscopy to confirm its position and to rule out any kinking that would prevent normal functioning. Catheter infusion (looking for impedance to inflow/infusion) and withdrawal (looking for interruption of flow on blood return) should be tested in the surgical suite prior to heparinization of the catheter lumen. A chest x-ray should be obtained in the recovery room to rule out complications and as a record of catheter position. Lastly, ultrasonography may be used during catheter placement to aid in vein localization for venous access and to determine the position of the catheter tip.

Placement of subcutaneous implanted ports

The procedure for placing a subcutaneous implanted port is similar to that for a tunneled external catheter, except for the creation of a subcutaneous port pocket. To prevent wound disruption, the subcutaneous port pocket should permit no tension in the placement of the port. The port is sutured to the muscular fascia to prevent port migration and is placed over the rib cage to provide easy access. Placement of a minimum of three separate sutures will help to prevent the implanted port from flipping over within the subcutaneous port pocket.

Device care

Subcutaneous implanted ports require flushing with a heparin solution (2-3 mL; 100 U/mL) after each use or monthly during periods of nonuse. During continuous infusion therapy, the noncoring (Huber) access needle should be replaced every third to fifth day.

Tunneled external catheters require more frequent care. The exit site is cleaned with an antiseptic agent, and an occlusive dressing is applied. This is generally done daily; however, some now advocate only biweekly cleanings and dressing changes. Hickman catheters are generally flushed daily with a heparin solution (2-3 mL; 100 U/mL) or after each use, and protective caps are replaced biweekly. However, some now advocate only biweekly flushing with a heparin solution (2-3 mL; 100 U/mL). Groshong catheters generally only require weekly flushing with 5 mL of a saline solution.

Complications

During device insertion

Complications during device placement are generally related to the method of insertion and the experience of the operator.

Pneumothorax is the most common complication of the percutaneous insertion technique, especially via the subclavian vein approach. The incidence of pneumothorax has been reported in most series to be approximately 1%-5%. It appears to be more frequently seen in nutritionally compromised and emaciated patients. Its incidence has also been thought to be related to the number of attempts required to access the vein and to the experience of the operator. Utilization of a venous cutdown approach eliminates the risk of pneumothorax.

Pneumothorax is usually recognized on a postoperative upright chest x-ray. The ability to detect a small pneumothorax on a chest x-ray can be aided by performing an expiratory film. Delayed pneumothorax can develop several hours to several days after attempted percutaneous device insertion. If the pneumothorax is small (< 5%), the patient can be followed with subsequent chest x-rays, and the air occupying the pneumothorax can be left in place to be reabsorbed. Use of 100% oxygen can aid in reabsorption of a pneumothorax. Patients with a larger pneumothorax are generally treated by placement of a chest tube that is connected to a closed suction system or a Heimlich valve (one-way valve).

Iatrogenic arterial puncture occurs most frequently with the percutaneous internal jugular approach and less frequently with the percutaneous subclavian vein approach. Pulsatile flow confirms an arterial puncture. In this instance, the venipuncture needle should be removed and the vessel compressed for 5-10 minutes. If an arterial puncture is initially unrecognized and the guidewire is passed into the vessel, a position of the guidewire to the left of the thoracic spine on fluoroscopy should alert the operator's suspicions for the occurrence of this complication. In a patient with a persistent left vena cava, the guidewire will also be seen to the left of the spine on fluoroscopy. An intraoperative venogram may help to confirm the diagnosis.

Hemothorax as a result of injury to major vessels is seen less than 1% of the time. It can be life-threatening, however, when it does occur. During the percutaneous approach, injury to one of the major vessels with the venipuncture needle, guidewire, or dilator and peel-away introducer sheath may result in a hemothorax. Careful attention to insertion technique and use of fluoroscopy will help to prevent this complication. Utilization of a venous cutdown approach is much less likely to injure a major vessel.

Most patients who develop a hemothorax can be treated with a large-bore, laterally placed chest tube connected to a closed suction system. Many of these closed suction systems have a blood re-infusion collecting system. Thoracotomy may be indicated in certain circumstances [in patients with ongoing bleeding (> 500 mL/h) or with a massive hemothorax (> 1,500 mL)].

Local hematomas can occur more frequently in thrombocytopenic patients or coagulopathic patients. They are best treated by local compression. Adequate replacement of platelets and clotting factors prior to device placement can help prevent these complications.

Catheter tip malposition is usually recognized and corrected at the time of catheter placement with the use of intraoperative fluoroscopy. However, catheters situated in the azygos vein or the right internal mammary vein can look strikingly similar to catheters situated in the superior vena cava in an anterior-posterior projection under intraoperative fluoroscopy. Frequently, these catheters do not withdraw blood easily and the catheter tip does not move with the cardiac rhythm. Lateral rotation of the intraoperative fluoroscope and utilization of intraoperative venography can help to differentiate this sometimes subtle finding.

Other device-related complications

Catheter compression, fracture, and embolization can occur when a catheter placed by the percutaneous subclavian approach is inserted too medially along the clavicle at the medial costoclavicular ligament. In such cases, the catheter may become chronically compressed between the clavicle and the first rib. This can be recognized radiographically as a "pinch-off sign." Chronic compression of the catheter may result in structural fatigue of the catheter wall that may eventually cause fracturing and distal embolization of the catheter. This can be prevented by ensuring that the venipuncture site is situated more laterally on the clavicle as well as 1-2 cm below the clavicle. If this problem is recognized during catheter placement, the catheter should be removed and then placed through a different venipuncture site.

Device malfunction can be divided into two types: (1) inability to withdraw blood from a device and (2) inability to infuse into a device. Inability to withdraw blood from a device, despite retaining the ability to infuse into the device, is most frequently caused by a fibrin sheath at the tip of the catheter that produces a one-way valve effect. Less frequently, it is due to a catheter tip positioned against the side wall of the vein. In patients with this problem, a Valsalva maneuver or repositioning of the patient can sometimes result in a successful blood withdraw.

Inability both to withdraw blood from and infuse into a device can result from many mechanical causes, such as catheter tip malposition, catheter kinking, catheter intraluminal thrombosis, intraluminal precipitation of medications, or venous thrombosis. A simple chest x-ray can identify some of these mechanical causes. Venography and venous duplex Doppler ultrasound imaging are also useful.

Thrombolytic therapy, using tissue plasminogen activator (tPA) or alteplase (recombinant tPA), can help to restore the ability to withdraw blood from a device or to clear a device from intraluminal thrombosis or intraluminal precipitation of medications. Usually 1-2 mg of tPA in 1-2 cc of sterile water is instilled into the device, left in place for 1-2 hours, and then aspirated. Alternatively, 2.5-cc aliquots (diluted to 1 mg/mL) of alteplase can be used in a similar fashion. This may be repeated daily for several days until total patency is restored. Likewise, chemical occlusion of a device resulting from precipitation of chemotherapeutic agents, poorly soluble salts (calcium, magnesium, or phosphates), or antibiotics (amikacin [Amikin], vancomycin) can be successfully treated with instillation of 0.2-1.0 mL of 0.1 N hydrochloric acid. The solution is irrigated in and out of the device for 2 minutes, left in place for 1 hour, and then aspirated. This may be repeated daily for several days until total patency is restored. No side effects or metabolic acidosis has been associated with hydrochloric acid at these doses.

External catheter damage External catheters can be damaged at the site of a catheter clamp or at a suture site. The use of needleless connections for infusions and irrigations should prevent needle damage to external portions of the catheter. Most external catheters have repair kits to replace any damaged external portion of the catheter.

Drug extravasation into the subcutaneous tissues can occur with subcutaneous implanted ports when there is inappropriate placement or accidental dislodgment of the Huber access needle from the implanted port. This may result in chemical cellulitis, tissue necrosis, and loss of soft tissue in the area of extravasation. Clinical signs of extravasation include pain, burning, soft-tissue swelling, skin erythema, and skin vesicle formation at the infusion site. If drug extravasation is suspected, the infusion should be stopped and the Huber access needle should be immediately withdrawn. Management depends on the type of drug infused and the amount of drug extravasated.

Venous thrombosis occurs more commonly than believed. The incidence of venous thrombosis varies in multiple studies, ranging from 0% to 65%. The incidence of venous thrombosis is higher in patients in whom the catheter tip is placed in the innominate vein or proximal superior vena cava as compared with the distal superior vena cava/right atrial junction. Ideally, the catheter tip should be positioned at the superior vena cava/right atrial junction and should be free floating. The incidence of venous thrombosis is higher in patients with multiple-lumen catheters than in those with single-lumen catheters. The incidence of venous thrombosis is higher in patients in whom the device was placed percutaneously than in those who underwent a venous cutdown approach. PICCs have been shown to be associated with a significant risk of upper extremity deep vein thrombosis. Preexisting hypercoagulable states predispose patients to the development of venous thrombosis.

Ipsilateral arm swelling, pain, and development of collateral veins in the skin overlying the chest wall should alert the clinician to the possibility of venous thrombosis. Venography, venous duplex Doppler ultrasound imaging, and CT/MRI scan can establish the diagnosis and the site of the obstruction.

Previous studies have suggested that the use of antithrombotic prophylaxis reduces the risk of central venous catheter-associated thrombosis in cancer patients. However, two double-blind, placebo-controlled, randomized trials assessing antithrombotic prophylaxis have now failed to show any such risk reduction within the time frame of those studies.

In one such trial by Verso et al, patients undergoing central venous catheter placement received either 6 weeks of subcutaneous low molecular weight heparin (LMWH; n = 155) or 6 weeks of subcutaneous placebo (n = 155). The overall incidence of central venous catheter-associated thrombosis was assessed at 6 weeks with upper extremity venography. Venography-proven thrombosis was observed in 14.2% (22 of 155) of the LMWH group and in 18.1% (28 of 155) of the placebo group ($P = .35$). Symptomatic thrombosis was observed in 1.0% of the LMWH group and in 3.1% of the placebo group. They concluded that the incidence of venography-proven thrombosis was lower than previously reported and that routine antithrombotic prophylaxis in cancer patients with central venous catheters should be reconsidered.

In one other such trial by Couban et al, patients undergoing central venous catheter placement received either 9 weeks of a 1-mg daily dose of warfarin (n = 130) or 9 weeks of a daily placebo (n = 125). The overall incidence of central venous catheter-associated thrombosis was assessed clinically, as defined as symptomatic central venous catheter-associated thrombosis. All symptomatic cases were then confirmed radiographically, first by compression ultrasonography, and then by venography, if ultrasonography results were normal. There was no statistically significant difference in the incidence of symptomatic central venous catheter-associated thrombosis between the two groups, with 4.6% (6 of 130) observed in the warfarin group and 4.0% (5 of 125) observed in the placebo group. They concluded that the incidence of symptomatic thrombosis was lower than previously reported and that administration of 1 mg/d of warfarin was not effective antithrombotic prophylaxis in cancer patients with central venous catheters. However, with the low rate of symptomatic central venous catheter-associated thrombosis, a much larger trial is required to address the issue definitively.

As a last point with regard to low-dose warfarin antithrombotic prophylaxis in cancer patients with central venous catheters, data have also shown a high incidence of INR (international normalized ratio) abnormalities in patients receiving 5-FU–based chemotherapy regimens who were maintained on 1 mg/d of warfarin, noted in 55 of 427 patients (12.8%), as reported by Magagnoli et al. In this regard, they recommended that such patients should undergo periodic monitoring of the prothrombin time and INR.

Treatment should be directed toward prevention of pulmonary embolism, avoidance of clot propagation, prevention of the postphlebitic syndrome, and preservation of the LTVA device, if possible. With these objectives in mind, the LTVA device should be removed only if it is no longer necessary or if initial therapy for venous thrombosis fails. The patient can be initially treated with systemic heparinization or subcutaneous LMWH followed by conversion to oral anticoagulation with warfarin. The LTVA device may be kept in place as long as the patient is asymptomatic and there is no contraindication to anticoagulation. According to NCCN guidelines, anticoagulant therapy should be continued for at least 1–3 months after device removal.

Device-related infections

Device-related infections can be divided into device-related bacteremia and site infections. Site infections consist of subcutaneous catheter tunnel infections and subcutaneous port pocket infections.

In general, device-related infections are thought to be greater for tunneled external catheters than subcutaneous implanted ports and greater for multiple-lumen catheters than single-lumen catheters. However, considerable controversy on this topic exists in the literature, since various studies examining device-related infection rates differ significantly with respect to patient characteristics, device maintenance schedules, and diagnostic criteria for defining a device-related infection. Differing device-use patterns and patient medical illness acuity are thought to explain the difference in device-related infection rates between tunneled external catheters and subcutaneous implanted ports and between multiple-lumen catheters and single-lumen catheters. Device-related infections of PICCs seem to occur more often in oncology patients than in non-oncology patients. Therefore, PICCs should be used with caution in oncology patients, except in cases of end-stage palliative comfort care.

It is controversial whether utilization of perioperative antibiotics for LTVA device placement decreases the incidence of device-related infections. Some studies have evaluated the addition of antibiotics (such as vancomycin) to the standard heparin-flush solution administered through LTVA devices to prevent device-related infections. Such results should be viewed with caution, however, in light of the increased incidence of vancomycin-resistant organisms in the hospital inpatient population.

Device-related bacteremia

Device-related bacteremia is a potentially life-threatening complication, especially in the immunocompromised patient. The infection generally is caused by gram-positive cocci (coagulase-negative staphylococci) or enteric gram-negative bacilli (*Enterobacteriaceae, Escherichia coli,* and *Pseudomonas* species). Less frequently, device-related bacteremia is caused by fungi (*Candida* species). The incidence of fungal infection is significantly higher in immunocompromised patients.

Criteria for diagnosis of device-related bacteremia vary among institutions. Some institutions utilize quantitative analysis of blood culture results, whereas others utilize qualitative analysis of blood culture results. Quantitative analysis involves comparing the number of colony-forming units seen in blood drawn through the device to blood drawn through the periphery. Usually, a 5- to 10-fold increase in the number of colony-forming units from blood drawn from the device as compared with concomitant peripheral cultures (or in the absence of positive peripheral cultures, > 1,000 colony-forming units from blood drawn from the device) signifies device-related bacteremia.

Qualitative analysis involves comparing positivity and negativity of blood cultures drawn from both the device and the periphery. Usually, simultaneous positive blood cultures drawn from both the device and the periphery, along with clinical relevance, signify device-related bacteremia.

Management If device-related bacteremia is suspected, appropriate systemic antibiotic coverage should be instituted after device and peripheral blood cultures are obtained. Antibiotic selection should be reassessed after organism identification and antibiotic sensitivities are available. Up to 70% of cases of device-related bacteremia can be successfully treated with a course of appropriate systemic antibiotics. The indications for device removal are the persistence of positive blood cultures after an appropriate course of systemic antibiotics, hypotension or severe systemic compromise, infections caused by *Candida* species, or recurrent infections caused by the same organism after successful systemic antibiotic therapy. (See chapter 45 on "Infectious Complications.")

Site infections

Site infections consist of subcutaneous catheter tunnel infections and subcutaneous port pocket infections. They can be superficial or deep. These infections are usually caused by gram-positive cocci (coagulase-negative staphylococci). Swelling, tenderness, and warmth over the site usually indicate a site infection. In the neutropenic patient, fever is often the only symptom. Swab culture of the skin exit site of the external catheter or the skin around the Huber access needle overlying the implanted port can sometimes identify the offending organism.

Management Local care at the skin exit site of the tunneled external catheter or removal of the Huber access needle from the subcutaneous implanted port and systemic antibiotics can be effective for most superficial site infections. Deep-seated subcutaneous catheter tunnel infections and subcutaneous port pocket infections may require device removal for successful eradication of the infection. Site infections caused by *Candida* species usually require device removal.

SUGGESTED READING

Abdullah BJ, Mohammad N, Sangkar JV, et al: Incidence of upper limb venous thrombosis associated with peripherally inserted central catheters (PICC). Br J Radiol 78:596–600, 2005.

Cheong K, Perry D, Karapetis C, et al: High rate of complications associated with peripherally inserted central venous catheters in patients with solid tumours. Intern Med J 34:234–238, 2004.

Couban S, Goodyear M, Burnell M, et al: Randomized placebo-controlled study of low-dose warfarin for the prevention of central venous catheter-associated thrombosis in patients with cancer. J Clin Oncol 23:4063–4069, 2005.

Estes JM, Rocconi R, Straughn JM, et al: Complications of indwelling venous access devices in patients with gynecologic malignancies. Gynecol Oncol 91:591–595, 2003.

Linenberger ML: Catheter-related thrombosis: Risks, diagnosis, and management. J Natl Compr Canc Netw 4:889–901, 2006.

Magagnoli M, Masci G, Castagna L, et al: Prophylaxis of central venous catheter-related thrombosis with minidose warfarin: Analysis of its use in 427 cancer patients. Anticancer Res 25:3143–3147, 2005.

Povoski SP: Eliminating the "pitfalls" of chronic indwelling central venous access device placement in cancer patients by utilizing a venous cutdown approach and be selectively and appropriately utilizing intraoperative venography. Int Semin Surg Oncol 4:16, 2007.

Povoski SP: External jugular vein cutdown approach for chronic indwelling central venous access in cancer patients: A potentially useful alternative. World J Surg Oncol 2:7, 2004.

Verso M, Agnelli G, Bertoglio S, et al: Enoxaparin for the prevention of venous thromboembolism associated with central vein catheter: A double-blind, placebo-controlled, randomized study in cancer patients. J Clin Oncol 23:4057–4062, 2005.

Dermatologic toxicities associated with targeted therapies

Mario E. Lacouture, MD

Improved cancer therapies have brought about unprecedented improvements in survival along with decreased hematopoietic toxicities, when compared to cytotoxic chemotherapy. Therefore, other components of the cancer experience have come forward, such as supportive care and psychological well-being. Most notably, dermatologic toxicities have gained considerable attention due to their high frequency, appearance in functional and cosmetically sensitive areas, association with symptoms of pain and pruritus–all of which lead to decreased quality of life and inconsistent dose intensity. In turn, clinical outcome may be affected with dose modifications in response to these untoward events.

Therapies targeting specific pathways or proteins in cancer cells are especially noted for dermatologic toxicities which affect up to 90% of treated patients. These toxicities are generally a class effect, and will occur with the use of monoclonal antibodies or small molecule kinase inhibitors with similar targets. Epidermal growth factor receptor (EGFR) inhibitors will lead to a papulopustular eruption, xerosis, pruritus, paronychia, alopecia, and hypertrichosis of the face with trichomegaly of the eyelashes. These effects will occur at different times during therapy, and not all patients will develop most toxicities. In a similar fashion, a number of dermatologic side effects have been associated with the small molecule multikinase inhibitors sunitinib (Sutent) and sorafenib (Nexavar), including hand-foot skin reaction (HFSR), xerosis, and subungual splinter hemorrhages.

On the following pages a number of photographs are provided to depict the various types of dermatologic reactions that may occur in patients receiving some of these agents.

FIGURE 1: Sensory disturbance (first) stage: Within the first few days of EGFR inhibitor drug initiation, a sensation of sunburn, associated with edema occurs in the central face.

FIGURE 2: Pustular (second) stage: Papules and pustules which may be tender or pruritic occurring with EGFR inhibitor therapy.

FIGURE 3: Papulopustular crust (third) stage: Crusting of papulopustules usually indicates resolving eruption to EGFR inhibitors.

FIGURE 4: Erythematous (fourth) stage: Upon resolution of the papulo-pustules, post-inflammatory erythema is a common sequelae, which may persist for several months.

Papulopustular Eruption, Phases 1-4 – Treatment of papulopustular eruption to EGFR inhibitors and multikinase inhibitors consists of a tetracycline antibiotic (tetracycline 500 mg bid, minocycline 100 mg qd, or doxycycline 100 mg bid). Topical corticosteroids of medium to low potency have also shown benefit.

FIGURE 5: Eyelash trichomegaly: Increased thickness and waviness of eyelashes and facial hair occurs in up to 33% of patients after 3-4 months of EGFR inhibitor therapy. Eyelashes may need to be trimmed, as they may grow inward causing corneal erosions or ulcerations.

FIGURE 6: EGFR inhibitor fissures: Fissures associated with tenderness in the fingertips and heels are a manifestation of severe xerosis to EGFR inhibitors. Treatment consists of liquid bandages and topical zinc oxide (20%-30%).

FIGURE 7: EGFR inhibitor inflammatory alopecia: Alopecia on the scalp as a result of EGFR inhibitor therapy induced follicular inflammation/superinfection. Treatment consists of topical steroid foams or solutions and oral antibiotics if infection is evidenced or suspected.

FIGURE 8: EGFR inhibitor xerosis: Dry skin develops in up to 58% of patients on EGFR inhibitor therapy, and usually occurs after the second month of drug initiation. Depending on the severity, treatment with topical emollients, ammonium lactate, and topical steroids is usually effective.

FIGURE 9: EGFR inhibitor photosensitivity: Increased sensitivity to ultraviolet radiation, manifested as sunburn, may occur when patients are receiving EGFR inhibitors. Therefore, it is critical for patients to apply broad spectrum sunscreens (containing zinc oxide or titanium dioxide) with an SPF >30.

FIGURE 10: EGFR inhibitor plus radiotherapy radiation dermatitis: Concurrent administration of EGFR inhibitors and radiation increases the risk of severe in-field radiation dermatitis. Tretament with high-potency topical steroids (mometasone) may be of benefit.

FIGURES 11A and 11B: Hand-foot skin reaction 1 and 2): Hand-foot skin reaction to the multikinase inhibitors sorafenib and sunitinib occurs in 30% of patients. Usually it develops within the first 2 weeks, and it is associated with blisters or hyperkeratosis overlying areas of pressure, which may impair activities of daily living in up to 10% of patients. Treatment with topical clobetasol and 40% urea, and pain control with non-steroidal anti-inflammatories or neurontin/pregabalin, may be necessary.

FIGURE 12: Docetaxel Periarticular thenar erythema with onycholysis (PATEO) syndrome: Docetaxel (Taxotere) induced tender or pruritic eryhtema in dorsum of the hands, along with subungual hemorrhages leading to nail separation and infection in up to 30% of treated patients. Therapy consists of high-potency topical steroids for erythematous areas, cold gloves, antiseptic soaks, and antibiotics for the nail changes and infection.

FIGURE 13: Pegylated doxorubicin (Doxil) and capecitabine (Xeloda) hand-foot syndrome: Painful erythema, edema, and sensation of tightness and cracking in the palms and soles occurs in up to 30% of patients. Treatment consists of topical ammonium lactate, and topical/oral steroids.

SUGGESTED READING

Jatoi A, Rowland K, Sloan JA, et al: Does tetracycline prevent/palliate epidermal growth factor receptor (EGFR) inhibitor-induced rash? A phase III trial from the North Central Cancer Treatment Group (N03CB). J Clin Oncol (abstract LBA9006)25:2007.

Lacouture ME: Mechanisms of cutaneous toxicities to EGFR inhibitors. Nat Rev Cancer 6:803–812, 2006.

Lacouture ME, Wu S, Robert C, et al: Evolving strategies for the management of hand-foot skin reaction associated with the multitargeted kinase inhibitors sorafenib and sunitinib. Oncologist 13:1001–1011, 2008.

Mitchell EP, Lacouture ME, Shearer H, et al: A phase II, open-label trial of skin toxicity (ST) evaluation (STEPP) in metastatic colorectal cancer (mCRC) patients (pts) receiving panitumumab (pmab) + FOLFIRI or irinotecan-only chemotherapy (CT as 2nd-line treatment (tx): Interim analysis. J Clin Oncol (abstract 15007)26:644s, 2008.

Robert C, Soria JC, Spatz A, et al: Cutaneous side-effects of kinase inhibitors and blocking antibodies. Lancet Oncol 6:491–500, 2005.

Scope A, Agero AL, Dusza SW, et al: Randomized double-blind trial of prophylactic oral minocycline and topical tazarotene for cetuximab-associated acne-like eruption. J Clin Oncol 25:5390–5396, 2007.

CHAPTER 44

Oncologic emergencies and paraneoplastic syndromes

Carmen P. Escalante, MD, Ellen Manzullo, MD, and Mitchell Weiss, MD

SUPERIOR VENA CAVA SYNDROME

Superior vena cava syndrome (SVCS) is a common occurrence in cancer patients and can lead to life-threatening complications such as cerebral or laryngeal edema. Although most commonly resulting from external compression of the vena cava by a tumor, SVCS can also stem from nonmalignant causes in cancer patients.

Etiology

Malignant causes

Primary intrathoracic malignancies are the cause of SVCS in approximately 87%–97% of cases. The most frequent malignancy associated with the syndrome is lung cancer, followed by lymphomas and solid tumors that metastasize to the mediastinum.

Lung cancer SVCS develops in approximately 3%–15% of patients with bronchogenic carcinoma, and it is four times more likely to occur in patients with right- versus left-sided lesions.

Metastatic disease Breast and testicular cancers are the most common metastatic malignancies causing SVCS, accounting for > 7% of cases. Metastatic disease to the thorax is responsible for SVCS in ~3%–20% of patients.

Nonmalignant causes

Thrombosis The most common nonmalignant cause of SVCS in cancer patients is thrombosis secondary to venous access devices (see chapter 43).

Other nonmalignant causes include cystic hygroma, substernal thyroid goiter, benign teratoma, dermoid cyst, thymoma, tuberculosis, histoplasmosis, actinomycosis, syphilis, pyogenic infections, radiation therapy, silicosis, and sarcoidosis. Some cases are idiopathic.

EMERGENCIES

Signs and symptoms

Classic symptoms Patients with SVCS most often present with complaints of facial edema or erythema, dyspnea, cough, orthopnea, or arm and neck edema. These classic symptoms are seen most commonly in patients with complete obstruction, as opposed to those with mildly obstructive disease.

Other associated symptoms may include hoarseness, dysphagia, head-aches, dizziness, syncope, lethargy, and chest pain. The symptoms may be worsened by positional changes, particularly bending forward, stooping, or lying down.

Common physical findings The most common physical findings include edema of the face, neck, or arms; dilatation of the veins of the upper body; and plethora or cyanosis of the face. Periorbital edema may be prominent.

Other physical findings include laryngeal or glossal edema, mental status changes, and pleural effusion (more commonly on the right side).

Diagnosis

It is important to establish the diagnosis and underlying etiology of SVCS, since some malignancies may be more amenable to specific treatment regimens than others. In the majority of cases, the diagnosis of SVCS is evident based on clinical examination alone.

The following diagnostic procedures may aid in establishing the diagnosis of SVCS and its etiology: chest x-ray, bronchoscopy, limited thoracotomy or thoracoscopy, contrast and radionuclide venography, Doppler ultrasonography, CT (especially contrast-enhanced spiral CT), and MRI.

Prognosis

The prognosis of SVCS depends on the etiology of the underlying obstruction. A review by Schraufnagel showed the average overall survival after the onset of SVCS to be 10 months, but there was wide variation ($\pm$ 25 months) depending on the underlying disease, with an average survival of 7.6 months. This duration was not significantly different from the survival duration of 12.2 months in patients presenting with SVCS as the primary manifestation of the disease. Thoracic malignancy, the most common cause of SVCS, had a poor prognosis of < 5 months.

Treatment

Treatment includes radiotherapy, chemotherapy, thrombolytic therapy and anti-coagulation, expandable wire stents, balloon angioplasty, and surgical bypass.

Most patients derive sufficient relief from obstructive symptoms when treated with medical adjuncts, such as diuretics and steroids (see section on "Adjunctive medical therapy"), so they can tolerate a work-up to determine the etiology of SVCS. In some instances, it is appropriate to delay treatment for 1–2 days if necessary to establish a firm tissue diagnosis.

Radiotherapy and chemotherapy

Both radiotherapy and chemotherapy are treatment options for SVCS, depending on the tumor type. The specific drugs and doses used are those active against the underlying malignancy.

Life-threatening symptoms, such as respiratory distress, are indications for urgent radiotherapy. A preliminary determination of the treatment goal (potentially curative or palliative only) is necessary prior to the initiation of treatment, even in the emergent setting.

Radiation therapy is the standard treatment of non–small-cell lung cancer (NSCLC) with SVCS. Recent studies suggest that chemotherapy may be as effective as radiotherapy in rapidly shrinking small-cell lung cancer (SCLC). Chemoradiation therapy may result in improved ultimate local control over chemotherapy alone in SCLC and non-Hodgkin lymphoma. Retrospective reviews of patients with SCLC have reported equivalent survival in patients with or without SVCS treated definitively with chemoradiation therapy.

Reasonable palliative courses can range from 2,000 cGy in 1 week to 4,000 cGy in 4 weeks. Curative regimens can range from 3,500 to 6,600 cGy based on histology. If indicated, more rapid palliation may be achieved by delivering daily doses of 400 cGy up to a dose of 800–1,200 cGy, after which the remainder of the appropriate total dose can be given in more standard daily fractions of 180 to 200 cGy. Some European investigators have used doses as high as 600 cGy 1 week apart in elderly patients.

Anticoagulation and thrombolysis

Anticoagulation for SVCS has become increasingly important due to thrombosis related to intravascular devices. In certain situations, the device remains in place. Both streptokinase and urokinase have been used for thrombolysis, although urokinase has been more effective in lysing clots in this setting. Urokinase is given as a 4,400-U/kg bolus followed by 4,400 U/kg/h, whereas streptokinase is administered as a 250,000-U bolus followed by 100,000 U/h. The use of thrombolytic therapy is controversial for catheter-related thrombosis, however.

Stenting

Placement of an expandable wire stent across the stenotic portion of the vena cava is an appropriate therapy for palliation of SVCS symptoms when other therapeutic modalities cannot be used or are ineffective. Use of stents is limited when intraluminal thrombosis is present. The Institut Catala d'Oncologia in Barcelona, Spain, published its results using endovascular stent insertion for the treatment of malignant SVCS. Stenting was performed in all 52 patients with lung cancer. Phlebographic resolution of the obstruction was achieved in 100% of cases, and symptomatic improvement was achieved in more than 80%

of patients. There was one major complication due to bleeding during antico-agulation. Reobstruction of the stent occurred in 17% of cases, mostly due to disease progression. Improvement of the obstruction allowed for delivery of full-dose systemic therapy for patients for whom this approach was indicated.

Other interventional treatments

Balloon angioplasty and surgical bypass have also been used in appropriate patients but are rarely indicated. Balloon angioplasty may be considered in patients with SVCS, significant clinical symptoms, and critical superior vena cava obstruction demonstrated by angiography. Surgical bypass is usually limited to patients with benign disease; however, for a select group of patients with SVCS, bypass may be an important aspect of palliative treatment. Other palliative efforts may be considered prior to bypass in this patient population.

Adjunctive medical therapy

Medications that may be used as adjuncts to the treatments described above include diuretics and steroids.

Diuretics may provide symptomatic relief of edema that is often immediate although transient. The use of diuretics is not a definitive treatment, and re-sulting complications may ensue, such as dehydration and decreased blood flow. Loop diuretics, such as furosemide, are often used. Dosage depends on the patient's volume status and renal function.

Steroids may be useful in the presence of respiratory compromise. They are also thought to be helpful in blocking the inflammatory reaction associated with irradiation.

Dosage depends on the severity of clinical symptoms. For severe and signifi-cant respiratory symptoms, hydrocortisone, 100–500 mg IV, may be admin-istered initially. Lower doses every 6–8 hours may be continued. Tapering of the steroid dosage should begin as soon as the patient's condition has stabilized. Prophylactic gastric protection is advised during steroid administration.

VENOUS THROMBOEMBOLIC COMPLICATIONS OF CANCER

Deep vein thrombosis (DVT) and pulmonary embolism (PE) are common and potentially serious clinical challenges. In the United States, the estimated inci-dence of DVT and PE is approximately 450,000 and 355,000 cases per year, respectively. The actual incidence is likely much higher than presently docu-mented due to often vague complaints and symptoms. PE may be associated with increased mortality and contributes to approximately 240,000 deaths an-nually in the United States.

Armand Trousseau noted the association between thrombosis and cancer more than 125 years ago. The risk of venous thromboembolism (VTE) in cancer patients depends upon the type and extent of the malignancy, the type of can-cer treatment, the existence and nature of comorbidities, and changes in hemostasis of the blood, which have been noted in more than 90% of cancer patients. The prevalence of clinically noted venous thrombosis in cancer patients is 15%; patients undergoing surgery, hormonal therapy, and chemotherapy have the highest risk. Venous thrombosis is the second leading cause of death in cancer patients.

Etiology of VTE in cancer patients

The etiology of VTE in cancer patients may be attributed to several factors, including hypercoagulable states, surgical interventions, chemotherapy, indwelling central venous catheters, and prolonged immobilization.

The mechanisms by which tumors cause a hypercoagulable state are not completely understood, but they may be attributed to abnormalities of blood composition (increased plasma levels of clotting factors, cancer procoagulant A, tissue factor, and cytokines) and increased release of plasminogen activator. Postoperative VTE was more common in patients with malignant disease (36%) than in those patients with benign disease (20%), according to recent analyses of several clinical trials in surgical patients.

Patients undergoing chemotherapy are at increased risk of venous thrombosis secondary to endothelial cell damage from drug toxicity. In the recent ATAC (Arimidex, Tamoxifen, Alone or in Combination) trial, the aromatase inhibitor anastrozole (Arimidex) was compared with tamoxifen for 5 years in 9,366 postmenopausal women with localized breast cancer. Forty-eight patients (1.6%) receiving anastrozole developed DVT events, compared with 74 patients (2.4%) in the tamoxifen arm $(P = .02)$. Anastrozole was associated with significant reductions in DVT events and should be considered for initial treatment in this population.

Indwelling central venous catheters predispose patients to upper extremity thrombosis and thrombosis of the axillary/subclavian vein. The catheters are also prone to occlusion. Increased venous stasis owing to immobility also promotes blood pooling into the intramuscular venous sinuses of the calf and may lead to thrombosis formation.

TUMOR TYPE ASSOCIATED WITH VTE

Several tumor types have been associated with higher rates of VTE, including those arising from the pancreas, lungs, and other mucin-secreting tumors. In general, tumor types associated with an increased incidence of thromboembolic events reflect the frequency of the tumors in the general population: In women, the most common tumors are breast, lung, gynecologic, and GI tumors; in men, prostate, lung, and GI tumors are most common. However, hematologic malignancies (multiple myeloma, lymphoma, and leukemia) also have significant rates of VTE.

Treatment

Several classes of agents have been used for prevention and treatment of VTE. Nonpharmacologic approaches to prophylaxis may include intermittent pneumatic compression, elastic stockings, and inferior vena cava filters. Commonly used pharmacologic agents for thromboprophylaxis and treatment of VTE include unfractionated heparin (UFH; standard, low-dose, or adjusted-dose), oral anticoagulants such as warfarin, and low molecular weight heparin (LMWH).

Initial treatment of DVT and PE includes inpatient UFH or LMWH and, more recently, outpatient LMWH for low-risk patients with DVT. (Although patients with PE have been treated with LMWH as outpatients, it is not the standard of care in the United States.)

UFH generally is administered as a bolus of 5,000 U followed by a continuous drip, usually initiated between 750–1,000 U/h. A baseline partial thromboplastin time (PTT) and prothrombin time (PT) are drawn prior to the initiation of treatment. PTT is then rechecked approximately 4–6 hours after treatment is begun, and the UFH is titrated to approximately 1.5 to 2 times control in most patients.

Warfarin is usually begun on day 1 or 2 of treatment; therapy is monitored to maintain an international normalized ratio (INR) between 2.0 and 3.0. (Patients with prosthetic valves require a higher INR.) It is standard practice to maintain UFH for 4–5 days while the warfarin is titrated to therapeutic levels. Most patients are maintained on warfarin for 3–6 months depending upon underlying risk factors. There is controversy regarding the duration of anticoagulation, and some investigators maintain that patients with active cancer should continue anticoagulation for as long as the cancer remains active. Patients with recurrent VTE are usually maintained on anticoagulants for the rest of their lives.

Patient response to warfarin depends on numerous factors, such as age, diet, alcohol consumption, and liver and GI function, as well as concomitant medications.

Recent studies have demonstrated the safety and efficacy of LMWH in the treatment and management of VTE. Several studies have demonstrated no appreciable differences in recurrent thromboembolism and an increased risk of bleeding with UFH and LMWHs. Because LMWHs do not require a continuous drip and frequent serum testing, some low-risk patients are now treated as outpatients. Studies are ongoing in the cancer patient population.

In the United States, enoxaparin (Lovenox) has received US Food and Drug Administration (FDA) approval for prevention and treatment of DVT. Tinzaparin (Innohep) also has FDA approval for the treatment of DVT. Dalteparin (Fragmin), another LMWH agent indicated for prophylaxis, has been approved by the FDA for cardiac use and for treatment of DVT/PE.

LMWH doses vary by product and are not equivalent. Enoxaparin is generally administered once or twice a day for treatment of VTE, whereas the indications for tinzaparin and dalteparin are for once-daily dosing. The commonly administered dose for treatment of DVT with enoxaparin is 1 mg/kg SC (subcutaneous) every 12 hours. Tinzaparin is given via SC injection at a dose of 175 IU/kg body weight once daily, and the dalteparin dose is 200 IU/kg SC once daily for the first month, followed by 150 IU/kg SC daily thereafter. Therapy with LMWH is continued for a minimum of 5 days during the acute phase of treatment. Generally, laboratory monitoring is unnecessary, although for individuals with renal insufficiency or those with < 50 kg body weight or obesity, plasma antifactor Xa concentrations may need to be monitored.

In an international study comparing the long-term treatment benefits of dalteparin versus warfarin in cancer patients with VTE, long-term dalteparin substantially reduced the rate of recurrent VTE, compared with warfarin therapy, without an increase in bleeding. Based on this trial, cancer patients requiring VTE treatment should continue dalteparin (or possibly another LMWH) during the chronic phase of treatment instead of switching to warfarin. Cost issues may require patients to remain on warfarin.

DIFFICULTIES IN ANTICOAGULATION

Often, therapeutic challenges arise in patients on anticoagulation therapy for VTE who require surgical interventions and, therefore, temporary discontinuation of their anticoagulation treatment.

Preoperative guidelines The timing of discontinuation of anticoagulation depends upon the type of treatment and the surgical intervention planned. For patients on continuous-drip heparin, the drip may be discontinued 4–6 hours prior to the procedure. A PTT should be drawn prior to the procedure to check for total reversal of the treatment. In cases where only partial reversal is noted or an emergency arises, fresh frozen plasma may be administered for rapid reversal.

Patients on warfarin may be advised to discontinue their medication 3–5 days prior to the planned procedure. This approach allows for a gradual reduction in the anticoagulation effect. An INR should be checked prior to the procedure. If partial reversal is noted or an emergency arises, vitamin K and/or fresh frozen plasma may be administered for acute reversal.

Postoperative guidelines Timing of postoperative therapy depends on the type of procedure undertaken and its associated risk of bleeding. Direct communication between the surgeon and the physician managing the anticoagulation treatment is necessary. When the surgeon believes that the risk of bleeding is at an acceptable level, anticoagulation should be restarted. It may be prudent to utilize UFH or LMWH prior to the initiation of warfarin, especially if a substantial risk of bleeding remains.

High-risk patients For high-risk patients (prosthetic valve, recurrent VTE), it may be reasonable to switch from warfarin to either UFH or LMWH, with appropriate discontinuation prior to the procedure. Both UFH and LMWH have shorter reversal times than does warfarin, although LMWHs are not fully reversible. Another option is to continue warfarin until shortly before the procedure, reversing treatment with vitamin K and/or fresh frozen plasma. The risk/benefit ratio should be considered when reviewing the options for the individual patient.

Surgery has long been known to be a risk factor for VTE. The nature of surgery in part determines the relative risk: Patients undergoing orthopedic surgery are at a particularly high risk. The risk is modified by the presence of other factors, such as underlying malignancy, age, obesity, and history of previous thromboembolism. Recent meta-analyses of clinical trials have shown there is a high overall risk of DVT during general surgery, based on rates observed in control subjects; there is a confirmed incidence of DVT of 25% noted by the fibrinogen uptake test. The risk is even higher (29%) in surgical patients with malignancy. Risk is also increased in those individuals with multiple risk factors (eg, age > 65 years, obesity, bed rest > 5 days). A comparison of commonly used prophylaxis in 160 clinical trials indicates that overall, low-dose UFH and LMWH are the most effective agents in reducing the incidence of DVT after general surgery. A higher dosage of the prophylactic agent may be needed for adequate prevention in patients with malignant disease.

Treatment alternatives for recurrence There are several treatment options for patients with recurrent VTE. Patients who develop recurrence of thrombosis while on therapeutic doses of anticoagulation should be considered for inferior vena cava filter placement. The filter will not prevent new clots from forming, but it does provide a physical barrier to prevent propagation of clots to the pulmonary bed. Alternatively, an inferior vena cava filter can be placed to avoid the need for long-term anticoagulant therapy if there are contraindications to anticoagulation. Or, another LMWH may be utilized prior to placement of an inferior vena cava filter, since there may be other complications related to filter placement (ie, postphlebitis syndrome, clotting of the filter).

Depending upon patient prognosis and tumor factors, other comorbidities, and propensity for bleeding, continued therapy with warfarin or LMWH may also be considered in addition to filter placement.

SPINAL CORD COMPRESSION

Spinal cord compression develops in 1%–5% of patients with systemic cancer. It should be considered an emergency, as treatment delays may result in irreversible paralysis and loss of bowel and bladder function.

Etiology

Compression of the spinal cord is due predominantly to extradural metastases (95%) and usually results from tumor involvement of the vertebral column. A tumor may occasionally metastasize to the epidural space without bony involvement.

Site of involvement The segment most often involved is the thoracic spine (70%), followed by the lumbosacral (20%) and cervical spine (10%).

Most common malignancies Spinal cord compression occurs in a variety of malignancies; the most common are lung, breast, unknown primary, prostate, and renal cancers.

Signs and symptoms

Early signs More than 90% of patients present with pain localized to the spine or radicular in nature (ie, not due to bony involvement but rather to neural compression). Pain, which is usually secondary to bony involvement, is often exacerbated with movement, recumbency, coughing, sneezing, or straining. The majority of patients experience pain for weeks to months before neurologic symptoms appear.

Intermediate signs If cord compression goes untreated, weakness often develops next. It may be preceded or accompanied by sensory loss.

Late signs Symptoms of autonomic dysfunction, urinary retention, and constipation are late findings. Once autonomic, motor, or sensory findings appear, spinal cord compression usually progresses rapidly and may result in irreversible paralysis in hours to days if untreated.

Physical findings may include tenderness to palpation or percussion over the involved spine, pain in the distribution of the involved nerve root, muscle weakness, spasticity, abnormal muscle stretch reflexes and extensor plantar responses, and sensory loss. Sensory loss occurs below the involved cord segment and indicates the site of compression. In patients with autonomic dysfunction, physical findings include a palpable bladder or diminished rectal tone.

Diagnosis

The first step in the diagnosis of spinal cord compression is an accurate neurologic history and examination.

X-rays More than 66% of patients with spinal cord compression have bony abnormalities on plain radiographs of the spine. Findings include erosion and loss of pedicles, partial or complete collapse of vertebral bodies, and paraspinous soft-tissue masses. Normal spine films are not helpful for excluding epidural metastases.

MRI The standard for diagnosing and localizing epidural cord compression is MRI. Gadolinium-enhanced MRI has been especially helpful in assessing cord compression secondary to spinal epidural abscesses, as gadolinium enhances actively inflamed tissues and defines anatomic boundaries. An abnormal signal within the disk space suggests the possibility of infection.

Primary or secondary neoplasms involving the vertebral bodies generally demonstrate a long T1, resulting in decreased signal intensity on a T1-weighted image, and a long T2, with increased signal intensity on the T2-weighted image.

CT and myelography If MRI is unavailable, a CT scan and/or myelogram may be used to diagnose and localize epidural cord compression.

Prognosis

Treatment outcome correlates with the degree and duration of neurologic impairment prior to therapy. In a prospective analysis of 209 patients treated for spinal cord compression with radiotherapy and steroids, Maranzano and Latini reported that of patients who were ambulatory, nonambulatory, or paraplegic prior to treatment, 98%, 60%, and 11%, respectively, were able to ambulate following therapy. Treatment outcome in the most radiosensitive malignancies (eg, lymphoma) was superior to that in the less sensitive cancers (renal cell carcinoma). Almost all ambulatory patients treated with either irradiation alone or laminectomy followed by postoperative irradiation remained ambulatory after treatment, whereas ~ 10% of patients whose lower extremities were paralyzed could walk after treatment.

Treatment

The goals of treatment of spinal cord compression are recovery and maintenance of normal neurologic function, local tumor control, stabilization of the spine, and pain control. Choice of treatment depends on clinical presentation, availability of histologic diagnosis, rapidity of the clinical course, type of malignancy, site of spinal involvement, stability of the spine, and previous treatment.

In general, radiation therapy has been the treatment of choice for these patients. This is based upon the belief that radiotherapy is as effective as surgery in terms of pain relief and maintaining neurologic function. In other words, the potential complications and convalescence associated with surgery can be avoided in this group of patients with a limited life expectancy.

This approach has been further investigated in a randomized clinical trial reported by Patchell et al. A total of 101 patients with spinal cord compression caused by metastatic cancer were randomized to undergo either surgery followed by adjuvant radiation therapy (n = 50) or radiation therapy alone (n = 51). Radiotherapy for both groups consisted of 10 fractions of 300 cGy each. The primary endpoint was the ability to walk.

The study was stopped after an interim analysis of the 101 patients revealed that 42 of 50 patients (84%) in the surgery group were able to walk after treatment, compared with 29 of 51 patients (57%) in the radiotherapy group ($P = .001$). Additionally, patients treated with surgery retained the ability to walk significantly longer than those patients treated with radiation therapy alone (median, 122 days vs 13 days; $P = .003$). Of the 32 patients who entered the trial unable to walk, 10 of 16 (62%) in the surgery arm regained the ability to walk, compared with 3 of 16 (19%) in the radiotherapy arm ($P = .01$). Based on the results of this trial, decompressive surgery followed by adjuvant radiation therapy should be considered in the treatment of patients with spinal cord compression.

The ability to regain ambulatory function after surgery had been recognized prior to this study. This finding represented the rationale for strong consideration of surgery in this group of patients. The authors advocated the wider use of surgery in most patients with spinal cord compression. Still, there are reasons to consider radiotherapy alone as appropriate initial treatment. They include the disappointing results in the radiotherapy-alone arm in this study compared with the experiences of previous studies and the possible reluctance to consider spinal surgery by patients and/or physicians (based upon limited life expectancy). These issues should, of course, be thoroughly reviewed during the process of informed consent.

Steroids

Dexamethasone should be administered if the patient's history and neurologic examination suggest spinal cord compression. There is controversy as to whether an initial high dose of intravenous (IV) dexamethasone (100 mg) followed by 10 mg of dexamethasone every 6 hours is necessary. Some studies have suggested lower doses are just as effective.

Radiation therapy

Radiation therapy alone is still usually the standard initial treatment for most patients with spinal cord compression due to a radiosensitive malignancy. Treatment outcome is contingent upon both the relative radiosensitivity of the malignancy and the neurologic status of the patient at the time radiotherapy is initiated.

Radiation portal In general, the treatment volume should include the area of epidural compression (as determined by MRI or myelography) plus two vertebral bodies above and below. Consideration should be given to including adjacent areas of abnormalities if feasible. Careful matching techniques should be employed in patients treated to adjacent vertebral levels, a situation that is not uncommon.

Radiation dose and fractionation The chosen regimen should take into account such factors as field size and normal tissue tolerance. Smaller fields are appropriately treated to 2,000–3,000 cGy over 1 or 2 weeks, respectively. Larger fields may occasionally necessitate longer courses, such as 4,000 cGy over 4 weeks, to minimize side effects.

The University Hospital Hamburg has reported their results on five fractionation schemes of radiation therapy for spinal cord compression. In this retrospective review, 1,304 patients were treated from January 1992 through December 2003. Radiation schedules included 1 x 8 Gy (n = 261), 5 x 4 Gy (n = 279), 10 x 3 Gy (n = 274), 15 x 2.5 Gy (n = 233), and 20 x 2 Gy (n = 257). Improvement in motor function was noted in 26% (1 x 8 Gy), 28% (5 x 4 Gy), 27% (10 x 3 Gy), 31% (15 x 2.5 Gy), and 28% (20 x 2 Gy). Motor function improvement and post-treatment ambulatory rates were not significantly different throughout all groups.

On multivariate analysis, age, performance status, pretreatment ambulatory status, and length of time motor deficits were present prior to the initiation of radiotherapy were all significantly associated with improved functional outcome, whereas the schedule of radiation therapy was not a significant indicator. Recurrence rates at 2 years were 24%, 26%, 14%, 9%, and 7%, respectively.

TABLE 1: Symptoms associated with hypercalcemia by organ system

General	CNS	Cardiac	GI	Renal
Dehydration	Weakness	Bradycardia	Nausea and vomiting	Polyuria
Anorexia	Hypotonia	Short QT interval	Constipation	Nephrocalcinosis
Pruritus	Proximal myopathy	Prolonged PR interval	Ileus	–
Weight loss	Mental status changes	Wide T wave	Pancreatitis	–
Fatigue	Seizure Coma	Atrial or ventricular arrhythmia	Dyspepsia	–

There was mild acute toxicity and no late toxicity. The authors concluded that shorter fractionation schemes should be considered for those patients with poor predicted survival.

In another study, the University Hospital Hamburg reported its prospective evaluation of 10 versus 20 fractions of radiation therapy for metastatic spinal cord compression. A total of 214 patients were irradiated with 30 Gy in 10 fractions (n = 110) or 40 Gy in 20 fractions (n = 104). Motor function improved in 43% of patients treated with 30 Gy and in 41% of patients treated with 40 Gy ($P = .799$). There was no significant difference in post-treatment ambulatory rates (60% and 64%, respectively; $P = .708$). As expected, being ambulatory prior to the initiation of treatment was associated with better functional outcome after irradiation ($P = .035$). Acute toxicity was mild, and no late toxicity was observed during the 12-month follow-up.

Retreatment may be entertained, particularly when no effective alternative exists. Usually, doses of 2,000 cGy over 2 weeks can be used for retreatment. It is important, however, to counsel the patient regarding the risk of radiation neuropathy. Furthermore, only those patients who had a lasting response to the initial treatment should be reirradiated, as tumors that were refractory to the first course or that recur within 3 months are unlikely to respond to subsequent courses.

Surgery

Vertebral body resection for a tumor anterior to the cord and posterior laminectomy for a tumor posterior to the cord may be appropriate treatment options for relieving spinal cord compression in patients who require spinal stability, have undergone previous radiotherapy in the area of the compression, require a tissue diagnosis of malignancy, or experience progression of the cord compression despite optimal treatment with steroids and irradiation.

In general, surgical decompression should be strongly considered in patients whose cord compression is caused by a relatively radioresistant cancer and who have a severe neurologic deficit (such as bowel or bladder dysfunction). Unfortunately, many patients in this situation are not candidates for aggressive surgery. In these cases, radiotherapy is offered, albeit with limited expectations for neurologic recovery.

Chemotherapy

Chemotherapy may be an effective treatment of spinal cord compression in select patients with a chemosensitive metastatic tumor. It also may be considered in combination with other treatment modalities, such as radiotherapy, or as an alternative if those modalities are not suitable options for relieving spinal cord compression.

HYPERCALCEMIA

Hypercalcemia is the most common metabolic emergency seen in individuals with cancer, occurring in an estimated 10%–20% of patients.

Etiology

The malignancies most commonly associated with hypercalcemia include myeloma, lung cancer (epidermoid tumors more often than small-cell tumors), and renal cancer. In some cases, the pathogenesis of hypercalcemia may relate to the release of parathyroidlike hormones, prostaglandins, and osteoclast-activating factor.

Signs and symptoms

Symptoms of hypercalcemia may involve various organ systems, including the central nervous, cardiac, GI, and renal systems (Table 1).

Bony metastasis versus paraneoplastic syndrome The signs and symptoms of hypercalcemia secondary to bony metastases are often indistinguishable from those of hypercalcemia as a paraneoplastic syndrome. The laboratory findings may vary. A tumor secreting an immunoreactive parathyroid hormone (iPTH)-like substance will have increased levels of cyclic adenosine monophosphate (cAMP), low levels of serum phosphorus, and variable levels of iPTH, depending on the specificity of the assay. Many patients with bony metastases also exhibit features consistent with "ectopic" hyperparathyroidism.

Diagnosis

An accurate history and physical examination are often the most helpful diagnostic tools to exclude correctable nonmalignant causes of hypercalcemia. Hypercalcemia in association with occult malignancies is rare. The presence of weight loss, fatigue, or muscle weakness should increase clinical suspicion of

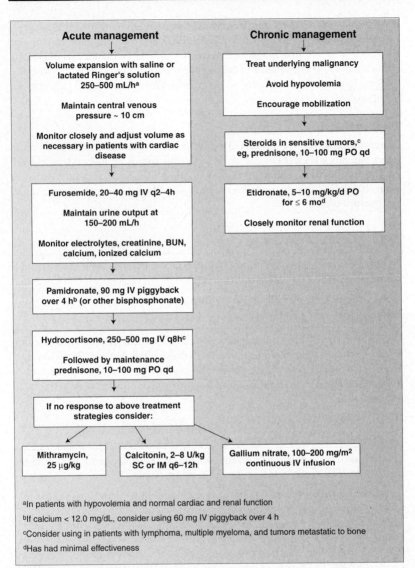

Acute management	Chronic management
Volume expansion with saline or lactated Ringer's solution 250–500 mL/h[a] **Maintain central venous pressure ~ 10 cm** **Monitor closely and adjust volume as necessary in patients with cardiac disease**	**Treat underlying malignancy** **Avoid hypovolemia** **Encourage mobilization**
	Steroids in sensitive tumors,[c] eg, prednisone, 10–100 mg PO qd
Furosemide, 20–40 mg IV q2–4h **Maintain urine output at 150–200 mL/h** **Monitor electrolytes, creatinine, BUN, calcium, ionized calcium**	**Etidronate, 5–10 mg/kg/d PO for ≤ 6 mo[d]** **Closely monitor renal function**

Pamidronate, 90 mg IV piggyback over 4 h[b] (or other bisphosphonate)

Hydrocortisone, 250–500 mg IV q8h[c]

Followed by maintenance prednisone, 10–100 mg PO qd

If no response to above treatment strategies consider:

Mithramycin, 25 µg/kg	**Calcitonin, 2–8 U/kg SC or IM q6–12h**	**Gallium nitrate, 100–200 mg/m² continuous IV infusion**

[a]In patients with hypovolemia and normal cardiac and renal function
[b]If calcium < 12.0 mg/dL, consider using 60 mg IV piggyback over 4 h
[c]Consider using in patients with lymphoma, multiple myeloma, and tumors metastatic to bone
[d]Has had minimal effectiveness

FIGURE 1: Algorithm for the treatment of hypercalcemia of malignancy

malignancy as the cause of hypercalcemia.

Laboratory findings In patients with hypercalcemia of malignancy, serum iPTH levels, determined by a double-antibody method, are extremely low or undetectable; levels of inorganic phosphorus are low or normal; and levels of 1,25-dihydroxyvitamin D are low or normal.

Use of additional tests to identify the underlying malignancy responsible for the hypercalcemia often depends on the history and physical findings.

Treatment

Asymptomatic patients with minimally elevated calcium levels (< 12.0 mg/dL) may be treated as outpatients, with close monitoring of calcium levels and symptoms. Encouragement of oral hydration, mobilization, and elimination of drugs that contribute to hypercalcemia are essential. Patients who are symptomatic or have calcium levels ≥ 12.0 mg/dL should be considered for inpatient management if medically appropriate. An algorithm for the acute and chronic treatment of hypercalcemia of malignancy is shown in Figure 1.

Volume expansion (eg, lactated Ringer's solution, 0.9% NaCl) Volume expansion and natriuresis increase renal blood flow and enhance calcium excretion secondary to the ionic exchange of calcium for sodium in the distal tubule. The volume required depends on the extent of hypovolemia, as well as the patient's cardiac and renal function. Often, infusion rates of 250–500 mL/h are needed. Typically, the onset of action is 12–24 hours.

Loop diuretics There is much controversy over the effectiveness of loop diuretics in the treatment of hypercalcemia. In theory, furosemide-induced natriuresis should enhance urinary calcium excretion. However, in most cases of significant hypercalcemia, hypovolemia is present. Thus, once euvolemia has been achieved with saline infusion, diuretics may be useful in preventing hypervolemia. Diuretic dosages depend on the patient's underlying renal function, and the dosing frequency should be based on hourly urine output. In patients with normal renal function, furosemide, 20–40 mg IV, may be initiated after volume expansion is achieved, with subsequent doses given when urine output is < 150–200 mL/h.

Bisphosphonates (etidronate, clodronate, pamidronate, and zoledronic acid [Zometa]) bind avidly to hydroxyapatite crystals and inhibit bone resorption. Their antiresorptive effects may be mediated by the inhibition of osteoclasts and activation by cytokines. Bisphosphonates also inhibit recruitment and differentiation of osteoclast precursors. They are poorly absorbed from the GI tract, have a very long half-life in bone, and appear to accumulate at sites of active bone turnover.

Pamidronate has been shown to be effective in restoring normocalcemia in 60%–100% of patients with hypercalcemia secondary to malignancy. The recommended dose is 90 mg IV over 4 hours. The single IV dose over 4 hours, lack of renal toxicity, and superiority over etidronate make pamidronate a logical choice for bisphosphonate therapy for hypercalcemia of malignancy. Side effects include low-grade fever and mild hypocalcemia and hypomagnesemia. Clodronate, another bisphosphonate indicated for cancer-associated hypercalcemia, is dosed at 300 mg IV daily for 5 consecutive days (infused over at least 2 hours) or 800–3,200 mg/d orally. Zoledronic acid (4 mg IV) is a newer bisphosphonate that can be infused quicker and has fewer systemic side effects than other bisphosphonates.

Corticosteroids In certain malignancies, such as lymphomas and hormone-sensitive breast cancers, corticosteroids may be of some value in producing a direct antitumor effect. In the majority of solid tumors, however, steroids are of limited or no value.

The onset of action is 3–5 days. Doses of prednisone (or its equivalent) may range from 10 to 100 mg/d.

Calcitonin inhibits bone degradation by binding directly to receptors on the osteoclast. It has few serious side effects (rare hypersensitivity) and can be given to patients with organ failure.

Calcitonin's onset of action is 2–4 hours, but its hypocalcemic effect is of short duration and peaks at 48 hours. There is little response to continued treatment. Doses range from 2 to 8 U/kg SC or IM (intramuscular) every 6–12 hours.

Plicamycin (Mithracin) has direct osteoclast-inhibitory effects and may also block the effects of vitamin D or parathyroid hormone. It reportedly is effective in ~80% of patients with hypercalcemia secondary to malignancy.

The onset of action of plicamycin is 24–48 hours. The duration of normocalcemia varies, but retreatment is required in 72–96 hours in most patients. The usual dose is 25 µg/kg (range: 10 to 50 µg/kg).

Significant toxicity increases with multiple injections and includes renal and liver toxicity. Thrombocytopenia is a common side effect.

Gallium nitrate (Ganite) directly inhibits osteoclasts and increases bone calcium without producing cytotoxic effects on bone cells. It successfully restores normocalcemia in 75%–85% of patients.

Gallium nitrates's onset of action is 24–48 hours. The dose range is 100–200 mg/m^2 given by continuous IV infusion for 5 days.

A study by Bertheault-Cvitkovic et al suggested that gallium nitrate may be superior to pamidronate for the acute normalization of cancer-related hypercalcemia. In other comparative trials, gallium nitrate proved to be more effective than both calcitonin and etidronate in patients with hypercalcemia that is secondary to malignancy.

There are some disadvantages to gallium nitrate therapy, including the need for inpatient care and daily IV infusions and potential nephrotoxicity. It has been recommended that the drug not be used in patients with creatinine levels > 2.5 mg/dL.

HYPERURICEMIA

Compared with hypercalcemia, hyperuricemia is a less common metabolic emergency in cancer patients.

Etiology and risk factors

Hyperuricemia occurs most often in patients with hematologic disorders, particularly leukemias, high-grade lymphomas, and myeloproliferative diseases (polycythemia vera). It may occur secondary to treatment of the malignancy.

Drugs Hyperuricemia is also associated with certain cytotoxic agents (eg, tiazofurin and aminothiadiazoles). Various other drugs can contribute to hyperuricemia by increasing uric acid production or decreasing its excretion. Diuretics (thiazides, furosemide, and ethacrynic acid [Edecrin]) cause acute uricosuria, and hyperuricemia may occur secondary to volume contraction. Antituberculous drugs, such as pyrazinamide and ethambutol (Myambutol), as well as nicotinic acid (niacin) are also associated with hyperuricemia.

Extensive or aggressive tumors Patients with extensive, anaplastic, or rapidly proliferating tumors are at greatest risk for hyperuricemia. These patients include those with bulky lymphomas and sarcomas, those with chronic myelocytic leukemia or chronic lymphocytic leukemia and extreme leukocytosis, and those undergoing remission-induction chemotherapy for acute leukemia.

Renal impairment Individuals with preexisting renal impairment are also at risk of becoming hyperuricemic.

Signs and symptoms

Patients with clinical syndromes caused by hyperuricemia present with significant elevations of serum uric acid. Gouty arthritis may be seen occasionally, but the most significant complication is renal dysfunction, particularly acute renal failure. Clinical symptoms associated with renal dysfunction vary depending on the degree of dysfunction and the timing of its development. In patients with acute renal failure, clinical symptoms may include abnormal mental status, nausea and vomiting, fluid overload, pericarditis, and seizures.

Diagnosis

The diagnosis of hyperuricemia is based on laboratory findings of high serum uric acid levels, hyperuricosuria, and increased serum creatinine and urea nitrogen levels.

Prognosis

Prognosis often depends on the etiology of the hyperuricemia.

Treatment

Prophylactic measures against the development of hyperuricemia should be undertaken prior to the initiation of chemotherapy. Drugs that increase serum urate levels or produce acidic urine (eg, thiazides and salicylates) should be discontinued if possible. Alkalinization of the urine should be initiated to maintain a urine pH > 7.0. Usually, sodium bicarbonate solution (50–100 mmol/L) is added to IV fluids and then adjusted so that an alkaline urinary pH is maintained. The carbonic anhydrase inhibitor acetazolamide (Diamox) may be used to increase the effects of alkalinization. It is important to remember that alkalinization is secondary to the overall goal of decreasing urinary uric acid concentration by increasing urinary volume.

Allopurinol, a xanthine oxidase inhibitor, is the mainstay of drug treatment and may be started 1–2 days prior to cytotoxic treatment. Dosages range from 300–600 mg/d, and therapy is usually continued for 1–2 weeks or until the danger of hyperuricemia has passed.

Rasburicase (Elitek) is an antihyperuricemia drug. It has been approved by the FDA for malignancy-associated hyperuricemia in pediatric patients but is also used in adults. The usual pediatric dose is 0.15 or 0.2 mg/kg IV over 30 minutes for 5 days. The usual adult dosage is 0.15–0.2 mg/kg/d in limited studies.

Acute oliguria In patients who develop acute oliguria, ureteral obstruction by urate calculi should be considered. This condition should be evaluated by ultrasonography or CT. Administration of IV contrast agents for pyelography should be avoided, as they may increase the risk of acute tubular necrosis.

Dialysis Patients with advancing renal insufficiency and subsequent renal failure may benefit from peritoneal dialysis or hemodialysis. Dialysis has been shown to be effective in reversing renal failure caused by urate deposition.

TUMOR LYSIS SYNDROME

Tumor lysis syndrome occurs due to the rapid release of intracellular contents into the bloodstream, leading to life-threatening concentrations. If the resulting metabolic abnormalities remain uncorrected, patients may develop renal failure and sudden death.

Etiology and risk factors

Tumor lysis syndrome most commonly develops during the rapid growth phase of high-grade lymphomas and leukemia in patients with high leukocyte counts; it is less common in patients with solid tumors. The syndrome is often iatrogenic, caused by cytotoxic chemotherapy. Because of clinicians' increased awareness of the tumor lysis syndrome during the past decade and the use of adequate prophylaxis prior to the initiation of chemotherapy, there are fewer cases currently. Occasionally, the syndrome occurs following treatment with irradiation, glucocorticosteroids, tamoxifen, or interferon.

Patients at risk The typical patient at risk for tumor lysis syndrome tends to be young (< 25 years of age) and male and has an advanced disease stage (often with abdominal disease) and a markedly elevated lactic dehydrogenase level.

Other predisposing factors include volume depletion, concentrated acidic urine pH, and excessive urinary uric acid excretion rates.

Signs and symptoms

The syndrome is characterized by hyperuricemia, hyperkalemia, hyperphosphatemia, hypocalcemia, and, often, oliguric renal failure.

Diagnosis

The diagnosis of tumor lysis syndrome is based on the development of increased levels of serum uric acid, phosphorus, and potassium; decreased levels of serum calcium; and renal dysfunction following chemotherapy.

Prognosis

Prognosis varies depending on the adequate correction of metabolic abnormalities and the underlying etiology of tumor lysis.

Treatment

Prophylactic measures Patients at risk for tumor lysis syndrome should be identified before the initiation of chemotherapy and should be adequately hydrated and given agents to alkalinize the urine. Treatment with allopurinol (IV or oral) may be instituted to minimize hyperuricemia. The recommended dosage of IV allopurinol ranges from 200 to 400 mg/m^2/d. This regimen should be started 24–48 hours before the initiation of cytotoxic treatment. The dose may be equally divided into 6-, 8-, or 12-hour increments, but the final concentration should not exceed 6 mg/mL. (For oral dosages of allopurinol and IV doses of rasburicase, see the section on "Hyperuricemia, treatment" earlier in this chapter.)

Serum electrolytes, uric acid, phosphorus, calcium, and creatinine levels should be checked repeatedly for 3–4 days after chemotherapy is initiated, with the frequency of monitoring dependent upon the clinical condition and the risk profile of the patient.

Established tumor lysis Once tumor lysis is established, treatment is directed at vigorous correction of electrolyte abnormalities, hydration, and hemodialysis (as appropriate in patients with renal failure).

SYNDROME OF INAPPROPRIATE SECRETION OF ANTIDIURETIC HORMONE

The syndrome of inappropriate secretion of antidiuretic hormone (SIADH) is a paraneoplastic condition that is associated with malignant tumors (particularly SCLC), CNS disease (eg, infection, intracerebral lesions, head trauma, and subarachnoid hemorrhage), and pulmonary disorders (eg, tuberculosis, pneumonia, and abscess).

Signs and symptoms

Hyponatremia is the most common presenting sign of SIADH. Patients who experience a rapid fall in plasma sodium levels are usually the most symptomatic.

Other presentations Patients with SIADH can also experience malaise,

TABLE 2: Criteria for the diagnosis of SIADH

Criterion	Definition
Hyponatremia	Serum sodium level < 135 mEq/L
Hypo-osmotic plasma	Plasma osmolality < 280 mOsm/kg
Hyper-osmotic urine	Urinary osmolality > 500 mOsm/kg
Hypernatremic urine	Urinary sodium level > 20 mEq/L (without diuretic therapy)

SIADH = syndrome of inappropriate secretion of antidiuretic hormone

altered mental status, seizures, coma, and, occasionally, death. Focal neurologic findings can occur in the absence of brain metastases.

Diagnosis

To make a diagnosis of SIADH, certain criteria must be met (Table 2). In addition to those criteria, patients should have normal renal, adrenal, and thyroid function, along with normal extracellular fluid status.

Drug history It is important to obtain a full list of the medications that the patient is taking, since certain drugs can impair free water excretion either by acting on the renal tubule or by inducing pituitary arginine vasopressin (AVP). These drugs include morphine, cyclophosphamide, vincristine, chlorpropamide (Diabinese), amitriptyline, and clofibrate (Atromid-S).

Treatment

The major focus of treatment for SIADH related to malignancy is successful treatment of the underlying cancer.

Acute treatment is indicated in patients who are symptomatic and who have severe hyponatremia (eg, serum sodium level < 125 mEq/L). The goals of therapy in these patients are to initiate and maintain rapid diuresis with IV furosemide (1 mg/kg body weight) and to replace the sodium and potassium lost in the urine. Usually, the latter goal can be achieved by administering 0.9% saline with added potassium.

This rapid correction should not exceed a 20-mEq/L rise in serum sodium concentration during the first 48 hours. Patients who experience too rapid a rise in serum sodium concentration may suffer neurologic damage and central pontine myelinolysis.

Chronic treatment The mainstay of chronic therapy is water restriction to 500–1,000 mL/d. When this measure alone is unsuccessful, demeclocycline (Declomycin), 300–600 mg orally bid, may be used in patients without liver disease. The onset of action may be > 1 week.

LAMBERT-EATON SYNDROME

The Lambert-Eaton syndrome is strongly associated with SCLC. It is caused by antibodies that interfere with the release of presynaptic acetylcholine at the neuromuscular junction.

Signs and symptoms

Fatigue/muscle weakness This syndrome is characterized by fatigue and proximal muscle weakness, particularly of the pelvic girdle and thighs.

Autonomic symptoms Many patients with this disorder have autonomic symptoms, one of the most common of which is dry mouth.

Other symptoms Other possible symptoms include diplopia or blurred vision, ptosis, dysarthria, dysphagia, and paresthesias.

Diagnosis

Patients with the Lambert-Eaton syndrome show an improvement in muscle strength with exercise.

Electromyographic (EMG) studies are helpful in making the diagnosis. These studies reveal an increase in the muscle action potential with repeated nerve stimulation at rates faster than 10 per second.

Edrophonium test In addition, in contrast to individuals with myasthenia gravis, patients with the Lambert-Eaton syndrome have a poor response to the edrophonium test.

Treatment

Chemotherapy is the first line of treatment, since 90% of patients with SCLC will respond to this measure. In fact, recovery from the Lambert-Eaton syndrome has been noted in some patients treated with chemotherapy.

Other therapies For patients in whom chemotherapy fails to improve symptoms or control the tumor, guanidine has been reported to be useful, as has 3,4-diaminopyridine.

Guanidine is taken orally beginning with a dosage of 5–10 mg/kg/d divided throughout the waking hours. The dosage may be increased to a maximum of 30 mg/kg/d on the basis of the patient's clinical response. However, side effects may be severe at dosages > 1 g/d. Also, the dose of guanidine should not be increased more often than every 3 days, since the maximum response to a dose may not be seen for 2–3 days. At dosages of 5–25 mg 3–4 times per day, 3,4-diaminopyridine can significantly improve symptoms. Side effects of this drug include perioral and acral paresthesias, insomnia, and epigastric distress.

In addition, plasmapheresis, steroids, immunosuppression, and IV gamma globulin are all of potential benefit.

POLYMYOSITIS/DERMATOMYOSITIS

The relationship between polymyositis/dermatomyositis and malignancy was established long ago. The most commonly associated malignancies are breast, lung, and ovarian cancers. An increased incidence of cancer patients with dermatomyositis (10%) has been observed, but the association of cancer with polymyositis is less clear.

Signs and symptoms

Muscle weakness Patients with this syndrome typically experience proximal muscle weakness that progresses over weeks to months. Weakness in the hips, thighs, and shoulder girdle may cause patients to have difficulties in getting out of a chair, climbing stairs, or combing their hair. Patients also may experience dysphagia as well as weakness of the flexor muscles of the neck.

In the majority of cases, the distal muscles of the extremities are not involved. Also, most patients do not have involvement of the extraocular muscles.

Rashes Patients with dermatomyositis can have involvement of the eyelids, forehead, cheeks, chest, elbows, knees, and knuckles with the classic heliotrope rash. A more diffuse rash may also occur.

Diagnosis

Muscle enzymes and erythrocyte sedimentation rate Patients with polymyositis/dermatomyositis usually have an elevation in their serum muscle enzyme levels and erythrocyte sedimentation rate (ESR).

EMG studies and muscle biopsies In addition, EMG tracings are abnormal, and muscle biopsies reveal minimal inflammatory changes, along with muscle fiber necrosis, in patients with polymyositis/dermatomyositis.

Treatment

Steroids In addition to treatment of the underlying malignancy, patients with polymyositis or dermatomyositis are treated with high-dose oral steroids (eg, prednisone, 60–80 mg/d). Other supportive measures, such as range-of-motion exercises, are also prescribed.

Immunosuppressives In patients who do not respond to steroid therapy, immunosuppressive therapy is often added. This type of therapy needs to be tailored to the individual patient, and consultation with a rheumatologist should be considered.

Therapy for skin disease The skin disease of dermatomyositis can be treated with a variety of measures, such as topical corticosteroids, antimalarials, photoprotection, and, at times, low-dose methotrexate.

SUGGESTED READING

ON SUPERIOR VENA CAVA SYNDROME

Mose S, Stabik C, Eberlein K, et al: Retrospective analysis of the superior vena cava syndrome in irradiated cancer patients. Anticancer Res 26:4933–4936, 2006.

Rice TW, Rodriguez RM, Light RW: The superior vena cava syndrome: Clinical characteristics and evolving etiology. Medicine (Baltimore) 85:37–42, 2006.

ON VENOUS THROMBOEMBOLIC COMPLICATIONS

Howell A, Cuzick J, Baum M, et al: Results of the ATAC (Arimidex, Tamoxifen, Alone or in Combination) trial after completion of 5 years' adjuvant treatment for breast cancer. Lancet 365:60–62, 2005.

Chew HK, Wun T, Harvey DJ, et al: Incidence of venous thromboembolism and the impact on survival in breast cancer patients. J Clin Oncol 25:70–76, 2007.

ON SPINAL CORD COMPRESSION

Patchell RA, Tibbs PA, Regine WF, et al: Direct decompressive surgical resection in the treatment of spinal cord compression caused by metastatic cancer: A randomised trial. Lancet 366:643–648, 2005.

Rades D, Stalpers LJ, Veninga T, et al: Evaluation of five radiation schedules and prognostic factors for metastatic spinal cord compression. J Clin Oncol 23:3366–3375, 2005.

Rades D, Veninga T, Stalpers LJ, et al: Outcome after radiotherapy alone for metastatic spinal cord compression in patients with oligometastases. J Clin Oncol 25:50–56, 2007.

ON HYPERCALCEMIA

Cvitkovic F, Armand JP, Tubiana-Hulin M, et al: Randomized, double-blind, phase II trial of gallium nitrate compared with pamidronate for acute control of cancer-related hypercalcemia. Cancer J 12:47–53, 2006.

ON HYPERURICEMIA/TUMOR LYSIS SYNDROME

Jeha S, Kantarjian H, Irwin D, et al: Efficacy and safety of rasburicase, a recombinant urate oxidase (Elitek), in the management of malignancy-associated hyperuricemia in pediatric and adult patients: Final results of a multicenter compassionate use trial. Leukemia 19:34–38, 2005.

ON SYNDROME OF INAPPROPRIATE SECRETION OF ANTIDIURETIC HORMONE

Flombaum CD: Metabolic emergencies in the cancer patient. Semin Oncol 27:322–334, 2000.

Raftopoulos H: Diagnosis and management of hyponatremia in cancer patients. Support Care Cancer 15:1341–1347, 2007.

ON LAMBERT-EATON SYNDROME

Dropcho EJ: Remote neurologic manifestations of cancer. Neurol Clin 20:85–122, 2002.

Wirtz PW, Smallegange TM, Wintzen AR, et al: Differences in clinical features between the Lambert-Eaton myasthenic syndrome with and without cancer: An analysis of 227 published cases. Clin Neurol Neurosurg 104:359–363, 2002.

ON POLYMYOSITIS/DERMATOMYOSITIS

Sparsa A, Liozon E, Herrmann F, et al: Routine vs extensive malignancy search for adult dermatomyositis and polymyositis: A study of 40 patients. Arch Dermatol 138:885–890, 2002.

Wakata N, Kurihara T, Saito E, et al: Polymyositis and dermatomyositis associated with malignancy: A 30-year retrospective study. Int J Dermatol 41:729–734, 2002.

CHAPTER 45

Infectious complications

James Ito, Jr., MD

Infections are among the most common, potentially serious complications of cancer and its treatment. This chapter discusses infections from a syndromic approach: that is, infections present as a complex of signs and symptoms to the clinician. The syndromes addressed include febrile neutropenia, pneumonia, catheter-associated infections, and gastrointestinal infections (*Clostridium difficile*-associated diarrhea and typhlitis). Special sections focus on fungal and viral infections.

INFECTION DURING FEBRILE NEUTROPENIA

It has long been recognized that the incidence of infection is high in patients who develop a fever during neutropenia and that empiric antimicrobial therapy is warranted in such patients.

Definitions

Fever is usually defined as a temperature $\geq 38.3°C$.

Neutropenia is defined as a neutrophil count of $500/\mu L$, although patients with a neutrophil count between 500 and $1,000/\mu L$ in whom a decrease is anticipated are considered to be neutropenic. Patients with a neutrophil count $< 100/\mu L$ are at greatest risk for infection, as are those with a rapid decrease in neutrophil count and those with protracted neutropenia.

Etiology

Bacteria Infections occurring during episodes of febrile neutropenia are caused predominantly by aerobic gram-negative bacilli (especially *Escherichia coli, Klebsiella pneumoniae,* and *Pseudomonas aeruginosa*) and gram-positive cocci (coagulase-negative staphylococci, β-hemolytic streptococci, viridans streptococci, enterococci, and *Staphylococcus aureus*). In recent years, gram-positive infections have become more prominent with the increasing use of indwelling IV catheters.

Fungi Fungal infections usually occur after a patient has received broad-spectrum antimicrobial therapy and/or steroids. The most common fungal pathogens are *Candida* species (predominantly *C albicans* and *C tropicalis*) and

Aspergillus species. Less common are *Fusarium, Scedosporium,* and *Zygomycetes* infections (see also section on "Fungal infections").

Viruses Viral infections occurring during neutropenia are caused predominantly by herpesviruses and respiratory viruses. The herpesviruses include herpes simplex virus (HSV), varicella zoster virus (VZV), cytomegalovirus (CMV), and Epstein-Barr virus (EBV). The respiratory viruses include adenovirus, respiratory syncytial virus, parainfluenza virus, influenza A and B viruses, and rhinovirus (see also section on "Viral infections").

Signs and symptoms

The most remarkable aspect of the febrile, neutropenic patient is the lack of physical findings. This is due to the neutropenia and the absence of an inflammatory response at the infection site. The patient may have only a fever with or without chills or rigors. Even if the patient has pneumonia, there may be few respiratory symptoms. Likewise, a perirectal abscess may be relatively asymptomatic.

Diagnosis

An initial evaluation and diagnostic work-up of any fever in a neutropenic patient should begin immediately but should not delay the initiation of empiric therapy (see below). A complete history (exposures, past infections, rashes, cough, abdominal pain, diarrhea) should be taken and a physical examination (skin lesions, exit site and tunnel of right atrial catheter, oropharynx, abdomen, perineum) should be performed.

Diagnostic work-up should include:

- at least two sets of blood cultures: one from a peripheral vein and one from each port of a central venous catheter. If fever persists in the face of negative cultures, blood cultures for fungi and acid-fast bacilli should be considered.
- culture of any drainage from a catheter exit site
- stool examination for *C difficile* and other bacterial/protozoal agents
- urine culture and urinalysis
- chest radiograph
- aspiration or biopsy of any skin lesions.

CT If indicated by signs or symptoms, CT scans of the brain (followed by lumbar puncture), chest, abdomen, and pelvis can be performed.

Laboratory tests Determination of serum transaminases, CBC, and serum creatinine is also recommended.

Treatment

INITIAL EMPIRIC ANTIBIOTIC THERAPY

Initial antibacterial therapy in the febrile, neutropenic patient should be broad-spectrum and should be based on the prevalence and susceptibility of bacterial isolates seen in the individual hospital setting (Figure 1). When choosing an antibiotic, the clinician also should take into consideration the patient's allergies, renal and hepatic function, and other drugs he or she is receiving that may interact with the empiric antimicrobial agent.

The choice of initial empiric antibiotic therapy for the febrile, neutropenic patient is dictated in part by the susceptibility pattern of blood isolates seen at a particular cancer center. If the prevalence of extended-spectrum beta-lactamase (ESBL) gram-negative bacteria is high, for example, one probably would not want to use a third-generation cephalosporin such as ceftazidime as initial empiric monotherapy. (Some data suggest that prolonged use of ceftazidime monotherapy in this setting promotes the emergence of ESBL bacteria.) City of Hope has been using ceftazidime as initial monotherapy for the past 15 years, however, without a significant rise in the incidence of resistant gram-negative infections, and this experience has been shared by other centers. Finally, any special circumstance, such as the suspicion of an indwelling IV catheter-associated infection, may influence the antibiotic choice.

Either single antibiotics or antibiotic combinations can be used for initial empiric therapy (see Table 1 for dosage regimens).

Monotherapy

Ceftazidime, cefepime (Maxipime), imipenem-cilastatin (Primaxin), or meropenem (Merrem), when used as monotherapy, avoids the potential for nephrotoxicity. However, none of these antibiotics covers coagulase-negative staphylococci, methicillin-resistant *S aureus* (MRSA), vancomycin-resistant or vancomycin-susceptible enterococci, some strains of penicillin-resistant *Streptococcus pneumoniae,* and viridans streptococci. Also, ceftazidime does not cover anaerobes well, and imipenem-cilastatin may have CNS toxicity at high doses.

Duotherapy

Aminoglycoside plus antipseudomonal β-lactam The aminoglycoside could be gentamicin, tobramycin, or amikacin (Amikin). The β-lactam could be ticarcillin (Ticar) or piperacillin (Pipracil), either alone or with a β-lactamase inhibitor (piperacillin/tazobactam [Zosyn]); mezlocillin (Mezlin); ceftazidime; or cefoperazone (Cefobid).

Advantages of the combination of an aminoglycoside and an antipseudomonal β-lactam include possible synergistic effects against gram-negative bacilli and decreased emergence of resistant strains. The major disadvantages of the combination are potential nephrotoxicity, ototoxicity, hypokalemia, and the need to monitor drug levels of the aminoglycoside. Also, gram-positive coverage is not ideal.

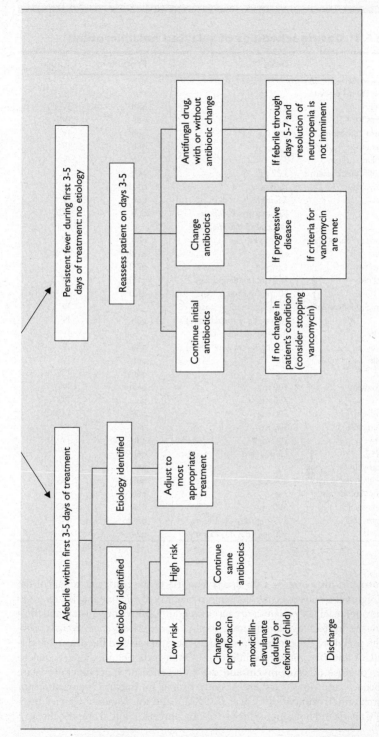

FIGURE 1: Guide to the initial management of the febrile neutropenic patient

Adapted, with permission, from Hughes WT, et al: 2002 guidelines for the use of antimicrobial agents in neutropenic patients with cancer. Clin Infect Dis 34:730-751, 2002.

TABLE 1: Dosing schedules of selected antimicrobials

Drug	Dose	Frequency	Route
Antibacterial agents			
Ceftazidime	2 g	q8h	IV
Cefepime	2 g	q8h	IV
Imipenem-cilastatin	500 mg	q6h	IV
Meropenem	1 g	q8h	IV
Piperacillin sodium	3 g	q4h	IV
Piperacillin/tazobactam	3.375 g	q6h	IV
Vancomycin	15 mg/kg	q12h	IV
	7.5 mg/kg	q6h	IV
	125 mg (for *C difficile*-associated diarrhea)	q6h	PO
Quinupristin/dalfopristin	7.5 mg/kg	q8h	IV
Linezolid	600 mg	q12h	IV/PO
Daptomycin	4 mg/kg	q24h	IV
Tigecycline	100 mg (loading dose)	q12h	IV
	50 mg (maintenance)	q12h	IV
Gentamicin/tobramycin	2 mg/kg (loading dose)		IV
	1.5 mg/kg (maintenance)	q8h	IV
Amikacin	8 mg/kg (loading dose)		IV
	7.5 mg/kg (maintenance)	q8h	IV
Cefazolin	2 g	q6h	IV
Nafcillin	2 g	q4h	IV
Ciprofloxacin	400 mg	q12h	IV
	750 mg	bid	PO
Levofloxacin	500 mg	q24h	IV/PO
Metronidazole	500 mg	q6h	IV
Clindamycin	900 mg	q8h	IV
TMP-SMZ	15 mg/kg/d	q6h	IV
Erythromycin	1 g	q6h	IV
Amoxicillin/clavulanate	500 mg	q8h	PO
Ampicillin/sulbactam	3 g	q6h	IV
Clarithromycin	500 mg	bid	PO
Azithromycin	500 mg (day 1), 250 mg	q24h	PO
	500 mg (day 1), 250 mg	q24h	IV

Vancomycin plus one or two drugs The use of vancomycin as part of the initial regimen is controversial. Certainly, a majority of documented bacteremias in neutropenic febrile patients are caused by gram-positive organisms, and most of them are due to coagulase-negative staphylococci. Also, vancomycin is probably the preferred drug for viridans streptococcal sepsis and the drug of choice for MRSA and *Corynebacterium* infections. On the other hand, there is concern for the overuse of vancomycin and the emergence of vancomycin-resistant enterococci (and now *S aureus*). A study by the European Organization for Research and Treatment of Cancer (EORTC) and the National Cancer Institute of Canada did not support the use of vancomycin in initial empiric therapy.

Drug	Dose	Frequency	Route
Antifungal agents			
Amphotericin B			
Therapy	0.5-1.0 mg/kg	daily	IV
Prophylaxis	0.1-0.2 mg/kg	daily	IV
Fluconazole	400 mg	daily	IV or PO
Itraconazole capsules	200 mg (loading dose)	tid × 4 d	PO
	200 mg (maintenance)	bid	PO
Itraconazole oral solution	(see capsules above)		
Itraconazole injection	200 mg (loading dose)	bid × 4 doses	IV
	200 mg (maintenance)	daily	IV
Amphotericin B			
Lipid complex	5 mg/kg	daily	IV
Cholesteryl sulfate	3-6 mg/kg	daily	IV
Liposome	3-5 mg/kg	daily	IV
Caspofungin	70 mg (loading dose)		IV
	50 mg (maintenance)	daily	IV
Voriconazole	6 mg/kg (loading dose) × 2	q12h	IV
	4 mg/kg (maintenance)	q12h	IV
	200 mg (maintenance) for > 40 kg	q12h	PO
	100 mg (maintenance) for ≤ 40 kg	q12h	PO
Micafungin	50 mg (for prophylaxis)	q24h	IV
	150 mg (treatment)	q24h	IV
Anidulafungin	200 mg (loading dose)		IV
	100 mg (maintenance)	daily	IV
Posaconazole	200 mg (prophylaxis)	tid	PO
	400 mg (treatment)	bid	PO
Antiviral agents			
Acyclovir			
For HSV	5 mg/kg	q8h	IV
For VZV	10 mg/kg	q8h	IV
For HSV encephalitis	15 mg/kg	q8h	IV
Ganciclovir	5 mg/kg (induction)	q12h	IV
	5 mg/kg (maintenance)	daily	IV
Valganciclovir	900 mg (induction)	q12h	PO
Foscarnet	60 mg/kg (induction)	q8h	IV for 14 d
	90 mg/kg (maintenance)	daily	IV
Cidofovir	5 mg/kg	q wk × 2	IV
	then	q2wk	
	or 1 mg/kg	qod	IV
Amantadine, rimantadine	100 mg	bid	PO
Zanamivir	5 mg	bid	inhalation
Oseltamivir	75 mg	bid	PO

HSV = herpes simplex virus; TMP-SMZ = trimethoprim-sulfamethoxazole; VZV = varicella zoster virus

It should be noted that the Centers for Disease Control and Prevention (CDC) advises against the use of vancomycin in initial empiric therapy for a febrile, neutropenic patient "unless initial evidence indicates that the patient has an infection caused by gram-positive micro-organisms (eg, at an inflamed exit site of a Hickman catheter) and the prevalence of infections caused by MRSA in the hospital is substantial."

Thus, it is recommended (in the 2002 guidelines for the use of antimicrobial agents in neutropenic patients with unexplained fever developed by the Infectious Diseases Society of America) that vancomycin be added to the initial regimen (eg, with ceftazidime) in selected patients, including:

- patients with clinically obvious, serious catheter-related infections

- patients undergoing intensive chemotherapy that produces substantial mucosal damage (ie, high-dose cytarabine [Ara-C], which increases the risk of penicillin-resistant streptococcal infections, particularly those due to viridans streptococci)

- patients receiving prophylaxis with quinolones before the onset of the febrile episode

- patients who have known colonization with pneumococci that are resistant to penicillin and cephalosporins or MRSA

- patients with a blood culture positive for gram-positive bacteria before final identification and susceptibility testing

- patients with hypotension or other evidence of cardiovascular impairment.

Double β-lactam therapy usually consists of a third-generation cephalosporin (ceftazidime or cefoperazone) and a ureidopenicillin (piperacillin, ticarcillin, or mezlocillin). The advantages of this regimen are low toxicity (mainly renal) and theoretical synergism. However, it is more costly (compared with monotherapy) and has the possibility of antagonism.

CHANGES IN INITIAL THERAPY

Defervescence If the fever subsides after 3 days of empiric therapy and a specific organism is identified, broad-spectrum antibiotic coverage can be modified to provide optimal treatment. Antibiotics can be discontinued after 7 days if all evidence of infection has been eradicated.

If no organism is isolated, treatment with the initial regimen should be continued for a minimum of 7 days. If the patient is clinically well, the regimen can be switched to an oral antibiotic, such as cefixime (Suprax) or a quinolone.

Persistent, unresponsive fever If the fever persists after 4-7 days of antibiotic therapy, reassessment is recommended. If no infectious etiology is determined, a change in or addition to the antibiotic regimen is recommended.

If vancomycin was not part of the initial empiric regimen, many physicians would consider adding it. However, because of the recent recommendation by the CDC against empiric vancomycin use, it probably should not be added unless there is a strong clinical or microbiologic reason to do so. Instead, cefazolin or nafcillin could be added for better gram-positive coverage. If the initial regimen did not provide anaerobic coverage, metronidazole could be added. Finally, if fever and neutropenia persist despite 3-5 days of antibiotic therapy, an antifungal agent (caspofungin [Cancidas], liposomal amphotericin B [AmBisome], amphotericin B lipid complex [Abelcet], itraconazole [Sporanox], voriconazole [Vfend]), or even fluconazole ([Diflucan] if the risk of

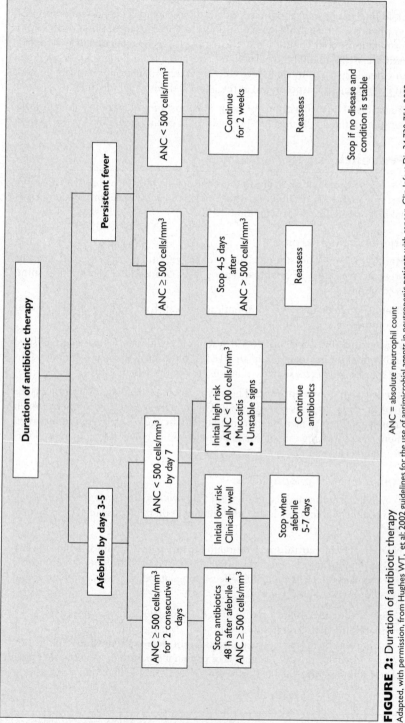

FIGURE 2: Duration of antibiotic therapy ANC = absolute neutrophil count

- Adapted, with permission, from Hughes WT, et al: 2002 guidelines for the use of antimicrobial agents in neutropenic patients with cancer. Clin Infect Dis 34:730-751, 2002.

mold infection is low) should be added. If the patient is already on antifungal prophylaxis with an azole or echinocandin, a polyene (an amphotericin B lipid formulation) should be started. If the patient is receiving a polyene as prophylaxis, the dose should be escalated, or, alternatively, a change can be made to an extended-spectrum azole (eg, voriconazole). Another alternative is to add an echinocandin (caspofungin) to the increased dosage of the polyene.

Duration of antimicrobial therapy The most important determinant of the duration of therapy is the absolute neutrophil count (Figure 2).

Prevention

Attempts to prevent infection in the neutropenic host focus on two broad areas: preventing acquisition of pathogenic organisms and suppressing or eradicating endogenous microbial flora.

Hygienic measures

Hand-washing The simplest, most effective, and least expensive way to prevent acquisition of potential pathogens is to institute strict hand-washing precautions.

Diet A cooked diet with elimination of fresh fruit and vegetables is also recommended.

Water and air Water purification systems (to eliminate *Legionella* organisms) and high-efficiency particulate air (HEPA) filtration systems (to eliminate fungal spores) can decrease rates of acquisition of these pathogens.

"Protective" environments The use of more "protective" environments for neutropenic patients is controversial. The total protective environment, which consists of a totally sterile environment and an aggressive antimicrobial regimen, can reduce the rate of infection but does not contribute to increased survival and is also costly.

Antibacterial prophylaxis

Prophylactic antibacterial therapy generally falls into three categories: oral nonabsorbable antibiotics, selective decontamination regimens, and systemic prophylaxis.

Nonabsorbable antibiotics Although the use of oral nonabsorbable antibiotics has demonstrated some reduction in infection rates, this option has become less popular due to its cost, side effects, unpalatability, poor compliance, and selection of resistant organisms.

Selective decontamination with trimethoprim-sulfamethoxazole (TMP-SMZ), ie, establishment of "colonization resistance" by preserving anaerobic flora while reducing aerobic bacteria, has not resulted in clear-cut reductions in infection rates. Moreover, the disadvantages of prolonged neutropenia and emergence of resistant organisms make this regimen less desirable than others.

Fluoroquinolones More recently, many studies have touted the value of anti-bacterial prophylaxis with fluoroquinolones (eg, ciprofloxacin [Cipro], ofloxacin [Floxin], and levofloxacin [Levaquin]) in neutropenic patients. However, no single study (except for a meta-analysis of 52 trials) has demonstrated a survival advantage. Thus, neither the National Comprehensive Cancer Network (NCCN) nor the Infectious Diseases Society of America (IDSA) guidelines recommend using antibacterial prophylaxis in neutropenic patients. The NCCN guideline recommends that bacterial prophylaxis (fluoroquinolones) be considered for high-risk patients (neutropenia < 100 μL for ≥ 7 days). Despite this lack of a strong recommendation, fluoroquinolone (mainly levofloxacin) prophylaxis is widely used at many cancer centers; the obvious downside of this trend is the emergence of resistant bacteria, which has already been observed in many institutions. Levofloxacin use has also been associated with the emergence of hypervirulent *C difficile* enterocolitis.

Pneumocystis carinii pneumonia In patients at risk for *P carinii* pneumonia (patients undergoing allogeneic hematopoietic cell transplantation [HCT], those with lymphoma, or those receiving steroids), TMP-SMZ, administered for only 2 or 3 days per week, can reduce the incidence of infection.

Antifungal prophylaxis

Fluconazole, itraconazole, micafungin (Mycamine), and posaconazole have all been shown to lower the incidence of invasive fungal infection when used as prophylaxis in the HCT setting. In a retrospective study, low-dose conventional amphotericin B has also been associated with a lower incidence of infection. Fluconazole, however, has no activity against molds. Itraconazole is limited by its gastrointestinal and hepatic toxicities. Posaconazole has been shown to prevent both *Candida* and *Aspergillus* infections in both neutropenic AML (acute myelogenous leukemia) and MDS (myelodysplastic syndrome) patients and the high-risk allogeneic HCT recipient with graft versus host disease (GVHD). Antifungal prophylaxis should be reserved for those patients at highest risk for invasive fungal infection—ie, HCT and high-risk leukemia patients undergoing high-dose chemotherapy (see also "Prevention" section under "Fungal infections").

Antiviral prophylaxis

Acyclovir Patients at risk for mucositis (ie, those undergoing induction therapy for leukemia or lymphoma or HCT) who have evidence of prior HSV infection (positive serology) can receive prophylaxis with twice-daily IV acyclovir (see Table 1 for dose).

The approach of using preemptive therapy in CMV infection/disease was developed because using the marrow-toxic antiviral agent ganciclovir as prophylaxis resulted in reduced survival rates due to more opportunistic infections, especially invasive fungal infections. A non-marrow-toxic antiviral would avoid this problem and could be used as effective prophylaxis. That ideal drug may be maribavir. In a phase II study, maribavir, used as prophylaxis in allogeneic HCT, prevented viremia in 80%–90% of patients and prevented CMV interstitial pneumonitis in all patients *(Blood 108:abstract 593, 2006).*

TABLE 2: Altered host defenses and associated respiratory pathogens in immunocompromised patients with cancer

Granulocytopenia

Gram-negative bacilli: *Pseudomonas aeruginosa, Klebsiella pneumoniae, Escherichia coli, Enterobacter* species

Gram-positive cocci: *Staphylococcus aureus, Staphylococcus epidermidis,* group D streptococci, α-hemolytic streptococci

Gram-positive bacilli: *Bacillus* species, *Clostridium* species

Fungi: *Aspergillus* species, *Zygomycetes, Fusarium* species, *Trichosporon beigelii, Candida* species, *Torulopsis glabrata*

Cellular (T-lymphocyte) immune defects

Bacteria: *Mycobacterium* species, *Nocardia asteroides, Legionella* species, *Listeria monocytogenes, Salmonella* species

Viruses: Cytomegalovirus, varicella zoster virus, herpes simplex virus, Epstein-Barr virus

Protozoa: *Pneumocystis carinii, Toxoplasma gondii*

Fungi: *Cryptococcus neoformans, Histoplasma capsulatum, Coccidioides immitis*

Helminths: *Strongyloides stercoralis*

Humoral (B-lymphocyte) immune deficiency

Bacteria: *Streptococcus pneumoniae, Haemophilus influenzae*

Impaired tracheobronchial clearance

Bacteria and fungi colonizing the lower respiratory tract

Invasive procedures: Mechanical disruption of epithelial barriers

Bacteria and fungi colonizing the respiratory tract and skin

Altered neurologic function

Bacteria and fungi colonizing the oropharynx and upper respiratory tract

Adapted, with permission, from Walsh TJ, Rubin R, Pizzo PA: Respiratory diseases in patients with malignant neoplasms, in Shelhamer J, Pizzo PA, Parillo JE, et al (eds): Respiratory Disease in the Immunosuppressed Host, p 640. Philadelphia, JB Lippincott, 1991.

Ganciclovir has been shown to be an effective "preemptive" antiviral in preventing CMV interstitial pneumonia in allogeneic HCT recipients who demonstrate evidence of viremia by polymerase chain reaction (PCR), antigen testing, or positive blood cultures (see section on "Viral infections").

PNEUMONIA

A significant number of infections in cancer patients are due to pneumonia. For example, 25% of documented infections in patients with nonlymphocytic leukemia are caused by pneumonia. Also, 50% of allogeneic HCT recipients will develop pneumonia.

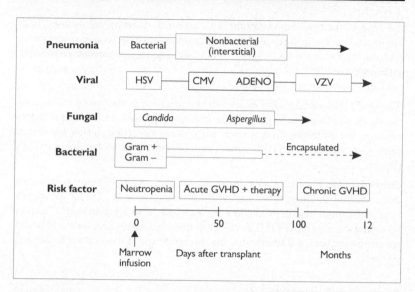

FIGURE 3: Timing of infectious syndromes after bone marrow transplantation

ADENO = adenovirus; CMV = cytomegalovirus; GVHD = graft-vs-host disease; HSV = herpes simplex
virus; VZV = varicella zoster virus

Adapted, with permission, from Meyers JD: Infections in marrow recipients, in Mandell GL, Doublas RG,
Bennett JE (eds): Principles and Practice of Infectious Diseases, 2nd ed, pp 1674-1676. New York,
Wiley, 1985.

Etiology and risk factors

Some of the risk factors that predispose cancer patients to pneumonia are cellular and humoral immune deficiencies, neutropenia, impaired tracheobronchial clearance, use of antibiotics and steroids, and surgery.

Etiologic agents The etiologic agents responsible for pneumonia in the cancer patient run the gamut of most bacterial, fungal, and viral organisms.

Noninfectious processes mimicking pneumonia Numerous noninfectious processes can mimic pneumonia in cancer patients. They include congestive heart failure, aseptic emboli, metastatic disease, adult respiratory distress syndrome, hemorrhage, radiation injury, hypersensitivity disorders and reactions, and trauma.

Pinpointing the pathogen Certain characteristics of each cancer patient may help predict the specific etiologic agent.

Type of immunosuppression One characteristic that is particularly useful is the type of immunosuppression that the patient is experiencing. This depends on the type of neoplastic disease (eg, lymphoma, leukemia) and, more importantly, the type of therapy (eg, chemotherapy, radiation therapy, allogeneic HCT). For example, certain gram-negative and gram-positive bacteria are more prevalent during neutropenia, whereas other bacteria (*S pneumoniae, Haemophilus influenzae*) are more common with a humoral immune deficiency, such as occurs after splenectomy (see Table 2).

Timing of pneumonia Another important characteristic is the timing of the pneumonia; in other words, the phase of the immunosuppression can help predict the etiology. For example, an interstitial pneumonia occurring during the first 30 days after allogeneic HCT would not be expected to be due to CMV (Figure 3).

Other factors Finally, other factors such as the duration of neutropenia, prior antimicrobial therapy, other agents (such as steroids) used, and the specific local microbiota help in prediction. For example, if an allogeneic HCT patient receiving steroids for GVHD develops nodular infiltrates after weeks of broad-spectrum antibacterial antibiotics, an *Aspergillus* species would be highly suspected.

Signs and symptoms

Cough Although a productive cough is almost always present in a normal host with pneumonia, often neither a cough nor sputum is seen in an immunocompromised cancer patient with such an infection.

Fever, however, is almost invariably present in the cancer patient with pneumonia and, by itself, should prompt a work-up for pneumonia.

Other possible symptoms include shortness of breath, pleuritic chest pain, and hemoptysis.

Diagnosis

Because pneumonia can progress rapidly and result in high morbidity and mortality in the compromised host, and because the etiologic agent is often difficult to ascertain, the clinician needs to be aggressive in diagnosing and treating these infections.

The diagnosis of pneumonia is most commonly made by a simple chest radiograph. However, there are rare occasions when a pulmonary infiltrate or small nodular lesion is seen only on a CT scan.

Etiologic diagnosis

An etiologic diagnosis is made by the following procedures: sputum (expectorated or induced), bronchoscopy with bronchoalveolar lavage and transbronchial biopsy, transthoracic needle biopsy/aspiration, and open lung biopsy.

Sputum An adequate sputum specimen is difficult to obtain from cancer patients, especially during neutropenia.

Bronchoscopy with bronchoalveolar lavage is a much more sensitive technique than sputum analysis but may miss the organism when the pulmonary disease is peripheral or nodular.

Transthoracic needle biopsy/aspiration under CT guidance may be helpful if the lesion is proximal but may be contraindicated in a severely thrombocytopenic patient. This procedure is indicated when there is a focal/nodular lesion in the periphery.

Open lung biopsy is the most definitive diagnostic procedure but also the most invasive. It is still not clear whether the information obtained by open biopsy improves overall survival. The less invasive thoracoscopic open lung biopsy is becoming more popular than open lung biopsy.

Smears and cultures Both fluid and tissue specimens should be sent for bacterial smears (including acid-fast bacilli and modified acid-fast bacilli) and cultures (including those for anaerobes, acid-fast bacilli, and *Legionella* organisms), fungal smears (potassium hydroxide) and cultures, cytology (for viral inclusions and silver stains for fungi and *P carinii*), and histopathology.

Treatment

The therapeutic approach to pneumonia in the cancer patient should take into consideration the category of immunosuppression (neoplastic disease and immunosuppressive therapy), as well as the timing of onset and pattern of the pneumonia.

EMPIRIC ANTIBIOTIC THERAPY

In neutropenic patients experiencing their first fever and localized pulmonary infiltrates, one can justify initiating empiric therapy similar to that used for febrile, neutropenic patients (see previous discussion), since the majority of pneumonias in this setting are caused by gram-negative bacteria. However, in other situations, such as pneumonia that has a later onset, develops after empiric antibiotics have been initiated, is more aggressive or severe, occurs in a more severely compromised host (eg, a patient who has had allogeneic HCT), or is characterized by a diffuse or interstitial infiltrate, one should proceed to immediate bronchoscopy with bronchoalveolar lavage (and possibly transbronchial biopsy).

ADDITIONS TO EMPIRIC THERAPY

If no diagnosis is forthcoming after bronchoscopy and bronchoalveolar lavage, additions to empiric therapy should be made.

Anaerobic, gram-positive, and *Legionella* coverage Certainly, anaerobic coverage should be considered, as well as gram-positive coverage. *Legionella* coverage should be added, especially if warranted by the epidemiologic setting.

Antifungal and antituberculous therapy Finally, antifungal therapy should be initiated if there is no response to antibacterial therapy and especially if

TABLE 3: Probable causes of and treatments for pulmonary infiltrates in granulocytopenic patients

Pattern of infiltrate	Probable organisms	Treatment
Localized		
Early[a]	*Klebsiella* species, other Enterobacteriaceae, *Pseudomonas aeruginosa*	Empiric antibacterial therapy
Refractory[b]	Resistant Enterobacteriaceae and resistant *P aeruginosa*	Modify according to susceptibility
	Pseudomonas maltophilia	
	Pneumocystis carinii[c]	TMP-SMZ
	Legionella species[c]	Macrolide (clarithromycin, azithromycin) with or without rifampin
	Mycoplasma species	Macrolide (clarithromycin, azithromycin)
	Mycobacterium tuberculosis[c]	Isoniazid, rifampin, and pyrazinamide
	Nocardia asteroides[c]	TMP-SMZ, minocycline, imipenem
	Cryptococcus neoformans[c]	Amphotericin B formulation
	Histoplasma capsulatum[d]	Amphotericin B formulation
	Aspergillus species[e]	Voriconazole, amphotericin B formulation, caspofungin, itraconazole[f]
Late[a,b]	*Aspergillus* species	Voriconazole, amphotericin B formulation, caspofungin, itraconazole[f]
	P carinii[c]	TMP-SMZ
	Trichosporon beigelii	Amphotericin B formulation[f]
	Scedosporium	Amphotericin B formulation, voriconazole
	Fusarium species	Amphotericin B formulation[f]
	Zygomycetes	Amphotericin B formulation
	Candida species	Amphotericin B formulation, fluconazole, itraconazole, caspofungin, voriconazole
	Resistant Enterobacteriaceae and resistant *P aeruginosa*	Modify according to susceptibility
	Xanthomonas maltophilia	TMP-SMZ
	Legionella species[c]	Macrolide (clarithromycin, azithromycin)

there are nodular or cavitary lesions. In addition, if such lesions are present and/or the epidemiologic setting is compatible, antituberculous therapy should be added.

Further diagnostic procedures If bronchoscopy with bronchoalveolar lavage does not reveal an etiology and the pneumonia is progressing despite empiric therapy, consideration should be given to transthoracic needle biopsy/aspiration and open lung biopsy. As mentioned previously, if there is a peripheral, focal lesion, transthoracic needle biopsy/aspiration can be attempted.

The ultimate diagnostic procedure is open biopsy, but because its contribution to increased survival is unknown, the decision to proceed with this most invasive procedure must be undertaken carefully.

Pattern of infiltrate	Probable organisms	Treatment
Late	N asteroides[c]	TMP-SMZ, minocycline, imipenem
	M tuberculosis[c]	Isoniazid, rifampin, and pyrazinamide
	H capsulatum[d]	Amphotericin B formulation
	Coccidioides immitis[d]	Amphotericin B formulation
Diffuse	P carinii[c]	TMP-SMZ
	Legionella species[c]	Macrolide (clarithromycin, azithromycin) with or without rifampin
	Chlamydia pneumoniae	Macrolide (clarithromycin, azithromycin) or tetracycline
	M tuberculosis[c]	Isoniazid plus rifampin
	H capsulatum[d]	Amphotericin B formulation
	Strongyloides stercoralis[d]	Thiabendazole
	Cytomegalovirus	Ganciclovir plus IV immune globulin, foscarnet
	If diagnostic procedure is not possible	Empiric therapy with macrolide and TMP-SMZ

TMP-SMZ = trimethoprim-sulfamethoxazole

Adapted, with permission, from Walsh TJ, Pizzo PA: Ann Intern Med 117:424–428,1992.

[a] The terms "early" and "late" refer to the time of development of pulmonary infiltrates during the course of granulocytopenia.

[b] Serial chest radiographs and, where appropriate, a baseline and follow-up CT scan of refractory and late focal infiltrates are recommended.

[c] Granulocytopenic patients who have concomitant defective cell-mediated immunity or who are receiving corticosteroids are at particularly high risk for these infections.

[d] Granulocytopenic patients from endemic areas who have concomitant defective cell-mediated immunity or who are receiving corticosteroids are at particularly high risk for these infections.

[e] Granulocytopenic patients with a previous episode of pulmonary aspergillosis have a high risk of developing recurrent pulmonary aspergillosis early in the course of subsequent cytotoxic chemo-therapy.

[f] These pulmonary fungal infections often develop in patients who are already receiving empiric amphotericin B (0.5 mg/kg/d). These pulmonary mycoses may be more responsive to higher doses of amphotericin B (1.0-1.5 mg/kg/d). Refractory infections may require investigational antifungal triazoles or lipid formulations of amphotericin B, depending on the organism.

SPECIFIC ANTIMICROBIAL THERAPY

The specific antimicrobial therapy suggested for each etiology is listed in Table 3.

Prevention

Methods to prevent pulmonary infections fall into the following categories: colonization prevention, antimicrobial prophylaxis (and preemptive treatment), vaccination, and immunomodulation.

Hand-washing The simplest method of colonization prevention is hand-washing.

Other colonization prevention methods, such as protective environments, are discussed in the previous section.

Air and water With regard to pulmonary pathogens, HEPA-filtered rooms can eliminate *Aspergillus* spores from the immediate environment. Water supplies can be checked for *Legionella* contamination and/or adequate disinfection maintained (eg, chlorination, copper/silver ionization, temperature [60°C]).

Antimicrobial prophylaxis is discussed in the previous section.

Active immunization The influenza and pneumococcal (killed) vaccines should be administered to cancer patients.

Immunomodulation Immunomodulators, such as granulocyte colony-stimulating factor (G-CSF, filgrastim [Neupogen]) and granulocyte-macrophage colony-stimulating factor (GM-CSF, sargramostim [Leukine]), may help reduce infection by decreasing the duration of neutropenia. (For more on growth factors, see chapter 40.)

CATHETER–ASSOCIATED INFECTIONS

Chronic indwelling right atrial catheters are commonly placed in cancer patients, as they permit frequent, long-term vascular access for drug and blood product administration, hyperalimentation, and blood drawing.

Hickman and Broviac catheters have an exit site on the skin surface, are anchored with a subcutaneous Dacron felt cuff, and have a subcutaneous tunnel entering the venous system (via the subclavian, external jugular, internal jugular, cephalic, saphenous, or femoral veins), where they lead into the superior or inferior vena cava or right atrium. These catheters can have single, double, or triple lumens. Another type of catheter has a totally implanted port (Port-A-Cath) that is accessed percutaneously.

There are four types of catheter-associated infections: exit-site infections, tunnel infections, catheter-associated bacteremia/fungemia, and septic thrombophlebitis.

There are approximately 0.4 infections per 100 catheter-days and 0.26 bacteremias per 100 catheter-days.

Etiology

It is assumed that catheter-associated infections are caused by tracking of organisms from the skin along the catheter, contamination of the lumen during manipulation, or direct seeding during bacteremia/fungemia.

Staphylococci By far, the most common micro-organisms associated with catheter-associated infections are coagulase-negative staphylococci. The next most common pathogen is coagulase-positive *S aureus*.

Less common pathogens include gram-negative bacilli, gram-positive bacilli (such as *Corynebacterium* JK and *Bacillus* species), fungi (especially *Candida* species), and rapidly growing mycobacteria.

Signs and symptoms

Exit-site infections may be manifested by local erythema, warmth, and tenderness. Purulent drainage may be present.

Tunnel infections are characterized by tenderness along the subcutaneous track.

Catheter-associated bacteremia/fungemia usually displays no local findings. A fever may be the only sign, but other signs and symptoms of sepsis or even full-blown septic shock syndrome may be present.

Septic thrombophlebitis Likewise, septic thrombophlebitis may have no findings, except those associated with sepsis or venous thrombosis (edema).

Diagnosis

In any cancer patient with a right atrial catheter who becomes febrile or is shown to be bacteremic or fungemic, a catheter-associated infection should be suspected. Without the signs or symptoms of an exit-site or tunnel infection, however, a diagnosis may be difficult.

Cultures Two blood cultures should be drawn: one from the catheter and one from a peripheral vein. There are two methods that may be helpful in making a diagnosis of right atrial catheter infection. Both depend upon drawing both (catheter and peripheral vein) blood cultures simultaneously. In the first method, quantitative colony counts are determined from both cultures. If the catheter colony counts are several-fold (3-10-fold) higher than the colony count from the peripheral vein, it suggests a catheter-associated infection. The second method, differential time to positivity (DTP), requires an automated continuously monitored blood culture system, which determines the time at which a blood culture turns positive. If the catheter culture turns positive at least 2 hours before the peripheral vein culture, it suggests a catheter-associated infection. A catheter infection should be assumed when the organism isolated is a coagulase-negative *Staphylococcus, Corynebacterium, Bacillus,* or *Candida* species or a mycobacterium.

If signs are consistent with an exit-site or tunnel infection, an attempt should be made to culture any exit-site drainage.

Treatment

Catheter removal

Although it was once believed that all catheters had to be removed to eradicate infection, it is now clear that many catheters can be salvaged. An exception to this guideline would be if the organism isolated is *Corynebacterium*JK, a *Bacillus* species, a *Candida* organism, or a rapidly growing mycobacterium. Some physicians would add to this list *S aureus*, vancomycin-resistant enterococci, *P aeruginosa*, polymicrobial bacteremia, and *Fusarium* species. The catheter also should be removed in patients with septic thrombophlebitis or evidence of septic emboli. A tunnel infection or pocket-space abscess should prompt catheter removal as well. Finally, fever or bacteremia that persists (> 72 hours) after therapy has been initiated necessitates removal of the catheter if there is no other source of infection.

Antibiotic therapy

Empiric therapy If a catheter-associated infection is suspected, vancomycin should be initiated empirically. If the patient is known to be colonized with vancomycin-resistant enterococci, empiric therapy with quinupristin/dalfopristin (Synercid) or linezolid (Zyvox) should be considered.

Two new antimicrobial agents with activity against MRSA and vancomycin-resistant enterococci (VRE) have been approved: daptomycin (Cubicin) and tigecycline (Tygacil). Both drugs have activity against MRSA and VRE, but they are approved only for MRSA infections. Although some of these new agents have shortcomings (eg, activity of daptomycin is neutralized by surfactant in the lungs and emergence of resistance while on this antibiotic), they enlarge our armamentarium for fighting these resistant gram-positive infections.

Specific therapy When a micro-organism has been isolated and tested for sensitivity, specific antimicrobial therapy should be added. If the catheter is left in place, a minimum of 14 days of parenteral (not oral) therapy should be administered through the catheter (rotating through each port), and follow-up cultures should be obtained. However, in the case of suspected severe hypervirulent *C difficile* enterocolitis, vancomycin may be the drug of choice.

The emergence of hypervirulent, resistant strains of *Clostridium difficile* continues. New drugs are being evaluated to meet this challenge, including nitazoxanide, tolevamer, ramoplain, and rifaximin, but none so far has emerged as being superior to vancomycin or metronidazole. Vancomycin may be superior to metronidazole in treating patients with severe *C difficile* enterocolitis (Zar FA, Bakkanagari SR, Moorthi KM, et al: *Clin Infect Dis* 45:302-307), 2007. Subtotal colectomy with ileostomy may be required in these severe cases (Adams SD, Mercer DW: *Curr Opin Crit Care* 13:450-455, 2007).

Search for infectious metastasis

Whether or not the catheter is removed, if the patient remains febrile, a search for sources of metastatic infection (lungs, liver, spleen, brain, heart valves) should be initiated.

Fibrinolytics and anticoagulants

The use of fibrinolytics and anticoagulation is controversial. Anticoagulation is indicated in cases of septic thrombophlebitis when the deep venous system is involved.

C DIFFICILE–ASSOCIATED DIARRHEA

Although many infectious complications involve the GI tract and abdomen in cancer patients, *C difficile*–associated diarrhea and typhlitis are the most important clinically.

Diarrhea is common in the cancer patient during chemotherapy. One of the most common causes of diarrhea is antibiotic-associated colitis. By far, the predominant etiology of antibiotic-associated colitis is *C difficile*.

Etiology and risk factors

Antibiotics The major risk factor for *C difficile*–associated diarrhea is treatment with antibiotics, especially broad-spectrum β-lactams with activity against enteric bacteria and clindamycin (Cleocin). Antibiotic therapy causes a disruption in the normal bacterial flora of the colon. This disruption allows for colonization with *C difficile*, a spore-forming anaerobe present in the hospital environment, via the oral-fecal route. Pathogenic strains then produce toxins that cause diarrhea and pseudomembranous colitis.

Other risk factors include surgery (primarily colonic, gastric, and pelvic), colon carcinoma, leukemia, and uremia. Obviously, the hospitalized cancer patient undergoing chemotherapy and/or surgery and receiving broad-spectrum antibiotics is most vulnerable to this infection.

Signs and symptoms

Infection with *C difficile* can be asymptomatic. When signs and symptoms do occur, they may range from mild to moderate diarrhea with lower abdominal pain, to antibiotic-associated colitis without pseudomembranous formation, to pseudomembranous colitis, to fulminant colitis. Fulminant colitis may be associated with toxic megacolon and even perforation of the viscus and peritonitis. On occasion, a patient may present with just abdominal pain or fever and no diarrhea.

Pseudomembranes may be absent in mild disease but usually are present in severe disease and are easily recognized on sigmoidoscopic or colonoscopic examination as adherent yellow plaques that may coalesce over large areas.

Diagnosis

The development of diarrhea or even abdominal pain or fever in a cancer patient should prompt a work-up for *C difficile*–associated diarrhea.

Stool cytotoxin test The laboratory diagnosis of *C difficile* infection depends on the demonstration of *C difficile* toxins in the stool. The gold standard is the stool cytotoxin test, a tissue-culture assay that demonstrates cell rounding by *C difficile* toxin B.

Enzyme immunoassay Another test that can demonstrate *C difficile* toxins (A and/or B) in the stool is an enzyme immunoassay. It is less expensive and faster than the cytotoxin test and does not need to be performed by specially trained laboratory personnel.

Stool culture Although a stool culture for *C difficile* may also be obtained, it has less significance in making the diagnosis.

Treatment

INITIAL MANAGEMENT

The initial step in the management of *C difficile*–associated diarrhea is to discontinue antibiotic therapy. Patients may not require any other therapy. However, stopping antibiotics in a cancer patient may not be possible or the patient may be severely ill from the colitis. In these instances, specific anti–*C difficile* therapy is required.

Specific antibiotic therapy

Metronidazole and vancomycin Metronidazole (250 mg PO qid) or vancomycin (125 mg PO qid), both given for 10 days, are the drugs of choice. Metronidazole is preferred because it is less expensive and the use of vancomycin may promote the emergence of VRE.

For the patient who cannot tolerate oral medications, IV metronidazole (500 mg q6h) can be given. IV vancomycin should not be used, as high intraluminal levels cannot be attained.

Other agents that might be used for treatment include bacitracin (25,000 U PO qid) and cholestyramine (4 g PO qid).

Surgical therapy Subtotal colectomy with ileostomy may be required for severe *C difficile* enterocolitis.

TREATMENT OF RELAPSE

Relapse occurs in 10%-20% of patients. Mild cases may not need to be treated. If treatment is indicated, a repeat 7- to 14-day course of either metronidazole or vancomycin may be administered. If the infection persists after repeated therapy, longer courses (4-6 weeks) followed by a gradual tapering of the dose may be helpful.

Prevention

Contact isolation Patients with *C difficile*–associated diarrhea and those who are known carriers should be placed in "contact isolation"; ie, the use of gloves, gowns, and careful hand-washing should be instituted.

Disinfection During outbreaks, the use of sodium hypochlorite to disinfect contaminated surfaces has been recommended.

Antibiotic prophylaxis of high-risk patients or carriers is not recommended.

TYPHLITIS

Typhlitis (necrotizing enterocolitis) occurs in patients who are severely neutropenic, usually in the setting of chemotherapy. Pathologically, the areas of involvement include the cecum and terminal ileum. Typhlitis is a broad-spectrum disease characterized by bowel wall edema, diffuse or patchy necrosis involving the mucosa alone or the full thickness of the bowel wall, mucosal ulcerations, hemorrhage, inflammatory infiltrates, and infiltration of the bowel wall by bacteria or fungi. Mild cases are self-limiting when treated with bowel rest/antibiotics. Death may occur in severe cases.

Signs and symptoms

Signs and symptoms of typhlitis can be nonspecific but usually include fever, abdominal pain (typically in the right lower quadrant), and abdominal distention. The patient may have diarrhea (sometimes bloody), nausea, and vomiting or may demonstrate signs and symptoms consistent with those of acute appendicitis.

Physical findings There may be abdominal guarding and rebound tenderness, diminished bowel sounds, or even a mass in the right lower quadrant of the abdomen.

Diagnosis

Radiographs or CT scans of the abdomen may demonstrate a thickened cecum, mass, or even gas within the colon wall.

Treatment

Mortality from typhlitis is high (> 50%) and therapy is controversial. However, broad-spectrum antibiotics covering both gut aerobes and anaerobes and resection of necrotic bowel are recommended.

FUNGAL INFECTIONS

Fungal infections are a leading cause of morbidity and mortality in cancer patients. These infections pose a formidable management challenge, in that diagnosis is often difficult to make at an early stage and, therefore, appropriate treatment may be delayed.

Etiology and risk factors

Candida **species** The most common fungal infections in cancer patients are caused by *Candida* species. Of the candidal pathogens found in these patients, *C albicans* is the most common. However, more recently other *Candida* species, such as *C tropicalis, C glabrata, C parapsilosis, C krusei,* and *C lusitaniae,* have become more prevalent. This finding is significant, as many of these species (*C krusei, C glabrata, C lusitaniae*) can be resistant to fluconazole and less susceptible to amphotericin B.

Major risk factors for candidal infections include neutropenia, a breakdown in physical defense barriers (such as mucositis induced by chemotherapy and radiation therapy), broad-spectrum antibiotics, immune dysfunction (caused by chemotherapy and steroids), surgery (especially GI surgery), long-term indwelling vascular catheters, and poor nutritional status/total parenteral nutrition.

Aspergillus species is a less common cause of infection in cancer patients than candidal organisms but is more virulent. The most common of the *Aspergillus* species is *A fumigatus*, followed by *A flavus, A niger,* and *A terreus.*

Risk factors for *Aspergillus* infections include severe immunosuppression (primarily allogeneic HCT), steroid therapy, GVHD, and environmental exposure.

Other fungi Other emerging fungal pathogens in the cancer patient include *Fusarium, Trichosporon, Zygomycetes,* and *Scedosporium* species; *Malassezia furfur;* and the dematiaceous/pigmented fungi (eg, *Bipolaris spicifera, Cladosporium bantianum).*

Finally, the endemic fungi, *Coccidioides immitis* and *Histoplasma capsulatum,* are often more virulent and aggressive than other fungi in the immunocompromised host.

Signs and symptoms

Candidiasis

Candidiasis can present as a wide spectrum of diseases, from mucosal infection to disseminated and invasive disease.

Local mucosal infection Oropharyngeal candidiasis can present as classic thrush with beige plaques. It may be painful, as there may be a concurrent mucositis due to the ablative chemotherapy. Oropharyngeal candidiasis may extend into the esophagus as esophagitis, which may manifest as odynophagia. Epiglottitis may present as odynophagia and laryngeal stridor.

Disseminated infection Candidemia may present simply as an asymptomatic fever or may result in a full-blown septic shock syndrome (acute disseminated candidiasis). In contrast, chronic disseminated candidiasis, which involves the chronic, indolent infection of different organs, such as the liver, spleen, and kidneys, may be manifested by fever alone.

Aspergillosis

Invasive aspergillosis most commonly involves the lungs and sinuses. However, it can also disseminate to the brain (and may be the most common cause of brain abscesses in HCT patients). Less commonly, aspergillosis can disseminate to other organs, including the skin.

Pulmonary aspergillosis Signs and symptoms of invasive pulmonary aspergillosis include pleuritic pain, pulmonary hemorrhage, hemoptysis, and cavitation. The chest radiograph or CT scan may demonstrate pulmonary nodular infiltration and/or cavitary lesions.

Sinusitis Patients with sinusitis may have few signs (swelling) or symptoms (pain), especially if they are neutropenic.

Brain abscess Patients with brain abscesses may have headaches and neurologic signs consistent with the specific site of the lesion.

Skin involvement may present as necrotizing skin nodules or ulcers.

Other infections

***Fusarium* infections** The signs and symptoms of *Fusarium* infections are similar to those of aspergillosis; ie; pulmonary infiltrates, sinusitis, and cutaneous lesions are prominent.

***Trichosporon* infections** are similar to *Candida* infections in that they can cause disseminated disease in multiple organs.

***Zygomycetes* infections** cause sinopulmonary disease.

***Scedosporium* species** are similar to *Aspergillus* species in their structure and predilection for the respiratory tract.

C immitis* and *H capsulatum also target the lungs but can disseminate to other organs.

Diagnosis

Diagnosis of fungal infection in the cancer patient requires documentation by culture or histologic examination.

Candidiasis Although the diagnosis of oropharyngeal candidiasis often is made on clinical grounds, the lesions should be scraped for microscopic examination and culture. Biopsy of esophageal lesions via endoscopy should be performed to confirm *Candida* (as opposed to HSV or CMV) as the etiology of the infection.

A positive blood culture for *Candida* (especially a species other than *C albicans)* should never be considered a "contaminant" and often implies a right atrial catheter infection. Less likely to result in positive blood cultures are chronic, deep-seated infections, such as hepatosplenic candidiasis. Such infections require biopsy for confirmation.

***Aspergillus* species,** like other species, such as *Zygomycetes* and dematiaceous fungi, is rarely found in the bloodstream and requires tissue sampling for diagnosis. Occasionally, bronchoalveolar lavage fluid or sinus drainage will yield *Aspergillus*, but often a lung biopsy is required. Recently, an *Aspergillus* galactomannan enzyme immunoassay test has become available for the diagnosis of invasive aspergillosis. Unfortunately, it is not clear that it is a sufficiently sensitive (especially in patients receiving antifungal agents) or predictive test for the disease. There are also two other diagnostic tests now available: the glucan assay (for [1,3]-β-D-glucan) and the *Aspergillus* DNA polymerase chain reaction. Unfortunately, there is a paucity of data and lack of experience with these assays to determine their utility in diagnosing and predicting invasive fungal infection in patients at highest risk.

Fusarium, Scedosporium, and Trichosporon species, in contrast to *Aspergillus* species, are often found in the bloodstream.

Skin lesions Any skin lesion should be suspected of being of fungal origin and should be biopsied, cultured, and examined histologically.

Search for sites of infection When a fungal infection is suspected or documented, a search for possible sites of infection should ensue. For a blood culture that grows a *Candida* species, the intravascular catheter should, in most cases, be removed for diagnostic as well as therapeutic reasons, and the catheter tip should be cultured. A CT scan of the abdomen should be obtained. In cases of suspected *Aspergillus* infection, in addition to a CT scan of the chest, a CT scan of the brain and sinuses should be performed.

Treatment

ANTIFUNGAL AGENTS

There are now three major groups of antifungal agents: 1) the polyenes (amphotericin B deoxycholate and its lipid formulations [amphotericin B lipid complex, liposomal amphotericin B, amphotericin B cholsteryl sulfate]); 2) the azoles (fluconazole, itraconzaole, voriconazole, posaconazole); and 3) the echinocandins (caspofungin, micafungin, anidulafungin).

Amphotericin B deoxycholate has been the standard therapy for invasive fungal infection for 50 years. It is fungicidal and has a broad spectrum of activity against yeasts and molds, including the *Zygomycetes*. It is thought to be less active against *C guillermondii* and *C lusitaniae*. However, it is limited by its nephrotoxicity and infusional toxicity. The lipid formulations are less nephrotoxic but much more expensive than the other formulations.

The azoles are not nephrotoxic. The first-generation azoles (fluconazole and itraconazole) are considered fungistatic, whereas the extended-spectrum azoles (voriconazole and posaconazole) are considered more fungicidal. Fluconazole is well absorbed orally and can be administered orally or intravenously but is not active against molds and certain *Candida* species (*C krusei*). Itraconazole is hepatoxic and is not well absorbed when orally administered. Voriconazole is well absorbed orally and can also be administered intravenously. It is broadly active against most *Candida* species and most molds, with the exception of the *Zygomycetes*. Posaconazole can only be orally administered and is well absorbed. It is broadly active against most *Candida* species and most molds, including the *Zygomycetes*.

The echinocandins are the least toxic of the antifungal agents. They can only be administered intravenously. They are said to be fungicidal against yeasts but fungistatic against molds.

Candidiasis

Local mucosal candidiasis In patients with local mucosal candidiasis (including esophagitis), oral fluconazole or itraconazole can be used. If the patient has difficulty in taking oral medication, IV fluconazole should be used. If the patient was receiving prophylactic fluconazole when candidiasis developed, there is a high likelihood that the causative *Candida* species may be azole-resistant, and either an echinocandin (caspofungin, micafungin, or anidulafungin) or a lipid formulation of amphotericin B should be used.

Candidemia If candidemia is documented, the intravascular catheter should be removed. This step should be followed by the administration of an antifungal for at least 2 weeks after the last positive blood culture is obtained and all signs and symptoms have resolved. Although fluconazole has been shown to be an effective and safe agent in the treatment of candidemia, there are certain circumstances in which an alternative (an echinocandin or a lipid formulation of amphotericin B) might be preferable. These situations would include hemodynamic instability, neutropenia, or high suspicion of azole resistance (eg, a patient who is colonized with a resistant *Candida* species or has been on recent fluconazole prophylaxis or treatment).

Disseminated, deep-seated candidiasis (eg, hepatosplenic infection). Although the standard of therapy for deep-seated candidiasis has been long-term therapy with amphotericin deoxycholate, it has been limited by nephrotoxicity. Thus, the lipid formulations of amphotericin B have allowed higher cumulative doses with a lower nephrotoxic potential. The azoles (fluconazole, voriconazole) have the advantage of convenient (ie, oral) administration and good absorption, with little toxicity. The echinocandins also have been shown to be effective against this infection.

Aspergillosis

Antifungal therapy Amphotericin B deoxycholate (1.0-1.5 mg/kg/d) had been the standard therapy for invasive aspergillosis. However, voriconazole led to better responses, improved survival, and fewer adverse events than did amphotericin B when used as initial therapy in patients with invasive aspergillosis.

> Posaconazole, another extended-spectrum azole joining voriconazole, has recently become available, and its advantages are broad activity against molds (including the *Zygomycetes*) and its oral administration with good absorption (when taken with food). Posaconazole has been shown to be an effective prophylactic agent (against *Candida* and *Aspergillus*) in neutropenic AML and MDS patients as well as high risk allogeneic HCT recipients with GVHD (*Cornely OA, Maertens J, Winston DJ, et al: N Engl J Med 356:348-59, 2007; Ullmann AJ, Lipton JH, Vesole DH, et al: N Engl J Med 356:335-347, 2007*). And now anidulafungin (*Reboli AC, Rotstein C, Pappas PG, et al: N Engl J Med 356:2472-2482, 2007*) and micafungin (*Pappas PG, Rotstein CM, Betts RF, et al: Clin Infect Dis 45:883-893, 2007*) have joined caspofungin as echinocandin therapy for candidemia and invasive candidiasis.

Thus, voriconazole is the standard therapy for invasive aspergillosis. In addition, new antifungals and new formulations of amphotericin B have been approved for use in invasive aspergillosis in patients who are intolerant of or refractory to conventional amphotericin B. They include amphotericin B lipid complex, amphotericin B cholesteryl sulfate, liposomal amphotericin B, itraconazole oral solution, IV itraconazole, and caspofungin. All of these formulations are less nephrotoxic than amphotericin B deoxycholate.

Surgical removal of infected sites In addition to antifungal therapy, it is important to attempt surgical removal of infected sites, if at all feasible. Sinus surgery should be performed. Resection of pulmonary lesions should be attempted if there are only one or two limited, discrete lesions.

Infections with other fungi

Although amphotericin B is the drug of choice for most invasive fungal infections, there are exceptions. *Scedosporium* and *Fusarium* species are often resistant to amphotericin B, and voriconazole may be the drug of choice for these infections. Voriconazole, however, is not active against *Zygomycetes* species, and if an infection with this organism is suspected or documented, amphotericin B deoxycholate, an amphotericin B lipid formulation, or posaconazole should be used. The dematiaceous/pigmented fungi also may be better treated with itraconazole. For *Trichosporon* infections, voriconazole may be more effective than amphotericin B.

Prevention

Because invasive fungal infection occurs with high frequency in the setting of HCT, most prophylactic studies have been performed in HCT recipients. Thus, the following recommendations apply mainly to this group, although prophylaxis can be justified when the incidence of these infections in any population is high enough.

Fluconazole Two randomized, placebo-controlled studies using prophylactic fluconazole (400 mg/d) have demonstrated a decrease in invasive and superficial *C albicans* infections. One study showed a reduction in mortality. As fluconazole is not active against *C krusei, C glabrata,* or *Aspergillus* species, there is concern that its prophylactic use will increase the incidence of these resistant fungi. Some authors have reported such an occurrence.

Micafungin has been approved for use as an antifungal (candidiasis) prophylactic agent in HCT. There was also a trend toward protection against *Aspergillus* infection with micafungin, although it was not significant.

Itraconazole has been shown to be an effective antifungal prophylactic agent in HCT, but no survival benefit has been demonstrated, possibly because of the toxic GI effects and hepatotoxicity associated with this agent.

Low-dose amphotericin B was observed, in a retrospective study, to decrease the incidence of *Candida* infection. However, this regimen only delayed the onset of *Aspergillus* infections.

Posaconazole has been shown to be effective antifungal prophylaxis in two settings: (1) neutropenic AML and MDS patients; and (2) allogeneic HCT recipients with GVHD.

Other prophylactic regimens have been used in small numbers of patients, with varying degrees of success. They include aerosolized amphotericin B, intranasal amphotericin B, and amphotericin B lipid complex. Voriconazole (vs fluconazole) is currently being studied as a prophylactic agent in HCT.

The prophylactic regimen of choice in HCT might be an echinocandin (eg, micafungin) intitially (while the patient is neutropenic and hospitalized) followed by an oral azole (eg, posaconazole) administered to those outpatients who remain at high risk for mold infections.

HEPA filtration Other than using prophylactic antifungals, there is little that can be done to prevent fungal infections in cancer patients. The one possible exception is the use of HEPA filtration, which can eliminate *Aspergillus* spores from the environment. However, most patients emerge from this environment still possessing the same risk factors (steroids, GVHD) for aspergillosis.

VIRAL INFECTIONS

Opportunistic viral infections are a particular problem in cancer patients who undergo HCT and those with hematologic cancers. Accurate diagnosis of viral infections is important, as treatment is available for many of them.

Etiology

As mentioned previously, viral infections in cancer patients are caused predominantly by herpesviruses (HSV, VZV, CMV, and EBV). The herpesvirus infections usually are reactivations of latent infections. Respiratory viruses that infect cancer patients include respiratory syncytial virus, influenza viruses A and B, parainfluenza virus, rhinovirus, and adenovirus.

Signs and symptoms

Although all of the herpesviruses can cause fever and a septic picture, HSV usually presents as mucositis or a vesicular rash, VZV presents as a vesicular rash in a dermatomal distribution, and CMV, in the HCT setting, presents as interstitial pneumonia. When HSV or VZV disseminates, each virus can cause disseminated cutaneous lesions or visceral (liver, lung, brain) involvement. VZV infection can present with GI symptoms, such as epigastric or general abdominal pain.

Diagnosis

To make a specific viral etiologic diagnosis, tissue or fluid must be obtained from the infected site and processed for histologic/cytologic examination and culture.

Vesicular skin lesions When a cancer patient presents with a vesicular rash, it is invariably due to either HSV or VZV. If the distribution of lesions is in a dermatomal pattern, a clinical diagnosis of VZV can be made. However, if there is cutaneous dissemination, the vesicular lesions should be aspirated (and sent for viral culture) or scraped down to the base, smeared on a glass slide, and sent for direct fluorescent antibody staining (for HSV and VZV).

Visceral involvement When there is visceral involvement with either HSV, VZV, or CMV, biopsy material is examined for inclusions and is submitted for culture.

Respiratory infection For the respiratory viruses, diagnosis is usually made by examination of bronchoalveolar lavage fluid (obtained by bronchoscopy) or biopsy (obtained by transbronchial, percutaneous thoracic, thoracoscopic, or open lung biopsy). In the special case of CMV interstitial pneumonitis in the HCT setting, diagnosis of infection (prior to disease onset) can be made by detection of antigens or virus in the bloodstream, in addition to evidence of the virus in bronchoalveolar lavage fluid.

CNS involvement can be determined by PCR performed on the cerebrospinal fluid for the following agents: HSV, VZV, human herpesvirus 6 (HHV-6), and adenovirus.

Antibody testing is of little use in the diagnosis of viral infection in the cancer patient.

Evidence of CMV viremia, which is utilized to initiate preemptive therapy, can be determined by PCR, antigen detection, or blood (shell-vial) culture.

Treatment

HSV infection Localized HSV infection is usually treated with acyclovir, 5 mg/kg IV q8h. If there is dissemination, a dose of 10 mg/kg q8h can be used, and if there is CNS involvement, up to 15 mg/kg IV q8h can be utilized. If acyclovir-resistant HSV is suspected, foscarnet (Foscavir) can be used (see Table 1 for doses). However, this is a nephrotoxic drug.

VZV infection is usually treated with acyclovir, administered at a dose of 10 mg/kg IV q8h.

CMV infection is treated with ganciclovir or foscarnet. Ganciclovir is the drug of choice but is toxic to bone marrow.

In the HCT setting, "preemptive" treatment (treatment to prevent disease after evidence of infection is obtained) consists of ganciclovir, 5 mg/kg IV bid for 7 days followed by 5 mg/kg/d IV for another 3-5 weeks. Actual treatment of

CMV interstitial pneumonia consists of ganciclovir, 5 mg/kg IV q12h, along with immunoglobulin, 500 mg/kg IV every other day for 21 days (induction phase). Maintenance therapy (for as long as immunosuppression is present) consists of ganciclovir, 5 mg/kg/d IV for 5 days each week, and immunoglobulin, 500 mg/kg IV every week.

Foscarnet can be used instead of ganciclovir if there is marrow toxicity but poses a potential risk of nephrotoxicity.

For CMV infection resistant to both ganciclovir and foscarnet, cidofovir (Vistide) can be used.

HHV-6 infection/disease can be treated with ganciclovir, foscarnet, or cidofovir.

Respiratory viral infection Among the respiratory viruses, there is specific antiviral therapy only for respiratory syncytial virus and influenza A. Ribavirin (Virazole), 1.1 g/d by aerosol (20 mg/mL), has been used for respiratory syncytial virus (but has not been shown to be effective) and rimantadine (Flumadine) or amantadine (Symmetrel), both 100 mg PO bid, for influenza A. Zanamivir (Relenza) and oseltamivir (Tamiflu, 75 mg PO bid) can be used for both influenza A and B. Finally, cidofovir has been used (but not FDA approved) for adenovirus infection.

Prevention

Herpesvirus infections

Acyclovir HSV and VZV reactivate with great frequency in cancer patients undergoing chemotherapy and/or radiation therapy. This finding is especially true in the HCT population, in which 80% of HSV-seropositive patients and up to 40% of VZV-seropositive patients have a reactivation of HSV or VZV. Therefore, in HSV-seropositive HCT patients, prophylactic acyclovir is indicated. However, prophylaxis may only delay the onset of infection. Any HSV infection that occurs during acyclovir prophylaxis should be considered resistant to acyclovir. Acyclovir has also been shown to reduce the incidence of CMV infection after HCT.

Ganciclovir is generally considered too (marrow) toxic to be used as universal prophylaxis against CMV. Thus, the preemptive approach was developed to focus on only treating those who had evidence of CMV infection (viremia) as determined by PCR, antigen detection, or blood (shell-vial) culture. This approach allowed treatment of viremia before it evolved into CMV disease (interstitial pneumonitis).

CMV-seronegative blood support In the small group of HCT recipients who are CMV-seronegative, the use of CMV-seronegative blood support has been shown to reduce CMV infection dramatically.

Varicella zoster immune globulin In any susceptible cancer patient exposed to VZV, varicella zoster immune globulin should be administered within 96 hours of exposure.

Varicella virus vaccine (Varivax) should not be given to those with hematologic malignancies, malignant neoplasms, or immunodeficiencies, with the exception of those with childhood leukemia in remission for 1 year, when selected criteria are met.

Influenza

Influenza vaccine Although the efficacy of the influenza vaccine is unknown in the HCT setting, it should be administered to all cancer patients.

Rimantadine, amantadine, zanamivir, or oseltamivir can be given prophylactically during an outbreak of influenza.

SUGGESTED READING

ON FEVER AND NEUTROPENIA

Freifeld AG, Segal BH, Baden LR, et al: National Comprehensive Cancer Network practice guidelines in oncology: prevention and treatment of cancer-related infections – v.1.2008. Available at: http://www.nccn.org/professionals/physicians_gls/PDF/infections.pdf. Accessed March 2008.

ON CATHETER-ASSOCIATED INFECTIONS

Raad I, Hanna H, Maki D: Intravascular catheter-related infections: Advances in diagnosis, prevention, and management. Lancet Infect Dis 7:645–657, 2007.

ON C DIFFICILE–ASSOCIATED DIARRHEA

Gerding DN, Muto CA, Owens RC Jr.: Treatment of Clostridium difficile infection. Clin Infect Dis 46(suppl 1):S32–S42, 2008.

Miller MA: Clinical management of *Clostridium difficile*-associated disease. Clin Infect Dis 45(suppl 2):S122–S128, 2007.

ON FUNGAL INFECTIONS

Pappas PG, Rex JH, Sobel JD, et al: Guidelines for treatment of candidiasis. Clin Infect Dis 38:161–189, 2004.

Segal BH, Almyroudis NG, Battiwalla M, et al: Prevention and early treatment of invasive fugal infection in patients with cancer and neutropenia and in stem cell transplant recipients in the era of newer broad-spectrum antifungal agents and diagnostic adjuncts. Clin Infect Dis 44:402–409, 2007.

Walsh TJ, Anaissie EJ, Denning DW, et al: Treatment of aspergillosis: Clinical practice guidelines of the Infectious Diseases Society of America. Clin Infect Dis 46:327–360, 2008.

CHAPTER 46

Fluid complications

Frederic W. Grannis, Jr., MD, Carey A. Cullinane, MD, and Lily Lai, MD

MALIGNANT PLEURAL EFFUSION

Malignant pleural effusion complicates the care of approximately 150,000 people in the United States each year. The pleural effusion is usually caused by a disturbance of the normal Starling forces regulating reabsorption of fluid in the pleural space, secondary to obstruction of mediastinal lymph nodes draining the parietal pleura. Tumors that metastasize frequently to these nodes, eg, lung cancer, breast cancer, and lymphoma, cause most malignant effusions. It is, therefore, puzzling that small-cell lung cancer infrequently causes effusions. Primary effusion lymphomas caused by human herpesvirus 8 and perhaps Epstein-Barr virus (EBV) are seen in patients with AIDS.

Pleural effusion restricts ventilation and causes progressive shortness of breath by compression of lung tissue as well as paradoxical movement of the inverted diaphragm. Pleural deposits of tumor cause pleuritic pain.

Pleural effusions commonly occur in patients with advanced-stage tumors, who frequently have metastases to the brain, bone, and other organs, physiologic deficits, malnutrition, debilitation, and other comorbidities. Because of these numerous clinical and pathologic variables, it is difficult to perform meaningful trials in patients with pleural effusions. For the same reason, it is often difficult to predict a potential treatment outcome for the specific patient with multiple interrelated clinical problems. Altundag and colleagues from M. D. Anderson Cancer Center performed a retrospective study of patients with "wet" IIIB non–small-cell lung cancer. Of the 37 patients who had no detectable distant metastasis at the time of diagnosis, 12 (32%) experienced improved survival. They concluded that selected patients with wet IIIB disease may benefit from aggressive local treatment strategies.

Diagnosis

The new onset of pleural effusion may herald the presence of a previously undiagnosed malignancy or, more typically, complicate the course of a known tumor.

Thoracentesis The first step in management in almost all cases is thoracentesis. An adequate specimen should be obtained and sent for cell count; determination of glucose, protein, lactic dehydrogenase (LDH), and pH; and appropriate cultures and cytology. A negative cytology result is not uncommon and does not rule out a malignant etiology.

The Light criteria (LDH > 200 U/L; pleural-serum LDH ratio > 0.6; and pleural-serum protein ratio > 0.5) help categorize pleural effusions as exudates. The majority of undiagnosed exudates are eventually diagnosed as malignant, whereas < 5% of transudates are shown to be caused by cancer.

Because it is sometimes difficult to prove the malignant nature of an effusion, many molecular tests on pleural fluid have been investigated. Multiple reports measure pleural tumor marker proteins, cadherins, matrix metalloproteins, cytokines, telomerase, mRNA, exosomes, and serum and pleural DN methylation patterns, but to date, no test or panel of tests can reliably diagnose malignant effusions.

Kwek et al, from Massachusetts General Hospital, reported that PET scans performed on nine patients, an average of 22 months following talc pleurodesis, showed focal nodular fluorodeoxyglucose uptake in the pleura (mean standard error of mean 5.4; range: 1.2-16.

Pleural biopsy If cytology of an exudative effusion is negative and malignant disease is still suspected (approximately 50% of cases), blind pleural biopsy has a low diagnostic yield that can be improved by computed tomography (CT) or ultrasonographic guidance.

Thoracoscopy Thoracoscopic examination performed under either general or local anesthesia and using rigid or partly flexible thoracoscopes with the patient offers very high sensitivity, specificity, and diagnostic accuracy with a low complication rate. It allows comprehensive visualization of one pleural cavity, coupled with the opportunity to biopsy areas of disease. This method provides a definitive diagnosis and allows the pathologist to suggest possible sites of primary disease based on the histopathology. There was no incidence of later development of a malignant pleural effusion following a benign thoracoscopic study in 25 patients at the Lahey Clinic. Furthermore, this technique permits the diagnosis and staging of malignant mesothelioma if it is the cause of the effusion. Thoracoscopy also offers the opportunity for simultaneous treatment.

Gaspari, et al of Milan, Italy, report an 89% success rate following video-assisted thoracic surgery (VATS) talc pleurodesis in breast cancer patients with malignant pleural effusion. Biopsies taken during VATS showed that receptor status and c-ErB-2 status changed from negative to positive in 15% of patients.

Bronchoscopy may be helpful when an underlying lung cancer is suspected, especially if there is associated hemoptysis, a lung mass, atelectasis, or a massive effusion. It may also be useful when there is a cytologically positive effusion with no obvious primary tumor.

Prognosis

Prognosis of patients with malignant pleural effusion varies by primary tumor. For example, median survival for patients with lung cancer is 3 months, whereas it is 10 months for patients with breast cancer. Median survival is also shorter in patients with encasement atelectasis (3 months).

Treatment

INITIAL TREATMENT

Because the specific clinical circumstances may vary markedly in different patients, treatment must be individualized to provide the best palliation for each patient. Generally, there are many different methods available for the treatment of malignant effusions, and there is little compelling evidence to guide clinicians in the choice of the best methods. Accordingly, treatment decisions must be made with careful reference to the status of the patient and the skills and equipment available in the local community. In general, malignant pleural effusion should be treated aggressively as soon as it is diagnosed. In most cases, effusion will rapidly recur after treatment by thoracentesis or tube thoracostomy alone. If the clinician decides to administer systemic chemotherapy for the underlying primary malignancy, in tumors such as breast cancer, lymphoma, and small-cell lung cancer, it is important to monitor the patient carefully for recurrent effusion and to treat such recurrences immediately. There are few published data to document the chance of success in clearance of malignant pleural effusions with systemic chemotherapy.

If a malignant pleural effusion is left untreated, the underlying collapsed lung will become encased by tumor and fibrous tissue in as many as 10% to 30% of cases. Once this encasement atelectasis has occurred, the underlying lung is "trapped" and will no longer reexpand after thoracentesis or tube thoracostomy. Characteristically, the chest x-ray in such cases shows resolution of the pleural effusion after thoracentesis, but the underlying lung remains partially collapsed. This finding is often misinterpreted by the inexperienced clinician as evidence of a pneumothorax, and a chest tube is placed. The air space persists and the lung remains unexpanded, even with high suction and pulmonary physiotherapy. Allowing the chest tube to remain in place can worsen the situation, resulting in bronchopleural fistulization and empyema. In some cases, a trapped lung on an initial chest x-ray will have delayed reexpansion following chest tube or small pleural catheter drainage.

Intrapleural alteplase (in doses between 10 and 100 mg diluted in 50 to 150 mL of saline) has been used with success in some patients with gelatinous or loculated effusions without systemic bleeding complications.

Physical techniques

To avoid encasement atelectasis, pleural effusion should be treated definitively at the time of initial diagnosis. Multiple physical techniques of producing adhesions between the parietal and visceral pleurae, obliterating the space, and preventing recurrence have been used. They include open or thoracoscopic pleurectomy, gauze abrasion, or laser pleurodesis. Surgical methods have not been demonstrated to have any advantage over simpler chemical pleurodesis techniques in the treatment of malignant effusions. Gauze abrasion can easily be employed when unresectable lung cancer with associated effusion is found at the time of thoracotomy.

A randomized, prospective study from Ljubljanska, Slovenia, of 87 patients with malignant pleural effusion secondary to breast cancer showed that the thoracoscopic mechanical abrasion pleurodesis was equivalent to talc pleurodesis in those with normal pleural fluid pH and superior in patients with a low pH.

Chemical agents

Multiple chemical agents have been used.

Tetracycline Tetracycline pleurodesis results in a lower incidence of recurrence when compared with tube thoracostomy alone but often causes severe pain. Tetracycline is no longer commercially available in the United States.

Doxycycline and minocycline are probably equivalent in efficacy to tetracycline.

Bleomycin Intrapleural bleomycin, in a dose of 60 U, has been shown to be more effective than tetracycline and is not painful, but it is costly. Absorption of the drug can result in systemic toxicity. Combined use of tetracycline and bleomycin has been demonstrated to be more efficacious than the use of either drug singly.

Talc pleurodesis was first introduced by Bethune in the 1930s. The first use of talc in malignant pleural effusion was by John Chambers in 1958. Talc powder (Sclerosol Intrapleural Aerosol) has demonstrated efficacy in numerous large studies, preventing recurrent effusion in 70% to 92% of cases. Talc is less painful than tetracycline. Cost is minimal, but special sterilization techniques must be mastered by the hospital pharmacy. Talc formulations may have significant differences in the size of particles. Smaller particles may be absorbed and disseminated systemically and may contribute to the increased incidence of adult respiratory distress syndrome (ARDS) or substantial hypoxemia. Talc has also been shown to cause decreases in forced vital capacity (FVC), forced expiratory volume in one second (FEV_1), and diffusing capacity long term.

Talc can be insufflated in a dry state at the time of thoracoscopy or instilled as a slurry through a chest tube. The dose should be restricted to no more than 5 g. A prospective phase III intergroup trial of 501 patients randomized to receive thoracoscopic talc versus talc slurry pleurodes is showed similar efficacy in each arm, with increased respiratory complications (14% vs 6%) but less fatigue and higher patient ratings in the insufflation group.

Multiloculated effusions may follow talc use. It is important to ensure that talc does not solidify and form a concretion in the chest tube, thus preventing the drainage of pleural fluid and complete reexpansion of the lung following pleurodesis. Such an event is more likely when small-bore chest tubes are used.

Pleurodesis technique With talc pleurodesis, a 24- to 32-French tube has customarily been inserted through a lower intercostal space and placed on underwater seal suction drainage until all fluid is drained and the lung has completely reexpanded. Because severe lung damage can be produced by improper chest tube placement, it is imperative to prove the presence of free fluid by a preliminary needle tap and to enter the pleural space gently with a blunt clamp technique, rather than by blind trocar insertion. If there is any question about the presence of loculated effusion or underlying adhesions, the use of CT or sonography may enhance the safety of the procedure. In the case of large effusions, especially those that have been present for some time, the fluid should be drained slowly to avoid reexpansion pulmonary edema.

Significant complications can occur with both thoracentesis and chest tube thoracostomy. These procedures should not be performed by inexperienced practitioners without training and supervision.

Premedications If doxycycline or talc is to be used, the patient should be premedicated with narcotics. Intrapleural instillation of 20 mL of 1% lidocaine before administration of the chemical agent may help reduce pain.

Following instillation of the chemical agent, the chest tube should remain clamped for at least 2 hours. If high-volume drainage persists, the treatment can be repeated. The chest tube can be removed after 2 or 3 days if drainage is < 300 mL/day.

Follow-up x-rays at monthly intervals assess the adequacy of treatment and allow early retreatment in case of recurrence.

Alternative approaches Use of fluid-sclerosing agents and outpatient pleurodesis has been advocated by some investigators and has the potential for reducing hospital stay and treatment cost. Patz performed a prospective, randomized trial of bleomycin vs doxycycline (72% bleomycin versus 79% doxycycline) pleurodesis via a 14-French catheter and found no difference in efficacy.

Other approaches that must be considered experimental at this time include quinacrine, silver nitrate, powdered collagen, and distilled water, as well as various biologic agents, including *Corynebacterium parvum,* OK-432, tumor necrosis factor, interleukin-2 (Proleukin), interferon-α (Intron A, Roferon-A), interferon-β (Betaseron), and interferon-γ (Actimmune).

TREATMENT OF ENCASEMENT ATELECTASIS

If encasement atelectasis is found at thoracentesis or thoracoscopy, tube thoracostomy and pleurodesis are futile and contraindicated.

Surgical decortication has been advocated for this problem. This potentially dangerous procedure may result in severe complications, however, such as bronchopleural fistula and empyema.

Pleuroperitoneal shunts The Royal Brompton Hospital, London, group reported experience with pleuroperitoneal shunts in 160 patients with malignant pleural effusion and a trapped lung. Effective palliation was achieved in 95% of patients; 15% of patients required shunt revisions for complications.

Intermittent thoracentesis, as needed to relieve symptoms, may be the best option in patients with a short anticipated survival.

Catheter drainage Another new option is to insert a tunneled, small-bore, cuffed, silicone catheter (PleurX pleural catheter, Denver Biomaterials, Inc.,

Denver, Colorado) into the pleural cavity. The patient or family members may then drain fluid, using vacuum bottles, whenever recurrent effusion causes symptoms.

Kakuda reported on placement of 61 PleurX pleural catheters in 50 patients with malignant pleural effusions at City of Hope. Thirty-four percent had lung cancer and 24% had breast cancer. There were no operative deaths. In cases where the catheter was placed under thoracoscopic control, 27 of 38 patients (68%) had encasement atelectasis visualized. Eighty-one percent had a good result with control of effusion, with subsequent catheter removal (19%) or intermittent drainage for > 1 month or until death (62%). Five percent of patients had major complications, including empyema and tumor implant. These catheters can also be inserted using the Seldinger technique with the patient under local anesthesia.

Chemotherapy options depend on the cell type of the tumor and the general condition of the patient. Although intrapleural chemotherapy offers the possibility of high-dose local therapy with minimal systemic effects, only a few, small pilot studies utilizing mitoxantrone, doxorubicin, and hyperthermic cisplatin have been published.

Ang and colleagues from Singapore reported longer mean survival (12 vs 5 months) when systemic chemotherapy was given to 71 patients who initially presented with malignant pleural/pericardial effusions. New studies in this area are much needed.

In Taiwan, Su et al treated 27 patients with non–small-cell lung cancer presenting with a malignant pleural effusion with a regimen of intrapleural cisplatin and gemcitabine (Gemzar), followed by radiotherapy (7,020 cGy in 39 fractions), and completed with IV docetaxel. Only two patients experienced recurrent pleural effusion. The median disease-free and overall survival rates were 8 and 16 months, respectively, and 63% of patients were alive at 1 year.

Radiation therapy may be indicated in some patients with lymphoma but has limited effectiveness in other tumor types, particularly if mediastinal adenopathy is absent.

Chylothorax (in the absence of trauma) is usually secondary to cancer, most frequently lymphoma. An added element of morbidity is conferred by the loss of protein, calories, and lymphocytes in the draining fluid. Chylothorax secondary to lymphoma is usually of low volume and responds to talc pleurodesis in combination with radiotherapy or chemotherapy.

PERICARDIAL EFFUSION

Pericardial effusion develops in 5% to 15% of patients with cancer and is sometimes the initial manifestation of malignancy. Most pericardial effusions in cancer patients result from obstruction of the lymphatic drainage of the heart secondary to metastases. The typical presentation is that of a patient with known cancer who is found to have a large pericardial effusion without signs of inflammation. Bloody pericardial fluid is not a reliable sign of malignant effusion.

The most common malignant causes of pericardial effusions are lung and breast cancers, leukemias (specifically acute myelogenous, lymphoblastic, and chronic myelogenous leukemia [blast crisis]), and lymphomas.

Not all pericardial effusions associated with cancer are malignant, and cases with negative cytology may represent as many as half of cancer-associated pericardial effusions. Such effusions are more common in patients with mediastinal lymphoma, Hodgkin lymphoma, or breast cancer. Other nonmalignant causes include drug-induced or postirradiation pericarditis, tuberculosis, collagen diseases, uremia, and congestive heart failure. Many effusions that initially have negative cytology will become positive over time.

Seto et al, from the Kyushu Cancer Center, reported a single-arm series of 80 patients with previously untreated malignant pleural effusions from non–small-cell lung cancer. The patients had a chest tube placed and were given 25 mg of cisplatin in 500 mL of distilled water intrapleurally. Toxicity was acceptable. Median time of drainage was 4 days. A total of 34% had a complete response and 49% had a partial response for an overall response rate of 83%. A striking finding in this study was that the median survival time of all patients was 239 days, a longer survival than seen in comparable patients treated with pleurodesis. The authors recommend a phase III study *(Seto T, Ushimima S, Yamamoto H, et al: Br J Cancer 95:717-721, 2006).*

Tamponade occurs when fluid accumulates faster than the pericardium can stretch. Compression of all four heart chambers ensues, with tachycardia and diminishing cardiac output. Fluid loading can counteract intrapericardial pressure temporarily. Reciprocal filling of right- and left-sided chambers with inspiration and expiration, secondary to paradoxical movement of the ventricular septum, is a final mechanism to maintain blood flow before death.

Diagnosis

A high index of suspicion is required to make the diagnosis of pericardial effusion.

Signs and symptoms Dyspnea is the most common symptom. Patients may also complain of chest pain or discomfort, easy fatigability, cough, and orthopnea or may be completely asymptomatic. Signs include distant heart sounds and pericardial friction rub. With cardiac tamponade, progressive heart failure occurs, with increased shortness of breath, cold sweats, confusion, pulsus paradoxus > 13 mm Hg, jugular venous distention, and hypotension.

Chest x-ray Chest radiographic evidence of pericardial effusion includes cardiomegaly with a "water bottle" heart; an irregular, nodular contour of the cardiac shadow; and mediastinal widening.

ECG The electrocardiogram (ECG) shows nonspecific ST- and T-wave changes, tachycardia, low QRS voltage, electrical alternans, and atrial dysrhythmia.

Pericardiocentesis and echocardiography An echocardiogram not only can confirm a suspected pericardial effusion but also can document the size of the effusion and its effect on ventricular function. A pericardial tap with cytologic examination (positive in 50% to 85% of cases with associated malignancy) will confirm the diagnosis of malignant effusion or differentiate it from other causes of pericardial effusion. Serious complications, including cardiac perforation and death, can occur during pericardiocentesis, even when performed with echocardiographic guidance by experienced clinicians.

Tumor markers or special staining and cytogenetic techniques may improve the diagnostic yield, but ultimately an open pericardial biopsy may be necessary. Szturmowicz, et al, from Warsaw, Poland, studied pericardial fluid carcinoembryonic antigen (CEA) and CYFRA 21-1 levels in 84 patients with pericardial effusion. There were significant differences in patients with malignant versus benign effusions with both tests. With cutoff points of > 100 ng/mL for CYFRA 21-1 and > 5 ng/mL for CEA, 14 of 15 patients with malignant pericardial effusion with negative cytologic results had a positive result on one or both tests.

CT and magnetic resonance imaging (MRI) as diagnostic adjuncts may provide additional information about the presence and location of loculations or mass lesions within the pericardium and adjacent structures.

Cardiac catheterization may occasionally be of value to rule out superior vena caval obstruction, diagnose microvascular tumor spread in the lungs with secondary pulmonary hypertension, and document constrictive pericarditis before surgical intervention. Pericardial fluid has been aspirated in experimental animals by femoral vein catheterization and needle puncture of the right atrial appendage from within. This technique has not been used in humans.

Pericardioscopy allows visualization and biopsy at the time of subxiphoid or thoracoscopic pericardiotomy and can improve the diagnostic yield.

Prognosis

In general, cancer patients who develop a significant pericardial effusion have a high mortality, with a mean time to death of 2.2 to 4.7 months. However, about 25% of selected patients treated surgically for cardiac tamponade enjoy a 1-year survival.

Treatment

GENERAL CONCEPTS

As is the case with malignant pleural effusion, it is difficult to evaluate treatments for pericardial effusion because of the many variables. Because malignant pericardial effusion is less common than malignant pleural effusion, it is more difficult to collect data in a prospective manner. Certain generalizations can, however, be derived from available data:

- All cancer patients with pericardial effusion require a systematic evaluation and should not be dismissed summarily as having an untreatable and/or terminal problem.

- Ultimately, both the management and natural course of the effusion depend on (1) the underlying condition of the patient, (2) the extent of clinical symptoms associated with the cardiac compression, and (3) the type and extent of the underlying malignant disease.

GENERAL TREATMENT APPROACHES

Asymptomatic, small effusions may be managed with careful follow-up and treatment directed against the underlying malignancy. On the other hand, cardiac tamponade is a true oncologic emergency. Immediate pericardiocentesis, under echocardiographic guidance, may be performed to relieve the patient's symptoms. A high failure rate is anticipated because the effusion rapidly recurs unless steps are taken to prevent it. Therefore, a more definitive treatment plan should be made following the initial diagnostic/therapeutic tap.

In patients with symptomatic, moderate-to-large effusions who do not present as an emergency, therapy should be aimed at relieving symptoms and preventing recurrence of tamponade or constrictive pericardial disease. Patients with tumors responsive to chemotherapy or radiation therapy may attain longer remissions with appropriate therapy.

There are two theoretical mechanisms for control of pericardial effusion: creation of a persistent defect in the pericardium allowing fluid to drain out and be reabsorbed by surrounding tissues or sclerosis of the mesothelium resulting in the formation of fibrous adhesions that obliterate the pericardial cavity.

Postmortem studies have demonstrated that both of these mechanisms are operative. The fact that effusions can recur implies that there is either insufficient damage to the mesothelial layer or that rapid recurrence of effusion prevents coaptation of visceral and parietal pericardium and prevents the formation of adhesions. This, in turn, would suggest that early closure of the pericardial defect can result in recurrence.

TREATMENT METHODS

Various methods can be used to treat malignant pericardial effusion.

Observation Observation alone may be reasonable in the presence of small asymptomatic effusions.

Pericardiocentesis is useful in relieving tamponade and obtaining a diagnosis. Echocardiographic guidance considerably enhances the safety of this procedure. Ninety percent of pericardial effusions will recur within 3 months after pericardiocentesis alone.

Pericardiocentesis and percutaneous tube drainage can now be performed with low risk and are recommended by some clinical groups. Problems that may occur include occlusion or displacement of the small-bore tubes, dysrhythmia, recurrent effusion, and infections. Mayo Clinic cardiologists recommend initial percutaneous pericardiocentesis with extended catheter drainage as their technique of choice.

Intrapericardial sclerotherapy and chemotherapy following percutaneous or open drainage have been reported to be effective treatments by some groups. Problems include pain during sclerosing agent treatments and recurrence of effusions. Good results have been reported with instillation of a number of agents, including bleomycin (10 mg), cisplatin (30 mg), mitomycin (2 mg), thiotepa (1.5 mg), and mitoxantrone (10 to 20 mg). Agents are selected based on their antitumor or sclerosing effect.

Martinoni et al, from Milan, Italy, reported on the use of intrapericardial administration of thiotepa (15 mg on days 1,3, and 5) following placement of a pericardial drainage catheter in 33 patients with malignant pericardial effusion. There were three recurrent effusions (9.1%). The medial survival was 115 days. They concluded that this protocol is safe, well tolerated, and improves quality and duration of life

> Marcy et al, of Nice Cedex, France reviewed multiple, well-illustrated percutaneous methods for management of malignant pericardial effusions *(Marcy PY, Bondiau PY, Brunner P: Eur Radiol 15:2000-2009, 2005).*

Pericardiocentesis and balloon pericardial window After percutaneous placement of a guidewire following pericardiocentesis, a balloon dilating catheter can be placed across the pericardium under fluoroscopic guidance and a window created by balloon inflation.

At the National Taiwan University, cardiologists performed percutaneous double-balloon pericardiotomy in 50 patients with cancer and pericardial effusion and followed their course using serial echocardiograms. Success without recurrence was achieved in 88%. Fifty percent of patients died within 4 months, and 25% survived to 11 months.

Subtotal pericardial resection is seldom performed today. Although it is the definitive treatment, in that there is almost no chance of recurrence or constriction, higher morbidity and longer recovery time render this operation undesirable in patients who have a short anticipated survival. Its use is restricted to cancer patients with recurrent effusions who are in good overall condition and are expected to survive for up to 1 year.

Limited pericardial resection (pericardial window) via anterior thoracotomy or a thoracoscopic approach has a lower morbidity than less invasive techniques, but recovery is delayed. There is a low risk of recurrence. Cardiac herniation is possible if the size of the opening in the pericardium is not carefully controlled.

At City of Hope, Cullinane et al reported on 62 patients with malignant disease who had surgical pericardial window for management of pericardial effusion. Windows were created either thoracoscopically (32) or by subxiphoid (12) or limited thoracotomy (18) approaches. Primary tumors included non–small-cell lung cancer (NSCLC), breast, hematologic, and other solid-organ malignancies. Three recurrent effusions (4.8%) required reoperations. Eight patients (13%) died during the same admission as their surgical procedure. Median survival was much shorter for patients with NSCLC (2.6 months) than for patients with breast cancer (11 months) or hematologic malignancy (10 months). Surgical pericardial window is a safe and durable operative procedure that may provide extended survival in certain subgroups of cancer patients.

Subxiphoid pericardial resection can be performed with the patient under local anesthesia and may be combined with tube drainage and/or pericardial sclerosis. Our group and others have noted recurrences following this technique.

Subxiphoid pericardioperitoneal window through the fused portion of the diaphragm and pericardium has been developed to allow continued drainage of pericardial fluid into the peritoneum. Experience with the procedure is limited, but recurrences may be less frequent than those associated with subxiphoid drainage alone.

Technical factors Prior pleurodesis for malignant pleural effusion makes an ipsilateral transpleural operation difficult or impossible. In lung cancer patients, major airway obstruction may preclude single-lung anesthesia and, thus, thoracoscopic pericardiectomy. Prior median sternotomy may prohibit the use of a subxiphoid approach.

Complications A 30-day mortality rate of 10% or higher has been reported for all of these modalities but is related more to the gravity of the underlying tumor and its sequelae. A small percentage of patients will develop severe problems with pulmonary edema or cardiogenic shock following pericardial decompression. The mechanisms of these problems are poorly understood. Late neoplastic pericardial constriction can occur following initially successful partial pericardiectomy.

Radiotherapy

External-beam irradiation is utilized infrequently in this clinical setting but may be an important option in specialized circumstances, especially in patients with radiosensitive tumors who have not received prior radiation therapy. Responses ranging from 66% to 93% have been reported with this form of treatment, depending on the type of associated tumor.

Systemic therapy

Chemotherapy Systemic chemotherapy is effective in treating pericardial effusions in patients with lymphomas, hematologic malignancies, or breast cancer. Long-term survival can be attained in these patients. If the pericardial effusion is small and/or asymptomatic, invasive treatment may be omitted in some of these cases. Data regarding the effectiveness of systemic chemotherapy or chemotherapy delivered locally in prevention of recurrent pericardial and pleural effusion are limited. New studies in this area are badly needed.

Biologic therapy with various agents is in the early stages of investigation.

MALIGNANT ASCITES

Malignant ascites results when there is an imbalance in the secretion of proteins and cells into the peritoneal cavity and absorption of fluids via the lymphatic system. Greater capillary permeability as a result of the release of cytokines by malignant cells increases the protein concentration in the peritoneal fluid. Recently, several studies have demonstrated higher levels of vascular endothelial growth factor (VEGF), a cytokine known to cause capillary leak, in the sera and effusions of patients with malignancies.

Signs and symptoms

Patients with malignant ascites usually present with anorexia, nausea, respiratory compromise, and immobility. Complaints of abdominal bloating, heaviness, and ill-fitting clothes are common. Weight gain despite muscle wasting is a prominent sign.

Diagnosis

A malignant etiology accounts for only 10% of all cases of ascites. Nonmalignant diseases causing ascites include liver failure, congestive heart failure, and occlusion of the inferior vena cava or hepatic vein. About one-third of all patients with malignancies will develop ascites. Malignant ascites has been described with many tumor types but is most commonly seen with gynecologic neoplasms (~50%), GI malignancies (20% to 25%), and breast cancer (10% to 18%). In 15% to 30% of patients, the ascites is associated with diffuse carcinomatosis of the peritoneal cavity.

Physical examination does not distinguish whether ascites is due to malignant or benign conditions. Patients may have abdominal fullness with fluid wave, anterior distribution of the normal abdominal tympany, and pedal edema. Occasionally, the hepatic metastases or tumor nodules studding the peritoneal surface can be palpated through the abdominal wall, which has been altered by ascitic distention.

RADIOLOGIC STUDIES

Radiographs Ascites can be inferred from plain radiographs of the abdomen. Signs include a ground-glass pattern and centralization of the intestines and abdominal contents.

Ultrasonography Abdominal ultrasonography has been shown to be the most sensitive, most specific method for detecting and quantifying ascites. It also permits delineation of areas of loculation.

Success at removing peritoneal fluid in patients was markedly better with ultrasonographic assistance, as demonstrated in a randomized trial. Ultrasonography improved the physician's ability to aspirate ascites from 67% (27 of 44 patients) to 95% (40 of 42 patients).

CT Abdominal and pelvic CT is effective in detecting ascites. In addition, CT scans may demonstrate masses, mesenteric stranding, omental studding, and diffuse carcinomatosis. Intravenous and oral contrasts are necessary, thus increasing the degree of invasiveness of this modality.

Paracentesis After the diagnosis of peritoneal ascites has been made on the basis of the physical examination and imaging, paracentesis should be performed to characterize the fluid. The color and nature of the fluid often suggest the diagnosis. Malignant ascites can be bloody, opaque, chylous, or serous. Benign ascites is usually serous and clear.

Analysis of the fluid should include cell count, cytology, LDH level, proteins, and appropriate evaluation for infectious etiologies. In addition, the fluid can be sent for the determination of tumor markers, such as CEA, CA-125, $p53$, and human chorionic gonadotropin-β (hCG-β). The hCG-β level is frequently elevated in malignancy-related ascites and has been combined with cytology to yield an 89.5% efficiency in diagnosis. The use of DNA ploidy indices allowed a 98.5% sensitivity and a 100% sensitivity in the identification of malignant cells within ascitic fluid. The use of the telomerase assay, along with cytologic evaluation of the ascitic fluid contents, has a 77% sensitivity in detecting malignant ascites.

Laparoscopy Several studies have utilized minimally invasive laparoscopy as the diagnostic tool of choice. The fluid can be drained under direct visualization, the peritoneal cavity can be evaluated carefully, and any suspicious masses can be biopsied at the time of the laparoscopy.

Prognosis

The presence of ascites in a patient with malignancy often portends end-stage disease. Median survival after the diagnosis of malignant ascites ranges from 7 to 13 weeks. Patients with gynecologic and breast malignancies have a better overall prognosis than patients with GI malignancies.

Treatment

Medical therapy

Traditionally, the first line of treatment is medical management. Medical therapies include repeated paracentesis, fluid restriction, diuretics, chemotherapy, and intraperitoneal sclerosis.

Repeated paracentesis, probably the most frequently employed treatment modality, provides significant symptomatic relief in the majority of cases. The procedure is minimally invasive and can be combined with abdomi-

> Laparoscopic instillation of hyperthermic chemotherapy has been shown to be successful in palliating patients with debilitating malignant ascites. Patients survived for an average of 6.7 months after the procedure and did not have recurrence of their ascites (Garofalo A, Valle M, Garcia J, et al: EJSO 32:682-685, 2006).

nal ultrasonography to better localize fluid collections. High-volume paracentesis has been performed without inducing significant hemodynamic instability and with good patient tolerance.

After paracentesis, 78% of all patients reported relief of their symptoms, especially in the areas of abdominal bloating, anorexia, dyspnea, insomnia, and fatigue. In addition, overall quality of life improved after paracentesis.

Significant morbidity occurs with repeated taps and becomes more severe with each tap necessary to alleviate symptoms. Ascitic fluid contains a high concentration of proteins. Routine removal of ascites further depletes protein stores. The removal of large volumes of fluid also can result in electrolyte abnormalities and hypovolemia. In addition, complications can result from the procedure itself. They include hemorrhage, injury to intra-abdominal structures, peritonitis, and bowel obstruction. Contraindications to repeated paracentesis are viscous loculated fluid and hemorrhagic fluid.

With the placement of an intraperitoneal port, used also for the instillation of intraperitoneal chemotherapy, removal of ascitic fluid is possible without the need for repeated paracentesis. Other possible catheters for use in repeated paracentesis include PleurX and Tenckoff catheters (used for intraperitoneal dialysis). Placement of a semipermanent catheter minimizes the risk of injury to intra-abdominal structures. However, the benefits are tempered by increased infectious risks as well as the possibility of a nonfunctioning catheter requiring removal and replacement.

Diuretics, fluid and salt restriction Unlike ascites from benign causes such as cirrhosis and congestive heart failure, malignant ascites responds poorly to fluid restriction, decreased salt intake, and diuretic therapy. The most commonly used diuretics (in patients who may have some response to diuretic treatment) are spironolactone (Aldactone) and amiloride (Midamor). Patients with massive hepatic metastases are most likely to benefit from spironolactone.

The onset of action for spironolactone is delayed (3 to 4 days), whereas the effects of amiloride are seen after 24 hours. The most common complications associated with these diuretics are painful gynecomastia, renal tubular acidosis, and hyperkalemia.

Chemotherapy, both systemic and intraperitoneal, has had some success in the treatment of malignant ascites. The most commonly used agents are cisplatin and mitomycin. Intraperitoneal hyperthermic chemotherapy has been used with some efficacy in GI malignancies to decrease recurrence of ascites as well as to prevent the formation of ascites in patients with peritoneal carcinomatosis.

Sclerotherapy Sclerosing agents include bleomycin (60 mg/50 mL of normal saline) and talc (5 g/50 mL of normal saline). Responses are seen in ~30% of patients treated with these agents.

Theoretically, intraperitoneal chemotherapy and sclerosis obliterate the peritoneal space and prevent future fluid accumulation. If sclerosis is unsuccessful, it may produce loculations and make subsequent paracentesis difficult.

Other systemic therapies There are several reports of the use of gold-198 or phosphorus-32 in patients with peritoneal effusions, with response rates of 30% to 50%. Experimental models and early clinical trials have shown that an intraperitoneal bolus of tumor necrosis factor (45 to 350 µg/m²) given weekly may be effective in resolving malignant ascites. Other cytokines, including interferon-α, had varying success. A randomized, prospective trial definitively addressing the role of cytokines and other biologic treatments in the management of malignant ascites has yet to be completed.

> The efficacy of peritoneovenous shunts in patients with malignant ascites was evaluated retrospectively. Overall, the morbidity rate was 36%, the occlusion rate was 12%, and postoperative survival after placement of the shunt was a mean of 54.5 days. A decrease in body weight and abdominal girth was shown. Most patients did not require further care for their ascites (Tomiyama K, Takahashi M, Fujii T, et al: Anticancer Res 26:2393-2395, 2006).

Surgery

Limited surgical options are available to treat patients who have refractory ascites after maximal medical management, demonstrate a significant decrease in quality of life as a result of ascites, and have a life expectancy of > 3 months.

Peritoneovenous shunts have been used since 1974 for the relief of ascites associated with benign conditions. In the 1980s, shunting was applied to the treatment of malignant ascites.

The LeVeen shunt contains a disc valve in a firm polypropylene casing, whereas the Denver shunt has a valve that lies within a fluid-filled, compressible silicone chamber. Both valves provide a connection between the peritoneal cavity and venous system that permits the free flow of fluid from the peritoneal cavity when a 2- to 4-cm water pressure gradient exists.

Success rates vary with shunting, depending on the nature of the ascites and the pathology of the primary tumor. Patients with ovarian cancer, for example, do very well, with palliation achieved in ≥ 50% of cases. However, ascites arising from GI malignancies is associated with a poorer response rate (10% to 15%).

Patient selection Candidates for shunt placement should be carefully selected. Cardiac and respiratory evaluations should be performed prior to the procedure. Shunt placement is *contraindicated* in the presence of the following:

- a moribund patient whose death is anticipated within weeks
- peritonitis
- major organ failure
- adhesive loculation
- thick, tenacious fluid.

Complications of shunting Initial concerns about the use of a shunt in the treatment of malignant ascites centered around intravascular dissemination of tumor. In practice, there has been little difference in overall mortality in patients with and without shunts.

Disseminated intravascular coagulation During the early experience with shunting, particularly in cirrhotic patients, symptomatic clinical disseminated intravascular coagulation (DIC) developed rapidly and was a major source of morbidity and mortality. However, overwhelming DIC occurs infrequently in the oncologic population.

The pathophysiology of DIC has been studied extensively and is thought to be multifactorial. The reinfusion of large volumes of ascitic fluid may cause a deficiency in endogenous circulating coagulation factors by dilution. Secondarily, a fibrinolytic state is initiated by the introduction of soluble collagen (contained within the ascitic fluid) into the bloodstream, leading to a DIC state. Infrequently, full-blown DIC results and requires ligation of the shunt or even shunt removal. Discarding 50% to 70% of the ascitic fluid before establishing the peritoneovenous connection may prevent this complication but may increase the risk of early failure due to a reduced initial flow rate.

Commonly, coagulation parameters are abnormal without signs or symptoms. In some institutions, these laboratory values are so consistently abnormal that they are used to monitor shunt patency. Abnormalities most commonly seen include decreased platelets and fibrinogen and elevated prothrombin time, partial thromboplastin time, and fibrin split products.

Other common complications include shunt occlusion (10% to 20%), heart failure (6%), ascitic leak from the insertion site (4%), infection (< 5%), and perioperative death (10% to 20% when all operative candidates are included).

Shunt patency may be indirectly correlated with the presence of malignant cells. One study found that patients with positive cytology results had a 26-day shunt survival, as compared with 140 days in patients with negative cytology results. Other studies have failed to demonstrate a correlation between ascites with malignant cells and decreased survival.

Clearly, shunting is not a benign procedure, but in carefully selected patients who have not responded to other treatment modalities and who are experiencing symptoms from ascites, it may provide needed palliation. Because of the limited effectiveness of peritoneovenous shunts, patients should be carefully selected prior to shunt placement.

Radical peritoniectomy Other surgical procedures used to treat malignant ascites have been proposed. They include radical peritoniectomy combined with intraperitoneal chemotherapy. This is an extensive operation with significant morbidity, although initial results appear to demonstrate that it decreases the production of ascites. To date, no randomized trial has demonstrated that radical peritoniectomy increases efficacy or survival.

SUGGESTED READING

ON MALIGNANT PLEURAL EFFUSION

Altundag O, Stewart DJ, Stevens C, et al: The risk of distant metastases in patients with non-small cell lung cancer (NSCLC) with cytologically proven malignant pleural effusion, stage IIIB: A retrospective analysis (abstract). J Clin Oncol 23(suppl):853s, 2005.

Dresler CM, Olak J, Herndon JE 2nd, et al: Phase III intergroup study of talc poudrage vs talc slurry sclerosis for malignant pleural effusion. Chest 127:909–915, 2005.

Gasparri R, Leo F, Veronesi G, et al: Video-assisted management of malignant pleural effusion in breast carcinoma. Cancer 106:271–276, 2006.

Haddad FJ, Younes RN, Gross JL, et al: Pleurodesis in patients with malignant pleural effusions: Talc slurry or bleomycin? Results of a prospective randomized trial. World J Surg 28:749–753, 2004.

Hsu LH, Soong TC, Feng AC, et al: Intrapleural urokinase for the treatment of loculated malignant pleural effusions and trapped lungs in medically inoperable cancer patients. J Thorac Oncol 1:460–467, 2006.

Ishida A, Miyazawa T, Miyazu Y, et al: Intrapleural cisplatin and OK432 therapy for malignant pleural effusion caused by non-small cell lung cancer. Respirology 11:90–97, 2006.

Kwek BH, Aquino SL, Fischman AJ: Fluorodeoxyglucose positron emission tomography and CT after talc pleurodesis. Chest 125:2356–2360, 2004.

Paschoalini Mda S, Vargas FS, Marchi E, et al: Prospective randomized trial of silver nitrate vs talc slurry in pleurodesis for symptomatic malignant pleural effusions. Chest 128:684–689, 2005.

Steger V, Mika U, Toomes H, et al: Who gains most? A 10-year experience with 611 thoracoscopic talc pleurodeses. Ann Thorac Surg 83:1940–1945, 2007.

Tan C, Sedrakyan A, Browne J, et al: The evidence on the effectiveness of management for malignant pleural effusion: A systematic review. Eur J Cardiothorac Surg 29:829–838, 2006.

Tremblay A, Mason C, Michaud G: Use of tunnelled pleural catheters for malignant pleural effusions in patients fit for pleurodesis. Eur Respir J 30:759–762, 2007.

Warren WH, Kalimi R, Khodadadian LM, et al: Management of malignant pleural effusions using the Pleur (x) catheter. Ann Thorac Surg 85:1049–1055, 2008.

ON PERICARDIAL EFFUSION

Bischiniotis TS, Lafaras CT, Platogiannis DN, et al: Intrapericardial cisplatin administration after pericardiocentesis in patients with lung adenocarcinoma and malignant cardiac tamponade. Hellenic J Cardiol 46:324–329, 2005.

Cullinane CA, Paz IB, Smith D, et al: Prognostic factors in the surgical management of pericardial effusion in the patient with concurrent malignancy. Chest 125:1328–1334, 2004.

Maisch B, Seferovic PM, Ristic AD, et al: Guidelines on the diagnosis and management of pericardial diseases executive summary: The Task Force on the Diagnosis and Management of Pericardial Diseases of the European Society of Cardiology. Eur Heart J 25:587–610, 2004.

Martinoni A, Cipolla CM, Cardinale D, et al: Long-term results of intrapericardial chemotherapeutic treatment of malignant pericardial effusions with thiotepa. Chest 126:1412–1416, 2004.

McDonald JM, Meyers BF, Guthrie TJ, et al: Comparison of open subxiphoid pericardial drainage with percutaneous catheter drainage for symptomatic pericardial effusion. Ann Thorac Surg 76:811–816, 2003.

Szturmowicz M, Tomkowksi W, Fijalkowska A, et al: Diagnostic utility of CYFRA 21-1 and CEA assays in pericardial fluid for the recognition of neoplastic pericarditis. Int J Biol Markers 20:43–49, 2005.

Tomkowski WZ, Wisniewska J, Szturmowicz M, et al: Evaluation of intrapericardial cisplatin administration in cases with recurrent malignant pericardial effusion and cardiac tamponade. Support Care Cancer 12:53–57, 2004.

Tsang TS, Enrique-Sarano M, Freeman WK, et al: Consecutive 1,127 therapeutic echocardiographically guided pericardiocenteses: Clinical profile, practice patterns, and outcomes spanning 21 years. Mayo Clin Proc 77:429–436, 2002.

ON MALIGNANT ASCITES

Becker G, Galandi D, Blum HE: Malignant ascites: Systematic review and guideline for treatment. Eur J Cancer 42:589–597, 2006.

Easson A, Bezjak A, Ross S, et al: Change in symptoms after paracentesis for symptomatic malignant ascites [abstract]. J Clin Oncol 23(suppl):16s, 2005.

Gushchin V, Demmy TL, Kane JM 3rd: Surgical management of metastatic peritoneal or pleural disease. Semin Oncol 34:215–225, 2007.

Nazeer SR, Dewbre H, Miller AH: Ultrasound-assisted paracentesis performed by emergency physicians vs the traditional technique: A prospective, randomized study. Am J Emerg Med 23:363–367, 2005.

Rosenberg SM: Palliation of malignant ascites. Gastroenterol Clin North Am 35:189–199, 2006.

AVASTIN® (Bevacizumab)

For Intravenous Use

WARNINGS

Gastrointestinal Perforations

Avastin administration can result in the development of gastrointestinal perforation, in some instances resulting in fatality. Gastrointestinal perforation, sometimes associated with intra-abdominal abscess, occurred throughout treatment with Avastin (i.e., was not correlated to duration of exposure). The incidence of gastrointestinal perforation (gastrointestinal perforation, fistula formation, and/or intra-abdominal abscess) in patients with colorectal cancer and in patients with non-small cell lung cancer (NSCLC) receiving Avastin was 2.4% and 0.9%, respectively. The typical presentation was reported as abdominal pain associated with symptoms such as constipation and vomiting. Gastrointestinal perforation should be included in the differential diagnosis of patients presenting with abdominal pain on Avastin. Avastin therapy should be permanently discontinued in patients with gastrointestinal perforation. (See **WARNINGS: Gastrointestinal Perforations** and **DOSAGE AND ADMINISTRATION: Dose Modifications**.)

Wound Healing Complications

Avastin administration can result in the development of wound dehiscence, in some instances resulting in fatality. Avastin therapy should be permanently discontinued in patients with wound dehiscence requiring medical intervention. The appropriate interval between termination of Avastin and subsequent elective surgery required to avoid the risks of impaired wound healing/wound dehiscence has not been determined. (See **WARNINGS: Wound Healing Complications** and **DOSAGE AND ADMINISTRATION: Dose Modifications**.)

Hemorrhage

Fatal pulmonary hemorrhage can occur in patients with NSCLC treated with chemotherapy and Avastin. The incidence of severe or fatal hemoptysis was 31% in patients with squamous histology and 2.3% in patients with NSCLC excluding predominant squamous histology. Patients with recent hemoptysis (≥1/2 tsp of red blood) should not receive Avastin. (See **WARNINGS: Hemorrhage, ADVERSE REACTIONS: Hemorrhage,** and **DOSAGE AND ADMINISTRATION: Dose Modifications**.)

INDICATIONS AND USAGE

Avastin®, in combination with intravenous 5-fluorouracil–based chemotherapy, is indicated for first- or second-line treatment of patients with metastatic carcinoma of the colon or rectum.

Avastin®, in combination with carboplatin and paclitaxel, is indicated for first-line treatment of patients with unresectable, locally advanced, recurrent or metastatic non-squamous, non-small cell lung cancer.

Avastin®, in combination with paclitaxel is indicated for the treatment of patients who have not received chemotherapy for metastatic HER2 negative breast cancer.

The effectiveness of Avastin in metastatic breast cancer is based on an improvement in progression free survival. Avastin is not indicated for patients with breast cancer that has progressed following anthracycline and taxane chemotherapy administered for metastatic disease.

Currently, no data are available that demonstrate an improvement in disease-related symptoms or increased survival with Avastin in breast cancer. (See CLINICAL STUDIES.)

CONTRAINDICATIONS
None.

WARNINGS

Gastrointestinal Perforations (See DOSAGE AND ADMINISTRATION: Dose Modifications)

Gastrointestinal perforation complicated by intra-abdominal abscesses or fistula formation and in some instances with fatal outcome, occurs at an increased incidence in patients receiving Avastin as compared to controls. In Studies 1, 2, and 3, the incidence of gastrointestinal perforation (gastrointestinal perforation, fistula formation, and/or intra-abdominal abscess) in patients receiving Avastin was 2.4%. These episodes occurred with or without intra-abdominal abscesses and at various time points during treatment. The typical presentation was reported as abdominal pain associated with symptoms such as constipation and emesis.

In post-marketing clinical studies and reports, gastrointestinal perforation, fistula formation in the gastrointestinal tract (eg. gastrointestinal, enterocutaneous, esophageal, duodenal, rectal), and/or intra-abdominal abscess occurred in patients receiving Avastin for colorectal and for other types of cancer. The overall incidence in clinical studies was 1%, but may be higher in some cancer settings. Of the reported events, approximately 30% were fatal. Patients with gastrointestinal perforation, regardless of underlying cancer, typically present with abdominal pain, nausea and fever. Events were reported at various time points during treatment ranging from one week to greater than 1 year from initiation of Avastin, with most events occurring within the first 50 days.

Permanently discontinue Avastin in patients with gastrointestinal perforation (gastrointestinal perforation, fistula formation, and/or intra-abdominal abscess).

Non-Gastrointestinal Fistula Formation (See DOSAGE AND ADMINISTRATION: Dose Modifications)

Non-gastrointestinal fistula formation has been reported in patients treated with Avastin in controlled clinical studies (with an incidence of <0.3%) and in post-marketing experience, in some cases with fatal outcome. Fistula formation involving the following areas of the body other than the gastrointestinal tract have been reported: tracheo-esophageal, bronchopleural, biliary, vagina and bladder. Events were reported throughout treatment with Avastin, with most events occurring within the first 6 months. Permanently discontinue Avastin in patients with fistula formation involving an internal organ.

Wound Healing Complications (See DOSAGE AND ADMINISTRATION: Dose Modifications)

Avastin impairs wound healing in animal models. In clinical studies of Avastin, patients were not allowed to receive Avastin until at least 28 days had elapsed following surgery. In clinical studies of Avastin in combination with chemotherapy, there were 6 instances of dehiscence among 788 patients (0.8%).

The appropriate interval between discontinuation of Avastin and subsequent elective surgery required to avoid the risks of impaired wound healing has not been determined. In Study 1, 39 patients who received bolus-IFL plus Avastin underwent surgery following Avastin therapy; of these patients, six (15%) had wound healing/bleeding complications. In the same study, 25 patients in the bolus-IFL arm underwent surgery; of these patients, one of 25 (4%) had wound healing/bleeding complications. The longest interval between last dose of study drug and dehiscence was 56 days; this occurred in a patient on the bolus-IFL plus Avastin arm.

AVASTIN® (Bevacizumab)

The interval between termination of Avastin and subsequent elective surgery should take into consideration the calculated half-life of Avastin (approximately 20 days). Discontinue Avastin in patients with wound healing complications requiring medical intervention.

Hemorrhage (See DOSAGE AND ADMINISTRATION: Dose Modifications)

Two distinct patterns of bleeding have occurred in patients receiving Avastin. The first is minor hemorrhage, most commonly NCI-CTC Grade 1 epistaxis. The second is serious, and in some cases fatal, hemorrhagic events.

In Study 6, four of 13 (31%) Avastin-treated patients with squamous cell histology and two of 53 (4%) Avastin-treated patients with histology other than squamous cell, experienced serious or fatal pulmonary hemorrhage as compared to none of the 32 (0%) patients receiving chemotherapy alone. Of the patients experiencing pulmonary hemorrhage requiring medical intervention, many had cavitation and/or necrosis of the tumor, either pre-existing or developing during Avastin therapy. In Study 5, the rate of pulmonary hemorrhage requiring medical intervention for the PC plus Avastin arm was 2.3% (10 of 427) compared to 0.5% (2 of 441) for the PC alone arm. There were seven deaths due to pulmonary hemorrhage reported by investigators in the PC plus Avastin arm as compared to one in the PC alone arm. Generally, these serious hemorrhagic events presented as major or massive hemoptysis without an antecedent history of minor hemoptysis during Avastin therapy. Do not administer Avastin to patients with recent history of hemoptysis (≥1/2 tsp of red blood). Other serious bleeding events occurring in patients receiving Avastin across all indications include gastrointestinal hemorrhage, subarachnoid hemorrhage, and hemorrhagic stroke. Some of these events were fatal. (See ADVERSE REACTIONS: Hemorrhage.)

The risk of central nervous system (CNS) bleeding in patients with CNS metastases receiving Avastin has not been evaluated because these patients were excluded fromlate stage clinical studies following development of CNS hemorrhage in a patient with a CNS metastasis in a Phase 1 study.

Discontinue Avastin in patients with serious hemorrhage (i.e., requiring medical intervention) and initiate aggressive medical management. (See ADVERSE REACTIONS: Hemorrhage.)

Arterial Thromboembolic Events (see DOSAGE AND ADMINISTRATION: Dose Modifications and PRECAUTIONS: Geriatric Use)

Arterial thromboembolic events (ATE) occurred at a higher incidence in patients receiving Avastin in combination with chemotherapy as compared to those receiving chemotherapy alone. ATE included cerebral infarction, transient ischemic attacks (TIAs), myocardial infarction (MI), angina, and a variety of other ATE. These events were fatal in some instances. In a pooled analysis of randomized, controlled clinical trials involving 1745 patients, the incidence of ATE was 4.4% among patients treated with Avastin in combination with chemotherapy and 1.9% among patients receiving chemotherapy alone. Fatal outcomes for these events occurred in 7 of 963 patients (0.7%) who were treated with Avastin in combination with chemotherapy, compared to 3 of 782 patients (0.4%) who were treated with chemotherapy alone. The incidences of both cerebrovascular arterial events (1.9% vs. 0.5%) and cardiovascular arterial events (2.1% vs. 1.0%) were increased in patients receiving Avastin compared to chemotherapy alone. The relative risk of ATE was greater in patients 65 and over (8.5% vs. 2.9%) as compared to those less than 65 (2.1% vs. 1.4%). (See PRECAUTIONS: Geriatric Use.)

The safety of resumption of Avastin therapy after resolution of an ATE has not been studied. Permanently discontinue Avastin in patients who experience a severe ATE during treatment. (See **DOSAGE AND ADMINISTRATION: Dose Modifications** and **PRECAUTIONS: Geriatric Use**.)

Hypertension (See DOSAGE AND ADMINISTRATION: Dose Modifications)

The incidence of severe hypertension was increased in patients receiving Avastin as compared to controls. Across clinical studies the incidence of NCI-CTC Grade 3 or 4 hypertension ranged from 8-18%.

Medication classes used for management of patients with NCI-CTC Grade 3 hypertension receiving Avastin included angiotensin-converting enzyme inhibitors, beta blockers, diuretics, and calcium channel blockers. Development or worsening of hypertension can require hospitalization or require discontinuation of Avastin in up to 1.7% of patients. Hypertension can persist after discontinuation of Avastin. Complications can include hypertensive encephalopathy (in some cases fatal) and CNS hemorrhage.

In the post-marketing experience, acute increases in blood pressure associated with initial or subsequent infusions of Avastin have been reported (see **PRECAUTIONS: Infusion Reactions**). Some cases were serious and associated with clinical sequelae. Permanently discontinue Avastin in patients with hypertensive crisis or hypertensive encephalopathy. Temporarily suspend Avastin in patients with severe hypertension that is not controlled with medical management. (See **DOSAGE AND ADMINISTRATION: Dose Modifications**.)

Reversible Posterior Leukoencephalopathy Syndrome (RPLS) (See DOSAGE AND ADMINISTRATION: Dose Modifications)

RPLS has been reported in clinical studies (with an incidence of <0.1%) and in post-marketing experience. RPLS is a neurological disorder which can present with headache, seizure, lethargy, confusion, blindness and other visual and neurologic disturbances. Mild to severe hypertension may be present, but is not necessary for diagnosis of RPLS. Magnetic Resonance Imaging (MRI) is necessary to confirm the diagnosis of RPLS. The onset of symptoms has been reported to occur from 16 hours to 1 year after initiation of Avastin.

In patients developing RPLS, discontinue Avastin and initiate treatment of hypertension, if present. Symptoms usually resolve or improve within days, although some patients have experienced ongoing neurologic sequelae. The safety of reinitiating Avastin therapy in patients previously experiencing RPLS is not known.

Neutropenia and Infection (See PRECAUTIONS: Geriatric Use and ADVERSE REACTIONS: Neutropenia and Infection)

Increased rates of severe neutropenia, febrile neutropenia, and infection with severe neutropenia (including some fatalities) have been observed in patients treated with myelosuppressive chemotherapy plus Avastin. (See **PRECAUTIONS: Geriatric Use** and **ADVERSE REACTIONS: Neutropenia and Infection**.)

Proteinuria (See DOSAGE AND ADMINISTRATION: Dose Modifications)

The incidence and severity of proteinuria is increased in patients receiving Avastin as compared to control. In Studies 1, 3 and 5 the incidence of NCI-CTC Grade 3 and 4 proteinuria, characterized as >3.5 gm/24 hours, ranged up to 3.0% in Avastin-treated patients.

Nephrotic syndrome occurred in three of 1459 (0.5%) patients receiving Avastin in clinical studies. One patient died and one required dialysis. In three patients, proteinuria decreased in severity several months after discontinuation of Avastin. No patient had normalization of

urinary protein levels (by 24-hour urine) following discontinuation of Avastin.
The highest incidence of proteinuria was observed in a dose-ranging, placebo-controlled, randomized study of Avastin in patients with metastatic renal cell carcinoma, an indication for which Avastin is not approved, 24-hour urine collections were obtained in approximately half the patients enrolled. Among patients in whom 24-hour urine collections were obtained, four of 19 (21%) patients receiving Avastin at 10 mg/kg every two weeks, two of 14 (14%) patients receiving Avastin at 3 mg/kg every two weeks, and none of the 15 placebo patients experienced NCI-CTC Grade 3 proteinuria (>3.5 gm protein/24 hours).

Discontinue Avastin in patients with nephrotic syndrome. The safety of continued Avastin treatment in patients with moderate to severe proteinuria has not been evaluated. In most clinical studies, Avastin was interrupted for ≥2 grams of proteinuria/24 hours and resumed when proteinuria was <2 gm/24 hours. Patients with moderate to severe proteinuria based on 24-hour collections should be monitored regularly until improvement and/or resolution is observed. (See **DOSAGE AND ADMINISTRATION: Dose Modifications.**)

Congestive Heart Failure
NCI-CTC Grade 2–4 left ventricular dysfunction, was reported in 25 of 1459 (1.7%) patients receiving Avastin in clinical studies. In Study 7, the rate of congestive heart failure (defined as NCI-CTC Grade 3 and 4) in the Avastin plus paclitaxel arm was 2.2 % versus 0.3% in the control arm. Among patients receiving anthracyclines, the rate of CHF was 3.8% for Avastin treated patients and 0.6% for patients receiving paclitaxel alone. Congestive heart failure occurred in six of 44 (14%) patients with relapsed acute leukemia (an unlabelled indication) receiving Avastin and concurrent anthracyclines in a single arm study.

The safety of continuation or resumption of Avastin in patients with cardiac dysfunction has not been studied.

PRECAUTIONS
General
Use Avastin with caution in patients with known hypersensitivity to Avastin or any component of this drug product.

Infusion Reactions
In clinical studies, infusion reactions with the first dose of Avastin were uncommon (<3%) and severe reactions occurred in 0.2% of patients. Infusion reactions reported in the clinical trials and post-marketing experience include hypertension, hypertensive crises associated with neurologic signs and symptoms, wheezing, oxygen desaturation, NCI-CTC Grade 3 hypersensitivity, chest pain, headaches, rigors, and diaphoresis. Adequate information on rechallenge is not available. Avastin infusion should be interrupted in all patients with severe infusion reactions and appropriate medical therapy administered.

There are no data regarding the most appropriate method of identification of patients who may safely be retreated with Avastin after experiencing a severe infusion reaction.

Surgery
Avastin therapy should not be initiated for at least 28 days following major surgery. The surgical incision should be fully healed prior to initiation of Avastin. Because of the potential for impaired wound healing, Avastin should be suspended prior to elective surgery. The appropriate interval between the last dose of Avastin and elective surgery is unknown; however, the half-life of Avastin is estimated to be 20 days (see **CLINICAL PHARMACOLOGY: Pharmacokinetics**) and the interval chosen should take into consideration the half-life of the drug. (See **WARNINGS: Gastrointestinal Perforations** and **Wound Healing Complications.**)

Cardiovascular Disease
Patients were excluded from participation in Avastin clinical trials if, in the previous year, they had experienced clinically significant cardiovascular disease. In an exploratory analysis pooling the data from five randomized, placebo-controlled, clinical trials conducted in patients without a recent history of clinically significant cardiovascular disease, the overall incidence of arterial thromboembolic events, the incidence of fatal arterial thromboembolic events, and the incidence of cardiovascular thromboembolic events were increased in patients receiving Avastin plus chemotherapy as compared to chemotherapy alone.

Laboratory Tests
Blood pressure monitoring should be conducted every two to three weeks during treatment with Avastin. Patients who develop hypertension on Avastin may require blood pressure monitoring at more frequent intervals. Patients with Avastin-induced or -exacerbated hypertension who discontinue Avastin should continue to have their blood pressure monitored at regular intervals.

Patients receiving Avastin should be monitored for the development or worsening of proteinuria with serial urinalyses. Patients with a 2+ or greater urine dipstick reading should undergo further assessment, e.g., a 24-hour urine collection. (See **WARNINGS: Proteinuria** and **DOSAGE AND ADMINISTRATION: Dose Modifications.**)

Drug Interactions
No formal drug interaction studies with anti-neoplastic agents have been conducted. In Study 1, patients with colorectal cancer were given irinotecan/5-FU/leucovorin (bolus-IFL) with or without Avastin. Irinotecan concentrations were similar in patients receiving bolus-IFL alone and in combination with Avastin. The concentrations of SN38, the active metabolite of irinotecan, were on average 33% higher in patients receiving bolus-IFL in combination with Avastin when compared with bolus-IFL alone. In Study 1, patients receiving bolus-IFL plus Avastin had a higher incidence of NCI-CTC Grade 3–4 diarrhea and neutropenia. Due to high inter-patient variability and limited sampling, the extent of the increase in SN38 in patients receiving concurrent irinotecan and Avastin is uncertain. In Study 6, based on limited data, there did not appear to be a difference in the mean exposure of either carboplatin or paclitaxel when each was administered alone or in combination with Avastin. However, 3 of the 8 patients receiving Avastin plus paclitaxel/carboplatin had substantially lower paclitaxel exposure after four cycles of treatment (at Day 63) than those at Day 0, while patients receiving paclitaxel/carboplatin without Avastin had a greater paclitaxel exposure at Day 63 than at Day 0.

Carcinogenesis, Mutagenesis, Impairment of Fertility
No carcinogenicity data are available for Avastin in animals or humans.

Avastin may impair fertility. Dose-related decreases in ovarian and uterine weights, endometrial proliferation, number of menstrual cycles, and arrested follicular development or absent corpora lutea were observed in female cynomolgus monkeys treated with 10 or 50 mg/kg of Avastin for 13 or 26 weeks. Following a 4- or 12-week recovery period, which examined only the high–dose group, trends suggestive of reversibility were noted in the two females for each regimen that were assigned to recover. After the 12-week recovery period, follicular maturation arrest was no longer observed, but ovarian weights were still moderately decreased. Reduced endometrial

proliferation was no longer observed at the 12-week recovery time point, but uterine weight decreases were still notable, corpora lutea were absent in 1 out of 2 animals, and the number of menstrual cycles remained reduced (67%).

Pregnancy Category C
Avastin has been shown to be teratogenic in rabbits when administered in doses that approximate the human dose on a mg/kg basis. Observed effects included decreases in maternal and fetal body weights, an increased number of fetal resorptions, and an increased incidence of specific gross and skeletal fetal alterations. Adverse fetal outcomes were observed at all doses tested.

Angiogenesis is critical to fetal development and the inhibition of angiogenesis following administration of Avastin is likely to result in adverse effects on pregnancy. There are no adequate and well-controlled studies in pregnant women. Avastin should be used during pregnancy or in any woman not employing adequate contraception only if the potential benefit justifies the potential risk to the fetus. All patients should be counseled regarding the potential risk of Avastin to the developing fetus prior to initiation of therapy. If the patient becomes pregnant while receiving Avastin, she should be apprised of the potential hazard to the fetus and/or the potential risk of loss of pregnancy. Patients who discontinue Avastin should also be counseled concerning the prolonged exposure following discontinuation of therapy (half-life of approximately 20 days) and the possible effects of Avastin on fetal development.

Nursing Mothers
It is not known whether Avastin is secreted in human milk. Because human IgG1 is secreted into human milk, the potential for absorption and harm to the infant after ingestion is unknown. Women should be advised to discontinue nursing during treatment with Avastin and for a prolonged period following the use of Avastin, taking into account the half-life of the product, approximately 20 days [range 11-50 days]. (See **CLINICAL PHARMACOLOGY: Pharmacokinetics**.)

Pediatric Use
The safety and effectiveness of Avastin in pediatric patients has not been studied. However, physeal dysplasia was observed in juvenile cynomolgus monkeys with open growth plates treated for four weeks with doses that were less than the recommended human dose based on mg/kg and exposure. The incidence and severity of physeal dysplasia were dose-related and were at least partially reversible upon cessation of treatment.

Geriatric Use
In Study 1, NCI-CTC Grade 3–4 adverse events were collected in all patients receiving study drug (396 bolus-IFL plus placebo; 392 bolus-IFL plus Avastin; 109 5-FU/LV plus Avastin), while NCI-CTC Grade 1 and 2 adverse events were collected in a subset of 309 patients. There were insufficient numbers of patients 65 years and older in the subset in which NCI-CTC Grade 1–4 adverse events were collected to determine whether the overall adverse event profile was different in the elderly as compared to younger patients. Among the 392 patients receiving bolus-IFL plus Avastin, 126 were at least 65 years of age. Severe adverse events that occurred at a higher incidence (≥2%) in the elderly when compared to those less than 65 years were asthenia, sepsis, deep thrombophlebitis, hypertension, hypotension, myocardial infarction, congestive heart failure, diarrhea, constipation, anorexia, leukopenia, anemia, dehydration, hypokalemia, and hyponatremia. The effect of Avastin on overall survival was similar in elderly patients as compared to younger patients.

In Study 3, patients age 65 and older receiving Avastin plus FOLFOX4 had a greater relative risk as compared to younger patients for the following adverse events: nausea, emesis, ileus, and fatigue.

In Study 5 patients age 65 and older receiving carboplatin, paclitaxel, and Avastin had a greater relative risk for proteinuria as compared to younger patients.

In Study 7, there were insufficient numbers of patients ≥65 years old to determine whether the overall adverse event profile was different in the elderly as compared with younger patients.

Of the 742 patients enrolled in Genentech-sponsored clinical studies in which all adverse events were captured, 212 (29%) were age 65 or older and 43 (6%) were age 75 or older. Adverse events of any severity that occurred at a higher incidence in the elderly as compared to younger patients, in addition to those described above, were dyspepsia, gastrointestinal hemorrhage, edema, epistaxis, increased cough, and voice alteration.

In an exploratory, pooled analysis of 1745 patients treated in five randomized, controlled studies, there were 618 (35%) patients age 65 or older and 1127 patients less than 65 years of age. The overall incidence of arterial thromboembolic events was increased in all patients receiving Avastin with chemotherapy as compared to those receiving chemotherapy alone, regardless of age. The increase in arterial thromboembolic events incidence was greater in patients 65 and over (8.5% vs. 2.9%) as compared to those less than 65 (2.1% vs. 1.4%). (See **WARNINGS: Arterial Thromboembolic Events.**)

ADVERSE REACTIONS
The most serious adverse reactions in patients receiving Avastin were:
- Gastrointestinal Perforations (see **WARNINGS**)
- Non-Gastrointestinal Fistula Formation (see **WARNINGS**)
- Wound Healing Complications (see **WARNINGS**)
- Hemorrhage (see **WARNINGS**)
- Arterial Thromboembolic Events (see **WARNINGS**)
- Hypertensive Crises (see **WARNINGS: Hypertension**)
- Reversible Posterior Leukoencephalopathy Syndrome (see **WARNINGS**)
- Neutropenia and Infection (see **WARNINGS**)
- Nephrotic Syndrome (see **WARNINGS: Proteinuria**)
- Congestive Heart Failure (see **WARNINGS**)

Adverse Reactions in Clinical Trials
Because clinical trials are conducted under widely varying conditions, adverse reaction rates observed in the clinical trials of a drug cannot be directly compared to rates in the clinical trials of another drug and may not reflect the rates observed in practice. The adverse reaction information from clinical trials does, however, provide a basis for identifying the adverse events that appear to be related to drug use and for approximating rates.

The data described below reflect exposure to Avastin in 1529 patients, including 665 receiving Avastin for at least 6 months and 199 receiving Avastin for at least one year. Avastin was studied primarily in placebo- and active-controlled trials (n=501, and n=1028, respectively).

Gastrointestinal Perforation
The incidence of gastrointestinal perforation across all studies ranged from 0–3.7%. The incidence of gastrointestinal perforation, in some cases fatal, in patients with

AVASTIN® (Bevacizumab)

mCRC receiving Avastin alone or in combination with chemotherapy was 2.4% compared to 0.3% in patients receiving only chemotherapy. The incidence of gastrointestinal perforation in NSCLC patients receiving Avastin was 0.9% compared to 0% in patients receiving only chemotherapy. (See **WARNINGS: Gastrointestinal Perforations** and **DOSAGE AND ADMINISTRATION: Dose Modifications.**)

Non-Gastrointestinal Fistula Formation
(See **WARNINGS: Non-Gastrointestinal Fistula Formation, DOSAGE AND ADMINISTRATION: Dose Modifications.**)

Wound Healing Complications
The incidence of post-operative wound healing and/or bleeding complications was increased in patients with mCRC receiving Avastin as compared to patients receiving only chemotherapy. Among patients requiring surgery on or within 60 days of receiving study treatment, wound healing and/or bleeding complications occurred in 15% (6/39) of patients receiving bolus-IFL plus Avastin as compared to 4% (1/25) of patients who received bolus-IFL alone. In the same study, the incidence of wound dehiscence was also higher in the Avastin-treated patients (1% vs. 0.5%).

Hemorrhage
Severe or fatal hemorrhages, including hemoptysis, gastrointestinal bleeding, hematemesis, CNS hemorrhage, epistaxis, and vaginal bleeding occurred up to five-fold more frequently in Avastin-treated patients compared to patients treated with chemotherapy alone. NCI-CTC Grade 3–5 hemorrhagic events occurred in 4.7% of NSCLC patients and 5.2% of mCRC patients receiving Avastin compared to 1.1% and 0.7% for the control groups respectively. (See **WARNINGS: Hemorrhage.**)

The incidence of epistaxis was higher (35% vs. 10%) in patients with mCRC receiving bolus-IFL plus Avastin compared with patients receiving bolus-IFL plus placebo. These events were generally mild in severity (NCI-CTC Grade 1) and resolved without medical intervention. Additional mild to moderate hemorrhagic events reported more frequently in patients receiving bolus-IFL plus Avastin when compared to those receiving bolus-IFL plus placebo included gastrointestinal hemorrhage (24% vs. 6%), minor gum bleeding (2% vs. 0%), and vaginal hemorrhage (4% vs. 2%). (See **WARNINGS: Hemorrhage** and **DOSAGE AND ADMINISTRATION: Dose Modifications.**)

Arterial Thromboembolic Events
The incidence of arterial thromboembolic events was increased in NSCLC patients receiving PC plus Avastin (3.0%) compared with patients receiving PC alone (1.4%). Five events were fatal in the PC plus Avastin arm, compared with 1 event in the PC alone arm. This increased risk is consistent with that observed in patients with mCRC. (See **WARNINGS: Arterial Thromboembolic Events, DOSAGE AND ADMINISTRATION: Dose Modifications,** and **PRECAUTIONS: Geriatric Use.**)

Venous Thromboembolic Events
The incidence of NCI-CTC Grade 3–4 venous thromboembolic events was higher in patients with mCRC or NSCLC receiving Avastin with chemotherapy as compared to those receiving chemotherapy alone. In addition, in patients with mCRC the risk of developing a second subsequent thromboembolic event in patients receiving Avastin and chemotherapy is increased compared to patients receiving chemotherapy alone. In Study 1, 53 patients (14%) on the bolus-IFL plus Avastin arm and 30 patients (8%) on the bolus-IFL plus placebo arm received full dose warfarin following a venous thromboembolic event. Among these patients, an additional thromboembolic event occurred in 21% (11/53) of patients receiving bolus-IFL plus Avastin and 3% (1/30) of patients receiving bolus-IFL alone.

The overall incidence of NCI-CTC Grade 3–4 venous thromboembolic events in Study 1 was 15.1% in patients receiving bolus-IFL plus Avastin and 13.6% in patients receiving bolus-IFL plus placebo. In Study 1, the incidence of the following NCI-CTC Grade 3 and 4 venous thromboembolic events was higher in patients receiving bolus-IFL plus Avastin as compared to patients receiving bolus-IFL plus placebo: deep venous thrombosis (34 vs. 19 patients) and intra-abdominal venous thrombosis (10 vs. 5 patients).

Hypertension
Fatal CNS hemorrhage complicating Avastin induced hypertension can occur.

In Study 1, the incidences of hypertension and of severe hypertension were increased in patients with mCRC receiving Avastin compared to those receiving chemotherapy alone (see Table 4).

Table 4
Incidence of Hypertension and Severe Hypertension in Study 1

	Arm 1 IFL+Placebo (n=394)	Arm 2 IFL+Avastin (n=392)	Arm 3 5-FU/LV+ Avastin (n=109)
Hypertension[a] (>150/100 mmHg)	43%	60%	67%
Severe Hypertension[a] (>200/110 mmHg)	2%	7%	10%

[a] This includes patients with either a systolic or diastolic reading greater than the cutoff value on one or more occasions.

Among patients with severe hypertension in the Avastin arms, slightly over half the patients (51%) had a diastolic reading greater than 110 mmHg associated with a systolic reading less than 200 mmHg.

Similar results were seen in patients receiving Avastin alone or in combination with FOLFOX4 or carboplatin and paclitaxel. (See **WARNINGS: Hypertension** and **DOSAGE AND ADMINISTRATION: Dose Modifications.**)

Neutropenia and Infection
An increased incidence of neutropenia has been reported in patients receiving Avastin and chemotherapy compared to chemotherapy alone. In Study 1, the incidence of NCI-CTC Grade 3 or 4 neutropenia was increased in patients with mCRC receiving IFL+Avastin (21%) compared to patients receiving IFL alone (14%). In Study 5, the incidence of NCI-CTC Grade 4 neutropenia was increased in patients with NSCLC receiving PC plus Avastin (26.2%) compared with patients receiving PC alone (17.2%). Febrile neutropenia was also increased (5.4% for PC plus Avastin vs. 1.8% for PC alone). There were 19 (4.5%) infections with NCI-CTC Grade 3 or 4 neutropenia in the PC plus Avastin arm of which 3 were fatal compared to 9 (2%) neutropenic infections in patients receiving PC alone, of which none were fatal. During the first 6 cycles of treatment the incidence of serious infections including pneumonia, febrile neutropenia, catheter infections and wound infections was increased in the PC plus Avastin arm [58 patients (13.6%)] compared to the PC alone arm [29 patients (6.6%)].

Proteinuria
(See **WARNINGS: Proteinuria, DOSAGE AND ADMINISTRATION: Dose Modifications,** and **PRECAUTIONS: Geriatric Use.**)

AVASTIN® (Bevacizumab)

Immunogenicity
As with all therapeutic proteins, there is a potential for immunogenicity. The incidence of antibody development in patients receiving Avastin has not been adequately determined because the assay sensitivity was inadequate to reliably detect lower titers. Enzyme-linked immunosorbent assays (ELISAs) were performed on sera from approximately 500 patients treated with Avastin, primarily in combination with chemotherapy. High titer human anti-Avastin antibodies were not detected.

Immunogenicity data are highly dependent on the sensitivity and specificity of the assay. Additionally, the observed incidence of antibody positivity in an assay may be influenced by several factors, including sample handling, timing of sample collection, concomitant medications, and underlying disease. For these reasons, comparison of the incidence of antibodies to Avastin with the incidence of antibodies to other products may be misleading.

Metastatic Carcinoma of the Colon and Rectum
The data in Tables 5 and 6 were obtained in Study 1. All NCI-CTC Grade 3 and 4 adverse events and selected NCI-CTC Grade 1 and 2 adverse events (hypertension, proteinuria, thromboembolic events) were reported for the overall study population. The median age was 60, 60% were male, 79% were Caucasian, 78% had a colon primary lesion, 56% had extra-abdominal disease, 29% had prior adjuvant or neoadjuvant chemotherapy, and 57% had ECOG performance status of 0. The median duration of exposure to Avastin was 8 months in Arm 2 and 7 months in Arm 3. Severe and life-threatening (NCI-CTC Grade 3 and 4) adverse events, which occurred at a higher incidence (≥2%) in patients receiving bolus-IFL plus Avastin as compared to bolus-IFL plus placebo, are presented in Table 5.

Table 5
NCI-CTC Grade 3 and 4 Adverse Events in Study 1
(Occurring at Higher Incidence (≥2%) in Avastin vs. Control)

	Arm 1 IFL+Placebo (n=396)		Arm 2 IFL+Avastin (n=392)	
NCI-CTC Grade 3–4 Events	295	(74%)	340	(87%)
Body as a Whole				
Asthenia	28	(7%)	38	(10%)
Abdominal Pain	20	(5%)	32	(8%)
Pain	21	(5%)	30	(8%)
Cardiovascular				
Hypertension	10	(2%)	46	(12%)
Deep Vein Thrombosis	19	(5%)	34	(9%)
Intra-Abdominal Thrombosis	5	(1%)	13	(3%)
Syncope	4	(1%)	11	(3%)
Digestive				
Diarrhea	99	(25%)	133	(34%)
Constipation	9	(2%)	14	(4%)
Hemic/Lymphatic				
Leukopenia	122	(31%)	145	(37%)
Neutropenia[a]	41	(14%)	58	(21%)

[a] Central laboratories were collected on Days 1 and 21 of each cycle. Neutrophil counts are available in 303 patients in Arm 1 and 276 in Arm 2.

NCI-CTC Grade 1–4 adverse events which occurred at a higher incidence (≥5%) in patients receiving bolus-IFL plus Avastin as compared to the bolus-IFL plus placebo arm, are presented in Table 6.

Table 6
NCI-CTC Grade 1–4 Adverse Events in Study 1
(Occurring at Higher Incidence (≥5%) in IFL+Avastin vs. IFL)

	Arm 1 IFL+Placebo (n=98)		Arm 2 IFL+Avastin (n=102)		Arm 3 5-FU/LV+Avastin (n=109)	
Body as a Whole						
Pain	54	(55%)	62	(61%)	67	(62%)
Abdominal Pain	54	(55%)	62	(61%)	55	(50%)
Headache	19	(19%)	27	(26%)	30	(26%)
Cardiovascular						
Hypertension	14	(14%)	23	(23%)	37	(34%)
Hypotension	7	(7%)	15	(15%)	8	(7%)
Deep Vein Thrombosis	3	(3%)	9	(9%)	6	(6%)
Digestive						
Vomiting	46	(47%)	53	(52%)	51	(47%)
Anorexia	29	(30%)	44	(43%)	38	(35%)
Constipation	28	(29%)	41	(40%)	32	(29%)
Stomatitis	18	(18%)	33	(32%)	33	(30%)
Dyspepsia	15	(15%)	25	(24%)	19	(17%)
GI Hemorrhage	6	(6%)	25	(24%)	21	(19%)
Weight Loss	10	(10%)	15	(15%)	18	(16%)
Dry Mouth	2	(2%)	7	(7%)	4	(4%)
Colitis	1	(1%)	6	(6%)	1	(1%)
Hemic/Lymphatic						
Thrombocytopenia	0		5	(5%)	5	(5%)
Nervous						
Dizziness	20	(20%)	27	(26%)	21	(19%)
Respiratory						
Upper Respiratory Infection	38	(39%)	48	(47%)	44	(40%)
Epistaxis	10	(10%)	36	(35%)	35	(32%)
Dyspnea	15	(15%)	26	(26%)	27	(25%)
Voice Alteration	2	(2%)	9	(9%)	6	(6%)
Skin/Appendages						
Alopecia	25	(26%)	33	(32%)	6	(6%)
Skin Ulcer	1	(1%)	6	(6%)	7	(6%)
Special Senses						
Taste Disorder	9	(9%)	14	(14%)	23	(21%)
Urogenital						
Proteinuria	24	(24%)	37	(36%)	39	(36%)

AVASTIN® (Bevacizumab)

The data in Table 7 were obtained in Study 3. Only NCI-CTC Grade 3–5 non-hematologic and Grade 4–5 hematologic adverse events related to treatment were reported. The median age was a 61 years, 40% were female, 87% were Caucasian, 99% received prior chemotherapy for metastatic colorectal cancer, 26% had received prior radiation therapy, and the 49% had an ECOG performance status of 0. Selected NCI-CTC Grade 3–5 non-hematologic and Grade 4–5 hematologic adverse events which occurred at a higher incidence in patients receiving FOLFOX4 plus Avastin as compared to those who received FOLFOX4 alone, are presented in Table 7. These data are likely to under-estimate the true adverse event rates due to the reporting mechanisms used in Study 3.

Table 7
NCI-CTC Grade 3–5 Non-Hematologic and Grade 4–5 Hematologic Adverse Events in Study 3 (Occurring at Higher Incidence (≥2%) with Avastin + FOLFOX4 vs. FOLFOX4)

	FOLFOX4 (n=285)		FOLFOX4 + Avastin (n=287)		Avastin (n=234)	
Patients with at least one event	171	(60%)	219	(76%)	87	(37%)
Gastrointestinal						
Diarrhea	36	(13%)	51	(18%)	5	(2%)
Nausea	13	(5%)	35	(12%)	14	(6%)
Vomiting	11	(4%)	32	(11%)	15	(6%)
Dehydration	14	(5%)	29	(10%)	15	(6%)
Ileus	4	(1%)	10	(4%)	11	(5%)
Neurology						
Neuropathy–sensory	26	(9%)	48	(17%)	2	(1%)
Neurologic–other	8	(3%)	15	(5%)	3	(1%)
Constitutional symptoms						
Fatigue	37	(13%)	56	(19%)	12	(5%)
Pain						
Abdominal pain	13	(5%)	24	(8%)	19	(8%)
Headache	0	(0%)	8	(3%)	4	(2%)
Cardiovascular (general)						
Hypertension	5	(2%)	26	(9%)	19	(8%)
Hemorrhage						
Hemorrhage	2	(1%)	15	(5%)	9	(4%)

Non-Squamous, Non-Small Cell Lung Cancer

The data in Table 8 were obtained in Study 5. Only NCI-CTC Grade 3–5 non-hematologic and Grade 4–5 hematologic adverse events were reported. The median age was 63, 46% were female, no patients had received prior chemotherapy, 76% had Stage IV disease, 12% had Stage IIIB disease with malignant pleural effusion, 11% had recurrent disease, and 40% had an ECOG performance status of 0. The median duration of exposure to Avastin was 4.9 months.

NCI-CTC Grade 3, 4, and 5 adverse events that occurred at a ≥2% higher incidence in patients receiving PC plus Avastin as compared with PC alone are presented in Table 8.

Table 8
NCI-CTC Grade 3–5 Non-Hematologic and Grade 4 and 5 Hematologic Adverse Events in Study 5 (Occurring at a ≥2% Higher Incidence in Avastin-Treated Patients Compared with Control)

	No. (%) of NSCLC Patients			
NCI-CTC Category Term[a]	PC (n=441)		PC + Avastin (n=427)	
Any event	286	(65%)	334	(78%)
Blood/bone marrow				
Neutropenia	76	(17%)	113	(27%)
Constitutional symptoms				
Fatigue	57	(13%)	67	(16%)
Cardiovascular (general)				
Hypertension	3	(0.7%)	33	(8%)
Vascular				
Venous thrombus/embolism	14	(3%)	23	(5%)
Infection/febrile neutropenia				
Infection without neutropenia	12	(3%)	30	(7%)
Infection with NCI-CTC Grade 3 or 4 neutropenia	9	(2%)	19	(4%)
Febrile neutropenia	8	(2%)	23	(5%)
Pulmonary/upper respiratory				
Pneumonitis/pulmonary infiltrates	11	(3%)	21	(5%)
Metabolic/laboratory				
Hyponatremia	5	(1%)	16	(4%)
Pain				
Headache	2	(0.5%)	13	(3%)
Renal/genitourinary				
Proteinuria	0	(0%)	13	(3%)

[a] Events were reported and graded according to NCI-CTC, Version 2.0. Per protocol, investigators were required to report NCI-CTC Grade 3–5 non-hematologic and Grade 4 and 5 hematologic events.

Metastatic Breast Cancer

The data in Table 9 were obtained in Study 7. Only NCI-CTC Grade 3–5 non-hematologic and Grade 4–5 hematologic adverse events were reported. The median age was 55 years (range 27 - 85); 76% were white; 36% had received prior hormonal therapy for advanced disease, and 66% had received adjuvant chemotherapy, including 20% with prior taxane use and 50% with prior anthracyclines use. The median duration of exposure was 9 months with Avastin plus paclitaxel and 5 months for patients receiving paclitaxel alone

Severe and life-threatening (NCI-CTC Grade 3 and 4) adverse events that occurred at a higher incidence (≥2%) in patients receiving paclitaxel plus Avastin compared with paclitaxel alone, are presented in Table 9.

AVASTIN® (Bevacizumab)

Table 9
NCI-CTC Grade 3–5 Non-Hematologic and Grade 4 and 5 Hematologic Adverse Events in Study 7 (Occurring at Higher Incidence (≥2%) in Paclitaxel + Avastin vs. Paclitaxel alone)

NCI-CTC Terminology	Paclitaxel (n=348)		Paclitaxel + Avastin (n=363)	
Patients with at least one event	176	(50.6%)	258	(71.1%)
Neuropathy—sensory	61	(17.5%)	88	(24.2%)
Cerebrovascular ischemia	0	(0%)	9	(2.5%)
Hypertension	5	(1.4%)	58	(16.0%)
Headache	2	(0.6%)	13	(3.6%)
Bone pain	6	(1.7%)	14	(3.9%)
Nausea	5	(1.4%)	15	(4.1%)
Vomiting	8	(2.3%)	20	(5.5%)
Diarrhea	5	(1.4%)	17	(4.7%)
Dehydration	3	(0.9%)	12	(3.3%)
Fatigue	18	(5.2%)	39	(10.7%)
Infection w/o neutropenia	16	(4.6%)	33	(9.1%)
Infection w/ unknown ANC	1	(0.3%)	11	(3.0%)
Neutrophils	11	(3.2%)	21	(5.8%)
Rash/desquamation	1	(0.3%)	9	(2.5%)
Proteinuria	0	(0.0%)	11	(3.0%)

Sensory neuropathy, hypertension, and fatigue were reported at a ≥5% higher absolute incidence in the paclitaxel+ Avastin arm compared with the paclitaxel alone arm.

Fatal adverse reactions occurred in 6/363 (1.7%) of patients who received paclitaxel plus Avastin. Causes of death were gastrointestinal perforation (2), myocardial infarction (2), diarrhea/abdominal pain/weakness/hypotension (2).

Other Serious Adverse Events
The following additional serious adverse events occurred in at least one subject treated with Avastin in clinical studies or post-marketing experience:
Body as a Whole: polyserositis
Cardiovascular: pulmonary hypertension
Digestive: intestinal necrosis, mesenteric venous occlusion, anastomotic ulceration
Hemic and lymphatic: pancytopenia
Respiratory: nasal septum perforation

OVERDOSAGE
The highest dose tested in humans (20 mg/kg IV) was associated with headache in nine of 16 patients and with severe headache in three of 16 patients.

Avastin®
(Bevacizumab)
For Intravenous Use
Manufactured by:
Genentech, Inc.
1 DNA Way
South San Francisco, CA 94080-4990

Genentech
BIO☉NCOLOGY™

7453210
4835703
Initial U.S. Approval: February 2004
Code Revision Date: March 2008
©2008 Genentech, Inc.

APPENDIX I

Response evaluation criteria and performance scales

RECIST: DEFINITION OF RESPONSE

In clinical studies, formal response criteria have been developed and have gained wide acceptance. The National Cancer Institute (NCI) has proposed and implemented newer standard response criteria called Response Evaluation Criteria in Solid Tumors (RECIST). In contrast, the World Health Organization (WHO) has a different standard for assessing response. Major differences between these guidelines are outlined below.

Comparison of RECIST and WHO guidelines

Characteristic	RECIST	WHO
Objective response (OR) (LD is the longest diameter)	**Target lesions** change in sum of LDs, maximum 5 per organ up to 10 total (more than one organ)	**Measurable disease** change in the sum of the products of LDs and greatest perpendicular diameters, no maximum number of lesions specified
Complete response (CR)	Disappearance of all target lesions, confirmed at ≥ 4 weeks	Disappearance of all known disease, confirmed at ≥ 4 weeks
Partial response (PR)	$\geq 30\%$ decrease from baseline, confirmed at ≥ 4 weeks	$\geq 50\%$ decrease from baseline, confirmed at ≥ 4 weeks
Progressive disease (PD)	$\geq 20\%$ increase over smallest sum observed or appearance of new lesions	$\geq 25\%$ increase in one or more lesions or appearance of new lesions
Stable disease (SD)	Neither PR nor PD criteria met	Neither PR nor PD criteria met (no change)

PERFORMANCE SCALES

The Karnofsky performance index and WHO (Zubrod) scale are commonly used as proxy measures for quality of life. Because they measure only one dimension of the construct, they would not be considered quality-of-life measures by today's standards. However, given their historic relevance and current high frequency of usage as proxy measures, we have included them here.

Karnofsky performance index

Definition

Able to carry on normal activity and to work	100	Normal; no complaints; no evidence of disease
	90	Able to carry on normal activity; minor signs or symptoms of disease
	80	Normal activity with effort; some signs or symptoms of disease
Unable to work; able to live at home, care for most personal needs; a varying amount of assistance is needed	70	Cares for self; unable to carry on normal activity or to do active work
	60	Requires occasional assistance but is able to care for most needs
	50	Requires considerable assistance and frequent medical care
Unable to care for self; requires equivalent of institutional or hospital care; disease may be progressing rapidly	40	Disabled; requires special care and assistance
	30	Severely disabled; hospitalization is indicated, although death is not imminent
	20	Very sick; hospitalization necessary; active supportive treatment necessary
	10	Moribund; fatal processes progressing rapidly
	0	Dead

From Karnofsky DA, Abelmann WH, Craver LF, et al: The use of the nitrogen mustards in the palliative treatment of carcinoma. Cancer 1:634–656, 1948.

WHO (Zubrod) scale

This scale is used to measure performance of which the patient is *capable*. For example, a patient in the hospital for metabolic studies may be fully capable of performing normal activities but will remain in bed through his or her own choice. Such a patient should be coded 0, "normal."

0	Normal activity
1	Symptoms but nearly fully ambulatory
2	Some bed time but needs to be in bed < 50% of normal daytime
3	Needs to be in bed > 50% of normal daytime
4	Unable to get out of bed

From Zubrod CG, Schneiderman M, Frei E III, et al: Appraisal of methods for the study of chemotherapy of cancer in man: Comparative therapeutic trial of nitrogen mustard and triethylene thiophosphoramide. J Chron Dis 11:7–33, 1960.

APPENDIX 2

Cancer information on the Internet

J. Sybil Biermann, MD

The Internet has become nearly indispensable for finding the latest information on cancer diagnosis, treatment, and prevention. This chapter highlights several websites that cater to oncology professionals, researchers, and patients.

American Cancer Society

www.cancer.org Basic resources including the American Cancer Society's Cancer Facts & Figures 2008 are readily available from the home page. Estimates of the numbers of new cancer cases and deaths for the current year are presented according to gender, site, and stage. Also presented is information on cancer mortality, the probability of developing cancer at certain ages, and cancer survival in adults and children.

American Society of Clinical Oncology

www.asco.org Health care professionals can access information on American Society of Clinical Oncology (ASCO) policies, clinical guidelines, publications, and a searchable database of abstracts from ASCO's annual scientific meetings dating back to 1995.

www.cancer.net ASCO launched cancer.net in 2008, a comprehensive, doctor-approved patient website that provides reliable, up-to-the-minute information on more than 120 types of cancer and cancer-related syndromes.

American Society of Hematology

www.hematology.org A comprehensive collection of articles and reviews on hematologic malignancies may be found at the American Society of Hematology's (ASH) website. The site also offers a direct link to the Society's official journal, *Blood*, where the full text of all articles dating back to January 1996 can be downloaded and printed.

Cancer Information Service

http://cis.nci.nih.gov/ Cancer Information Service (CIS) is a nationwide network of 14 regional offices supported by the National Cancer Institute (NCI). Reliable information on cancer causes and prevention and a collection of recently issued NCI Cancer Facts fact sheets and the new What You Need To Know About™ series of patient guides are also available online by following links from the CIS home page. CIS also offers a toll-free phone service and provides accurate, up-to-date information on cancer to the public in English and Spanish. The phone number is 1-800-4-CANCER.

Cancernetwork.com

www.cancernetwork.com An excellent source of reliable cancer information is cancernetwork.com The site features free access to the full text of over 6,000 peer-reviewed medical journal articles from the pages of *ONCOLOGY* and news reports from *Oncology News International*; selected text of this handbook, *Cancer Management: A Multidisciplinary Approach*; free CME based on review articles, cancer-related news stories, and background material online, and more.

Centers for Disease Control and Prevention

http://www.cdc.gov/ The Centers for Disease Control and Prevention (CDC) maintains several websites for both health professionals and researchers, as well as the public.

www.cdc.gov/nccdphp/ Information on CDC cancer prevention programs may be accessed at the National Center for Chronic Disease Prevention and Health Promotion's website.

CenterWatch

www.centerwatch.com CenterWatch offers a worldwide directory of more than 41,000 active industry and government-sponsored trials with independent review board (IRB) approval. Each listing contains a brief summary of the study, the general inclusion/exclusion criteria, and contact information. The database is easily searched, even by a newcomer, and the website has become a major influence for patient recruitment into active clinical trials.

Coalition of National Cancer Cooperative Groups

http://www.CancerTrialsHelp.org/ The Coalition of National Cancer Cooperative Groups was founded in 1997 by the Cancer and Leukemia Group B (CALGB), Eastern Cooperative Oncology Group (ECOG), North Central Cancer Treatment Group (NCCTG), National Surgical Adjuvant Breast and Bowel Project (NSABP), Pediatric Oncology Group (POG), and Radiation Therapy Oncology Group (RTOG). The Coalition's website provides details on the Coalition's initiatives in many areas and features a software tool, TrialCheckSM, for locating ongoing clinical trials among the Coalition's cooperative groups.

National Cancer Institute

http://cancer.gov The NCI's vast website provides information suitable to clinical practitioners, researchers, patients, and the general public. Among the cancer resources available from the home page are:

http://cancer.gov/cancerinfo/pdq/ Peer-reviewed, frequently updated summaries on cancer treatment, screening, prevention, genetics, and supportive care; **http://www.clinicaltrials.gov** A registry of approximately 25,000 clinical studies sponsored by the National Institutes of Health, other Federal agencies, and private industries and conducted in all 50 states and in more than 120 countries plus up-to-date information for locating these trials; **http://researchportfolio.cancer.gov/** A comprehensive database of NCI-supported basic and clinical research programs; **http://cancer.gov/researchandfunding** A directory of NCI research tools and funding opportunities (human, animal, and genomic) for cancer researchers; **http://cancer.gov/statistics** Statistical databases and resources, including cancer incidence by gender, race, ethnicity, and type of cancer; 5-year survival rates; frequencies of childhood cancers; and cancer mortality in the United States by gender and race patient information.

National Comprehensive Cancer Network

www.nccn.org The National Comprehensive Cancer Network (NCCN) website provides access to the NCCN's current Clinical Practice Guidelines, links to ongoing clinical trials at member institutions, and a directory of physicians for referrals. Recent additions include treatment guidelines for patients in both Spanish and English as well as NCCN drugs and biologic companions.

National Institute of Dental and Craniofacial Research

www.nidcr.nih.gov/oralhealth/topics/cancertreatment Resources on cancer treatment and oral health for health professionals and patients including, in English and Spanish, information for preventing and managing oral health complications of cancer treatment.

PubMed.gov

http://pubmed.gov/ PubMed a service of the National Library of Medicine (NLM), provides access to over 12 million Medline citations in abstract form dating back to the mid-1960s. **http://www.cancer.gov/search/pubmed/** In addition, PubMed offers selected cancer topic searches for more than 100 different cancer topics.

SearchMedica

Searchmedica.com SearchMedica's index contains well over 1,000 websites organized into numerous therapeutic categories, including cancer. Searches may also be refined by clicking one of the therapeutic category links to narrow results to that area. SearchMedica also allows users to refine results by content category such as Research/Reviews, Practical Articles and News, Patient Education Materials, and Practice Guidelines.

Surveillance, Epidemiology, and End Results Program

http://seer.cancer.gov/ The NCI's Surveillance, Epidemiology, and End Results (SEER) program collects and publishes cancer incidence and survival data from population-based cancer registries covering approximately 26% of the

US population. Trends in age-adjusted SEER cancer incidence and mortality, by race and gender, are presented, as well as 5-year survival rates, by race and gender, and much more.

Other Internet sources of cancer information

www.apos-society.org Psychological services/counseling from the American Psychosocial Oncology Society (APOS). APOS provides a helpline for patients in addition to other tools and resources for oncologists and other health professionals involved in the care of cancer patients.

www.mdlinx.com/HemeOncLinx/ MdLinx provides daily summaries of hematology/oncology articles culled from a wide variety of professional publications. Articles can be accessed by linkage from the web page. Registered users (registration is free) can also have synopses sent daily to e-mail accounts on general or specified topics within hematology and oncology.

www.mskcc.org/aboutherbs Alternative therapies: An excellent resource for information on commonly used herbs and botanicals is the Memorial Sloan-Kettering Cancer Center site. General information on health-related frauds can be found at www.quackwatch.org.

www.oncolink.com OncoLink is a popular website maintained by the University of Pennsylvania, offering a broad variety of news articles, fact sheets, and annotated links to cancer-related information at other websites. The site includes multimedia slide shows, video films, and audio lectures on a wide range of topics.

Additional resources

www.aacr.org American Association for Cancer Research

www.acr.org The American College of Radiology

www.astro.org The American Society for Therapeutic Radiology and Oncology

www.leukemia-lymphoma.org The Leukemia & Lymphoma Society

www.ons.org Oncology Nursing Society

Links to the web pages of state and other regional cancer registries may be found at **www.askcnet.org/dataq/cancer.htm**. This site also includes links to cancer registries around the world. Other places to look for cancer registries and statistical data in the United States and Canada are the websites maintained by the North American Association of Central Cancer Registries **(www.naaccr.org)**, and the International Agency for Research on Cancer **(www.iarc.fr)**.

European sites, the sites maintained by the International Union Against Cancer **(www.uicc.org)**, CancerBACUP **(www.cancerbacup.org.uk)**, and the European Organisation for Research and Treatment of Cancer **(http://www.eortc.be/)** are extensive, information-rich resources designed primarily for health care professionals.

Selected cancer drugs and indications

**NEWLY APPROVED BY THE
US FOOD AND DRUG ADMINISTRATION,
MAY 2007 – NOVEMBER 2008**

Bendamustine (Treanda): For the treatment of chronic lymphocytic leukemia. Approved March 2008; For the treatment of indolent B-cell non-Hodgkin lymphoma. Approved November 2008.

Bevacizumab (Avastin): For use in metastatic breast cancer in combination with paclitaxel chemotherapy. Accelerated approval for this indication granted February 2008.

Bortezomib (Velcade): For patients with previously untreated multiple myeloma. Approved for this indication June 2008.

Dalteparin (Fragmin): To reduce the recurrence of symptomatic venous thromboembolism (VTE) in patients with cancer. Approved May 2007.

Denileukin Diftitox (Ontak): Treatment of CD25+ CTCL. Full approval October 2008.

Dexrazoxane (Totect): Treatment of extravasation symptoms (pain, burning, swelling, and redness near infusion site) resulting from intravenous anthracycline chemotherapy. Approved September 2007.

Docetaxel (Taxotere): Induction treatment in combination with cisplatin and fluorouracil of locally advanced squamous cell carcinoma of the head and neck. Approved September 2007.

Doxorubicin HCl liposome injection (Doxil): Treatment in combination with bortezomib of previously untreated multiple myeloma patients or those who have received at least one prior line of therapy. Approved May 2007.

Fosaprepitant dimeglumine for injection (Emend): Intravenous therapy for the prevention of chemotherapy-induced nausea and vomiting. Injectable formulation approved January 2008.

Granisetron (Sancuso): Treatment of chemotherapy-induced nausea and vomiting. Approved September 2008.

Human Papillomavirus (HPV) vaccine (Gardasil): For the prevention of vaginal and vulvar cancer caused by HPV types 16 and 18 in girls and women aged 9 to 26 years. Approved for this indication September 2008.

Ixabepilone (Ixempra): For the treatment of breast cancer. Approved October 2007.

Nilotinib (Tasigna): For the treatment of chronic myelogenous leukemia. Approved October 2007.

Oxymorphone HCl (Opana): An opioid analgesic for the relief of moderate-to-severe pain in patients requiring continuous, around-the-clock, opioid treatment for an extended period of time. Three new dosage strengths, 7.5 mg, 15 mg, and 30 mg, approved March 2008.

Pemetrexed (Alimta): Treatment of first-line non-small-cell lung cancer. Approved September 2008.

Romiplostim (Nplate): For patients with chronic immune thrombocytopenic purpura (ITP) who do not respond sufficiently to current treatments. Approved August 2008.

Raloxifene hydrochloride (Evista): For reducing the risk of invasive breast cancer in postmenopausal women with osteoporosis and in postmenopausal women at high risk for invasive breast cancer. Approved September 2007.

Sorafenib (Nexavar): For the treatment of patients with unresectable hepatocellular carcinoma (HCC). Approved for this indication November 2007.

Temsirolimus (Torisel): Treatment of renal cell carcinoma. Approved May 2007.

Topotecan (Hycamtin): For the treatment of small-cell lung cancer. Approved October 2007.

Chemotherapeutic agents and their uses, dosages, and toxicities

Chris H. Takimoto, MD, PhD, and Emiliano Calvo, MD, PhD

The chemotherapeutic agents included in this Appendix are classified by mechanism of action and are organized as follows:

- alkylating agents;
- antimetabolites;
- natural products;
- targeted agents
    - monoclonal antibodies
    - molecularly targeted therapies

FDA-approved uses and dose-limiting effects are set in italic type for emphasis.

For a complete discussion of these mechanisms of action, see chapter 3 on "Principles of oncologic pharmacotherapy."

> Abbreviations: ALL = acute lymphoblastic leukemia; AML = acute myelogenous leukemia; AUC = area under the curve; BMT = bone marrow transplantation; CLL = chronic lymphocytic leukemia; CML = chronic myelogenous leukemia; CMML = chronic myelomacrocytic leukemia; EGFR = epidermal growth factor receptor; 5-FU = fluorouracil; GFR = glomerular filtration rate; GIST = gastrointestinal stromal tumor; HL = Hodgkin lymphoma; MDS = myelodysplastic syndromes; MOPP = mechlorethamine, Oncovin, procarbazine, and prednisone; NHL = non–Hodgkin lymphoma; NSCLC = non–small-cell lung cancer; SCLC = small-cell lung cancer; SIADH = syndrome of inappropriate antidiuretic hormone secretion; WBC = white blood cell

Alkylating agents

Drug and its uses	Dosages	Toxicities
Nitrogen mustards		
Bendamustine *CLL*	IV: 100 mg/m^2 on d 1 and d 2 of a 28 d cycle, up to 6 cycles	*Bone marrow depression, fever, nausea, and vomiting*
Chlorambucil *CLL, HL, NHL, ovarian cancer, choriocarcinoma, lymphosarcoma*	0.1-0.2 mg/kg PO daily for 3-6 wk as required (usually 4-10 mg/d) or intermittent 0.4 mg/kg every 3-4 wk; increase by 0.1 mg/kg until control of disease or toxicity	*Bone marrow depression, gonadal dysfunction, leukemia, hyperuricemia, pulmonary fibrosis*
Cyclophosphamide *AML, ALL, CLL, HL, and NHL, multiple myeloma, mycosis fungoides, neuroblas-toma, ovarian and breast cancers, retinoblastoma, lung, testicular, and bladder cancers, sarcoma*	40-50 mg/kg IV in divided doses over 2-5 d to start, followed by 10-15 mg/kg IV every 7-10 d; or 3-5 mg/kg IV twice weekly; or 1-5 mg/kg/d PO	*Bone marrow depression, hemorrhagic cystitis, immunosuppression, alopecia, stomatitis, SIADH*
Estramustine *Prostate, renal cell carcinomas*	14 mg/kg/d PO in 3-4 equally divided doses; 300 mg/d IV for 3-4 wk, followed by 300-450 mg/wk IV over 3-8 wk	*Bone marrow depression, ischemic heart disease, thromboembolism, thrombophlebitis gynecomastia, nausea and vomiting, hepatotoxicity*
Ifosfamide *Germ-cell testicular cancer, sarcoma, NHL, lung cancer*	1.2 g/m^2/d via slow IV infusion for 5 consecutive days; repeat every 3 wk; give with mesna	*Bone marrow depression, hemorrhagic cystitis, confusion, somnolence*
Mechlorethamine *HL NHL, CML, CLL, mycosis fungoides, bronchogenic carcin-oma, lymphosarcoma, polycythemia vera, malignant effusions (intracavitary)*	0.4 mg/kg ideal body weight given as single dose or in divided doses of 0.1-0.2 mg/kg/d	*Bone marrow depression, nausea and vomiting,* local phlebitis, severe skin necrosis if extravasated, gonadal dysfunction
Melphalan *Multiple myeloma, breast and ovarian cancers, sarcoma, testicular and lung cancers*	<u>Continuous therapy:</u> 6 mg PO daily for 2-3 wk, no therapy for 2-4 wk, then maintenance with 2-4 mg PO daily <u>Pulse:</u> 10 mg/m^2 PO daily for 4 d every 4-6 wk	*Bone marrow depression,* anorexia, nausea and vomiting, gonadal testicular dysfunction, leukemia

Alkylating agents

Drug and its uses	Dosages	Toxicities
Aziridine		
Thiotepa *Ovarian, breast, and superficial bladder cancers, HL, CML, CLL, bronchogenic carcinoma, malignant effusions (intra-cavitary), BMT for refrac-tory leukemia, lymphomas*	IV: 0.3-0.4 mg/kg by rapid IV infusion Intravesical: 60 mg/60 mL sterile water instilled and retained in bladder for 2 h; repeat weekly for 4 wk Intracavitary: 0.6-0.8 mg/kg	*Bone marrow depression, nausea and vomiting, mucositis, skin rashes*
Alkyl sulfonate		
Busulfan *CML, BMT for refractory leukemia, lymphomas*	2-8 mg PO daily for remission induction; adjust dosage to WBC count; 1-3 mg PO daily for maintenance; withhold induction if WBC count < 15,000/µL; resume therapy when WBC count > 50,000/µL	*Bone marrow depression, pulmonary fibrosis, aplastic anemia, amen-orrhea, gynecomastia, skin hyperpigmentation*
Nitrosoureas		
Carmustine *Brain tumor, multiple myeloma, HL, NHL, melanoma, BMT for refractory solid tumors and lymphomas*	150-200 mg/m² IV every 6-8 wk	*Delayed bone marrow depression, nausea and vomiting, reversible hepato-toxicity, local phlebitis, pul-monary and renal damage (high dose)*
Gliadel wafers *Glioblastoma multiforme*	Up to 8 wafers placed in the brain cavity created by tumor removal	Fever, pain, and abnormal healing
Lomustine *Brain tumors, HL, GI carcinomas, NSCLC*	130 mg/m² PO every 6 wk; adjust dose in combination chemotherapy	*Delayed bone marrow depression, nausea and vomiting, reversible hepato-toxicity, pulmonary and renal damage, neurologic reactions, leukemia*
Streptozocin *Pancreatic islet-cell, carcinoid, colon, hepatoma, NSCLC, HL*	Daily: 500 mg/m² IV for 5 d every 6 wk until maximum benefit or toxicity Weekly: 1,000 mg/m² IV weekly for first 2 wk, then escalate dose to response or toxicity, not to exceed a single dose of 1,500 mg/m²	*Renal damage, nausea and vomiting, diarrhea, altered glucose metabolism, liver dysfunction*

Alkylating agents

Drug and its uses	Dosages	Toxicities
Platinum complexes		
Carboplatin *Ovarian cancer,* endometrial, head and neck, lung, testicular, and breast cancers, relapsed acute leukemia, NHL	<u>Single agent:</u> 360 mg/m^2 IV every 4 wk <u>Combination:</u> 300 mg/m^2 IV every 4 wk <u>Calvert formula:</u> Total dose (mg) = Target AUC $\times$ (GFR + 25)	*Bone marrow depression,* nausea and vomiting, peripheral neuropathy ototoxicity
Cisplatin *Testicular, ovarian, bladder,* uterine, cervical, and lung cancers, squamous cell cancer of the head and neck, sarcoma, NHL	50 mg/m^2 IV or more every 3 wk; or 20 mg/m^2 IV daily for 4-5 d every 3-4 wk; give vigorous hydration before and after chemotherapy	*Renal damage,* nausea and vomiting, electrolyte disturbance, peripheral neuropathy, bone marrow depression, ototoxicity, radiosensitizer
Oxaliplatin *Colorectal,* ovarian cancers	85 mg/m^2 oxaliplatin and 200 mg/m^2 leucovorin (IV) IV infusion over 120 min on d 1 followed by 400 mg/m^2 5-FU IV bolus, then 600 mg/m^2 5-FU by IV infusion over 22 h. On d 2, 200 mg/m^2 IV over 120 min IV, followed by 400 mg/m^2 5-FU IV bolus, 600 mg/m^2 5-FU IV infusion over 22 h. Repeat every 2 wk	*Bone marrow depression, diarrhea,* nausea and vomiting, neuropathies exacerbated by cold exposure, pharyngolaryngeal dysesthesia
Nonclassic alkylators		
Altretamine *Ovarian,* lung, breast, and cervical cancers, NHL	4-12 mg/kg/d or 260 mg/m^2, PO divided in 3-4 doses for 14-21 d of a 28-d regimen	*Nausea and vomiting,* bone marrow depression, paresthesias, CNS toxicity
Dacarbazine *Malignant melanoma, HL,* soft-tissue sarcomas, neuroblastoma	<u>Melanoma:</u> 2.0-4.5 mg/kg/d IV for 10 d every 4 wk; or 250 mg/m^2/d IV for 5 d every 3 wk <u>HL:</u> 375 mg/m^2 IV on d 1, repeated every 15 d (single agent); 150 mg/m^2/d IV for 5 d every 4 wk (combination therapy)	*Bone marrow depression,* nausea and vomiting, flu-like syndrome, transient hepatotoxicity, local irritation, facial flushing, alopecia
Procarbazine *HL* NHL, brain tumors, lung cancer	<u>Single agent:</u> 4-6 mg/kg/d PO until maximum response <u>HL (MOPP):</u> 100 mg/m^2/d PO for 14 d	*Bone marrow depression,* nausea and vomiting, lethargy, depression, paresthesias, headache, flu-like symptoms
Temozolomide *Anaplastic astrocytoma (relapsed),* renal cell cancer, melanoma	150 mg/m^2/d PO for 5 d every 28 d	*Bone marrow depression,* nausea and vomiting

Antimetabolites

Drug and its uses	Dosages	Toxicities
Folate analog		
Methotrexate *Breast, head and neck, GI, and lung cancers, ALL, CNS leukemia (intrathecal), gestational trophoblastic tumors, NHL (advanced stage), Burkitt lymphoma, osteosarcoma, mycosis fungoides*	Numerous dosing schedules with combination therapy: <u>Low dose:</u> 2.5-5.0 mg PO daily; or 5-25 mg/m^2 PO, IM, IV twice weekly; or 50 mg/m^2 IV every 2-3 wk <u>High dose:</u> 1-12 g/m^2 IV with leucovorin rescue every 1-3 wk <u>Intrathecal:</u> 5-10 mg/m^2 (up to 15 mg) every 3-7 d	*Mucositis, GI ulceration (may produce hemorrhage or perforation), bone marrow depression, pulmonary fibrosis (previously irradiated area),* nerve root irritation and convulsion (intrathecal), liver cirrhosis and osteoporosis (chronic therapy), renal damage (high dose), diarrhea, skin erythema
Pemetrexed *Mesothelioma, NSCLC*	500 mg/m^2 IV over 10 min every 21 d	*Bone marrow depression,* stomatitis/pharyngitis, rash/skin desquamation
Purine analogs		
Fludarabine *CLL, AML, NHL (low-grade)*	25 mg/m^2/d IV over 30 min for 5 d; repeat every 28 d	*Bone marrow depression,* nausea and vomiting, fever, malaise, pulmonary infiltrates, tumor lysis syndrome, CNS effects (high dose)
Mercaptopurine *ALL, CML, AML*	1.5-2.5 mg/kg/d PO (100-200 mg in average adult) until response or toxic effects are seen; may increase dose to 5 mg/kg/d; adjust for maintenance dose; reduce dose by 50%-75% if given with allopurinol or if renal or hepatic insufficiency ensues	*Bone marrow depression,* nausea and vomiting, anorexia, diarrhea, cholestasis
Thioguanine *AML, ALL, CML, advanced colorectal cancer, multiple myeloma*	2 mg/kg/d PO until response or toxic effects are seen; may cautiously increase to 3 mg/kg/d	*Bone marrow depression,* liver damage, stomatitis
Adenosine analogs		
Cladribine *Hairy-cell leukemia, NHL, mycosis fungoides, AML, CML, CLL*	0.09 mg/kg/d (4 mg/m^2/d) by continuous IV infusion for 7 consecutive days	*Bone marrow depression,* febrile episodes, rash, infections, septicemia
Pentostatin *Hairy-cell leukemia, ALL, CLL, lymphoblastic lymphoma, mycosis fungoides*	4 mg/m^2 IV over 30 min every other wk or for 3 consecutive wk; give vigorous hydration before and after chemotherapy	*Nephrotoxicity, CNS depression,* bone marrow depression, nausea and vomiting, conjunctivitis

Antimetabolites

Drug and its uses	Dosages	Toxicities
Pyrimidine analogs		
Capecitabine *Breast cancer (relapsed), colorectal cancer, and other GI malignancies*	1,250 mg/m^2 bid PO with food (2 wk on drug, 1 wk of rest)	*Diarrhea, stomatitis,* nausea and vomiting, fatigue, hand-foot syndrome, bone marrow depression (minimal)
Cytarabine *AML, ALL, CML, NHL, CNS leukemia (intrathecal)*	<u>AML induction:</u> 100 mg/m^2/d by continuous IV infusion on days 1-7; or 100 mg/m^2 IV every 12 h on days 1-7 <u>Relapsed ALL:</u> 3 g/m^2 IV over 1-3 h every 12 h for 4 doses	*Bone marrow depression,* nausea and vomiting, diarrhea, arachnoiditis (intrathecal), stomatitis, hepatic dysfunction, fever, conjunctivitis, confusion, somnolence, cerebellar toxicity
DepoCyt (liposomal cytarabine) *CNS leukemia/lymphoma*	<u>Intrathecal:</u> DepoCyt, 50 mg over 1-5 min every 14 d, with dexamethasone, 4 mg PO bid × 5 d	
Floxuridine *GI adenocarcinomas metastatic to liver, including oral, pancreatic, biliary, colon, and hepatic cancers, and metastatic breast cancer*	0.1-0.6 mg/kg/d over several days via continuous arterial infusion supplying well-defined tumor; treatments given over 1-6 wk	*Stomatitis and GI ulcers, bone marrow depression,* abdominal pain, nausea and vomiting, diarrhea, liver dysfunction (transient)
Fluorouracil *Colon, rectal, stomach, pancreatic, breast, head and neck, renal cell, prostate, and ovarian cancers, squamous cell carcinomas of esophagus, basal and squamous cell carcinoma of skin (topical), hepatic cancer (intra-arterial)*	Numerous dosing schedules with combination therapy: <u>Loading dose:</u> 300-500 mg/m^2; or 12 mg/kg IV daily for 3-5 d, followed by weekly maintenance <u>Maintenance:</u> 10-15 mg/kg IV weekly, as toxicity permits <u>Infusion:</u> 20-25 mg/kg by continuous IV infusion over 24 h daily for 4-5 d, every 4 wk	*Stomatitis and GI ulcers (infusion)* bone marrow depression *(bolus),* diarrhea, nausea and vomiting, esophagitis, angina, cerebellar ataxia, radiosensitizer
Gemcitabine *Pancreatic, lung, breast, ovarian,* and bladder cancers	1,000 mg/m^2 IV over 30 min, once weekly for up to 7 wk (or until toxicity necessitates reducing or withholding a dose), followed by 1 wk of rest <u>Subsequent cycles:</u> Infusions once weekly for 3 consecutive wk out of every 4 wk	*Bone marrow depression,* transient fever, flu-like syndrome, skin rash, mild nausea and vomiting
Substituted urea		
Hydroxyurea *CML, acute leukemia (emergent treatment), head and neck cancer, ovarian cancer, melanoma,* essential thrombocytosis, polycythemia vera	<u>Intermittent:</u> 80 mg/kg PO every third day <u>Continuous:</u> 20-30 mg/kg PO daily	*Bone marrow depression,* mild nausea and vomiting, skin rashes, radiosensitizer

Natural products

Drug and its uses	Dosages	Toxicities
Antitumor antibiotics		
Bleomycin *Testicular cancer, HL, reticulum cell sarcoma, lymphosarcoma, squamous cell cancer of the head and neck, skin, cervix, vulva, and penis*	10-20 U/m^2 given IV, IM, or SC weekly or twice weekly; maximum total dose, 400 U; <u>a 2-U test dose should be given because of a possible anaphylactoid reaction</u>	*Pneumonitis and pulmonary fibrosis,* fever and allergic reactions, anaphylaxis, hyperpigmentation, Raynaud's phenomenon, alopecia
Dactinomycin *Testicular cancer, gestational trophoblastic tumors, Wilms' tumor, rhabdomyosarcoma, Ewing's sarcoma*	0.010-0.015 mg/kg IV daily for 5 d every 3 wk (usual adult dose, 0.5 mg) or 2 mg/m^2 IV as a single dose every 3-4 wk	*Stomatitis, bone marrow depression,* anorexia, nausea and vomiting, diarrhea, alopecia, skin changes, anaphylactoid reaction
Daunorubicin *AML, ALL*	<u>Remission induction:</u> 30-45 mg/m^2/d IV for 3 d in combination therapy; total cumulative dose, 550 mg/m^2	*Bone marrow depression,* cardiotoxicity, alopecia, nausea and vomiting, diarrhea, stomatitis, fever, dermatitis at previously irradiated sites, red urine, anaphylactoid reaction
DaunoXome (liposomal daunorubicin) *Kaposi's sarcoma*	<u>Liposomal preparation:</u> 40 mg/m^2 IV every 2 wk	
Doxorubicin *ALL, AML, breast, ovarian, bladder cancers, HL, NHL, SCLC, gastric cancer, sarcoma, Wilms' tumor, neuroblastoma, thyroid cancer*	60-90 mg/m^2 single IV injection every 21 d, 20-30 mg/m^2/d IV for 3 d every 3-4 wk, or 20 mg/m^2 IV weekly; total cumulative dose of 550 mg/m^2; reduce dose for liver dysfunction	*Bone marrow depression, cardiotoxicity, stomatitis (continuous infusion),* alopecia, nausea and vomiting, fever, dermatitis at previously irradiated sites, red urine, anaphylactoid reaction
Doxil (liposomal doxorubicin) *Ovarian cancer (refractory to paclitaxel- and platinum-based regimens), Kaposi's sarcoma*	50 mg/m^2 IV every 4 wk 20 mg/m^2 IV every 3 wk	*Bone marrow depression,* hand-foot syndrome
Epirubicin *Breast cancer*	100 mg/m^2 IV on day 1 or 60 mg/m^2 IV on days 1 and 8 in combination therapy	*Bone marrow depression, cardiotoxicity, stomatitis,* alopecia
Idarubicin *AML, CML (blast phase), ALL*	12 mg/m^2/d IV for 3 d every 3 wk in combination therapy	*Bone marrow depression,* nausea and vomiting, stomatitis, alopecia, cardiotoxicity

Natural products

Drug and its uses	Dosages	Toxicities
Mitoxantrone *AML, prostate, ALL, CML, breast and ovarian cancers*	<u>Remission induction:</u> 12 mg/m^2/d IV for 3 d, in combination with Ara-C	*Bone marrow depression, cardiotoxicity, alopecia, stom- atitis, nausea and vomiting, blue urine and sclera*
Mitomycin *Gastric, colorectal, pancreatic adeno- carcinomas, NSCLC, breast, uterine, cervical, and head and neck cancers*	20 mg/m^2 IV every 6-8 wk as a single agent or 5-10 mg/m^2 IV every 6 wk in combination therapy	*Bone marrow depression (cumulative), nausea and vomiting, anorexia, alopecia, stomatitis, fever, pulmonary fibrosis*
Valrubicin *Bladder*	800 mg IV once a wk for 6 wk	*Local bladder symptoms*

Epipodophyllotoxins

Etoposide *Testicular cancer (refractory), SCLC, HL, NHL, AML, gestational tropho- blastic tumors*	<u>Testicular:</u> 50-100 mg/m^2/d IV for 5 d or 100 mg/m^2/d IV on days 1, 3, and 5 <u>Lung:</u> 35-50 mg/m^2/d IV for 5 d or 100 mg/m^2/d PO for 5 d For both indications, given with combination therapy and repeated every 3-4 wk	*Bone marrow depression, nausea and vomiting, diarrhea, fever, hypotension with rapid infusion, alopecia, rash*
Teniposide *Relapsed ALL in children, SCLC*	<u>ALL:</u> 100 mg/m^2 once or twice weekly or 20-60 mg/m^2/d for 5 d in combi- nation with Ara-C <u>Lung:</u> 80-90 mg/m^2/d for 5 d as a single agent	*Bone marrow depression, nausea and vomiting, alopecia, hypotension with rapid infusion, increased liver enzymes*

Microtubule agents

Docetaxel *Breast (relapsed), NSCLC prostate, ovarian, pancreatic, head and neck, esophagus, stomach, cervical, Kaposi's sarcoma, uterine, and bladder cancers*	60-100 mg/m^2 IV over 1 h every 21 d or up to 42 mg/m^2 IV every wk	*Bone marrow depression, fluid retention, hypersensitivity reaction, paresthesias, rash, alopecia, myalgias*
Paclitaxel *Ovarian cancer, (relapsed), NSCLC (in com- bination with cisplatin), Kaposi's sarcoma, breast cancer (relapsed), head and neck, gastric, colon, esophagus, uterine, prostate, bladder cancers and melanomas*	135-175 mg/m^2 by IV infusion (ranging from 3-96 h) every 3 wk or 80 mg/m^2 IV every wk	*Bone marrow depression peripheral neuropathy, alopecia, mucositis, anaphylaxis, dyspnea, myalgias*

Natural products

Drug and its uses	Dosages	Toxicities
Vinblastine *HL, NHL, gestational trophoblastic tumors, testicular and breast cancers, mycosis fungoides, Kaposi's sarcoma, histiocytosis X, bladder and renal cancers, NSCLC, CML (blast crisis)*	4-12 mg/m^2 IV as a single agent every 1-2 wk; titrate dose to myelosuppression; adjust for hepatic insufficiency	*Bone marrow depression, nausea and vomiting, ileus, alopecia, stomatitis, myalgias, vesication*
Vincristine *ALL, HL, NHL, rhabdomyosarcoma, neuroblastoma, Wilms' tumor, multiple myeloma, sarcomas, breast cancer*	0.4-1.4 mg/m^2 IV weekly; maximum total dose, 2 mg/wk; reduce dose for hepatic insufficiency	*Peripheral neuropathy, ileus, abdominal pain, SIADH, bone marrow depression (mild)*
Vinorelbine *NSCLC, breast, ovarian, head and neck cancers, HL*	30 mg/m^2 IV over 10 min; repeat weekly	*Peripheral neuropathy, bone marrow depression, nausea and vomiting, hepatic dysfunction*

Camptothecin analogs

Drug and its uses	Dosages	Toxicities
Irinotecan *Colorectal cancer,* lung, ovarian, and cervical cancers	125 mg/m^2 IV over 90 min once weekly for 4 wk; then 2 wk rest; or 350 mg/m^2 every 21 d	*Bone marrow depression, diarrhea, nausea and vomiting anorexia, weight loss*
Topotecan *Cervical cancer, ovarian cancer (relapsed), SCLC (relapsed),* MDS, CMML	1.5 mg/m^2 IV over 30 min for 5 consecutive days at 21-d intervals	*Bone marrow depression, fever, flu-like symptoms, nausea and vomiting*

Enzyme

Drug and its uses	Dosages	Toxicities
Asparaginase *ALL, CML, AML*	6,000 IU/m^2 IM 3 times weekly for 9 doses or 100 IU/kg/d IV for 10 continuous days, starting on day 22 of treatment; usually given with vincristine and prednisone	*Allergic reactions (fever, chills skin rash, anaphylaxis), nausea and vomiting, anorexia, liver dysfunction, CNS depression, coagulopathy, hyperglycemia*

Targeted therapies: Monoclonal antibodies

Drug and its uses	Dosages	Toxicities
Alemtuzumab *Chemotherapy-refractory* *B-cell CLL*	Rapid daily dose escalation, until tolerated, from 3 mg/d, and then 10 mg/d, to the recommended maintenance dose of 30 mg IV over 120 min, three times per wk on alternate days for up to 12 wk	*Pancytopenia,* infusion reaction, opportunistic infections, skin rash, nausea/vomiting
Bevacizumab *Breast cancer,* *colorectal cancer,* *NSCLC*	5 mg/kg IV over 60-90 min every 14 d	Asthenia, headache, epistaxis, proteinuria, GI perforations/ wound-healing complications, hypertension/hypertensive crisis; hemoptysis[a]
Cetuximab *EGFR-expressing* *colorectal cancer,* *head and neck cancer*	400 mg/m^2 IV over 120 min, loading dose, and 250 mg/m^2 IV over 60 min every 7 d, as maintenance	*Skin rash, infusion reaction,* asthenia, diarrhea, nausea
Panitumumab *EGFR-expressing* *colorectal cancer*	6 mg/kg IV over 60 minutes every 14 days	Skin rash, hypomagnesemia, paronychia, fatigue, infusion reactions, nausea/vomiting, diarrhea
Rituximab *CD20-positive B-cell NHL*	375 mg/m^2 IV infusion (50-100 mg/h) once weekly	Infusion reactions, asthenia, headache, skin rash/pruritus, leukopenia/infection, nausea, tumor lysis syndrome
Trastuzumab *HER2-overexpressing* *breast cancer*	4 mg/kg IV over 90 min, loading dose, and 2 mg/kg IV over 30 min every 7 d, as maintenance	Cardiac failure, infusion reaction, diarrhea

[a] Some patients with NSCLC receiving bevacizumab with chemotherapy experienced hemoptysis.

Molecularly targeted therapies

Drug and its uses	Dosages	Toxicities
Bortezomib *Multiple myeloma*	1.3 mg/m^2 d 1, 4, 8, and 11 every 3 wk	*Diarrhea, peripheral neuropathy,* asthenia, fever, anorexia, nausea and vomiting, rash, headache, thrombocytopenia
Dasatinib *CML, ALL*	140 mg/d (divided doses; 70 mg BID)	Fluid retention events (eg, pleural effusion); GI events: diarrhea, nausea, abdominal pain, vomiting; bleeding events; hematologic toxicities: neutropenia, thrombocytopenia, anemia
Erlotinib *NSCLC, pancreas*	150 mg/d PO	*Acne-form skin rash, diarrhea,* anorexia, fatigue, dyspnea
Gefitinib *NSCLC*	250 mg/d PO	*Acne-form skin rash, diarrhea,* transaminitis, asthenia, mild nausea and vomiting
Imatinib *CML, GIST*	400 mg/d PO in chronic-phase CML and GIST and 600 mg/d PO for CML in accelerated phase or blast crisis	Nausea and vomiting, edema and fluid retention, myalgias, diarrhea, myelosuppression, transaminitis
Lapatinib *HER2-positive metastatic breast cancer*	1,250 mg PO qd × 21 d in combination with capecitabine 2,000 mg/m^2/d PO (divided doses) on d 1-14 of a repeating 21-d cycle	*Diarrhea,* hand-foot syndrome, nausea, rash, vomiting, fatigue
Nilotinib *CML*	400 mg bid PO	*Myelosuppression, hyperbiliru-binemia,* rash, pruritus, nausea, headache, fatigue, constipation, elevated lipase, QTc prolongation
Sorafenib *Renal cell cancer*	400 mg bid PO	Diarrhea, nausea, stomatitis, asthenia, cardiac ischemia, hand-foot syndrome, hypertension, bleeding, anorexia
Sunitinib *Renal cell cancer, GIST*	50 mg/d PO for 4 wk, then 2-wk rest period	Diarrhea, nausea, stomatitis, asthenia, skin discoloration, hand-foot syndrome, hypertension, bleeding, anorexia
Temsirolimus *Renal cell cancer*	25 mg IV weekly	Rash, asthenia, mucositis, edema, dyslipemia, hyperglicemia, elevated serum creatinine. Rarely, interstitial lung disease

Index

signs and symptoms, 500
staging and prognosis, 502
treatment, 503
 adjuvant radiation therapy, 506
 adjuvant systemic therapy, 512
 definitive radiation treatment, 511
 surgery, 503
Esophageal cancer
 advanced disease
  chemotherapy in, 284
  treatment of, 283
 diagnosis, 271
 epidemiology, 269
 etiology and risk factors, 270
 localized disease, treatment of, 275
 pathology, 272
 screening and surveillance, 272
 signs and symptoms, 270
 staging and prognosis, 274
 treatment, 275

F

Fatigue
 assessment, 954
 clinical features, 952
 management, 955
 mechanism, 951
Fluid complications (*see* Ascites, malignant; Pleural effusion, malignant; Pericardial effusion)

G

Gallbladder cancer
 diagnosis, 349
 epidemiology, 348
 etiology and risk factors, 349
 pathology, 352
 signs and symptoms, 349
 staging and prognosis, 352
 surgery, 353
Gastric cancer
 adjuvant therapy, 300
 advanced disease, medical treatment of, 303
 epidemiology, 291
 etiology, risk factors, and prevention, 292
 localized disease, primary treatment of, 296
 neoadjuvant therapy, 299
 pathology, 294
 screening and diagnosis, 293
 signs and symptoms, 293
 staging and prognosis, 295

treatment, 296
unresectable tumors, treatment of, 301
Gastrointestinal cancer (*see* Anal canal carcinoma; Bile duct cancer; Carcinoid tumors, GI tract; Colorectal cancer; Esophageal cancer; Gallbladder cancer; Gastric cancer; Hepatocellular cancer; Pancreatic cancer; Pancreatic endocrine tumors)
Gestational trophoblastic diseases
 clinical presentation, 521
 diagnostic studies, 522
 metastatic disease
  low-risk, 524
  high-risk, 524
 salvage therapy, 524
 treatment, 523

H

Hairy-cell leukemia (*see also* Leukemia)
 differential diagnosis, 856
 epidemiology and etiology, 856
 treatment, 856
Head and neck tumors
 anatomy, 39
 epidemiology, 35
 etiology and risk factors, 37
 follow-up of long-term survivors, 58
 pathology, 44
 recurrent cancer, 81
 screening and diagnosis, 40
 signs and symptoms, 39
 staging and prognosis, 46
 treatment approaches, 46
 treatment of the neck, 57
 tumor regions, 58
  glottis, 74
  hypopharynx, 68
  larynx, 69
  lips, 60
  mouth floor, 63
  nasopharynx, 77
  oral cavity, 59
  oropharynx, 64
  subglottis, 75
  supraglottis, 73
  tongue, 62
  tongue base, 66
  tonsils and tonsillar pillar, 67
  unknown head and neck primary site, 76
Hematopoietic cell transplantation
 allogeneic transplantation, 879
 autologous transplantation, 880